a LANGE medical book

Review of
General
Psychiatry

fifth edition

Howard H. Goldman, MD, MPH, PhD
Professor of Psychiatry
Institute of Psychiatry and Human Behavior
University of Maryland, Baltimore

Research Associate
Center for Health Services Research and Development
School of Hygiene and Public Health
Johns Hopkins University, Baltimore

Lange Medical Books/McGraw-Hill
Medical Publishing Division

New York St. Louis San Francisco Auckland Bogotá Caracas Lisbon London
Madrid Mexico City Milan Montreal New Delhi San Juan
Singapore Sydney Tokyo Toronto

McGraw-Hill

A Division of The **McGraw·Hill** *Companies*

Review of General Psychiatry, Fifth Edition

4567890 CUS CUS 098765

ISBN: 0-8385-8434-9
ISSN: 0894-2404

Notice

Medicine is an ever-changing science. As new research and clinical experience broaden our knowledge, changes in treatment and drug therapy are required. The authors and the publisher of this work have checked with sources believed to be reliable in their efforts to provide information that is complete and generally in accord with the standards accepted at the time of publication. However, in view of the possibility of human error or changes in medical sciences, neither the authors nor the publisher nor any other party who has been involved in the preparation or publication of this work warrants that the information contained herein is in every respect accurate or complete, and they disclaim all responsibility for any errors or omissions or for the results obtained from use of the information contained in this work. Readers are encouraged to confirm the information contained herein with other sources. For example and in particular, readers are advised to check the product information sheet included in the package of each drug they plan to administer to be certain that the information contained in this work is accurate and that changes have not been made in the recommended dose or in the contraindications for administration. This recommendation is of particular importance in connection with new or infrequently used drugs.

This book was set in Times Roman by Rainbow Graphics, LLC.
The editors were Janet Foltin, Harriet Lebowitz, and Jeanmarie Roche.
The production supervisor was Rohnda Barnes.
The cover designer was Elizabeth Schmitz.
The manager of art services was Eve Siegel.
The illustrator was Wendy Jackelow.
The index was prepared by Katherine Pitcoff.

Phoenix Book Technologies was printer and binder.

This book was printed on acid-free paper.

Contents

SECTION I. THEORY & CONCEPTS

SECTION II. PSYCHIATRIC ASSESSMENT

SECTION III. MENTAL DISORDERS

SECTION IV. TREATMENT MODALITIES

Authors

Bruce Africa, MD, PhD
Former Associate Clinical Professor of Psychiatry, University of California, San Francisco.

David Anderson, MD
Senior Staff Physician, Henry Ford Hospital, Detroit, Michigan.

Kenneth L. Appelbaum, MD
Associate Professor of Clinical Psychiatry; Director, Correctional Mental Health, University of Massachusetts Medical Center, Worcester.

Paul S. Appelbaum, MD
AF Zeleznik Professor and Chairman, Department of Psychiatry, University of Massachusetts Medical School, Worcester.

Renée Binder, MD
Professor of Psychiatry, Director, Psychiatry and Law Program, University of California, San Francisco.

Linda Cahill, MD
Associate Professor of Clinical Pediatrics, Albert Einstein College of Medicine; Medical Director, Child Protection Center, Division of Community Pediatrics, Children's Hospital at Montefiore, Bronx, New York.

H. Westley Clark, MD, JD, MPH
Associate Clinical Professor, Department of Psychiatry, University of California, San Francisco.

James David, MD
Associate Professor for Students; Associate Dean for Students, Albert Einstein College of Medicine, Bronx, New York.

Glenn C. Davis, MD
Corporate Vice President, Academic Affairs, Henry Ford Health System, Detroit, Michigan; Professor of Psychiatry, Case Western Reserve University; Clinical Professor of Psychiatry, University of Michigan.

Kathryn N. DeWitt, PhD
Private practice, Palo Alto, California.

Stuart J. Eisendrath, MD
Professor of Clinical Psychiatry and Director of Adult Psychiatry Clinic, University of California, San Francisco.

Howard L. Fields, MD, PhD
Professor of Neurology, Physiology, and Psychiatry, University of California, San Francisco.

Michael B. First, MD
Associate Professor of Clinical Psychiatry, Columbia University College of Physicians & Surgeons; Editor, *DSM-IV* Text and Criteria, American Psychiatric Association, Washington, DC; Research Psychiatrist, New York State Psychiatric Institute, New York.

Frederick G. Flynn, DO, COL, MC
Chief, Neurology Service, Program Director, Neurology Residency, and Chief, Neurobehavior, Madigan Army Medical Center, Tacoma, Washington; Associate Professor of Neurology, University of Washington School of Medicine, Seattle; Associate Professor of Neurology, Uniformed Services University of Health Sciences, Bethesda, Maryland.

Steven A. Foreman, MD
Assistant Clinical Professor, Department of Psychiatry, University of California, San Francisco.

Allen Frances, MD
Professor, Department of Psychiatry and Behavioral Sciences, Duke University Medical Center, Durham, North Carolina.

Oliver Freudenreich, MD
Graduate Assistant in Psychiatry, Massachusetts General Hospital; Clinical Fellow in Psychiatry, Harvard Medical School, Boston, Massachusetts.

Richard J. Goldberg, MD
Professor, Department of Psychiatry and Human Behavior and Department of Medicine, Brown University; Psychiatrist-in-Chief, Rhode Island Hospital and The Miriam Hospital, Providence, Rhode Island.

Beth Goldman, MD, MPH
Private practice, Birmingham, Michigan; Medical Consultant, Center for Healthcare Quality and Evaluative Studies, Blue Cross Blue Shield of Michigan.

Howard H. Goldman, MD, MPH, PhD
Professor of Psychiatry, Institute of Psychiatry and Human Behavior, University of Maryland, Baltimore; Research Associate, Center for Health Services Research and Development, School of Hygiene and Public Health, Johns Hopkins University, Baltimore.

Gary L. Gottlieb, MD, MBA
Professor of Psychiatry, Harvard Medical School; Chairman, Partners Psychiatry and Mental Health System, Boston, Massachusetts.

John H. Greist, MD
Clinical Professor of Psychiatry, University of Wisconsin Medical School; Distinguished Senior Scientist, Madison Institute of Medicine, Inc., Madison, Wisconsin.

Phillip Grob, MD
Assistant Professor, University of Maryland School of Medicine, Baltimore.

Gemma G. Guillermo, MD
Clinical Instructor of Psychology, Division of Psychosocial Medicine, University of California, San Francisco.

Ellen Haller, MD
Associate Adjunct Professor, Department of Psychiatry, University of California, San Francisco.

Rona J. Hu, MD
Assistant Professor of Psychiatry, Stanford University School of Medicine, Palo Alto, California.

Roberta Huberman, MD
Assistant Clinical Professor of Psychiatry, Mt. Sinai Medical Center, New York, New York; Private practice, Princeton, New Jersey.

Gerard J. Hunt, PhD
Senior Psychotherapist, Resource Group, Towson, Maryland.

James W. Jefferson, MD
Clinical Professor of Psychiatry, University of Wisconsin Medical School; Distinguished Senior Scientist, Madison Institute of Medicine, Inc., Madison, Wisconsin.

Nick Kanas, MD
Professor and Director, Group Therapy Training Program, Department of Psychiatry, University of California, San Francisco; Associate Chief, Psychiatry Service, Department of Veterans Affairs Medical Center, San Francisco.

Ralph J. Kiernan, PhD
Clinical Assistant Professor of Psychology in Psychiatry, Stanford University Medical Center, Palo Alto, California.

Ellen S. Krantz, PhD
Postdoctoral Fellow, Kennedy Krieger Institute, Johns Hopkins University, Baltimore, Maryland.

J.W. Langston, MD
President, The Parkinson's Institute, Sunnyvale, California.

Mim J. Landry
Freelance medical writer, Silver Spring, Maryland.

Gregory K. Lehne, PhD
Assistant Professor of Medical Psychology, Department of Psychiatry and Behavioral Sciences, The Johns Hopkins University School of Medicine, Baltimore, Maryland.

Hanna Levenson, PhD
Clinical Professor, Department of Psychiatry, University of California Medical School, San Francisco; Director, Levenson Institute for Training (LIFT), San Francisco.

Richard J. Loewenstein, MD
Clinical Associate Professor, Department of Psychiatry and Behavioral Sciences, University of Maryland School of Medicine, Baltimore.

David Lorreck, MD
Assistant Professor, University of Maryland Medical School; Director, Baltimore Veterans Affairs Medical Center Alzheimer's Program.

Shane MacKay, MD
Staff Psychiatrist, Alta Bates Medical Center, Berkeley, California.

Charles R. Marmar, MD
Professor and Vice Chairman, Department of Psychiatry, University of California, San Francisco; Chief, Mental Health Service, Acting Chief of Staff, San Francisco Veterans Affairs Medical Center.

Terry Michael McClanahan, MA
University of California, San Francisco.

Laurie E. McQueen, MSSW
DSM Project Manager, American Psychiatric Association, Washington, DC.

Edward L. Merrin, MD
Medical Director, Psychstrategies, Inc., Santa Rosa, California.

Aubrey W. Metcalf, MD
Clinical Professor of Psychiatry, University of California, San Francisco; Senior Supervising Child and Adolescent Psychiatrist, LPPI, University of California, San Francisco.

Jonathan Mueller, MD
Associate Clinical Professor, Department of Psychiatry, University of California, San Francisco.

Kim Norman, MD
Clinical Professor, Department of Psychiatry, University of California, San Francisco; Director, Eating Disorder Clinic, Langley Porter Psychiatric Institute.

Jacqueline B. Persons, PhD
Director, San Francisco Bay Area Center for Cognitive Therapy; Associate Clinical Professor, Department of Psychiatry, University of California Medical School, San Francisco.

Harold A. Pincus, MD
Executive Vice Chair, Department of Psychiatry, University of Pittsburgh School of Medicine.

S. Michael Plaut, PhD
Associate Professor of Psychiatry, University of Maryland School of Medicine, Baltimore.

Kenneth S. Pope, PhD
Private practice, Norwalk, Connecticut.

Steven D. Prakken, MD
Senior Resident, Department of Psychiatry, University of California, San Francisco.

David Preven, MD
Clinical Professor, Department of Psychiatry and Behavioral Sciences, Albert Einstein College of Medicine, New York, New York; Chief of Psychiatry, Weiler Hospital, Bronx, New York.

Stephen D. Purcell, MD
Associate Clinical Professor, Department of Psychiatry, University of California, San Francisco.

David E. Reiser, MD
Associate Clinical Professor of Psychiatry, University of Colorado Health Sciences Center, Denver.

Victor I. Reus, MD
Professor, Department of Psychiatry and Senior Investigator, Center for Neurobiology and Behavior, University of California, San Francisco, School of Medicine.

Gary M. Rodin, MD
Head, Mental Health Program, University Health Network, Toronto, Canada; Professor of Psychiatry, University of Toronto, Canada.

Jeffrey Rowe, MD
Assistant Clinical Professor of Psychiatry, University of California, San Francisco.

Stuart R. Schwartz, MD
Professor of Psychiatry; Vice Chairman of Educational Programs at UMDNJ Robert Wood Johnson Medical School, Piscataway, New Jersey.

Rodney J. Shapiro, PhD
Clinical Professor of Psychiatry, University of California, San Francisco; Director, Networks Family Counseling Center, San Francisco.

David Smith, MD
Founder and Medical Director, Haight Ashbury Free Medical Clinics; Associate Clinical Professor of Occupational Health and Clinical Toxicology, University of California, San Francisco.

Lonnie Snowden, PhD
Director, Center for Mental Health Services Research; Professor, School of Social Welfare, University of California, Berkeley.

Craig Van Dyke, MD
Professor and Chair, Department of Psychiatry, University of California, San Francisco.

Robert S. Wallerstein, MD
Professor Emeritus and Former Chair, Department of Psychiatry, University of California, San Francisco, School of Medicine.

Daniel S. Weiss, PhD
Professor of Medical Psychology, Department of Psychiatry, University of California, San Francisco; Director of Research, PTSD Research, Veterans Affairs Medical Center, San Francisco.

Mitchell D. Wilson, MD
Assistant Clinical Professor of Psychiatry, University of California, San Francisco; Faculty Member, San Francisco Psychoanalytic Institute; Private practice in Psychoanalysis and General Psychology, Berkeley, California.

Mary Witt, MD, MPH
Assistant Clinical Professor of Psychiatry and Pediatrics, Albert Einstein College of Medicine; Psychiatrist, Children's Evaluation and Rehabilitation Center, Rose F. Kennedy Center University Affiliated Program, Bronx, New York.

Preface

Review of General Psychiatry, 5th edition, is designed for medical students—for course adoption, to supplement course syllabus materials, to complement readings in the literature, and to use as a companion text with more comprehensive works. Written by psychiatric educators, this text serves the needs of medical students in most settings. In addition, it can serve as a review text for psychiatric residents and other trainees, and as a reference for physicians and other health professionals.

Psychiatry is a discipline of observation and probing inquiry, a basic science of behavior, and a clinical science of mental disorder and emotional responses to physiological change, somatic illness, and life events. Critics in neuroscience characterize psychiatry as brainless; critics within psychological medicine fear that psychiatry will become mindless. Students everywhere are concerned that the medical curriculum not be witless. Our aim is to present psychiatry with the proper mix of brain, mind, and wit.

NEW TO THIS EDITION

This edition welcomes 15 new authors, many of whom are co-authors working with contributors to earlier editions of *Review of General Psychiatry.*

Seven chapters have been extensively revised:

Neurochemistry in Psychiatry
Social & Cultural Aspects of Health, Illness, & Treatment
Dementia, Delirium, & Amnestic Disorders
Schizophrenic Disorders
Somatoform & Dissociative Disorders
Childhood Mental Disorders & Child Psychiatry
Somatic Therapies

CONTINUING FEATURES

- Material on basic biological and psychosocial science as well as clinical material on diagnosis and treatment.
- Full range of disorders with complete diagnostic criteria as described in the *Diagnostic and Statistical Manual of Mental Disorders,* Fourth edition (*DSM-IV*).
- Updated neuroscience and psychopharmacology.
- Clinical vignettes illustrating the features of most mental disorders and comprehensive clinical assessment.
- Glossary of psychiatric signs and symptoms.
- Six chapters on psychiatric assessment.
- Diagnostic and treatment algorithms.
- Consistent, readable format, permitting efficient use in multiple clinical settings.
- Selected references for further investigation.
- Information useful to the nonpsychiatrist physician and the medical student and resident in psychiatry.

ACKNOWLEDGMENTS

Review of General Psychiatry represents more than the work of its title page editor and its named contributors. I would like to acknowledge the assistance of other contributors to our text.

Although the fifth edition bears little resemblance to the original course materials prepared at UCSF prior to the first edition, I wish to thank my predecessors and colleagues in San Francisco for setting the initial direction for this text. I would also like to thank the publisher, the editorial staff at McGraw-Hill, especially David Barnes and Harriet Lebowitz, and the manuscript copyeditor, Arline Keithe. A special debt of gratitude is extended to Jim Ransom, whose outstanding editorial work on the first edition continues to make the text readable.

The contributors, the publisher, and I are grateful to the American Psychiatric Association for permission to quote directly from *Diagnostic and Statistical Manual of Mental Disorders*, Fourth edition (*DSM-IV*), in this work. Descriptive matter is enclosed in quotation marks in the text exactly as it appears in *DSM-IV*. Tabular matter is modified slightly as to form only in accordance with the publisher's editorial usage.

We are still interested in soliciting comments and recommendations for future editions of this textbook. Correspondence should be addressed to us at McGraw-Hill, Medical Publishing Division, Lange Medical Books, Two Penn Plaza, 12th Floor, New York, NY 10121.

Howard H. Goldman, MD, MPH, PhD
Baltimore, Maryland
June, 2000

Section I.
Theory & Concepts

Review of General Psychiatry: Introduction

1

Howard H. Goldman, MD, MPH, PhD

Review of General Psychiatry examines and discusses the two major domains of the medical specialty field of psychiatry: mental disorder and individual behavior in health and sickness. Both areas are characterized by a degree of scientific uncertainty. Psychiatry uses models of behavior and mental activity to reduce uncertainty by organizing what is known into a conceptual framework.

THE BIOPSYCHOSOCIAL MODEL

The biopsychosocial model is a defense against uncertainty, an approach to thinking about mental disorder and individual behavior. The psychiatrist may view both domains from biomedical and psychosocial perspectives and consider specific problems and potential solutions from each viewpoint. The biopsychosocial model is a perspective, not a theory—a way of organizing disparate data that permits clinicians and scientists to consider various points of view and integrate them into a coherent approach to the patient. For example, the busy medical student with migraine headache is not viewed as the passive victim of familial defects in neurovascular function *or* the angry combatant in a competitive profession, living a stressful life-style. *Both* views are correct, potentially helpful, and not mutually exclusive. The model, championed by George Engel and discussed again in other chapters, is introduced below in a clinical case and in a summary of some current research in neuroscience to demonstrate its scope and utility.

What do the aged couple in the following illustrative case and the animal model of anxiety in the snail *Aplysia* have in common? How does the biopsychosocial model enable us to appreciate these shared features? There is substantial agreement that clinical biomedical problems, such as heart attacks, are in part influenced by psychosocial factors, for instance, the sudden death of a loved one. It also is generally accepted that biomedical problems (eg, a stroke) may

cause secondary behavioral and psychosocial problems (eg, loss of a job or dissolution of a marriage). It is more difficult to appreciate the specific effect of social and psychological factors on anatomic structures and physiological functions. The clinical case of an aged couple will show how the biopsychosocial model facilitates understanding of the interactions of biomedical and psychosocial factors. The animal model of anxiety in *Aplysia* illustrates the use of the biopsychosocial model in basic research. In particular, it examines the mechanism by which learned responses (eg, anxiety) may cause specific neurochemical and neuroanatomic changes.

Illustrative Case

A couple in their mid-80s had been married for 65 years and continued to live together in an apartment in spite of their increasing infirmities. The husband had severe emphysema and cardiac arrhythmia and was becoming forgetful; his wife had mild hypertension and was becoming impaired by senile dementia. On the eve of his 85th birthday, the old man became acutely short of breath and anxious. Fearful that he was going to die, he called his married daughter and was taken to the hospital in acute respiratory distress. He was later found to have inoperable lung cancer for which only palliative treatment could be offered.

While the patient was hospitalized, his wife went to live with their daughter and son-in-law. At night she wandered the rooms of the house, looking for her husband. She was argumentative and confused, not seeming to know where she was or what she should do. Her children and grandchildren had been aware of her increasing mental problems, but she was much more disturbed than they had realized or perhaps had wanted to realize.

Her apparently dramatic change could be explained in two ways: (1) she was undergoing a period of acute situational stress; and (2) her deterioration had not been obvious as long as she was part of a functioning couple. Her husband had been helping her at home, nursing her, and covering up her deficits so that the family would not see them. He was no longer available to do these things. Plans were made to discharge him to a nursing home, where he could continue to live with his wife in a double room. Although he was depressed, he adjusted to the nursing home, accepting the fact that this was where he would live out his days. He lived to see his granddaughter married, and then he died. The wife never adjusted, and her mental condition continued to deteriorate. She still expected her husband to come home each evening, concluding that she never saw him because he left each day before she awakened and returned while she was asleep.

The interaction of biomedical and psychosocial factors in disease and illness is illustrated by this case. The husband's illness had precipitated a change in the delicate balance of the couple's independence. The wife needed nursing care, and his illness kept him from providing it. Many people die or become ill on achieving certain milestones—an anniversary, a holiday, or, as in this case, a birthday. This man's 85th birthday had special significance. His driver's license, the key to his independence and his ability to care for his wife at home, expired on his birthday. He had been preparing for the test with great difficulty and was afraid he would not pass. Going to a nursing home gave him the comfort of knowing that when he died, his wife would be taken care of without being a burden to the family. His cancer had been developing for a long time, but clinically obvious illness began on his birthday.

A keen awareness of the interplay between biomedical and psychosocial factors is the essence of clinical medicine. Knowledge of the nuances of this interaction can help to answer two of the most important questions in medicine: Why did the patient become ill *now* (and not yesterday or a week or month ago)? And how can we treat this individual with an established diagnosis (that may be incurable)?

The mechanisms by which stress precipitates and exacerbates illness, lowers host resistance, and perhaps causes some diseases are currently being investigated. It would also be useful to examine how coping and adaptation work to prevent illness or reduce its severity. Learning how symbolic events, thoughts, and feelings influence behavior and initiate pathological processes in humans is a challenge for future research. Some early work in this area has been reported by Eric Kandel and his associates studying an animal model of anxiety in the marine snail *Aplysia,* whose nervous system is simple, well understood, and accessible to investigation.

Research Example: Animal Model of Anxiety

Using the sea snail *Aplysia* as a research subject, Kandel describes an animal model of anticipatory anxiety and chronic anxiety reflected in two forms of learned fear produced by classic conditioning and sensitization. Each form of fear is associated with distinguishable cellular and molecular changes.

Aplysia demonstrates a defensive "fear response" when presented with a noxious stimulus such as an electric shock to its head. The response includes an increase in movement away from the stimulus ("escape locomotion"), an increase in other defensive behaviors (eg, withdrawal of the head and siphon into the shell, releasing ink), and a decrease in feeding behavior. This fearful response may be learned by the snail in two ways: *Aplysia* may be conditioned, like Pavlov's dog (see Chapter 2), to respond fearfully to a neutral stimulus, such as shrimp extract, without the electric shock. If the snail is repeatedly given an electric shock each time shrimp extract is presented to it, the snail eventually responds with fear to the shrimp extract alone. This classic conditioning is similar to human anticipatory anxiety (and phobic anxiety). *Aplysia* can also be sensitized by random, unpredictable electric shocks, resulting in generally heightened responsiveness, so that almost any stimulus produces fearful behavior, as seen in chronic anxiety in humans.

In a series of elegant experiments, Kandel and his colleagues explored the cellular and molecular mechanisms associated with these two forms of learned fear. The sensitization model of chronic anxiety has been studied more extensively and appears to be related to presynaptic facilitation. The repeated head shocks lead to an "enhancement of the connections made by the sensory neurons on their target cells: the interneurons and the motor neurons" (Kandel, 1983, p 1285), resulting in increased escape behavior.

This enhancement is caused by increases in a serotonin-like neurotransmitter in the presynaptic sensory neurons, which produces an increase in cyclic adenosine monophosphate (cAMP). In turn, cAMP leads to an increase in neurotransmitter release from terminals in the synapse connecting the sensory neurons and motor neurons. The resulting neurotransmission activates "escape locomotion" and other defensive behaviors in response to a wide array of stimuli.

The investigators found that the molecular mechanism involved enhanced protein phosphorylation and increased influx of calcium, resulting in morphological changes in the presynaptic neurons, detectable by electron microscopy. They speculate that the functional and structural changes associated with sensitization may be caused by alterations in gene expression: "the possibility of gene regulation by experience suggests a class of molecular regulatory defects that might be caused by learning" (Kandel, 1983, p 1287).

The conditioning model for anticipatory anxiety is not as well described but seems to be similar in many ways to sensitization. Also producing presynaptic facilitation, conditioned fear appears to "augment" the process by "activity-dependent enhancement." This means that the learned association between the conditioned stimulus (the shrimp extract) and the fear response is produced by the increased release of neurotransmitter when the snail senses the presence of shrimp extract. The increased neurotransmission in response to the conditioned stimulus then sets in motion the same enhanced fear response mechanism seen in the sensitization model of chronic anxiety.

This research suggests that "normal learning, the learning of anxiety and unlearning it through psychotherapeutic intervention, might involve long-term functional and structural changes in the brain" (Kandel, 1983, p 1291). Investigations such as these demonstrate the interaction of biomedical and psychosocial phenomena, brain and behavior, in everyday life and clinical medicine.

Fifteen years and countless experiments after these early studies on an animal model of anxiety, neurobiology has evolved so much that Kandel has articulated a new intellectual framework for psychiatry. This new conceptual framework, grounded in neuroscience, may be summarized in five principles about the relationship of mind to brain (Kandel, 1998, p 460).

"Principle 1. All mental processes . . . derive from operations of the brain."

"Principle 2. Genes and their protein products are important determinants of the patterns of interconnections between neurons in the brain and the details of their functioning."

"Principle 3. Altered genes do not, by themselves, explain all of the variance of a given major mental illness."

"Principle 4. Alterations in gene expression induced by learning give rise to changes in patterns of neuronal connections."

"Principle 5. Insofar as psychotherapy or counseling is effective and produces long-term changes in behavior, it presumably does so through learning, by producing changes in gene expression."

THE PLAN OF THE TEXTBOOK

Review of General Psychiatry is divided into four sections: theories and concepts, psychiatric assessment, the mental disorders, and treatments and special interventions.

The first section presents the basic science of psychiatry, material usually included in first-year psychiatry courses. This section introduces the biopsychosocial model and explores its various aspects. The section concludes with an introduction to psychopathology, the clinical science of psychiatry, the study of mental disorder, and a glossary of psychopathology terminology.

The second section concerns clinical assessment. It can serve as a basic text for introductory courses in interviewing and clinical psychiatry, including a clerkship in psychiatry.

The third and fourth sections may be used as a text for introductory courses in clinical psychiatry and for the core clerkship in psychiatry. Some of the chapters are also designed for use in a consultation-liaison psychiatry course and for courses in the psychiatric aspects of medical practice. The third section presents the mental disorders, for the most part as they are classified in the fourth edition of *Diagnostic and Statistical Manual of Mental Disorders* (*DSM-IV*). An illustrative case is provided for many of the disorders presented in each chapter. The fourth section discusses methods of psychiatric treatment and presents some material on special topics in psychiatry. Although the text was designed for use in general medical and psychiatric education, we hope that trainees and practitioners in other health, mental health, and social welfare disciplines will find *Review of General Psychiatry* helpful and stimulating.

REFERENCES & SUGGESTED READINGS

American Psychiatric Association: *Diagnostic and Statistical Manual of Mental Disorders,* 4th ed. American Psychiatric Association, 1994.

Dubos R: *Man Adapting.* Yale University Press, 1980.

Eisenberg L: Psychiatry and society. N Engl J Med 1977; 296:903.

Engel G: The need for a new medical model: A challenge for biomedicine. Science 1977;196:129.

Kandel E: From metapsychology to molecular biology: Explorations into the nature of anxiety. Am J Psychiatry 1983;140:1277.

Kandel ER: A new intellectual framework for psychiatry. Am J Psychiatry 1998;155:457.

Kandel ER, Schwartz JH, Jessell TM (editors): *Essentials of Neural Science and Behavior.* Appleton & Lange, 1995.

2

Theoretical Foundations of Psychiatry

James David, MD, & David Preven, MD

This chapter includes a brief history of prefreudian psychiatry and a discussion of the major theories and treatment methods that comprise modern practice. These subjects are discussed in greater detail in later chapters. The purpose is to provide a skeletal framework of the field that can be expanded by further readings and clinical experiences.

The field of psychiatry, in concert with the allied mental health professions, has come to encompass a wide spectrum of human mental, instinctual, and behavioral experience—mood disorders, eating disorders, sexual disorders, phobias, etc. Considering the number and diversity of mental disorders encompassed, it is not surprising that a great many conflicting theories have evolved about their causes, mechanisms, and proper treatment. The student in search of a unifying conceptual framework—a unified field theory of psychiatry—will be disappointed. It is necessary to take on trust that each of the various theories that comprise modern psychiatry has its own place in the unfinished mosaic of knowledge in this field.

HISTORY OF PSYCHIATRY BEFORE FREUD

Early civilizations frequently attributed madness to magical or divine forces. Attempts at treatment were administered mostly by clergy and were grounded in religious beliefs and ritual.

Greek and Roman societies began to apply the medical beliefs of their day to psychiatric symptoms, hypothesized to result from imbalances of the essential humors (blood, phlegm, yellow bile, and black bile) and other derangements of vital processes. Hippocratic doctrine considered hysteria (derived from the Greek word for womb: *hysterus*) a consequence of a physically wandering uterus. Galen (c 130–c 201) attributed melancholia to an excess of black bile.

Asylums for the mentally ill were first established in medieval times. In the Renaissance the insane, believed to be possessed by the devil, were condemned by ecclesiastical authorities and tortured as witches. Even the greatest physicians of the day advocated that they be burned. This age-old stigmatization of the mentally ill, with its attendant fear and discrimination, is, unfortunately, still very much with us.

Seventeenth- and eighteenth-century asylums, with some exceptions, were dreadful places where patients were kept in chains and whipping was a common form of treatment. Toward the latter part of this period—notably around the time of the French Revolution—reforms in treatment of the insane began. Phillipe Pinel (1745–1826) in France and William Tuke (1732–1822) in England were influential advocates for humane treatment of the mentally ill. The chains and cruelty began to give way to decent living conditions and to attempts at rehabilitation.

In the late 1700s, Franz Mesmer (1734–1815), an Austrian physician, pioneered work now considered by some to be the earliest example of psychotherapy. He would establish rapport with and work with individual patients, practicing what was at the time called mesmerism—later modified and renamed hypnosis.

The nineteenth century heralded the beginning of a more scientific approach to psychiatry. Many detailed descriptions of psychiatric syndromes were recorded, and the basis of the modern classification of mental disorders was established. Emil Kraepelin (1856–1926) is best known for his contribution to differential diagnosis in psychiatry. He suggested two major categories of severe mental disorders: manic-depressive illness and dementia praecox. Kraepelin's manic-depressive category generally corresponds to the modern classification of mood disorders (bipolar disorder, recurrent major depression, and other disorders, discussed in Chapter 20); he noted the cyclical course of this type of illness, with recovery following symptomatic episodes. Dementia praecox is the forerunner to the current classification of schizophrenia and related syndromes (Chapters 20 and 21). Furthermore, Kraepelin noted the long-term deteriorating course of this type of illness, in contrast to the fluctuating course of manic-depressive illnesses. Eugen Bleuler (1857–1939), a Swiss psychiatrist, further studied and described dementia praecox and renamed the syndrome schizophrenia to distinguish it from true dementia.

In the latter part of the nineteenth century, Jean Charcot (1825–1893), a French neurologist, was treating hysteria with hypnosis. This treatment technique was, for a time, adopted by an obscure Austrian physician who had been impressed with Charcot's work. The emergence (under hypnosis) of psychic material not readily ascertained in the normal waking state contributed to this practitioner's later revelations regarding mental functioning. His name was Sigmund Freud.

FREUD'S CONTRIBUTION

Few twentieth-century individuals loom as large as Sigmund Freud (1856–1939), both as a founder of modern psychiatry and as a cultural force. His impact on the arts, literature, and education was profound and far-reaching. Much of his wide appeal can be attributed to the masterful way he described his theories and case histories, often linking them to references in the Bible, classical literature, and Renaissance culture. In the United States his influence on the development of psychiatry and culture in the mid-twentieth century was such that every student of medicine should know something about Sigmund Freud and his theories—regardless of recent controversies about their place in contemporary psychiatric treatment.

Although Freud trained as a neurologist, he was barred from practicing traditional neurology in Vienna in part because of anti-Semitism. That professional crisis provided Freud with an unexpected opportunity. He began to consult with patients whose symptoms were not explained by the traditional approaches of the discipline. Freud's work with these patients inspired him to formulate the theories and practice of psychoanalysis. The word psychoanalysis, then and now, refers both to the theory Freud developed and the treatment itself (see Chapter 31).

Psychoanalysis as Theory

Psychoanalysis as a theory provides a comprehensive approach to understanding psychic development, emotion, and behavior as well as psychiatric illness. As Freud developed his ideas, he posited a **psychic apparatus** with three parts: **id, ego,** and **superego.** This **structural theory,** as it was called, defined the superego as the conscience, the id as the repository of raw impulses and drives such as sex and aggression, and the ego as the rational mediator between the expectations of the superego and the pressures for gratification of the id. Freud believed that the three structures related to each other in a dynamic equilibrium. If the ego failed to keep the demands of the id and superego in balance, the individual experienced psychological symptoms and distress.

Another fundamental concept of psychoanalysis—the **psychosexual stages of development**—postulated that a person must accomplish a series of tasks or achievements from infancy to adulthood to achieve psychological health (see Chapter 4). Freud associated each of these psychosexual stages with a part of the anatomy as well as with physiological and psychological functions. For example, the **oral stage,** from birth to 18 months, was anatomically represented by the mouth, with eating (symbolically sucking at the breast) as the physiological function and being loved and nurtured as the psychological task. The **anal phase,** which begins at around 2 years, focused on the anus anatomically, with bowel control as the physiological function and autonomy and self-control as the psychological task. Finally, the **genital phase,** at ages 3–5, defined the genitals as pleasure-providing organs physiologically and linked them psychologically to the then-prevalent notion that males were active (phallic) and females passive (receptive). As Freud listened to his patients' childhood histories, he hypothesized that failure to complete the task of a certain psychosexual phase would impair adult psychological health and functioning. For example, problems of inadequate nurturing during the oral stage could produce an adult who feels unloved and suffers dependency problems in relationships.

It is implicit in the concept of psychosexual stages that early experience shapes the adult's self-image and potential for success in work and relationships. It is one of Freud's pivotal contributions to modern understanding of mental disease that trauma during development causes psychopathology in adult life. Therefore, a successful psychoanalysis must include a detailed history of the patient's early life as well as a complete exploration of current difficulties.

Psychoanalysis as a Form of Treatment

Psychoanalysis is not synonymous with psychotherapy. It is a type of psychotherapy practiced by a minority of therapists who must receive specialized analytic training in addition to their more generalized therapeutic training. Psychoanalysis as a specific treatment method requires some explanation because its techniques are unusual and often misunderstood. The patient lies on a couch and the analyst sits out of the patient's line of sight. The analyst attempts to represent, as much as possible, a neutral figure. To proceed with the major task of analysis—an examination of the patient's inner life—the analyst responds to many of the patient's comments with silence or with an explanation (**interpretation**) aimed at uncovering their deeper, latent meaning. Called the **rule of abstinence,** this seemingly asocial means of communication is designed to help patients overcome a natural reluctance to expose intimate details of their lives.

As unnatural as this technique appears, Freud felt it was essential to achieve the major objective of a psychoanalysis: uncovering the patient's hidden psychic life, which he called **the unconscious.** He defined the unconscious as a layer of mental life that exists outside of awareness but still influences emotions and behavior. Freud emphasized that the analyst's central task was to help patients discover the secrets of their unconscious. Once aware of these hidden feelings and thoughts, patients would be able to examine the role they played in the development of symptoms.

Symptom Formation

Freud hypothesized that symptoms of mental disorder arose when conflicting emotions such as hate and love or assertiveness and passivity produced unmanageable distress. Borrowing from popular scientific notions about conservation of energy, he posited that psychic conflict created an energy imbalance in the psychic apparatus. The patient was alerted to this imbalance of psychic energy by experiencing anxiety. This psychological alert, called **signal anxiety,** induced the psychic apparatus to relieve distress by transferring awareness of the conflict into the unconscious. This mechanism of movement from the conscious to the unconscious is called **repression.** However, repression often fails to bury the conflict entirely. Elements of awareness leak into consciousness, again causing anxiety. Then, in another attempt to diminish distress, the psychic apparatus further disposes of the anxiety by transforming it into a neurotic symptom (**symptom formation**). Freud posited the creation of **psychic defenses** as protection against intrapsychic conflict and anxiety and considered symptom formation largely a consequence of the failure of the **mechanisms of defense** (Table 2–1).

Working with Unconscious Material

In his intensive work with patients, Freud discovered phenomena and developed techniques that allowed the analyst to observe the workings of the unconscious. These include slips of the tongue, dream analysis, free association, transference, and resistance. These subjects will be described and illustrated by means of clinical material.

A. Slips of the Tongue: Slips of the tongue, commonly called **freudian slips,** were one of Freud's earliest discoveries. Clues to unconscious material were evident when a person misused a word resulting in a trivial error that in fact revealed the patient's inner feelings. A typical freudian slip is demonstrated by the following:

> An unattached young man, envious of a couple who are in love, remarks as they go off to the beach, "Have a nice lay" (instead of "nice day"). Before this slip, if asked directly, the young man would have been unaware that he had a fantasy about the couple's love life. But the slip suggests otherwise.

Table 2–1. Mechanisms of defense.

Denial
The unconscious literally deletes from awareness an unpleasant or anxiety-provoking reality. A patient told of a terminal diagnosis has "forgotten" being so informed.

Sublimation
The redirection of an unacceptable impulse into an acceptable form of behavior. An individual with intense unconscious voyeuristic impulses becomes a sex therapist.

Reaction formation
The redirection of an unacceptable impulse into its opposite. A former smoker zealously enforces the new "no smoking" law.

Displacement
An impulse toward a given person or situation is redirected toward a "safer" less distressing object. A resident is humiliated by an attending physician and becomes enraged at his subordinate interns and medical students.

Projection
An unacceptable or anxiety-provoking impulse or affect is transplanted to another individual or situation. It is then "out there" rather than in oneself. A parent becomes preoccupied with his adolescent daughter's alleged promiscuity, thereby projecting his own impulses onto the teenager.

Rationalization
An acceptable explanation for a feeling or behavior is used to camouflage the unacceptable underlying motive or impulse. An obese man thinks he overate at the party so as not to offend his hostess.

Intellectualization
The avoidance of "feeling" by taking refuge in "thinking." A defeated quarterback avoids feelings of self-reproach and inadequacy by meticulously and logically explaining the details of his strategic errors.

Repression
Disturbing psychological material is secondarily removed from consciousness or primarily prevented from becoming conscious. Repressed memories and feelings associated with childhood sexual abuse are unleashed into consciousness when, as an adult, the patient is taken to a movie about a woman who had been raped.

Isolation of affect
The removal of disturbing affect from an idea or event, with the dispassionate details or description remaining. A combat veteran recounts seeing a friend killed but speaks in a cold and distant tone. He has "isolated" and "repressed" the intense fear and horror (affect) that might accompany the memory.

Suppression
Intentional repression of unpleasant conscious material. A medical student exits the Part I examination with a sense that he has failed. He decides not to worry about it until the scores arrive in the mail because it will accomplish nothing to do so.

Humor
A conscious and unconscious defense that allows material that stirs unpleasant affects to be better tolerated in consciousness. A screaming patient is the subject of laughter and mimicry in the privacy of the doctor's lounge.

B. Dreams: Dreams have been described as the "royal road" to the unconscious. Freud believed they had a manifest or apparent content that disguised their latent or unconscious content. According to analytic theory, dream work allows sleep to be uninterrupted by transforming the distressing **latent content** of the dream into the merely perplexing **manifest content.**

For example, an adolescent describes a dream in which an angel appears and holds his arm. In discussing the dream, the teenager reveals he is troubled by the angel's presence. An exploration of the dream through **free association**—the process of allowing random thoughts to come to mind and be expressed verbally—reveals that the young man associates the dream image with hands, sheets, and ultimately masturbation. When fully analyzed, the angel holding his arm, preventing masturbation, symbolically represents religious values that conflict with his sexual impulses. Thus, the analysis of the dream makes him aware of conflicts about masturbation that can then be explored therapeutically. With this insight, he can then decide how to manage the conflict between sexual impulses and religious rules.

C. Vignette of an Analysis: The following vignette of an analysis illustrates **free association, transference, resistance,** and **symptom formation.**

A 33-year-old single woman consults an analyst because her right arm is paralyzed and anesthetic. Previous neurological examinations have failed to explain her disability. Although the patient's family expresses concern about the symptoms, the patient appears remarkably calm about it (*la belle indifférence*). In the course of treatment, the analyst discovers that the patient's elderly father, a widower, has suffered a paralytic stroke, leaving him unable to feed himself. The patient's two older sisters decide that all three should take turns feeding their father. Hours before the patient was to take her first turn, the paralysis occurred. Given that the patient's impairment is not explained physically, the analyst attempts to uncover its psychological origins. He instructs the patient to verbalize whatever comes to mind (**free association**) and to report any dreams. These techniques of free association and **dream interpretation** enable the analyst to glimpse the patient's unconscious. The data obtained from free association and dreams will be pieced together like the parts of a puzzle to construct a picture of the relevant unconscious material.

Over several sessions, the analyst learns that the patient has conflicting emotions about her father. For example, while free associating, the patient reports the suspicion that the analyst is staring at her breasts and wishes to touch them. Exploration of this fantasy leads to her long-term feelings of sexual vulnerability in the presence of an older man. The analyst now—and her father in her past—are thus linked (**transference**). With considerable distress, the patient recalls episodes as a teenager when her father teased her about and playfully touched her developing breasts. This memory was recovered with so much reluctance and pain by the patient that she considered discontinuing treatment. This phenomenon, called **resistance,** occurs when a patient attempts to avoid a topic that may lead to awareness of unconscious material. Such material is shunned because of the emotional pain caused by its discovery.

As the treatment progresses using free association, dreams, transference, and resistance, the analyst discovers that the patient is unconsciously in conflict about caring for her dying father. She speaks about him with hostility as she recalls his teasing behavior but remembers him warmly for his support in later life. Now aware that she harbors the heretofore unconscious impulse to vengefully torment her now defenseless father, she understands how her **conflict** between nurturing and aggression has produced a paralysis that allowed reprieve from a difficult situation. The nature of this conflict was unconscious and, therefore, unknown to the patient before the analysis.

Once the patient has been able to recall her adolescent trauma in the safe environment of the analysis, she resolves to work through her conflicting feelings of hostility and love. In other words, her incompletely repressed feelings about caring for her father were converted to a paralysis. Now, with insight into these conflicts, she can work through or accept the fact that ambivalent feelings are a nonthreatening part of human experience. Once she is unburdened of the conflict, the anxiety disappears, the conversion symptom resolves, and her arm functions again.

In summary, the paralysis provides an escape from an unresolved dilemma. The symptom eliminated her anxiety (now converted to a paralysis) because it precluded either striking or feeding her father (**primary gain**). The conversion disorder also elicits support and sympathy from the family (**secondary gain**) (see Chapter 22).

Hysterical paralysis is a particularly dramatic symptom; however, an intrapsychic paralysis (eg, in the areas of intimacy or sexual functioning) will be less conspicuous but perhaps no less distressing to the afflicted patient. Unresolved unconscious conflicts may lead to a multitude of symptoms.

Mind & Body

Students in the preclinical phase of medical school often find it difficult to accept the concept that mental states can influence bodily functions. The intriguing phenomenon of hypnosis provides a familiar example of the power of the mind over the body. During a state of hypnotic suggestion, a subject, asked to make his arm "as stiff as a board," finds that the arm cannot be passively flexed by another person. A subject not in a hypnotized state would be unable to resist such forceful flexion. Moreover, hypnotized persons can experience standardized painful stimuli without apparent distress.

SCHOOLS OF PSYCHOANALYSIS & LATER PSYCHOTHERAPIES

Psychoanalytic theory was for a time virtually synonymous with the writings and teachings of Sigmund

Freud. However, over the years, divergent schools of psychoanalytic theory and psychotherapy evolved. An inner circle of practitioners had gathered around Freud, and, ironically, it was these disciples who broke with strict freudian principles to found the major nonfreudian schools of psychoanalytic psychology.

Carl Jung and Alfred Adler are perhaps the best known of this group and are briefly discussed below. Other early psychoanalysts influential in the history of psychiatry and psychology include Wilhelm Reich, Otto Rank, Erik Erikson, Anna Freud, and Karen Horney.

Carl Jung (1875–1961) differed with and ultimately left Freud to found a separate school of psychology and psychotherapy. One of the numerous concepts for which he is well known was his division of the unconscious into the personal unconscious and the collective unconscious. The **collective unconscious** was posited as an inherited commonality of all humankind, the repository of **archetypes**—universal images and concepts found repeatedly in the mythologies of diverse cultures. It is contrasted with the **personal unconscious,** which is based on the individual's early experience and individual memories. Jung postulated that all humans face life with a common heritage of images and preprogrammed patterns, that is, the collective history of the human race.

Jung is also known for his schema that describes personality types according to three axes: extroversion-introversion, sensation-intuition, and thinking-feeling. He believed that individual personality styles tend toward one of the two polarities in each of these three axes and that there is benefit in reclaiming one's capacity for wholeness, that is, to actualize personality characteristics that are less developed. He asserted the importance of integrating the opposing aspects found within oneself.

Alfred Adler (1870–1937) also split with Freud after years of collaboration to found his own school of psychology. He was the first of the inner circle to do so. Adler gave less weight to unconscious psychosexual material, focusing rather on socially mediated phenomena. He discussed **feelings of inferiority,** grounded in the infant's experience of helplessness, and of a **will to power** (as a compensatory drive) influencing one's social interactions. Adler is also known for his observations regarding the role of **birth order** in personality development, and he described personality styles typical of first-born, middle, and youngest siblings.

Karen Horney (1885–1952) was an influential analyst who also founded her own school. Her views emphasized the cultural context in which we develop, in particular with regard to sex roles. She felt that character traits commonly considered feminine (dependency, submissiveness, etc) were derived from cultural rather than biological influences. Horney, in general, reflected a move away from the more individualized, psychosexual origins of mental illness toward an emphasis on social and interpersonal forces in development.

Harry Stack Sullivan (1892–1949), an American who did not train with Freud, founded a school of psychoanalytic psychology that focused on **interpersonal relations**—with less emphasis on Freud's psychosexual stages. He introduced theories of stages that were later than those of Freud, placing importance on **preadolescence** and the **juvenile** stages and viewing **peer relations** as critical to individual development. Sullivan believed that close friendships ("chumships") during preadolescence and early adolescence laid the essential groundwork for the later development of love relationships with the opposite sex.

The **humanistic/existential** schools of psychology emerged later in the twentieth century and represented the field's increasing eclecticism and gradual broadening of theories away from the original freudian principles. Axiomatic to these schools is a more philosophical bent, with attention to concepts such as authenticity, taking responsibility for one's life, successful individuation, and the attainment of self-actualization. These schools contended that people have great potential for mental health and the capacity to live vigorously and "with meaning."

The progression has been from Freud to the schools of his followers and colleagues and to a widening array of psychological theories, until most practicing psychotherapists consider themselves somewhat eclectic with regard to the nonsomatic treatments and apply an amalgam of psychological constructs in their work with patients. Many psychotherapists continue to identify themselves with a specific technique or school of thought, but this is becoming the exception rather than the rule.

SOCIAL LEARNING THEORY

Social learning theory asserts that behaviors (even complex behaviors) are **externally determined** and are maintained more by environmental consequences, such as reward and punishment, than by internal psychological processes.

The development of the theories and principles underlying modern behavioral treatments and the historic development of psychoanalytic treatments took place concurrently. Yet the two schools of thought evolved independently, with seemingly little common ground. The pivotal distinction arises from the early behaviorist's primary focus on **observable events,** with little, if any, attention paid to the subjective reporting of nonobservables such as feelings or thoughts. In time, behavioral theories and treatments expanded to encompass less easily quantified phenomena such as cognition and anxiety. Yet the central dogma of the behaviorists and the behavioral model remains focused on behavioral change and not on insight, self-reflection, or unconscious mental activity.

The history of behavioral theory begins with the experiments of Ivan Pavlov (1849–1936), best known for his paradigm of **classical conditioning,** wherein a dog that naturally salivates at the sight of meat is then conditioned to salivate at the sound of a bell when no food is present. This example illustrates several key terms in social learning theory. The **unconditioned stimulus** (the food) is the original **stimulus** that led to the **response** of salivation. This unconditioned stimulus is then **paired** with a **conditioned stimulus,** the sound of a bell. In time, response (salivating) is elicited by the conditioned stimulus (the bell) even in the absence of the unconditioned stimulus (the food). This simple classical conditioning process has a role in more complex human behaviors.

Modern addictionologists know that their patients are at special risk for relapse when exposed to stimuli that were at one time closely associated with the substance of abuse. The sight of a familiar liquor store or a dealer-haunted street corner can elicit a powerful craving for the abused substance in individuals whose "high" was closely associated with these stimuli. The abused substance in this example is the unconditioned stimulus, which elicits craving in a drug-dependent person—craving being the homologue of Pavlov's dog's salivating.

J. B. Watson (1878–1958), an American psychologist influenced by Pavlov, conducted a famous experiment in which an 11-month-old boy, Albert B., was the subject. Albert would cry and become frightened in response to loud noises, an **unconditioned stimulus.** Watson paired the loud noise with the sight of a white rat, the **conditioned stimulus.** Albert quickly learned to avoid the rat, which he had not previously feared. Furthermore, Albert also avoided other objects with appearances similar to the white rat, an example of **stimulus generalization.**

Edward Thorndike (1874–1949) and B. F. Skinner (1904–1990) were prominent pioneers in the field of behaviorism. Thorndike postulated the **law of effect:** the consequences of a behavior determine the frequency of that behavior. Skinner, a central figure in the development and exposition of behavioral theory, is known particularly for his work in operant conditioning.

Operant conditioning is the manipulation of behaviors through consequences structured to **follow** the targeted behaviors. **Positive reinforcers** increase the frequency of a behavior, and, conversely, **punishment** decreases the frequency of a behavior. This behavioral definition of punishment requires an accompanying decrease in target behavior frequency. If scolding a child does not lead to a decrease in the targeted behavior, it is not technically defined as punishment. **Negative reinforcement** is reward by the removal or avoidance of an undesirable consequence

and serves, as does positive reinforcement, to **increase** the frequency of a targeted behavior. These terms are illustrated in the following example:

A pigeon may peck at a bar in its cage every now and then. If pecking on the bar is now **positively reinforced** by immediately rewarding the behavior with food, the frequency of pecking the bar increases; this is **operant conditioning.** If, subsequently, pecking the bar no longer leads to a food reward, the conditioned increase in the frequency of the behavior will gradually be **extinguished.** The time course of this **extinction** of a conditioned response varies considerably depending on the nature of the conditioning that initiated the behavior.

In the case of the pigeon, if food was forthcoming every time the bar was pecked (**continuous reinforcement**), the behavior would be extinguished rather quickly after the food reinforcement is discontinued. If food was given only *some of the times* the bar was pecked (**intermittent reinforcement**), extinction of the pecking behavior would occur much more slowly. The power of **intermittent positive reinforcement** is graphically demonstrated at casinos and race tracks; the relatively rare jackpot drives a high frequency of unrewarded plays despite the cost of each play. This is an example of the importance of the **schedule of reinforcement** on the persistence of behaviors. Behaviors conditioned by strong positive reinforcers on an intermittent reinforcement schedule are slow to extinguish.

Complex behaviors can be conditioned through **shaping,** wherein successive approximations of the desired behavior are reinforced in turn. Encouraging a withdrawn, hospitalized patient to interact with peers might involve initially rewarding simply sitting near peers, then rewarding an occasional "thank you" or "excuse me," the intervention moving in stepwise fashion toward the desired complex behavior of interacting fully with peers.

Behavioral principles are often used in the treatment of phobias and frequently employ both **relaxation training** and **systematic desensitization,** a combination of techniques pioneered by Joseph Wolpe (1915–). The patient is trained to self-induce a relaxed state by serially tensing and then relaxing muscles, working through the major muscle groups, usually from head to toe or vice versa. The patient is then instructed to imagine the phobic situation, beginning with only a mild stimulus, and simultaneously to remain in the relaxed state.

For example, a man with a fear of flying would first learn the relaxation exercise and then be directed to imagine purchasing a plane ticket while maintaining the relaxed state. The next step might be remaining relaxed while imagining arriving at the airport with his luggage, and so on, until the relaxed state can persist even while vividly imagining a turbulent flight in a crowded aircraft. The patient is thus **systematically desensitized** to a stimulus that once elicited a *phobic* response. A more comprehensive discussion of behavioral treatments is found in Chapters 33 and 36.

NEUROBIOLOGY & SOMATIC TREATMENTS

Somatic treatments (Chapter 30) are considered nonpsychological in nature and consist essentially of the administration of psychotropic medications and the use of electroconvulsive therapy (ECT). The history of somatic treatments is one of empirical and at times fortuitous advances. Medications not specifically targeted for treatment of psychiatric conditions were in several instances discovered to have efficacy in the treatment of a mental disorder. The clinically observed effect of this medication on a psychiatric syndrome would inevitably lead to hypotheses regarding the neurobiological basis of the drug effect.

If, for example, a medication originally introduced to treat nausea but also effective in treating delusional thinking is discovered to decrease central nervous system dopamine neurotransmission, a hypothesis implicating excessive dopamine neurotransmission as the cause of delusional thoughts is generated. This example is somewhat oversimplified but illustrates the concurrent evolution of somatic treatments and the science of neurobiology. The medications have helped elucidate biological mechanisms of mental illness, as has research with chemical probes structurally similar to the medications. Modern psychopharmacology is the science of influencing central nervous system neurotransmission.

As yet, the detailed mechanisms mediating most psychiatric illnesses are not fully understood, but modern theories are centered primarily around dysfunctional neurotransmission. For example, the medications used to treat the symptoms of schizophrenia are thought to do so primarily via their effect on dopaminergic neurotransmission. Antidepressant medications and electroconvulsive therapy affect neurotransmission mediated by norepinephrine and/or serotonin, obsessive-compulsive disorder is treated with medications that affect serotonergic neurotransmission, and so on. These treatments and their hypothesized mechanisms of action are discussed in greater detail in Chapters 6 and 30 and in the chapters devoted to specific types of mental disorder.

Further light is shed on the neurobiology of mental illness by research in the fields of genetics and molecular biology. As illustrated in the following discussion and examples, it is generally accepted that with regard to mental illness the answer to questions about the relative influence of nature versus nurture is that both contribute to the development of psychiatric disorders. It is often stated, in discussions of the causes of the major psychiatric disorders, that they result from the confluence of an inherited genetic vulnerability to the disorder plus environmental factors, that is, developmental experiences (the so-called **stress-diathesis model**).

A powerful tool in evaluating genetic versus environmental factors in mental illness is the study of family pedigrees and especially the study of twins. Monozygotic (identical) twins have virtually identical genomes, whereas dizygotic (fraternal) twins, on average, share only half their genes. It can therefore be predicted that genetically based illnesses will show a higher concordance rate in monozygotic than in dizygotic twins.

For example, in schizophrenia, the **concordance** rate in monozygotic twins is approximately 50%. This indicates that if one member of a pair of monozygotic twins has schizophrenia, there is a 50% likelihood that the other twin will also have the illness. In dizygotic twins the concordance rate is approximately one-fourth that found in monozygotic twins, thus supporting the role of heredity in this illness. This 50% concordance rate in genetically identical individuals argues eloquently for both the genetic contribution to the illness and for the nongenetic, environmental contribution because the **discordance** rate is also 50%. Studies suggest that schizophrenic patients with the worst long-term outcome may have greater genetic loading for schizophrenia (ie, genetic relatives also have the disorder) than do schizophrenics with more favorable outcomes (Keefe et al, 1987).

THE CHALLENGE OF INTEGRATION

The preceding sections have covered considerable ground—from primitive religion to genetics, from Freud to Skinner, from the collective unconscious to electroconvulsive therapy. At some point, it is necessary to acknowledge and grapple with the difficulty of integrating this body of information across disciplines and across theoretical frameworks within the field of psychiatry.

Quality patient care is ultimately an interdisciplinary and integrative endeavor. Throughout this text, several case studies will be presented to illustrate the principle that solutions to all problems involving the complexity of human beings require a broadly based integrative approach. The application of medical science and psychology and the simultaneous appreciation of the sociological context of a patient's illness are needed to build that broad base.

Specialization is the reality of modern medicine and contemporary society in general. Even within the traditional medical and surgical specialties there are subspecialties. In the face of a burgeoning biomedical data base, this trend is both rational and inevitable with one proviso: All specialists and subspecialists must avoid thinking that an effective, compassionate doctor-patient relationship falls into the realm of "someone else's specialty."

It must be emphasized that any effective clinical

relationship involves more than treating a disease or symptom. Treating a complex person requires attention to the psychological aspects of the situation and to the social context of the patient's life (family, work, etc). The following case is reported as a narrative delivered by the patient, a 41-year-old construction foreman.

> "I had to go for an insurance physical because I got a new job. This young doc noticed something suspicious on one of my testicles, and he said it was probably nothing but that I should go see a urologist to get it checked out. He says this to me and is out the door 10 seconds later. Busy guy.
>
> "So I get home, and I start to worry, but I couldn't feel anything wrong down there. So I wonder if whatever it was might be serious, like cancer, and it crosses my mind that, God forbid, I might need surgery and that I'd lose my testicles or never get hard-ons, or something. Now that really scared me so I didn't tell my wife and just tried to forget the whole thing. She was trying to get pregnant and I figured I'd wait until after that.
>
> "Nearly 2 years go by, and she's not pregnant. My wife's gynecologist sends home a plastic container for me to give a sperm sample, and then drop it off at a lab. Okay. I've been checking myself, and my testicles feel just like always, so I tell myself not to worry. But I do anyway.
>
> "To make a long story short, it turns out that she's not getting pregnant because my sperm count is too low. I go to a urologist and he says I have an extra vein that's causing the problem, that he can fix it, and maybe my sperm count will get higher.
>
> "He tells me that it's not cancer even though I didn't even ask him that. He says there's basically no chance I'd lose anything, and he drew some pictures on a piece of paper. He was great and I said okay to the operation. He said the insurance doctor made a good pick-up and that a lot of doctors would've missed it. My wife was pregnant about 4 months after the operation. I just wish sometimes that I would've gotten it checked out sooner."

Comment: As noted by the urologist, the original discovery of the varicocele was a "good pick-up" from a biomedical viewpoint, but the doctor-patient contact was nonetheless inadequate and allowed for significant distress in the psychological and social spheres of the patient's life.

In a landmark article in 1977, George Engel elucidated the **biopsychosocial model,** a framework based on an integrative, whole-person approach to patient care. Engel coined this term with the intent of distinguishing this more holistic approach from the more prevalent **biomedical model.** As the field of medicine evolves, so must our awareness of the body-mind interface. Eric Kandel writes, in a 1998 article chronicling the entwined arenas of neurobiology and psychodynamics:

> the years since 1980 have witnessed major developments in the brain sciences, in particular in the analysis of how different aspects of mental functioning are represented by different regions of the brain [and in psychopharmacology]. Thus, psychiatry is now presented with a new and unique opportunity. When it comes to studying mental function, biologists are badly in need of guidance. It is here that psychiatry, and cognitive psychology, as guide and tutor, can make a particularly valuable contribution to brain science. One of the powers of psychiatry, of cognitive psychology, and of psychoanalysis lies in their perspectives. Psychiatry, cognitive psychology, and psychoanalysis can define for biology the mental functions that need to be studied for a meaningful and sophisticated understanding of the biology of the human mind. In this interaction, psychiatry can play a double role. First, *it can seek answers to questions on its own level,* questions related to the diagnosis and treatment of mental disorders. Second, it can pose the behavioral questions that biology needs to answer if we are to have a realistically advanced understanding of human higher mental processes. (Kandel, 1998)

REFERENCES & SUGGESTED READINGS

Alexander F, Selesnick S: *The History of Psychiatry.* New American Library, 1966.

American Psychiatric Association: *Diagnostic and Statistical Manual of Mental Disorders,* 4th ed. American Psychiatric Association, 1994.

Bandura A: *A Social Learning Theory.* General Learning Press, 1971.

Benson H: *The Relaxation Response.* Morrow, 1976.

Bloom F et al (editors): *Psychopharmacology: The Fourth Generation of Progress.* Raven Press, 1994.

Cavener JO et al (editors): *Psychiatry.* Lippincott/Basic Books, 1986.

Engel GE: *Psychological Development in Health and Disease.* Saunders, 1962.

Engel GE: The need for a new medical model: A challenge for biomedicine. Science 1977;196:129.

Engel GE: The clinical application of the biopsychosocial model. Am J Psychiatry 1978;137:535.

Farber SL: *Identical Twins Reared Apart: A Re-analysis.* Basic Books, 1981.

Fine R: *A History of Psychoanalysis.* Columbia University Press, 1979.

Freud A: *The Ego and the Mechanisms of Defense,* rev. ed. International University Press, 1967.

Freud S: *Standard Edition of the Complete Psychological Works of Sigmund Freud.* Hogarth Press, 1959.

Goodman L et al (editors): *Goodman & Gilman's The Pharmacological Basis of Therapeutics,* 9th ed. McGraw-Hill, 1996.

Hall C et al: *Theories of Personality,* 4th ed. Wiley, 1997.

Horney K: *The Neurotic Personality of Our Time.* Norton, 1937.

Jung CG: *Memories, Dreams, and Reflections.* Random House, 1961.

Kandel ER: A new intellectual framework for psychiatry. Am J Psychiatry 1998;155:457.

Kaplan HI, Sadock BJ (editors): *Comprehensive Textbook of Psychiatry*/VI, 6th ed. Williams & Wilkins, 1995.

Keefe RSE et al: Characteristics of very poor outcome schizophrenia. Am J Psychiatry 1987;144:889.

Leigh H, Reiser MF: *The Patient: Biological, Psychological, and Social Dimensions of Medical Practice,* 3rd ed. Plenum Press, 1992.

Piel G et al (editors): *The Brain: A Scientific American Book.* Freeman, 1979.

Reich W: *Character Analysis,* rev. ed. Straus & Young, 1980.

Tasman A et al (editors): *Psychiatry.* W.B. Saunders, 1996.

Thorndike EL: *The Psychology of Learning.* Teacher's College, 1913.

Vaillant G: *Adaptation to Life.* Little, Brown, 1977.

Weiner H: *Psychobiology and Human Disease.* Elsevier-North Holland, 1977.

Wolpe J: *The Practice of Behavior Therapy,* 4th ed. Pergamon, 1992.

Yalom I: *Existential Psychotherapy.* Basic Books, 1980.

The Mind & Somatic Illness: Psychological Factors Affecting Physical Illness

3

Stuart J. Eisendrath, MD, & Steven D. Prakken, MD

A 60-year-old woman entered a hospital emergency room complaining of light-headedness and chest palpitations. Shortly thereafter, she suffered a cardiac arrest that was successfully treated and she was transferred to the coronary care unit. When examined, the woman was anxious and depressed. On questioning, she revealed that the date of her cardiac arrest was the 1-year anniversary of her husband's death from cardiac arrest.

A 40-year-old businessman underwent a traumatic divorce and became seriously depressed. His ex-wife, to whom he had been devoted, had left him for a 25-year-old tennis instructor. Two months later the businessman was found to have an aggressive lymphoma; he died 3 months later after several unsuccessful trials of chemotherapy.

A 4-year-old boy had always had excellent health. Two weeks after his only sibling was born, however, he developed persistent cough and fever. He eventually required hospitalization for treatment of pneumonia.

The above are examples of typical clinical situations in which attentive and alert clinicians may see the influence of psychosocial factors on physical health. Physicians have been aware of this relationship since ancient times. The study of this relationship, usually termed psychosomatic medicine, has undergone marked conceptual shifts during the past decades. Today, theorists believe that there are no "psychosomatic" diseases per se and that all physical diseases have psychosocial components. These components may predispose to, initiate, or maintain illness.

Of note, the expansion of the category "Psychological factors affecting medical condition" in the *Diagnostic and Statistical Manual of Mental Disorders,* 4th edition (*DSM-IV*) as compared with *DSM-III-R* reflects the increasing appreciation of the complexity of interactions between psychological factors and medical conditions. The new classification includes factors that influence the course of illness, interfere with treatment, constitute additional health risks, or elicit stress-related physiological responses, which may worsen illness. These include existing mental disorders, psychological symptoms, personality traits or coping styles, maladaptive health behaviors, and other possible psychological factors. This chapter focuses on the development of theories of psychosomatic medicine in the twentieth century.

Mind/Body & Stress

Before the 1900s, the philosophy of Cartesian dualism viewed the mind and the body as separate entities. Organized religions claimed the mind and spirit as their domain, while physicians were ceded the body. This dichotomy was heightened by scientific progress in the late 1800s. The discovery that bacteria caused disease emphasized the physical aspects of medicine and led to the concept of linear causality: one type of bacterium directly causes one disease. This oversimplified concept—that one factor directly causes one specific disease—influenced the development of psychosomatic theory for several decades.

Cannon, one of psychosomatic medicine's pioneers, performed intricate laboratory experiments that studied the effects of fear and rage on animals. He observed that animals responded to emergencies with adaptive changes in physiology that prepared them for "fight or flight." Cannon theorized that the mechanism involved an inhibition of anabolic (parasympathetic; cholinergic) functions and an activation of catabolic (sympathetic; adrenergic) functions. This supplied the animals with energy needed to meet the emergency.

Extending the work of Cannon, Selye (1974) postulated that the entire organism responded to stress; eg, blood flow might be shunted from the gastrointestinal tract to the heart, brain, and musculature during stress. Such an adaptation would help the organism deal with stress over the short term, but if the stress was prolonged, the adaptation might result in increased friability of the gastrointestinal mucosa and eventual ulceration. Selye proposed that responses to stress could be triggered in inappropriate situations if the organism had become accustomed to reacting in that way. Later research in autonomic conditioning suggests that such inappropriate reactions may be difficult to extinguish.

Personality & Medical Illness

In the 1940s, Dunbar (1942, 1946) began developing her "personality profiles" of specific diseases. She felt that each disease was associated with a specific cluster of symptoms. Dunbar reviewed psychological data about patients with diseases such as hypertension, diabetes, rheumatoid arthritis, and myocardial infarction. From these data she formulated typical behavior patterns, family histories, and patterns of onset of illness that seemed to be associated. She suggested, for example, that people with myocardial infarction tend to be compulsive and to overwork and that the infarction tends to follow exposure to shock, particularly at work.

The idea that a specific personality may be associated with a certain disease is most evident in current research into the behavior of people with coronary disease. Friedman and Rosenman (1974) labeled the behavior of these patients type A. Their work suggested that these patients chronically feel the pressure of time and a sense of hostile competitiveness.

A major deficit in the "specific personality" approach to understanding the relationship between psychological makeup and disease is that almost all of the data rely on retrospective analysis. Researchers study people who have a certain disease in an attempt to discern whether certain personality traits caused the disease, but specific psychological profiles are of limited value. Investigators following the model of direct linear causation derived from Koch's postulates tended to adopt the approach in the 1930s and 1940s that personality might "cause" disease. Treatment techniques (chiefly psychoanalysis) that tried to eradicate the precipitating psychological factor were notably unsuccessful, however.

It therefore became clear that direct, unitary causation did not operate in the development of diseases. Dunbar herself was careful to avoid implications of cause and effect in her work. Alternative explanations of the behavior associated with certain diseases were formulated. Perhaps the behavior resulted from the disease, or perhaps the behavior and the physical illness were both phenotypic expressions of some common gene. These theories suggested that psychological treatments that attempted to change behavior might not "cure" disease.

In contrast to Dunbar's personality-specific research, Alexander (1950) explored the relationship between specific psychological conflicts and disease states. He investigated seven diseases regarded as classic psychosomatic disorders: peptic ulcers, bronchial asthma, rheumatoid arthritis, ulcerative colitis, essential hypertension, thyrotoxicosis, and neurodermatitis. His work attempted to answer the main question in psychosomatic medicine in the 1930s and 1940s—why does the individual have these specific symptoms?

Alexander believed that psychosomatic diseases developed out of "visceral neurosis." Physiological changes accompanied unresolved emotional conflicts and eventually resulted in pathological derangements in the organ system. For example, Alexander hypothesized that individuals with peptic ulcer disease suffered from infantile desires for others to supply love, support, advice, and money. These desires intensified when the individuals became frustrated, but then patients felt guilt and shame because they wanted to appear as capable, independent adults. The desire to be cared for was equivalent to the infantile wish to be fed, and conflicting drives for independence and dependence were expressed as increased gastric secretions. The secretions in turn led to ulcers.

Alexander advanced the theory of psychosomatic medicine significantly by abandoning a model of disease based on unitary, direct causation. He postulated a three-part constellation of factors necessary to produce disease:

1. The individual must have a specific set of psychological conflicts.
2. A specific situation that triggers the onset of disease must occur; in ulcer disease, this might be the loss of a person on whom the patient depended.
3. The individual must have a constitutional vulnerability, an "X factor," that biologically predisposes the patient to that specific illness.

Alexander's work suffered because it was based on retrospective analysis. Mirsky (1958) investigated Alexander's ideas in an ingenious prospective study that used army recruits who were entering basic training. The recruits were divided into two groups on the basis of high or low levels of serum pepsinogen, a genetically determined trait that correlates with some types of ulcer formation. Those recruits with high levels of serum pepsinogen were found to have the infantile features suggested by Alexander. Moreover, they could be identified from their responses to psychological testing by independent raters who did not know their serum pepsinogen levels. The recruits who subsequently developed ulcers associated with the stress of basic training proved to be from the group who had high levels of serum pepsinogen.

Further Development of Theories of Psychosomatic Medicine

The Mirsky study tended to confirm many of Alexander's ideas but left many questions unanswered. How did stress lead to precipitating disease? Why did psychotherapeutic approaches have such variable success in treating psychosomatic disorders?

Mirsky's study opened a new area of inquiry in psychosomatic medicine. Could an inherited biological tendency toward gastric hypersecretion lead to psychological sequelae? For example, a newborn with high rates of gastric secretion might biologically require hourly feedings to diminish gastric acidity. If the mother fed the newborn at "average" intervals of once every 3 hours, conflict concerning dependence on others for attention and nurturance might be created in the newborn's personality. The genetic predisposition to gastric hypersecretion could lead to somatopsychic effects. Personality development could therefore be a result of physiological events, rather than the reverse.

Grinker (1973) began integrating such possibilities into a unified field theory of psychosomatic medicine, basically a general systems model of illness. This theory emphasized that each element of the human "system" (eg, personality or genetic constitution) had multiple reverberating connections throughout the system. Biological and psychosocial forces could interact with each other to produce disease. This theory clearly pointed out the inadequacy of the unitary, direct causation model of disease.

At the same time, Engel directed psychosomatic theory toward less specific but broader concepts. Engel (1975) noted that loss of an important person in the patient's life frequently preceded the onset or exacerbation of illness. Engel described how he suffered a myocardial infarction when mourning the death of his twin brother.

Engel (1967) believed that the loss of any important relationship led to several phases of response. First was arousal to search for the lost relationship. If the search failed, the individual entered a state of "conservation withdrawal" and ceased to search; physiological processes (eg, gastric secretion) became hypoactive. Engel believed that such a sequence could lead to a "giving up-given up" state, in which individuals felt helpless to change their situation and hopeless about receiving aid from others. Engel did not believe that this sense of powerlessness was in itself sufficient to cause illness, nor that this condition had to exist before illness occurred. Such a condition could predispose a person to illness, however.

Animal experiments lent support to Engel's position. Kaufman and Rosenblum (1969) used different species of monkeys to study the physiological response of an infant who was separated from its mother. The infant's patterns of behavior tended to follow the series of responses outlined by Engel, and the incidence of illness increased. Among certain species, however, the pattern was moderated if the deprived young monkey was provided with social support.

Epidemiologic studies have also supported Engel's work. Holmes and Rahe (1967) evaluated the effects of stressful events on the occurrence of physical illness. In both retrospective and prospective studies, they found that the number and magnitude of life changes (eg, bereavements, new jobs, moving to another place) correlated with the onset and severity of disease. Their work suggests that changes in life may encourage the development of disease, but in a nonspecific way.

Other researchers have evaluated bereavement as one specific and powerful type of life change. Rees and Lutkins (1967) noted that the number of deaths among relatives of patients who had died was seven times higher than that in the general population. Parkes and Brown (1972) found similarly elevated mortality rates in another population of bereaved individuals. These findings have been reproduced in many countries. It is clear that loss of an emotionally important person is associated with increased incidence of both illness and death, particularly in young widowers.

Reiser (1975) believed that there are three phases related to illness. During the period before illness develops, the patient is shaped by genetic constitution and early psychosocial experiences. When the illness appears, the prior "programming" is activated by nonspecific psychosocial stresses, such as bereavement. Other factors, such as environmental exposure to viruses or malignant transformation in cells, may then challenge the stressed individual and produce disease. In the third phase, after the onset of disease, psychosocial forces operate to modulate the course of the disease.

Biopsychosocial Model of Disease

Engel (1977) synthesized the advances in psychosomatic medicine by developing the biopsychosocial model of disease, which recognizes that all diseases have biological, psychological, and social components. Engel's model emphasizes that each individual comprises systems and is in turn part of larger outside systems. Each person is composed of molecules, cells, and organs; each person is also a member of a family, community, culture, nation, and the world. Every individual has a biological, psychological, and social structure that may affect other levels of the system and vice versa. As an example, Engel (1980) described a patient undergoing cardiac arrest, an account paraphrased here and used to illustrate how Engel's theory may be applied:

> A patient suffers chest pain and goes to a hospital emergency room. Because he has had one previous myocardial infarction, he suspects that he is having another. He is examined by a new intern, who also suspects an infarction and attempts to insert an intravenous line. After several unsuccessful attempts, the intern leaves the patient alone in his cubicle and goes to get assistance. While unattended, the patient continues to feel pain and also feels alone and worried about the competence of his caretakers. He suffers a cardiac arrest and is immediately resuscitated successfully by the emergency team.

If the viewpoint adopted by the clinician is a biomedical model based on linear causality, the successful resuscitation of the patient is a laudable event. If psychosocial factors are taken into account, however, important information is revealed about the patient and the incident, namely, that the patient's pain, fear, and doubts most likely affected the physical disease process, possibly through direct vagal effects, increased levels of circulating catecholamines, or other physiological responses. If medical personnel had considered psychosocial factors and started appropriate treatment (eg, ensuring constant attention by the nursing staff or using anxiolytic medications), the cardiac arrest might not have occurred. The biopsychosocial model does not simplistically assert that the myocardial infarction was a direct result of the patient's state of mind. It does provide a broader understanding of disease processes, and it encourages physicians to think about truly comprehensive treatment that considers both the physical and the psychosocial elements of disease.

The model also includes sociocultural factors in its conception of disease. It has been widely demonstrated, for example, that pain as a presenting symptom is affected by gender, race, and ethnic origin. The biopsychosocial model holds that a stoic New England Yankee may be experiencing as much pain as an expressive Italian patient with the same disease.

CURRENT CONCEPTS IN PSYCHOSOMATIC MEDICINE

The biopsychosocial model provides one approach to study the relationship between disease and psychosocial factors. Current research in psychosomatic medicine has shifted from the "why" questions so common in earlier decades to the "how" questions, eg, how does the bereavement experience become translated into physical illness? In other words, how are psychological experiences transduced into bodily changes?

Work in the fields of type A behavior (TAB) and psychoimmunology highlights current approaches aimed at understanding the transduction process. In addition to Friedman and Rosenman's work, a number of prospective studies have demonstrated that TAB is indeed a risk factor for coronary artery disease (CAD). These studies corrected a major weakness of the earlier retrospective research. In individuals with already diagnosed CAD, Brackett and Powell (1988) found that type A personality increases the risk of sudden cardiac death but does not increase the risk of other cardiac events or nonsudden cardiac death.

More recent studies have investigated the components of TAB that are most related to CAD and other illnesses. Early reviews (Goldstein and Niaura, 1992) noted that expressive hostility and antagonistic interactions were the key toxic elements of the type A personality, but this has been refined even further with some very intriguing results. In a study by Price et al (1995) it was found that insecurity was the underlying motivator of the two primary overt components of TAB, time urgency and free floating hostility. In a review by Hart (1997) it was noted that the time urgency/impatience component of TAB is predictive of both illness incidence and severity, even for noncoronary illness, whereas the hard-driving/competitive component had no effect on illness but had a positive influence on achievement. That there may be protective elements of TAB was documented by Carmelli and Swan (1996) where the lowest all-cause mortality incidence in a population were the type A individuals who had a nonhostile, sociable, and emotionally expressive style.

The number of studies investigating the effects of psychological treatment of type A personality on CAD is still small. Nunes et al (1987), in their meta-analysis of existing controlled studies, found that psychological treatment significantly reduces type A personality measures. Although it improves clinical outcome of CAD at 1 year only marginally, psychological treatment may significantly improve outcome at 3 years. In addition, other studies found that lack of social support predicts severity of CAD and mortality in subjects with type A personality (Niaura and Goldstein, 1992).

In attempting to understand how TAB might produce CAD, several studies investigating physiological changes in type A individuals found that these individuals show higher increases in blood pressure, heart rate, and catecholamines when challenged with stressful tasks (Goldstein and Niaura, 1992). This evidence was supported by Sundin et al (1995) in a study comparing healthy and postmyocardial infarction (MI) groups with both type A and type B profiles. They found that when mental and physical stressors were applied in both the healthy and post-MI groups of type A individuals there was an increase in systolic and diastolic blood pressure reactivity, compared to the type B groups. There were also hemodynamic changes consistent with β-adrenergic activation. More studies are needed to clarify further what behavioral, hemodynamic, and neuroendocrine mechanisms may contribute to the development of atherosclerosis.

Psychoimmunology and psychoneuroimmunology are related areas of research in which the relationship between psychological processes and physiological events is being elucidated. Numerous research studies have already proven the hypothesis that psychological events have profound physical effects on individuals. Schliefer et al (1983) studied the spouses of women dying of breast cancer. They discovered depressed lymphocyte response to mitogens peaking at 2 months postbereavement and gradually returning to normal over the remainder of the postbereavement year for most subjects. This carefully designed study demonstrated that the abnormalities in the immune system were a direct result of the bereavement process and not a result of factors such as nutrition, activity, or sleep. Other losses, such as marital separation and divorce, can also lead to changes in the immunity (Kiecolt-Glaser and Glaser, 1986).

Animal experimentation has also demonstrated marked effects of stress on illness. Riley (1975) exposed two groups of mice to the tumor-causing Bittner virus. The group in a stress-free environment had a 7% incidence of tumor, whereas the stressed group had a 92% incidence of tumor.

The effects of psychological stress are not limited to just the immune system. There are also documented stress-related changes in the cardiovascular, metabolic, and neurological systems of humans. A perceived lack of control, added to high psychological stress in the work site, produces elevated ambulatory blood pressures, increased left-ventricular mass index (Schnall et al, 1992), and increased atherosclerosis (Everson et al, 1997). Chronic stress and hostility are linked to activation of the fibrinogen system and platelets, both risk factors for myocardial infarction (Raikkonen et al, 1996; Markowe et al, 1985). Atrophy of the hippocampus has been seen by magnetic resonance imaging studies in posttraumatic stress disorder, recurrent depressive disorders, and Cushing's disease (Sapolsky, 1996; McEwen and Magarinos, 1997). Some of these hippocampal changes may be related to an increase in cortisol levels.

Although the negative effects of stress on the immune system have been documented, whether this dysfunction of the immune system has any direct effects on production of illness has yet to be determined. Prospective trials have shown that the number of episodes of illness (documented by viral cultures) is related to daily stress scores, and that the stress from "rigid and chaotic" families increases the incidence of influenza B fourfold (Cohen, 1995). In a viral challenge study, Cohen (1995) found a dose-response relationship between psychological stress and clinical illness across five different viruses. In stressed (restrained) mice, Bonneau et al (1991) were able to show a suppression of a specific herpes simplex virus (HSV) immune response and a commensurate increase in that virus at the site of the infection.

Several surprising studies have looked at the effects of conditioning on the immune system and have demonstrated the relationship among the immune system, mind, and brain. These experiments began with an innovative study by Ader and Cohen (1975), who induced immunosuppression in rats as a conditioned response. They exposed rats to saccharin along with the immunosuppressant drug cyclophosphamide. Subsequent reexposure of the rats to saccharin alone produced immunosuppression at significant levels and demonstrated that immunosuppression can be a learned behavior.

Extending this approach, Smith and McDaniel (1983) examined the possibility of a similar conditioned response in humans. They performed tuberculin skin tests on one arm of subjects monthly for 5 months, injecting saline into the opposite arm. On the sixth trial, without informing either the subject or the nurse administering the test, the injections were reversed. Researchers discovered a markedly decreased cutaneous reaction in the arm where the tuberculin skin test antigen had been injected but where subjects and nurses had expected saline to be administered. Such studies demonstrated that psychological states, including expectations, can affect the immune response. This could have interesting implications in regard to the etiology of the placebo effect.

Potential clinical applications of conditioned alterations of the immune response have also been studied. Olness and Ader (1992) were able to reduce the total dose of cyclophosphamide to half the dose in the treatment of an adolescent with severe lupus erythematosus by initially pairing the drug with taste (cod liver oil) and subsequently offering the taste alone on some treatments. The patient improved clinically and 5 years later continued to do well. Recent animal experiments have demonstrated that conditioning can attenuate the development of arthritis in rats, prolong skin graft survival in mice, and extend survival of heart transplants in rats (Ader, 1992). Ader highlighted the potential clinical significance of such studies because they may allow the development of treatment regimens that reduce the cumulative effects of certain immunosuppressive drugs.

It is now clear, even from the small sampling of studies noted above, that there is a documented link between psychological states and physiological changes, and that these changes produce true clinical diseases. How this actually occurs has been the subject of intense research that has now shown a virtual net of mind-brain interconnections.

There are three primary sets of evidence for mind-brain interconnections. The first involves the documented direct autonomic innervation of lymphoid tissue. This includes the visualization of "synapticlike" terminals seen in association with lymphocytes and other lymphatic organs such as bone marrow, thymus, spleen, tonsil, and gut-associated lymphoid tissue (Romano et al, 1994). The second is that both systems share common receptors and messengers. High concentrations of binding sites for many neuropeptides and neurotransmitters, the primary messengers of the central nervous system (CNS), are found on the surface of white blood cells, thus permitting the blood-borne communication of the CNS with the immune system. At the same time immune cells have been found to produce not only cytokines (immune system messengers such as interleukins and interferons) but also neurohormones, neuropeptides, and neurotransmitters such as catecholamines and acetylcholine (the messengers of the CNS) (Haas, 1997). As would be expected in this two-way communication, there are widely distributed cytokine receptors in the brain, much of which is concentrated in the mid brain and limbic system. This permits the corresponding return flow of information and feedback from the immune system to the CNS. Third, significant changes in cellular functions are found to occur in response to messengers from the opposing system. Ader et al (1990) reviewed numerous animal studies that illustrated the varied effects of anterior pituitary and adrenal hormones on the immune system, affecting processes such as lymphocyte proliferation and production of lymphokines. Conversely, cytokines affect neural tissue. One example shows that interleukin I increases the activity of the autonomic nervous system input to the thymus, adrenal, kidney, and spleen.

Limbic structures are well known for their modulation and processing of emotion, memory, and diverse cognitive functions. It has been clearly shown that there are afferent and efferent connections between this "seat of emotion" and adrenal steroids, gonadal hormones, thyroid hormone, the hypothalamic-pituitary-adrenal (HPA) axis, and the immune system. These effects can be as diverse as unilateral limbic lesions causing impairment of spelling lymphocyte proliferation, prenatal immune challenges inducing abnormal HPA function in adults, or peripheral interleukin administration causing increased norepinephrine turnover in the hypothalamus and hippocampus and 5-hydroxytryptamine (serotonin) turnover in the hippocampus and prefrontal cortex (Hass, 1997).

The effects noted above are but a few of the hundreds that have been documented, pointing to the complexity of this marginally explored overarching system. In the next generation it will likely become obvious that the psychoneuroimmunological system is fundamental to the health and healing of the human organism.

Now that research has proven that these diverse intercommunications exist, how does this inform our clinical work? Initially it leads us to understand that classical treatments with antidepressants and neuroleptics may well have wider effects than is commonly considered, although this has yet to be well studied. It also supports new directions in treatment, such as the possibility of treating some depression by affecting persistently elevated levels of cortisol with agents such as ketoconazole. But psychotherapeutically, can some intervention targeted at a "common pathway" in this psychoneuroimmunological system move a human system closer to homeostasis and similarly, improve mental and physical health?

There have been some intriguing studies pointing to the "felt sense of control" as one of the possible candidates for this type of central "common pathway." Many of the studied mechanisms causing dysregulation of the psychoneuroimmunological (PNI) system can be reframed as having the issue of "sense of control" at their core. An example is TAB, with hostility and time pressure being used as counterproductive coping strategies to compensate for insecurity. Here, the insecurity contains a clear lack of a sense of agency in the world. It can be seen as an abiding fear of not being able to affect the world in the desired way. In the studies cited earlier, the central theme of lack of control can also be noted: in depression (decrease in hippocampal size), in chaotic families (susceptibility to viral infection), or in the simple expectation of normalcy (decrease in tuberculin reaction when sites of injection are switched).

Others have directly studied the lack of control and found a wide variety of effects, including increased circulating catecholamines and corticosteroids, significantly increased morbidity and mortality, depression, anxiety, malaise, distrust, and demoralization (Mirowsky, 1997). Still others have shown that the presence of control is associated with fewer and less severe physical symptoms, faster recovery from illness, and greater longevity (Lachman and Weaver, 1998). In a study designed to clarify the factors leading to the well-known differences in health in varying social classes it was found that those in the lowest income group who had a high sense of control showed levels of health and well-being comparable with the higher income group. This is in contrast to the usual finding of low income and low sense of control corresponding with poor health (Lachman and Weaver, 1998).

Further studies are needed to clarify the role of the "felt sense of control" and other possible common pathways in the PNI system. This would be instrumental in helping to direct us as we search for powerful clinical applications of this new knowledge.

SUMMARY

The field of psychosomatic medicine has shifted from theories of unitary psychogenic causes of disease to an approach that integrates psychosocial and biological factors. Current research is even revealing the mechanisms by which psychological factors are transduced into physiological changes.

The biopsychosocial model is important in all diseases and is especially useful in helping to decide which treatments to use; eg, treatment based only on biological considerations may be useless in coronary artery disease unless the patient's psychosocial characteristics are taken into account. In addition to their possible type A behaviors and the influence that hostility or time pressure may have on their disease course, other factors may also play a role. These include their sense of control, their compliance with medication, and their ability to effect changes in behaviors such as smoking, diet, and exercise. As Lipowski (1977) noted, the complete cause of the disease should remain the focus of our interest. It is hoped, as research continues to accumulate, that the health field will acknowledge the centrality of mind-brain interactions and begin uniformly to apply integrated treatments to diseases in both the medical and psychological arenas.

REFERENCES & SUGGESTED READINGS

Ader R: On the clinical relevance of psychoneuroimmunology. Clin Immunol Immunopathol 1992;64(1):6.

Ader R, Cohen N: Behaviorally conditioned immunosuppression. Psychosom Med 1975;37:333.

Ader R, Cohen N: Psychoneuroimmunology: Conditioning and stress. Annu Rev Psychol 1993;44:53.

Ader R, Felten D, Cohen N: Interactions between the brain and immune system. Annu Rev Pharmacol Toxicol 1990; 30:561.

Alexander F: *Psychosomatic Medicine. Its Principles and Applications.* Norton, 1950.

Bonneau RH et al: Stress-induced suppression of herpes simplex virus (HSV)-specific cytotoxic T lymphocyte and natural killer cell activity and enhancement of acute pathogenesis following local HSV infection. Brain Behav Immunol 1991;5:170.

Brackett CD, Powell LH: Psychosocial and physiologic predictors of sudden cardiac death after healing of acute myocardial infarction. Am J Cardiol 1988;61:979.

Carmelli D, Swan GE: The relationship of type A behavior and its components to all-cause mortality in an elderly subgroup of men from the Western Collaborative Group Study. J Psychosom Res 1996;40(5):475.

Cohen S: Psychological stress and susceptibility to upper respiratory infections. Am J Respir Crit Care Med 1995; 152:S53.

Dunbar HF: The relationship between anxiety states and organic disease. Clinics 1942;1:879.

Dunbar HF: *Emotions and Bodily Change,* 3rd ed. Columbia University Press, 1946.

Engel GL: A psychological setting of somatic disease: The giving up-given up complex. Proc Roy Soc Med 1967; 60:553.

Engel GL: The death of a twin: Mourning and anniversary reactions. Fragments of 10 years of self-analysis. Int J Psychoanal 1975;56:23.

Engel GL: The need for a new medical model: A challenge for biomedicine. Science 1977;196:129.

Engel GL: The clinical application of the biopsychosocial model. Am J Psychiatry 1980;137:535.

Everson AS et al: Interaction of workplace demands and cardiovascular reactivity in progression of carotid artherosclerosis: Population based study. Br Med J 1997;314:553.

Felten DL et al: Noradrenergic sympathetic neural interaction with the immune system; structure and function. Immunol Rev 1987;100:225.

Friedman M, Rosenman RH: *Type A Behavior and Your Heart.* Knopf, 1974.

Goldstein MG, Niaura R: Psychological factors affecting physical condition: Cardiovascular disease literature review. Part I: Coronary artery disease and sudden death. Psychosomatics 1992;33:134.

Grinker RR: *Psychosomatic Concepts,* 3rd ed. Jason Aronson, 1973.

Hart KE: A moratorium on research using the Jenkins Activity Survey for Type A behavior? J Clin Psychol 1997; 53(8):905.

Hass HS, Schauenstein K: Neuroimmunomodulation via limbic structures—the neuroanatomy of psychoimmunology. Prog Neurobiol 1997;51(2):195.

Holmes TH, Rahe RH: The social readjustment rating scale. J Psychosom Res 1967;11:213.

Kaufman IC, Rosenblum L: Effects of separation from mother on the emotional behavior of infant monkeys. Ann NY Acad Sci 1969;159:601.

Kiecolt-Glaser JK, Glaser R: Psychological influences on immunity. Psychosomatics 1986;27:621.

Lachman ME, Weaver SL: The sense of control as a moderator of social class differences in health and well-being. J Personality Social Psychol 1998;74(3):763.

Lipowski ZJ: Psychosomatic medicine in the seventies: An overview. Am J Psychiatry 1977;134:233.

Locke SE: Stress adaptation and immunity. Gen Hosp Psychiatry 1982;4:49.

Locke SE et al: *The Influence of Stress on the Immune Response: Preliminary Report of the Annual Meeting.* American Psychosomatic Society, March 31, 1978.

Markowe HL et al: Fibrinogen: A possible link between social class and coronary heart disease. Br Med J 1985; 291:1312.

McEwen BS, Magarinos AM: Stress effects on morphology and function of the hippocampus. Ann NY Acad Sci 1997; 821:271.

Mirowsky J: Age, subjective life expectancy, and the sense of control: The horizon hypothesis. J Gerontol Ser B 1997; 52(3):S125.

Mirowsky J, Ross CE: Fundamental analysis in research on well-being: Distress and the sense of control. Gerontologist 1996;36(5):584.

Mirsky IA: Physiologic, psychologic, and social determinants in the etiology of duodenal ulcer. Am J Dig Dis 1958;3:285.

Niaura R, Goldstein MG: Psychological factors affecting physical condition: Cardiovascular disease literature review. Part II: Coronary artery disease and sudden death and hypertension. Psychosomatics 1992;33:146.

Nunes EV, Frank KA, Kornfeld DS: Psychologic treatment for the type A behavior pattern and for coronary heart disease: A meta-analysis of the literature. Psychosom Med 1987;48:159.

Olness K, Ader R: Conditioning as an adjunct in the pharmacotherapy of lupus erythematosus. J Dev Behav Pediatr 1992;13(2):124.

Parkes CM, Brown RJ: Health after bereavement: A controlled study of young Boston widows and widowers. Psychosom Med 1972;34:449.

Price VA et al: Relation between insecurity and type A behavior. Am Heart J 1995;129(3):488.

Raikkonen K et al: Association of chronic stress with plasminogen activator inhibitor-1 in healthy middle-aged men. Arterioscler Thromb Vasc Biol 1996;16:363.

Rees WD, Lutkins SG: Mortality or bereavement. Br Med J 1967;4:13.

Reiser MF: Changing theoretical concepts in psychosomatic medicine. In: *American Handbook of Psychiatry,* 2nd ed. Vol 4, pp 477–500. Basic Books, 1975.

Romano TA et al: Noradrenergic and peptidergic innervation of the lymphoid organs in the beluga, *Delphinapterus leucas:* An anatomical link between the nervous and immune systems. J Morphol 1994;221:243.

Rose RM: Endocrine responses to stressful psychological events: advances in psychoneuroendocrinology. Psychiatr Clin North Am 1980;3:251.

Schliefer SJ et al: Suppression of lymphocyte stimulation following bereavement. JAMA 1983;250:374.

Selye H: *Stress Without Distress.* Lippincott, 1974.

Smith RG, McDaniel SM: Psychologically mediated effect on the delayed hypersensitivity reaction to tuberculin in humans. Psychosom Med 1983;45:65.

Sundin O et al: Cardiovascular reactivity, type A behavior, and coronary heart disease. Psychophysiology 1995; 32(1):28.

Weiner H et al: Etiology of duodenal ulcer. Psychosom Med 1957;19:1.

Wolff HG, Wolf S, Hare CE (editors): *Life Stress and Bodily Disease.* Williams & Wilkins, 1950.

Child, Adolescent, & Adult Development

4

Aubrey W. Metcalf, MD, & Jeffrey Rowe, MD

DEVELOPMENT & THE LIFE CYCLE

An understanding of the processes of normal growth and development is indispensable for the study of human biology and behavior. The field is now a basic science in all clinical curricula. Continuous advances in knowledge confirm a striking orderliness, coherence, and continuity in the immensely complicated, mysterious, and beautiful transformations that occur from conception to old age. These advances are providing rich information on how we come to be the way we are. Much detailed study has yet to be done, but the main mechanisms of biological development are well understood in animals and young humans, and their links to behavior are rapidly being clarified. As research on personality in later life accumulates, it has become apparent that behavioral reorganizations and age-related developmental tasks are characteristic not only of the early years but of the entire life cycle. For the clinician, an understanding of the orderliness of development serves as a framework within which each individual patient can be assessed and understood.

THE HISTORY OF INQUIRY INTO GROWTH & DEVELOPMENT

Phylogeny is the study of the successive forms of life that have come into being on the earth. Not only the physical form but many of the behaviors that evolved over 60 million years to ensure the survival of young mammals are directly carried over into human life—particularly the first few months and years of it. This mammalian heritage appears to affect development, with decreasing influence, throughout the life cycle.

Ontogeny is the study of the successive forms each individual passes through in its lifetime. The ancients were aware of the continuous and progressive changes in the organism from earliest life through maturity, but their concept was not "developmental" as the word is used today. Their idea of embryology was founded on the homunculus theory of "preformationism," first proposed by a Greek philosopher in the fifth century BC. This was a linear model of development—what we now call growth, ie, increase in the number and size of cells (hyperplasia and hypertrophy). This notion was unchallenged for more than 2000 years until microscopic study revealed that younger embryos lacked some of the organs and tissues present in older ones of the same species. This established that development was not simple linear enlargement but a progression through successive stages, with the emergence of new forms.

THE CAUSES OF DEVELOPMENT

In the physical ontogeny of any young organism, when the initial organic substrate and the expectable environment interact they form a new genetic substrate ready for the next developmental step. In the ontogeny of behavior, the genetic constitution brings into being primitive reflex actions and patterns on a controlled timetable, some in utero and others as late as adolescence, and perhaps even later. This process is called **epigenesis.** As a result the organism develops and learns the necessary behaviors for survival.

For some functions, there are *critical periods* after which behavioral differentiation is incomplete or impossible. For example, cats blindfolded from birth lose the ability to see properly if their eyes are not uncovered before the end of the critical period. These timetables are more or less fixed genomically, depending on the species and the age of the organism, and many of them apply to human development as well.

Individual Development

When we consider the forces that drive individual development, it is obvious that ontogeny does not rely entirely on chance conditioning by the required environmental stimuli. Examples are numerous of animals (including primates) acting in ways they have had no opportunity to learn. We ordinarily call such behavior instinctive (unlearned) and conclude that it represents some internal system conveyed by inheritance.

For every organism, there is an environment within which its physiological and behavioral systems operate best at any point in its ontogeny. This was called the "environment of evolutionary adaptedness" by John

Bowlby. The causes of individual development, for all animals, from the one-celled to the infant human, are those environmental stimuli to which the young organism is sensitive at each level of its maturational cycle. The natural environment of infants is the **caregiving situation** within which development and learning occur. A normal result can be expected so long as the experiences are not too discrepant from the environment of evolutionary adaptedness. The infant's delight at seeing the mother* is not at first connected to the conscious experience of needing her physical or nutritional support, but is a response to specific signals for which the infant is primed by evolution. It is an instinctive mechanism for achieving the vital attachment between infants and caregivers that is necessary for survival.

Human Behavior: Instinctual & Noninstinctual

Physical activity in the human fetus begins with characteristic spontaneous movements and simple reflex responses to internal processes and external sensory input. After birth, and within the environment of evolutionary adaptedness, these constitutional tendencies extend to form the first-step behaviors of normal development: eye and head orientation, rooting, sucking, grasping, and swallowing. The new behaviors become the substrates for the next step in development. Physical and social experience affects the way in which genes are expressed and promote the further development of brain connections and structures, leading to new behaviors. This is **epigenetic** development (Lombroso, 1998). The infant's actions may themselves evoke the environmental response necessary for the succeeding developmental step. The baby's smile, for example, provokes and sustains the positive social responses needed for a normal outcome.

Behavioral maldevelopment may result from heritable defects, noxious intrauterine influences, maternal illnesses, prematurity, or birth trauma; however, the primary cause of infant-onset behavioral disorders is interference with the interpersonal exchanges necessary for normal behavior to emerge. Social interaction is as essential as physical development in the making of an intact child.

In humans, as with other mammals, complex instinctive behavior is not present at birth as it is in insects. What is inherited is the marked *potential* for developing certain sorts of behavioral systems needed for survival in varied settings, given the expectable experiences of the young of that species. This capac-

ity permits greater individual adaptability than other animals possess, but it also imposes a risk of distorted or destructive behavior if the environment during development differs significantly from the environment to which the species is adapted. For this reason there are limits to the capacity of human infants to adjust to variations in their caregiving environment.

The interpersonal experience of infants is conveyed by the caregivers' nurturing attention. For humans, the primary motivators of attachment are the social and interpersonal interactions with the caring person rather than the secondary role of the caregiver in assuaging of pain, hunger, or physical danger. From the first bond with the caregiver, interpersonal connections are major factors in the growth of personality, and disturbed or inadequate relationships at an early age underlie much unhappiness and mental illness in childhood and later.

THE DEVELOPMENTAL PERSPECTIVE

Almost all modern theories of personality and psychopathology now have what is called a *developmental perspective,* whose main characteristics were well described by Breger (1974): (1) the progression of behavioral maturation is from the less complex to the more complex; (2) what emerges in the immediate (and even the distant) future is relatively dependent on what has already arisen; and (3) above all, the effect of any experience will often depend on the stage at which it occurs in the development of the individual.

The third characteristic is most important in understanding the ontogeny of personality and mental functioning. Environmental stresses, such as the death of a mother, vary greatly depending on a person's stage of development: the consequences are very different for a daughter who is a 4-month-old baby, a 4-year-old child, or a 40-year-old adult. The birth of a sibling has different consequences for a 1-year-old or 6-year-old than for a 2-year-old child. A knowledge of the normal progression of the individual's ability to understand and cope with the environment helps the clinician differentiate pathological social maturation from normal variations and will help the therapist decide what treatment is likely to be beneficial.

For medical practice the most important aspect of any theory of psychology or psychopathology is its usefulness in predicting future development and in suggesting means of altering the course of existing illness or maldevelopment in the direction of health. Unfortunately, no single theory is adequate to explain the diversity of human individuals and cultures, although neurophysiological, behavioral, and ethological research is beginning to merge with more sophisticated observations of human feelings and behavior.

---

* To avoid constant repetition, reference to parents, mothers, or fathers is to be understood as meaning any consistent caregivers to whom the child has formed a primary or important attachment, such as spousal partners of either sex, other adults in the home, adoptive or foster parents, and sometimes other caring personnel.

THEORIES OF DEVELOPMENT

Valid theories of human development must be derived from a combination of clinical experience and systematic, scientific observation. Many hypotheses in use at present contribute workable perspectives, and several aspire to the status of general theories of human psychology. The two best known systems used by clinicians today are those derived from classic psychoanalysis and from piagetian developmental psychology. Criticism has been justly leveled against the former for being excessively intrapsychic and unyielding to systematic validation and against the latter for taking no account of emotions or the biological mechanisms of development. Both theories are closed systems and products of western culture, but they have long histories of clinical usefulness and can serve as appropriate instruments for further research and validation. A third approach, that of attachment, is a modern attempt to update the first two using recent findings in general systems theory and animal ethology.

Three influential explanations of human psychology are discussed at length here because of their special relevance to child development: Piaget's *épistemologie génétique,* Erikson's psychoanalytic view, and Bowlby's attachment theory. Lack of space prevents discussion of the consequences for development of problems of parenthood, social and economic class, poverty, family cultural context, and other important topics.

JEAN PIAGET (1896–1980)

Piaget is the best known child psychologist in the world, and his theory of cognitive development has been the most influential. He was born in Geneva, Switzerland, and spent his entire career there. For Piaget, the intellectual functions are the core of personality formation and serve to coordinate development in all spheres. He acknowledged the importance of emotional life in childhood, but did not speculate about its development.

Piaget was the first modern theorist to emphasize that from the beginning the infant is active in exploring the world and striving to master it. He held that the process is genomically inherited and proceeds in all children through a series of fixed developmental phases and subphases. It is epigenetic in that mastery of each phase depends on success in mastering the elements of the preceding phase and forms the basis for future refinement.

For Piaget there are two fundamental processes by which the organism adapts: assimilation and accommodation. *Assimilation* is the absorption ("taking in") of an experience as a whole, insofar as the individual understands it. It consists of fitting an experience into an existing cognitive structure. An analogy is assimi-

lation of food by the gut, which is limited by the extent to which the organism is able to digest what it takes in. *Accommodation* is the process of changing the existing cognitive structure to adjust to and use new experiences. The digestive tract of a species may evolve so that individuals can use new foods, or a theory may be modified to explain contradictory data. Learning proceeds by assimilating new perceptions in terms of the existing cognitive capacity and restructuring the cognitive apparatus to accommodate new perceptions.

Piaget describes four stages in the development of cognition (Table 4–1): the **sensorimotor stage** and **stage of preoperational thought** (prelogical thought) in early childhood; the **stage of concrete operations,** roughly the grammar school years; and the **stage of formal operations,** the teenage years. Some children reach and master the oncoming stage a bit sooner than others, but this is not a function of intelligence. Very intelligent children in the preoperational stage are unable to perform ordinary tasks of the concrete stage even though they may be able to read, write, and speak far in advance of their peers. Each stage reinterprets previous understanding and experience according to new ways of thinking and organizing information (Singer and Revenson, 1996).

Regression During Stress & Illness

Physicians and others caring for sick or injured people have noted that stress is often accompanied by regression of cognitive functioning. An adult is apt to become as "concrete" and egocentric as a child of 8 when health or love relationships are threatened. Even well-functioning adolescents and adults may have ideas about illness that fall short of their cognitive mastery of other nonstressful subject matter. Piaget's special importance has been his emphasis on clinical developmental psychology. He insisted, decades before it became popular, that children understand the world differently from adults and learn in a different way. Everyone who works with children (and with adults under stress) is in Piaget's debt for these insights.

ERIK ERIKSON (1902–1994)

There are many offshoots from Freud's original theories about human development, the best known of which is still that of Erik Erikson. He was born in Germany and trained in Vienna as the first male Montessori teacher. He then became a lay psychoanalyst with special interest in the problems of children. He emigrated to the United States in 1933 and had a distinguished career as a writer on anthropology, personality development, and psychohistory. His first book, *Childhood and Society* in 1950, provided a synthesis of human development from his unique point of view (Roazen, 1997).

Table 4-1. Summary of human development from multiple perspectives.[a]

Age	DEVELOPMENTAL LANDMARKS Performance Levels (A. Gesell, etc)	PSYCHOSEXUAL STAGES (S. Freud) Ego Defense Mechanisms (G. Vaillant)	Psychodynamic Development		INTELLECTUAL DEVELOPMENT Cognitive Stages (J. Piaget)
			PSYCHOSEXUAL STAGES Psychosocial Modes *Tasks and VALUES* (E. Erikson)	ATTACHMENT THEORY (J. Bowlby) *Psychologic Characteristics* (A. Freud)	
Birth	Reflex smile/grimace	ORAL *"Narcissistic" defenses* Projection (delusional in older persons) Denial (psychotic in older persons) Distortion	ORAL-RESPIRATORY-SENSORY-KINESTHETIC Incorporative model *Trust versus mistrust* HOPE	I. PREATTACHMENT (0 TO 8–10 WEEKS) Orientation to signals without discrimination of a figure	SENSORIMOTOR STAGE I. Reflex (0–2 months)
2 months	Develops eye/hand control				II. Primary circular reaction (2–6 months)
3 months	Social smile; 180° visual pursuit			II. ATTACHMENT-IN-THE-MAKING (8–10 WEEKS TO 6 MONTHS) Orientation and signals directed toward one (or more) discriminated figure	III. Secondary circular reaction (2–8 months)
6 months	Reaches for objects; rolls over Transfers objects; raking grasp			III. CLEAR-CUT ATTACHMENT (6 MONTHS TO END OF LIFE) Maintenance of proximity to a discriminated figure by means of local motion as signals	IV. Secondary schemes (8–12 months)
9 months	Sits up well; purposeful release; prehension deft; cruises at rail				V. Tertiary circular reaction (12–16 months) VI. Invention of new means through mental combinations (16 months on)
Infancy 1 year	Walks unassisted; uses 3–4 words; builds towers of 2 cubes	ANAL *"Immature" defenses* Projection Schizoid fantasy Hypochondriasis *Passive-aggressive behavior* Acting out	ANAL-URETHRAL-MUSCULAR Retentive-eliminative mode *Autonomy versus shame and doubt* WILL	*Exuberant exploration* *Realizes omnipotence is limited, becomes conservative* *Oppositional behavior* *Messiness* *Parallel play* *Pleasure in looking and being looked at*	
18 months	Scribbles with crayon; uses 10–20 words; builds towers of 5–6 cubes; names a few pictures			IV. GOAL-CORRECTED PARTNERSHIP *Disgust* *Orderliness possible* *Fantasy play* *Masturbation begins* *Curiosity heightened*	STAGE OF PREOPERATIONAL THOUGHT (PRELOGICAL) 1. Development of symbolic functions 2. Differentiation between signs and symbols 3. Use of language 4. Observational learning, representation versus direct action 5. Egocentrism 6. Thinking by intuition
2 years	Runs and falls; uses 3-word sentences; names several body parts; uses appropriate personal pronouns				
Preschool 3 years	Rides tricycle; copies a circle; can stand on one foot; talks of self and others	PHALLIC/INFANTILE GENITAL *"Neurotic" defenses* Intellectualization Repression Displacement Reaction formation Dissociation	GENITAL/OEDIPAL Intrusive-inclusive mode *Initiative versus guilt* PURPOSE	*Cooperative play* *Imaginary companion* *Task perseverance* *Rivalry with parent of same sex* *Problem solving* *Games with rules begin*	
4 years	Buttons clothes; throws ball overhand; copies square; draws a person; says ABCs				
5 years	Copies triangle and diamond; ties knots in string; complete toilet self-help				

Age		Defenses (Vaillant)	Psychosocial (Erikson)	Social behavior	Cognitive stage (Piaget)
School age		LATENCY *Continues "neurotic" defenses (see Preschool) and begins "mature" defenses (see Adolescence)*	PSYCHOSEXUAL MORATORIUM Industry versus inferiority SKILL	LATENCY *Hobbies* *Ritualistic play* *Rational attitudes about foods* *Enjoys friends and "best friends"* *Invests self in teachers and older leaders*	STAGE OF CONCRETE OPERATIONS Child begins to be rational and more stable in thought; an orderly conceptual framework is applied in understanding the world; physical quantities such as weight and volume are now viewed as constants despite changes in shape and size
6 years	Can roller-skate; prints name; ties shoelaces				
7 years	Knows seasons of year; rides 2-wheeled bike				
8 years	Shares ideas; names days of week; repeats 5 digits forward				
9 years	Can define such words as sympathy and foolish				
10 years	Able to rhyme; repeats 4 digits in reverse				
Preadolescence		PREADOLESCENCE			
11 years	Understands pity, grief, surprise; knows where sun sets				
Adolescence		EARLY ADOLESCENCE *"Mature" defenses* *Altruism* *Humor* *Suppression* *Anticipation* *Sublimation*	PSYCHOSOCIAL MORATORIUM *Identity versus role confusion* FIDELITY	ADOLESCENCE *Rebelliousness* *Loosens family ties* *Runs in cliques* *Responsible independence emerges in fragments* *Work habits solidify* *Obvious heterosexual interests (girls usually before boys)*	STAGE OF FORMAL OPERATIONS Child can now deal deductively not only with the reality the child sees but also with abstractions and propositional statements The adolescent uses deductive reasoning and can evaluate the logic and quality of his or her own thinking; increased powers of abstraction enable him or her to deal with laws and principles; although egocentrism is still evident, balanced idealistic attitudes emerge in late adolescence Some "normal" people do not advance this far in intellectual development; many do not lose their essential egocentrism at all Egocentrism returns at senescence
12 years	Can comprehend definitions of scientific words of great complexity such as entropy				
13 years					
14 years	Can divide small number in head		YOUNG ADULTHOOD (age 20–30) *Intimacy versus isolation* LOVE		
15 years	Can repeat 6 digits forward and 5 digits backward	MIDDLE ADOLESCENCE			
16 years					
17 years		LATE ADOLESCENCE	ADULTHOOD (age 30–65) *Generativity versus self-absorption or stagnation* CARE		
18 years			LATE MATURITY (65 and older) *Integrity versus despair* WISDOM		

a In each of the three center columns on psychodynamic development, the different styles of printing are vertically matched to the names and systems of the theorists in the heading box.

Erikson expands freudian theory to include social and cultural dimensions. In his restructuring of psychoanalytic developmental psychology he sees two basic drives working in opposite directions—one, an outgoing vector, tending toward expansion and life, and the other, a backward-turning vector, tending toward retreat from life. The tension between these drives gives rise to the normal crises of the life cycle. In his description of emotional development Erikson gives prominence to the ego as well as to the id. He was the first analyst to garner wide public interest for the then-modern idea that *interpersonal* relationships are important in the foundation of emotional life and one of the principal forces shaping development. The child affects the parents and through them the society. Thus, development is psycho*social* as well as psycho*sexual*.

Erikson has distilled **modes of operation** from the psychosexual **zones** and phases of classical psychoanalysis and shows how these modes are reflected in typical behaviors throughout life (Table 4–1). Although we quickly outlive the "oral" phase of psychosexual development, for example, we never outlive the need for food or the performance of tasks mastered during this phase of development. Our mode of "getting" or "taking in" reflects the adequacy of our resolution of that phase, and provides a pattern of functioning that may include regression to infantile behaviors.

Erikson conceives of normal development as a succession of eight stages from birth to old age. These stages are **epigenetic** in that the success of each subsequent stage is partially dependent on how well the previous one has been mastered. Each stage is represented by a personal, intrapsychic balance (the psychosexual) and an outer, interpersonal balance (the psychosocial). The balance is dynamic and much affected by personal relationships and by the culture in which the child is reared. Each successive stage presents a new challenge to be met if normal development is to continue, but each stage also presents opportunities for new and more adaptive solutions to inadequately mastered previous stages. This is true because all modes of operation are still potentially present in each stage.

Erikson retains the classic concept of "secondary drive" (that the infant becomes attached to the caregiver because of the more primary gratification of feeding), but he uses terms somewhat different than Freud's to characterize the psychosexual stages. These terms appear (in capitals) at the top of each stage in Table 4–1. Underneath (in regular type) is what Erikson considers the **mode** of that stage (incorporative mode for the oral stage, retentive-eliminative mode for the anal stage, etc), followed (in italic type) by the polarity implicit in that stage (eg, trust versus mistrust for the oral stage). These are the **psychosocial** tasks of the stage. Finally, Erikson characterizes his view of development as a crucible for fundamental human

values. In each stage, one of the eight human values (in italic capitals in Table 4–1) is established or lost (eg, **hope** in the oral stage, **wisdom** in late adult life).

JOHN BOWLBY (1907–1990)

The body of thought that has come to be called **attachment theory** began with a paper by British child psychoanalyst John Bowlby in 1958. In his subsequent major works, Bowlby dispenses with the secondary drive theory of how infants become attached to their caregivers and reinterprets psychoanalytic understanding of early development in terms of animal ethology and modern evolutionary theory. In addition, he takes into account the newer ideas of control systems and the model of information processing embraced by cognitive psychology.

Bowlby emphasizes Darwin's explicit view that every feature of anatomy, physiology, and behavior in an animal species contributes to or once contributed to the survival of that species in its natural environment. The behaviors underlying mating, the care of infants, and the attachment of young to their caregivers are obviously of the greatest importance to survival and are so stable across human cultures that they have come to be numbered among the few instinctual systems of the species. Survival through years of comparative dependency is not left to chance or to the dedication of caregivers alone. An intrinsic and primary behavioral system evolved to make certain that the infant would be motivated to remain with its caregivers.

In general, attachment behaviors are those observable actions of a child that promote an appropriate nearness to the primary caregiver so that dangers may be avoided. From the first, strong stimuli are distressing, as are looming figures or a sudden sensation of being dropped from a safe (held) position. By age 2 or 3 months, being alone or in strange surroundings elicits obvious distress. By the time attachment to specific caregivers begins (between 3 and 6 months), fearful behavior and attachment behavior are aroused by the same stimuli; the child is alarmed by the danger, and this alarm precipitates action (attachment behavior) to increase proximity to the caregiver. If adequate nearness cannot be achieved quickly, the child will feel distress that is both more severe than, and qualitatively different from, the original sense of alarm or fear. Bowlby called this different kind of distress **anxiety.**

The infant experiences minor degrees of anxiety (awareness of not being close enough to the attachment figure) repeatedly and learns to master it if ready access to familiar people is maintained. After about 6 months, the infant will anticipate the discomfort of anxiety on seeing its caregiver preparing to leave and will activate its own attachment behaviors and protests in an attempt to prevent the departure. The more consistent the caregiver's behavior is in the mind of the child, the more separation the child is likely to tolerate. In the presence of the attachment figure, the child feels the opposite of anxiety—**security**—unless fearful that that person will unexpectedly leave or become unresponsive.

The very young baby first explores the mother's body; here the attachment and exploration systems coincide. This favors the development of a strong bond. Later, the mother or primary caregiver serves as a secure base from which to explore at some distance; here attachment behavior is balanced by exploratory behavior. A child who feels secure is able to move away from the mother for play and discovery. When security is threatened by alarm or too much separation, attachment behavior predominates. If security is uncertain much of the time, the child's capacity for learning and for developing social relationships will be distorted and possibly impaired.

Attachment **behavior** must be distinguished from the attachment **bond** implied by the behavior. Once formed, the attachment bond persists and is manifested by the behavior resulting from the emotional consequences of separations, which may result in very different personal exchanges than before, or apparently none at all. A child separated for a significant period from its attachment figure, without an adequate substitute, may exhibit anger, seeming indifference, or cold behavior. These are signs of emotional and cognitive reaction to the trauma of separation and not of absence of attachment.

Bowlby's approach to the dawn of interpersonal relations has clarified the essentially social origins of the child's tie to its caregiver. The attachment system is the first and most important psychological schema to develop. It shares some behaviors with the nutritional system initially, and the sexual system later, but it is an entirely separate and essentially social behavioral system (Karen, 1997).

SUMMARY OF THEORIES OF CHILD DEVELOPMENT

Table 4–1 summarizes five perspectives on human development. They are, of course, not the only views on the subject. Psychodynamic approaches are heavily represented in this table because they are most used in clinical psychiatric practice. For a modern psychoanalytic view of child and adolescent development, informed by other disciplines, see Lewis (1997). A recent synthesis of cognitive psychology, neuroscience, and psychodynamics is found in Horowitz (1998). An excellent integration of developmental neurobiology, attachment research, and psychotherapy is available in Siegel (1999) and in Lewis, Amini, and Lannon (2000). Theories of personality and psychopathology derived from nonanalytic psychology and philosophy, particularly the modern humanistic theories, are discussed in Chapters 2 and 3 in this text.

CHILD DEVELOPMENT FROM BEFORE BIRTH TO ADOLESCENCE

THE PREPSYCHOLOGICAL PERIOD: CONCEPTION THROUGH AGE 2 MONTHS

Prenatal Life

It is not known whether the fetus must have any specific *sensory* experiences to develop properly, nor do we know what (if any) noxious sensory input distorts or impedes that development. Excess or deficiency of maternal circulating hormones (eg, thyroid, pituitary, adrenocortical, and sex hormones) is known to affect physical development adversely, particularly the central nervous system. Damage to the fetus can occur as a result of direct causes, such as physical agents (trauma, genetic abnormality, inadequate blood supply, and disease) and chemical agents (eg, pesticides and mercury from contaminated fish). Indirect damage may be caused by illness in the mother or the mother's use of drugs, alcohol, and tobacco, or other destructive habits, many of which lead to prematurity, a risk whatever the cause. In addition to prematurity and obstetric complications, the primary dangers to the fetal nervous system are maternal viral infections, substance abuse, and severe protein malnutrition. Central nervous system metaplasia (increases in number and complexity of cells) is maximal during the first 3 months of pregnancy, and protein starvation during this period is devastating for future intellectual development. Brain tissue that fails to receive adequate nourishment in this phase of pregnancy cannot, unlike other parts of the body, be repaired by proper feeding later. This vulnerability continues, but to a lesser extent, throughout gestation and the first few years of life. There is no evidence that the mother's emotional state, attitudes, thoughts, or conflicts have any direct psychological effect on the fetus (Lecanuet et al, 1995). Attention to the fetus and then to the newborn, as well as to family psychosocial factors, is very important in the prevention and treatment of prematurity and other at-risk conditions at birth. Multimodal interventions can significantly improve later outcomes (Zeanah et al, 1998).

Birth & the Neonatal Period

Much creative energy has been expended in speculation about birth as a factor in emotional development. Despite plausible conjectures, current evidence indicates that the physical act of delivery has little psychological importance for the infant. However, it is of major psychological importance for the mother and her supporters, which means that even if it is never shown that specific favorable conditions at delivery are crucial to the *child's* psychological future, they certainly may be to the mother and others, and thus indirectly to the child. A satisfied mother and father and a smiling baby are more likely to form early and strong bonds with each other. This common sense assumption has led progressive obstetric units to provide a more homelike atmosphere in labor and delivery rooms and to allot a more active role to the parents, including the presence of the father or other supporting adult during the birth process and afterward. LeBoyer or Lamaze methods can reduce the fear and pain of the mother and make delivery a more positive experience.

One thing is certain, the infant, even at the moment of delivery, is not a "tabula rasa" on which experience writes all. In the delivery room some infants are observed tracking certain colors and shapes of light with their eyes while ignoring others. Within a few days, and without much experience, this skill improves markedly. What appears to be happening is that the infant is already seeking patterns. At this point the patterns are relatively nonspecific, but the attempt is definitely not indiscriminate. With time, what infants seek becomes shaped by what they actually get and how satisfying it is, but from the first there are inclinations to react in predictable ways to certain expectable patterns of sight, sound, and touch.

Mutually satisfying caregiver-child interactions, the result of the caregiver's speedy and contingent responses to the infant's signals, consolidate the rhythms of the baby's life and lead to more awake-alert times within which learning takes place before physical tensions such as hunger or other discomforts stimulate restlessness or crying. The act of being satisfied serves as an early prototype of a future feeling of trust or security. If needs are filled efficiently and empathetically, a sense of trust and security begins to take form; if needs are not met in a timely manner, the result is distress, and eventually mistrust, the forerunners of insecurity, anxiety, and psychic conflict in the later months of infancy and in childhood.

The Dawn of Psychological Awareness

The prenatal and early neonatal period appears to be dominated by biological needs and responses. The mother or other caregiver is the "auxiliary ego" who makes life not only bearable but possible, and it is mostly through her—the rhythms of her body during gestation and her care and social stimulations after birth—that the child experiences the world. The mother's physical ministrations bridge the enormous changes that delivery creates in the physiological needs of oxygenation, nutrition, elimination, regulation of body temperature, etc.

Because the normal infant behaves so naturally in the caregiving situation, it is tempting to believe that the newborn appreciates experiences in a psychological way. But this is doubtful. For an event to have psy-

chological meaning in the first few hours and days of life, rather sophisticated evaluative processes and the ability to discriminate between external and internal stimuli must exist, but there is no evidence for this. Unless tissue damage is sustained, a physically difficult labor—or even discomfort, cruelty, or neglect in the first several weeks—does not limit the child's potential for future development. In fact, the gravest congenital abnormalities requiring multiple surgical procedures and other painful methods of treatment ordinarily do not result in psychological maldevelopment if the attachment situation is adequate. It is only later, when the child's psyche is organized by the quality and frequency of the caregiver's social responses, that it is possible to speak of a truly psychological life in a child. Nevertheless, future research may reveal that certain early stimuli have epigenetic importance for optimal development later, and this possibility should be borne in mind in handling the youngest of infants.

We assume that "awareness" in neonates consists only of being comfortable or not, and that infants differentiate only vaguely between the outer and inner environments. The fixed-action patterns present at birth—rooting, sucking, postural adjustment, looking and listening, grasping, and crying—stimulate the caregiver to provide what is needed to relieve discomfort. Although infants will seek to escape from unpleasant stimulation, the usual salient experience consists of repeated exposure, in a decidedly social context, to pleasurable and tension-relieving stimuli. (This assimilation of external stimuli, or "coming inside" of the external world, through the mouth in feeding but through other sensory modalities as well, has given rise to the concept of orality in psychoanalytic theory.)

The Role of the Father

The role of the father or spousal partner, from birth on, can be as important to the infant as that of the mother. If the mother is the primary caregiver, the father can be the first alternative caregiver. The relationship between fathers and infants is only now being examined closely, but it appears that fathers and other persons can serve as primary caregivers just as well as mothers. It is an advantage for both infants and caregivers if there is more than one attachment figure in the home and this person need not be the child's parent. The commonly held conviction that infants develop best in a home with both a father and a mother may be true, but it is based on convention and tradition rather than research data (Lamb, 1997).

Temperament

In the first weeks or months of life, infants begin to show characteristic styles of behavior that develop into consistent patterns. Caregivers react to this style for better or worse according to their expectations and tolerance, and their responses tend to shape subsequent behavior. This constancy in pattern is usually stable until about 2 years of age, after which time traits of individual diversity start to appear, reflecting that child's innate temperament as well as environment. There is no question that "difficult babies" can be a great trial to their caregivers, some of whom are not able to fulfill these demands. Even with "easy" babies the family's ability to provide a good emotional environment may be inadequate, and these deficiencies immediately begin to influence the epigenetic progress of development so that a child's competence at age 2 or age 6 may fall short of the potential that was present at birth.

There is still considerable disagreement about how temperament and attachment are related, but it is clear they influence each other in a reciprocal way. The *quality* of attachment is shown by the way behavior is organized with any one partner. Temperament is the *style* of behavior with all partners. At present the consensus is that temperament influences the way the security of attachment is expressed, but does not determine it. Normal infants adapt to caregiving by "organizing" their responses, that is, they spontaneously knit together early fragments of behavior (eg, looking, crying, calling) to summon and retain the services of their attachment figure. If the caregiving is "good enough," the child will have a "secure attachment" as can be judged in a simple but elegant classic research procedure called the "Strange Situation." If in ordinary circumstances at home the response of the caregiver is less than optimal, infants will organize a set of behaviors that can be objectively judged "insecure." These are of two main types, "avoidant" and "ambivalent-resistant." Both types of "insecure" attachment are, at present, considered within the normal range, although "less-than-optimal" (Sroufe et al, 1996).

Aberrations of infant development that result from physical defects, extremes of constitutional style, etc, may be noted at or soon after birth. If dealt with skillfully by the caregiver, they may resolve, or they may persist despite ideal nurturing. If the caregiver continues to function without guilt, rage, or rejection, and there is no further insult, the child will develop to the limits of its constitutional potential, which still may be compromised. However, ideal nurturing in needy cases is not as common as might be wished. Some infants' requirements are overwhelming, and caregivers being human may have their own problems, stemming from suboptimal rearing or current failure of social support systems.

Considering the variations in environments, certain behavioral extremes or "deficiencies" may result, despite the absence of any genomic predispositions. An example would be a passive infant born to a very dependent woman with little formal education and low self-esteem. In the absence of contrary influences, this infant could exhibit borderline retardation, even though there were no indications of subnormal intellectual potential early in life. Such situations contribute to the diversity of humankind and, although unfortunate, need not be considered pathological.

Of all the characteristics of newborns that stimulate parental responses and affect what the child learns, the most striking is whether the infant is a girl or a boy. The gender of the child elicits responses from the parents congruent with their hopes, fears, identifications, and preconceptions. These parental responses shape the direction of the child's reactions and, later, the child's feelings about himself or herself. Those who deal with newborns and infants often hear parents subjectively attribute qualities to their children that are not objectively obvious to others.

Precursors of Attachment

At birth the infant has simple attachment behaviors, but attachment itself is as yet nonexistent. Dependence on nurturing caregivers is complete. This begins what may be called the "prepsychological period" of attachment.

What brings children and caregiving persons together for these protective and nurturing ends is **attachment behavior.** Although from the start infants orient themselves toward external signals emanating from human beings, they do not at first discriminate between one person and another but seem to be scanning for patterns and for things that move. Very young infants respond preferentially to soft, high-pitched voices and soothing, cooing sounds; however, the impetus to orient to the caregiver is so strong that as early as the fourth week of life the infant will turn toward its primary caregiver's voice, whether soft or loud, high or deep, while ignoring others. The infant's smile and its first gurgles and coos are powerful "social releasers" that elicit attention and affection from the caregivers. As yet, however, the smile, vocalization, and general excitement at the appearance of a human face and the sound of a human voice are still fixed-action responses similar to the palmar grasp reflex. The social smile becomes distinguishable from the reflex "smile" between the fourth and eighth weeks.

The infant makes a ready and positive response to strangers up to about the eighteenth week. The pleasure in these interactions is not simply related to anticipated relief of hunger or physical discomfort, but is the result of primary social behaviors present at or soon after birth. These uncoordinated actions mature and coalesce into a system as the child associates socially with the caregiver. The close child-caregiver bond provides protection and physical sustenance and is a necessary preparation for relationships in later life. The appearance of the promiscuous social smile and the beginning of discrimination between the primary attachment figure and others signal the end of the prepsychological stage and the beginnings of attachment proper.

THE PERIOD OF ATTACHMENT: THE INFANT AT 2–9 MONTHS

The Positive Phase of Attachment

During the third month an infant recognizes the primary caregiver and soon begins to reserve its most vivacious smiles and kicks for that person. Mothers and fathers will say, "He sees me now" or "She knows it's me." By 6 months, infants are alert, attentive to the environment, and eager to move into it. They grasp purposefully at whatever comes into view as long as they can see their own hands in the field. They try to sit up and to watch or follow anything that moves, as long as it does not approach too fast or make too much noise. They are particularly eager to get at and stay close to their primary caregiver or mother, holding onto and exploring her. They have no mental image of objects out of sight and quickly lose interest, after a brief moment of perplexity, if a toy they have been playing with suddenly disappears under a blanket. However, by this time they have begun to associate certain objects with activities that have provided gratification, such as holding a bottle.

Between 4 and 6½ months, most home-reared children narrow their attachment behavior to focus on the figure of their primary emotional caregiver, usually the mother, and, to a lesser extent, other social respondents in the home, particularly the father. Weakly attached infants are more likely to confine their social behavior to a single person. Interaction with one or a few constant people is essential for the formation of secure attachments. It is not known how much social exchange is necessary, and it probably varies depending on the child's constitution. Between the fifth and seventh months, the inclination to focus on a particular figure is strongest, and when this connection has been achieved, the tendency to seek other figures for attachment declines dramatically. This change is reminiscent of the critical periods for imprinting in animals. The sensitive phase within which attachment can be formed normally ends as early as the sixth or as late as the eighth month. In the unusual event that the infant has not had consistent access to a figure on which to focus, the ability to form attachments wanes after about the eighteenth month, and thereafter it is extremely difficult to accomplish.

Although the complexity and richness of relations with attachment figures continue to grow, the endearing positive response to strangers, which is maximal at 14–18 weeks, gives way to a sobering demeanor and staring at 18–24 weeks. This shift in attitude about strangers signals completion of the positive phase of attachment.

The Limiting Phase of Attachment

After 6 months, conditions for the development of attachment in home-reared children are furthered by the emergence of fear responses. **Separation anxiety** is the sense of discomfort a child feels when experiencing, or being threatened by, a separation from the attachment figure. When this happens the normal child abandons exploration and begins attachment signals and behavior. As noted previously, becoming sober and staring at strangers start around the eighteenth week. **Stranger anxiety** is manifest at variable times, even in the absence of bad experience. It begins at about 26 weeks in home-reared infants, but is usually not well established until the eighth month. This response is distress at seeing the stranger and not merely separation anxiety because it occurs while infants are securely in the arms of their primary caregivers. It is important to note that these two types of behavior, although interrelated, are differentiable and either one may appear before the other.

Naturally, stranger fear and separation anxiety often function together; the child tries *to move away from* a frightening situation and *go toward* the person or place that offers protection and safety. Since stranger distress reinforces attachment behavior, it functions to enhance the already well-developed attachment drives, thus bringing to a close the positive phase of primary attachment. Thereafter, the infant may go to others and be friendly, but will not develop the same emotional attachments accorded to his or her own primary caregivers. This focus on the immediate family provides an apprenticeship in human relations that must be mastered before the child can move comfortably outside the family circle.

When painful experience, or the threat of it, consistently comes from attachment figures themselves, as in abusive families, it drives the child *toward* rather than away from those figures. The result is a strong attachment bond that is insecure and often masochistic. This can be the nidus of much later psychopathology.

Screening for Attachment Adequacy

Since the most important achievement of the first year is a secure attachment to one or more caregivers, pediatricians and others involved with children must watch for the normal development of that phenomenon and be alert to its deviations. Attachment behavior can be roughly assessed early in the first year primarily by noting the infant's response to the human face peering down. During the third and fourth months, the **social smile** is fully developed. Anyone can elicit such a smile in a healthy baby of this age by approaching slowly and presenting his or her face for inspection. Soft vocalizing helps. If the infant is well and not distracted, it will smile when the observer smiles. Although this smile may be a response to other cues as well, the human face, smiling, nodding, and cooing, is the strongest stimulus. Absence of such a characteristic reaction at this age warrants investigation for some physical or psychological abnormality.

Beginning in the seventh month, attachment to the primary caregiver can be easily screened in the clinic or elsewhere. As the stranger, such as the doctor or other unfamiliar adult, approaches the child and its mother, the child shows apprehension at the intrusion of a strange face. While safely on its mother's lap, a child not otherwise distressed will continue to smile broadly at her, reaching for her and playing with her hair, but will immediately become sober when looking at the doctor and will not return a smile but will turn back with concern to the mother instead. This is the beginning of active discrimination between familiars and strangers that a fully attached infant will normally show. At 7 or 8 months, the child may cry when put on the examining table and protest vigorously when taken off the mother's lap. The child's distress at the strange face of the examiner and separation from the mother is an indication that the attachment system is in good order.

Cognitive Advances

Piaget called the time from birth to the point of full attachment and beyond (age 0 to 16–24 months) the **sensorimotor stage,** in which the biological apparatus determines the cognitive experience of the child. The senses receive stimuli, and the motor apparatus responds in a stereotyped or reflexive way: stimulus in, response out. A feedback loop is formed, and the result is the first cognitive structure beyond the reflexes. For example, as the reflex grasp becomes purposeful, what is grasped finds new uses beyond simply being mouthed. As development proceeds in this manner, children become aware that they can influence the environment.

At 6–9 months, when fear of strangers is developing, the first cognitively intentional acts are observed. In Piaget's charming phrase, the child learns to initiate "procedures calculated to make interesting spectacles last." Deliberate and planned action begins. Since some kinds of behavior produce engaging results, such as the noise of a rattle or the movement of a toy activated by a string, interest shifts from the action itself to its repeatable consequences. Still, the infant is inclined to equate the movement or gesture with the result, an essentially magical procedure.

THE INFANT AT 9–12 MONTHS

Physical & Cognitive Abilities

Near the end of the first year children can sit, crawl toward attractive objects and away from repugnant or fearsome ones, walk a few steps without support or more steps using one hand to steady themselves, fixate and track with their eyes, grasp with either hand, and convey what is grasped to their mouth. They have command over their motor systems, mental representations of familiar people and objects in the environment, and rudimentary devices for securing and retaining things and people that are wanted or needed. Objects now have an existence that survives loss of visual or tactile contact, so that children may search for a toy that has recently disappeared. If a ball is placed

under a blanket and they can see a bulge, they will reach under the blanket and retrieve the ball. However, if the ball is taken from under the first blanket and put under another one, even though they see this happen, they will not search at the second site. This illustrates Piaget's assertion that infants do not distinguish an object from the motor action with which the object is associated.

Attachment & Stranger Fear Responses

Even before objects have an existence for the infant separate from the actions with which they are associated, the affiliations with loved persons have formed, and the infant has durable internal models of them. By 12 months attachment to the primary caregivers has been completed. If they are separated, the infant is distressed; if they are permanently parted, the infant mourns. The ability to discriminate among people as well as the fear of strangers bind the child to the nuclear family and serve to protect it from other dangers. Sustained by the active social relationships formed, the young child is now equipped to venture into the world of experience beyond the caregiver's embrace, and most children navigate this period more or less successfully. However, if the attachment of their caregiver in childhood to his or her primary caregiver was insecure, the chances are heightened that these children will experience difficulty in social relations and other aspects of the wider world (Main, 1995).

Negative Effects of Overlong Separation

Since attachment is necessary for healthy physical and emotional development, and since separation is tolerable only in moderation, overlong separation in early life can be expected to have morbid consequences. Bowlby and the Robertsons described and filmed the response of young, well-attached children to long separation from their parents when no adequate substitutes are available (for example, a 20-month-old child left in a residential nursery because his or her mother has been hospitalized). The result is protest, despair, and detachment. The **protest phase** begins after about 3 days of separation, with crying, calling, and searching for the attachment figure. The child clamors for the attention of caregiving adults but knows they are only substitutes. Anger develops and shows in the child's ambivalence when the mother does return; the child may avert his or her face, reject the mother's offers of affectionate hugging, and cling to an attendant instead. If the separation continues too long a **despair phase** follows. The child is still attached to the absent mother but communicates an air of hopelessness, which requires skill and time to overcome. If the mother returns in the despair phase, before detachment occurs, the child may *appear* to be quite indifferent to her. This does not mean the child is no longer attached, but that *the se-*

curity of that attachment has been dealt such a blow that the child has adapted mentally by changing its internal model of the mother. All this puts a great strain on the child's ability to trust the caregiving environment. If the primary caregiver, out of disappointment or anger at the rebuff, responds to the child's ambivalence or apparent indifference by rejection, disastrous disaffection and estrangement may result. Finally, if there is no reunion, the child becomes **detached.** In this phase he or she begins to be progressively reinterested in the environment, although more in material objects than in people, and a discriminated and functional attachment is very hard to reestablish.

Children placed for adoption can move from a foster home to an adoptive home with little difficulty until they are about 6 months of age; after that age many children become visibly upset, and by the eighth month, all children show serious distress when moved from one foster home to another, or from a foster home to an adoptive home—particularly if the foster home was a socially stimulating one in which the child had developed strong affiliations. The distress is caused by rupture of the attachment bond that begins to strengthen during the sixth month, and the sequence of protest, despair, and detachment occurs as just described, and requires sensitive handling in the new foster or adoptive home.

In all situations of long separation *without adequate substitute,* some form of stress takes place, regardless of the circumstances necessitating the separation and despite attention from skillful but unfamiliar caregivers. The presence of a sibling, grandparent, or other secondary attachment figure can greatly reduce the stress of separation, and special attention by a trained and patient substitute caregiver, who does not rotate with others on a workshift schedule, will minimize the potential damage. It can be seen that the disposition to form attachment and its normal phases are a biological given. How secure they are depends on the child's experience.

Many adults with moderate to severe emotional problems seem to have had insecure attachments in childhood. However, this is not to say that all children who make these less-than-optimal primary attachments, or endure painful separations, will have such problems. For children who have not yet reached the stage of detachment, initiation or resumption of affectionate care may reverse the process and limit developmental damage.

Early Infant Daycare

Research on nonparental care for children above the age of 2 (or even 12 months) has shown benign or even optimal effects for children if "good" care can be obtained. The most important criteria of such care are, for children, a well-trained, sensitive, stable staff and a high worker-to-child ratio, and, for parents, availability, affordability, and collaboration. Research has shown that excellent infant out-of-home care, as

financed and monitored by the Swedish government, has not posed a risk factor there. However, these findings cannot be compared to infant daycare practices often found in the United States, where spiraling costs, undertrained caregivers, and crowded conditions threaten the quality of care. Here there are apparent risk factors in daycare initiated before the first birthday, even in relatively good care.

Although many infants do well in very early nonparental daycare (and some do better than they would at home), statistics from several studies (reviewed by Belsky et al, 1995) continue to show that extensive (more than 20 hours per week) daycare in the first year increases the risk of developing an attachment that is not secure. Good daycare is not a cause of less-than-optimal attachment during this period, but a marker that indicates an increased likelihood of it. Most observers believe that *low quality* daycare *is* often the cause of insecurity in small children. All parents want to make decisions that are in the best interests of their children, but in regard to daycare, most often they must base these decisions on pressing financial and personal issues. Since there is no solid agreement by experts on whether parents should use or not use good quality daycare in the first year of their child's life, parents must assess their individual situation and choose the solution that best takes both the infant's needs and their own needs into consideration (Leach and Eyer, 1997).

THE SECOND YEAR: MASTERY OF THE BODY

Physical & Social Advances

The child's second year is characterized by increasingly vigorous autonomous behavior and a corresponding ready distress at separation from attachment figures. To be with someone who is familiar is of the utmost importance at this age. The fear of separation, however, is not the only fear experienced. As with younger infants, sudden sounds, the appearance of strange objects and unfamiliar people, and the rapid approach of large objects initiate the fear response and stimulate attachment behavior. There is little indication that imagination or fantasy plays any part in such distress; children are innately fearful of these things, and they learn to avoid other situations that have been associated with pain or frightening experiences, such as large animals or noisy machinery. They also learn to be aware of fear in their parents and siblings and to express it as their own.

This year of life has been called the period of mastery of the body, since exploration of the child's own body, particularly the erogenous zones, is a primary preoccupation. However, children have an irrepressible tendency to explore the outside world as well, just for the enjoyment and problem solving involved, particularly if their new motor skills are accompanied by the parents' praise and pleasure. Because motor development outpaces the emergence of rationality and discretion, conflicts with what the parents consider appropriate behavior inevitably arise. When the child's demands are thwarted, frustration and rage may result, and the child sets out to test the limits of the parents' tolerance. Since the child is small, the parents are usually successful in controlling him or her by removal or restraint; however, there are areas of physiological function over which parents cannot exert control—sleeping, eating, drinking, and excretion—and this produces conflict.

By the eighteenth month, the child is able to use spoons, cups, and other simple household items in appropriate ways. By age 2, small toys, cars, dolls, and playhouse furniture are beginning to be used in imaginative play.

At this point in life, both boys and girls are likely to have established an exuberant relationship with the world. As social skills emerge, shyness with strangers lessens, and children resume the search for further friendly associations. This imposes new demands on the primary caregivers to keep up with their children and protect them from harm.

Parental Example & Intervention

During the second year, two major influences exert an increased effect on the child's behavior and personality: parental example (modeling) and parental intervention (positive and negative reinforcement). Even before this time, children are eager to imitate and identify with one or both parents; the peek-a-boo, patty-cake, and baby-talk games of the first 6 months are common examples. Later, toddlers will delight in imitating complex parental behaviors based on observation, without having grasped the purpose of the behavior. The cat is petted or its tail pulled, teddy bears punished or rewarded, and all manner of familiar adult behaviors are put into action. This propensity to imitate adults and to absorb their emotions reinforces the child's inclination to respond with fear, anxiety, or distress to the same stimuli that evoke these responses in the parents.

The shaping effect of parental intervention assumes more importance as language becomes the chief means of interaction between parents and children. Although this influence may start to have some effect as early as the third month, it is maximal after age 1, when the child becomes able to divine the parents' intentions, see through their plans, and accurately assess some of their emotions. This awareness makes for conflict and the internalization of conflict. The child wants to do something, and the parents object. Their opposition is "internalized" as the child modifies its behavior in order to please them and avoid being discountenanced or punished. A common example is the absorption of the concept of "No!" Toddlers often act as if "no" were still external. They may reach for the television knobs and then, hand poised in the air, say

"No!" firmly and pull away. Once internalized, the powerful concept of "No!" can be turned against the parents as the child realizes they can be thwarted in some ways. The well-known oppositionism of this age group has resulted in its characterization as "the terrible twos."

During this period, toilet training depends partly on maturation of the nervous system. Bowel and bladder control is important to the extent the parents think it is. Overconcern about "accidents" focuses the child's attention on these physiological activities and confers an unwarranted importance on struggles between parent and child about matters over which neither has full mastery.

The child's interest in his or her body at this time emphasizes the parts that give pleasure and are under some kind of control. Excretory products are not repulsive at first. A little boy enjoys directing his stream of urine, and fecal play is a transient phenomenon in some children. A general tendency to "make a mess" is often noted, as are all physical activities that have some semblance of attempts to master the environment. Since fine motor control is not yet achieved and judgment is immature, life, limb, and household items are at risk. Since this is also the time when the child has the power to expel or retain feces—and perhaps is engaged in a contest with the caregiver over who is to control that pleasurable activity—it has been called the anal-sadistic stage in psychoanalytic descriptions of development.

Cognitive Advances

During the second year, the child can be observed studying situations and devising experiments to create new experiences. Newly acquired skills are perfected by repetition and practice. Consolidation by repetition is a recognized feature of mentation and shows that the function itself is a source of enjoyment, apart from any need to relieve boredom or tension or derive libidinal pleasure. During this period, the child uses action, which eventually will be superseded by language, as the chief means of dealing with the world and conforming to its social requirements. For this reason Piaget calls the first 2 years of life the "sensorimotor" stage and considers it preintelligent (ie, a time prior to verbal conceptual thinking).

By about 16 months, as cognition matures, sensorimotor activity is slowly replaced by increasingly conceptual processes. The child is able to maintain a mental image of an object, can imagine its simple displacement, and can search for it in places where it might be hidden. Piaget calls this "object permanence." Studies have shown that the primary caregiver is usually the first "object" to acquire such permanency in the child's mind and that children whose attachments are strong and positive are better able to develop mental images of other things.

The child's experiences in communicating with his or her parents serve as inner directives concerning which cognitive impulses can be openly entertained and which must remain unconscious; that is, without the child's awareness of the process, they are kept from consciousness because of their forbidden content. By this process, the "unconscious mind" begins to take form. The parents' own unconscious sanctions are sensed by the child and received as authoritative along with their overt and conscious directives. As long as the parents are relatively free of conflict about their values, the child can, if necessary, tolerate rather strict conscious and unconscious instructions about what may or may not be thought and done. However, sexual and assertive inclinations are strong, and their force will sometimes be exerted against any opposition.

Parents are best advised to tactfully help children gratify as many of their impulses as reasonably possible within acceptable social and cultural bounds. When necessary frustration produces rage and tantrums, children should be given a firm explanation of where, when, how, and with whom the sought-for gratification can be achieved, rather than an angry or anxious negative response. Parents should cultivate a habit of nonretaliatory acceptance of their children's anger but should not hesitate to use gentle physical restraint if children try to hurt the parents or themselves.

THE CHILD AT AGE 2–4

Cognitive Advances

Age 2–4 is the time when children, having mastered the sensorimotor mechanisms of their bodies, begin to use symbols and syntax in dealing with the world. However, they still "reason" by intuition rather than by logic. All things are judged by surface appearance and interpreted by post hoc rationalizing. Children at this age are confused by causality, attributing effects to the loudest, most recent, or most impressive preceding event. For example, a 3½-year-old boy might assume that a thunderstorm has caused his sore throat and that the doctor's examination cured it.

During this period, the piagetian stage of **preoperational thought** (age 2–4 to 6), children maintain a relative egocentrism; they personalize their observations and experiences. (In some children egocentrism wanes as early as age 4.) Although many secure toddlers show a spontaneous empathy for the distress of others, even at as young an age as 1 year, they cannot be objective about why they feel that way, and they either do not comprehend at all or, at best, repeat without understanding what they are told.

They are also unable to reverse a thought process. Shown a picture of a result, they cannot reconstruct the starting point from other scenes depicting it. They do not rank things relatively except in terms of opposites, eg, "bad" or "good." Moral laws exist as indivisible parts of certain types of behavior. To obey adults is to be "good"; to disobey is to be "bad," even if doing so is accidental or unavoidable.

Physical & Social Advances

The expansion of mental life is most striking during the third and fourth years. There is an enormous increase in the ability to use words and symbols (pictures and gestures) and to combine them in new ways to enrich the inner life with fantasy and to explore and control the outside world. Although there is great variation in the age at which children master language, in American culture by age 2 most children have a speaking vocabulary of 100–300 words and are able to understand several hundred more. Ingenious experiments have demonstrated that with certain supports some children can recognize up to 1000 words.

If their attachments are secure, boys and girls begin to spend less time with the parents and look outward for amusement and stimulation, particularly in the company of other children. **Parallel play** comes first, in which young children are observed playing "together" but not yet "with each other." Between ages 2½ and 3 **associative play** evolves, with elements of peer interaction and cooperation; during the fourth year **cooperative play** with one other child is possible. It is not until the fifth year that cooperative play in a group becomes a regular feature of childhood behavior.

Fantasy

Fantasy play is one means by which children aged 2–4 master the world. In fantasy, they can retaliate, set right, modify, and improve their condition in ways that are beyond their control in real life. The child can relive unpleasant or frightening experiences in fantasy and play and often revise and master them. This is one basis of playroom psychotherapy (see Chapter 28).

Sibling Rivalry

Age 2–4 is the time when a child is most likely to be presented with a baby brother or sister. Next to long separation from the primary attachment figure or other catastrophe, the arrival of a sibling is the most frequent and important psychological event in early childhood; its effects, particularly in shaping attitudes about competitors and dependents, continue to be felt throughout life. The arrival of a sibling provides a special opportunity to develop important social skills and to learn to handle aggression, but it is also the nucleus around which neurotic distortion may collect.

Most commonly, the child who has enjoyed the mother's undivided love and attention for several years now has to share these with a competitor. The child may respond with babyish activity and demands for attention and may regress to other behavior characteristics of an earlier stage of development. The parents' response to the child's behavior will determine whether the child will adapt to the new situation with few residual effects or whether, for the child, it will remain a focus of anxious concern and bitterness. The new mother should respond by allowing some regression in her 2-year-old child and by expressing her understanding of why it is happening. The father or some other family adult not directly responsible for the care of the new baby should spend more time with the older child.

For the infant, an older sibling is a figure for possible attachment and identification. For the much older child the new baby may be less a competitor than a playmate, or the object of behavior in imitation of the admired parents, for good or ill. Systematic effects of birth order have been shown for each member of the sibship (Sulloway, 1997).

Transitional Objects

Many parents are annoyed when their children—even up to the school-age years—have some object they like to hold and carry about with them, usually a blanket, stuffed animal, or other article of soft material that they seek out in times of disappointment, fatigue, or pain. To explain this the concept of the **transitional object** was introduced by D. W. Winnicott, a pediatrician turned child analyst. His psychodynamic explanation of this phenomenon remains a subject of debate, but there is no evidence that the practice has any pernicious effect so long as the child does not *prefer* the transitional object to the attachment figure.

Gender Identity

During the third and fourth years (if not earlier) children discover the difference between boys and girls and have a natural curiosity about it. There is an increasing interest in bathroom matters and in the genitals and genital play, although this is usually forbidden by the adults in the family, who do not tolerate genital exhibitionism as they may have tolerated and encouraged other types of showing off. The restriction does not lead to conflict if the parents accept the impulse as natural but indicate that social tradition calls for privacy in these matters.

This is also the age at which awareness of being male or female occurs. How parents act in their own gender roles and what behavior they expect and demand from their sons and daughters determine how children internalize their gender. In our society mothers are more accepting of crossgender behavior than are fathers and brothers.

Great controversy currently surrounds the psychology of gender identity and later sexual partner preference (heterosexual, bisexual, or homosexual). As with all behaviors, it is likely that genomic influence, through structure and hormones shaped by evolution, initially provides for a (limited) range of possible outcomes, in line with species survival. Starting with this given, the life experience of every child, over years of epigenetic change, selects and shapes the viable possibilities, resulting in the diversity of sexual partner preference in the human race. Personal convictions color the acceptance and interpretation of the available scientific evidence. At present the opinions of expert students of development are mixed, but most feel that the influence of life experience accounts for a preponderance of the variance in these exceedingly complex matters. Of course, in any single individual, the genomic and/or environmental elements can be far from the average expectable ones, and the resulting behavior may not conform to the statistical "norm" (Bradley and Zucker, 1997).

Sexual behavior adds a complicated emotional dimension to the child's relationship with the family. Children's understanding of sexual impulses is determined largely by the sophistication of their cognitive processes. Parental disapproval of sexual behavior by a small boy may arouse fears about potential harm to his penis, which he perceives as central to his sexual feelings. When he discovers that girls do not have penises, the immature little boy may wonder where the missing penises might be and how they came to be lost or hidden. Children of this age are not far removed from the phase of development in which they dealt with the world only through their bodies, and they are greatly concerned about bodily integrity and any possible threats to it.

The little girl at age 2 or 3 may also become concerned when she discovers she lacks a penis and may not be fully satisfied by reassurances that she has not lost hers, that she has something of equivalent value inside her body, and that she will someday be able to produce a baby. Despite the fear and doubts resulting from sexual thoughts and fantasies at this age, children's self-respect still rests on how the parents behave toward them and how the parents behave toward each other. The mother's security as a female adult and the respect she receives from her husband provide the daughter's best source of reassurance that she is a worthy and fully equal member of the family. Although both boys and girls at ages 2 and 3 are very impressed with the penis, girls of 4 or 5 can easily grasp the idea that they have internal organs of comparable value. Also at 4 or 5, when the mystery of procreation becomes comprehensible, both girls and boys are fascinated by that process. Later, in the school-age years, some of the aggressive behavior boys direct toward girls—and their bragging and self-aggrandizing—can be traced to a wish that they could have the female's procreative abilities (Linday, 1994).

THE CHILD AT AGE 4–6

Cognitive Advances

During the preschool years, the time of preoperational (prelogical) thought (ages 2/4–6), the child's thinking is largely egocentric, as it was during the sensorimotor period. At this age it is still not possible to retain both the concept of a thing in its entirety and the individuality of its parts. Appearance dominates judgment, so that something very long and thin may be considered "larger" than something that is not as long or tall but that has much more bulk. Most things are seen in terms of absolutes: best/worst, bad/good, etc. The 5-year-old child is not adept at comparisons or basic mathematical concepts. If candy is spread out, a child may know that there are 10 pieces; if the candy is then lumped into a mound or put into a paper sack, the child is no longer sure and must count the pieces again.

Words are particularly important in this very egocentric stage. Because words are perceived as concrete things and have a magical capacity to stand as accomplished facts, children are often deeply hurt by being called names; it is as if the name caller were actually transforming them into the derogated thing.

Children of this age have only a vague concept of time. Today, yesterday, and tomorrow may be clear enough, but the 4- to 5-year-old child has difficulty envisioning how long it will be from now until 2 or 3 days from now, and the distant past and recent past may be lumped together as "day before yesterday." A physical illness may be described as the result of some aspect of the child's personal experience, usually a single sensory experience. "How did you get sick?" "It was the night, at night," or "I played with John." Toward the end of this period, a grasp of impersonal causality begins to appear, and egocentrism weakens.

Childhood Sexual Experience

Sexuality is extremely complex, extremely important, and extremely interesting. It develops slowly and diversely and changes with age and sophistication. It is linked to attachment and loving relationships, but also to fear, anxiety, and masochism. Every person has a somewhat different experience and only the most common elements can be described here.

During the years from age 4 to age 6 overt sexual behavior can be differentiated from attachment behavior. Most adults cannot remember their own sexual preoccupations during this time, and many prefer to believe that children are innocent of such thoughts. Whether this overtly sexual behavior constitutes the emergence of a new instinctual system or is an outgrowth of the physical sensuality characteristic of attachment is still being debated. It is clear, however, that the forms taken by new eroticized initiatives will be affected by what is acceptable in the family and will reflect parental attitudes, particularly unconscious ones. A father is often pleased by his daughter's coquettishly "feminine" behavior and a mother by her son's "manly" behavior, and both will respond positively to it. Their responses to the incestuous content of the children's repertoire will be limited, however, so that in the long run, the child must endure some disappointment. But the need for parental nonsexual love, attention, and direction—the attachment needs—continues for many years.

Research on gender identity and sexual preference indicates that there are prenatal hormonal effects and likely genetic influences as well, in seamless combination with specific personal life experience. What percentage of the variance can be ascribed to each of these influences in any one case is imponderable. However, current childrearing practices that deemphasize sexual stereotypes are unlikely to derail appropriate development of a solid gender identity so long as the basic love and attachment are secure (Tasker and Golombok, 1997).

Children's sexuality emerges in stages that are not coalesced into an organized set at first. Sexualized attachment behavior is normal in prekindergarten children and is directed toward both parents. During these years, depending on the response of the adults, the children learn what is acceptable and what is not. (At this age children, still innocent, respond with alacrity to sexuality imposed on them by abusing parents or others.) By age 3½ most children know that they are girls or boys and that they are expected to act in certain ways in terms of their gender and sexual behavior. The most common experience in western culture is that between ages 4 and 6 years boys and girls go through a phase of immaturely perceived sexual love for the parent of the opposite sex, followed by the inevitable disappointment when it becomes clear that competition with the father or mother for exclusive possession of the other parent is a lost cause. However, this experience is reassuring as well, since they need not risk what they expect would be the loss of love of the parent of the same sex should they succeed.

To be capable of mature sexuality later, all children face the task of relinquishing their parents as primary sexual objects, at least in reality, without losing that parent's support and love. How well the three parties handle the renunciation will determine to some extent the child's emotional stability and maturity in later life. If the parents are themselves free of conflicts about the child's incestuous impulses and are careful to avoid any semblance of participation in such behavior, the child will eventually learn to select sexual respondents outside the family that are appropriate to their age and stage of development. The result will be increased self-respect and even pride in having taken a step toward growing up, and, for most people, a forgetting of the erotic feelings formerly directed toward family members.

The differences between sexual behavior in developing boys and girls may depend in part on the fact that although the first love object for both is usually a woman (their mother), the boy must renounce the sexual elements of this love, and much of the nonsexual closeness as well, while preserving the possibility of a full relationship with another woman later. Although the girl must also give up the sexual attachment she feels for her mother, she does not have to experience this painful separation of love as completely as boys, because, in our society, her physically close attachment to her mother can continue, along with the development of her sexual interest in her father and other males. Later, a girl's physical expression of love for her mother, in nonsexual embraces, confidences, girl-talk, etc, is the rule in happy families in our society. A boy does not usually have this type of intimate relationship with his mother or father but turns instead to other boys for his (mis)information and discussions about sex. Later, boys often show their eroticized feelings about their mothers by reaction formation: arguing with her passionately while they divert their attention to girls their age. How much of these differences are due to culture and how much to nature is unknown.

Many girls between ages 4 and 6 go through a phase of wishing they had a penis (not necessarily wishing they were boys), and some girls experience a sense of deficiency about this, particularly in families in which boys are more highly valued by the parents. In such cases girls may dress like boys (or *be* dressed like boys) and engage in activities traditionally associated more with boys than with girls, such as rough competitive play, all the way up to mid-adolescence. (Today, however, the unisex dressing of both boys and girls has mooted this point somewhat.) Although being a "tomboy" may be a repudiation of femininity for some girls, more often it is simply an exploration of more physical forms of play. The same reversal of traditional gender activities may occur with boys. However, a much greater percentage of school-age girls are free to be "tomboys" than boys are free to be "sissyboys." No doubt this is because other boys do not condone any deviation in this regard (nor do their fathers), whereas girls and their mothers usually tolerate it well. Aside from these few, girls who otherwise identify wholly with their mothers and other females and have no problems with their femininity may seek assertive goals as much as boys do simply because of the physical mastery and competitive gratifications that can be achieved. In most societies girls, as a group, are not as assertive as boys, particularly just after puberty. The reasons for this are obscure. Most certainly culture is involved, but genetic inclinations, augmented by hormones, must also play a part. Popular American culture is narrowing the behavioral dimorphism for all ages, and both men and women now are freer to explore what formerly was considered opposite-gender–specific behavior. It is a sign of social progress and health that young women are taking to the outdoors and athletic sports so readily, and that it is not considered unfeminine to be physical and even competitive.**

** Controversy over the psychology of female sexual development has continued ever since Freud advanced his first tentative conclusions 100 years ago. At present, opinion is widely diverse among psychoanalysts and other developmentalists, male and female.

If the child's sexual feelings during this early period of discovery and experimentation with romance within the family are accepted by the parents as natural and dealt with by means of simple redirection, explanations, and reassurance, the child will turn his or her attention to things in which success is possible while quietly continuing to explore sexuality when alone or secretly with other children. If this period of life in which conflict is normal is disrupted by separation or by illness or injury of the child or parents, or if covert erotization of the child-parent relationship, reversal of the child-parent role, vicarious encouragement of cross-dressing, or intensive sibling sexual play occur, anxiety will be experienced in the context of the child's sexual preoccupations and may leave psychic stains that will persist as dominant themes in psychological symptoms and treatment later (Metcalf, 1991).

Guilt

The rudimentary moral sense developing in children during this period engenders guilt about sexual and aggressive impulses toward parents and siblings. At this stage of prelogical thought children recognize unconsciously that these impulses would be opposed by the parents and assume that by having these impulses they deserve draconian punishment on the level of "an eye for an eye." Because children also love and need the parents they seek to redress these transgressions. Such secret behavior or thoughts and fantasies must remain unconscious because they are so dangerous, but the guilt remains operant, if vague, and can be relieved by punishment and forgiveness. Parents need to be aware that some provocative behavior toward them by the child may be unconsciously calculated to elicit punishment to relieve guilt about sexual, hostile, or destructive fantasies. For most people this inclination to punish themselves for real or supposed transgressions continues to some degree throughout life, in proportion to the dominance of any unconscious residue from this early stage of life.

The Role of Fantasy

One of the most remarkable human traits is the capacity for fantasy and the use of words and symbols and directed memories to enhance fantasy. Children try to make sense out of experiences; they hypothesize, engage in research, and reach conclusions on the basis of imperfect understanding, and they attempt to control and change what they find unsatisfactory. When humans fail, they have recourse to imagination and rationalization in which problems yield to magical solutions and disappointments can be relived as victories. All this is explicit in children's games, the stories they invent, and the fairy tales they love. Some of the fantasies of childhood survive in the unconscious and reappear in adult life in the form of dreams, in the free association of patients in psychiatric treatment, and in the waking lives of psychotic patients. The ability to fantasize increases as the cognitive skills gain sophistication. At each succeeding level of development, earlier conscious preoccupations are reworked. Through this process, some unconscious distortions, formed in childhood and resurfacing in psychotherapy, can be examined and corrected.

The Effects of Illness in Childhood

A child's reaction to illness or injury is conditioned by three factors: (1) the specifics of the disorder (severity, duration, signs and symptoms), (2) the stage of psychological development already achieved and its stability, and (3) the response of parents and siblings. The most obvious reaction is regression, eg, clinging, whining, thumb-sucking, and bed-wetting, in a child who has outgrown such "babyish" behavior. The younger child is most fearful of separation; an older preschooler may also fear pain or mutilation (if surgery is necessary) or may perceive the illness as punishment for misdemeanors committed or contemplated.

Children also tend to take cues from their parents. If the parents are horrified, paralyzed with fear, disgusted, or angered by the child's misfortune, and if they withdraw, they will compound the psychological and physical damage. Psychological trauma can be minimized if the parents are able to maintain a compassionate and supportive attitude and are particularly attentive during the most stressful phase without being overindulgent.

THE SCHOOL-AGE YEARS: AGE 6–12

During the sixth or seventh year, almost all children have matured enough that they can spend a part of each day in some kind of educational experience and apart from their attachment figures. They have the cognitive abilities and controls that are needed to conduct themselves well away from home. By this time, children have renounced incestuous preoccupations and have turned toward relationships with peers and interests in how the world works.

However, what may appear to be independent functioning at this age still depends on reliable adult continuity of care for its consolidation and continuance. Under conditions of social deprivation, when children of this age are left to their own devices, a premature and pathological spirit of independence and self-reliance may develop. Although perhaps permitting survival in abnormal circumstances such as war or social deprivation, too much independence too early almost always hinders the full development of the individual.

Cognitive Advances

During the school-age years maturation of the central nervous system and cumulative life experiences enable children to relate the parts of an object to its whole and to retain a concept of the whole while considering the parts. Children learn not only to conceive a course of events from the beginning to the end but also to understand it back from the end to the beginning, as in rearranging pictures to form a coherent story. Piaget calls this **operational** or **logical thought.** In the early (**concrete**) stage of operational thinking, the logic still depends on the child's perception of how things appear to be. Later, during adolescence, abstract (**formal**) thinking begins: thinking about thought.

In the stage of **concrete operations** (age 6–12) impressionistic and intuitive thinking is augmented by the possibility of taking small, logical steps in reasoning, and the results are more constant, reproducible, and communicable. Children begin to understand systems of classification. For example, "nesting" is descriptive of all classes that are additive; each larger category sums up all of the previous parts. It is only now, in the concrete stage, that they can understand the question, "Are there more birds or more crows in the world?" With this ability, children can conceptualize experiences individually and then organize them as parts of a larger whole. The change is from an inductive to a deductive way of understanding the world and from magical thinking to a more scientific approach. This knowledge precedes the ability to apply it very well or to put it into words—a 7-year-old child has difficulty explaining *why* she knows there are more birds than crows—and the new skills are used mostly in the service of the social and gratification aims characteristic of earlier phases of development, such as defeating others in competition or getting more attention and advantages.

Because the child at this age is better able to perceive cause and effect, there is a shift from categorical judgments learned by rote toward cognitive manipulation of rules and reasons. As the ability to understand and handle the outside world increases, the environment becomes more stimulating and comprehensible. Cooperative play in groups occurs, since intrafamilial competitiveness can now be expressed through games and fantasies. As the child proceeds through the elementary school years, rules become more reasonable and ideas of punishment less strict. Right and wrong begin to lose their absolute qualities.

Since his time, many students have noted Piaget's invariable and distinct stages do not always fit the broader range of developmental pathways. Also, the social context seems to have more influence than he thought. Vygotsky has pointed to the "zones of proximal development" just beyond the child's present level, where children can solve the piagetian problems somewhat earlier if they have sufficient support.

Sexual Latency or Moratorium

The disappearance of observable erotic behavior in most children in western society at this age (and the disinclination of adults to acknowledge such behavior in children of any age) first suggested that this period was one of sexual latency and diminished sex drive. What seems more likely is that the energies formerly expended on incestuous competition within the family are now turned outward (**sublimated**). Internally, eroticism continues in clandestine forms.

Despite frequent regression in the face of disappointment and frustration, school-age children are resourceful in their own behalf and are beginning to be less rigid in their moral judgments. It is natural, beginning at this time and continuing for a lengthy period, to conform to the mores and "dress codes" of schoolmates, and there is often also a general disillusionment—at least overtly—with the parental image. If the parents continue to offer loving support and guidance, the child will continue to identify with their general characteristics, usually emphasizing those of the parent of the same sex. During the elementary school years and adolescence, when issues of self-esteem are so important, the child needs the help of parents, older siblings, and particularly teachers in gradually acquiring skills that call for patience and practice. The support system that these people provide by their developmentally appropriate feedback and guidance is called "scaffolding" by Bandura.

During this period, there is an obvious voluntary separation of the sexes. Protestations of contempt by each group for the other may be an effort to control uncomfortable libidinal interests. Preference for playmates of the same sex appears to be primarily a natural rather than a cultural phenomenon, since it occurs in almost all societies during the preteen years.

School

Going to school is the single most significant developmental event of middle childhood. When children leave their families and even their neighborhood groups to go to school for the greater part of most days, all of the deficiencies of social and behavioral interaction that have been tolerated or gone unnoticed in the home environment come to light. There are many causes of trouble in school, but the most prevalent problems are the result of cultural or economic deprivation. These, along with specific learning disabilities and emotional disorders, are at the root of most school difficulties and suboptimal achievement.

ADOLESCENCE

Describing the extraordinarily complex and variable adolescent experience is challenging, so the following acts only as an outline and summary of the broad spectrum of middle-class teen development. Studies of other societies and of different social classes in the western world indicate vast differences in the range of behavior and difficulty experienced during this period.

The major tasks of adolescence are (1) establish-

ment of a firm individuality (a sense of self or ego identity) and (2) integration of the pubertal surge of sexual and assertive impulses. Both of these tasks, already familiar from other periods of childhood, are the psychological concomitants of the physical developments of puberty. The maturing motor system of the body approaches adult strength and adeptness; the hormonal shift and spurt announce the capacity for fertilization; and the increase in neuronal complexity in the brain makes adult thinking and judgment possible. Social skills developed in relationships with family members, playmates, and others determine whether the transition to adulthood will be turbulent or smooth, short or long.

Adolescence begins with the recognizable physical changes of puberty. The subsequent stages of psychological advance, regression and regrouping, partial fixation, and further advance are diverse and may occur simultaneously or in alternating fashion in any one young person. The end point of adolescence is defined by social rather than physical criteria and is the subject of much dispute between the generations. Eventually, however, the press of physical maturation carries the young person out of adolescence and into adulthood.

For our purposes, the end of adolescence is defined as that point in young life when the major social investiture for the given social class is complete. At this point the obligations and privileges of adulthood are assumed, postponed, or rejected. The duration of this process will be short or long in direct relation to local conditions of survival, ie, the need to augment the procreative, work, or fighting forces. In many societies it is quite short; in some classes of western society, it is an extended period and blends with a special, postadolescent phase that has been called "youth," where the individual no longer is an adolescent physically or cognitively but still has not become a full adult in society. This is a period complicated by irresolution or enhanced by refinements of education, travel, pleasure-seeking activity, or volunteer service for others.

Cognitive Advances

During the elementary school-age years, problem-solving activity is mostly limited to actual situations in the real or fantasy world. At some time between ages 12 and 15—usually in the stage described here as early adolescence—some young people develop the ability to deal with abstractions, to think about improbables. Piaget calls this the **stage of formal operations** to emphasize that the *form* of the proposition is what is important, not the content (as in the formulas of mathematics, which can be applied to an infinite variety of numbers). In formal-stage thinking, the individual extracts the key elements and then is able, through mental processes, to combine, reverse, and recombine them into possibilities that perhaps never were or may never be actualized in the real world.

This capacity contributes to the adolescent's propensity toward moral abstraction, grandiosity, idealism, and dedication to things that "might be but are not." Although Piaget described this development as the final stage in normal cognitive growth, it should be regarded as a special achievement rather than a universal expectation. Only about one-third of adults function to any large degree in the formal stage; another third do so some of the time but have little need for it in their daily lives; and the rest seem never to achieve it at all. Although the capacity for formal thought is correlated with normal intelligence, it is not directly related to it. Failure to progress to the concrete stage from preoperational thinking is evidence of mental deficiency or disorder: a failure of development. This is not necessarily the case with failure to achieve the formal stage in adolescence. Most people move on from the concrete stage to learn workaday techniques for solving life's problems and have no practical use for the skills of the formal stage.

The Structure of Adolescence

Those who have studied and written about normal adolescence in North America commonly perceive three stages: early, middle, and late. Some add a foregoing preadolescent phase and a succeeding youth phase, which helps to emphasize that adolescence proper is inextricable from what went before and what follows. In most instances it is clear that in the year or so before the onset of puberty a restless increase in motor and psychological needs begins, typical of the same individual during age 2–4. The young person may be harder to get along with, the activities of the school years are no longer as satisfying, and parental control becomes difficult to sustain. A characteristic of this period is that children, boys more than girls, turn away from their mothers to their circles of close friends. These changes intensify as physical development proceeds.

A. Early Adolescence: Adolescence begins with the advent of pubertal change, when new ways of self-expression (sexual and social) and new skills appear. These emerging interests are noticeable because people outside the family become the objects of sometimes passionate connection. The relationships available within the family can no longer properly suffice to gratify the new aspirations of a progressively more vigorous and sexual person. Early adolescents usually start by exercising these drives within the home environment, and the result may severely test the family relationships. If demands for growing space and sexual expression can be recognized and progressive emancipation allowed, the family will remain a source of support and guidance during these experimental sallies into a widening world.

Much has been written of the turbulence or "Sturm und Drang" of adolescence in western society. However, it is only when the youngster's behavior is primarily antiself, antifamilial, or antisocial that one must suspect pathogenic forces at work, particularly within the family. These potentially destructive forces sometimes lead young people to seek support and remedial experiences elsewhere. If a benevolent outside environment meets the need, the troubled youngster may be able to continue normal development and make a successful adult adjustment. More often, however, such conflicts lead to stalling at an intermediate stage, premature rupture of family relationships, or partial regression to inadequate earlier adaptations.

Despite the risks, and their own fears, most young people are irresistibly drawn toward the satisfactions and prerogatives adults seem to enjoy, particularly in the area of sexual experience. Even in what is perceived to be a permissive modern society, adolescents continue to experience conflict over erotic impulses and their expression. Childhood fantasies about sexual anatomy and function may persist into these years in spite of free access to accurate information about sex and procreation.

Certainly the preoccupation with sexual themes in all types of entertainment and advertising has increased the intensity and hurried the onset of active erotic life in recent decades in all social classes. Still, for a significant portion of youngsters, overt sexual behavior during early and middle adolescence is suppressed, deflected, or repressed. Premature experience is eluded through the escape channels of romanticism, masturbation, and verbalization with peers of the same sex.

Early adolescence is characterized by increased introspection and self-absorption; exciting but indescribable new sensations and changes in physical proportions occur such that the body image established through the school years is destabilized. Since they feel that much of what is happening cannot be discussed with their parents, young people at this age form intense personal relationships with one or two friends of the same age and gender. Transient identification with adolescent or adult groups or media stars provides opportunities for young people to try various roles. The first contact with drugs usually occurs at this time—mostly alcohol, marijuana, and cigarettes, but often a variety of proprietary mood elevators or depressants and sometimes harder drugs. The influence of respected peers is of great importance in the pursuit or avoidance of destructive drug use. Positive friendships, sexual fantasy and masturbation, and growing pleasure in physical and intellectual activity are in most cases the preferred alternatives to hazardous sexual experimentation or drug abuse.

The attention of adolescents fluctuates back and forth from friend to self, to idealized heroes and back again to self. Bursts of activity alternate with seemingly interminable periods of passive absorption in music, reading, video games, the Net, and television. A wish to be different is paradoxically combined with a passionate insistence on sameness, so that having the same designer jeans or jacket or the same earrings as their special friends becomes an urgent necessity. Adolescents seem to form a subculture—a world apart to which only the young can belong.

It was once assumed that a turbulent adolescence was essential to full development. However, only about one-fifth of normal adolescents have a stormy time; about the same proportion proceed smoothly to adulthood. The remainder show turmoil and anxiety in surges, with spurts of development and periods of stress and stalled progress (Bukowski et al, 1996).

B. Middle Adolescence: Eventually, after consolidation through relationships with peers has occurred and experience with fantasy loses its appeal, boys and girls become overtly interested in each other as the objects of sexual behavior, and middle adolescence holds sway. The boy has commonly focused until now on male identification models, whereas the girl has in most cases maintained an active interest in boys and in both male and female idols. In early adolescence such interest is usually free of conscious erotic content, although overt sexuality is increasing in the age group 11–13 in the West. With the beginning of focused heterosexual interest in middle adolescence, the preoccupation with intimate friendship, masturbation, and sexual play with members of the same sex is replaced by identifications with *groups.* The demanding, argumentative, dependent relationship with the father or (most often) mother suddenly resolves as young persons invest more of their energies outside the family. School clubs, athletics, and social activities of all kinds now provide opportunities to add a physical dimension to relationships with young people of the opposite sex. Access to cars, later hours, more money, and less adult supervision have the same effect.

During this period of increasing libidinal preoccupation, it continues to be obvious how private conversations with peers of the same sex protect against premature heterosexual activity. Excessive modesty (or its equivalent, teasing exhibitionism or nervous flirting) reflects the strength of the sexual impulses and the energy being expended on their control. Undoubtedly, some adolescents accelerate their development during this phase, but others, feeling hopelessly outclassed, self-conscious, or frightened, falter and stop in some fixated state. Still a third group, inconsistently guided or ignored by their parents at earlier stages, take license for freedom and attempt by extreme behavior to provoke parents and other authority figures to set needed limits.

In early mid-adolescence, as the search for self-mastery and satisfying sexual relationships reaches its apex, we see all the forward, backward, and lateral movement that characterizes the adolescent in our society. The object of "first love" usually resembles in some way the parent of the opposite sex, or—if the conflict over renouncing the parent as a sexual goal was too intense—he or she may seek diametrically opposite physical traits in the early love choice. The young person usually identifies with the parent of the same sex at this time, often in open imitation of dress and mannerisms. The boy becomes suddenly more integrated, genuinely masculine, as compared with earlier strutting and posing. The girl becomes more womanly, as compared with her former vanities and affectations. This accomplishment marks the end of the middle adolescent period.

C. Late Adolescence: In late adolescence, a consolidation of personality occurs, with relative stability and consonance of feelings and behavior. There is often a decrease in introspection and the creative imagination characteristic of earlier adolescence. By the end of this period, young people's styles of behavior show striking similarities to those they may have formerly repudiated in their parents. The admired and respected parental values have been made their own—for better or for worse—and in this way the generations are linked. The gender and libidinal struggles of mid-adolescence yield center stage to the search for vocational choice and a satisfying position in the social group. Students who have done poorly in grades 8–11 suddenly, with the close of the major developmental press of the first two adolescent phases, may take up their studies with dedication and qualify for college.

For many young people in the middle and working classes, late adolescence means that school is finished and work and spousal choices are made or are imminent. They pass immediately into adulthood. For some, particularly in the projects and barrios of metropolitan areas, a limbo of unemployment, aimlessness, and petty (if not major) crime supervenes between dropping out of high school and pregnancy or prison, with perhaps later entry into the labor market. This track, although it cannot be called "normal," is certainly not unusual under such disadvantaged circumstances. For others more fortunate, late adolescence marks the beginning of long years of further schooling and professional training—a phase of adulthood beyond adolescence but short of the full investiture of adulthood. In this "youth" phase, some of the hallmarks of adolescent student status persist.

Psychologically speaking, however, normal adolescence comes to a close in the college years (at about age 20) for those continuing in school. Adolescent-type conflicts may linger, but adolescence is over. A 24-year-old graduate student with identity diffusion or antisocial behavior, which might be normal for some 16 year olds, is not a person with prolonged adolescence but an adult with problems.

Along with the maturing cognitive abilities, people in late adolescence usually become less preoccupied with themselves and more concerned with cultural values and ideologies. They often become seriously interested in religion, ethics, or politics, but usually still in a tentative, reversible way, expecting that bad outcomes can be expunged, amnesty granted, and records sealed. Commitment to a formal cause may also represent some of the energy loosened from family ties and is an outlet for energies not yet invested in vocation and love-partner choice and other usual adult preoccupations.

Attachment

Dependence on the primary attachment figures characteristic of the first decade—being cared for—gives way gradually to a measured independence in the second decade. This is the time of life when people learn how to care for themselves in the world. Physical and emotional separation from the parents occurs, sexual identity is consolidated, and erotic interest is more solidly focused on eligible peers. By the close of adolescence, love relationships reflect the quality of the old attachments, this time including, if all has gone well, tender and satisfying genital sexuality with an emotionally valued partner.

When this process is accomplished, usually early in the third decade, young adults are prepared, without precluding their own further development, to undertake the primary care of others. The attachment cycle completes itself in the quality of care provided to a new generation. At this point, young adults can begin to return to their parents on a basis of equality. Old attachments continue to express themselves in attenuated form in letters, telephone calls, and visits, and attachment figures are sought out in times of sadness or adversity, giving structure and continuity to personal relationships over a lifetime.

ADULT DEVELOPMENT

At the beginning of this chapter, development was defined as lawful, qualitative change toward greater capacity for adapted living. It has been easy to see that the march through childhood and adolescence meets this formal definition of development, and these changes are so pronounced—and so rapid—that much space has been devoted to describing them. Despite the fact that the remainder of the life cycle is often three or four times as long as the 20 years it takes to reach adulthood, whether the changes that occur during the years of adult life remaining can be correctly deemed "development," corresponding to the definition above, is an unresolved question.

Freud thought that development was primarily a function of the first decade. However, most of the well-known theorists who have written about life-span psychology, though having their roots in psychoanalysis, have disagreed with Freud on this point. Jung went against the flow and introduced the idea of life stages, including the concept of midlife crisis. Erikson was also a pioneer in maintaining that development proceeds throughout life, and, more recently, Vaillant, Gould, Levinson, and Colarusso and Nemiroff have made significant contributions. Central to these theories is the further evolution of **personal identity** or **self-concept.** These writers sought to describe how individuals come to think of themselves, and how this identity changes and evolves over time.

Despite the lack of conclusive empirical data it seems reasonable—even self-evident—that the changes that occur over an adult's lifetime—love, career, marriage, children, retirement, proximity of death—must also force the achievement of developmental steps, just as the major changes of childhood do. In the remainder of this chapter, adulthood will be discussed in terms of how adults think (cognition), how they represent themselves (traits), and finally, the developmental tasks most adults face as they age.

Cognition in Adulthood

After achievement of the formal stage of intelligence in middle adolescence, there is evidence of a specific "postformal" stage that some people manage to develop. Many adults use a different logical path from the one characterized by Piaget, which is at once more complicated, relativistic, and context specific. Research is proceeding on this issue and may some day explain why some well-functioning adults do not primarily use formal logic.

Beyond any shift of quality in adult cognition, there is also considerable controversy about whether there is a significant decline in intelligence and other basic cognitive processes during adulthood and, if so, when it first appears and in what processes. The answers to these questions have come in principal part from empirical research using batteries of cognitive tasks with large samples of healthy subjects.

It is generally conceded that from age 30 to 60 years, there is a variable decline in a variety of memory tasks, even when motivation and psychological factors are considered. There are multiple and conflicting hypotheses to account for this finding. It is agreed, however, that although ability to learn slows, persons of all ages can benefit from training and experience.

In addition, depending on the measures used, there are contradictions in the data on intelligence. On the Wechsler-Bellvue Intelligence Scales, a linear decline of up to 30 points has been demonstrated in the level of general intellectual functioning during the decades after age 30. Yet, as reflected in one valid and reliable test of mental abilities, intelligence appears to remain stable into the 50s, after which there is a progressive decline. In another instrument, the subject's ability to apprehend relationships in puzzles does not deteriorate with age, but it takes about twice as much time for a healthy 80-year-old to achieve the same score as a 20-year-old. Thus, no simple explanation seems to account for the observed change in cognitive functioning that occurs with aging. One promising new approach to investigation of the relationship of age and IQ is to correlate stability or decline in intelligence with general and specific health factors—conditions known to affect mental functioning.

What must be borne in mind is that any age differences in adult abilities described here are statistical, referring to whole groups or subgroups. Understanding any one person requires a knowledge of age-related factors for that person and the realization that anyone's current abilities are inextricably bound to the context of their life experience and their current potential.

Traits in Adulthood

Trait psychology is a discipline that views personality as a collection of internal attitudes influencing thought, behavior, and self-representation. Reliable cross-sectional research data have been produced showing many significant changes in traits, but no clear patterns have emerged. A summary of such research shows—rather than characteristic development and change—an impressive degree of stability of traits over long intervals.

This tendency to stability in personality seems to contradict the idea that life-span development occurs according to graded steps and in epigenetic progression. Neugarten has offered one explanation for the paucity of evidence that there is development in adulthood. She suggests that there is stability of socioadaptational processes, as reflected externally in traits, and development in intrapsychic processes, as observed in psychoanalytic treatment or open-ended life-span interviews.

DEVELOPMENTAL TASKS OF ADULTHOOD

Although personality traits may remain stable over the course of adulthood, there clearly are certain challenges, or tasks, that must be faced as the adolescent matures into the young adult (20–40 years old), the middle-aged adult (40–65 years old), and the older adult. These include development of one's career, altering the relationship with one's parents, achieving intimacy in love relationships, coping with pregnancy and parenthood, suffering through divorce, stabilizing one's identity, coping with illness and disability, and preparing for death (Aiken, 1998).

Career

As adolescence gives way to adulthood, individuals begin to move out of the "student" role and into that of the "worker." Work activities take on a central role in the younger adult's life. There is a period of experimentation of styles and identification of mentors after whom to model new and different work behavior. Job shifts, seeking higher salary, or pursuing interesting and prestigious work gradually must be integrated with concerns for job security, availability of life and health insurance, and planning for retirement. Individual achievement must be blended with the needs of other employees and employer. Success brings with it the opportunity to supervise and help others and pass on wisdom. For the middle-aged and older adult, preparations must be made to give up work as a major source of pleasure and self-esteem.

Relationship with Parents

Children and adolescents' dependence on their parents for financial support, advice, and psychological support often continues into the early years of young adulthood. Each struggles with how to support and allow the young adult to have independent thought, authority and responsibility over decision making, and the opportunity to lead a separate life. For some this is a natural extension of the family's pattern of granting developmentally appropriate independence, for others it is a source of great intergenerational conflict (McAdams and de St. Aubin, 1998).

As the young adult grows into the middle-aged adult there is a sense of equality and mutuality to the relationship with their parents. At the same time there is a shift in understanding of their parents' lives. Choices made that may have seemed baffling to the adolescent or young adult become more understandable in the light of experience. Appreciation for the intelligence, perseverance, or commitment to ideals or mores of their parents can bring the two generations emotionally closer.

At some point in middle adulthood the caretaking of sick or disabled parents becomes an issue. The dependency the young adult used to have on his parent now becomes reversed as preparations for the parents aging, and later death, become necessary. Feeding, cleaning, and guiding one's parents through the last stage of their lives can be a touching experience or a great drain on emotional and financial resources. Leadership of the extended family is passed on as the older adults defer family decision making to their children and grandchildren.

Intimacy in Relationships

Earlier in this chapter the work of Bowlby and Erikson is summarized. Their ideas about the need for attachment to meaningful others and the need to establish loving and intimate relationships are basic to the understanding of courtship and marriage in young adulthood. During adolescence objects of affection are identified, some dating occurs, but rarely does mature intimacy develop. This task of realistic connection to another marked by caring for and understanding of another's needs and desires without the loss of one's own sense of self is a major life challenge. Young adults spend a significant portion of their time, income, and effort trying to achieve this intimacy (Brennan et al, 1998).

Initial rounds of dating are often attempts to sort out an individual's feelings about becoming intimate. These activities also help to determine which feelings are overidealizations and which are based more in reality. "Living together" prior to marriage can be an attempt at either of these tasks.

Entering a commitment to marry is seen by some as the end of a long process of achieving intimacy but is actually only the beginning. Finding an intimate relationship, developing an identity as a couple, maintaining individuality, weathering crises, and learning to argue are ongoing tasks throughout adulthood. Career pressures, child rearing, and diminishing sexual function are challenges to maintaining this intimacy.

Pregnancy

The decision to have children is another step in the adult development of an individual. It signals the readiness of the young adult to give up being mainly self-concerned and become responsible for the care of another. Financial difficulties and lack of stable and mature intimacy between the parents can become worse with the stress of pregnancy. The amount of attention and adoration shared within the couple now must make room for the expected child. Mothers notice the physical and emotional changes going on inside their bodies and focus inward. Fathers do not have the same internal changes and may deny the reality of the pregnancy until they feel the baby move. Failure to understand the inward focus of the mother can leave the father feeling rejected and angry and the mother abandoned and resentful. Both need to work toward maintaining intimacy throughout the process to guard against misunderstanding.

The last trimester of pregnancy is often the time when first-time parents consolidate their identities as parents. Selecting the child's name, preparing a room for the child, and purchasing clothing and supplies are clear signs parents are preparing to become a family. The child is given a "spot in the family" before birth as it becomes real to its parents.

Parenthood

With childbirth comes huge changes in the couple's daily routine and pattern of interaction. New allocations of roles and responsibilities are necessary. Decisions about childcare, finances, and relationships with extended family have to be made. The new child's helplessness coupled with the mother's physical and psychological changes, begun in pregnancy, support the development of bonding by the mother. This shift in affectionate attention can threaten the parents' intimacy unless they are able to empathize with each other while they nurture the new child.

Parents' activities must also change to provide the appropriate holding environment. At first the focus will be providing for the child's physical needs, fostering basic trust and self-soothing, and building a secure attachment. Later, facilitation of separation, encouragement of independence, teaching of social rules and morality, setting of appropriate behavioral limits, as well as fostering development of self-regulation and ability to inhibit are all parental responsibilities.

As parents help their children through various developmental stages they often relive memories of their own childhood. Identification with certain struggles and successes, attempts to come to resolution about old conflicts with their own parents, and new discoveries about how parents feel about children's behavior are some of the things that help to increase empathy in new parents. Parents need to recognize which issues concern their child and which ones concern their own childhood to prevent disruption of the child's development (Lieberman, 1997).

Helping to guide a child's choices and behavior decreases as the child reaches late adolescence and prepares to strike out on its own. Encouraging growth and development, which leads to autonomy and separation from the family, is the goal of parenting. This separation results in the parents having to adjust to "an empty nest" and confront any unresolved or unattended issues of intimacy.

Divorce

Unfortunately, many couples have conflicts that interfere with intimacy and provoke anger. Sometimes these conflicts overpower the need for social connection or the hope of resolution. Divorce of a couple is a complicated action that results in a variety of feeling states. It is usual for the young or middle-aged adult to experience guilt, sadness, sense of failure, fear of loneliness, sense of loss of identity, and depression no matter who requested the divorce. Too-rapid remarriage, continuing depression, substance abuse, superficial sexual relationships, and irrational behavior can be a result of these feeling states.

The consequences of divorce include loss of socioeconomic status (particularly for women), loss of social group, estrangement from in-laws, and loss of the friendship of the ex-spouse. When children are part of the family the results can include ongoing parental conflict over custody, visitation, and financial support. In addition there is the stress of single parenting, conflictual emotional reactions by the children, and emotional impact on relatives and friends. Benefits of divorce can include reduced interspousal conflict, freedom to reestablish intimacy with a different partner, and enhanced opportunity for personal identity.

Identity Consolidation

At some point in young adulthood a sense of "finally feeling like an adult" develops. For many this occurs around the mid-point of young adulthood as career is progressing, intimacy is being achieved, pregnancy and parenthood have been experienced, and relationships with parents are maturing. Both success and failure have been experienced. Loss of family members or job or unexpected events have tempered adolescent omnipotence. There is a realistic sense about the possible courses one's life might follow.

By middle adulthood the individual has experienced much of this and now has less focus on life's potential and more on the success or failure of one's efforts. Many develop a desire to pass on "lessons learned" to the next generation. Writing books, teaching courses, and donating money are all examples of what Erikson labeled *generativity.*

There is also a loss of illusions. One cannot have absolute safety nor provide it for another. Hard work and perseverance do not always lead to success. Life cannot be controlled; bad things happen despite all preparations and precautions. These life lessons often lead to a reworking of identity, which can result in increased confidence and creativity or depression and despair (Colarusso, 1997).

Illness & Disability

As adults age they notice changes in their functional abilities. Memory and cognition decline, physical strength decreases, and the ability to heal from injury or illness becomes less vigorous. These changes often come as a surprise to later-stage adults because their view of themselves tends to advance less rapidly than do these physical changes.

Chronic or degenerative illness, failure to completely recover from injury, and the occurrence of diseases caused by life-style can result in disability. This comes as a narcissistic blow to the middle-aged adult.

Usually the individual has had enough life experience to realize that full recovery is not possible. Adjusting to not being able, and never again being able, to do a usual activity is a depressing thought for many. Illness or disability coupled with retirement from career are significant risk factors for the development of hopelessness and suicidal ideation, particularly in men. The disabled middle to late adult must find meaning and value in life to avoid the occurrence of despondency and depression (Colarusso, 1998).

Death

Life has a beginning and an end. Adults spend most of their lives avoiding this fact. For most older adults, reviewing their life, reconciling the successes with the failures, and preparing themselves for the end of life are the last tasks, but not necessarily depressing or fearful ones (see also Chapters 37 and 38). Many older adults come to some resolution about the kind of life they have had and are ready for the end. They put great effort into clarifying last wills, passing on important mementos or information, or resolving old conflicts. Others make sure their passing will not cause their families undo confusion or hardship. *Ego integrity* is the term Erikson used to describe successful participation in these processes.

REFERENCES & SUGGESTED READINGS

Aiken LR (editor): *Human Development in Adulthood.* Plenum, 1998.

Belsky J, Rosenberger K, Crnic K: The origins of attachment security: "Classical" and contextual determinants. In: *Attachment Theory: Social, Developmental, and Clinical Perspectives.* Goldberg S, Muir R, Kerr J (editors). Analytic Press, 1995.

Bradley SJ, Zucker KJ: Gender identity disorder: A review of the past 10 years. J Am Acad Child Adolesc Psychiatry 1997;36:7.

Breger L: *From Instinct to Identity: The Development of Personality.* Prentice-Hall, 1974.

Brennan KA, Clark CL, Shaver PR: Self-report measurement of adult attachment: An integrative overview. In: *Attachment Theory and Close Relationships.* Simpson JE et al (editors). Guilford, 1998.

Bukowski WM et al (editors): *The Company They Keep: Friendship in Childhood and Adolescence.* Cambridge University Press, 1996.

Colarusso CA: Separation-individuation processes in middle adulthood: The fourth individuation. In: *The Seasons of Life: Separation-Individuation Perspectives.* Akhtar S, Kramer S (editors). Aronsen, 1997.

Colarusso CA: Development and treatment in late adulthood. In: *The Course of Life: Completing the Journey.* Vol 7. Pollock GH, Greenspan SI (editors). International Universities Press, 1998.

Horowitz MJ: *Cognitive Psychodynamics: From Conflict to Character.* Wiley, 1998.

Karen R: *Becoming Attached.* Oxford University Press, 1997.

Lamb ME (editor): *The Role of the Father in Child Development,* 3rd ed. Wiley, 1997.

Leach P, Eyer DE: Women's behavior: Do mothers harm their children when they work outside the home? In: *Women, Men & Gender.* Walsh MR (editor). Yale University Press, 1997.

Lecanuet J-P et al (editors): *Fetal Development: A Psychobiological Perspective.* Erlbaum, 1995.

Lewis M: Overview of infant, child, and adolescent development. In: *Textbook of Child and Adolescent Psychiatry,* 2nd ed. Weiner J (editor). American Psychiatric Press, 1997.

Lewis TB, Amini F, Lannon RA: *A General Theory of Love.* Random House, 2000.

Lieberman AF: Negative maternal attributions: Effects on toddlers' sense of self. In: *Attachment and Psychopathology.* Atkinson L, Zucker KJ (editors). Guilford, 1997.

Linday L: Maternal reports of pregnancy, genital, and related fantasies in preschool and kindergarten children. J Am Acad Child Adolesc Psychiatry 1994;33:416.

Lombroso PJ (editor): Development and neurobiology (Section). J Am Acad Child Adolesc Psychiatry 1998; 37:1.

Main M: Attachment: Overview, with implications for clinical work. In: *Attachment Theory: Social, Developmental and Clinical Perspectives.* Goldberg S, Muir R, Kerr J (editors). Analytic Press, 1995.

McAdams DP, de St. Aubin E (editors): *Generativity and Adult Development: How and Why We Care for the Next Generation.* American Psychological Association, 1998.

Metcalf A: Childhood: From process to structure. In: *Hysterical Personality,* 2nd ed. Horowitz M (editor). Aronson, 1991.

Roazen P: *Erik H. Erikson: The Power and Limits of a Vision.* Aronson, 1997.

Siegel DJ: *The Developing Mind: Toward a Neurobiology of Interpersonal Experience.* Guilford, 1999.

Singer DG, Revenson TA (editors): *A Piaget Primer: How a Child Thinks,* rev. ed. Plume, 1996.

Sroufe LA et al: *Child Development: Its Nature and Course,* 3rd ed. McGraw-Hill, 1996.

Sulloway FA: *Born to Rebel: Birth Order, Family Dynamics, and Creative Lives.* Vintage Books, 1997.

Tasker FL, Golombok S: *Growing Up in a Lesbian Family: Effects on Child Development.* Guilford, 1997.

Zeanah CH et al: Infant development and developmental risk. In: *Reviews in Child and Adolescent Psychiatry.* Dulcan MK (editor). American Academy of Child and Adolescent Psychiatry, 1998.

Brain & Behavior

Frederick G. Flynn, DO, COL, MC, Jonathan Mueller, MD, & Howard L. Fields, MD, PhD

Practitioners of psychiatry require a working knowledge of brain structure and function as well as of individual psychology. Knowledge about psychodynamic concepts complements and strengthens the clinician's understanding of behavioral and intrapsychic changes associated with alterations in the structure and function of the central nervous system. In this chapter, a review of the gross anatomy of the brain is followed by descriptions of disorders of the central nervous system that illustrate the role of the brain in human behavior.

Until recently, psychiatric education has emphasized the diagnosis and management of schizophrenia, depression, and anxiety disorders. It has just recently begun to include the study of memory disorders, aphasias, head trauma, and epilepsies.

In evaluating and managing patients with brain lesions, several factors must be taken into account: personalities, intellectual gifts, and cognitive processes prior to brain injury are highly individual; lesions that produce changes in behavior and cognition are themselves never exactly the same; and social support networks and the motivation to improve following brain damage vary tremendously. Nevertheless, many characteristics are shared by brain-injured patients, and a knowledge of common syndromes aids the clinician in developing an individualized approach. The psychiatrist who is unaware of neurobehavioral syndromes will miss those diagnoses, to the detriment of the patient's care. For example, altered behavior (eg, inattention or diminished language comprehension) due to organic causes may be mistakenly interpreted as a problem in psychodynamic motivation. The clinician must distinguish behavioral and cognitive changes caused by brain lesions from psychological reactions caused by acquired deficits in mental and motor abilities. Since intact portions of the brain compensate for damaged portions, this task may be difficult.

GROSS ANATOMY OF THE BRAIN

An appreciation of neuroanatomy requires a knowledge of three different levels of the brain and the manner in which they are connected. MacLean (1969) used the term "triune" to describe three brains (Figure 5–1) essentially working as one: (1) a neomammalian brain (the neocortical mantle); (2) a paleomammalian brain (limbic or visceral brain); and (3) an ancient reptilian brain ("R complex"). These three levels will be discussed under the headings of neocortical surface anatomy, limbic system anatomy, and brainstem anatomy.

Neocortical Surface Anatomy
(See Figures 5–2 and 5–3)

The adult human brain weighs about 1350 g and contains over 10 billion nerve cells. The surface of the four cerebral lobes (Figure 5–2) is irrigated by three major blood vessels: the anterior, middle, and posterior cerebral arteries. Major boundaries are formed by the longitudinal (interhemispheric) cerebral fissure, which separates the left from the right hemisphere at the midline; the central sulcus (fissure of Rolando), which separates the frontal from the parietal lobe; and the lateral cerebral sulcus (fissure of Sylvius), which forms the superior margin of the temporal lobe.

A. Organization of the Cortex: The cortex consists of motor, sensory, and association areas. Although traditional anatomic locations of motor and sensory function will be discussed, recent evidence from electrocorticography suggests that motor actions and sensory perceptions can be elicited by stimulation of the cortex outside of these traditional areas.

1. Motor cortex—The motor cortex lies anterior to the central sulcus and may be subdivided into motor, premotor, supplemental motor, and frontal eye field areas.

2. Sensory cortex—The primary sensory cortex consists of regions that receive projections from thalamic relay nuclei. (Note that olfactory stimuli have no thalamic relay stations.) Auditory stimuli activate the eighth cranial nerve, and the messages traverse brainstem pathways and are conveyed by auditory fibers from the medial geniculate body of the thalamus to Heschl's gyrus (the primary auditory cortex) in the superior temporal lobe. Surrounding Heschl's gyrus is the auditory association cortex. In the dominant hemisphere the receptive association cortex for language, known as Wernicke's area, is located in the posterior third of the superior temporal gyrus. Visual input is transmitted from the retina via the optic nerve and tract to reach the lateral geniculate body of the thalamus; the messages are then conveyed by fibers that sweep backward after a slight forward loop to reach the banks of the calcarine fissure (the primary

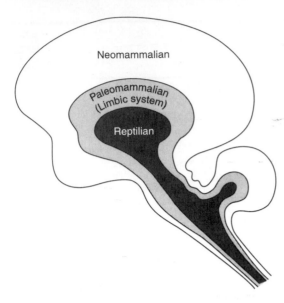

Figure 5–1. MacLean's "triune" brain. (Reproduced, with permission, from MacLean PD: The brain, empathy and medical education. J Nerv Ment Dis 1967;144:374. Copyright 1967 by Williams & Wilkins.)

visual cortex) on the medial aspect of the occipital lobe. Somatosensory input is carried via spinal and trigeminal thalamic tracts to the ventral posterior thalamus. Projections from the thalamus terminate in the primary sensory cortex along the postcentral gyrus. Somatosensory association cortex lies in the posterior, inferior, and superior parietal lobules.

3. Sensory association cortex—The sensory association cortex may be divided into unimodal, polymodal, and supramodal regions. The unimodal association cortex receives input exclusively from its respective sensory modality. Polymodal or heteromodal association cortex receives input from multiple sensory association areas. Supramodal association cortex performs the highest level of sensory integration. It receives no input from primary sensory cortices, but integrates information from both unimodal and polymodal, as well as limbic regions. Supramodal association cortex is believed to be located in the inferior parietal, prefrontal, and superior temporal regions.

B. Lobe Divisions: In addition to the functional division of the frontal lobe into motor, premotor, and prefrontal regions, three horizontal gyri—the superior, middle, and inferior frontal gyri—constitute major landmarks. In a similar fashion, the lateral as-

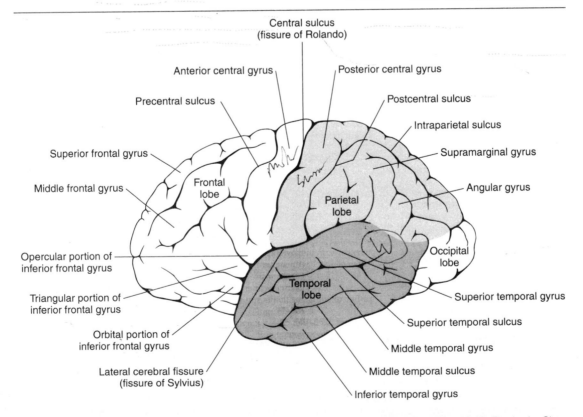

Figure 5–2. Lateral view of left cerebral hemisphere. (Reproduced, with permission, from Chusid JG: The brain. Chapter 3 in: *Correlative Neuroanatomy & Functional Neurology,* 19th ed. Lange, 1985.)

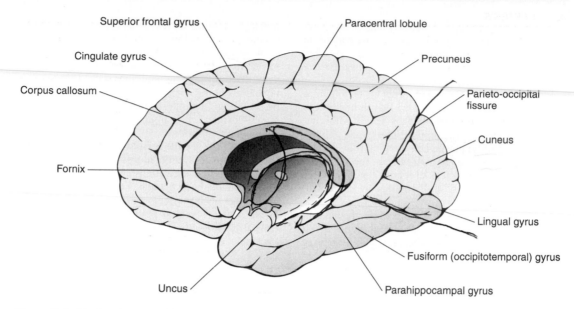

Figure 5–3. Medial view of right cerebral hemisphere. (Reproduced, with permission, from Chusid JG: The brain. Chapter 3 in: *Correlative Neuroanatomy & Functional Neurology,* 19th ed. Lange 1985.)

pect of the temporal lobe is also divided into superior, middle, and inferior gyri. Major divisions of the parietal lobe are the postcentral gyrus, the superior parietal lobule, and the inferior parietal lobule. The occipital lobe, also divided into superior and inferior gyri, contains the cuneus and lingual gyrus, respectively.

C. Sensory Cortex-Limbic System Connections: Through the sensory cortex-limbic system connections, the sensory information reflecting experience in the "outer world" is communicated to the "inner world" of emotions and drives, which are presumed to be governed by the limbic system.

Since the 1960s, it has been recognized that visual association fibers travel forward from the occipital region through the inferior and middle temporal gyri to reach the temporal pole. Fibers then sweep backward and medially to impinge on the amygdala, a component of the limbic system. The amygdala has been conceptualized as a gate, bridge, or way station between the sensory cortex and the hypothalamus. The amygdala plays an important role in conditioned fear responses, autonomic modulation, emotional memory, motivational drive, and recognition of emotional facial expression.

D. Frontal Lobe-Limbic System Connections: Pathways that arise in the orbitomedial and dorsolateral prefrontal regions impinge on the hypothalamus and brainstem directly. Since these fiber systems are bidirectional, they offer a pathway whereby the frontal lobes can not only monitor but also actually modulate core brain or autonomic system activity.

Limbic System Anatomy

The term "limbic system" refers to a group of structures anatomically situated between the diencephalon and telencephalon. Functionally, these structures mediate transactions between the extracorporeal world (as elaborated in the sensory association cortex) and primitive internal or visceral drives and responses integrated through the hypothalamus. To the extent that learning is a process whereby sensory experience achieves meaning or attains permanence in memory by being paired with the experience of pleasure or pain at the core brain or "visceral" level, all learning may be said to be influenced by the limbic system.

A. Limbic Circuits: Despite the fact that Willis in the seventeenth century and Broca in the nineteenth century used the term "limbic" to describe the ring of tissue on the medial surface of the hemispheres, it was not until 1937 that the notion of limbic circuitry had a major impact on psychiatry. In that year, Papez published "A Proposed Mechanism of Emotion," in which he suggested that a group of structures participated in transferring information from the hypothalamus to the cortex and back to the hypothalamus. Specifically, the Papez circuit (Figure 5–4) involves the transfer of information from the hippocampus over the fornices to the mamillary bodies of the hypothalamus and then via the mamillothalamic tract to the anterior thalamus. From the anterior thalamus, fibers ascend through the anterior limb of the internal capsule to reach the cingulate gyrus, where they sweep posteriorly via the retrosplenial cortex to once again reach the hippocampus. Today the fornix is known to be a bidirectional pathway largely involving cholinergic pathways. It is believed to be part of an intrinsic or obligatory pathway involved in registering new information, and its role in emotional experience continues to be examined.

Eleven years after Papez published his now famous paper, Yakovlev (1948) suggested that in addition to the medial structures described by Papez, three lateral cortical regions (the orbitofrontal cortex, temporal pole, and insula) played an important role in motivation. Yakovlev also highlighted the strategic position of two subcortical structures that Papez had not included in his circuit, the amygdala and dorsomedial thalamus.

In 1952, MacLean explicitly linked the medial limbic circuit of Papez with the basolateral limbic circuit of Yakovlev, referring to them as the limbic system, or visceral brain. The following is a brief summary of the major limbic system connections: (1) Both circuits exert powerful downward and presumably regulatory effects on the brainstem. (2) Both circuits have intrinsic connections, and the Papez circuitry has been described as "reverberating." (3) The basolateral limbic circuit has particularly strong upward connections to the sensory and frontal cortex, whereas the hippocampus (medial limbic circuit) receives sensory and frontal lobe input via multisynaptic pathways that converge on the entorhinal area before entering the hippocampus itself.

B. Limbic System-Neocortex Connections: Fibers arising from limbic structures in the medial temporal lobes travel to prefrontal regions by two distinct routes: a direct pathway via the uncinate fasciculus and an indirect pathway via the dorsomedial nucleus of the thalamus. Another example of limbic system-neocortex connections is the diffuse cholinergic projection system that arises from the nucleus basalis of Meynert in the basal forebrain and travels to widespread areas of the neocortex, as well as to the hippocampus and amygdala. Degeneration of neurons in the nucleus basalis of Meynert is one of the pathologic hallmarks of Alzheimer's disease and is responsible for a large part of the cholinergic deficit in the illness.

C. Limbic System-Basal Ganglia Connections: Many conventional anatomy texts fail to describe the intricate relationship between the limbic system and the basal ganglia. The ventral striatum, including the nucleus accumbens septi, the olfactory tubercle, and the ventral pallidum receive limbic circuits from the amygdala, the prefrontal cortex, and the ventral tegmental area. In addition, other contributions to this region arise from the hippocampus and cingulate cortex. The major efferent fiber projections from the ventral striatum include the amygdala, the medial dorsal nucleus of the thalamus, and the lateral habenular nucleus. There is additional efferent output to the hypothalamus and ventral tegmental area, as well as more caudal regions of the midbrain. Emotional influence in motor movement and gesture can be appreciated from examples ranging from a simple smile to a violent outburst. It is also important to note that movement disorders are frequently accompanied by neurobehavioral changes and psychiatric disease is often accompanied by changes in movement.

Some Features of Brainstem Anatomy

Coursing through the tegmentum of brainstem is a dense network of projection neurons and interneurons that comprises a reticular core. Ascending fibers aris-

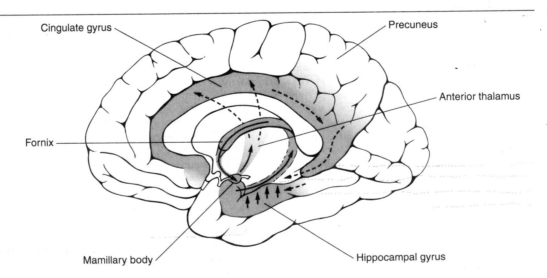

Figure 5–4. The Papez circuit, as described by MacLean. (Reproduced, with permission of Elsevier Science Publishing Co., Inc., from MacLean PD: Psychosomatic disease and the "visceral brain." Psychosom Med 1949;11:340. Copyright 1949 by The American Psychosomatic Society, Inc.)

ing from this core form the reticular activating system. From the reticular formation in the midbrain, fibers ascend both to the ventral forebrain and to the intralaminar and reticular nuclei of the thalamus. Thalamic fibers, in turn, project to diffuse areas of the cortex. Nauta (1958) coined the term septo-hypothalamo-mesencephalic continuum to describe a central core containing multiple neural tracts that connect (1) the septal region (the most anterior portion of the reticular activating system), (2) the hypothalamus, and (3) the midbrain. This continuum is roughly synonymous with MacLean's reptilian brain ("R complex") (Figure 5–1).

The septal region consists of a group of nuclei located beneath, in front of, and medial to the head of the caudate nucleus. In the 1960s, it was found that electrical stimulation of the septal region in both animals and humans resulted in a strong sensation of pleasure, and the septal area thus was labeled a "pleasure center."

The hypothalamus consists of multiple nuclei located behind and above the optic chiasm, beneath the thalamus, and above the pituitary. The hypothalamus forms the floor and part of the lateral wall of the third ventricle with the mamillary bodies as its posterior border. The hypothalamus functions as an outflow pathway for autonomic discharge and plays a major role in regulation of pituitary function. It also contains regions central to the expression of drive states and appears to function as a homeostatic control device for maintenance of the internal milieu.

The midbrain (mesencephalon), a region of the upper brainstem, is of special importance to psychiatrists, since it is the site of origin of two major ascending dopaminergic pathways. Fibers arising from the substantia nigra and traveling to the neostriatum (caudate nucleus and putamen) form the nigrostriatal pathway. The mesolimbic pathway consists of fibers that arise from the ventral tegmental area of the midbrain and ascend to the frontal and limbic regions of the forebrain, as well as the ventral striatum. (The antipsychotic effects of neuroleptic agents appear to be mediated by postsynaptic dopamine blockade in the mesolimbic pathways, while parkinsonian symptoms are produced by dopamine blockade at the level of the neostriatum.) Animal studies have implicated the mesolimbic dopaminergic pathway in the brain reward networks. There is evidence that the reinforcing properties of addicting drugs such as heroin and cocaine depend in part on activation of this system. In addition to these dopaminergic pathways, noradrenergic pathways and serotonergic pathways arising from the locus ceruleus and the dorsal raphe, respectively, together with dopaminergic pathways, constitute the medial forebrain bundle.

In summary, the septo-hypothalamo-mesencephalic continuum has extensive intrinsic connections and exerts a powerful upward influence on the cortex via the ascending reticular network and the numerous pathways of the medial forebrain bundle. In addition, the continuum is itself subject to downward influences from the medial and basolateral limbic circuits.

DRIVES & DRIVE DISORDERS

At its most elemental level the human organism, like crawling life, has a mouth, digestive tract, and anus, a skin to keep intact, and appendages with which to acquire food. Existence, for all organisms, is a constant struggle to feed—a struggle to incorporate whatever other organisms they can fit into their mouths and press down their gullets without choking. . . . If at the end of each person's life he were to be presented with the living spectacle of all that he had organismically incorporated in order to stay alive, he might well feel horrified by the living energy he had ingested. The horizon of a gourmet, or even the average person, would be taken up with hundreds of chickens, flocks of lambs and sheep, a small herd of steers, sties full of pigs, and rivers of fish. The din alone would be deafening.

This quotation from Becker (1975) illustrates the pivotal role of drives—in this case, the drive to eat. Philosophers have long debated the meaning of universal and innate biological forces or drives manifested in all forms of life. Scientists have tried to translate these concepts into considerations of matter and energy, brain tissue, and nerve transmission.

Freud's (1895) "Project for a Scientific Psychology" represented an attempt to consider how energy manifests itself and is transmitted in the brain and how objects in the external world begin to assume a particular charge or meaning for the observer. After hypothesizing the transfer of electrical energy (cathexis) from one neuron to another, Freud extended his model to include objects invested with or deprived of cathexis. For example, he spoke of infants as extending libidinal pseudopodia toward objects in the world.

Although reflex behavior is fully predictable, other more complex forms of behavior do not correlate as precisely with external stimulus conditions but are still far from voluntary. Students of behavior have invoked as hypothetical mechanisms the concept of motivational states that determine the intensity and direction of complex behaviors. Reflexes, drive behaviors, and fully voluntary behaviors thus seem to exist not as sharply demarcated features but along a continuum.

Theories of Drive

Various approaches to understanding drives can be seen in the work of ethologists, developmental psychologists, and anatomists.

A. Innate Capacities: Ethologists such as Lorenz and Tinbergen have made important discoveries about what they term "innate capacities." Turning away from the complexity of human behavior, ethologists have studied instinct or drive by working with animals such as fish, birds, and insects.

Tinbergen's work with the male stickleback fish is a good example of this approach. Whereas the presence of male fish with bright red bellies during mating season provokes fighting or attack behavior in other males, it provokes approach or mating behavior in females. Colorless models resembling stickleback fish fail to elicit this behavior in either males or females. On the other hand, crude pieces of wood painted with a patch of red elicit only male approach. From this sort of work arose the notion of a "sign stimulus," or "releaser"—a particular configuration or feature embedded in a complex stimulus—that triggers instinctual behavior such as eating, mating, or attack. Since these stereotyped response behaviors occur even in animals raised in total isolation, ethologists speak of them as operating through "innate releasing mechanisms."

The following example illustrates the types of behavior arising from triggered innate release mechanisms. When parent thrushes alight on the nest of newborns and shake the nest, the mouths of the newborn chicks gape upward. A few days later, touching the side of the young thrush's mouth produces the same response. Shortly thereafter, the sight of the parent bird (or even of a human finger) elicits gaping behavior that is still vertically oriented. Still later, gaping behavior is directed toward the visual stimulus. Two distinct types of behavior are seen: (1) a response initially elicited and controlled by proximal (vestibular or tactile) stimuli and (2) a response gradually recruited by more distal, such as visual, stimuli.

B. Human Reflexes: Early reflex behaviors such as sucking, grasping, and turning the head toward a stimulus (eg, a nipple or a finger touching the infant's cheek) occur not only in awake infants but also in infants who are asleep or in coma. Sucking behavior also occurs in anencephalic infants. Although the extensor plantar response may persist for a year, most of these primitive reflexes disappear by the age of 4–6 months. However, they often reemerge in human adults with frontal lobe disorders (eg, tumor or advanced Alzheimer's dementia). Thus, these primitive behaviors appear to have been held in check by the frontal neocortex.

C. Anatomy of Specific Drive Behaviors:
1. Rage—In the 1890s, it was noted that cerebral decortication in dogs caused them to respond to trivial stimuli (pinching of the tail, being removed from the cage, or even having a fly land on the animal's nose) with disinhibited rage.

In the 1920s, Cannon studied adrenal medullary sympathetic discharge in decorticated cats and described their massive reaction to trivial stimuli (eg, touching the cat's back) as "sham rage," consisting of the following behavior: (1) pupils dilating and hair standing on end, (2) hissing and growling, (3) baring the teeth and fangs, and (4) arching the back and

lashing the tail. In 1928, Bard pointed out that this entire sequence depended on the integrity of the posterior hypothalamus.

2. Eating—Feeding and eating have been studied in rather fine detail. Following initial observations that destructive lesions in the ventromedial hypothalamus resulted in hyperphagia and obesity, other reports began to document profound anorexia and weight loss following destruction of the lateral hypothalamus.

Thus, there arose the concepts of a ventromedial "satiety center" and a lateral "feeding center," or "appetite center." Reports of stereotactic surgery of the hypothalamus in animals, along with a few dramatic case reports of humans with lesions in these areas, have supported these initial observations. However, several lines of inquiry—as shown in the examples below—suggest that it may be inappropriate to conceptualize hypothalamic areas as "centers" for eating or satiety.

Lesions in the hypothalamus interrupt ascending dopaminergic pathways of the medial forebrain bundle. Severing these fibers outside the hypothalamus also produces the diminished arousal and aphagia seen with lateral hypothalamic lesions. In fact, animals with lesions in the hypothalamus do not have an isolated or selective loss of interest in food. Rather, they appear to manifest syndromes of multimodal sensory inattention—ie, reduced responsiveness to visual, auditory, tactile, and olfactory stimuli presented to the side opposite the lesion.

Although animals with ventromedial hypothalamic lesions usually eat more food than animals without lesions, if the food is adulterated (eg, made bitter with quinine), they actually eat less than normal animals do. Thus, they seem to show an exaggerated response to both noxious and pleasant stimuli.

Animals starved prior to destruction of the lateral hypothalamus will eat and gain weight immediately after the lesion is produced—apparently in an attempt to bring their weight to a "set point."

These observations point to the difficulties in conceptualizing "centers" for activities as complex as eating.

A hierarchical network approach to eating behavior recognizes contributions from three levels of control: (1) the hypothalamus, with its "hard-wired circuitry," regulates glucose levels, monitors fullness of the stomach (satiety versus hunger), and determines the "set point," ie, how much to eat; (2) the limbic system, in concert with the sensory systems, governs the selection of foods appropriate to appease the appetite, ie, what to eat; and (3) the prefrontal regions, which are involved in decisions about table manners, ie, when, where, and how to eat.

Disturbances at each of these levels can be seen. (1) Tumors of the diencephalic region may disrupt carbohydrate metabolism and lead to hyperphagia, rage, and obesity. Patients with dysfunction of appetite regulation may even tear doors off refrigerators to satisfy the carbohydrate drive. This is termed "appropriate megaphagia," since the items ingested are not qualitatively different from what is normally eaten. (2) Patients with medial temporal lobe disorders (eg, Klüver-Bucy syndrome) may ingest items such as tea bags or cigarette butts. This "inappropriate hyperphagia" has been interpreted as reflecting sensory-limbic disconnection with consequent visual agnosia, manifested in this case by the inability to recognize and discriminate between the edible and inedible items. (3) Dementia or frontal lobotomy may lead to disruption of social behavior with loss of table manners.

3. Pleasure—Animal experiments begun in the 1960s have shed light on the neural substrates for "pleasure." After electrodes were implanted in certain regions of the medial forebrain bundle, the animal could press a bar to receive an electric current to the brain (pleasure stimulus). Animals were observed to press the bar repeatedly—even to the point of neglecting water and food or to the point of exhaustion—and to cross an electric grid to receive further pleasure stimulation. It is now clear that a major component of the brain pathway for reinforcement is the mesolimbic dopaminergic projection from the ventral tegmental area of the midbrain to the nucleus accumbens, located near the septal area. This same pathway contributes to the rewarding effects of food, fluids, and certain drugs of abuse, such as cocaine.

Modulation of Drives

Drives depend on neural circuits whose developmental maturation is vulnerable to chemical and structural insults. Structurally intact circuits are themselves subject to modification and modulation by numerous forces. The following are examples of factors that shape and modulate the circuitry from which drives arise.

A. Genetics: Individuals with Down syndrome (trisomy 21) appear to have a biological disinclination to violent behavior.

B. Circadian Rhythms: Cortisol secretion, motor activity, and body temperature are all subject to 24-hour cycles. A pathway from the retina to the supraoptic nucleus of the hypothalamus plays a major role in adjustment to changes in the light-dark cycle, and circadian rhythmicity.

C. Hormones: Castration and antiandrogens are used to treat sex offenders in Europe. The human brain itself may have a "sexual identity": A region of the anterior hypothalamus (preoptic nucleus) has been termed "dimorphic" in rats, since its gross anatomy is shaped by exposure to circulating estrogens. α-Fetoprotein produced by the fetal liver protects the developing human fetal brain of both sexes from masculinization by circulating maternal estrogens. The third or fourth month of human gestation appears to be a "critical period" for the development of sexuality. Histopathological evaluation of the anterior hypothalamus demonstrated a difference in the cellular density and volume of the interstitial nucleus between homosexual men, heterosexual men, and heterosexual women. The volume of this nucleus was much larger in the heterosexual men, and the volume and cellular density in homosexual men were more similar to that of the size of the female interstitial nucleus (LeVay, 1991). Unfortunately, all the patients that LeVay studied had died from AIDS and, therefore, it is unknown whether this is a representative model of differentiating hypothalamic anatomy. Although this may support a biological theory of sexual preference, it does not negate the role of environmental and social forces on sexual behavior.

Clinical Disorders Affecting Drive

Psychiatrists and neurologists seldom see isolated drive disorders. Constellations of drive disorders, however, are seen frequently in the context of neuropsychiatric disorders. The following are examples of human drive disorders.

A. Anorexia Nervosa: This disorder is characterized by loss of 25% of baseline ideal weight; altered body perception and fear of obesity; amenorrhea; lanugo; hypotension; bradycardia; and peculiar behavior associated with eating and weight control, such as hoarding food, abusing laxatives, binge eating (bulimia), and vomiting. Anorexia occurs more frequently in females than in males (20:1) and is most common at age 15–25 years. The role of psychodynamic factors in this disorder is unclear. Behavioral regimens (eg, confinement to bed until satisfactory weight gain occurs) in conjunction with psychotherapy appear to be the most successful approach to treatment (see Chapter 28).

B. Kleine-Levin Syndrome: Episodic hypersomnia (up to 20 hours) alternates with hyperphagia, gorging of food, and hypersexuality (masturbation and aggressive sexual behavior) in this syndrome in adolescent boys. Patients are amnesic for these episodes, which recur at intervals of 3–6 months, last 1–3 weeks, and remit spontaneously.

C. Depression: Major depression is associated with the following neurovegetative signs.

1. Sleep—The amount of sleep is classically diminished in depression. Early morning awakening and rumination are prominent manifestations, but prolonged sleep with frequent arousals can also characterize major affective disorders. Hypersomnia is well recognized in "atypical depressions."

2. Eating—Anorexia with weight loss is common, but overeating is often seen in "atypical depressions."

3. Sex drive—Diminished interest in sex is often seen as one manifestation of anhedonia (inability to find pleasure in events that previously afforded enjoyment).

4. Motor activity—Psychomotor retardation is common in depression.

Secondary depression can be seen as a result of

organic brain disease (eg, cerebral infarct, tumor, Parkinson's disease). Left-hemisphere lesions (particularly frontal) are more likely to produce secondary depression than right-hemisphere lesions. Subcortical basal ganglia disease (eg, caudate lesions, Parkinson's disease, Huntington's disease) also more commonly produce depression than diffuse or multifocal cortical disease (eg, Alzheimer's disease).

D. Mania: Diminished need for sleep, hyperactivity, pressure of speech, and hypersexuality are common in manic states. Secondary mania can be seen following right peridiencephalic or subcortical lesions.

E. Klüver-Bucy Syndrome: Manifestations include placidity (tameness), visual agnosia, lack of sexual inhibitions, and a tendency to place objects in the mouth. Klüver-Bucy is usually associated with bilateral anteromedial temporal lesions, particularly when both amygdala are involved. This may be secondary to ischemic-hypoxic disease, cardiopulmonary arrest, herpes encephalitis, and Pick's disease.

F. Complex Partial Seizures: Although a few patients with long-standing complex partial seizures may manifest the interictal personality disorder referred to previously, it is more common that only one or two elements of this personality syndrome are manifested. Many patients with complex partial seizures will manifest none of the personality traits seen in this disorder.

G. Wernicke-Korsakoff Syndrome: Korsakoff's amnestic syndrome is preceded by the characteristic triad of Wernicke's encephalopathy, ie, confusion, ataxia, and eye movement disorders (nystagmus or ophthalmoplegia). Part of Korsakoff's syndrome may involve profound apathy in which neither sex nor alcohol interests the patient. Korsakoff's syndrome is a useful model for a drive disorder, with lesions distributed in strategic midline structures: (1) mamillary bodies in the posterior hypothalamus (part of Papez circuit); (2) the periaqueductal region (from the third to fourth ventricles), with lesions interrupting the ascending fibers of the medial forebrain bundle and the reticular activating system; and (3) the dorsomedial nucleus of the thalamus, which is a crucial bridge between multiple limbic regions and the frontal lobes.

ANATOMY & PHYSIOLOGY OF PAIN

Pain is a subjective experience with sensory, emotional, and behavioral components. Each individual perceives and copes with pain in a very personal manner. The International Association for the Study of Pain defines pain as "An unpleasant sensory and emotional experience associated with actual or potential tissue damage, or described in terms of such damage." The transmission of nociceptive impulses has a complex anatomy. Signals are constantly being integrated and modulated along the pain pathways.

This is particularly true at the injury site, the dorsal horn in the spinal cord, throughout the brainstem reticular core, and at limbic, thalamic, and cortical levels. Descending supraspinal tracts modify the perception of pain and produce efferent responses. Therapeutic strategies can be directed at any one or a number of these anatomical sites.

Primary afferent fibers subserving nociception include the small myelinated Aδ (delta) and the small unmyelinated C fibers. The Aδ fiber responds to mechanothermal stimuli whereas the C fiber is a polymodal nociceptor. These are high threshold fibers, which makes sense, because if they were low threshold fibers (eg, Aβ fibers for touch) we would all be walking around in constant pain. When trauma injures tissues where these nociceptive fibers reside, a number of cellular, vascular, and chemical events take place that result in the firing of these neurons. Cell damage results in mobilization of mast cells and platelets secreting histamine and serotonin. Bradykinin, thromboxane, prostaglandins, and cytokines produce increased excitability and stimulation of C fibers. Inflammation perpetuates this cycle. Sprouting at the nerve ending results in increased sensitivity to mechanical stimulation and spontaneous firing. Ectopic firing of adjacent neurons also occurs. All of these processes result in a lowered threshold to mechanical stimuli and vigorous discharges in usually silent nociceptors. In other words, under such circumstances ordinary movement and touch elicit pain.

Afferent fibers enter the dorsal horn where they ascend or descend a few levels in Lissauer's tract before participating in a complex interaction with local intrinsic spinal neurons as well as descending supraspinal fibers. Dorsal horn integration of nociceptive fibers occurs at nociceptive specific neurons in the lateral dorsal horn (Rexed Lamina I) and at wide dynamic range (WDR) neurons in the medial dorsal horn (Lamina V, X). The former field functions on an "all or none" basis, receives Aδ input, and projects through the submedius nucleus of the thalamus to the anterior cingulate. This pathway is felt to convey information regarding the affective, emotional, and motivational components of pain. Wide dynamic range neurons are not nociceptive specific. They receive input not only from Aδ and C fibers, but from Aβ fibers as well. These WDR neurons demonstrate a graded increase in the frequency of response. Fibers converge on WDR neurons from a number of adjacent levels. These neurons are therefore involved in referred pain. Projections are to multiple sensory thalamic nuclei. The two best known tracts that serve this function are the contralateral lateral and anterior spinothalamic tracts. These pathways carry information about sensory discrimination as well as localization of the stimulus. The Aβ fibers act on interneurons that secrete γ-aminobutyric acid (GABA), an inhibitory neurotransmitter. GABA acts on the WDR neuron to modulate the nociceptive C and Aδ input on the WDR neuron. Hence stimulation of Aβ fibers will increase GABA release and decrease the effects of nociceptive input on the WDR neuron. This is the principle used in transcutaneous electrical nerve stimulation (TENS) and dorsal column stimulation to suppress pain. When injury results in increased frequency of firing and lowering the threshold of C and Aδ fibers their input will override the protective effect of the Aβ fibers. C fibers secrete substance P, glutamate, and calcitonin gene-related peptide (CGRP). This depolarizes the WDR neuron and results in its firing and conveying of pain perception to the brain. With repetitive and faster stimulation of C fibers the phenomena of progressive facilitation occurs (wind up). Fibers in the adjacent noninjured area become hyperexcitable and collaterally stimulate WDR neurons. This results in low threshold touch fibers eliciting a painful response (when a wound is lightly touched it still elicits a painful response). This central facilitation persists despite general anesthesia. It may be avoided with preemptive analgesia with a local anesthetic block proximal to the injury site.

Supraspinal anatomy of pain is very complex and beyond the scope of this chapter. However, it is important to understand some of the major pathways and neurotransmitters involved in pain. Direct spinothalamic pathways terminate in the ventroposterior lateral (limbs) and medial (face), as well as the centrolateral nuclei of the thalamus. Other ascending pathways originate in various cell groups of the dorsal horn. The majority of these tracts cross at the spinal level, but some may have bilateral modulation at the reticular core. Different tracts project to the periaqueductal gray (PAG) region of the midbrain, the nucleus gigantocellularis (medulla), parabrachial and locus ceruleus (pons), hypothalamus, amygdala, cingulate, and septal nuclei (limbic regions). Cortical and limbic regions in turn project to brainstem nuclei, which in turn descend to modulate C fiber and WDR neuron activity in the cord. The PAG (a rich opiate region of dynorphin and β-endorphin) stimulates neurons in the locus ceruleus and the nucleus raphe magnus. Each of these regions sends descending inhibitory input to the nociceptive cells of the dorsal horn. These bulbospinal neurons secrete 5-hydroxytryptamine (serotonin, 5-HT), norepinephrine (NE), and enkephalin, which have an inhibitory effect on C fiber firing and tend to hyperpolarize WDR firing. This functional anatomy helps us understand how "positive" emotions and motivation emanating from cortical and limbic regions may actually result in a reduction of perceived pain. On the other hand "negative" emotions, such as those seen in depression, may result in enhanced perception of pain. It is of interest to note that central NE and 5-HT activity is diminished in depression, both critical to supraspinal inhibition of nociceptive input. Failure to treat the depression may set in play a continuous cycle of pain–depression–more pain–more depression. Recent thoughts on chronic pain suggest that it may result in N-methyl-D-aspartate (NMDA) receptor-mediated long-term potentiation (LTP) of WDR neurons with induction of immediate early genes (c-*fos* expression). This process results in increased prostaglandin synthesis and nitric oxide formation, both of which feed back and facilitate C fiber firing, creating an unchecked cycle of nociceptive fiber firing.

Pharmacotherapy of pain includes targeting the injury site (anti-inflammatories, cyclooxygenase inhibitors, local anesthetics, and sympatholytics), the spinal level (opiates, GABA drugs, cyclooxygenase inhibitors, nitric oxide synthetase inhibitors, NMDA receptor antagonists), and the brainstem and limbic levels (opiates, serotoninergic and norepinephrine agents, eg, antidepressants).

Chronic pain is a malignant process that has dire consequences. Increased autonomic nervous system activity, hypertension, myocardial stress, diminished gastrointestinal motility, diminished immune competency, and depression all lead to an increased cycle of pain. Pharmacotherapy should never be used alone in these patients. A multidisciplinary pain team approach should be instituted involving medication, physical and occupational therapy, psychiatric therapy, and on occasion anesthetic blocks and neurosurgery. The pain team should include spouses and family members in the counseling sessions so that a better understanding of the patient's condition and proper emotional support can be rendered.

Headache

One of the most common clinical syndromes in which primary pain mechanisms and cortical-limbic interaction play such an important role is migraine. Classic and complicated migraine is often accompanied by neurobehavioral sequelae. Migraine aura is often accompanied by feelings of dissociation and mood change. Focal neurological signs (eg, visual field defects, hemiparesis, aphasia) are the hallmark of complicated migraine. Some migraine syndromes may be manifested by confusion, transient amnesia, and illusionary or hallucinatory events (particularly visual), which may lead clinicians to inaccurately diagnose epilepsy or a primary psychiatric disorder. Treatment with antimigraine drugs may prove to be beneficial in ameliorating the cognitive changes as well as the headache.

EPILEPSY

Seizure disorders illustrate the most basic relationship between the brain and behavior. These disorders result in intermittent paroxysmal dysfunction of the brain, which is manifested by synchronous high-voltage electrical discharges and by a variety of motor, sensory, and behavioral phenomena. Once called "the sacred disease," because it was thought that epileptics were possessed by "spirit," epilepsy has served as a scientific model for understanding the role of the brain in human behavior.

Classification of Epilepsy

There have been many attempts to classify the epilepsies. Difficulties are encountered because a single underlying pathological process can produce various manifestations in different patients and because a variety of processes (eg, tumor, infarct, vascular malformation) can result in clinically indistinguishable seizures. There are several diseases whose sole manifestation is a seizure disorder. Each of these diseases has a somewhat different clinical and electroencephalographic manifestation. Thus, the epilepsies have two distinct aspects. First, epilepsy can be a general (nonspecific) response of the brain to a variety of metabolic and structural insults. Second, the epilepsies include a group of clinically distinct nervous system diseases.

Table 5–1 represents one clinically useful empirical classification scheme. The two major divisions are primary epilepsies, in which there is no known brain abnormality other than the clinical paroxysmal dysfunction; and secondary epilepsies, in which there is a known structural or metabolic abnormality of the brain.

Most primary epilepsies are generalized at onset—ie, there are electroencephalographic and clinical signs of widespread bilateral involvement of brain areas—with no preceding focal discharge. Impairment of consciousness and symmetric motor manifestations are seen. Primary generalized epilepsies usually appear before adolescence, are usually associated with normal intelligence, respond well to medical management, and may resolve, so that medication can be withdrawn.

Seizures that often have a focal or multifocal onset and then generalize may have an obvious underlying cause (eg, birth trauma or lipidoses) and are termed secondary generalized epilepsies (previously called symptomatic epilepsies). If the underlying disease can be treated, the seizures will stop; if not, seizure control may be difficult or impossible.

In partial epilepsies, the seizure discharge is limited to part of the brain, usually one hemisphere. If there is any alteration of consciousness during the seizure, it is referred to as a complex partial seizure. Partial seizures may spread and become generalized. They are then classified as secondary generalized epilepsy. Partial epilepsies are usually produced by structural lesions involving the limbic cortex, often originating in the temporal or frontal lobe. Partial epilepsy includes temporal lobe or psychomotor seizures.

Complex partial seizures are of importance in psychiatry because the manifestations during seizures may resemble those seen in psychiatric illness. For example, visual and auditory hallucinations (including hearing voices) are not rare. Objects in the environment may appear to shrink (micropsia), enlarge

Table 5–1. Classification of epilepsies.

Primary generalized epilepsies
Absence seizures
 Classic absence seizures of childhood, with diffuse 3-Hz spike-and-wave complexes
 Absence seizures of juvenile myoclonic epilepsy, characterized by staring and diffuse 3- to 6-Hz multi-spike-and-wave complexes during adolescence
 Juvenile absence seizures with diffuse 8- to 12-Hz rhythms
 Myoclonic absence seizures, with diffuse 3- to 6-Hz multi-spike-and-wave complexes
 Myoclonic absence seizures, characterized by staring, fragmentary myoclonus, automatisms, and diffuse 12-Hz rhythms
Myoclonic seizures
 Myoclonic seizures of early childhood, with 3- to 6-Hz multi-spike-and-wave complexes without mental retardation (Doose's syndrome)
 Juvenile myoclonic seizures of Janz or benign myoclonic seizures of adolescence and late childhood, with diffuse 4- to 6-Hz multi-spike-and-wave complexes
Clonic-tonic-clonic (grand mal) seizures
Tonic-clonic (grand mal) seizures
Partial epilepsies
Simple partial
Complex partial
 Simple partial at onset followed by impairment of consciousness automatisms
 Impairment of consciousness at onset
  Motionless stare and impaired consciousness followed by automatisms (temporal lobe epilepsy)
  Complex motor automatisms at start of impaired consciousness (frontal lobe, somatosensory, or occipital lobe epilepsy)
  Drop attack with impaired consciousness and automatisms (temporal lobe syncope)
Secondary generalized epilepsies
Simple partial evolving to tonic-clonic (secondary tonic-clonic)
Infantile spasms (propulsive petit mal, infantile myoclonic encephalopathy with hypsarrhythmia, or West's syndrome)
Myoclonic astatic or atonic epilepsies (epileptic drop attacks of Lennox-Gastaut in children with mental retardation)
Progressive myoclonic epilepsies in adolescents and adults with dementia (myoclonic epilepsies of Lafora, Lundborg, Hartung, Hunt, or Kuf)
Unclassified epilepsies

Source: Modified from the classification of the International League Against Epilepsy and the World Health Organization.

(macropsia), or move. Of particular interest are subjective changes such as a feeling of familiarity (déjà vu), of strangeness (jamais vu), or significant affectual changes such as fear, anxiety, or euphoria. Other manifestations include automatisms such as lip smacking or chewing movements; more complex behavior including incoherent speech, driving, or running (cursive), laughing (gelastic), or crying (dacrystic) may occur during the seizure, and the patient will have no memory of these acts. Strange smells, tastes, visceral sensations, or vertigo may occur and should raise the suspicion of complex partial seizures. In addition to these seizure phenomena, patients with complex partial seizures involving the temporal lobe may have an increased incidence of psychopathological manifestations between seizures. One of the most common is depression. Rarely aggressive behavior as well as schizophrenic-like psychosis have also been described. Long-standing complex partial seizures have, on occasion, been associated with distinct personality changes ("interictal personality," Geschwind's syndrome). These include humorlessness, hyperreligiosity or nascent philosophical thinking, hyposexuality, hyperviscosity (the tendency to "stick to" an individual or follow them wherever they go), hypergraphia, circumlocuotous verbosity, tangentiality, and depressed mood.

In cases of complex partial epilepsy that are refractory to anticonvulsant medication, epilepsy monitoring, including electrocorticography, leading to the identification and surgical excision of the seizure focus can lead to complete seizure control and some amelioration of the behavioral disturbance.

Mechanisms of Epilepsy

Partial epilepsies have been studied in a variety of animal species in which focal cortical lesions lead to paroxysmal discharge. In patients with partial epilepsy, the origin of the seizure can often be located between seizures by recording intermittent focal spikes on the electroencephalogram. In animals, such spikes can be produced by certain experimental focal cortical lesions. It is now clear that these surface spikes are generated by synchronous activity in cortical neurons. Intracellular recording has demonstrated that individual cortical neurons generate massive depolarizations that are synchronous with the spikes recorded at the cortical surface. These massive depolarizations are called paroxysmal depolarization shifts and are thought to represent a failure of normal synaptic inhibitory mechanisms. A variety of insults could produce this, including a reduction in the amount or efficacy of the inhibitory transmitter GABA, variable changes in ionic channel conductors (eg, Na^+, Ca^{2+}, K^+, and Mg^{2+}) and enhanced excitatory neurotransmission (eg, glutamate), as well as changes seen in the postsynaptic receptor complex (eg, NMDA receptors). Anticonvulsants are manufactured considering these principles. Many of the anticonvulsants in present use decrease Na^+ and Ca^{2+} conductance, increase K^+ and Mg^{2+} conductance, and increase central GABA activity. Current research is also focusing on developing drugs that will inhibit glutaminergic activity and/or selectively block NMDA receptors. The latter has been fraught with significant neuropsychiatric complications including psychosis.

In animals with induced focal cortical lesions, intermittent focal spikes may increase in frequency until they produce a prolonged depolarization with continuous repetitive firing of cortical neurons. Under these circumstances, the seizure activity may spread to adjacent cortex or across the corpus callosum to become generalized.

Whether results in animal models are relevant to human partial epilepsy is uncertain; however, paroxysmal depolarization shifts have been recorded in human cortical tissue taken from a seizure focus.

SLEEP & SLEEP DISORDERS

Sleep has many of the attributes of a drive. Sleep deprivation leads to an increased "urge" to sleep and to extended periods of sleep immediately following the deprivation. After several days of sleep deprivation, a confusional state may occur with disordered attention, emotional lability, reduced memory, delusions, and even hallucinations. The physiological purpose of sleep is actively being investigated.

Physiology of Sleep

Most animals experience a daily cycle of changes in levels of alertness and arousal as well as sleep and waking. Sleep was originally thought to be a passive process (ie, essentially a functional deafferentation) based on observations of animals falling into continual sleep or coma if the forebrain is deafferented by transection of the brainstem at the mesencephalic level. It has been observed, however, that lesions of the pons just in front of the trigeminal nerve cause animals to be hyperalert and sleep much less than normal. This indicates that normal sleep is an active process that requires activity of neurons in the brainstem. In fact, neurophysiological studies have demonstrated that nerve cells in the pontine reticular formation begin to discharge minutes prior to the onset of certain stages of sleep.

The sleep cycle consists of several distinct stages defined by the appearance of certain wave patterns on the electroencephalogram. The time required to pass through the complete sequence of sleep stages is about 90 minutes, and the cycle is repeated three to five times each night. There are two distinct states of sleep: slow-wave sleep and rapid eye movement (REM) sleep.

Slow-wave sleep—also called non-rapid eye movement (NREM) sleep—is divided into four stages (Figure 5–5): stage 1 is characterized by an electroencephalogram (EEG) in which the alpha rhythm has disappeared and the electroencephalographic background consists of low-voltage fast activity. In stages 2–4, the electroencephalogram becomes more synchronized (lower frequency, higher amplitude) and the subject becomes more difficult to arouse. Stage 2 sleep is primarily characterized by the onset of "sleep spindles" and "K complexes" seen on EEG. The longest and deepest period of slow-wave sleep each night is the first period of stage 3 and 4 sleep, usually within 2 hours after falling asleep. During this period, subjects are aroused with great difficulty and frequently demonstrate a transient confusional state. Stage 4 sleep, the deepest stage of slow-wave sleep, resembles hibernation in that blood pressure, pulse, respiratory

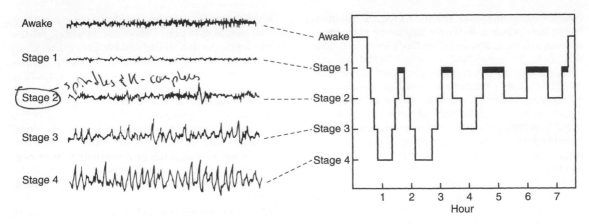

Figure 5–5. Left: Electroencephalographic recordings during different stages of wakefulness and sleep. Each line represents 30 seconds. The top recording of low-voltage fast activity is that of an awake brain. The next four tracings represent successively deeper stages of non-rapid eye movement (REM) (slow-wave) sleep, characterized by lower-frequency, higher-amplitude waves. **Right:** A typical night's pattern of sleep (hours 1–7) staging in a young adult. The time spent in REM sleep is represented by a dark bar. The first REM period is usually short (5–10 minutes), but periods tend to lengthen in successive cycles. Conversely, stages 3 and 4 dominate the NREM periods in the first third of the night, but they are often completely absent later. (Reproduced, with permission, from Kelly DD: Physiology of sleep and dreaming. Chapter 40 in: *Principles of Neural Science.* Kandel ER, Schwartz JH [editors]. Elsevier, 1981. Copyright 1981 by Elsevier Science Publishing Co., Inc.)

rate, and body temperature all drop and the consumption of oxygen by the brain is very low. It is not known where in the brain slow-wave sleep is initiated, but its electrical manifestations can still be observed in cortex that is disconnected from the brainstem.

After the initial slow-wave sleep stages, the electroencephalographic pattern usually shifts abruptly to the desynchronized (higher frequency, lower amplitude) pattern seen in stage 1 sleep. Despite some similarity with the "waking" electroencephalographic pattern, it is difficult to waken subjects in this stage of sleep. This is sometimes referred to as "paradoxic sleep." Because one of the most striking features of this stage is intermittent rapid eye movements, this stage is termed REM sleep. This represents 20–25% of sleep per night with the majority of REM sleep occurring during the later hours of sleep. During REM sleep, there is also a striking loss of limb muscle tone, which resembles paralysis. In normal subjects, REM sleep occurs only after a preceding period of deeper (stages 2–4) sleep. Studies indicate that dreaming occurs mainly during REM sleep. More than 80% of subjects aroused during REM sleep report vivid and colorful visual imagery. Subjects aroused 10 minutes after the REM period has terminated seldom report complete dream imagery. Since subjects usually have several REM episodes each night, they probably have several dreams, although they rarely remember more than one. If REM sleep is selectively blocked by wakening the subject at the beginning of REM sleep, a specific "REM debt" builds up, and the subject does not feel adequately rested. REM sleep is apparently

triggered by neurons in the dorsolateral midbrain and pontine reticular formation.

Sleep Disorders

Several of the drive disorders described previously are characterized by abnormalities of sleep. Excessive daytime sleepiness as well as insomnia may be secondary to medical illness, primary psychiatric diagnosis, or, in the normal population, based on age, daily schedules, stress, caffeine intake, and use of over-the-counter medication.

A. Insomnia: Insomnia is usually considered to be sleep deprivation or a marked change in the perceived sleep pattern. Factors contributing to insomnia include (1) situational problems such as transient stress, job pressures, and marital discord; (2) aging; (3) medical disorders that inevitably include pain and physical discomfort; (4) drug-related episodes, including withdrawal from alcohol or sedatives; and (5) psychological conditions, particularly the major mental illnesses such as schizophrenia and affective disorders.

Schizophrenic patients vary markedly in the degree of sleep disturbance they endure. In acute episodes, the disruption is severe, even to the point of total insomnia. The chronic schizophrenic or the patient in remission often has no complaints, and an electroencephalographic pattern is not remarkably abnormal.

Sleep disturbance is one of the most common symptoms of affective disorders. Some patients with bipolar disorder sleep more when they are depressed and less when they are manic, but there is much variation. Primary depressions usually show sleep continuity disturbances, shortened REM stage latency, more REM sleep at the beginning of the night than in early morning hours, and a marked reduction in sleep stages 3 and 4. In the manic phase, REM sleep is decreased, but there are varying reports on slow-wave sleep. In both unipolar and bipolar disorders, patients in the depressed phase usually have a decreased total sleep time. There is no correlation of particular types of depression with specific types of sleep problems. The treatment of insomnia should be directed at the underlying cause. When pharmacotherapy is warranted the use of short- to intermediate-acting benzodiazepines can be effective. Although short-acting benzodiazepines (eg, triazolam) will avoid "hangover" or daytime hypersomnolence seen with longer acting benzodiazepines (eg, flurazepam), they may cause rebound insomnia and are more prone to developing tolerance. Zolpidem, a nonbenzodiazepine, actually acts very selectively on the benzodiazepine 1 subreceptor exclusively. It effectively treats insomnia without affecting muscle relaxation. Melatonin, a neuromodulator secreted from the pineal gland, may also effectively treat insomnia, particularly in the elderly, and that associated with jet lag. Insomnia associated with psychosis or depression may best be treated with sedating neuroleptics and antidepressants, respectively. There is a rare but particularly lethal form of insomnia known as fatal familial insomnia. Onset is in middle age with the course usually lasting between 7 and 36 months. The disease results in the total incapacity to sleep as well as to generate EEG sleep patterns. It is associated with dementia and significant neurobehavioral changes. There is profound loss of neurons in thalamic nuclei, particularly the dorsal medial and anteroventral nuclei. It is felt to be a prion disease. The course is progressive, resulting in death within a few years.

B. Hypersomnia:

1. Narcolepsy—The sleep disturbance usually occurs before the age of 40 and includes excessive daytime hypersomnolence manifested by frequent daily attacks of sleep, lasting on average from 5 to 30 minutes each. In addition, it may include cataplexy, sleep paralysis, and hypnagogic or hypnopompic hallucinations. All individuals with narcolepsy will have the sleep attacks; close to 70% manifest cataplexy; approximately 33% will have hallucinations; and 25% will have sleep paralysis. The syndrome of narcolepsy is often associated with the HLA type grouping, DR2 or DQw1. Multiple sleep latency tests may demonstrate shortened latencies to REM onset. In some patients, sleep may begin with REM onset. Cataplexy is a sudden loss of muscle tone, with effects ranging from weakness of specific small muscle groups to general muscle weakness that causes the person to slump to the floor, unable to move. Cataplexy is often initiated by an emotional outburst (laughing, crying, anger) and lasts from several seconds to 30 minutes. Sleep paralysis involves acquisition of flaccid muscle

tone with full consciousness, either during awakening or while falling asleep. There may be associated fear with sleep paralysis. The attack is terminated by touching or calling the patient. Hypnagogic hallucinations, either visual or auditory, usually occur during the transition from wakefulness into REM onset sleep; hypnopompic hallucinations occur during awakening, and represent a transition from REM sleep to awakening. Treatment of the sleep attacks includes the use of central nervous system stimulants, such as *d*-amphetamine or methylphenidate. Effective treatment of cataplexy has been demonstrated with selective use of tertiary tricyclic antidepressants such as imipramine or clomipramine.

2. Kleine-Levin syndrome—This is a rare but clinically significant syndrome manifested by hypersomnic attacks that may last up to 20 hours and occur infrequently (3–4 times per year). There is confusion upon awakening. It is often associated with bulimia during these periods. Although its pathophysiology is not well established, tremors and other lesions of the ventromedial hypothalamus share some of the clinical features of this syndrome.

3. Sleep apnea—Apneic episodes occur in both REM and NREM sleep and often are accompanied by stertorous snoring. Hypersomnolence the next day also is common. Intellectual and personality changes include decreased attention span, decreased memory, and hyperirritability. There are two main types of sleep apnea: central apnea, in which there is a cessation of respiratory movement with loss of airflow; and obstructive apnea, in which there is persistent respiratory effort but upper airway blockage. Medical complications of sleep apnea include hypoxia, hypercapnia, hypertension, cardiac arrhythmia, cor pulmonale, right heart failure, and sudden death. Obstructive sleep apnea is often associated with obesity, upper airway infections, hypothyroidism, sedative hypnotics, and alcohol use. Workup includes all night polysomnography with oximetry. Treatment includes discontinuation of drugs that may be contributing to the disorder, weight loss, and continuous positive airway pressure (CPAP). Rarely uvulopalatopharyngoplasty or tracheostomy is warranted.

4. Other causes of hypersomnolence— These include sedating medications, alcohol, illicit drugs, encephalitic diseases, metabolic/endocrine disease, infectious mononucleosis, head trauma, neurodegenerative disease, and idiopathic hypersomnolence.

C. Parasomnias: Included are movements or autonomic activity at the onset or during any stage of sleep. Movements at the onset of sleep include hypnic jerks (sleep starts), which can be found in normal individuals. Deeper stages of NREM sleep may be associated with myoclonus, bruxism, head banging, restless leg syndrome, periodic movements of sleep, and paroxysmal sleep dystonia. Somnambulism, enuresis, and pavor nocturnus (night terrors) usually occur in children, predominantly during stages 3 and 4 of sleep. There may be associated autonomic changes with these movements. An interesting REM-associated parasomnia is the REM sleep behavioral disorder. Paradoxically, rather than having muscle atonia, these patients have increased muscle tone and literally move or thrash about, acting out their dreams. In some cases, the behavior may be aggressive and bed partners or patients themselves have been injured. Clonazepam can be an effective treatment for this disorder.

SYNDROMES OF DENIAL, NEGLECT, & INATTENTION

The parietal lobe receives and integrates tactile, visual, and auditory associative information. As it has grown through evolution, the brain has (1) pushed the motor area anteriorly, (2) pushed the visual cortex backward and downward, and (3) led to the development of an operculum (flap) composed of temporal, parietal, and frontal cortex.

The right parietal lobe region and the prefrontal region used to be referred to as "silent areas," since lesions in these regions may not produce gross disturbances of motor or sensory function. These regions have since been demonstrated to play an important role in higher cognitive functions.

ASSESSMENT OF PARIETAL LOBE DISORDERS

Several factors complicate assessment of parietal lobe disorders. Patients with lesions of the left parietal lobe frequently have receptive aphasia and, therefore, may be unable to understand the examiner's statements and questions. Patients with lesions of the right parietal lobe have problems sustaining and directing attention and may be only marginally cooperative. Since patients with parietal lobe disorders may be either unaware of their deficits or unable to communicate with the examiner, the history obtained from friends and family becomes invaluable.

During the mental status examination, extreme care must be taken to avoid overlooking any of the following: (1) language problems (see Language Disorders, below); (2) problems with the distribution of attention; (3) visual, spatial, or constructional deficits (see Apraxia & the Callosal Syndromes, below); (4) body image distortions; (5) tactile problems; (6) motility disturbances; and (7) other neuropsychiatric disturbances.

Denial of, Neglect of, & Inattention to Illness

In 1914, Babinski coined the term anosognosia to denote neglect of left hemiplegia following right cerebral infarction. He observed that his patients either were unaware of or seemed to ignore their deficits. His first patient was a woman who, despite an otherwise excellent recovery, never once over a period of years complained of or even alluded to her hemiplegia. When asked to move her arm, she behaved as if the examiner were talking to someone else. A second patient not only failed to move her paralyzed arm when asked to do so but would sometimes say, "There, it's done" without having moved at all. Babinski noted that each of these patients had left-sided weakness with sensory deficits in the affected limb. He speculated that anosognosia might be peculiar to patients with lesions of the right hemisphere. It is important to note that "denial of illness" is a somewhat clumsy translation of Babinski's original term, since it implies that patients have some level of awareness of their deficit but either repress or suppress this knowledge. Because most cases of anosognosia occur in association with right parietal lobe disorders and because neglect or inattention can also be produced in animals by surgically manipulating the parietal lobes, it seems unlikely that psychodynamic factors play a primary causative role in most neglect syndromes.

Right hemispheric lesions in at least five different areas can each produce striking neglect syndromes both in animals and in humans. These areas include the inferior parietal lobule, the prefrontal convexity, the cingulate gyrus, the thalamus, and the hypothalamus. It has been postulated that each of these areas is part of an anatomic loop connecting cortical, limbic, and reticular structures. Lesions at any level of this loop might thus produce attentional deficits. It is of particular interest that structures in the left parietal lobe play a role in the distribution of attention to objects and events in the right hemispace, whereas homologous structures in the right parietal lobe appear to play a role in the distribution of attention not only to the contralateral but also to the ipsilateral hemispace. Neglect may be the result not only of diminished "attention," but of diminished "intention" as well. Right frontal and anterior cingulate lesions result in a diminished motivational drive to act. Hence, what is often interpreted as an "attention" problem is actually not an interference with sensory input, but rather interference with the drive or desire to act in response to the sensory stimulus. This is more accurately described as a deficit of motor intention.

Body Image Distortions

Patients with lesions of the parietal lobe may deny the existence of a paralyzed limb or may admit its existence but repudiate ownership, claiming that it belongs to someone else. One male patient with left hemiplegia constantly lay on his right side, protesting that he had a paralyzed brother beside him. He explained that because this situation was offensive to him, he preferred to turn his back on his brother. On one occasion, without being aware that he was being observed, the patient was overheard addressing his "brother": "How are you?" "Do you want a cigarette?" In another case, a physician observed a male patient searching under the bed for his left arm, which he felt was missing. A patient whose limb is paralyzed secondary to parietal lobe disorder may adopt a facetious or condescending attitude toward the compromised limb, referring to it as a "piece of meat" or "dumb slob" or giving the offending body part a pet name. Critchley (1979) used the term "misoplegia" to describe a violent dislike for the paralyzed limb.

Tactile Sensory Disturbances

Patients with parietal lobe disorders may have tactile sensory disturbances despite the absence of gross sensory deficits. Their response to a tactile stimulus may be delayed, or they may have a distorted perception of the stimulus. Patients may experience tactile (haptic) hallucinations, such as the hallucination of a three-dimensional object in the hand or of a "phantom limb." Persistence of tactile experience or displacement of sensory experiences from one side of the body to the analogous contralateral side (allochiria) or from one body area to another (allesthesia) may also occur. More commonly, however, careful examination discloses striking deficits in the synthesis, interpretation, and differentiation of primitive sensory experiences. Astereognosis (tactile agnosia) refers to the inability to recognize a three-dimensional object by palpation. Disorders of tactile discrimination are not limited to the appreciation of shape and may occur with reference to texture (hylognosis), size (macro- or microstereognosis), or weight (barognosis) and writing (graphesthesia). Finally, impaired ability to recognize the posture of an extremity (statagnosia) tends to be associated with bizarre subjective experiences and may play a major role in determining a patient's mental attitude toward the disability.

Motility Disturbances

Patients with parietal lobe disorders manifest greater unilateral incapacity than would be expected on the basis of their motor weakness. Unilateral diminution in spontaneous movements and wasting of the hand muscles and shoulder girdle muscles suggest the importance of intact sensory pathways to motor activity and to the maintenance of muscle mass.

LANGUAGE DISORDERS

Aphasia usually suggests pathological changes in the left hemisphere. Aphasic patients with posterior lesions may present with acutely disorganized and incoherent speech that is sometimes mistaken for schizophrenic "word salad," whereas patients with anterior lesions are often noted to be severely depressed, frustrated, or irritable. Aphasia-like disorders may be induced by medications; lithium toxicity, for instance, may produce dysnomia (word-finding difficulty). Management of patients with organic brain disease, and particularly those with language disorders, requires an appreciation of both the functional deficits and preserved skills of the patient. Without assessing a patient's ability to comprehend, name, repeat, read, or write, the clinician's ability to help either the patient or the patient's family is severely limited.

Language Versus Speech Disorders

Although combinations of speech and language disorders may be seen, it is important to distinguish these two types of disorders. Dysarthrias (disorders of speech) are due to pathological changes in the neuromuscular apparatus responsible for the mechanical production of speech. Dysarthria may be seen either with lower brainstem lesions affecting the cranial nerves subserving motor speech outflow or with disruption of corticobulbar fibers traveling from the cortex to the brainstem. In speech disorders, articulation is characterized as spastic, flaccid, ataxic, or hypo- or hyperkinetic. In contrast, aphasias (disorders of language) are due to disruption of the neural machinery responsible for the reception, processing, and production of language-dependent ideas. Aphasic patients may demonstrate abnormalities not only in spoken but also in written communication and reading comprehension.

Language Circuitry of the Left Hemisphere

Since the 1860s—based on the work of Pierre Paul Broca, a French surgeon and anthropologist—it has been known that the vast majority of language disorders occur following damage to the left hemisphere. Ninety-seven percent of right-handed people have left hemispheric dominance for propositional language (the ability to use semantics and syntax to convey an idea or proposition). Ten percent of the population are left-handed, and over two-thirds of left-handed individuals have left hemispheric dominance for language skills.

The language circuitry of the left hemisphere (Figure 5–6) involves regions of the temporal, parietal, and frontal cortex surrounding the lateral cerebral (sylvian) fissure. Damage to the perisylvian region produces major aphasic syndromes whose features depend on the size, extent, and location of the lesion. Auditory fibers travel from the medial geniculate body of the thalamus to Heschl's gyrus in the superior temporal plane. Surrounding Heschl's gyrus is the auditory association cortex known as Wernicke's area. Fibers from Wernicke's area project forward to Broca's area in the inferior frontal lobe via the arcuate fasciculus and probably other white matter pathways such as the extreme capsule. Broca's area can be thought of as a motor association cortex. As an ex-

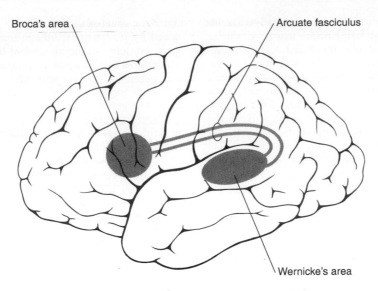

Figure 5–6. Perisylvian language circuitry.

tension of premotor cortex, it serves as an encoder that generates articulatory programs for the region of the motor cortex subserving the mouth, tongue, and larynx.

Since the entire perisylvian area is supplied by the middle cerebral artery, varieties of aphasia reflect which branch or branches of this artery are occluded.

Aphasias Due to Lesions in the Perisylvian Area (Table 5–2)

The three major aphasias discussed below all result from pathological changes in the perisylvian area of the left hemisphere, and all three are characterized by an inability to repeat spoken language. Patients with Wernicke's aphasia cannot repeat because they are unable to decode auditory messages. Those with Broca's aphasia fail to repeat because they cannot encode messages for motor output that have been understood. Patients with conduction aphasia cannot repeat because they are unable to transfer information from an intact auditory decoding apparatus (Wernicke's) to an intact language encoding apparatus (Broca's). If the entire perisylvian area is destroyed, patients lose both spontaneous speech and auditory comprehension. These unfortunate individuals have global aphasia. This is most often the result of internal carotid or proximal middle cerebral artery occlusion.

A. Broca's Aphasia: Broca's aphasia ("motor" aphasia) is characterized by poor articulation and severe impairment of verbal fluency (the ability to produce spontaneous, effortless speech) and is often accompanied by paralysis of the right face and arm. Comprehension is relatively unimpaired, and follow-ing recovery, patients often report that they knew precisely what they wanted to say but were unable to say it.

Because the speech of these patients consists mainly of nouns and hackneyed phrases or cliches, with omission of connecting words such as conjunctions and prepositions, it is often described as "telegraphic" and "agrammatical." Despite severe impairment in fluency, patients are sometimes capable of serial speech such as counting or reciting. Cursing and singing may also be preserved. Patients with Broca's aphasia tend to be angry, depressed, and frustrated. Surprisingly, however, suicide attempts in this population are extremely rare.

B. Wernicke's Aphasia: Wernicke's aphasia often occurs in the absence of motor impairment. Speech is fluent and effortless but devoid of meaning (often referred to as empty speech), and comprehension is grossly impaired. Lesions producing this "fluent" aphasia are located in or near Wernicke's area. Since the auditory association cortex functions as an auditory decoder or phonetic analyzer for spoken language, destruction of this area leads to inability to extract meaning from spoken language.

The affective behavior of patients with Wernicke's aphasia ranges from euphoric indifference to paranoid agitation. Management is complicated by patients' lack of insight into their illness. Rehabilitation therapy can be frustrating, if not futile, until they become aware of their deficits. Individuals with Wernicke's aphasia are at risk for suicide at two points in the course of their illness: (1) following sudden onset of a comprehension deficit, when their lack of insight and misinterpretation of others' actions may lead to

Table 5–2. Classification of aphasic syndromes.

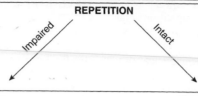

REPETITION

Impaired / Intact

Perisylvian Syndromes			Nonperisylvian Syndromes
	Fluency	Comprehension	
1. Broca's asphasia	–	+	1. Anomic aphasias
2. Wernicke's aphasia	+	–	2. Transcortical aphasias
3. Conduction aphasia	+	+	Motor
4. Global aphasia	–	–	Sensory
			Mixed ("isolation of the speech area")
			3. Subcortical aphasias
			Basal ganglia/internal capsule
			Thalamus
			Marie's quadrilateral space

chaotic paranoid behavior; and (2) as they begin to become aware of their impairment.

C. Conduction Aphasia: In conduction aphasia, spontaneous speech and comprehension are both preserved, but the patient has almost no ability to repeat spoken language. This condition results from lesions that spare both Broca's area and Wernicke's area, but disrupt the fibers that connect these two regions.

D. Aphemia: Aphemia is sometimes inappropriately referred to as verbal apraxia. It is a nonfluent or mute state resulting from disconnection between an intact Broca's area and the primary motor cortex controlling laryngeal muscles. Like Broca's aphasia, it is often associated with some degree of contralateral hemiparesis. Unlike Broca's aphasia, aphemic patients have a normal ability to communicate in writing.

Resolution usually is partial, leaving the patient with dysarthric speech, and infrequently the characteristic feature of sounding as though they are speaking with a foreign accent.

E. Pure Word Deafness: Lesions of the left middle superior temporal lobe or bilateral lesions that disconnect auditory association cortex for language, but not for nonverbal input, cause this syndrome. These patients are often felt to be partially deaf, yet when they respond to nonverbal auditory stimuli (eg, telephone or doorbell), even when volume is not increased, many are inappropriately labeled as malingerers or hysterics. These patients can speak well spontaneously and can write without deficit. Like Wernicke's patients, they may be paranoid. Resolution is usually incomplete.

Aphasias Due to Lesions Affecting Nonperisylvian Language Areas

The following language disorders result from lesions in nonperisylvian areas of the left hemisphere.

Patients with these disorders are able to repeat spoken language.

A. Anomic Aphasias: Anomic aphasias are characterized by severe impairment of word-finding ability. (As a general rule, all aphasias are accompanied by some difficulty with word finding.) Patients with anterior lesions appear to have problems with word production, whereas patients with posterior lesions have difficulty either with selection of the correct word or with access to their "central word lexicon." The most severe anomic aphasia is associated with lesions in the region of the dominant inferior parietal lobule. Damage to either the angular or supramarginal gyrus can produce anomia of such severity that patients not only fail to benefit from phonemic or semantic cues but may also be unable to recognize the name of a common item when presented with a list containing the word.

Word-finding difficulty may occur in the absence of a structural lesion, eg, with physical exhaustion, dehydration, fever, or metabolic encephalopathy. Thus, care should be taken to differentiate true anomic aphasia from transient language disorders that merely reflect physiological disequilibrium.

B. Transcortical Aphasias: These aphasias are characterized by impairment of either fluency (transcortical motor aphasia) or comprehension (transcortical sensory aphasia), depending on whether the lesion is anterior or posterior. The aphasias are termed transcortical because they typically result from infarctions at the border zone between the middle cerebral artery and either the anterior or the posterior cerebral artery.

Common causes include hypotension, blood loss, or failure to adequately perfuse through a more proximally stenotic artery. Transcortical motor aphasia usually involves a region of the prefrontal lobe, high on the convexity near the supplementary motor area. Because this area is preparatory for movement, transcortical motor aphasia is often felt to be a deficit in initiating the drive or motivation to speak. When words are provided for these patients, repetition is far better than spontaneous speech. Transcortical sensory aphasia disconnects receptive areas of phonemic appreciation from association areas of language comprehension. This association cortex is located in the posterior temporal and inferior parietal areas. Hence a patient can repeat, but has no understanding of what they are repeating. This is not dissimilar from a healthy individual repeating a phrase in a foreign language and phonemically doing a respectable job, but semantically having no idea what is actually said. When both transcortical areas are affected, this is called a mixed transcortical aphasia. These patients neither understand nor speak spontaneously, but can repeat what is heard (echolalia or "parroting").

C. Subcortical Aphasias: The third group of language disorders in which repetition is relatively preserved is referred to as the subcortical aphasias. Three types have been described. The anterior type results from vascular disorders (particularly hemorrhage) in the basal ganglia or anterior limb of the internal capsule. The posterior type results from vascular disorders in the thalamus. Both of these are characterized by an initial period of mutism. Paraphasic errors are common in subcortical aphasias. The third type of subcortical aphasia arises from pathological changes in the area known as Marie's quadrilateral space, and in this type, initial mutism persists as global aphasia. Several theories suggest that these subcortical regions may serve a primary language function, whereas other theories suggest that lesions in subcortical areas produce diaschisis of cortical language areas, which eventually result in functional language impairment.

Disturbances of Prosody

The "expressive" ability to modulate pitch, melody, and rhythm to impart emotional coloring (prosody) to one's own speech and the receptive ability to detect prosody in the speech of others are important "non-propositional" aspects of language. Patients with Broca's aphasia, Parkinson's disease, and moderately advanced dementia have difficulty with the inflection, rhythm, and melody of their speech. Recent evidence suggests that patients with damage to the right frontal region homologous to Broca's area may lose the ability to impart prosody to their speech, whereas patients with posterior right hemispheric lesions in areas homologous to Wernicke's area may lose the ability to decode or perceive affective coloring in the speech of others. The possibility of dissociations between felt inner emotion and affective expression is clearly of significance to psychiatrists, since it confounds the diagnosis of depression in patients with organic brain disease and may also represent an underrecognized complication of neuroleptic drug administration.

APRAXIA & THE CALLOSAL SYNDROMES

The term "apraxia" has been used in a confusingly large number of ways. In fact, many clinicians still use the term to denote disorders of movement they are unable or unwilling to characterize in some other way. The clinician who accepts another's diagnosis of apraxia without personally examining the patient adopts the ambiguity and uncertainty of the previous examiner. Thus, clinicians are advised to ask the previous examiner to specify what has been observed and then to examine the patient personally.

Constructional Apraxia

The term "constructional apraxia" is a somewhat awkward means of denoting difficulty with "constructions," eg, copying a simple drawing or reproducing a pattern. Constructional ability may be assessed in several ways (see Chapters 11 and 12). Since the earliest reports of constructional difficulty appeared, debate has continued about whether the deficit reflects (1) a perceptual problem with the spatial aspects of visual and tactile experience or (2) a motor disorder of programming complex movements in space. It now seems that the right and left hemispheres make separate and distinct contributions to performing complex constructional tasks. The right hemisphere appears to play a largely perceptual role, whereas the left hemisphere is instrumental at the executive or planning level of motor constructions. Thus, differences in constructional deficits are based on whether lesions are right or left sided.

Patients with right-sided lesions draw energetically and often add extra strokes. Their productions tend to be scattered and fragmented; boundaries are not observed, and virtually all aspects of spatial relations appear to be lost. These patients may also have difficulty dressing themselves and show hemispatial neglect (for the left side of space).

Patients with left-sided lesions draw slowly and seem to benefit from having a model to copy (this does not help patients with right-sided lesions). Their drawings tend to be somewhat more coherent but are simplified and lack inner detail. The coexistence of language disturbances and elements of Gerstmann's syndrome—acalculia, agraphia, right-left confusion, and finger agnosia—may be seen. Gerstmann's syndrome is usually localized to the dominant inferior parietal lobe. When Gerstmann's syndrome is associated with anomia, localization to the angular gyrus is most common (angular gyrus syndrome).

Apraxia for Dressing

Difficulty in orienting articles of clothing with reference to the body can be seen in patients with dementia or right parietal lobe disorders, but is probably most common in confusional states. "Dressing apraxia," when used to describe a patient with a right parietal lesion, is frequently a misnomer. In this case, the patient has no problem with praxis for dressing the unaffected side of the body (usually the right side), but does not dress the left side of their body because of neglect, not because of apraxia.

Apraxia of Gait

Patients with expanding frontal lobe lesions or lesions in the region of the supplemental motor area and patients with normal-pressure hydrocephalus may have great difficulty in initiating gait. Because they look as if their feet are glued to the floor, they are sometimes said to have a "magnetic gait." Patients with apraxia of gait are unable to use their limbs properly despite unimpaired strength and intact sensation. Their deficits are not limited to walking and appear to reflect a diffuse problem with the initiation of movements in the lower extremities. These patients may, for example, be unable to perform on command acts such as kicking an imaginary ball or drawing a circle with their feet while lying supine.

Apraxia of Speech

Apraxia of speech is a communication disorder intermediate between true aphasia and dysarthria. It is characterized by prolongation and segregation of syllables. Apraxia of speech, along with dysarthria, is often a component of Broca's aphasia. Apraxic "groping for articulatory postures" lends a plaintive quality to patients with Broca's aphasia. For the speech pathologist, however, it suggests that a particular therapeutic strategy (melodic intonation therapy) may be helpful.

Ideational Apraxia

Ideational apraxia denotes disturbance in the planning of a complex gesture or act even though each of its component parts can be executed singly without difficulty. The problem involves sequencing and integration of motor behavior over time. Heilman (1973) suggested that ideational apraxia was often inappropriately used to describe an actual dissociation apraxia. These patients, when asked to pantomime a movement, would simply look at their hands or move their limbs randomly. Their ability to imitate the examiner or use actual objects, however, was accurate. This can be explained by left hemisphere or callosal lesions that interrupt verbally driven commands (comprehended by the left hemisphere), from the right hemisphere, which moves the left limbs. Because this pathway is not necessary to imitate the examiner or use objects appropriately, these later capabilities remain intact.

Ideomotor Apraxia

Ideomotor apraxia denotes a disconnection syndrome wherein certain skilled movements cannot be performed in response to commands, although they can be performed spontaneously. Ideomotor apraxia should be diagnosed only if the following criteria are met: (1) Motor systems are intact, ie, no paralysis, paresis, slowing of movements, incoordination, or other movement disorder; (2) there is no sensory loss in the limbs; and (3) the disorder is not the result of inattention, lack of cooperation, poor comprehension, or intellectual deterioration.

The patient with ideomotor apraxia classically makes the most profound error when asked to pantomime an overlearned act. The performance will then typically improve after imitating the examiner or with the use of actual objects. Heilman (1992) classifies praxis errors as those of either content or production.

Ideomotor apraxic patients usually make production but not content errors. A content error would include substituting a completely different pantomime for the target pantomime. An example of a content error would be a patient who was asked to mimic opening a door and instead mimics hammering a nail. Patient's with ideomotor apraxia are much more inclined to have production errors, however, which may be either spatial or temporal. Although the pantomime that they are asked to carry out will often have at least some degree of resemblance to the target pantomime, they will have difficulties with orienting pantomime objects in the proper plane, or they may actually use body parts to represent parts of tools that they are to pantomime. An example would be using the index and middle finger as the two blades of a scissors. Patients with ideomotor apraxia will also have timing errors for start and stop movements through what should normally be a smooth-moving pantomime. The pathophysiology of ideomotor apraxia is usually the result of left hemispheric lesions in right-handed individuals, and may be due to right hemispheric lesions in left-handed individuals.

Major sites that may induce ideomotor apraxia are the corpus callosum, the inferior parietal lobe, and the supplementary motor area. Watson and Heilman (1985) proposed that representations and formulas for movement were a left parietal function in right-handed individuals. Lesions of the dominant parietal lobe produced not only a production deficit, known as ideomotor apraxia, but also a gesture comprehension or discrimination deficit. When a command is given, the inferior parietal lobe deciphers the conceptual memory for how the act is to be performed. This information is then sent forward to the region of the supplementary motor area, which is known to be involved in skilled movements and motor programming.

Neurons of the supplementary motor area are known to discharge before neurons in the motor cortex that actually result in the execution of a motor act. Because this area in right-handed individuals also controls motor preparation for movement in the right hemisphere, in response to a command, lesions of the left supplementary motor area may result in an ideomotor apraxia of the left limb. Because the anterior body of the corpus callosum is the anatomical structure used to communicate between the supplementary motor area in the left hemisphere and its connection with the right hemisphere motor areas, lesions of the body of the corpus callosum will often result in an apraxia of the left limb. These patients will often have more difficulty in imitating or using actual objects.

Since left middle cerebral artery infarctions are not rare, ideomotor apraxia might be expected to be common. In fact, it is infrequently reported. There appear to be several reasons for this: (1) Apraxia may be a transient phenomenon that disappears as edema diminishes or as alternative pathways are recruited. (2) Patients themselves are usually unaware of ideomotor apraxia, since they can perform volitional acts spontaneously. (3) Patients with apraxia are sometimes considered to be simply confused or to have comprehension problems. (4) Those testing for apraxia may fail to utilize strict criteria.

It is important to remember that one of the criteria for apraxia is intact comprehension. Comprehension can be tested in aphasic patients (1) by asking them questions of graded difficulty that require head nodding, head shaking, or yes-or-no responses and (2) by asking them to perform movements involving use of the axial muscles (movements that can be executed with extrapyramidal motor systems whose origins appear to arise from diffuse areas of the cortex) or eye movements. Intact comprehension is demonstrated if the patient can perform these tasks.

Conceptual Apraxia

Heilman (1992) utilizes the term conceptual apraxia to describe defects in the knowledge needed to make use of tools and objects. These patients will often commit errors of content as well as tool selection. They may actually lose the capacity to recall the type of action associated with specific tools or objects. It is important not to confuse this with a visual object agnosia or an object anomia. The lesion producing conceptual apraxia is felt to be located in the caudal parietal lobe or the temporoparietal junction.

Callosal Syndromes

The corpus callosum, composed of 200 million fibers, is the largest of several nerve fiber bundles connecting the hemispheres. Three other telencephalic interhemispheric pathways are the anterior commissure, hippocampal commissure, and massa intermedia. In addition, there are two midbrain commissures: the posterior and habenular commissures.

When surgical section of the corpus callosum was first performed in patients with intractable convulsions, behavior did not appear to be affected by the procedure. Large-scale studies in the 1940s led researchers to comment jokingly that the corpus callosum served only to transmit seizures from one hemisphere to the other or to keep the hemispheres from collapsing onto themselves. After Sperry's pioneer-

ing work on animals whose interhemispheric pathways had been surgically sectioned, Geschwind and Kaplan (1962) were able to document symptoms of callosal syndrome in a patient whose corpus callosum had been severed to control seizures. Since that time, a uniform clinical picture has been described in patients whose corpus callosum has been surgically transected or damaged by disease. These patients behave as if their two hemispheres were functioning autonomously. For example, the patient may open a drawer with one hand and immediately close it with the other or may button a shirt with the left hand and then unbutton it with the right hand (the "alien hand syndrome"). From observations that patients who wrote in a normal fashion with the right hand were unable to write with the left and were unable to name (although they could demonstrate recognition of) pictures of items that had been seen exclusively by the right hemisphere, researchers have gained insight into hemispheric specialization. Particularly important was the recognition that even though the right hemisphere was essentially mute, it was still able to process things in complicated ways. Geschwind's research on disconnection syndromes in animals and humans, published in 1965, has become a cornerstone of behavioral neurology. Even though the apraxias were not the first disorders of higher cortical dysfunction to be conceptualized as disconnection syndromes, they have served as a prototype for the study of mind-brain relations.

MEMORY DISORDERS

Memory is a very complicated process. Long-term remote memories are highly processed pieces of information that represent long standing knowledge of our personal worlds (eg, autobiographical knowledge, knowledge of family, and childhood memories). Short-term memory represents the new learning that goes on in our day-to-day lives. This is often referred to as declarative or explicit memory (ie, information that we consciously access). Declarative memory is further divided into episodic and semantic memory. Episodic memory is the memory of personally experienced events. Semantic memory is the memory of facts, principles, and rules that make up general knowledge of the world. Long-term remote memories are felt to be represented in diffuse cortical association areas. It is highly resistant to loss except in diseases affecting large areas of association cortex (eg, late stage dementia). By the time this degree of loss occurs the patient will have long since experienced loss of new learning (amnesia). When long-term remote memories appear to be lost in the face of intact new learning, psychogenic amnesia is suspected. The hippocampus appears to be the center of processing of new information that will be laid down in memory, although lesions in other limbic areas may also result in declarative memory problems (eg, fornix, basal forebrain, mammillary bodies). Declarative memory also incorporates other elements of memory that contribute to providing personal value and valence to the memories. Emotional memory, felt to be centered in the amygdala, contributes autonomic and emotional tone to the declarative memory. The prefrontal cortex contributes "source" (the "where" and "under what circumstance" the learning took place), "temporal" ("when" the learning occurred), working memory (the ability to hold pieces of information in immediate memory while manipulating other pieces of information), and the capacity to modulate emotional responses when memories are repeatedly recalled. Implicit memory (learning without conscious awareness) and procedural memory have different anatomical substrates than declarative memory, and are often spared in amnestic syndromes.

Korsakoff's (Amnestic) Syndrome

Wernicke's encephalopathy constitutes the acute phase of two distinct disorders—Wernicke's syndrome and Korsakoff's syndrome—both of which are caused by thiamine deficiency. Confusion, ataxia, and eye signs (nystagmus or ophthalmoplegia) comprise the traditional triad of symptoms in patients with Wernicke's encephalopathy. Because these patients are profoundly inattentive, it is inappropriate to characterize them as having a memory disorder. In the chronic stages of thiamine deficiency, however, apathy and memory disorder are the two most salient features.

The hallmark of Korsakoff's syndrome is a dissociation between immediate recall and short-term memory. In addition to significant problems registering new information (anterograde amnesia), these patients demonstrate memory problems that predate the onset of the syndrome (retrograde amnesia).

Unless formal testing of memory is performed routinely (see Chapters 11 and 16), the memory deficits associated with thiamine deficiency are easily missed, since these patients often converse in what appears to be a normal or even glib fashion. Moreover, their performance on tests of intellectual functioning is not significantly impaired by their amnestic state. Confabulation (the filling-in of memory blanks with what may appear to be fanciful information) is not an invariable part of the syndrome but tends to occur in the earlier stages and during recovery. Although confabulation has been construed as intentional misleading of the examiner, it is probably best viewed as an attempt by the prefrontal cortex to make sense of immediate information presented to the patient in the face of depleted information stores regarding the topic at hand.

Because lesions in Korsakoff's syndrome are localized to specific anatomical sites, the syndrome provides a model for the study of amnesia and brain localization. Petechial hemorrhagic lesions stretch from the third to the fourth ventricle in the midline along the cerebral aqueduct. Lesions in the mamillary bodies and in the dorsomedial nucleus of the thalamus are also predictable findings. Whereas the periventricular lesions lie in the ascending reticular network, lesions in the mamillary bodies lie in the medial limbic circuit described by Papez. The dorsomedial thalamus is a prominent way station for fibers passing from medial limbic structures, such as the amygdala, to the prefrontal cortex.

Alcoholic Memory Blackouts

In contrast to Korsakoff's syndrome, in which both the anatomy and pathophysiology are reasonably well understood, alcoholic blackouts represent a common occurrence whose pathogenesis is poorly understood. Two types of blackouts have been described: en bloc and fragmentary.

The onset of en bloc blackouts is abrupt, and the duration is from minutes to days. During blackouts, patients are incapable of registering new information and may ask the same question or tell the same story repeatedly. Despite their anterograde amnesia, these patients may have unimpaired ability to move about, drive an automobile, and perform routine tasks. In an en bloc blackout forgetting is complete and memory cannot be recovered for a period of time despite attempts to "jog the memory" with cues, hypnosis, or amobarbital interviews.

Fragmentary blackouts are more common than en bloc blackouts. Patients with fragmentary blackouts have "spotty" recall for events that happened during the blackout and sometimes report that events happened "as in a dream" or "a picture out of focus." During recovery, islands of recall seem to coalesce, and retrieval of information is facilitated by "jogging the memory." Casual observers cannot distinguish behavior of patients during alcoholic blackouts from their behavior during mild states of inebriation.

Transient Global Amnesia

The typical picture of transient global amnesia is that of a 50- or 60-year-old man who experiences a sudden onset of apparent confusion with loss of ability to learn new information. Although the term "confusion" is often used to describe these individuals, they do not have attention or vigilance problems, which are the hallmark of the acute confusional state. Attacks last hours, rarely days, and during this period patients tend (in contrast to patients having an alcoholic blackout) to be concerned that a problem exists. They may, for example, repeatedly ask questions such as "Where am I?" or "What is happening?" although they do not fail to recognize, by name, people whom they have known. Complex partial seizures, migraine, transient ischemia of the medial temporal lobes, sedative intoxication, and cerebral neoplasm have all been associated with transient global amnesia. Precipitating factors may include sudden alteration in body temperature or orgasm. Usually an attack occurs only once in any individual; however, when repeated attacks occur, the most common underlying cause is cerebrovascular disease. Spreading neuronal depression (commonly seen with migraine aura) has been suggested as a possible underlying pathophysiological mechanism.

Traumatic Amnesia

Following nontrivial head injury, memory problems are common. Traumatic amnesia refers to loss of memory both for a period of time preceding the head injury (retrograde amnesia) and for events following the injury (anterograde amnesia). Posttraumatic amnesia prevents the patient from registering new information. For example, a hospitalized patient may recognize visitors and talk with them, but have no recollection of the visit the next day. In general, posttraumatic amnesia lasts minutes to hours following return of consciousness; if it exceeds 24 hours, the patient usually has sustained severe and permanent neurological deficits such as those associated with prolonged coma. Termination of posttraumatic amnesia tends to be abrupt and often occurs after a period of sleep or following some emotionally meaningful event such as the visit of a close friend. Because the extent of retrograde amnesia immediately following injury may initially encompass years of the patient's life but later shrinks to within minutes to a few days of the injury, the term "shrinking retrograde amnesia" is appropriate. The patient with bifrontal lesions may manifest reduplicative paramnesia as well. This is the delusion of being convinced that one is in a specific geographic location despite all evidence to the contrary.

Amnesia Following Seizures

Following generalized major motor seizures, patients are invariably amnestic for the seizure itself as well as for a variable period of time after the seizure. In general, the same is true of complex partial seizures, although some patients remain conscious during such seizures. During the confusional period that follows seizures, patients may respond with agitation or aggression to gentle attempts to assist them, but will later be amnestic for this period of abnormal behavior. Continuous absence ("petit mal") is a rare condition in which patients lose touch with the environment for prolonged periods of time and thus are amnestic for events. Complex partial status epilepticus should be considered in patients with a known history of epilepsy who suddenly develop a prolonged amnestic or confusional state.

Acute Confusion with Associated Amnesia

Although acute confusion of toxic, metabolic, or infectious origin is not considered a true amnestic state, patients with acute confusion may be unable to register new information over prolonged periods of time. If examined following resolution of their confusion, they will often be "amnestic" for the confu-

sional period. Toxic states for which a person has no recall can occur with phencyclidine (PCP) abuse. This drug is a known "dissociative/amnestic" agent, and a person under its influence may commit crimes of violence for which he or she later has no recall.

Memory Impairment

Memory impairment unaccompanied by other evidence of intellectual deterioration is termed an amnestic syndrome. Early problems with memory become increasingly more severe in dementia of the Alzheimer type. The term "benign senile forgetfulness" has now been replaced with the term "age-associated memory impairment." This has been used to designate a modest decline in memory function only in the presence of no other dementing features. It occurs in adults of at least 50 years of age; however, most are in their seventh, eighth, or ninth decades.

Unlike the true amnestic state of Alzheimer's disease, this forgetfulness is often improved with memory cueing or reminders. Patients with moderately advanced dementia are usually unaware of their memory dysfunction and therefore not concerned about it. Depressed patients with complaints of cognitive deficits (depressive pseudodementia) are preoccupied with what they take to be memory deterioration and may seek help for this complaint. Thus, even though some patients in the earliest stages of dementia may be aware of and upset by their memory problems, patients who present with complaints of memory problems are more likely to have an affective illness. Some degenerative dementias may present initially with an affective disorder. One should cautiously follow patients with memory disorders associated with depression to determine if a degenerative dementia will later become unmasked.

Differential Diagnosis of Organic & Functional Amnestic Disorders

Nonorganic (psychogenic) memory disorders include dissociative episode (fugue state), feigned amnesia (malingering), factitious amnesia (a variant of Ganser's syndrome), and conditions in which thought processes are disrupted by intrusive thoughts or images (major affective illness, schizophrenia, posttraumatic stress disorder). Although the latter are psychiatric conditions, their "biological" features suggest that the term "psychogenic" is used here in a somewhat strained sense.

In differentiating organic from functional amnestic disorders, the clinician should consider the following factors: age; medical history (particularly history of neurological disorders); psychiatric history; the presence or absence of psychosocial precipitants (in what environment or under what circumstances the amnestic episodes occur); affective behavior during the episode; the patient's desire for recovery; what type of information is forgotten (loss of personal identity implies functional illness); evidence that the patient is registering some types of information while selectively ignoring others; the patient's response to cueing techniques (eg, hypnosis, use of amobarbital); and where the patient is when memory function is recovered. It is not uncommon in functional memory loss to have patients profess to have total loss of memory, only to objectively observe that they are capable of laying down new information on a day-to-day basis.

VISUAL PERCEPTUAL DISTURBANCES

Visual Object Agnosia

In visual agnosia, the recognition and function of a perceived stimulus, previously known to the patient, are impaired. There are two main types of visual object agnosia.

A. Aperceptive Visual Agnosia: Aperceptive visual agnosia is a deficit of visual analysis at the boundary between perception and recognition. Affected patients have difficulty distinguishing one form from another, and objects that are presented to them are not only misidentified visually, but cannot be drawn to confrontation. Identification, however, can be made through other sensory modalities, such as auditory, tactile, olfactory, or taste. These patients are felt to have extensive visual association cortex lesions bilaterally.

B. Associative Visual Agnosia: Associative visual agnosia is a deficit of recognition in the presence of intact visual perception. Affected patients are capable of drawing objects to confrontation quite accurately, but are unable to identify them by name or function. Associative visual agnosias can be distinguished from a visual anomia. The pure anomic patients are able to select the correct name when given a list of choices; agnosic patients are not. The anomic patients also can accurately demonstrate the functional use of a familiar object. Patients with associative visual agnosia usually have bilateral medial occipitotemporal lesions, and it is not uncommon to see other impairments associated with this, such as color agnosia, alexia, and prosopagnosia.

Color Abnormalities (Agnosia, Anomia, Imagery, Achromatopsia)

Color agnosia is loss of the ability to retrieve color knowledge about a given stimulus with no deficit of color perception. The patient will have difficulty matching colors or matching color names with objects, but still be able to name colors to confrontation. It is a rare condition, but has been described with left or bilateral occipitotemporal lesions. Color anomia is also rare. Naming colors to confrontation or pointing to a specific color when the name of the color is given may be impaired. Matching colors remains intact. Lesions in the left medial occipitotem-

poral area are seen in patients with color anomia. Color imagery deficits result in the inability to visually image color in the "mind's eye" (eg, imagining the color of one's car or a traffic sign). Bilateral fusiform gyrus lesions (left greater than right) have been associated with color imagery problems. Central achromatopsia is a defect of color perception. It more often occurs in a hemifield, but may be full field. Hemifield achromatopsia is due to a lesion in the contralateral occipitotemporal junction. Bilateral lesions in the occipitotemporal area occur with full field achromatopsia. Colors can neither be named nor matched. Visual agnosia, alexia, and/or prosopagnosia may accompany central achromatopsia.

Prosopagnosia

Although originally believed to be an inability to recognize familiar faces, with preserved ability to recognize through alternate means (ie, tactile sense or auditory recognition of voice), this condition has been expanded to include deficits of identifying the specific members of a class. For example, a canine expert may still be able to recognize a dog, but would no longer be able to differentiate a collie from a shepherd; or a car salesman would no longer be able to tell a Mercury from a Buick, despite the ability to still identify both vehicles as cars. Despite the inability to recognize a familiar face or a member of a specific class, detailed descriptions of the individual or the member of the class can be made by the patient. Patients with prosopagnosia may be able to match faces when given a choice of pictures; however, they cannot learn new faces and recognize them by name at a later time. Lesions in prosopagnosia are believed to be in the bilateral medial occipitotemporal areas; however, there have been some isolated cases suggesting that unilateral, right-sided, posteromedial occipitotemporal lesions are sufficient to produce this syndrome. Lesions most often involve occipitotemporal projections and are commonly associated with achromatopsia.

Topographagnosia

With topographagnosia (also referred to as environmental agnosia), patients are incapable of finding their way around a previously familiar environment, although they can verbally describe the environment around them. They can often utilize maps correctly and adapt verbal strategies, such as remembering street names and numbers in order to maneuver properly through their environment. Patients may have bilateral medial occipital lesions and, in these cases, environmental agnosia may be associated with prosopagnosia and achromatopsia. Unilateral, right-sided, occipitotemporal lesions have also been described, however. It is postulated that there is a disconnection between the ability to link current visual perception with stored visual environmental memories.

Anton's Syndrome

Anton's syndrome represents the denial of blindness. These patients often bump into objects in their environment and fail to make eye contact with individuals speaking with them. Yet, when confronted with their disability, they often make excuses and vehemently deny that they have any difficulty with their vision. This appears to be a form of anosagnosia and, although due to bilateral occipital lobe lesions, it is believed that the syndrome is actually caused by a disconnection of higher order association cortex that provides feedback for self-modulation and self-assessment. Fibers projecting from visual association cortex to prefrontal cortex may be involved in this condition.

Balint's Syndrome

Balint's syndrome involves a triad of features, including optic ataxia, ocular apraxia, and simultanagnosia. Optic ataxia is manifested by an inability to execute visually guided manual movements. This execution actually improves when patients close their eyes. Ocular motor apraxia, commonly referred to as "psychic paralysis of visual fixation," is manifested by the inability of the patient to quickly saccade to a target area in an intact visual field. It results in the inability to rapidly shift gaze from one object to another. Finally, simultanagnosia is the inability of patients to simultaneously perceive more than one item at a time in a picture or within their environment. These patients cannot simultaneously integrate more than one visual component of their environment with other visual components of the environment. It has been speculated that there are deficits of visual fixation; as soon as one part of the environmental image falls on the macula of the retina, there are sudden shifts in visual refixation to other elements of the environment. This occurs in such rapid fashion that synthesis of information required to understand the entire environment or a picture cannot be made. Although the components of Balint's syndrome may appear individually, the full triad is seen with bilateral parietooccipital lesions. There have been some reports of the syndrome occurring with unilateral right parietooccipital lesions.

FRONTAL SYSTEMS ABNORMALITIES

Understanding the behavioral manifestations of frontal lobe disease requires a basic knowledge of frontal lobe functions and of frontal connections to the rest of the central nervous system.

Frontal Lobe Connections

A. Sensory Input: Sensory input to the prefrontal region does not arise from primary sensory regions but rather from the high-level (polymodal and supramodal) association cortices of the temporal, parietal, and occipital lobes. Sensory information presented to the frontal lobes is therefore already highly processed. Input to the frontal convexities from the inferior parietal lobule serves as one example of such highly processed sensory input.

B. Motor Output: The frontal lobe contains four motor areas: (1) the motor strip containing giant pyramidal (Betz) cells, (2) the premotor region, (3) the frontal eye fields, and (4) the supplemental motor area. The frontal cortex, along with much of the neocortex, projects to the basal ganglia. Primary motor regions project to the putamen, and prefrontal and other neocortical association areas project to the caudate. Projections to the head of the caudate nucleus (which are not bidirectional) are particularly prominent. The importance of these frontostriatal ("psychomotor") pathways is suggested by the fact that the head of the caudate nucleus also receives limbic system input from such regions as the hippocampus and the amygdala. Thus, the basal ganglia can be seen as a point of convergence for frontal lobe and limbic system information.

C. Limbic System Input: As mentioned in the discussion of limbic system anatomy in this chapter, there are numerous links between prefrontal and limbic areas. These may conveniently be subdivided into four categories: (1) direct pathways from the medial temporal lobe structures to the frontal cortex via the uncinate fasciculus; (2) indirect fibers connecting frontal and limbic system regions via the dorsomedial nucleus of the thalamus; (3) indirect fibers passing from the hippocampus to prefrontal regions via the cingulate gyrus; and (4) mesocortical projection fibers from the ventral tegmental area to the prefrontal cortex.

D. Septo-Hypothalamo-Mesencephalic Continuum Input: There are direct pathways from the dorsolateral convexities and orbitomedial portions of the prefrontal area to the septo-hypothalamo-mesencephalic continuum.

Behavioral Changes in Frontal Lobe Lesions

Behavioral changes following frontal lobe damage may be grouped into three broad categories: personality, higher cortical functions, and motor function disturbances.

A. Personality Disturbances: The case of Phineas P. Gage, a 25-year-old construction foreman working on a railroad bed in Vermont, is perhaps the most famous example of personality disturbance associated with frontal lobe syndromes. According to the case report of Harlow (1868), Gage was using a tamping iron to pack blasting powder into a hole when the powder exploded. The explosion drove the tamping iron through his face and out the top of his skull, transacting his frontal lobes. After the accident, he became, in the words of his physician:

fitful, irreverent, indulging at times in the grossest pro-
fanity (which was not previously his custom), manifesting but little deference to his fellows, impatient of restraint or advice when it conflicts with his desires, at
times pertinaciously obstinate yet capricious and vacil-
lating, devising many plans for future operation which
are no sooner arranged than they are abandoned in turn
for others appearing more feasible. . . . His mind was
radically changed, so that his friends and acquaintances
said he was no longer Gage.

Studies of individuals who suffered penetrating
head injuries during World War I showed personality
disturbances of two distinct types. Individuals with
orbitomedial disorders appeared puerile, disinhibited,
and euphoric ("pseudopsychopathic"). Those with
brain injury limited to the dorsolateral convexities appeared apathetic and indifferent ("pseudodepressed").
Since patients rarely have lesions limited to either of
these regions, it is more common to see admixtures of
these two personality types. Geschwind has described
patients with irritability, apathy, and euphoria as manifesting "the impossible triad of frontal lobe pathology."

B. Higher Cortical Disturbances: Characterization of intellectual deficits following frontal
lobe damage has been a vexing problem. In the late
1940s (10 years after psychosurgery had come into
use), essentially no neuropsychological changes had
been consistently noted in postsurgical patients even
though psychologists searched diligently for signs of
intellectual deterioration. Failure to correlate intellectual deficits with prefrontal lobe damage called into
question the established view that the frontal lobes
were the highest seat of human intelligence and suggested that they might even be superfluous structures,
since they could apparently be removed with relative
impunity. Since that time, the consequences of
frontal lobe damage have been somewhat clarified,
largely as a result of the work of Luria, a Russian
neurologist and neuropsychologist (see Luria, 1980).
After seeing thousands of patients personally, Luria
concluded that the frontal lobes have four functions:
(1) generating plans for action; (2) programming the
components, or subroutines, of actions; (3) monitoring ongoing activity with reference both to the goal
and to environmental shifts; and (4) correcting the
course of activity already in progress.

Obviously, the frontal lobes do not act independently. They depend on high-level sensory input from
the temporal, parietal, and occipital lobes. Patients
with frontal lobe damage may have the following
problems: (1) difficulty suppressing irrelevant associations or intrusions; (2) inability to anticipate the
consequences of their actions, ie, physical damage to
property, self, or others and emotional consequences
for self and others; (3) inability to formulate an approach to complex problems that extend over time;
(4) remarkable dissociation of speech from action
(eg, a patient told to "squeeze a ball when the light

goes on" may say "I must squeeze the ball" when he
or she sees the light but will fail to carry out the action); and (5) difficulty understanding metaphors,
similes, and parables (the "inability to assume the abstract attitude" described by Goldstein in the 1940s
as the hallmark of organic disease).

Patients with frontal lobe damage have been said
to manifest "frontal amnesia." In actuality, these patients do not have amnestic problems similar to those
of patients with Korsakoff's psychosis. They are,
however, sometimes unable to hold in conscious
awareness the various pieces of information required
for a specific action. It has been speculated that these
individuals fail to generate mnemonic associations;
thus, their forgetting may reflect not so much a retrieval blockade as a disinclination to remember or a
failure to generate "limbic tags" for events.

Intelligence tests do not appear to be a good measure of the type of deficits seen following frontal lobe
damage. The Wisconsin Card-Sorting Test (in which
patients are asked to infer from the examiner's responses whether they are shifting cards by the appropriate criterion) and various maze-learning tasks have
proved helpful in neuropsychological assessment of
frontal lobe damage. Tests that measure the ability to
sustain, shift, or direct attention might be expected to
be most sensitive to frontal lobe lesions.

C. Motor Function Disturbances: The motor changes following frontal lobe damage may include the appearance of primitive reflexes such as
grasping, sucking, and snouting. However, in many
patients with significant prefrontal lobe damage (eg,
lobotomized psychiatric patients), these reflexes cannot be elicited. The grasp reflex is most frequently observed in patients over age 60, but its presence does
not correlate well either with gross brain damage or
with intellectual deterioration. Disturbances associated with difficulty in overcoming motor inertia are
seen in patients with frontal lobe damage. These include apraxia of gait, characterized by difficulty initiating gait; decreased "ocular palpation of the environment," which may contribute to the patient's tendency
to make judgments on the basis of incomplete information; and palilalia, characterized by repetition of
the last elements of an utterance (either the entire last
word or the last syllable). Difficulty "changing sets"
has long been recognized as a problem following
frontal lobe damage. Patients asked to draw a series of
geometric shapes such as a circle, triangle, and square
may perseverate the production of one of these three
elements. Luria has recommended the use of a simple
bedside test in which patients are asked to perform a
three-step command—striking the top of a table with
the edge of an open hand ("cut"), then striking the
table with a closed fist ("pound"), and finally striking
the table with an open palm ("slap")—as one index of
frontal lobe function.

Many of these problems with inertia and perseveration resemble symptoms that arise from *disorders of*

the basal ganglia. Because there are strong frontostriatal connections, it becomes difficult and even somewhat meaningless to attempt to separate frontal (cortical) from striatal (subcortical) symptoms.

CLINICAL ANATOMICAL SYNDROMES MANIFESTED BY FRONTAL LOBE LESIONS

There are three major anatomic regions of the frontal lobes—the frontal convexities, the orbitofrontal region, and the medial frontal region—that, when injured, produce characteristic abnormalities. Features from all three syndromes may overlap; however, there are characteristic traits that clinically distinguish these three syndromes.

A. Frontal Convexity Syndrome: Patients with frontal convexity syndrome are characteristically apathetic, although there may be intermittent impulsive or aggressive behavior. They tend to be slow and indifferent. They manifest perseveration, yet may be impersistent. They have problems changing rapidly from one set of tasks to another, tend to have significant motor programming deficits, have poor planning and strategy formulation, and manifest a fragmented approach to visual/spatial problem solving.

B. Orbitofrontal Syndrome: Damage to the orbitofrontal region often results in disinhibited and impulsive behavior. Social decorum is lost, and patients often demonstrate inappropriate affect (eg, laughing at tragic news). They tend to show poor judgment and insight, may easily be distracted by trivial stimuli, and are prone to antisocial behavior, including impulsive aggression, loss of empathy, proneness for substance abuse, and loss of self-monitoring.

C. Medial Frontal Syndrome: Medial frontal syndrome is associated with varying degrees of akinetic muteness or transcortical motor aphasia, paraparesis, incontinence, and loss of motivational drive.

D. Treatment: Dopaminergic agents, such as *d*-amphetamine or bromocriptine, have been reported to be helpful in the frontal convexity and medial frontal syndromes. Drugs such as carbamazepine, lithium, or neuroleptics have been used in the orbital frontal syndrome. Rarely are the higher cognitive problems amenable to pharmacotherapy.

MOVEMENT DISORDERS

Although almost all neurological diseases have psychological correlates, the movement disorders serve as striking prototypes of neuropsychiatric disorders. The connections between neurology and psychiatry are particularly strong in Parkinson's disease, Huntington's disease, tardive dyskinesia, Gilles de la Tourette syndrome, and Wilson's disease. Therefore, each of these disorders will be considered here.

Parkinson's Disease & Other Extrapyramidal Motor Disorders

A. Pathological Physiology: Tremor, muscular rigidity, and bradykinesia (the parkinsonian triad) are due to pathological changes in the posterior portion of the septo-hypothalamo-mesencephalic continuum—specifically, in the substantia nigra of the midbrain. This darkly pigmented area lies at the junction between the cerebral peduncles and the tegmentum of the midbrain. Dorsal and medial to the substantia nigra lies the ventral tegmental area, which is the origin of the mesolimbic dopaminergic pathways projecting to the limbic and frontal cortices. Destruction of the dopaminergic neurons in the substantia nigra leads to a decrease in the dopamine content of the neostriatum (caudate nucleus and putamen) and alters the cholinergic-dopaminergic balance. This imbalance of acetylcholine and dopamine may be treated with either dopamine precursors, dopamine agonists, or anticholinergic drugs.

B. Dementia in Parkinson's Disease: For many years, it was thought that intellectual deterioration was not an intrinsic feature of Parkinson's disease. It now appears that parkinsonian patients are at high risk (10 times that of age-matched controls) of developing dementia. The dementia of Parkinson's is clinically of the subcortical type, but there is also an increased incidence of pathological changes of the Alzheimer's type when compared to normal controls. Because so many symptoms of dementia in parkinsonian patients seem to involve a slowing of both mentation and motor activity, it has been suggested that the basal ganglia may play an important role in cognitive activity. Since dopaminergic pathways that ascend from the ventral tegmental region of the midbrain also travel to the frontal lobe cortex, damage to these mesolimbic and mesofrontal pathways may play a role in the dementia of Parkinson's disease. "Parkinson's Plus" syndromes may also be associated with dementia and major depression. These syndromes include striatonigral degeneration, progressive supranuclear palsy, Shy-Drager syndrome, and multiple system atrophy. These syndromes involve more widespread areas of the brain than Parkinson's disease and do not respond well to conventional anti-Parkinson drugs.

C. Drug-Induced Parkinsonism: Drug-induced parkinsonism may occur within 5–30 days after starting neuroleptic treatment. Although the parkinsonian triad of symptoms is present, the severity of symptoms in drug-induced parkinsonism differs from that in Parkinson's disease in that bradykinesia is often the most prominent feature, muscular rigidity is less pronounced, and tremor may be insignificant.

Acute dystonia, if present, usually appears in the first 5 days of neuroleptic treatment and is very painful. Dystonic reactions may be seen in the eyes, neck, tongue, jaw, or trunk and are frequently misdiagnosed as hysteria, malingering, or seizures. A drug such as benztropine mesylate, diphenhydramine, or diazepam should be administered intravenously. If dystonic reactions recur or persist, a neuroleptic agent of lower potency such as thioridazine or chlorpromazine may be indicated. Serum calcium levels should be measured to rule out hypocalcemia.

Akathisia, an inner sense of restlessness that may or may not be accompanied by gross motor restlessness, may occur 5–60 days after initiating treatment with dopamine blockers. Antihistamines and propranolol are more effective than purely atropinic substances in treating akathisia.

"Rabbit syndrome," a fine perioral tremor, may appear months after starting an antipsychotic agent. It is frequently misdiagnosed as tardive dyskinesia, but is actually a parkinsonian phenomenon that responds to treatment with anticholinergic agents.

Huntington's Disease

Movement disorder and dementia are the two major features of Huntington's disease. The age at onset of this autosomal dominant disorder ranges roughly from 25 to 50 years, with peak onset in the fourth decade. A DNA marker has been identified on the terminal short arm of chromosome 4 close to the Huntington's disease gene. Lymphocytes from family members can be used to map this DNA marker. Recently the gene mutation has been identified as an expansion trinucleotide repeat of the CAG base pairs. The younger the patient is at the onset of the disease the longer the expansion is. Although testing all family members is still somewhat controversial, early detection and possible treatment may be forthcoming. For patients who have been on neuroleptics it may be impossible to distinguish tardive dyskinesia from Huntington's disease, except on the basis of a family history of Huntington's disease or genetic testing. Multiple neurotransmitters are affected including diminished GABA, substance P, and enkephalin. Central dopamine, choline acetyltransferase, and glutamate activity is increased. Somatostatin, neuropeptide Y, and nitric oxide appear resistant in Huntington's disease.

Although patients may present with either motor or psychiatric symptoms, the former are more likely to bring the patient to medical attention. Initially, patients may fidget, twitch, grimace, and speak in a slurred fashion. As the disorder progresses, movements become conspicuously clumsy, of greater amplitude, and assume a bizarre and grotesque quality.

Personality disorder, thought or affective disorder, and dementia may occur. Violence and hypersexuality (often of a bizarre nature) are among the striking behavioral abnormalities that Huntington noted but are not common in all cases.

In patients with Huntington's disease, atrophy of the caudate nucleus leads to ballooning of the lateral ventricles, which can be seen on magnetic resonance imaging (MRI) or computed tomography (CT) scan in the late stages of illness. Metabolic changes in the head of the caudate nucleus can be demon-

strated early with positron emission tomography (PET) or single-photon emission computed tomography (SPECT).

Since the mean life expectancy of patients with Huntington's disease is 16 years following diagnosis, it is important to realize that symptomatic relief is available. The movement disorder, the agitation, and the violent behavior described above can be treated with dopamine blockers. For disturbances of affective behavior, treatment with lithium or tricyclic antidepressants should be considered.

Tardive Dyskinesia

In 1956, two years after approval of chlorpromazine as an antipsychotic agent, the first cases of persistent abnormal movements following discontinuation of the drug were reported.

A. Pharmacological Factors Affecting Onset and Treatment: Tardive dyskinesia is a late-onset disorder that occurs months to years after initiation of treatment with dopaminergic blocking agents. Suggested mechanisms for a functional dopaminergic excess have included (1) increased circulating blood levels of dopamine, (2) increased dopamine release by dopaminergic neurons, (3) increased responsiveness to dopamine at the postsynaptic receptor sites, and (4) synthesis of new, low threshold dopamine receptors. The precise pharmacological basis remains unclear. In all likelihood, tardive dyskinesia involves an imbalance of neurotransmitters (eg, dopamine, acetylcholine, and γ-aminobutyric acid) and perhaps neuropeptides such as cholecystokinin and somatostatin, as well.

Discontinuing dopamine-blocking agents is desirable but may not always be possible if psychosis is poorly controlled. Temporary worsening of the movement disorder is to be expected following cessation of these agents. Drug holidays (weeks or months) are indicated to determine whether patients continue to require antipsychotic medications.

Increasing the dose of dopamine-blocking agents is not suitable treatment for tardive dyskinesia, since it will only mask the symptoms while pathophysiological changes continue.

If patients are being treated with anticholinergic agents such as tricyclic antidepressants or with antihistamines, discontinuing these agents may produce dramatic alleviation of the movement disorder.

Although lecithin and choline have been used for treatment of dyskinesia, these agents do not appear efficacious. Lecithin causes a fishy odor, and choline must be given in massive doses. Change in antipsychotic to a predominant serotonergic form, such as clozapine or olanzapine, may be very beneficial in ameliorating the symptoms.

B. Types of Tardive Dyskinesia: Patients may present with one or more of the types of tardive dyskinesia described below. Older patients tend to have the buccolingual-masticatory and orofacial syndromes, whereas adolescents and young adults are more likely to develop choreiform movements, primarily of the extremities.

1. Buccolingual-masticatory dyskinesia— The movements for this type include twisting, turning, protruding, and smacking the tongue and lips.

2. Orofacial dyskinesia—This form is characterized by facial tics, grimacing, and blinking.

3. Axial dyskinesia—Truncal movements such as shoulder shrugging, lordotic posturing, and pelvic thrusting may all be seen in patients with axial dyskinesia.

4. Appendicular chorea—Choreiform movements of the fingers, hands, arms, or legs have a rapid, dancelike quality. Since these choreiform movements are usually accompanied by some degree of athetosis (slow, writhing movements), the term choreoathetosis is often employed. Ballistic movements, eg, a throwing movement of the arm, are occasionally seen.

C. Differential Diagnosis: It is impossible to distinguish tardive dyskinesia from Huntington's disease clinically. This leads to a particular problem. If a patient with a psychotic behavioral disturbance is treated with antipsychotic agents and years later develops a movement disorder, the clinician seeing the patient for the first time is likely to attribute the movement disorder to prior neuroleptic drug treatment. Thus, Huntington's disease can be masked unless a family history is determined.

Gilles de la Tourette Syndrome

This syndrome is characterized by chronic multiple motor and vocal tics. The age at onset is 2–15 years. Motor tics frequently consist of sniffing, snorting, or blinking; vocal tics consist of clicks, grunts, barks, coughs, or yelps. Coprolalia (the compulsive uttering of obscenities) is said to occur eventually in 60% of cases. Comorbidity, including obsessive-compulsive disorder (OCD), attention-deficit disorder (ADD), and affective disorders, may be seen with Tourette's syndrome. Suicide may occur secondary to profound social disruption produced by the disorder. Tourette's disease may exist for many years before the diagnosis is made. The cause and pathogenesis are unknown, but administration of central nervous system stimulants such as methylphenidate may precipitate the disorder. This poses a problem for those with comorbid ADD. Dopamine-blocking neuroleptic agents usually afford some symptomatic relief of the tics, and selective serotonin reuptake inhibitors can be used for OCD traits.

Wilson's Disease (Hepatolenticular Degeneration)

Wilson's disease is an autosomal recessive disorder caused by a mutation in a copper transporter gene on chromosome 13. Copper is deposited in the liver and lenticular nucleus (putamen and globus pallidus) of the basal ganglia. The defect in copper metabolism consists of diminished levels of ceruloplasmin, which may be documented by serum assay and increased urinary copper excretion. The neurological manifestations of the disease reflect progressive extrapyramidal dysfunction accompanied by deterioration of personality (eg, irritability, depression, psychosis) and intellect. Early signs include tremor, bradykinesia, dysarthria, and dysphagia. However the psychiatric features may precede the extrapyramidal features by months. Eventually, the patient develops a characteristic picture—a "vacuous smile," great difficulty chewing and swallowing, constant drooling, and a coarse "wing-flapping" tremor when the arms are outstretched. In advanced stages deposition of copper in the cornea (Kayser-Fleischer ring) may be seen with a slit lamp. There have been more than a few cases of documented Wilson's disease with neurological and liver involvement in which Kayser-Fleischer (K-F) rings were not present. When the diagnosis is strongly suspected but the patient is K-F ring negative, a liver biopsy can be diagnostic. Treatment consists of reduction in dietary copper, screening for copper in the patient's water supply, and administration of a copper chelating agent. D-Penicillamine is the most common first line chelating agent used. Because penicillamine may have significant side effects, alternate drugs include trientine and zinc acetate. Family members should be screened once the diagnosis is made because left untreated the disease is progressively fatal.

Cortical Degenerative Dementias

Because 10% of dementias are potentially reversible with treatment, appropriate diagnostic evaluation should be undertaken in all patients.

A. Alzheimer's Disease: Alzheimer's is the most common dementing disease, being responsible for 65% of all adult dementias. Alzheimer's is usually manifested throughout its course with impairments of memory, language, visual/spatial, and executive functions. Apraxia, agnosia, and personality change develop. Neuropsychiatric features are also prominent. Delusions occur in about 50% of patients, and hallucinations and depression in 20–30% of patients. Anxiety and catastrophic reactions are common. Motor system problems usually occur later in the disease. Rarely patients develop seizures and myoclonus.

Despite tremendous advances over the past 10 years, absolute diagnosis can be made only by biopsy or autopsy. Recent genetic advances have resulted in increased accuracy of diagnosis during life. At present genes on four chromosomes causing Alzheimer's disease (AD) have been defined. Others have been named as candidate genes. The most common, responsible for late life (greater than 55 years) familial autosomal dominant or sporadic AD, is linked to a gene on chromosome 19 that codes for apolipoprotein E (Apo E). This is a cholesterol transporter that has three alleles—2, 3, and 4. Everyone possesses apolipoprotein alleles. They may be homogenetic (eg, 3/3) or heterogenetic (eg, 2/3). The number 4 allele carries the highest risk and the 2 allele the least risk for AD. Seventy percent of the population has the 3 allele. Although only 14% of the general population has the 4 allele, over 75% of patients with Alzheimer's disease are found to have the number 4 allele. Rare early forms of familial autosomal dominant AD are linked to chromosome 21 (gene-amyloid precursor protein), 14 (gene-presenilin 1), and 1 (gene-presenillin 2). Candidate genes for other forms have been linked to chromosomes 12 and 17. Pathological changes in the brains of Alzheimer's patients include neurofibrillary tangles, senile plaques, amyloid angiopathy, and neuronal loss of cholinergic neurons. The greatest risk factors for Alzheimer's disease are age and Apo E4. Maternal age, head injury, low educational level, postmenopausal women off estrogen, and family members with Alzheimer's disease are all additional risk factors.

At this time the mainstay of therapy is directed at restoration of central cholinergic function. Drugs such as tacrine, donepizil, and metrifonate have demonstrated improvement in cognitive function (albeit transient), prolonged time period to further decline, and some improvement in behavioral features, such as apathy and wandering. Nonsteroidal anti-inflammatories have demonstrated benefit based on the premise that amyloid deposition elicits a profound inflammatory response. Oxidative stress plays a role in neuronal death. Vitamin E, because of its antioxidant properties, may help delay the cognitive decline. Estrogen in postmenopausal women has also been shown to be protective. Target symptom therapy (eg, neuroleptics, antidepressants, anxiolytics), as well as environmental manipulation, can be used for the treatment of neurobehavioral features. Development of other cholinergic agents, antioxidants, secretase inhibitors, growth factors, and Apo E2-like agents are presently underway.

B. Vascular Dementia: This clinically presents with a mix of cortical and subcortical features. Treatment is directed at the underlying cause and target symptoms.

C. Pick's Disease: This is a rare dementia manifested by marked personality change, including social dysdecorum, disinhibition, lack of insight and judgment, and anomic aphasia early in the course. Occasionally these patients may manifest characteristics of the Klüver-Bucy syndrome, mania, aggressiveness, irritability, emotional lability, and inappropriate jocularity. Intraneuronal inclusions known as Pick bodies are the pathological hallmark. Treatment is symptomatic. The disease is progressively fatal.

D. Frontotemporal Dementia: These patients present with many of the same clinical features of Pick's disease, but lack the pathological characteristics of Pick's disease, namely the Pick bodies. Frontotemporal dementia may not be one specific disease but possibly represented by multiple mutant genes.

E. Primary Progressive Aphasia: Neuronal loss and cortical gliosis focally confined to perisylvian language areas have been described in patients who exclusively demonstrated progressive aphasia, as well as patients who went on to pathological confirmation of Pick's disease or a spongiform encephalopathy.

F. Diffuse Lewy Body Disease: This disease has many of the cortical features of Alzheimer's disease but patients also develop extrapyramidal features of rigidity and bradykinesia. Visual hallucinations, delusions, and waxing/waning confusion is common even in the early stages. These patients have particular sensitivity to neuroleptics, which sometimes induce catatonia, even in very small doses. This can make treatment of the psychosis seen in this disease very problematic. Pathologically these patients demonstrate Lewy bodies throughout the cortex as well as brainstem areas.

G. Prion Disease: These were once considered to be infectious diseases. Most present as cortical dementias. Once thought to be caused by a slow virus, because of the long latency between infection and onset of symptoms, they are now believed to be caused by point mutations in a prion protein gene. Once symptoms begin there is a rapidly progressive dementia often accompanied by seizures and myoclonus. Pathologically the brains of these patients demonstrate variable spongiform changes. Creutzfeldt-Jakob and Gerstmann-Straussler-Scheinker diseases are examples. The latter disease also has prominent cerebellar findings.

REFERENCES & SUGGESTED READINGS

Adams, RD, Victor M, Ropper AH: *Principles of Neurology,* 6th ed. McGraw-Hill, 1997.

American Psychiatric Association: *Diagnostic and Statistical Manual of Mental Disorders,* 4th ed. American Psychiatric Association, 1994.

Ader R: Psychoneuroimmunology: Interactions between the Brain and the Immune System. In: *Neuro-Psychiatry.* Fogel BS, Schiffer RB (editors), Rao SM (assoc. editor). Williams & Wilkins, 1996.

Babinski MJ: [No title.] Rev Neurol (Paris) 1918;34:365.

Babinski MJ: Contribution a letude des troubles mentaux dans l'hemiplegie organique (anosognosie). Rev Neurol (Paris) 1914;27:175.

Bard P: A diencephalic mechanism for the expression of rage with special reference to the sympathetic nervous system. Am J Physiol 1928;84:490.

Basbaum AI: Memories of pain. Sci Med 1996;Nov/Dec: 22.

Becker E: *Escape From Evil.* Free Press, 1975.

Benson DF: *Aphasia, Alexia and Agraphia.* Churchill Livingstone, 1979.

Bogousslavsky J, Fisher M: *Textbook of Neurology.* Butterworth-Heinemann, 1998.

Borsook D, LeBel AA, McPeek B: *The Massachusetts General Hospital Handbook of Pain Management.* Little, Brown, 1996.

Brass LM: Cerebrovascular diseases and epilepsy. Clinical neuroimaging. American Academy of Neurology Annual Course Number 442 1993;7:107.

Broca P: Perte de la parole: Ramollissement chronique et destruction partielle du lobe anterieur gauche du cerveau. Paris Bull Soc Anthropol 1861;2:219.

Broca P: Anatomie comparee des circonvolutions cerebrales: Le grand lobe limbique et la scissure limbique dans la serie des mammiferes. Rev Anthropol [Series 2] 1878;1:385.

Brodal A: *Neurological Anatomy,* 3rd ed. Oxford University Press, 1981.

Critchley M: Misoplegia, or hatred of hemiplegia. In: *The Divine Banquet of the Brain.* Raven Press, 1979.

Critchley M: *The Parietal Lobes.* Hafner, 1953.

Cummings JL: Frontal-subcortical circuits and human behavior. Arch Neurol 1993;50:873.

Cummings JL, Benson DF: *Dementia: A Clinical Approach,* 2nd ed. Heinemann-Butterworth, 1992.

Cummings JL, Victoroff JI: Noncognitive neuropsychiatric syndromes in Alzheimer's disease. Neuropsychiatry Neuropsychol Behav Neurol 1990;3:140.

D'Esposito M, Alexander MP: The clinical profiles, recovery and rehabilitation of memory disorders. Neurorehabilitation 1995;5:141.

DeMoranville BM, Jackson I: Psychoneuro-endocrinology. In: *Neuropsychiatry.* Fogel BS, Schiffer RB (editors), Rao SM (assoc. editor). Williams & Wilkins, 1996.

Eisenach JC: New understanding and treatment of acute pain. Sem Anesth 1992;11:106.

Elliott KJ: Taxonomy and mechanisms of neuropathic pain. Sem Neurol 1994;14:195.

Enna SJ, Coyle JT: *Pharmacological Management of Neurological and Psychiatric Disorders.* McGraw-Hill, 1998.

Feinberg TE, Fara MJ: *Behavioral Neurology and Neuropsychology.* McGraw-Hill, 1997.

Flynn FG, Cummings JL, Gornbein J: Delusions in dementia syndromes. J Neuropsychol Clin Neurosci 1991; 3:364.

Flynn FG, Cummings JL, Tomiyasu U: Altered behavior associated with damage to the ventromedial hypothalamus. A distinctive syndrome. Behav Neurol 1988;1:49.

Freud S: Project for a scientific psychology (1895). In: *Standard Edition of the Complete Psychological Works of Sigmund Freud,* Vol. 1. Hogarth Press, 1966.

Galasko D et al: High cerebrospinal fluid tau and low amyloid beta-42 levels in the clinical diagnosis of Alzheimer's disease and relation to apolipoprotein E genotype. Arch Neurol 1998;55:937.

Garcia J, Altman RD: Chronic pain states: Pathophysiology and medical therapy. Sem Arth Rheum 1997;27:1.

Geschwind N: Disconnexion syndromes in animals and man. (2 parts.) Brain 1965;88:237, 585.

Geschwind N: The apraxias: Neural mechanisms of disorders of learned movements. Am Sci 1975;63:188.

Geschwind N, Kaplan E: A human cerebral disconnection syndrome. Neurology 1962;12:675.

Harlow JM: Recovery from the passage of an iron bar through the head. Mass Med Soc Publ 1868;2:329.

Heilman KM: Ideational apraxia—A redefinition. Brain 1973;96:861.

Heilman KM: Limb apraxia, behavioral neurology. American Academy of Neurology Annual Courses 1992; 340:31.

Kaplan HI, Sadock BJ: *Pocket Handbook of Primary Care Psychiatry.* Williams & Wilkins, 1996.

Kaplan HI, Sadock BJ: *Pocket Handbook of Psychiatric Drug Treatment,* 2nd ed. Williams & Wilkins, 1996.

Kaplan HI, Sadock BJ: *Synopsis of Psychiatry-Behavioral Sciences/Clinical Psychiatry,* 8th ed. Williams & Wilkins, 1998.

LeVay S: A difference in the hypothalamic structure between heterosexual and homosexual men. Science 1991; 253:1034.

Luria AR: *Higher Cortical Functions in Man,* 2nd ed. Basic Books, 1980.

MacLean PD: Some psychiatric implications of physiological studies on the frontotemporal portion of the limbic system (visceral brain). Electroencephalogr Clin Neurophysiol 1952;4:407.

MacLean PD: The brain, empathy and medical education. J Nerv Ment Dis 1967;144:374.

MacLean PD: *A Triune Concept of Brain and Behavior.* University of Toronto Press, 1969.

Masters CL, Beyreuther K: Science, medicine and the future: Alzheimer's disease. Br Med J 1998;316:446.

Mayeux R et al: Utility of the apolipoprotein E genotype in the diagnosis of Alzheimer's disease. N Engl J Med 1998;338:506.

Mesulam MM: Slowly progressive aphasia without generalized dementia. Ann Neurol 1982.

Mesulam MM: *Principles of Behavioral Neurology.* Davis, 1985.

Mesulam MM: Large scale neurocognitive networks and distributed processing for attention, language, and memory. Ann Neurol 1990;28:597.

Mueller J: Neuroanatomic correlates of emotion. Chapter 10 in: *Emotions in Health and Illness.* Temoshok L, Van Dyke C, Zegans LS (editors). Grune & Stratton, 1983.

Natelson BH: Clinical neuropharmacology: Depression and anxiety. American Academy of Neurology Annual Course Number 240 1993;7:15.

Nauta WJH: Hippocampal projections and related neural pathways to the midbrain in the cat. Brain 1958;81:319.

Papez JW: A proposed mechanism of emotion. Arch Neurol Psychiatry 1937;38:725.

Pfaf DW: *The Physiologic Mechanisms of Motivation.* Springer, 1982.

Plum F, Posner J: *The Diagnosis of Stupor and Coma,* 2nd ed. Davis, 1972.

Riggs JE (editor): *The Neurology of Aging—Neurologic Clinics.* Saunders, 1998.

Sperry R: Some effects of disconnecting the cerebral hemispheres. Science 1982;217:1223.

Watson RT, Heilman KM: Callosal apraxia. Brain 1983; 106:391.

Willis T: *Cerebri Anatome.* Martzer and Alleftry (London), 1664.

Yakovlev PI: Motility, behavior and the brain: Organization and neural coordinates of behavior. J Nerv Ment Dis 1948;107:313.

Yaksh TL: Pain after injury: Some basic mechanisms. J Florida Med Assoc 1997;84:16.

6 Neurochemistry in Psychiatry

Rona J. Hu, MD, & Victor I. Reus, MD

Biological psychiatry today faces the challenge of translating the vast amount of basic research in neuroscience into practical, clinical applications in humans. Research on specific neurotransmitters, their receptor subtypes, and the molecular biology of these systems has already revolutionized the development of new generations of psychiatric medications. There is promise for better understanding of the causes and mechanisms of psychiatric illnesses, and better diagnostic tools as well. It is an exciting time for researchers in the biological aspects of psychiatry. Clinicians, too, must now be familiar with at least the basic concepts of neurotransmission in order to understand and critically evaluate the recent literature, and choose intelligently among new treatments for their patients.

The focus of this chapter will be on the neurotransmitter systems in the central nervous system that are most relevant to psychiatry. Some of the technological advances that have contributed to a better understanding and treatment of psychiatric illnesses will also be discussed.

TRANSMISSION OF NERVE IMPULSES IN THE CENTRAL NERVOUS SYSTEM

The most fundamental unit of impulse transmission in the central nervous system is the synapse, a specialized area of contact between neurons that enables communication between them. There are three types of synapses: chemical, electrical, and conjoint. The most important are **chemical synapses,** in which the presynaptic neuron releases a chemical messenger when stimulated. The chemical messenger can then act on receptors on the postsynaptic neuron or on autoreceptors on the presynaptic neuron. **Electrical synapses** transmit their impulses by direct electrical means, and **conjoint synapses** operate via both chemical and electrical transmission. We will focus on the role of chemical synapses, whose communication through neurotransmitters has been extensively studied.

Nonsynaptic areas of neuronal membranes can also play a role in the functioning of neurons. Concentrations of electrolytes (such as calcium), changes in pH, and chemicals such as prostaglandins in the extracellular fluid of the brain can have major regulatory effects in the transmission of nerve impulses.

There are three general categories of neuroregulatory messengers responsible for chemical transmission: neurotransmitters, neuromodulators, and neurohormones. We focus first on the **neurotransmitters,** the "classical" chemical signals. They are synthesized in the presynaptic neuron, released into the synaptic cleft quickly (1–2 msec), bind to receptors, and transmit the impulse. **Neuromodulators** also bind to specific receptors, but they modify the response of the receptor to the neurotransmitter rather than directly transmitting the impulse. They may be released by presynaptic neurons or by nonneuronal tissue. **Neurohormones** are released by nerve cells into the systemic circulation rather than into the synapse. They therefore travel to sites far from the release point, and can affect peripheral organs as well as the central nervous system.

At one time it was thought that a given neuron would release only one chemical messenger, but now the **coexistence of neuroregulators**—the presence of more than one neurotransmitter, neuromodulator, or neurohormone within a single neuron—appears to be extremely common in the central nervous system, allowing more complex communication capabilities. Many synapses that use one neurotransmitter—for example, dopamine—can be shown to use another, such as γ-aminobutyric acid (GABA) or glutamate, as well.

Steps in Synaptic Transmission

A. Presynaptic: In the presynaptic neuron—the cell initiating the signal—the first three steps in synaptic transmission are the **synthesis, transport, and storage** of the chemical messenger. Each of these steps typically involves a myriad of enzymes and structures that can be altered by drugs or other signals. The synaptic vesicle containing the neurotransmitter can then fuse with the membrane and release its contents through exocytosis.

B. Postsynaptic: On the cell membrane of the postsynaptic neuron—the cell receiving the signal—sits the receptor. The **receptor** is a large protein or assemblage of proteins with a binding site that exhibits specificity for the particular neurotransmitter or **ligand** and causes the signal to be transduced (passed along). A ligand is a small molecule that can fit into pocket-like binding sites on the three-dimensional protein structure of the receptor, much as a key fits into a specific lock. Classical neurotransmitters are small molecules, such as monoamines or amino acids, that act as ligands for specific receptors. Many psychiatric medications work by acting as ligands that fit into the same binding sites as naturally occurring neurotransmitters.

Characteristics of the ligand-receptor interaction include saturability, specificity, and reversibility. **Saturability** means that the finite number of receptors on a cell surface is eventually filled up. (Using the lock-and-key analogy: if there are 10 locks available, 10 keys can open 10 locks, but 20 or 50 keys will still open only 10 locks.) **Specificity** is one of the most important criteria for receptors, since many biological small molecules can bind avidly to various tissues or even inert surfaces such as glass. A receptor should bind to specific ligands rather than to a random assortment of substances. A subset of specificity is **stereoselectivity:** if the ligand has stereoisomers, the receptor should bind to one much more avidly than to its mirror image. A putative receptor that binds both equally, like a glove that fits either hand, would have its receptor candidacy gravely questioned. **Reversibility** means that a neurotransmitter should bind reversibly to its receptor without permanently altering it. Although some drugs can alter a receptor's structure or functioning irreversibly, naturally occurring neurotransmitters generally function by binding to and dissociating from receptors in an ever-changing dance of temporary partnerships. Any newly discovered endogenous substance that purports to be a ligand for a receptor should fulfill at least these three criteria.

After the ligand binds, the receptor needs to effect a biological response—this "effector" component can be on the same protein as the binding site or on a closely associated protein. Receptors are generally classified into "superfamilies" based on their effector strategy. All known postsynaptic neurotransmitter receptors belong to one of two families: the ion channel receptors and the G-protein–coupled receptors. The difference in strategy between these receptors is of clinical relevance because drugs acting at fast, ion channel receptors can be expected to have immediate effects (eg, benzodiazepines acting at the GABA$_A$ receptor quickly quelling convulsions), whereas drugs acting at slow G-protein–coupled receptors cannot be expected to have effects in the time it takes the ligand to bind to the receptor (eg, most antipsychotics and antidepressants acting at dopamine and serotonin receptors).

Ion channel receptors (also known as ionophores or ionotropic receptors) can be called class I or "fast" receptors because binding by the neurotransmitter directly activates an ion pore and can mediate millisecond responses. Structurally, all ion channel receptors are made up of four or five protein subunits, like little barrels arranged in a tight rosette, forming a "pore" in the membrane. When activated by a ligand, the receptor changes its conformation to increase or decrease passage of a specific ion through the pore. An inhibitory neurotransmitter allows a negative ion such as chloride to enter the neuron, making the cell interior more electrically negative and therefore less likely to fire. An excitatory neurotransmitter allows a positive ion such as sodium or calcium to enter the cell. The ligand-gated ion channel superfamily includes the GABA$_A$ and N-methyl-D-aspartate (NMDA) receptors, activated by the most common inhibitory and excitatory neurotransmitters, respectively, in the central nervous system.

G-protein–coupled receptors (also known as metabotropic receptors) can be called class II or "slow" receptors, because of the number of steps involved from ligand binding to signal transduction. Structurally, all these receptors consist of a single protein whose polypeptide chain folds back and forth across the cell membrane seven times: for this reason, these receptors are also known as **seven-transmembrane receptors.** The intracellular "tail" of the receptor binds to a G-protein, from a class of proteins whose activity is controlled by guanine nucleotides (conversion of guanosine trisphosphate [GTP] to guanosine diphosphate [GDP]). These G-proteins then act on **nucleotide cyclases,** which catalyze the conversion of a nucleotide triphosphate to a "second messenger." The most common example is adenylate (or adenylyl) cyclase, which catalyzes the conversion of adenosine triphosphate (ATP) to cyclic adenosine monophosphate (cAMP), which travels through the cytoplasm spreading the message. G-proteins can act by stimulating (G$_s$-proteins) or inhibiting (G$_i$-proteins) the adenylate cyclase system, or by working through other second messenger systems such as phospholipase C. Second messengers then cause a host of other effects: activating protein kinases, phosphorylating ion channel receptors, affecting microtubular assembly and cytoskeletal structure, or changing gene expression by inducing synthesis of messenger RNA. Obviously, these changes can have longer lasting effects on neurons. G-protein–coupled receptors of interest to psychiatry include receptors for dopamine, norepinephrine, and serotonin, as well as opiates and most of the neuropeptides.

The difference in strategy between these two superfamilies can be compared to the difference between a telephone call and a television show. Ion channel receptors provide immediate, one-to-one communication that requires no further processing, like a telephone call. G-protein–coupled receptors are not as fast or direct, but their multiple steps in processing allow the signal to be amplified, just as a single speech, televised, can reach millions of viewers.

C. Termination: Termination of neurotransmitter activity may occur through three mechanisms. For most neurotransmitters, the primary mechanism is through active **reuptake** by specific transporters back into the presynaptic neuron. So far, these **transporter proteins** exhibit a structure similar to one another, with 12 transmembrane domains. Second, the neurotransmitters may be degraded by **specific enzymes within the synaptic cleft:** for example, acetylcholine is metabolized by acetylcholinesterase. Third, some of the neurotransmitter may simply diffuse away, into surrounding glial cells or into the extracellular fluid of the brain.

The steps in synaptic transmission are a dynamic flow: changes in one step affect other steps. A drug that initially exerts its specific action by causing increased neurotransmitter release, for example, can eventually cause the postsynaptic receptors to decrease their number or sensitivity. Acute effects may differ markedly from chronic effects once the central nervous system has attained a new state of equilibrium in the presence of the drug.

Regulation of Synaptic Transmission

As should be evident from the preceding description, chemical transmission can be regulated at each step, from presynaptic to postsynaptic to termination. **Synthesis** of a neurotransmitter can be controlled by varying the amount of precursors or by altering the activity of enzymes, particularly the **rate-limiting enzyme** (the pacesetter for the whole conveyor belt of synthetic steps). **Transport** and **storage** of neurotransmitters are subject to regulation by changes in microtubule, microfilament, and vesicle assembly. Regulation of **reuptake** of the neurotransmitter from the synapse back into the presynaptic neuron can be an effective way to control amounts of the transmitter in the synapse, as the popular antidepressant serotonin reuptake inhibitors can attest.

But much of the emphasis in research has been on the synapse itself: the release of the neurotransmitter into the synaptic cleft, alterations that can occur within the cleft, and then binding to the receptors on the other side. **Release** can be affected by presynaptic and postsynaptic inhibition, both directly and indirectly. In **presynaptic inhibition,** the released neurotransmitters may bind to autoreceptors on the same neuron or may feed back by an independent inhibitory presynaptic neuron. **Postsynaptic inhibition** may occur directly, as when an inhibitory neurotransmitter generates an inhibitory postsynaptic potential, or indirectly, during the refractory period after the action potential in the postsynaptic cell.

Within the cleft, specific enzymes may work to degrade the neurotransmitter before and after it reaches the postsynaptic neuron. We mentioned acetylcholinesterase, which degrades acetylcholine—a drug that inhibits this enzyme would increase the amount of acetylcholine available.

At the postsynaptic neuron, specific **receptors** are the site of action of many drugs. Since most neurotransmitters have several receptor subtypes, each with its own anatomic distribution and physiologic role, compounds that bind specifically to one subtype could have more specific effects than the neurotransmitter itself would have. Development of drugs with **specificity** or **selectivity** for a receptor subtype could therefore have fewer side effects than a less selective drug.

A compound being tested as a potential medication can be an agonist, antagonist, or inverse agonist at a particular receptor, depending on how the signal is transduced after the compound binds to the receptor. An **agonist** mimics or supports the actions of the naturally occurring neurotransmitter at the receptor. For example, the benzodiazepines are agonists at the $GABA_A$ receptor by increasing the efficacy of GABA. An **antagonist** blocks the effect of the endogenous neurotransmitter at the receptor, without causing a signal to be transduced. It can antagonize the neurotransmitter either by competing for the same binding site or by changing the conformation of the protein to make binding unfriendly. An example of competitive antagonism would be the dopamine-blocking actions of most antipsychotics. An example of noncompetitive antagonism would be the change in conformation that occurs when phencyclidine (PCP) binds to the NMDA receptor. (In general, agents developed for psychiatric use prefer competitive versus noncompetitive antagonism, because an equilibrium can be reached between the drug and the endogenous neurotransmitter.) A receptor that is activated at baseline can also be regulated by an **inverse agonist** that causes effects directly opposite to those of the neurotransmitter. Rather than simply preventing the neurotransmitter from binding, the inverse agonist causes an opposing signal to be transduced. Not all receptor systems have inverse agonists, since it requires the system to already be activated constitutively. To add to the complexity, drugs can have a combination of activities at specific receptors—for example, an antagonist that has weak, partial agonist activity.

Note that the **affinity** of the compound for the receptor—how avidly it binds—does not indicate what the next step of signal transduction will be. A compound with high affinity for a receptor could be an agonist or antagonist depending on its effect on the subsequent steps in signal transduction. A compound's affinity does indicate whether the compound requires high or low concentrations to compete with the naturally occurring neurotransmitter, so drugs are often compared with one another by their binding affinities at a particular receptor subtype. Affinity is typically expressed as the concentration of drug needed to occupy half of the available receptors: thus a lower number would indicate a drug with higher affinity, since it would need only a low concentration to saturate half the receptors. These concepts are now common enough that pharmaceutical companies prominently feature affinity data for receptor subtypes in advertisements for their new agents.

But as we have cautioned, the immediate effects of drug binding to receptor are often not enough to explain their effects. Long-term changes in postsynaptic **sensitivity** (degree of neuronal response) may occur through a change in the absolute number of available receptors or through a change in the function of the receptor complex. It is this change in receptor sensitivity that is thought to be involved in the development of drug tolerance and dependence.

Because the proteins of the receptor complex exist in the cell membrane, the fluidity of the lipid bilayer is also a site of regulation of neuronal activity. Localized areas of the membrane may rapidly become less or more fluid, primarily as a function of phospholipid methylation, which could then force more receptors into the synapse or could separate the receptors more widely.

After receptor binding, there can be a whole cascade of events subject to regulation. Medications acting on the cascade could have wide-ranging regulatory effects. As we discussed in our description of G-protein–coupled receptors, signal transduction in this superfamily requires a complex cascade of steps and systems, with each step in each system a potential target for drug action. Signal transduction and second messenger systems use a diverse array of strategies and substances: protein kinases and phosphorylation, phosphatidylinositol, arachidonic acid metabolites such as prostaglandins, ions such as calcium, and even gases such as nitric oxide and carbon monoxide.

NEUROTRANSMITTERS

Neurotransmitters can be classified into three general categories: monoamines, amino acids, and peptides. **Monoamines,** also known as biogenic amines, include dopamine, norepinephrine, and epinephrine (collectively known as the catecholamines for their common chemical structure), serotonin, acetylcholine, and histamine. **Amino acids** include GABA, glycine, and glutamate. **Peptides** include the endorphins (or endogenous opioids) and many hormones important to other organs in addition to the brain, such as cholecystokinin, angiotensin II, neurotensin, and corticotropin-releasing hormone. We will focus first on the neurotransmitters most commonly referenced in psychiatry, some of the monoamines, and amino acid neurotransmitters. Neurohormones and peptides are discussed separately in the section on psychoneuroendocrinology because of major conceptual differences between their function and that of the classical neurotransmitters.

We have organized the neurotransmitter section in a consistent manner, with categories of interest to both clinicians and researchers. Each neurotransmitter's description begins with a short summary of its major role in the normal brain. The **synthesis** and **degradation** or metabolism of each neurotransmitter are of interest for both diagnosis and treatment: neurotransmitter activity can be measured indirectly through the activity of its synthetic enzymes or its products of metabolism, and medications can target both synthesis and metabolism. Since synthesis is usually a series of steps using multiple enzymes, we highlight the role of the rate-limiting enzyme, which sets the pace for synthesis. The anatomic **pathways** or distribution of a neurotransmitter in the brain—where it works—are important in understanding how it works. Most neurotransmitters have multiple **receptors** or receptor subtypes, each differing in its sensitivity, distribution, and response to specific medications. Next, there are short discussions of the role each neurotransmitter is thought to play in **psychiatric illnesses** and the actions of **psychiatric medications.** Table 6–1 is a quick aid for studying and organization, but both the table and text are, of necessity, simplified for conciseness. Students interested in a more complete picture are referred to some of the references at the end of this chapter.

Dopamine

Dopamine, together with its close relative norepinephrine, mediates motivation, arousal, and the reward-reinforcement system. Alterations in dopamine neurotransmission contribute to the pathogenesis of schizophrenia and Parkinson's disease. Many drugs of abuse appear to increase amounts of dopamine in the synapse: some investigators have proposed dopamine as a final common pathway in addictions and novelty-seeking behavior.

A. Synthesis and Degradation: Dopamine is synthesized through a number of enzymatic steps from the amino acid tyrosine. The rate-limiting enzyme is tyrosine hydroxylase. Dopamine is metabolized primarily by monoamine oxidase (MAO) and then catechol-O-methyltransferase (COMT) to homovanillic acid (HVA, whose levels in blood and cerebrospinal fluid can therefore provide an indirect measure of dopamine levels). There are two types of monoamine oxidase in the central nervous system, with MAO-A more selectively metabolizing norepinephrine and serotonin and MAO-B more selectively metabolizing dopamine. In the synapse, dopamine neurotransmission is also terminated by reuptake into the presynaptic neuron by a selective **dopamine transporter,** a protein with 12 transmembrane domains. Drugs such as cocaine that inhibit this transporter therefore increase the amount of dopamine in the synapse.

B. Dopaminergic Pathways: There are multiple dopaminergic pathways in the central nervous system, whose neuronal cell bodies are mainly found in the substantia nigra and ventral tegmental areas. The pathways can be classified by the length of their projections from cell body to target. The major pathways of interest to psychiatry have long projections: the nigrostriatal, mesolimbic, and mesocortical pathways.

1. The nigrostriatal pathway—The nigrostriatal pathway has cell bodies in the substantia nigra that project to the striatum (caudate nucleus and putamen).

Table 6–1. Guide to neurotransmitters.[a]

Neurotransmitter	Made from (Enzyme)	Metabolized to (Enzyme)	Where Mainly Found	Receptor Types	Neuropsychiatric Disorders	Psychiatric Medications
Dopamine (DA)	Tyrosine (*TH*)	HVA (*MAO-B, COMT*)	Nigrostriatal mesolimbic	D_1 and D_5 D_2, D_3, D_4	Schizophrenia, Parkinson's	Antipsychotics
Norepinephrine (NE)	Dopamine (*DβH*)	MHPG (*MAO-A, COMT*)	Locus ceruleus, lateral tegmental	$\alpha_{1(A-D)}$ $\alpha_{2(A-D)}$ β_1 β_2	Depression, mania, panic	MAOIs, TCAs, amphetamines, clonidine
Serotonin (5-HT)	Tryptophan	5-HIAA (*MAO-A*)	Raphe nuclei	$5\text{-HT}_{1(A-F)}$ $5\text{-HT}_{2(A-C)}$ 5-HT_3 5-HT_{4-7}	Depression, suicide, impulse control	SSRIs
Acetylcholine (ACh)	Choline, acetyl-CoA (*CAT*)	Choline, acetyl-CoA (*AChE*)	Nucleus basalis of Meynert	Nicotinic, muscarinic (M_{1-5})	Alzheimer's	Selegiline, side effects of many medications
GABA	Glutamate (*GAD*)	Succinic acid (*GABA-T*)	Ubiquitous, inhibitory interneurons	$GABA_A$ (multi subtypes) $GABA_B$	Anxiety disorders, alcoholism	Benzodiazepines, barbiturates
Glutamate	Multi: glutamine, aspartate	Multi: GABA	Ubiquitous	NMDA, non-NMDA (kainate, AMPA, etc) $mGluR_{1-8}$	Schizophrenia, stroke, brain injury	Ketamine

[a] This oversimplified table does not include many important neurotransmitter and neurohormone systems, such as opioids, glycine, histamine, neurotensin, and CCK. In the second and third columns, the substrate or metabolite is listed first, with the rate-limiting enzyme in italics.
Abbreviations: HVA, homovanillic acid; MAO, monoamine oxidase; MAOI, MAO inhibitors; COMT, catechol-O-methyltransferase; DβH, dopamine-β-hydroxylase; MHPG, 3-methoxy-4-hydrox-yphenylglycol; TCAs, tricyclic antidepressants; 5-HIAA, 5-hydroxyindoleacetic acid; SSRIs, selective serotonin reuptake inhibitors; GABA-T, γ-aminobutyric acid transaminase; NMDA, N-methyl-D-aspartate; AMPA, α-amino-3-hydroxy-5-methylisoxazole-4-propionic acid; mGluR, metabotropic glutamate receptors.

This pathway is involved in initiation and coordination of muscle movement. For psychiatrists, this pathway is of interest because of its importance in neuroleptic-induced movement disorders and tardive dyskinesia. Dopamine and acetylcholine share a dynamic balance in this pathway: patients with diseases characterized by increased abnormal movements, such as Huntington's chorea and Tourette's syndrome, appear to have a relative excess of dopamine and deficiency of acetylcholine; with diseases characterized by difficulty initiating voluntary movements, such as Parkinson's disease, the reverse imbalance exists. Tardive dyskinesia may be due to the development of tolerance in the nigrostriatal system to chronic treatment with haloperidol and other antipsychotic drugs, which does not appear to develop in mesocortical dopamine systems.

2. The mesolimbic pathways—In the mesolimbic pathways cell bodies near (medial and superior to) the substantia nigra project to the limbic system (including the nucleus accumbens, amygdala, and piriform cortex). These neurons appear to respond to drug administration in a manner similar to nigrostriatal neurons. Dopaminergic activity in the nucleus accumbens, considered by some researchers to be the "reward center" of the brain, may mediate the addictive effects of many illicit drugs.

The **mesocortical pathways** project from the same area to the cortex (medial prefrontal, cingulate, and entorhinal areas). Specific subsets of these pathways (eg, mesoprefrontal, mesocingulate) may be distinguishable by their higher rate of physiological activity (bursts of firing) and their lack of tolerance to chronic antipsychotics, possibly mediated by a lack of autoreceptors on their neurons. The mesolimbic and mesocortical pathways are of particular interest to psychiatrists because of their involvement with emotions and complex behaviors. Schizophrenia may involve relative excesses of dopamine or hypersensitivity in these pathways.

3. Other dopaminergic pathways—Other dopaminergic pathways have shorter projections from cell body to target. The **tuberoinfundibular** (or tuberohypophyseal) pathway has cell bodies in the arcuate nuclei and periventricular area that project to the hypothalamus and posterior pituitary. This pathway mediates release of prolactin, which can cause side effects such as galactorrhea and menstrual irregularities in patients taking neuroleptic medications. The **medullary periventricular** pathway has cell bodies in the motor nucleus of the vagus nerve and the nucleus tractus solitarii. The projections are not well defined, but this pathway may be involved in the control of food intake. A group of **incertohypothalamic** neurons projects from the dorsal and posterior hypothalamus to the dorsal anterior hypothalamus and the lateral septal nuclei. The role of these dopaminergic neurons is unknown.

C. Dopaminergic Receptors: Five types of dopamine receptors have been characterized. All are members of the G-protein–coupled receptor family. They are defined as D_1-like or D_2-like depending on their effect on adenylate cyclase activity, although there are other distinguishing features as well.

Stimulation of the D_1-**like receptors**—D_1 and D_5—increases the activity of adenylate cyclase, increasing amounts of cyclic AMP. They can also increase phosphoinositide turnover. D_1-like receptors have dramatically decreased affinity for antagonists than D_2-like receptors, and have been thought to be less important in antipsychotic function. D_1 receptors appear to be found extensively as exclusively postsynaptic receptors, playing little or no role as presynaptic autoreceptors. D_5 is very similar to D_1 in its molecular biology and pharmacology, but has a 10-fold higher affinity for dopamine and is found in a narrower distribution in the brain, primarily in limbic regions.

Stimulation of the D_2-**like receptors**—D_2, D_3, and D_4—either inhibits or has no effect on activity of adenylate cyclase. The gene for D_2, the first dopamine receptor to be cloned, contains a very large first intron, a likely target for recombination or mutation. This could increase the likelihood of its involvement in hereditary forms of human disease. D_2 receptors are found both pre- and postsynapses, and are rich in both nigral and striatal regions. The D_3 receptor is not as well characterized but it has a particularly high affinity for dopamine. Its messenger RNA (mRNA) is expressed prominently in the nucleus accumbens. The D_4 receptor first attracted considerable attention because it is found primarily in the frontal cortex and because clozapine—the first of the "atypical" antipsychotics—demonstrated a high affinity for this receptor. Interest intensified when some researchers found a selective increase in the D_4 receptor subtype in the brains of schizophrenic patients, fueling hope that this new receptor type could be the key to schizophrenia. However, the lack of selectivity of the ligand used in the study (which had high affinity for D_2 and D_3 as well as D_4) and the failure of other groups to replicate the findings dampened enthusiasm somewhat. Pharmaceutical interest in D_4 sagged further when D_4-selective antagonists did not demonstrate particular antipsychotic efficacy. The D_4 receptor gene is highly polymorphic in human populations, with perhaps dozens of different alleles (alternate forms of the gene). This has inspired intense efforts to correlate different D_4 alleles with various psychopathologies.

These subtypes are important in the development of medications. With traditional antipsychotic drugs, their affinity for D_2 receptors correlates almost perfectly with their antipsychotic efficacy. However, the more recently developed "atypical" antipsychotics such as clozapine and olanzapine have lower D_2 affinities and might exert some of their therapeutic effects at D_3, D_4, or serotonin receptors. The newer drugs appear to be more effective for some patients refractory to traditional antipsychotics, and have a different side effect profile, with less risk of movement disorders.

D. Dopamine and Psychiatric Illnesses: The dopamine hypothesis of schizophrenia proposes that patients with this illness have excessive activity in the dopamine system, particularly the D_2 receptors in the mesolimbic or mesocortical pathways. The major supports for this hypothesis are that the clinical potency of most antipsychotics correlates strongly with their ability to block D_2 receptors and that many drugs such as amphetamine and cocaine that can cause psychotic behaviors are known to increase the amount of dopamine in the synaptic cleft. Some schizophrenic patients appear to have low monoamine oxidase activity, which would reduce the rate of degradation of dopamine and thus increase its amount in the synapse. Postmortem examination of the brains of patients with schizophrenia has revealed an increased number of D_2-like binding sites; however, this may be partially attributed to the effects of neuroleptic medications.

Dopamine also plays a role in mood disorders, although to a lesser extent than norepinephrine. Dopamine levels have been found by some investigators to be low in some depressed patients and high in some manic patients.

E. Dopamine and Psychiatric Medications: Antipsychotics are the major drugs used to treat schizophrenia and other psychotic conditions. As discussed, these drugs are potent antagonists of dopamine receptors; however, other neurotransmitter systems are likely to be important as well. Many antipsychotics also significantly block serotonergic, α-adrenergic, histaminergic, and cholinergic receptors. Research continues into which of these pharmacological actions are therapeutic and which are responsible for specific side effects.

The major adverse side effects associated with traditional antipsychotics are movement disorders and the potential development of tardive dyskinesia. Although the balance with other neurotransmitters may play a role, tardive dyskinesia seems to result when chronic dopamine blockade by antipsychotics causes postsynaptic dopamine receptor hypersensitivity. As mentioned, newer antipsychotics, often with lower affinity at the D_2 receptors, appear to have a much lower incidence of these debilitating movement disorders.

Norepinephrine

Norepinephrine (also known as noradrenaline) plays a major role in regulation of mood, anxiety, and vigilance or arousal. In physiology it is often discussed together with its close relative epinephrine (also known as adrenaline), which is important in systemic autonomic arousal but appears to play a relatively minor role in the central nervous system.

A. Synthesis and Degradation: Norepinephrine, like its catecholamine relatives dopamine and epinephrine, is synthesized from tyrosine, initially sharing a common synthetic pathway, until dopamine is converted to norepinephrine by dopamine-β-hydroxylase (DβH). Epinephrine can then be produced from norepinephrine by phenylethanolamine-*N*-methyltransferase. Norepinephrine is metabolized by MAO (more selectively by MAO-A) and COMT to 3-methoxy-4-hydroxyphenylglycol (MHPG). In the synapse, the activity of norepinephrine is terminated primarily by reuptake by a 12-transmembrane presynaptic protein, in a process analogous to that of dopamine.

B. Noradrenergic Pathways: There are two large groups of noradrenergic neurons. Most are found in the **locus ceruleus** in the upper pons. These neurons project to the cerebral cortex, hypothalamic and thalamic nuclei, and limbic system. The **lateral tegmental neurons** are loosely scattered within the lateral ventral tegmental fields and may be an important source of noradrenergic fibers to the basal forebrain, hypothalamus, and amygdala.

C. Noradrenergic Receptors: Norepinephrine and epinephrine both bind to a common pool of receptors, which could therefore be called either noradrenergic or adrenergic receptors. All are G-protein–coupled receptors and are grouped into three major classes based on second messenger coupling. α_1-Receptors are coupled to phospholipase C, α_2-receptors to G_i (inhibiting cAMP production), and β-receptors to G_s (stimulating cAMP production). α_1-Receptors are primarily postsynaptic whereas α_2-receptors are presynaptic, reducing norepinephrine synthesis in the presynaptic neuron. Both α_1- and α_2-receptors can be divided into three subclasses of receptors, the functional roles of which are poorly understood. β-Receptors are mostly postsynaptic and activate adenylate cyclase when stimulated, with β_1-receptors binding more strongly to norepinephrine and β_2-receptors to epinephrine. Both β_1- and β_2-receptors predominate at the ends of locus ceruleus tracts and may regulate the α-receptor system. Understanding of the localization and function of β_3-receptors is still incomplete.

D. Norepinephrine and Psychiatric Illnesses: The first monoamine hypotheses of affective illness stated that underactivity of norepinephrine or serotonin may cause depression and that increased activity in these pathways could result in mania. This hypothesis first arose when researchers noted that reserpine, which depletes and inhibits storage of catecholamines and serotonin, causes depression. They then noted that effective antidepressant drugs increased the amount of catecholamines and serotonin in the synapse either by blocking their presynaptic reuptake or by blocking their degradation. This hypothesis has been revised to account for chronic changes in receptor activity and sensitivity in antidepressant therapy. Studies of patients after 1–3 weeks of antidepressant drug treatment have shown increased α_1-receptor sensitivity, increased norepinephrine release, and decreased postsynaptic β- and presynaptic α_2-receptor activity and sensitivity. Current models of mood disorder highlight the importance of disequilibrium in the noradrenergic system, rather than a simple overall increase or decrease in noradrenergic activity.

Norepinephrine is also involved in panic disorder. Yohimbine, a selective α_2-receptor antagonist, reproduces panic symptoms immediately in susceptible individuals. Research in schizophrenia has focused on the role of dopamine, but overactivity of norepinephrine may play a role as well.

E. Norepinephrine and Psychiatric Medications: The tricyclic antidepressants (TCAs) and the monoamine oxidase inhibitors (MAOIs) are strongly, although nonselectively, noradrenergic. As discussed, they are thought to exercise their therapeutic effects through this mechanism. They also have major side effects through the adrenergic system: tricyclic antidepressants and MAOIs can cause postural hypotension, dizziness, and reflex tachycardia, primarily mediated by α_1-receptors. Because MAOIs inhibit not only central nervous system MAO but liver and intestinal MAO as well, they have a unique side effect. The inability to break down tyramine in foods such as aged cheese, beer, or wine can cause a surge in adrenergic activity and possibly a dangerous hypertensive crisis.

Serotonin

Serotonin plays a key role in mood, the perception of pain, and basic activities such as feeding, the sleep-wake cycle, motor activity, sexual behavior, and temperature regulation. Serotonin is involved in the presynaptic regulation of the release of other transmitters and affects many endocrine functions, including prolactin, cortisol, growth hormone, and possibly β-endorphin release.

A. Synthesis and Degradation: Serotonin, also known as 5-hydroxytryptamine (5-HT), is synthesized through a number of enzymatic steps from the amino acid tryptophan. The first enzyme in this pathway is tryptophan hydroxylase, but the primary regulatory factor is the concentration of tryptophan available as precursor. Serotonin is metabolized by MAO (preferentially MAO-A) to 5-hydroxyindoleacetic acid (5-HIAA). Although only about 1–2% of serotonin is found in the brain (for example, platelets contain serotonin), it cannot cross the blood-brain barrier, so brain cells must synthesize their own.

B. Serotonergic Pathways: Serotonergic systems have extraordinarily widespread projections, suggesting a broad regulatory function. Serotonergic neurons are concentrated in the area of the median and the dorsal raphe nuclei, caudal locus ceruleus, area postrema, and interpeduncular area. Both the medial and dorsal neurons project to the thalamus, hypothalamus, and basal ganglia. The medial neurons also project to the amygdala, piriform cortex, and cerebral cortex. Descending fibers from this group of serotonergic neurons innervate the spinal cord and modulate sensitivity to pain input. Serotonergic antidepressants have been widely used clinically to control chronic pain.

The pineal body contains 50 times as much serotonin per gram as the whole brain and contains all the enzymes required for the synthesis of serotonin. Because melatonin is produced from serotonin, and because both undergo a daily rhythm driven by environmental lighting patterns, the serotonin content of the pineal body has been of considerable interest in the control of circadian rhythms. However, the pineal body also contains a number of neuropeptides and is innervated by the sympathetic nervous system, making it likely that other neurotransmitters also influence circadian rhythms.

C. Serotonergic Receptors: Currently, there are 14 known subtypes of serotonin receptors (5-HT$_{1A}$, 5-HT$_{1B}$, 5-HT$_{1D}$, 5-HT$_{1E}$, 5-HT$_{1F}$, 5-HT$_{2A}$, 5-HT$_{2B}$, 5-HT$_{2C}$, 5-HT$_3$, 5-HT$_4$, 5-HT$_{5A}$, 5-HT$_{5B}$, 5-HT$_6$, and 5-HT$_7$). They are grouped into classes and subclasses based on molecular structure and second messenger coupling, and differ in tissue distribution. All except 5-HT$_3$ are G-protein–coupled receptors. The major classes of current interest to psychiatry are 5-HT$_1$, 5-HT$_2$, and 5-HT$_3$.

The **5-HT$_1$ receptors** are negatively coupled to adenylate cyclase. 5-HT$_{1A}$ postsynaptic receptors are markedly localized within the hippocampus. 5-HT$_{1A}$ receptor agonists decrease anxiety and aggression in animals. In humans, 5-HT$_{1A}$ receptors may be involved in response to antidepressant treatment. 5-HT$_{1A}$ receptors are also thought to be involved in sexual behavior. 5-HT$_{1B}$ receptors are presynaptic autoreceptors that are located most densely in the substantia nigra and globus pallidus. As autoreceptors they work in a negative feedback manner to inhibit serotonin release. What were formerly called 5-HT$_{1C}$ receptors are now classified as 5-HT$_{2C}$, because they are coupled to phospholipase C. 5-HT$_{1D}$ receptors can be autoreceptors that inhibit serotonin release or postsynaptic receptors in the striatum.

The **5-HT$_2$ receptors** are coupled to phospholipase C. They are postsynaptic in the hippocampus, frontal cortex, and spinal cord. Psychotic symptoms seem to be associated with 5-HT$_2$ receptors, since 5-HT$_2$ agonists such as lysergic acid diethylamide (LSD) produce psychiatric symptoms and antagonists include atypical antipsychotics. One of the most consistent changes observed after antidepressant treatment is down-regulation of 5-HT$_2$ receptors, suggesting a possible role in depression, but neither 5-HT$_2$ agonists nor antagonists are established antidepressants, indicating that the down-regulation is not essential for the antidepressant effect.

The **5-HT$_3$ receptors** are ligand-gated ion channels, the only serotonergic receptors with this structure. They are found in the central nervous system in the entorhinal cortex and the area postrema and in peripheral neurons. In vivo and in vitro studies have shown that 5-HT$_3$ receptors inhibit the release of acetylcholine in the cortex but increase the release of dopamine in the striatal and mesolimbic system.

Thus, there has been some interest in the use of selective 5-HT$_3$ antagonists in the treatment of schizophrenia, anxiety, drug addiction, and pain.

The roles of 5-HT$_4$, 5-HT$_5$, 5-HT$_6$, and 5-HT$_7$ are currently under investigation. 5-HT$_4$, 5-HT$_6$, and 5-HT$_7$ are positively coupled to adenylate cyclase. 5-HT$_6$ may be involved in antidepressant action.

D. Serotonin and Psychiatric Illnesses: Serotonin is involved in regulation of mood, anxiety, and aggression. A simplified overview would state that low serotonin levels correlate with increased depression, aggression, suicide, and impulsivity. The actual situation is more complex, as serotonin has broad regulatory functions and low levels can destabilize many neurotransmitter systems.

Some researchers have also postulated a role for the serotonin system in schizophrenia. Major support for this hypothesis comes from the study of the potent hallucinogenic drug LSD, which has a very high affinity for 5-HT$_{2C}$ receptors. In addition, many of the atypical antipsychotics are potent blockers of serotonin receptors, particularly the 5-HT$_{2A}$ and 5-HT$_{2C}$ subtypes.

E. Serotonin and Psychiatric Medications: The first antidepressant drugs, the tricyclics, increased serotonergic function through the blockade of catecholamine and serotonin reuptake. The next generation of antidepressants was designed to be selective serotonin reuptake inhibitors (SSRIs), which became the most commonly prescribed antidepressants shortly after their introduction. The success of these agents as antidepressants has lent support to the connection between low synaptic serotonin levels and depression. They subsequently became useful in the treatment of panic disorders, obsessive-compulsive disorder, anorexia, and other related anxiety disorders.

Lithium, used in manic-depressive illness or bipolar depression, shifts the relationship between uptake and synthesis in the 5-HT system, making the system more "stable." The clinical observation that it takes at least a week for the therapeutic effects of lithium to appear, during which time the serotonergic systems are shifting to a new equilibrium, lends support to this hypothesis.

Acetylcholine

In the normal central nervous system, the cholinergic neurons are thought to modulate arousal, learning, memory, rapid eye movement sleep, pain perception, and thirst. It is the main neurotransmitter for the parasympathetic system. Perhaps the most significant role of the cholinergic system in disease occurs in Alzheimer's dementia.

A. Synthesis and Degradation: Acetylcholine is synthesized from choline and acetyl-coenzyme A by the enzyme choline acetyltransferase. Synthesis is regulated mostly by the availability of choline and somewhat by the concentration of acetyl-choline, which feeds back to the choline acetyltransferase enzyme. Acetylcholine is rapidly metabolized within the synaptic cleft by acetylcholinesterase without requiring initial reuptake. About half of the choline produced by this degradation is taken back into the presynaptic neuron.

B. Cholinergic Pathways: There are a large number of cholinergic pathways in the brain, some entirely within a particular brain structure and some projecting across regions. Of the projection pathways, the two most relevant to psychiatry are part of a large ascending system of cholinergic neurons originating in the reticular formation and projecting to the hypothalamus, thalamus, hippocampus, and neocortex. A specific concentration of cholinergic cells in the nucleus basalis of Meynert projects to the cerebral cortex.

C. Cholinergic Receptors: Acetylcholine receptors include structurally very different classes: muscarinic receptors in the G-protein–coupled family and nicotinic receptors in the ion channel family. The muscarinic receptors are named after their selectivity for the agonist muscarine (derived from poisonous mushrooms). Five subtypes (M_1, M_2, M_3, M_4, and M_5) have been identified and all are coupled to G-proteins. Nicotinic receptors are named for their selectivity for their agonist nicotine. They are much less common than muscarinic receptors in the central nervous system, but they are important in attention and cognition. These receptors belong to the ion channel receptor superfamily, with multiple subunits gathered around a central pore. Sixteen different subunits have been identified: α_{1-9}, β_{1-4}, δ, γ, and ε. They can cluster into different combinations to form a myriad of structurally unique receptors.

D. Acetylcholine and Psychiatric Illnesses: Acetylcholine plays an important role in learning and memory, and derangements in the cholinergic system are associated with Alzheimer's dementia. A specific destruction of the cholinergic neurons of the nucleus basalis of Meynert has been observed in at least a subgroup of patients with this disorder. Dementia in general is associated with a decrease in concentrations of acetylcholine in the temporal neocortex, hippocampus, and amygdala. Attempts to facilitate cholinergic function by increasing amounts of choline precursors, such as lecithin, in the diet have been disappointing, but clinical research on cholinergic agonists is continuing.

Dopamine and acetylcholine share a dynamic balance in the nigrostriatal pathway involved in the initiation and coordination of muscle movement. Parkinson's, characterized by inhibited voluntary movement, is associated with a relative deficiency of dopamine and an excess of acetylcholine, whereas Huntington's chorea and Tourette's syndrome, characterized by increased abnormal involuntary movements, are associated with a relative excess of dopamine and a deficiency of acetylcholine in this pathway. Recent research also implicates a genetic polymorphism in a nicotinic receptor subunit in a subset of schizophrenic patients.

E. Acetylcholine and Psychiatric Medications: Many commonly used psychiatric medications are anticholinergic and can cause a number of adverse side effects due to their blockade of the parasympathetic system. Many psychotropic drugs, including tricyclic antidepressants, monoamine oxidase inhibitors, and neuroleptics, have anticholinergic effects at the **muscarinic receptors** that lead to side effects such as blurred vision, dry mouth, sinus tachycardia, constipation, and urinary retention. Since antipsychotic medications block dopamine and can cause Parkinson's disease–like side effects in patients, these side effects can be treated with anticholinergic agents.

γ-Aminobutyric Acid

γ-Aminobutyric acid (GABA) is the most common inhibitory amino acid neurotransmitter, present in perhaps 60% of the synapses in the human central nervous system. In the normal brain, GABA systems are crucial to the moment-to-moment interactions of neurons, the braking system of the brain, in a sense. The GABAergic systems are important in anxiety, seizures, and in the actions of benzodiazepines, barbiturates, and alcohol.

A. Synthesis and Degradation: GABA is synthesized from glutamic acid (glutamate) by the enzyme glutamic acid decarboxylase (GAD). It is metabolized to an assortment of amino acids, including glutamate, and then eventually to succinic acid by GABA transaminase (GABA-T). Both GAD and GABA-T require pyridoxal phosphate as a cofactor for activity.

B. GABA-Containing Pathways: GABAergic neurons do not occur in discrete pathways, per se, but are widely distributed throughout the brain. High concentrations occur in inhibitory interneurons and in the substantia nigra, globus pallidus, hypothalamus, and cerebral and cerebellar cortices.

C. GABA Receptors: There are two families of GABA receptors in the central nervous system, $GABA_A$ and $GABA_B$. The $GABA_A$ receptor is more prevalent and has been extensively studied. It belongs to the family of ligand-gated ion channel receptors; when activated, it opens a chloride channel, inhibiting the firing of neurons by causing hyperpolarization. The $GABA_A$ receptor is made up of five subunits around a central pore. So far, at least 14 subunit subtypes have been identified (α_{1-6}, β_{1-3}, γ_{1-3}, δ, and ρ). In mammalian brain, most functional $GABA_A$ receptors consist of two α, one or two β, and one or two γ subunits. Different combinations of α, β, and γ subtypes could therefore form hundreds or thousands of unique receptors (for example, a receptor consisting of α_1, α_5, β_2, β_3, and γ_2). What is particularly exciting about the subtypes is their distinct distribu-

tion in the brain. For example, α_6 is found only in the cerebellum, whereas α_5 is found primarily in the hippocampus. This suggests targets for medications with selected actions and fewer side effects.

The $GABA_B$ receptor is present in lower levels in the central nervous system than the $GABA_A$ receptor and is a G-protein–coupled rather than an ionotropic receptor. Its physiological role should be better characterized soon, as it was recently cloned.

D. GABA and Psychiatric Illnesses: GABA is the most abundant inhibitory neurotransmitter in the brain and coexists in neurons with a wide range of neurotransmitters, including serotonin, dopamine, acetylcholine, glutamate, glycine, histamine, and peptides such as endorphins. GABA is postulated to have a direct role in anxiety disorders and alcoholism. Because of its wide-ranging regulatory role, GABA has also been implicated in the pathophysiology of schizophrenia, Huntington's disease, Parkinson's disease, epilepsy, tardive dyskinesia, and senile dementia. GABA is not likely to provide a "single-bullet" explanation for these disorders, but could be involved through its extensive interactions with other neurotransmitters.

E. GABA and Psychiatric Medications: Benzodiazepines, barbituates, and alcohol are all agonists at different sites on the $GABA_A$ receptor. As GABA agonists, they have widespread inhibitory effects, including inhibition of arousal, anxiety, memory, coordination, seizures, and respiration. Because they act at different, noncompeting sites, they are potentially synergistic when taken together, increasing the likelihood of dangerous side effects. Since current $GABA_A$ agonists are not selective for the subunit subtypes described, researchers hope to develop compounds targeting specific subunits.

A selective benzodiazepine antagonist, flumazenil, is useful clinically to treat overdoses, because it quickly and readily reverses the sedation and many other effects of benzodiazepine drugs. This compound has few effects when administered alone, as would be expected from a relatively pure antagonist drug.

Glutamate

Like GABA, glutamate is an amino acid neurotransmitter; but whereas GABA is inhibitory (the "brakes"), glutamate is the major excitatory neurotransmitter (the "gas pedal"). Studies of amino acid neurotransmitters are complicated by the widespread presence of these amino acids in blood and cerebrospinal fluid. Studies of glutamate have been particularly difficult because it is an important building block in the synthesis of proteins, plays an important part in the detoxification of ammonia in the brain, and serves as a precursor for GABA. Thus, although glutamate occurs in particularly high concentrations in the brain, it is not easy to estimate how much of this is functioning as a neurotransmitter and how much is serving in metabolic and other roles.

A. Synthesis and Degradation: Glutamate can be synthesized from a number of different immediate precursors and amino acids: it can be synthesized from 2-oxoglutarate and aspartate by aspartate aminotransferase, from glutamine by phosphate-activated glutaminase, or from 2-oxoglutarate by ornithine aminotransferase. Synthesis can by regulated by the accumulation of precursors such as glutamine or by end-product inhibition.

B. Glutamatergic Pathways: Like GABA, glutamate is widely distributed in the central nervous system, rather than existing in discrete pathways. As mentioned previously, glutamate serves an important metabolic role in addition to its role as a neurotransmitter. Glutamate receptors are particularly enriched in the hippocampus and cerebral cortex.

C. Glutamate Receptors: Like GABA receptors, glutamate receptors include members of the metabotropic (G-protein–coupled) and ionotropic superfamilies. Glutamate is an agonist at all of these receptors. Eight metabotropic glutamate receptors, divided into three groups, have been identified, but have not been as well studied as the ionotropic receptors. Group I, including $mGluR_1$ and $mGluR_5$, is linked to phospholipase C, whereas groups II and III are negatively coupled to adenylate cyclase. Group I is under intense investigation for possible roles in neurological and psychiatric disorders.

The ionotropic glutamate receptors are divided into NMDA and non-NMDA receptors. The NMDA receptor binds to the amino acid N-methyl-D-aspartate. It has received much attention because it has been implicated in diverse processes such as memory acquisition, developmental plasticity, epilepsy, and ischemic brain injury. As an ion channel receptor, it is made up of subunits that appear to have distinct binding sites for glutamate, glycine, phencyclidine (PCP), magnesium, and zinc.

Non-NMDA ionotropic glutamate receptors include receptors that bind kainate and α-amino-3-hydroxy-5-methylisoxazole-4-propionic acid (AMPA, also known as quisqualate). AMPA receptors and kainate receptors have a distribution in the brain parallel to that of NMDA receptors.

D. Glutamate and Psychiatric Illnesses: As mentioned, much of the attention surrounding glutamate and excitatory amino acids has been directed at the specific subtype of glutamate receptor known as the NMDA receptor. In normal brain, the NMDA receptor mediates long-term potentiation, an increase in synaptic efficiency that underlies memory and learning. However, NMDA receptor hyperfunction, like a gas pedal applied during a traffic jam, causes an excitotoxic "glutamate cascade," magnifying the cell damage caused by hypoglycemia, hypoxia, and seizures. Conversely, NMDA hypofunction, such as that produced by NMDA antagonists, can cause hallucinations and dissociation from reality. Some investigators believe that the behavioral and cellular effects of PCP and other NMDA receptor antagonists could serve as a model for schizophrenia and psychotic illnesses (see discussion below).

E. Glutamate and Psychiatric Medications: Although there was initially some hope that antagonists to excitatory amino acids could be neuroprotective, this approach has turned out to have problems of its own. A class of NMDA receptor antagonists (including the anesthetic drug ketamine and the illicit hallucinogen phencyclidine) stops the glutamate cascade but causes damage to cortical neurons in animals.

PSYCHONEUROENDOCRINOLOGY

Psychoneuroendocrinology is a subspecialty of endocrinology that takes into account the fundamental relationships among central nervous system biology, behavior, and the endocrine system. Reciprocal interactions between immune and neuroendocrine systems indicate that a complete understanding of biological and behavioral relationships between the central nervous and endocrine systems is dependent on immune function as well. Although beyond the scope of this review, receptors for hormones, neurotransmitters, and neuropeptides exist on immune cells, as do receptors for cytokines in the nervous system and in endocrine glands. Each system can affect the regulation of another, in both immediate and more extended time frames. The classical chemical messengers of the endocrine system are the hormones, which are released into the systemic circulation and may exert effects in the body far distant from their site of release. The three major structural classes of hormones are the steroids, peptides, and amino acids; it is the peptide class that has attracted the most interest in psychoneuroendocrinology, although recently, neuroactive steroids are receiving increased attention. These compounds, which include allopregnanolone and tetrahydrodeoxycorticosterone (THDOC), rapidly alter CNS excitability and are anxiolytic, theoretically through their effects on $GABA_A$ and NMDA receptor complexes.

As mentioned previously, the peptides coexist with the biogenic amines in presynaptic terminals and are released along with the biogenic amines when the neurons containing them are stimulated. They therefore function as cotransmitters; formerly, it had been thought that only one neuroregulator existed in any one type of cell. Given the importance of the biogenic amines in human behavior, the relationship between the two classes of compound is thought to be important and is the subject of ongoing research. Peptides can act as neuromodulators and neurohormones at distant sites or may have local effects similar to those of classical neurotransmitters. Many of these peptides are also involved in regulation of the traditional hormonal axes: for example, corticotropin-releasing hormone and adrenocorticotropic hormone are peptides that regulate the cortisol axis. Others, such as neurotrophins, are signaling molecules that regulate neuronal development and potentiate synaptic function throughout life, possibly serving as key factors in learning-induced synaptic plasticity.

An important quality distinguishing peptides from classical neurotransmitters is their polymorphism: at least nine endogenous opioids and five forms of cholecystokinin are now known.

Synthesis & Degradation of Peptides

The synthesis of neuropeptides involves transcription of DNA in the cell nucleus to form RNA, whose translation guides the production of proteins in the cytoplasm. Both transcription and translation are under multiple regulatory controls. The product of translation is a precursor protein that is metabolized into active components by peptidases, a step also subject to regulatory control. This system allows many peptides to be derived from a single gene product. The peptides are then transported, stored, and released in a manner similar to that described for conventional neurotransmitters. The action of the peptides is terminated by the action of peptidases.

Peptides & Psychiatric Illnesses

In contrast to monoamines and amino acids, peptide neuroregulators can act at sites more distant from their site of release, can affect neuronal function over a longer period of time, can modulate rather than directly transmit messages, and can coordinate complex behaviors rather than simply activate single cells.

The basic role of neuroendocrine systems (and the peptides in particular) in psychiatric disorders is still largely unknown. Neuroendocrine abnormalities have been identified in some psychiatric disorders; these may represent markers of dysfunction or may themselves be directly responsible for pathophysiological changes.

Central Nervous System–Hypothalamic–Anterior Pituitary Axis

The basic organization of the central nervous system–hypothalamic–anterior pituitary axis involves input from the limbic system and cortex to the hypothalamus, which in turn releases releasing factors and inhibitory factors affecting the pituitary. The pituitary then releases trophic hormones that may stimulate the peripheral glands to release hormones. All of the released products have the potential to provide feedback regulation to previous components of the axis. Although the following sections discuss the hypothalamic factor and pituitary trophic hormones under the heading of the final hormones of their systems, many of the substances have been found to exist elsewhere than in the hypothalamus, and many may have direct effects unrelated to their hormonal action.

A. Cortisol: The cortisol axis is important in the physiological response to stress and may be involved in the control of mood and behavior. In addition to its direct hormonal actions, cortisol also regulates protein synthesis and modulates production of synthetic enzymes in the central nervous system.

The regulatory controls in the levels of cortisol are corticotropin-releasing hormone (CRH) and adrenocorticotropic hormone (ACTH). A diurnal variation in ACTH and cortisol levels occurs in humans, with peak cortisol levels occurring around 6:00–7:00 AM. Both ACTH and CRH exist in the central nervous system outside the hypothalamus. Extrahypothalamic ACTH is found in the brainstem, thalamus, and limbic system, where it may play a modulating role in attention, memory, and learning. The role of extrahypothalamic CRH is not clear.

Because of the crucial role of the cortisol axis in the stress response, it is not surprising that it also has a role in mood and behavior. Patients with hypercortisolism (Cushing's syndrome) may have depression, mania, confusion, and psychotic symptoms. Apathy, fatigue, and depression are common symptoms in hypocortisolism (Addison's disease). High cortisol levels with loss of the usual diurnal variation in levels have been reported mainly in patients with depression, but also in some patients with mania, obsessive-compulsive disorder, schizoaffective disorder, or eating disorders. A subgroup of depressed patients has also demonstrated an attenuated ACTH response to CRH stimulation. When CRH is administered centrally in animals, it causes behavioral effects similar to those observed in animal models of anxiety and depression. Exposure to severe stress or experimentally induced exposure to glucocorticoids at critical stages in early development can cause lifelong alterations in stress responsivity and affect growth, and development and immune system function in adulthood. If stress-induced elevations in glucocorticoid level are sustained, neuronal survival may decrease; some studies have shown a relationship between high levels of glucocorticoids and hippocampal atrophy in both animal models and illnesses such as depression and posttraumatic stress disorder. CRH antagonists are currently being evaluated as possible therapeutic agents in the treatment of anxiety and depressive disorders.

B. Gonadal Regulatory Steroids: The primary role of the gonadal regulatory system is the regulation of gonadal steroid hormone production, with specific reference to puberty, the menstrual cycle, and menopause.

The peptides involved in the regulation of production of estrogens, progesterone, and androgens are gonadotropin-releasing hormone (GRH), luteinizing hormone (LH), and follicle-stimulating hormone (FSH). GRH exists primarily in the hypothalamus, but is also found in the amygdala and midbrain. It is structurally similar to thyrotropin-releasing hormone. There is evidence that GRH functions as a neuromodulator and that it has both inhibitory and excitatory effects on postsynaptic cells. Its primary effect is on sexual behavior; however, it may also be involved in the general control of alertness and anxiety as well as in early development of the central nervous system.

The gonadal regulatory system is involved in several psychiatric illnesses. Disturbances in regulation are undoubtedly involved in premenstrual syndromes and there is evidence for dysregulation of the hypothalamic–pituitary–gonadal axis and peri- and postmenopausal women with endogenous depression and in postpartum depression. Anorexia nervosa is characterized by a reversion to prepubertal patterns of secretion of the gonadal regulatory system, with low levels of GRH and no circadian or monthly variation in hormone levels. There is evidence that estrogens have an antidepressant effect in some women, and antiandrogens have been used in the treatment of male sex offenders to decrease aggression as well as sexual drive. The observation that many serious mental illnesses have their onset at puberty may be related to the dramatic changes in the gonadal regulatory system that occur at this time. Estrogens may also have a protective effect in delaying age-related decrements in cognition. A relative testosterone deficiency has been linked to decreased libido in both men and women, but it is unclear at present whether testosterone supplementation provides behavioral benefits to men in the context of normal aging-related declines in function.

C. Thyroid Hormones: In addition to its traditional endocrine functions, the thyroid regulatory system may play a role in the regulation of mood, since the regulatory peptides and hormones of the thyroid system are able to regulate the number of available central nervous system β-adrenergic receptors. The thyroid regulatory system is known to play a critical role in central nervous system development, as shown by the profound neurological and other abnormalities seen in perinatal hypothyroid states.

The peptides involved in the regulation of triiodothyronine (T_3) and thyroxine (T_4) production are thyrotropin-releasing hormone (TRH) and thyrotropin. Thyrotropin-releasing hormone is widely distributed outside the hypothalamus in the cerebral cortex, brainstem, spinal cord, periventricular area, amygdala, and basal ganglia. It is released from neurons on stimulation and therefore has neurotransmitter-like properties. It generally has an inhibitory effect on postsynaptic cells. It is thought that thyrotropin-releasing hormone is involved in the regulation of mood and behavior in addition to and independently of its traditional endocrine role.

A number of psychiatric symptoms can be associated with thyroid system dysfunction. In adults, hyperthyroidism may cause anxiety, restlessness, and irritability, although an "apathetic" hyperthyroidism characterized by depression and withdrawal may also occur, especially in geriatric patients. Hypothyroid states are characterized by depression, cognitive impairment, confusion, and psychosis. A blunted thyrotropin response to infusions of thyrotropin-releasing hormone has been noted in about one-third of patients with major depression, and abnormal augmented responses have been found in many depressed women. In these women, there is frequently an increase in antithyroid antibody titers. Addition of T_3 and T_4 as supplements to antidepressant treatment has been shown to accelerate response in some patients, particularly women, and can be effective in treating patients who have failed to respond to antidepressants alone. Some studies have documented a poor response to antidepressants in patients who have preexisting thyroid abnormalities and others have documented a relationship between normalization of thyroid function and beneficial response to antidepressant treatment.

D. Growth Hormone: The peptides regulating the release of growth hormone are growth hormone–releasing factor and somatostatin (growth hormone–inhibiting factor). Recently, another receptor has been identified indicating an additional endogenous regulatory factor. Obviously, gross disorders of growth hormone regulation result in acromegaly or dwarfism; less obvious are behavioral effects associated with more subtle variations in growth hormone–releasing factor or somatostatin.

Release of growth hormone increases with exercise and in times of stress; there is also a sleep-associated release pattern. The growth hormone response to growth hormone–releasing factors is altered in depression and in anorexia nervosa, as is the normal sleep-associated release pattern.

Somatostatin is found in high concentrations outside the hypothalamus, particularly in the cerebral cortex and amygdala, but it is also found in the brainstem, basal ganglia, and hippocampus. It has been demonstrated that somatostatin is released from neurons on stimulation and serves as a potential neurotransmitter or neuromodulator; it may also have an inhibitory effect on postsynaptic neurons. The behavioral effect of somatostatin is to decrease activity and increase sedation. A significant alteration in somatostatin regulation may account for many of the neuroendocrine changes noted in major depressive illness, and the role of somatostatin as a possible neuromodulator of acetylcholine may be important in the mechanism of Alzheimer's disease.

E. Prolactin: The controls regulating the release of prolactin are prolactin-inhibiting hormone, prolactin-releasing hormone, TRH, vasoactive intestinal peptide, and GABA. Prolactin bears certain structural similarities to growth hormone. Prolactin levels are increased during pregnancy and nursing as well as during sleep and exercise. Neuroleptic antipsychotic medications cause a marked increase in circulating prolactin because they block the tuberoinfundibular receptors for dopamine, which may function physiologically as prolactin-inhibiting hormone. Hyperactivity of the prolactin regulatory system may lead to lethargy, irritability, and increased thirst, all of which can sometimes be side effects of neuroleptic medications.

F. Melanocyte-Stimulating Hormone: The regulatory peptides for melanocyte-stimulating hormone are melanocyte-stimulating hormone release-inhibiting hormone and melanocyte-releasing hormone. Little is known about the role of these substances in the central nervous system; however, melanocyte-stimulating hormone may be involved in learning and memory, and there have been a few reports that melanocyte-stimulating hormone and melanocyte-stimulating hormone release-inhibiting hormone have an antidepressant effect.

Central Nervous System– Hypothalamic–Posterior Pituitary Axis: Vasopressin & Oxytocin

Vasopressin (also known as antidiuretic hormone) and oxytocin are two very similar peptides, each made of nine amino acids with internal 1,6-disulfide bridges. They differ from each other in only two amino acids in their sequences. Both are synthesized in the supraoptic nuclei and paraventricular nuclei of the hypothalamus, which send projections to the posterior pituitary, from which the hormones are released into the circulation. Both have well-known peripheral hormonal effects: vasopressin increases blood pressure and facilitates water reabsorption in the distal tubules of the kidney, and oxytocin stimulates uterine muscle contractions. Both have also been identified as neurotransmitters in the central nervous system, where they may have a variety of behavioral effects. The two hormones are derived from two different precursors, which also produce two specific carrier proteins. These carrier proteins may themselves have independent effects on the central nervous system.

Vasopressin is thought to play a role in attention, memory, and learning. Neurons containing vasopressin project to the anterior pituitary and into the cerebrospinal fluid through cells ending in the third ventricle. Release of vasopressin is increased by pain, stress, exercise, morphine, nicotine, and barbiturates and is decreased by alcohol. Inappropriate secretion of vasopressin can be induced by various psychopharmacological agents but, for unclear reasons, can also occur spontaneously in psychiatric patients. A number of specific agonists and antagonists of vasopressin have been developed, and their use in experimental animals has suggested possible antidepressant effects of vasopressin as well as what appears to be a key role in mammalian bonding behavior. Elevations in central vasopressin have also been associated with a life history of aggressive behavior in humans and aggression in rodents.

Oxytocin has been shown to be released by neurons and may function as a neurotransmitter. It appears to have an inhibitory effect on postsynaptic cells. Intriguingly, oxytocin has also been implicated in mammalian bonding behavior, particularly in the initiation and maintenance of maternal behavior, social bonding, and sexual receptivity.

Central Nervous System–Pineal Gland Axis: Melatonin

Melatonin seems to be central to the regulation of circadian rhythms and sexual maturation. It is synthesized from serotonin in the pineal gland by the action of serotonin-*N*-acetylase and 5-hydroxyindole-*O*-methyltransferase. The major regulator of melatonin synthesis is the light-dark cycle, with synthesis increased during darkness. Regular fluctuations in the production of melatonin occur even without light-dark cues, but the cycle is longer. Because the pineal gland also contains many other peptides, including vasopressin and luteinizing hormone–releasing hormone, it is likely that melatonin interacts with many other hormones and transmitters in complex ways. The pineal gland appears to be regulated by a major β-adrenergic mechanism, and β-antagonists such as propranolol decrease melatonin synthesis. The fact that melatonin has both synchronizing and phase-shifting properties in the regulation of biological rhythms has led to its usage in treatment of "jet lag" and insomnia.

Other Central Nervous System Peptides

A. Endogenous Opioids: These are peptides found endogenously in the body that have pharmacological properties similar to morphine, with its well-known effects on pain perception, behavior, and various physiological responses. There are now known to be three major branches of the endogenous opioid peptide family, classified by their precursor proteins: the proopiomelanocortin (POMC)-derived peptides, the proenkephalin-derived peptides, and the prodynorphin-related peptides.

The **POMC-derived peptides** include β-endorphin, the most potent of the natural opioids, which is approximately 50–100 times as potent as morphine in its behavioral effects. The POMC precursor is a large nonopioid protein that can be processed different ways in different regions of the brain: in the corticotropin-secreting cells of the anterior pituitary, POMC is processed largely to corticotropin and to an inactive form of β-endorphin, while in the intermediate lobe cells and arcuate neurons, POMC is processed to melanocyte-stimulating hormone and active β-endorphin. That the same precursor is processed variously into opioids and hormones involved in the cortisol axis and the pineal gland–melatonin axis suggests that opioids are involved in regulation of pain, anxiety, and memory; indeed, β-endorphin release is shown to be increased by stress. Neurons containing β-endorphin have long projections and are mostly found within the endocrine-oriented systems of the medial hypothalamus, diencephalon, and pons.

The **proenkephalin-derived peptides** are expressed in neuronal systems wholly separate from the POMC neurons. Met-enkephalin and Leu-enkephalin are two very similar five-amino-acid peptides that differ only in their fifth amino acid. Both are widely distributed throughout the central and peripheral nervous systems. Their precursor, proenkephalin, produces the two peptides in a 6:1 ratio of Met- to Leu-enkephalin.

The **prodynorphin-derived** peptides include four major peptides, called dynorphin A, dynorphin B, and two neoendorphins, α and β. All are potent opioid agonists. As with the proenkephalin-derived peptides, the prodynorphin-derived peptides are widely distributed in neurons with short projections.

Opiate receptors are classified by their specificity for agonists and antagonists as well as by their effects. The μ receptor has morphine, opiate alkaloids, β-endorphin, and enkephalins as agonists. The δ receptor is the receptor for enkephalins, while the κ receptor is the receptor for dynorphin. The σ receptor is different from the other opiate receptors in that naloxone does not reverse agonist activity. Phencyclidine, haloperidol, and steroids are agonists at the σ receptor and indicate that σ receptors play a role in motor function and possibly drug abuse.

The general role of the endogenous opioids includes the regulation of pain, anxiety, and memory. Other likely effects include regulation of sexual activity, feeding, temperature, and blood pressure. A variety of endogenous opioid abnormalities have been reported in schizophrenia, affective illnesses, and eating disorders. Treatment of psychiatric disorders with both opioid agonists and antagonists (eg, naloxone in the treatment of childhood autism) have thus far yielded conflicting results.

B. Substance P: Substance P appears to modulate pain perception and possibly motor control. It may be the principal neurotransmitter for the primary afferent sensory fibers from the dorsal root ganglion to the substantia gelatinosa of the spinal cord. Substance P is found in particularly high concentrations in the hypothalamus, median eminence, and basal ganglia; it is also found in the brainstem, amygdala, hippocampus, and cerebral cortex. Substance P is released from neurons on stimulation and serves as a possible neurotransmitter, with excitatory effects on postsynaptic cells. Levels of substance P have been reported to be markedly reduced in patients with Huntington's chorea.

C. Cholecystokinin: In addition to its role as a gastrointestinal hormone, cholecystokinin (CCK) has been shown to be released from central nervous system neurons and appears to function as a neurotransmitter. This peptide is found in high concentrations in the hippocampus and cerebral cortex as well as in the brainstem, basal ganglia, hypothalamus, and amygdala. It may partially mediate the sensation of satiety, although the role of peripheral CCK, which is released from distended intestines, needs to be carefully distinguished from the role of central nervous system CCK. It may play a role in anxiety, since it is shown to exist within many GABA-containing intracortical neurons. CCK antagonists have shown some efficacy in animal models of anxiety and in preventing panic attacks precipitated by CCK analogs. Its coexistence with dopamine in the nucleus accumbens septi argues for a role in the pathophysiology of schizophrenia. Some researchers have also found an apparent opioid antagonist action of CCK without direct effects at the opiate receptors; this action could be used to enhance opioid analgesia with inhibitors of CCK.

D. Vasoactive Intestinal Peptide: Vasoactive intestinal peptide is another gastrointestinal peptide hormone that appears to function in the central nervous system as a neurotransmitter, although its role in the central nervous system is not known. It is structurally similar to glucagon.

Vasoactive intestinal peptide is found in particularly high concentrations in the hippocampus and the cerebral cortex; it is also found in the brainstem, basal ganglia, hypothalamus, and amygdala.

E. Angiotensin II: In addition to its role in the peripheral modulation of blood pressure, the angiotensin system appears to be active in the central nervous system. Angiotensinogen is converted by renin into angiotensin I (a decapeptide), which is then cleaved by a converting enzyme to angiotensin II (an octapeptide), which can then be converted to angiotensin III (a seven-amino-acid peptide). All of these substances and the enzymes for their conversions are present in the brain, although angiotensin II has received the most attention. The angiotensin system in the brain is concentrated in the periventricular region. Behavioral effects are being investigated; thus far the main effect discovered is a dramatic stimulation of water drinking when small amounts of angiotensin II are injected into the third ventricle. Angiotensin-converting enzyme inhibitors have been very useful in controlling hypertension; they have also been reported, through unknown central effects, to have antidepressant properties.

F. Neurotensin: Neurotensin is thought to regulate pain, sensitivity, arousal, and body temperature; it may also regulate inhibitory modulation of dopaminergic activity. It is found in the highest concentration in the hypothalamus and substantia nigra as well as in the nucleus accumbens septi, septal area, spinal cord, brainstem, interneurons of the substantia gelatinosa, and the motor trigeminal nucleus. Neurotensin may have reward-enhancing effects in the central nervous system through its antidopaminergic actions in the prefrontal cortex and possesses some neuroleptic activity through its decreasing affinity of the D_2 agonist binding site.

DIRECTIONS IN RESEARCH

The changes within one generation in psychopharmacology and drug development strategy have been dramatic: from serendipitous discovery to rational drug design. For example, to current medical students it is almost unimaginable that not long ago, antipsychotic efficacy in new compounds could be inferred only if a drug caused extrapyramidal symptoms in animals. In other words, before neurotransmitters and their receptor systems were characterized, it was impossible to identify a likely anti-psychotic except by the presence of one of its most dreaded side effects. The rapid acceleration in development of new medications is made possible by numerous advances in technology and neuroscience.

The revolution in **molecular biology,** gathering speed from its beginning, is now poised to explode. Three basic techniques of molecular biology, cloning (reproducing a selected segment of genetic information), sequencing (identifying and reading the molecular structure of a gene), and genetic engineering (controlling and altering gene expression) have developed and interacted to produce powerful methods of neuroscientific exploration.

Cloning short sequences of DNA and amplifying them into large quantities, in a process called polymerase chain reaction, makes it possible to obtain genetic information from tiny amounts of blood or even hair follicles. This technology has found widespread applications, from medicine to the criminal justice system. Cloning of an entire genome to produce genetically identical organisms has now been achieved in complex mammals such as sheep and mice.

Genetic sequencing has advanced at a dizzying rate. Studies of quantitative trait loci (using selective breeding for a quantifiable trait or behavior) have allowed us to identify previously unsuspected genes that may govern these traits. Obviously, this technique cannot be used in humans. The human genome project, scheduled for completion soon, will identify the sequence of the entire human genetic code. It is estimated that there are on the order of 100,000–140,000 genes, approximately 70% of which are expressed in the central nervous system. One-third of the genes appear to be expressed only in the brain. As newly discovered sequences are homologous to genes for known receptors, we are already discovering new neurotransmitter systems. Elucidation of their function will clearly have profound implications for psychiatry. The challenge will be to correlate these genes to illnesses or behaviors in the human population. Two complementary approaches are being used. Linkage analysis compares the entire genome of two phenotypically different groups. The candidate gene approach starts with a known receptor or protein and looks for differences between two populations.

Early genetic engineering, in which recombinant DNA was introduced into cells not normally expressing a specific protein, was vital to the isolation and characterization of neurotransmitter receptors. Targeted mutations of a single nucleotide helped demonstrate the specific sites important to receptor function. Genetic engineering has now progressed to germ line alterations in complex animals such as mice. Transgenics (in which a particular gene is added or overexpressed) and knockouts (in which a particular gene is inactivated) now include animals lacking entire receptor subtypes, such as 5-HT_{2C}. This technology has even progressed to inducible knockouts in which a gene can be turned off in a particular stage of development or a particular brain structure.

The advances in molecular biology have generated vast quantities of information. What has made it possible to interpret and use this information are advances in **computer technology.** Computer-aided drug design, systematically substituting different R groups around a molecular backbone, can predict possible medications based on three-dimensional models of neurotransmitter-receptor interactions. Large libraries of compounds can then be produced using high-speed automated synthesis. These compounds can be tested in high-throughput screening for binding to known neurotransmitter receptors. Genetic information can also undergo highly automated screening, using two-dimensional "gene chip" arrays, whose assembly is borrowed from microchip manufacture. Computers are obviously vital to processing information, but are also important to communicating it. The internet and web-based genome scans allow scientists, instantaneously and regardless of geography, to check new sequences against the accumulated knowledge of the worldwide scientific community.

One challenge of translating neuroscience to clinical applications has been studying brain function in humans without excessively invasive techniques. **Neuroimaging** has progressed from exclusively structural descriptions to investigating brain function during active tasks. Positron emission tomography (PET) and single-photon emission computed tomography (SPECT) use radioactively labeled compounds such as glucose or neurotransmitters to look at activated brain regions. Functional magnetic resonance imaging (fMRI) uses the different magnetic properties of oxyhemoglobin and deoxyhemoglobin to monitor cerebral blood flow and thus areas of activation without using radioactive compounds. Magnetic resonance spectroscopy (MRS), a technology in early development, can be used to study many compounds and neurotransmitters using their magnetic resonance, potentially combining some of the advantages of PET and fMRI. Clearly neuroimaging will continue to be a dynamic area of research.

It is a truly amazing era for research in neuroscience and psychopharmacology. The study of neurotransmitters and their receptors has fueled much of the current revolution in psychopharmacology. The next step could be a paradigm shift from palliative treatment to potential cures for major mental illnesses.

REFERENCES & SUGGESTED READINGS

General References

Barondes SH: *Molecules and Mental Illness.* Scientific American Library, 1999. A lively and lavishly illustrated introduction to neurochemistry suitable for all backgrounds.

Blum K, Noble EP (editors): *Handbook of Psychiatric Genetics.* CRC Press, 1997. A useful guide for understanding background, methods, and recent findings in psychiatric genetics.

Cooper JR, Bloom FE, Roth HR (editors): *The Biochemical Basis of Neuropharmacology,* 7th ed. Oxford University Press, 1996. The definitive textbook on neuropharmacology.

Hardman JG et al (editors): *Goodman & Gilman's The Phar-macological Basis of Therapeutics,* 9th ed. Mc-Graw-Hill, 1996. The classic clinically oriented pharmacology reference, which has been updated to include molecular pharmacology.

Kandel ER, Schwartz JH, Jessell TM (editors): *Essentials of Neural Science and Behavior.* Appleton & Lange, 1995. An excellent textbook in neuroscience with emphasis on relevant neurophysiology.

Original Sources and Other References

Biggio G et al: *GABA-A Receptors and Anxiety, From Neurobiology to Treatment: Advances in Biochemical Psychopharmacology.* Vol 48. Raven Press, 1995. A comprehensive guide to GABA-A receptors, part of a multivolume series in psychopharmacology.

Bunzow JR et al: Cloning and expression of a rat D2 dopamine receptor cDNA. Nature 1989;342(6252):865. A landmark paper heralding an era of cloning and characterizing neurotransmitter receptors.

Freedman R et al: Linkage of a neurophysiological deficit in schizophrenia to a chromosome 15 locus. Proc Natl Acad Sci USA 1997;94:587. An intriguing finding that potentially links nicotinic receptor subunits to a subset of patients with schizophrenia.

Jacobs BL (editor): Special Supplement Issue Serotonin 50th Anniversary. Neuropsychopharmacology 1999;21. Numerous articles focusing on the latest in serotonin research, including an excellent introductory overview.

Koob GF, Nestler EJ: The neurobiology of drug addiction. J Neuropsychiatry 1997;9:482. A descriptive overview of the neurobiological effects of drug use that may contribute to addiction.

Lieberman JA, Sheitman BB, Kinon BJ: Neurochemical sensitization in the pathology of schizophrenia: Deficits and dysfunction in neuronal regulation and plasticity. Neuropsychopharmacology 1997;17(4):205. A relevant overview of the neuropathophysiology of schizophrenia.

Mossner R, Lesch KP: Knockout mice in neuropsychopharmacology: Present and future. Int J Neuropsychopharmacol 1998;1:87. A good introduction to an exciting new technique used in understanding the central nervous system.

Palfreyman PG, Reynolds IJ, Skolnick P (editors): *Direct and Allosteric Control of Glutamate Receptors.* CRC Press, 1994. A definitive guide to the glutamate receptor; part of a multivolume series in pharmacology and toxicology.

Tang YP et al: Genetic enhancement of learning and memory in mice. Nature 1999;401(6748):63. Intriguing research on NMDA receptor subunit NR2B, demonstrating the therapeutic potential of genetic engineering.

Wisden W et al: The distribution of 13 GABA-A receptor subunit mRNAs in the rat brain. I. Telencephalon, diencephalon, mesencephalon. J Neurosci 1992;12(3):1040. A pivotal paper demonstrating the distinct distribution of GABA-A subunits in the brain.

Social & Cultural Aspects of Health, Illness, & Treatment

7

Gerard J. Hunt, PhD, & Lonnie Snowden, PhD

This chapter will discuss a number of social factors that influence (1) the etiology and course of illness, (2) the decision to seek treatment and the kind of treatment sought, (3) the treatment itself, and (4) the patient's response to treatment and its outcome. The social factors that will be considered include age, sex, race, socioeconomic status, marital status, family situation, ethnicity, and cultural beliefs. The following case illustrates how social factors interact with biological and psychological aspects of people's lives to produce specific outcomes.

ILLUSTRATIVE CASE

Mrs V, a 45-year-old, married, Mexican-American woman, comes to the emergency room at 11:00 AM following a fall in her home at 3:00 AM. She reports that she got up to go to the bathroom and, in the dark, instead of turning left to go down the hall, walked straight ahead and fell down a half flight of stairs, hitting her head and knocking herself unconscious. She had lived in this house for 14 years and had walked to the bathroom at night many times.

Mrs V was born in Mexico. She has been living in the United States as a citizen for the past 15 years with her husband, who is American born and owns his own small business. Recently, Mrs V's mother died in Mexico, and Mrs V returned there for the funeral and a visit with her family. She has no relatives in the United States.

Her husband, who accompanied her to the emergency room, reports that he heard her fall; when he found her she was alert but she lost consciousness twice as he attempted to help her back up the stairs to bed. He called 911; Mrs V was examined by the paramedics but refused hospitalization.

The following morning she was still dizzy and somewhat nauseated and at the urging of her physician, who was contacted by her husband, she went to the emergency room. Over the next 8 hours vital signs were taken every half-hour, blood work was done, she was x-rayed for possible spinal injury, and a CT scan of the head was performed. Her husband remained with her the entire time.

Although all tests proved negative, she was admitted overnight for observation, and in the morning the attending neurologist making rounds agreed with the resident's preliminary diagnosis of "postconcussive syndrome." She was released and returned home.

Comment: A household fall that could have produced serious injury fortunately ended without major sequelae. However, some salient questions remain unanswered. Why did Mrs V fall? Why did she fall on this particular night? What was going on in her life at the time of the accident, and how likely is it that she will be at risk for another accident or illness?

And whose responsibility is it to ask these questions? The emergency room physician? The neurology resident who saw Mrs V in the emergency room? The attending neurologist? The internist who was called by her husband? If you were one of these physicians, what questions would you ask Mrs V? What hypotheses would you have about her fall?

SOCIAL FACTORS & THE BIOPSYCHOSOCIAL MODEL

It is difficult to deal with social factors apart from biological and psychological ones. Could Mrs V have had a transient disruption in brain functioning that caused momentary disorientation as she walked to the bathroom? Could she have been under some psychological stress that influenced the operation of her central nervous system response? Could that stress have been connected to the recent death of her mother and her visit to Mexico? Could all of these factors be interacting with each other simultaneously to produce the fall?

Although we do not have complete answers to these questions, evidence is accumulating that the biological, psychological, and social factors in people's lives interact to influence every aspect of the phenomena of health and illness, the treatment of illness, and the response to treatment.

THE INFLUENCE OF SOCIAL FACTORS ON THE ETIOLOGY & COURSE OF ILLNESS

Age, Sex, Race, Socioeconomic Status, & Ethnicity

A. Age: Persons in different age groups are at risk for different illnesses and health problems. Congenital abnormalities and premature birth contribute to most deaths of infants during their first year. Many of these are related to maternal risk factors during pregnancy such as poor nutrition, smoking, the use of alcohol and other drugs, pregnancy after age 38, and lack of prenatal care. Young persons die mostly from accidents (primarily automobile accidents) and suicide. People over the age of 65 suffer predominantly from chronic illnesses such as arthritis, hypertension, and heart disease. Rates of severe cognitive impairment are higher than those found in younger age groups, but rates of other mental illnesses appear to be lower, perhaps the result of underreporting and lower rates of detection (Scott-Lennox and George, 1996).

Life expectancy for all Americans has been increasing over the past 100 years and by 2050 about 22.8% of the population will be 65 years old or older. In 1900, life expectancy in the United States was 47 years, compared to 75 years at present. This improvement and the decline in the rate of infant mortality from 16% in 1900 to approximately 1% at present can be attributed to a number of social factors including improvements in the standard of living for all Americans and the improved quality and quantity of available health care services (Treas, 1995).

B. Sex: American women live longer than men. In 1990, the average life expectancy for white women was 79 years compared to 72 years for white men. Nonwhite women live to be about 74 years on average and nonwhite men to about 66 years (National Center for Health Statistics, 1996).

The differences in longevity between men and women appear to result from an interaction of physiological, psychological, and social processes. Prenatal and neonatal death rates for boys are higher than for girls, indicating a physiological vulnerability. Men typically die in greater numbers from accidents and under violent circumstances and, until recently, may have experienced greater cultural pressure to succeed, with the stress that accompanies such a mandate.

Women have been reported to utilize medical care in greater numbers than men (National Center for Health Statistics, 1996), with at least one study finding many of these visits to be for gynecological and obstetrical problems as well as for preventive care (Gijsbers van Wijk et al, 1992).

There are also differences in the kinds of mental illness suffered by men and women. Survey research shows that women tend to suffer from anxiety and depressive disorders, whereas men are more prone to substance abuse disorders (National Center for Health

Statistics, 1996; Kessler et al, 1994). The total prevalence of mental illness seems to be about the same in men and women, although, again, women are more likely than men to seek help for it (National Center for Health Statistics, 1996).

C. Race: Of the 15 leading causes of death at present in the United States, differences in the death rates between African-Americans and whites have been found in 14. Racial differences are particularly pronounced in the higher rates of death among African-Americans from AIDS, homicide, kidney diseases, diabetes, and conditions of newborns (Collins, 1995). Thus, African-American infants have twice the mortality rate of white infants (2% compared to 1%). Differences in social position account partly, but not entirely, for differences in disease-specific and overall mortality rates (Lillie-Blanton et al, 1996). African-Americans are more likely than whites to lack insurance coverage and a usual source of health care (Weinick et al, 1997) and, as a consequence, are less likely during a given year to have received any health care (Snowden et al, 1997).

Despite relatively high levels of stress and high mortality rates among African-Americans, few racial differences have been documented in the prevalence of mental illness or substance abuse (Zhang and Snowden, in press). They do, however, experience high rates of homelessness and institutional confinement, particularly confinement to mental hospitals and prisons. Furthermore, African-Americans who are mentally ill and suffer from chemical dependency reside disproportionately outside of households surveyed in epidemiologic studies.

D. Social Class: Social class is expressed in terms of occupational rank, income, education, and social status. Increasingly, the concept is understood to apply not only to individual people, but also to the households and neighborhoods in which they live (Krieger et al, 1997). In the United States, social class is a major factor in the development and course of many illnesses. In general, for all age groups, high social class is correlated with increased life expectancy and low social class is correlated with increased vulnerability to illness and death. Persons of lower socioeconomic status have been shown to be more susceptible to illnesses such as hypertension, arthritis, upper respiratory infections, speech difficulties, and eye diseases (Krieger et al, 1997).

Breast cancer may not follow the general rule that the lower the social class, the higher the incidence of illness and mortality. Krieger (1990) found the rate to be higher among non–working-class women in a study controlling for age and race.

In the United States and other "Western" countries death rates from cardiovascular disease have been declining since the mid-1960s. The decline has been greater for younger age groups, whites, and persons of higher socioeconomic status (Weiss and Lonnquist, 1997). Men and women of lower occcupational status have been shown to suffer from significantly elevated rates of hypertension (Waitzman and Smith, 1994).

Socioeconomic factors are powerful contributors to the risk of coronary heart disease and cardiac death. Williams et al (1992) found that patients with chest pain and those with documented coronary heart disease showed decreased survival if they had yearly incomes of $40,000 or less, were unmarried, and were without a confidant. Similarly, Case et al (1992) reported that patients who survived a myocardial infarction and who had less than 12 years of education or who were living alone showed an increased risk of both fatal and nonfatal heart attacks following discharge from a coronary care unit. In both these studies, the results were independent of a number of medically relevant factors. The two studies also indicate that social support may play a positive role in recovery from coronary heart disease. More will be said below about the importance of family and social support in treatment outcomes and rehabilitation.

Mental illnesses are also strongly associated with social class, with the highest rates of mental illness consistently being found among the lowest social classes (Kessler et al, 1994). People at low levels of income or education, for example, had rates of psychiatric disorder almost four times the rates found among people at high levels of income or education (Basic Behavioral Science Task Force, 1996). Living under adverse conditions increases the numbers of social stressors, which increases the incidence of mental illness among the poor; in turn, the resulting downward social mobility, or "social drift," leads persons with mental illness to become increasingly poor (Dohrenwend, 1992).

E. Ethnicity: Susceptibility to disease varies among ethnic groups in the United States. High rates of alcoholism have been reported for persons of Irish and Scandinavian descent and for Native Americans and low rates for persons of Asian background. Ashkenazi Jews have a higher incidence of diabetes, Tay-Sachs disease, and a variety of other metabolic diseases and African-Americans have a higher incidence of hypertension and sickle cell disease than the general population. More will be said later about the important role of ethnicity in health, illness, and the treatment of illness.

This information about the effect of social factors on the etiology and course of illness and mortality is valuable to a physician because, when a patient arrives for treatment, the major social categories into which the patient falls provide clues to the kinds of disease(s) that might be present. Even if a "typical" disease is not found for a particular patient, knowing the potential vulnerabilities of that patient prompts the doctor to educate the patient in preventive measures—particularly the benefits and methods of early detection.

On the basis of the above information, to what illness(es) might Mrs V in the illustrative case be susceptible, and what preventive counseling would you provide to her?

The Effect of Family on the Development & Course of Illness

Family influences the development and course of illness in at least three ways. First, a family's lifestyle strongly defines a person's patterns of eating, drinking, and use of tobacco, alcohol, and other drugs. Attitudes toward body size, cleanliness, and preventive health measures are learned at an early age and reinforced within the family context. If all members of a family are overweight, or if all smoke or abuse alcohol, the chances increase that new members will incorporate these behaviors to the detriment of their present and future health (Must et al, 1992).

Second, a family can influence the health and illness of its members by its patterns of interaction. Family therapy interventions into the ways in which family members interact have been shown to improve treatment outcomes for children with problems of conduct disorder and aggression, and for adults with phobias and with schizophrenia (Shadish et al, 1993).

Third, a family may act as a buffer against certain kinds of illnesses. Several studies have demonstrated a higher risk of myocardial infarctions and cardiac death in coronary heart disease patients who were unmarried, lived alone, or lacked a confidant (Case et al, 1992; Williams et al, 1992; Malcolm and Dobson, 1989). King et al (1993) found that the perception of support on the part of coronary artery patients and their spouses was related to emotional and functional outcomes. In a number of studies access to emotional support has been linked to a better adjustment among persons diagnosed with various forms of cancer (Helgeson and Cohen, 1996).

The mechanisms by which family interaction assists in lowering its members' vulnerability to illness are not completely clear. However, there is considerable evidence that the presence of various social supports has a positive influence on psychological states as well as on less severe infectious diseases, possibly through the influence of increased immune functioning (Cohen, 1996). Conversely, there is evidence that perceived psychosocial stress, particularly in the absence of social supports, contributes to both physical and psychological illness (Cohen, 1996). What questions might you ask Mrs V about her relationship with her family in Mexico, her marriage, and the social supports in her life at present?

THE INFLUENCE OF SOCIAL FACTORS ON THE DECISION TO SEEK TREATMENT & THE TYPE OF TREATMENT SOUGHT

Physical Illness

Because physicians and patients experience sickness differently, it is helpful to distinguish between "disease" and "illness." Disease can be defined as a malfunctioning in the physiological operation of the organism (Weiss and Lonnquist, 1997). It is disease that is usually identified by the physician. Illness is a morbid subjective state experienced by the patient. Clearly, there can be disease without illness, as in the case of hypertension, which exhibits no symptoms, and there can be illness without disease, as when a patient complains of not feeling well and the physician can find no organic malfunction.

This distinction is important in considering what people do when they experience illness. Age, sex, race, and socioeconomic class all influence a person's reactions to symptoms of illness. The leading cause of death for adult males between 30 and 60 years is myocardial infarction. However, what people do when they experience chest pain varies. Although 56% arrive at the hospital within 4 hours after the occurrence of symptoms, 16% arrive more than 14 hours after they have noticed chest pain. Problems with transportation account for only about 10% of these cases (Cohen-Cole, 1990).

Becker and his colleagues (1993) found that although emergency medical response time was the same for both whites and African-Americans experiencing cardiac arrests, African-Americans were less likely to have a "witnessed" cardiac arrest and were less likely to receive CPR from a bystander. They were also less likely to be admitted to a hospital and about three times more likely than whites to die from the heart attack.

Older people tend to seek help less readily than younger patients, and older women are particularly slow in seeking help for chest pain, most probably because they are less likely than men to believe that their symptoms are connected with heart disease.

Lower-class persons are also slower to seek treatment than their upper-class counterparts. Financial problems and difficulties with transportation may account for some of these variations. Medicaid and Medicare have reduced, to some extent, financial obstacles to medical care for the elderly, the disabled, and the poor (Cohen et al, 1994). Although minorities may have gained ground in access to medical care during the 1980s, research indicates that African-Americans, Asians, and Hispanic-Americans do not fare as well as whites on measures of access (Cornelius, 1993).

Mental Illness

As with physical illness, social factors play an important role in a person's decision to seek treatment for mental or emotional illness. A widely used framework to understand factors that promote or deter mental health services use is that of Anderson (1995). According to Anderson, seeking treatment occurs because of three kinds of determinants: population determinants, including factors that predispose services use (eg, gender, low sense of shame), enable services use (eg, health insurance), and indicate a need for

treatment (eg, occurrence of panic attacks); determinants related to the mental health care delivery system; and determinants existing in larger political, economic, and physical environments.

Some people seek help for emotional and mental illnesses on their own; others must be manipulated or even coerced into treatment by family and friends. The more bizarre and disruptive the symptoms, the more likely it is that the person will seek care or be forced to accept it.

Social variables seem to exert their strongest influence on *where* rather than *whether* a person seeks help for an emotional illness (Cockerham, 1986). Social networks have been found to be instrumental at times in guiding people to professional help for physical as well as emotional problems. This network is often composed of small groups of friends and/or relatives who have received help for the kind of problem the person is facing (Pescosolido, 1992; Worthington, 1992; Ballard et al, 1993).

INFLUENCE OF SOCIAL FACTORS ON TREATMENT & ITS OUTCOME

To provide effective treatment, physicians, in addition to the required technical skills, must possess skills in generating healing exchanges between themselves and their patients. Because virtually all forms of medical care involve interaction between two or more people, an understanding of how social factors influence treatment will assist the physician in developing and honing these skills.

Patients want two things from their doctors: technical competence and an indication of caring. Regarding the first, patients insist that their physician make an accurate diagnosis and implement or recommend an effective treatment regimen (Robbins et al, 1993; Hill et al, 1992; Sanchez et al, 1992).

However, these studies also indicate that patients want to know that the physician is interested in them and their ideas and beliefs about their illness. It is here that problems arise. One study indicated that physicians interrupted their patients within the first 18 seconds of their interview, leaving the patients feeling that the physician did not get to hear their story and therefore did not understand their most important problems (Beckman and Frankel, 1984). The devotion by the physician of enough time to obtain a shared understanding with patients and to involve them in the management of their illness has been associated with positive views of the encounter by both doctor and patient (Arborelius and Dremberg, 1992). However, increased time may be a necessary but not a sufficient condition to produce effective communications between physicians and patients. Some physicians' styles of relating to patients may not change even when more time is available (Ridsdale et al, 1992).

Compliance

Noncompliance with medical advice has been documented to vary between 15% and 93%, with studies showing that about one-third to one-half of all patients are noncompliant (Weiss and Lonnquist, 1997). Morris and Schulz (1993) found that patients evaluate and use medication not simply on the basis of its clinical effectiveness, but on how it affects all aspects of their lives including physical, economic, psychological, and social influences.

Sherbourne et al (1992) found that patient satisfaction with the interpersonal quality and financial aspects of their care was positively related to their adherence to a physician's advice. However, satisfaction with only the technical quality of care was negatively associated with how patients with heart disease adhered to their physicians' recommendations.

Patients with mental illness who formed a therapeutic alliance with their therapists within the first 8 months of treatment were significantly more likely than those who did not make this connection to remain in treatment, to comply with prescribed recommendations for medication, and to achieve better overall outcomes after 2 years (Frank and Gunderson, 1990). When treating persons suffering from depression, mental health specialists are more likely than general medical practitioners to permit shared decision making about treatment (Wells et al, 1996). Physicians may be able to improve their patients' compliance by taking their patients' perspectives into account when prescribing medications and making other recommendations for treatment (Rost et al, 1989). Training in these areas has assisted physicians in developing skills that have produced improved patient outcomes (Cohen-Cole and Bird, 1986).

With this as a background, the next section examines how interactions between physicians and patients have been conceptualized. The more physicians appreciate the social context of the patients' lives, the better they will be able to understand their patients' world view including their attitudes toward and beliefs about their illnesses. Communicating this understanding to patients will make them feel that the physician is interested in them and cares about them as persons and not just as "subjects" or "cases."

Patient & Physician Roles: Complementary or Conflicting?

Parsons (1951) outlined the general norms that govern being sick in this society. Essentially, two "expectations" and two "privileges" accompany this "sick role." Sick people are expected (1) to be motivated to get well and (2) to seek competent help for their problem. In return, they (1) are not held responsible for their illness and (2) are exempted from their customary social duties and responsibilities.

For the physician, Parsons similarly notes two privileges and five obligations. Privileges include (1) access to physical and emotional intimacy with the patient and (2) professional dominance. Obligations include (1) acting for the welfare of the patient, (2) being guided by standards of ethical professional behavior, (3) applying professional skills and knowledge as competently as possible, (4) being objective and emotionally detached, and (5) engaging in professional self-regulation.

Extending Parsons' thinking, Szasz and Hollander (1956) outline three models within which they believed physicians and patients might interact: (1) activity-passivity, (2) guidance-cooperation, and (3) mutual participation. Acting within the first model, the doctor does something to the patient, who usually is a passive recipient. Clinically, this is illustrated by emergency medical illness or acute trauma. In the second type of interaction, the physician tells the patient what to do, and the patient cooperates by doing it. The treatment of acute illness is an example of this type of interaction. In the third instance, the physician helps patients to help themselves—each is a partner in the effort to get well. Rehabilitation of the patient with chronic disabilities is the applicable clinical situation.

Although these models provide a beginning in conceptualizing the interaction between physicians and patients, they have been criticized for not fully exploring the complexity of the encounter and for attributing too much power and control to the doctor. According to Parsons, the imbalance in the relationship is caused by the difference in competencies between physicians and patients. In matters of health, physicians are said to have more learning and technical expertise than patients. Furthermore, when ill, an emotional dependency may arise that might place a patient in a subordinate role vis-à-vis the doctor. Thus, Parsons and his colleagues argued for a "professional dominance" in the encounter between physician and patient.

Although the preceding may be an accurate description of the connection between physician and patient in acute and emergency care conditions, it might not apply so readily in chronic care situations. In the latter cases, the patient may indeed know more about his or her condition than the physician and may actually be more adept at handling it. Under these conditions, the physician may become a *consultant* to the patient, seeking to add knowledge and expertise to what the patient has already acquired. For example, an athlete with chronic musculoskeletal impairments may know more than the physician about what warm-up exercises to perform, what activities will exacerbate pain and limit motion, and when to rest. However, he or she may need consultation on the effects of a medication or an intercurrent illness on the musculoskeletal system.

Critics have also pointed out that these models fail to deal with interactions between physician and patient in which patients do not define themselves as ill (eg, alcoholism, some forms of mental illness, hypertension) or are ambivalent about their motivation to get well. Under these circumstances, the relationship between the doctor and the patient may be strained. However, competent medical care that includes being interested in and caring about the patient is still required.

Perhaps the most important criticism of Parsons' model for the physician is that it assumes too much complementarity. It views physicians and patients as operating in the same ways toward the same ends and ignores important differences that may exist between them. In the next section more will be said about the influences of cultural beliefs on health, illness, and treatment, but it can be noted here that at least three sets of cultural beliefs, often unspoken, influence the interaction between the patient and the physician: (1) the physician's personal values and beliefs, (2) the values and beliefs of the patient, and (3) the values and beliefs of the institution of medicine as currently practiced in the local social context.

Under what beliefs might Mrs V have been operating when she first refused to be taken to the hospital by the paramedics? Were these different from her husband's beliefs? What personal beliefs did the physician have about household falls when he called Mrs V? What might his medical beliefs have been? How much complementarity or difference might there have been between these views?

Role of the Family in Treatment

The role of a family member in treatment is highlighted in the case of Mrs V. It appears that her beliefs about household falls and blows to the head that cause unconsciousness were not sufficient to convince her to seek treatment. However, when her physician called and urged her to go the emergency room, she did so. The interaction of the physician and the husband helped Mrs V to obtain care.

The role of the family can be seen by the physician from three perspectives. First, family support can be an important factor in improving treatment outcomes. Second, family members can be useful therapeutic allies of the physician. Third, family members may need assistance as a consequence of the disease, disability, or death of another family member. These three perspectives can be examined for acute, chronic, and terminal illnesses.

A. Family Support and Treatment Outcomes: Just as family support acts to protect members from morbidity and mortality, evidence indicates that family and/or social support can improve the outcome of patients' treatment. Family interventions have been shown to be effective in the treatment of schizophrenia when based on a model that reduces psychophysiological arousal, and instructs family members in methods that help them to manage problematic behavior and communicate effectively (Dixon and Lehman, 1995). Social support, or the perception of it, contributed to improved rehabilitation in stroke patients (Glass and Maddox, 1992) and those suffer-

ing from head and neck cancer (Baker, 1992). Adolescents being treated for drug and alcohol abuse and patients in a smoking cessation program had improved lengths of abstinence under conditions of social support (Myers et al, 1993; Spiegel et al, 1993).

B. The Family and Acute Illness: Family members are a rich source of information for the physician regarding any acute or emergent problem. What are the circumstances under which the problem arises? Why did the problem arise at the present time? Has it ever occurred before? What were the circumstances then? What has been done in the past by the patient, the family, or other doctors to treat this problem? Answers to these questions can be of great use to the physician, particularly when the patient is unable or unwilling to respond.

The family can also be useful to the physician in providing information about cultural behaviors that support the health of its members or contribute to their developing illness. Depending on the problem confronting the physician, questions about diet, use and abuse of alcohol, use of tobacco, and views about dangerous life-styles or behaviors may be helpful.

Families may need assistance from the physician to deal with the acute illness of one of its members. For example, information about areas such as diet and activity—particularly sexual activity—may be helpful to a family of a patient recovering from a myocardial infarction. Information regarding the potential dangers of specific dietary patterns or social activities (heavy drinking or riding a motorcycle without a helmet) may be necessary. In a review regarding both acute and chronic cardiac disease, Sirles and Selleck (1989) found that cognitive, emotional, and material support were needed to prevent maladaptive coping by both patients and their families.

The physician may also wish to ask the family about the effect of the patient's illness on them. One trauma surgeon was surprised to see the devastating effect on the family of an injury to a young man he was treating for a broken leg. To the surgeon, the problem was minor compared with his usual fare. To the family, it meant shattered dreams. Their son was a local track star, and his success meant a lot to them. They deeply appreciated the surgeon's empathy and counsel at that time.

C. Family and Chronic Illness: A member of the family with a chronic illness or disease or physical disability changes the structure of a family and the dynamics of its interactions (Subramanian, 1991). Special dietary and other environmental considerations must be provided for those with diabetes, asthma, or hypertension. Even greater accommodations must be made for the family member with paraplegia or quadriplegia or for those with chronic mental illness such as schizophrenia. Families often wish to know as much as possible about the illness and how they can help their loved one. Often of greater importance is what they can do to help prevent a recurrence of the illness once it has been brought under control.

However, the role of ally is not always an easy one. Although it may be of great use to the doctor to have a dedicated family member at home helping to take care of a chronically ill patient, that responsibility often represents a great burden to the family member and can distort the normal structure and functioning of a family in ways that are detrimental to its members (Floyd and Gallagher, 1997; Lefley, 1996). The physician treating a chronically ill patient must take precautions to see that this does not happen. By determining the extent of the burden carried by a family member or members and developing alternatives, if possible, the physician can ensure that each member of the family will be able to develop and function in as normal a manner as possible.

A second way in which the doctor can assist family members of chronically ill patients is by assuring them that they are neither the cause of the patient's illness or disability nor the agent of its recurrence. Families often carry great guilt and—with certain chronic illnesses—shame concerning their role in the patient's illness. For these reasons, explanations of the etiology of the illness can help family members greatly.

Family members have become more assertive in calling attention to their needs. Family members of persons suffering from severe and persistent mental illness came together in 1979 to form a grassroots advocacy group, the National Alliance for the Mentally Ill (NAMI) (Lefley, 1996). With over 1000 affiliates and more than 150,000 members, NAMI organizes family support groups and public education campaigns, seeks representation on local and national governance bodies, and advocates for research and training in effective methods of treatment.

D. Family and Terminal Illness: Dying, like living, is complex. Many factors affect the experiences of terminally ill patients and their families. Will the death be sudden or prolonged? What kind of illness or event will cause the death? Where will the patient die? What is the relationship of the family to the dying patient? What is the role of the patient within the family? How much social, psychological, and financial support is available for both patient and family? What will the family situation be following the death? The answers to these and similar questions will greatly determine the quality of a patient's dying and his or her family's reactions to it. To be maximally effective, the physician must take the answers to these questions into consideration (see Chapter 37).

The complexity of the dying process is illustrated in a study by Sonneblick et al (1993) of the offspring of terminally ill patients, in which the vast majority (66–78%) of patients' adult children requested the continuation of fluid, nutrition, and medication and a significant minority (25–29%) requested the initia-

tion of mechanical supports, even when these may not have been their parents' wishes. The authors found that religious values and the degree of closeness of their relationship influenced the offspring's requests. Again, in situations such as these, to be helpful, physicians must be aware of their own feelings and beliefs, those of the patient, and those of the patient's family.

Acquired immunodeficiency syndrome and the terminal illnesses associated with it provide a further illustration of the complexity of the dying process and the patient's and the family's experiences with it. Patients, their significant others, and both sets of families may experience grief and shock over the diagnosis and its implications. Sadness, anxiety, helplessness, and anger are often observed. Because of the nature of this illness, stigmatization, fear, shame, and isolation often complicate grieving for physicians, patients, and those close to them. Nonjudgmental counseling, information, and education by the physician can be a great help (Lippman et al, 1993).

Collaboration among the physician, the patient, and the family is a worthwhile goal. Providing physical and psychological comfort to the dying patient is a role physicians and families share. Arrangements can be made among the family, the physician, and the patient regarding "heroic measures" to prolong life and when to allow death to come without intervention. These are sensitive issues, and compassion, openness, and tact are required from the physician working with a patient and the patient's family.

Expressions of grief are also complex and, as will be shown below, are influenced to a great extent by cultural prescription. Family members may express their grief in a variety of ways. Granting the permission to experience whatever feelings might be present and providing a safe context for their expression may be one way in which a doctor can help a family deal with its loss. Since there is significant variation in the way people experience and express the loss of a loved one, physicians must avoid institutionalized methods or preconceived notions about how family members "should" grieve (Leon, 1992). Maintaining an attitude of acceptance and understanding is most helpful (Van Dongen, 1991).

The loss of any member of the immediate family unbalances the delicate structure of family relations, and assistance may be necessary from the physician and other medical staff in helping the family reorganize in new ways (Birenbaum and Robinson, 1991).

In the beginning of this section, it was suggested that one of the privileges of the physician was access to both physical and psychological intimacy with patients. Many physicians may be more skilled at physical than with psychological interventions. However, the latter can be as helpful to patients as the former, and, although they do require skill, they are within the reach of most physicians.

THE INFLUENCE OF CULTURE

The most powerful social influence on human behavior is the culture in which the individual lives, works, procreates, and dies. Culture can be viewed as the aggregate of all beliefs, customs, language, history, and technological achievements of a people. Culture contains not only directly observable behavior but also the values and beliefs that govern that behavior. It provides us with the notions of what is right and wrong and gives meaning to our actions.

As part of their culture, all societies have a medical system that assists its people in dealing with the universal experience of disease and death. These systems contain a theory explaining the causes of illness as well as techniques for diagnosis and treatment. Some of these medical systems are closely connected to the culture's system of religious beliefs, and some, such as those in the United States, are not (Weiss and Lonnquist, 1997). As Kleinman et al (1978) have noted, we learn appropriate ways of being ill and what to do about it.

As noted above, interactions between physician and patient are influenced by (1) the personal culture of the physician, (2) the personal culture and subculture of the patient, and (3) the culture of the institution of medicine itself (Burkett, 1991).

The Influence of Culture on the Physician

Medicine exists as a part of a wider culture and, as such, is influenced by the values and beliefs of that social context. What is defined as a disease and what is to be done about it are factors influenced by culture. For example, patients in Great Britain are only about one-sixth as likely to have coronary bypass surgery as their American counterparts and only about one-half as likely to have an x-ray for any reason. French physicians prescribe lactobacillus (derived from yogurt) to counteract stomach upsets from antibiotics, a practice that is not routine in other Western countries (Payer, 1988).

Culture also influences the definition of psychological health, illness, and treatment. The *DSM-IV* (*Diagnostic and Statistical Manual of Mental Disorders,* 4th edition) and the ICD10 (*Manual of the International Statistical Classification of Diseases, Injuries and Causes of Death*) each contains both verifiable signs and symptoms as well as subjective culture-based judgments about what is normal and abnormal behavior and what appropriate methods of treatment are.

In an effort to assess the impact of a patient's culture on his or her psychiatric illness and its treatment, *DSM-IV* includes an appendix offering practitioners guidelines for making a "cultural formulation" to accompany the other five diagnostic assessments or "axes" that make up a complete clinical evaluation. Included is an appraisal of the patient's (1) cultural identity, (2) cultural explanation of the illness, (3) environment, including culturally specific social stressors and supports, and (4) relationship with the clinician and how this may be affected by the cultural differences between them. Also included is an overall assessment of the influence of the above cultural considerations on the diagnosis and care recommended for the patient.

Science itself is not exempt from the influence of culture since it exists as part of a wider context. What is important to study, what will be supported by government agencies as well as citizens, and how the results will be received (front page or "buried" in obscure journals) are all culturally determined.

Since antiquity, healers have known and utilized the powerful effects of patients' beliefs in assisting them in recovering from illness. With the advent of Hippocratic medicine, this "placebo effect" emerged as a major adjunct to the physician's arsenal. Currently it is seen as a powerful ally as physicians realize that what they and their patients believe about a medication or a treatment intervention can greatly influence the effectiveness of that remedy (Frank, 1975; Chopra, 1993).

The Influence of Culture on Patients

Kleinman et al (1978) expanded our understanding of the influence of culture on transactions between physicians and patients by examining the "explanatory model" that patients bring to the interaction. Patients do not arrive with a blank slate concerning medical care, nor do their beliefs and values necessarily correspond to those of the treating physician. Rather, patients arrive with their own model, which may contain an etiological explanation of why they got sick, how this illness is likely to affect them, what course it might take, and what should be done about it.

With this in mind, the physician can consider that for every difference in social characteristic (age, sex, social class, ethnicity), there may be a corresponding difference in beliefs and values between doctor and patient. Thus, if Mrs V, a Mexican-American woman in her 40s, is being treated by an emergency room physician who is African-American, male, and in his 30s, there might well be differences between them even with regard to the seriousness and treatment of a fall!

How is the physician to determine and deal with these differences? Kleinman et al (1978) provide the following questions that can be incorporated into the medical interview.

1. What do you think has caused your problem?
2. Why do you think it started when it did?
3. What do you think your sickness does to you?
4. How severe is your sickness? Will it last a long or a short time?
5. What kind of treatment do you think you should receive?

6. What are the most important results you hope to receive from this treatment?
7. What are the chief problems your sickness has caused you?
8. What do you fear most about your sickness?

These questions can be of great help to the physician in seeking to determine how the patient views his or her illness. However, at least two problems may arise in their use. First, physicians may feel uncomfortable in asking the patient what is wrong and what should be done about it. The physician may feel—and the patient may agree—that under the cultural norms of this society, the physician is responsible for determining these. This problem can be handled by prefacing the questions with a comment such as, "I have my ideas about what your problem is and what to do about it, and I am aware that patients sometimes have their own ideas about their illnesses, and I was wondering about what you were thinking." Friendly overtures of this nature let the patients know that the physician is interested in how they view the problem and may contribute to their perception of the physician as someone who cares about them.

The second problem in eliciting the patient's model is that it may be different from the physician's model. If there are no direct conflicts between the two in terms of treatment, the patient's model, or elements of the patient's model, can be respectfully incorporated into the physician's treatment regimen, thereby strengthening it.

However, sometimes the patient's model may differ from the physician's model in regard to important issues of treatment. Patients may want or expect a form of treatment that the physician deems harmful or useless, or the patient may consider the physician's recommendations as useless or in conflict with important cultural beliefs. When models clash, *negotiation* is an important tool, and in many cases *time* can be the element negotiated. Would the patient be willing to try the physician's prescription for a specified period of time, and then, if the desired results are not forthcoming, switch to the patient's remedy? Would the patient prefer to try his or her own prescription first and then the physician's?

Again, negotiating these issues requires some skill and a small investment of time. However, eliciting the patient's model allows physicians to determine whether their patients' cultural beliefs are in harmony with their own. If done with sensitivity and respect, this should improve patient compliance.

The above discussion is intended to assist physicians in dealing with their individual patients. Is general information available that the practitioner can use as guidelines in determining the differences that may exist between patients and doctors? The answer is yes, with an important caution about stereotypic thinking.

ETHNICITY & STEREOTYPING

Avoid Stereotyping

Physicians can make use of known characteristic similarities within racial or ethnic groups without stereotypically assuming that each individual patient will be like every other patient from the same group. An African-American patient may be quite different from a white patient on certain specific variables, and still be equally different from another patient who is African-American. If the physician can avoid the temptation to stereotype the patient, information about different racial and ethnic groups may be useful as guidelines for diagnosis and treatment. Some of this information is presented below.

Hinton and Kleinman (1993) suggested guidelines for treating patients from different cultures. The physician should take special care to show empathy and to elicit the patients perspective on the problem. The patient's experience should then be assessed in the context of his or her family, workplace, and community. Diagnosis is rendered both in terms of categories given in *DSM-IV* as well as any applicable culturally based idiom of distress.

African-Americans

African-Americans constitute the largest ethnic minority group in the United States, comprising approximately 12% of the population. They have a higher incidence of hypertension, renal disease, stroke, and diabetes than whites and thus have a higher mortality rate in different age classifications. They also are more likely to die from trauma and violence.

African-Americans are a very heterogeneous group that includes a large and growing middle class, and any generalizations about their family structure, health beliefs, and attitudes toward health and illness are bound to suffer from stereotyping and racial bias. It is important for the physician to realize that characteristics often attributed to racial factors (or sometimes to biological factors) may instead be a product of social class and the disadvantaged position that many African-Americans have experienced in the United States.

Although research has indicated that African-American women are more likely than white women to believe that home remedies are better than prescription medicines, most African-Americans utilize orthodox biomedicine almost entirely for their health care (Snowden et al, 1997). In general, African-Americans are religious and believe in the restorative power of prayer (Broman, 1996), and may minimize or disregard the occurrence of stressful events (Johnson and Crowley, 1996). Folk illnesses having symptoms resembling problems conventionally understood as anxiety related and as somatization are recognized in certain locales (Snowden et al, 1997).

Hispanic-Americans

Spanish-speaking people from Puerto Rico, Mexico, Cuba, as well as from countries in Central and South America and the Caribbean constitute what is referred to as the Hispanic population in the United States. At present they are the fastest growing minority in the United States. Although this group is extremely diverse, as a whole they tend to be at risk for diabetes, hypertension, tuberculosis, HIV infection, alcoholism, cirrhosis, and violent deaths (Anonymous, 1991). They are more likely than the white population to live in poverty, be unemployed, and have little education or private insurance. Their use of health care services is affected by insurance status, income, and difficulties in communicating in English. Problems associated with migration and with ethnic discrimination in jobs and education have also been part of the heritage of these groups in the United States (del Pinal and Singer, 1997).

Overall norms and beliefs include placing a high value on the extended family as well as idealized concepts of what constitutes manliness and feminine virtue. Many groups have both natural and folk beliefs regarding health, illness, and treatment, and folk healers are utilized in many communities along with orthodox medical practitioners. Collaboration with indigenous practitioners can aid in the physician's ability to assist Hispanic patients (Weiss and Lonnquist, 1997).

One of the most widely known idiomatic expressions of distress is conveyed by the term "nervios" used by Mexican-Americans and Puerto Ricans (Lewis-Fernandez, 1996). "Nervios" reflects an underlying tendency to suffer in an anxious, depressed, or dissociative state, or to exhibit unconventional or impulsive behavior, due to interpersonal frustration. "Nervios" is attributed to an alteration, whether acquired or inherited, of the nervous system.

Other Ethnic Americans

Asian-Americans and people from the Middle East, as well as Native Americans, constitute other heterogeneous ethnic groups within our society. Each has culturally derived beliefs about health, illness, and its treatment that influence the way they view illness and what they do about it.

For example, Iranian patients attempt to mask expressions of dysphoria, which may be exhibited in other ways such as sulking or not eating (Pliskin, 1992). Ethiopian patients consider the frank disclosure of bad news inappropriate and insensitive. They prefer that a family member be told, who then will relate the information to the patient in the proper context and in a culturally approved manner (Beyene, 1992). Native Americans' definitions of health often incorporate spiritual values emphasizing a harmonious balance among the individual, the community, and nature (Weiss and Lonnquist, 1997).

Cultural differences also influence the ability of patients to benefit from mental health services. Despite great gains in adapting to the culture of Western countries, including the United States, many Vietnamese refugees continue to suffer from the traumas of their wartime experiences, culture shock, the loss of loved ones, and economic hardship. Cultural differences between the patient and practitioner, in addition to communication problems, often diminish the effectiveness of psychotherapy (Gold, 1992). Recent research has also suggested that the pharmacokinetic and pharmacodynamic profiles of some psychotropic medications may be different in Asian than in non-Asian patients. This would lead to differences in recommended dosages as well as differences in side effects features (Lin and Shen, 1991).

Sensitive and respectful inquiry by the physician may reveal beliefs and values that can be utilized in the overall care of the patient. However, members of some groups may be reticent to share their views with even the most open and compassionate practitioner who is not of their background. Under these circumstances, when the outcome of treatment is involved, the use of indigenous consultants may be appropriate. The use of native persons may also be useful when problems of language arise.

REFERENCES & SUGGESTED READINGS

Adams WL et al: Alcohol-related hospitalizations of elderly people. JAMA 1993;270:1222.

Anderson RM: Revisiting the behavioral model and access to health care: Does it matter? J Health Soc Behav 1995; 36:1.

Anonymous: Hispanic health in the United States. JAMA 1991;265:248.

Arborelius E, Dremberg S: What can doctors do to achieve a successful consultation? Fam Pract 1992;9:81.

Baker CA: Factors associated with rehabilitation in head and neck cancer. Cancer Nurs 1992;15:395.

Ballard EL et al: Recruitment of black elderly for clinical research studies of dementia. Gerontologist 1993;33:581.

Basic Behavioral Sciences Task Force of the National Advisory Mental Health Council: Basic behavioral science research for mental health: Sociocultural and environmental processes. Am Psychol 1996;51:722.

Becker LB et al: Racial differences in the incidence of cardiac arrest and subsequent survival. N Engl J Med 1993; 329:600.

Beckman HB, Frankel RM: The effect of physician behavior on the collection of data. Ann Intern Med 1984;101:692.

Beyene Y: Medical disclosure and refugees: Telling bad news to Ethiopian patients. West J Med 1992;157:328.

Birenbaum LK, Robinson MA: Family relationships in two types of terminal care. Soc Sci Med 1991;32:95.

Broman CL: Coping with personal problems. In: *Mental Health in Black America.* Neighbors HW, Jackson JS (editors). Sage, 1996.

Burkett GL: Culture, illness and the biopsychosocial model. Fam Med 1991;23:287.

Case RB et al: Living alone after myocardial infarction. JAMA 1992;267:515.

Chopra D: *Ageless Body, Timeless Mind.* Harmony Books, 1993.

Cockerham WC: *Medical Sociology,* 3rd ed. Prentice Hall, 1986.

Cohen J et al: *Use of Services and Expenses for Noninstitutionalized Population under Medicaid.* Agency for Health Care Policy and Research Pub. No. 94-0051, 1994.

Cohen S: Psychological stress, immunity, and respiratory infections. Curr Direct Psychol Sci 1996;5:86.

Cohen-Cole SA: The biopsychosocial model in medical practice. In: *Human Behavior: An Introduction for Medical Students.* Stoudemire A (editor). Lippincott, 1990.

Cohen-Cole SA, Bird J: Interviewing the cardiac patient. III. A practical guide to educate patients and to promote cooperation and treatment. Qual Life Cardiovasc Care 1986;3:101.

Collins CA: Mortality outlook: An overview of African American health. African Am Res Perspect 1995;2:17.

Cornelius LJ: Ethnic minorities and access to medical care. J Assoc Academic Minority Physicians 1993;4:16.

del Pinal J, Singer A: Generations of diversity: Latinos in the United States. Popul Bull 1997;52:1.

Dixon LB, Lehman AF: Family interventions in schizophrenia. Schiz Bull 1995;21:631.

Dohrenwend BP: Socioeconomic status and psychiatric disorders: The causation-selection issue. Science 1992;255:947.

Floyd FJ, Gallagher EM: Parental stress, care demands, and use of support services for school-age children with disabilities and behavior problems. Fam Relations 1997;46:359.

Frank AF, Gunderson JC: The role of the therapeutic alliance in the treatment of schizophrenia. Arch Gen Psychiatry 1990;47:220.

Frank JD: The faith that heals. Johns Hopkins Med J 1975;137:127.

Gijsbers van Wijk CM et al: Male and female morbidity in general practice: The nature of sex differences. Soc Sci Med 1992;35:665.

Glass TA, Maddox GL: The quality and quantity of social support stroke recovery as psycho-social transition. Soc Sci Med 1992;34:1249.

Gold SJ: Mental health and illness in Vietnamese refugees. West J Med 1992;157:290.

Helgeson VS, Cohen S: Social support and adjustment to cancer. Health Psychol 1996;15:135.

Hill J et al: Survey of satisfaction with care in a rheumatology outpatient clinic. Ann Rheum Dis 1992;51:195.

Hinton L, Kleinman A: Cultural issues and international psychiatric diagnosis. In: *International Review of Psychiatry.* Costa de Silva J, Nadelson C (editors). American Psychiatric Press, 1993.

Johnson RE, Crowley CE: An analysis of stress denial. In: *Mental Health in Black America.* Neighbors HM, Jackson JS (editors). Sage, 1996.

Kessler RC et al: Lifetime and 12-month prevalence of *DSM-III-R* psychiatric disorders in the United States. Arch Gen Psychiatry 1994;51:8.

King KB et al: Social support and long-term recovery from coronary artery surgery. Health Psychol 1993;12:56.

Kleinman A et al: Culture, illness and care: Clinical lessons from anthropologic and cross-cultural research. Ann Intern Med 1978;88:251.

Krieger N: Social class and the black/white crossover in the age specific incidence of breast cancer. Am J Epidemiol 1990;131:804.

Krieger N, Williams DR, Moss NE: Measuring social class in US public health research: Concepts, methodologies, and guidelines. Annu Rev Public Health 1997;18:341.

Lefley HP: *Family Caregiving in Mental Illness.* Sage, 1996.

Lefley HP: Synthesizing the family caregiving studies: Implications for service planning, social policy, and further research. Fam Relations 1997;46:443.

Leon IG: Perinatal loss. A critique of current hospital practices. Clin Pediatr 1992;31:366.

Lewis-Fernandez R: Diagnosis and treatment of nervios and ataques in a female Puerto Rican migrant. Cult Med Psychiatry 1996;20:155.

Lillie-Blanton M et al: Racial differences in health: Not just black and white but shades of gray. Annu Rev Public Health 1996;17:411.

Lin KM, Shen WW: Pharmacotherapy for southeast Asian psychiatric patients. J Nerv Ment Dis 1991;179:346.

Lippman SB et al: AIDS and the family. AIDS Care 1993; 5:71.

Malcolm JA, Dobson AJ: Marriage is associated with a lower risk of ischaemic heart disease in men. Med J Aust 1989;151:185.

Matthews KA et al: Educational attainment and behavioral and biological risk factors for coronary heart disease in middle-age women. Am J Epidemiol 1989;129:132.

Morris LS, Schulz RM: Medication compliance: The patient's perspective. Clin Ther 1993;15:593.

Must A et al: Long-term morbidity and mortality of overweight adolescents. N Engl J Med 1992;327:1350.

Myers MG et al: Coping as a predictor of adolescent substance abuse treatment outcome. J Subst Abuse 1993; 5:15.

National Center for Health Statistics: *Health, United States, 1995.* Public Health Service, 1996.

Parsons T: *The Social System.* Free Press, 1951.

Payer L: *Medicine and Culture.* Holt, 1988.

Pescosolido BA: Beyond rational choice: The social dynamics of how people seek help. Am J Sociol 1992; 97:1096.

Pliskin KL: Dysphoria and somatization in Iranian culture. West J Med 1992;157:295.

Ridsdale L et al: Doctors' interviewing techniques and its response to different booking time. Fam Pract 1992;9:57.

Robbins JA et al: The influence of physician practice behaviors on patient satisfaction. Fam Med 1993;25:17.

Rost K et al: Introduction of information during the initial medical visit: Consequences for patient follow-through with physician recommendations for medication. Soc Sci Med 1989;28:315.

Ruberman W: Psychosocial influences on mortality of patients with coronary heart disease. JAMA 1992;267:559.

Sanchez MC et al: Patient expectations and satisfaction with medical care for upper respiratory infections. J Gen Intern Med 1992;7:432.

Scott-Lennox JA, George LK: Epidemiology of psychiatric disorders and mental health services use among older

Americans. In: *Mental Health Services: A Public Health Perspective.* Levin BL, Petrila J (editors). Oxford University Press, 1996.

Shadish WR et al: Effects of family and marital therapies: A meta analysis. J Consult Clin Psychol 1993;61:992.

Sherbourne CD et al: Antecedents of adherence to medical recommendations. J Behav Med 1992;15:447.

Sirles AT, Selleck CS: Cardiac disease and the family: Impact, assessment and implications. J Cardiovasc Nurs 1989;3:23.

Snowden LR, Libby A, Thomas K: Health care-related attitudes and utilization among African American women. Womens Health: Res Gender Behav Policy 1997;3:301.

Sonnenblick M et al: Dissociation between the wishes of terminally ill parents and decisions by their offspring. J Am Geriatr Soc 1993;41:599.

Spiegel D et al: Predictors of smoking abstinence following a single-session restructuring intervention with self-hypnosis. Am J Psychiatry 1993;150:1090.

Subramanian K: The multidimensional impact of chronic pain on the spouse. Soc Work Health Care 1991;15:47.

Szasz T, Hollander M: A contribution to the philosophy of medicine: The basic models of the doctor & patient relationship. AMA Arch Intern Med 1956;97:585.

Treas J: Older Americans in the 1990s and beyond. Popul Bull 1995;50:1.

Van Dongen CJ: Experiences of family members after a suicide. J Fam Pract 1991;33:375.

Waitzman N, Smith K: The effects of occupational class transitions on hypertension: Racial disparities among working age men. Am J Public Health 1994;84:945.

Weinick RM, Zuvekas SH, Drilea SK: *Access to Health Care—Sources and Barriers.* MEPS Research Finding No. 3, Agency for Health Care Policy and Research Pub. No. 98-0001, 1997.

Weiss GL, Lonnquist LE: *The Sociology of Health, Healing, and Illness,* 2nd ed. Prentice Hall, 1997.

Wells KB et al: *Caring for Depression.* Harvard University Press, 1996.

Williams RB et al: Prognostic importance of social and economic resources among medically treated patients with angiographically documented coronary artery disease. JAMA 1992;267:520.

Worthington RC: Family support networks: Help for children with special needs. Fam Med 1992;24:41.

Zhang AY, Snowden LR: Prevalence of mental disorders in ethnic minority groups in five communities nationwide. Cult Diversity Mental Health, in press.

Psychopathology: Psychiatric Diagnosis & Psychosocial Formulation

8

Howard H. Goldman, MD, MPH, PhD, & Steven A. Foreman, MD

Psychopathology is the study of mental disorders and abnormal thoughts, feelings, and behavior. Clinical psychiatry is thus concerned with two related processes: (1) diagnosing mental disorder and (2) assessing psychiatric factors in health and illness. Psychopathology is a specialized domain, defined by concern for particular disorders (eg, schizophrenia, depression). Clinical psychiatry is a generic process common in evaluating all patients regardless of diagnosis and may extend beyond the traditional boundaries of medicine to include assessment of "problems in living" and normal human behavior. It shares this two-dimensional approach with other medical specialties. Cardiologists, for example, are concerned not only with diagnosing cardiac disease but also with assessing cardiovascular function in all patients. Although they share important similarities, with the objectives of both being patient assessment, psychiatry and other medical specialties have some important differences.

The basic processes of diagnosis are quite similar in the various branches of clinical medicine. The clinician observes patterns of signs and symptoms in a patient that are similar to patterns characteristic of a syndrome or specific disorder and decides on a name or diagnosis. The diagnostic label implies that *this* patient's pattern of signs and symptoms is similar to the pattern observed in other patients with the same diagnosis. The pattern of signs and symptoms may have the same cause or may develop in the same way (pathogenesis) or may be associated with the same abnormalities (pathology). The diagnostician observes the patient and tries to answer two questions:

1. Does the patient have frank [mental, cardiac, etc] disease?
2. Does the patient have signs or symptoms of . . . [mental, cardiac, etc] dysfunction that suggest the onset of disease or suggest that the patient's clinical status would be compromised or deteriorate under stress such as an intercurrent illness, surgery, or death of a loved one?

The clinician may also look for evidence of special skills or strengths or signs of abundant health that may enable the patient to adapt well to a particular situation or stress.

For most purposes of clinical assessment, it is sufficient to say that there *is* or *is not* evidence of disease. In some cases, however, the diagnostician may want to speculate about the circumstances (tolerance limits) under which the patient can be expected to function within "normal limits." In clinical psychiatry, the diagnostician first determines if mental disorder is present (**diagnosis**) and then proceeds to assess the patient's mental function, behavior, social circumstances, and personality—a process called **psychosocial formulation.** Each patient is described uniquely, and the description is expanded to include personal information useful in patient care. To conclude that a patient's psychiatric status is "within normal limits" is generally unsatisfactory. Psychodynamic formulation is one type of psychosocial formulation based on psychoanalytic theories of mental function and dysfunction. It is the most common formulation encountered in clinical psychiatry and is discussed later in this chapter.

There is a growing body of knowledge about the impact of behavior, emotion, personality, social circumstances, life-style, and stressful life events on health and illness. Clinical evaluation is incomplete without an assessment of these factors (psychosocial formulation). Unlike the diagnostic process, which explains how one patient is similar to others, psychosocial formulation shows how each patient is unique. It attempts to explain why a patient presents at a particular time with a specific set of complaints. For example, a man with hemoptysis who waited 2 months before seeking treatment presented with vague complaints of chest pain. The physician found the chest pain to be benign, and hemoptysis proved to be the clue to malignant disease. Questioning the patient revealed that he presented with complaints on the anniversary of the death of his child following cardiac surgery; and because his mother had died of lung cancer, he had denied the significance of the cough out of fear. The psychosocial formulation made on each patient can help the physician understand the patient's psychological defenses and personality, so an individualized approach to treatment can be planned.

How can the physician help the patient understand the illness and cooperate in making informed decisions about treatment? What psychosocial factors will affect compliance with treatment? What are the patient's social and family resources in coping with the illness? Is special assistance needed at times of stress? The process of psychosocial formulation parallels the diagnostic process both in medicine and in psychiatry. Its goal is to enable the therapist to understand and assess each patient individually.

THE BIOPSYCHOSOCIAL MODEL

Current thinking in clinical psychiatry is that no *single* or *unitary* theory of psychopathology is adequate to explain all that needs to be explained about mental disorders. Instead, psychiatry has embraced a biopsychosocial model, recommended by George Engel and others before him, that attempts to integrate three perspectives into a comprehensive view of human behavior in health and illness. Drawing on biomedical, psychological, and social theories of psychopathology, the biopsychosocial model distinguishes the two major patient assessment processes in clinical psychiatry and, for that matter, in general medicine: (1) diagnosis and (2) individual psychosocial formulation. In the absence of a widely accepted theory of psychopathology that explains the pathogenesis of mental disorder, diagnosis becomes a process of categorizing signs and symptoms that occur together in recognizable patterns. This descriptive, phenomenological process seeks to define disease entities carefully enough so that similarities of underlying pathogenesis or causes can be discerned.

The following are criteria for inclusion or exclusion from a diagnostic category:

1. Verifiable signs and symptoms with a specified duration and intensity.
2. Common natural history.
3. Prognosis.
4. Response to treatment.

Once a diagnosis has been made and the patient is placed in a particular diagnostic category, the process of individual psychosocial assessment can begin. As previously noted, whether the diagnosis is psychiatric or somatic, individual psychosocial assessment is essential for evaluating patients comprehensively. As Francis Scott Smyth, former Dean of the School of Medicine, University of California (San Francisco), once noted, "To know what kind of a person has a disease is as essential as to know what kind of disease a patient has" (Smyth, 1962).

For the present, at least, the search for a unitary theory of psychopathology can be said to have intellectual appeal but no urgent utility. We do not need a theory linking diagnosis and pathogenesis to arrive at a correct diagnosis, a realistic individual psychosocial assessment, and an effective plan of treatment. Furthermore, it is not essential to associate psychological development or personality in a causal relationship with a diagnosis of depression, schizophrenia, or ulcerative colitis. As a practical matter, it is sufficient to diagnose mental illness in a biomedical mode and to assess our patients individually in a psychosocial mode. The diagnostic process enables clinicians to select a known category of dysfunction or disorder that fits the patient's symptoms and signs—ie, to define how the patient is similar to other patients. The more difficult process of psychosocial assessment helps clinicians to understand the meaning and expression of this disorder in each individual.

CLINICAL USE OF THE BIOPSYCHOSOCIAL MODEL

In *Ordinary People,* a popular novel and successful movie, Conrad Jarrett, the young protagonist, is portrayed as being depressed. The character will serve as a clinical example to illustrate two important points: (1) the utility of the biopsychosocial model to guide clinical assessment and (2) the benefit of both diagnosis and psychosocial (in this case, psychodynamic) formulation for patient evaluation and treatment. This example was selected because the young man had a disorder—a major depressive episode—that may be explained and treated both biomedically and psychosocially. The case demonstrates the need to diagnose a disorder for its biomedical benefits and to formulate the individual psychodynamics for its psychosocial benefits. Occasionally, patients can be treated successfully from only one perspective. Generally, a biopsychosocial perspective encouraging both diagnosis and formulation is optimal.

Conrad Jarrett was hospitalized and treated with electroconvulsive therapy after he attempted suicide following an extended period of depressed mood with guilt feelings marked by self-reproach, hopelessness, and thoughts of death. He was socially withdrawn and seemed to have lost all sense of pleasure. He also experienced difficulty sleeping, agitation, and poor appetite. He had nightmares in which he reexperienced a boating accident in which his older brother died. With the help of a psychiatrist, he eventually came to realize that his guilt over having survived the accident might explain his depression.

Conrad felt neglected by his mother and had always resented his brother because he was the favorite. He suspected that some part of him wanted the brother to die and that he did not try hard enough to rescue the drowning boy. The feelings left him despondent and angry. His suicide attempt represented an unconscious wish both to be punished and to punish his mother.

It is useful to examine these events from both a biomedical-diagnostic and a psychosocial perspective. Understanding Conrad and the approach to his treatment will be influenced by both points of view. From the biomedical-diagnostic perspective, Conrad is suffering from a major depressive episode characterized by depressed mood and a pattern of behavior including withdrawal from pleasurable activities; he is haunted by guilt and self-reproach, hopelessness, and suicidal thoughts. Conrad is also suffering from sleep and appetite disturbance. Such an illness usually responds to biomedical treatments such as antidepressant medication or electroconvulsive therapy. The psychodynamic formulation, developed during psychotherapy, provides an individualized understanding of the psychosocial forces contributing to this patient's depression. The formulation helps in understanding the unique presentation of this young man undergoing a major depressive episode.

As is often the case in practice, it is not known whether the biomedical-diagnostic or the psychosocial perspective contributes more to the understanding of the cause and pathogenetic mechanism of Conrad's illness. Furthermore, it is not known if some still unidentified constitutional predisposition must be present for major depressive disorder to occur. Also, it is uncertain if the physiological findings (such as a depletion of catecholamines in the brain) are the cause of the depressive episode or the result of psychodynamics. However, it is known that not all patients with major depressive episodes have the same psychodynamic formulation, and not all individuals with the same personality structure and similar life experiences suffer major depressive episodes.

Because we have agreed not to seek unitary explanations for this and other types of mental disorder, we need not restrict ourselves to any one therapeutic resource. Controlled clinical trials have demonstrated that electroconvulsive treatment or antidepressant medication is usually necessary for optimal control of severe depressive symptoms in major depressive episodes and that psychotherapy (especially focused on social adaptation) is indicated for maximal recovery of social function. Insight psychotherapy is intellectually satisfying for some patients and may help prevent the painful repetition of depressive episodes. Such treatment enables patients to recognize their mixed feelings toward loved ones, even after the loved ones are lost through death, divorce, or other separation. Medication has also been shown to prevent recurrences of depressive symptoms, even without psychodynamic understanding of the disorder.

Continuing research may someday clarify the connection between the psychodynamics of depression and the psychobiology of major depressive episodes. Meanwhile, a dual perspective—biomedical and psychosocial, diagnostic and individualized—is essential for comprehensive patient care.

DIAGNOSIS & PSYCHOPATHOLOGY

Diagnosis in psychiatry is a complex and challenging process, even though it may require less experience than psychodynamic or psychosocial formulation. Diagnosis serves several purposes, some of benefit to the patient and others of benefit to the provider of care, the patient's family, or society. A diagnosis of a mental disorder is a type of "shorthand" for defining an individual's problems in a way that will be recognized by patients, doctors, and society. It enables clinicians to communicate more reliably and effectively with one another about a certain class of problems. In addition, it officially classifies the patient as "sick," granting exemption from certain responsibilities and giving the patient permission to engage in certain types of behavior and to expect certain types of behavior from others.

A diagnosis also implies a degree of understanding of a pattern of illness, suggesting a specific treatment and an expected outcome or prognosis. Establishing a diagnosis may also make the physician or other care provider feel better about dealing with the uncertainties of illness, human suffering, and death. Sometimes the process of diagnosis is all the physician can offer, but it should be offered even so. The danger that a psychiatric diagnosis may function as a social label or stigma is a risk that must be accepted. The benefits of specific treatment may depend on specificity and precision in diagnosis. Leprosy, syphilis, lung cancer, tuberculosis, and mania are all stigmatizing diagnoses. Failure to make the diagnosis could deprive a patient of both specific treatment and general supportive care.

Precision in diagnosis is important for research. To understand illness, physicians must be able to describe it reliably enough to achieve a degree of homogeneity in a study population; this might facilitate the discovery of a common cause for the pattern of illness or dysfunction. Communication, research, and treatment are three important reasons why phenomenological descriptions and classification into specific disorders are important, even without a full understanding of underlying causes and pathophysiological mechanisms.

Diagnosis involves three processes that will be discussed in turn in the following sections. The diagnostician begins by organizing a set of **symptoms and signs** elicited from the patient history and from the physical and mental status examinations. These observations are then grouped into **syndromes.** Further specification produces diagnoses of **mental disorders.** Mental disorders are characterized by abnormalities in thoughts, perceptions, mood, and behavior that deviate from a socially defined norm enough to impair social functioning. As noted above, psychopathology is the study of these deviations, the symptoms and signs of mental disorders, their etiology, and their pathogenesis.

Symptoms are subjective complaints, and signs are

objective evidence of a pathological state. A symptom could be a headache, a fear, or a report of auditory hallucinations. A sign may be nystagmus, tachycardia, or loosening of associations. Symptoms and signs frequently occur in recognizable patterns called syndromes.

A disorder is more specific than a syndrome. A disorder is also a set of symptoms and signs, but with a specified course of the illness, premorbid history, and pattern of familial occurrence. It is assumed that every disorder has a specific pathogenesis, although the pathogenesis may be unclear. The same syndrome can occur in many different disorders or diseases. In psychiatry, the term "disorder" is occasionally distinguished from "disease." A disease is even more specific than a disorder in that a known cause and a specific pathogenesis are implied.

The goal of medicine is to understand pathological processes so they can be prevented or treated effectively. Most medical treatment is symptomatic or syndromic in nature. Physicians prefer to base all treatment on an etiological diagnosis, as done with antibiotic drugs for specific infectious diseases or for vitamin therapy for vitamin deficiencies, but in most cases clinicians treat symptoms (pain), signs (fever, inflammation), or syndromes (congestive heart failure, hypercortisolism [Cushing's syndrome], dementia, depression). Therapy differs, depending on the level of diagnostic specificity. For example, fever can be treated with aspirin, but it is important to know whether the fever is part of a syndrome along with productive cough that might respond to antibiotic therapy, in contrast to a syndrome of fever, joint pain, and rash, which might suggest a different therapy.

A syndrome consisting entirely of fever and productive cough might represent either a bacterial or fungal disorder. To help the clinician make the distinction, further historical details, physical examination, x-ray studies, and laboratory procedures are needed. If the sputum cultures grow *Streptococcus pneumoniae* and the chest x-ray shows a patchy density in the right lower lobe, it is possible to diagnose a specific disease—pneumococcal pneumonia. For the patient with this diagnosis, specific antibiotic treatment is indicated.

In psychiatric disorders, the pathological features are rarely shown on x-ray films. No bacillus or enzymatic defect has been shown to cause schizophrenia or bipolar affective disorder. For this reason, physicians rarely speak of **diseases** with known causes and pathophysiological mechanisms. Instead, clinicians speak of **disorders** that may represent particular underlying, but as yet unknown, disease processes. In some cases, the disorders are little more than **syndromes**—clusters of symptoms and signs.

The fourth edition of *Diagnostic and Statistical Manual of Mental Disorders* (*DSM-IV*), now the standard diagnostic text in psychiatry, attempts to formalize the nomenclature by organizing psychopathology into a series of disorders. In most instances, *DSM-IV* makes no assumptions about the causes or the pathophysiological mechanisms underlying the disorders. It recognizes limitations in the understanding of psychopathology. *DSM-IV* defines disorders by means of **inclusion and exclusion criteria,** which were discussed previously in this chapter. For further details on psychopathology and psychiatric diagnosis, see Chapter 15 for a discussion of the *DSM-IV* and see the Glossary of Psychiatric Signs & Symptoms, which immediately follows.

GLOSSARY OF PSYCHIATRIC SIGNS & SYMPTOMS

The diagnostic process in psychiatry begins with a careful history, physical examination, and mental status examination. Observations take the form of signs and symptoms. This section is a glossary of terms used to define and describe these signs and symptoms.

Affect: Emotions or feelings as they are expressed by the patient and observable by others. Affect is an objective sign observable on mental status examination, in contrast to Mood (see definition), which is a subjective experience reported by the patient. Affect is characterized in several ways: (1) By the type of emotion expressed and observed such as anger, sadness, or elation. (2) By the intensity and the range of emotion expressed, ie, flat, blunted, constricted, or broad. In flat affect, there is no expression of feeling; the face is immobile, and the voice is monotonous. In blunted affect, the expression of feeling is severely reduced. In constricted affect, the expression of feelings is clearly reduced but to a lesser degree than in the case of blunted affect. Broad affect is the normal condition in which a full range of feelings is expressed. (3) By its appropriateness, ie, inappropriate affect is apparent emotion discordant with accompanying thought or speech (eg, laughing while telling a story most people would find horrifying). (4) By the consistency of emotion; labile affect shifts rapidly among different emotional states such as crying, laughing, and anger.

Ambivalence: The condition of having two strong but opposite feelings or ideas. The individual cannot decide which way to respond, and therefore has difficulty in taking any action. A feature of obsessive-compulsive disorder and schizophrenia.

Anhedonia: Loss of interest in pleasure-seeking activities. A feature of depressive disorder.

Anorexia: Loss of or diminished appetite. A feature of depressive disorder.

Anxiety: A dysphoric (unpleasant) state similar to fear with no accompanying apparent source of danger. A feeling of apprehension, anticipation, or dread of possible danger. Anxiety is sometimes defined by the physiological state of autonomic arousal, alertness, vigilance, and motor tension. Free-floating anxiety is anxiety in the absence of an identifiable object of dread. Phobia (see definition) is severe anxiety aroused by a specific object or circumstance even though the subject knows the feeling "doesn't make sense."

Autistic thinking: Thought derived from fantasy. External reality is accorded subjective and fantasied meanings. Preoccupation with the private world may lead the autistic individual to withdraw from external reality.

Automatic obedience: Obedience to commands without exercising critical judgment. A feature of catatonia.

Blocking: Disruption of thought evidenced by an interruption or momentary disruption of speech. The individual appears to be trying to remember what he or she was thinking or saying.

Catalepsy: A condition in which the subject "freezes" in almost any abnormal posture that he or she is placed (left arm extended, etc). A feature of catatonia.

Catatonia: A syndrome characterized by cataleptic posturing, stereotypy, mutism, stupor, negativism, automatic obedience, echolalia, and echopraxia. There are two subtypes: excited and retarded. The excited subtype is characterized by dramatic increases in motor behavior, occasionally to the point of physical collapse; the retarded subtype is characterized by slowed motor behavior, occasionally to the point of immobility. Catatonia was formerly thought to be a subtype of schizophrenia. It is now thought to be a feature of affective disorders (chiefly mania), schizophrenia, organic mental disorder, and other psychoses.

Cerea flexibilitas ("waxy flexibility"): A specific type of catalepsy in which the examiner encounters resistance ("like bending a soft wax rod") when attempting to move parts of the subject's body. A feature of catatonia.

Circumstantiality: A disturbance of communication in which the train of associations is interrupted by frequent digressions before the central idea is finally presented. The digressions are irrelevant or marginally relevant to what is being said. Seen in a wide variety of pathological states, or may be a normal if annoying language habit.

Clang associations: The rhyming or punning associations of one word with another with no logical connection: "My head is rock candy. Dandy. Randy. Sandy. Piece of the rock. Mutual of Omaha." Seen in manic episodes, schizophrenia, and other psychotic states.

Clouding of consciousness: Impaired awareness of the environment. The least severe impairment of consciousness on the continuum from full alertness to coma.

Compulsion: The need to repeat some action in a ritualistic, stereotyped manner, uncontrollable by an act of will. The act frequently has symbolic meaning. The subject knows there is no true connection between performing the motor behavior and fulfilling or alleviating the fantasied wish or fear. The compulsive act may seem unpleasant, tedious, or distressful, but resistance is associated with mounting anxiety that can be relieved only by performing the act. Seen in obsessive-compulsive disorder and schizophrenia.

Concrete thinking: Thinking characterized by diminished capacity to form abstractions. The subject is unable to think metaphorically or hypothetically. Thought is limited to one dimension of meaning. Words and figures of speech are taken literally, and the nuances of implied meaning are not used or not appreciated. Common in organic mental disorder and schizophrenia.

Confabulation: The fabrication of events or data that either fill in gaps in a story or constitute entire fictions in response to questions that cannot be factually answered because of organic memory impairment. A feature of amnestic syndrome.

Confusion: A disturbance of consciousness with loss of orientation to person, place, or time (see Disorientation). Confusion may result from impaired memory loss (as in dementia) or a deficit in attention (as in delirium).

Delirium: A disturbance of consciousness resulting from organic brain disease (usually acute) and characterized by clouding of consciousness, restlessness, confusion, psychomotor retardation or agitation, and affective lability. It has a rapid onset and a fluctuating, waxing and waning course, and there is an associated disturbance of sleep.

Delusion: (See also Hallucination, Ideas of reference, and Paranoia.) A false belief or idea firmly held despite abundant contradictory evidence. A defect of reality testing. (A belief may not be delusional if it is shared by other members of a culture or large group.) A delusion is always evidence of psychosis. *Examples:* (1) Delusions of being controlled, ie, thoughts, feelings, or behaviors are controlled by external forces. (2) Delusions of grandeur, ie, being influential and important, perhaps having occult powers, or actually being some powerful figure out of history (Napoleonic complex). (3) Delusions of persecution, ie, being followed, harassed, threatened, or plotted against. (4) Delusions of reference, ie, external events or "portents" have personal significance, such as special messages or commands. A person with delusions of reference believes that strangers on the street are talking about him or her, the television commentator is sending coded messages, etc.

Dementia: Deterioration (caused by organic brain syndrome) from a previous level of intellectual functioning involving personality change and resulting in impairment of memory, abstract thinking, judgment, and impulse control. Clouding of consciousness does not occur. Dementia may be chronic (with insidious onset) or acute and reversible or irreversible.

Depersonalization: The experience of feeling strange, unreal, and detached from the environment or from oneself, ie, of being outside one's body, or feeling that parts of the body are very large, very small, or not under one's control, etc. Seen in a wide variety of disorders, including depression, anxiety, schizophrenia, epilepsy, and hypnagogic states. It may be a normal finding in adolescents (see Derealization).

Derailment: "Getting off the track" with respect to speech, volition, or thought. Moving in random fashion from one topic, thought, or behavior to another.

Derealization: The experience of feeling that the immediate environment is unreal or changed. (Depersonalization and derealization occur together and are probably aspects of the same phenomenon.)

Dereistic thinking: Failure to take the facts of reality into account, so that thoughts derive mainly from fantasy rather than experience and logical inference.

Disorientation: (1) Not oriented to time, ie, not knowing what day, month, season, or year it is; (2) not oriented to place, ie, not knowing the name of the building, the kind of building, or the city, state, or country in which one is presently located; or (3) not oriented to person, ie, not knowing who one is. Disorientation is one of the diagnostic criteria for delirium and is seen in delirium and organic memory disturbances.

Echolalia: Repetition of another person's speech (see Echopraxia).

Echopraxia: Imitation of another person's movements. (Echolalia and echopraxia are seen in pervasive developmental disorders, organic mental disorders, catatonia, and other psychotic disorders.)

Flight of ideas: A series of thoughts verbalized rapidly with abrupt shifts of subject matter for no apparent logical reason. Flight of ideas is associated with Pressure of speech (see definition). It is often difficult to differentiate flight of ideas from Loosening of associations (see definition). Classically, the connections between associations in flight of ideas are thought to be more coherent than in loosening of associations. However, in its severe form, flight of ideas can result in complete disorganization and incoherence. Seen in mania as well as in organic mental disorders, schizophrenia, and other psychotic and nonpsychotic states.

Folie à deux ("madness for two"): A disorder characterized by the sharing of delusional (usually persecutory) ideas by two or more (folie à plusieurs) individuals living in close association, usually in a family relationship. One member of the pair (or group) seems always to influence and dominate the other(s). The delusional ideas may lead to strange types of behavior such as preparing for the end of the world.

Formication: See Hallucination, tactile.

Fugue: Sudden, unexpected "flights" or wandering away from home or workplace and assumption of a new identity. There is amnesia for the previous identity and no memory of the fugue when it is over.

Hallucination: A false sensory perception of something that is not there. An Illusion (see definition) differs in being a perceptual distortion of something that is there. A delusion differs in being a disorder of thought. A delusion is always a sign of psychosis, because it represents a defect in reality testing. A hallucination is not always a sign of psychosis: one who "sees" pink elephants but knows they are not really there is not psychotic; one who "feels" bugs crawling on his or her skin and believes the bugs are really there is not only hallucinating but is also psychotic. *Examples:* (1) Auditory hallucinations—false perceptions of sounds (voices, music, buzzing, motor noises, murmuring). (2) Gustatory hallucinations—false perceptions of taste. (3) Olfactory hallucinations—false perceptions of smell. (4) Somatic hallucinations—false sensations of something happening in or to the body such as the sensation of knives piercing the body or a feeling of electricity in the arms. (Usually associated with a delusion consistent with the feeling.) (5) Tactile hallucinations—false sensations of touch. (Usually associated with a delusion consistent with the sensation.) Formication (from *L formica,* "ant"), a particular type of tactile hallucination, is the sensation of bugs crawling on or under the skin. (6) Visual hallucinations—false visual perceptions with eyes open in a lighted environment. (Visual images with the eyes closed are not true hallucinations. Hypnagogic and hypnopompic hallucinations—images experienced during the "twilight" stages while falling asleep and waking up, respectively—are not true hallucinations.) All of the above hallucinations can occur in schizophrenia, affective disorders, and organic mental disorders. Auditory and somatic hallucinations are common in functional disorders. Visual hallucinations are suggestive of organic mental disorders but are seen in functional disorders. Gustatory, olfactory, and tactile hallucinations strongly suggest organic mental disorders. Tactile hallucinations are common in drug and alcohol withdrawal and intoxication states.

Ideas of reference: Similar to Delusions of reference (see definition) but held with less conviction.

Illusion: (See also Hallucination.) A distorted perception of a material object.

Incoherence: Speech that is incomprehensible because of severe loosening of associations, distortions of grammar or syntax, or the use of idiosyncratic word definitions.

Insomnia: Difficulty sleeping—either initial insomnia, difficulty in falling asleep; middle insomnia, waking up in the middle of the night and going back to sleep with difficulty; or terminal insomnia, awakening early without being able to go back to sleep.

Loosening of associations: (See also Flight of ideas and Tangentiality.) A disorder of thinking and speech in which ideas shift from one subject to another with remote or no apparent reasons. The speaker is unaware of the incongruity. A classical sign of schizophrenia but may also be seen in any psychotic state.

Mood: The subjective experience of feeling or emotion as described by the patient in the history. Mood is a pervasive and sustained emotion. It is distinct from Affect (see definition), which is a feeling state noted by the examiner during the mental status examination. Mood is characterized by the type of emotion the patient describes, eg, sadness, feeling blue, happiness, elation, anger, and anxiety. Mood is dysphoric if the experience is unpleasant, eg, characterized by irritability, anger, or depression. Mood can be elevated, expansive, or euphoric, eg, characterized by increasing feelings of well-being, energy, and positive self-regard.

Mood-congruent: A term applied to hallucinations or delusions whose content is consistent with the predominant mood. Mood-congruent hallucinations or delusions in mania, for example, typically involve grandiosity, inflated self-esteem, confidence of one's personal powers, and identifications with famous persons or deities. Mood-congruent hallucinations or delusions in depression involve themes of worthlessness, guilt, defectiveness, disease, death, nihilism, and deserved punishment.

Mood-incongruent: A term applied to hallucinations or delusions whose content has no apparent relationship to the predominant mood. Examples are persecutory delusions, delusions of reference, delusions of control, thought insertion, thought withdrawal, and thought broadcasting, in which the content has no apparent relation to the mood-congruent themes mentioned above. Mood-incongruent hallucinations and delusions are seen in schizophrenia and sometimes in mania and depression.

Mutism: Not speaking. A feature of catatonia.

Negativism: Extreme opposition, resistance to suggestion. A feature of catatonia.

Neologisms: Invented "new words" with new meanings, often formed by combining elements of other words. A feature of schizophrenia and other psychotic disorders.

Obsession: Recurring ideas, images, or wishes that dominate thought. The content may be unacceptable and actively resisted but intrudes into consciousness again and again. A feature of obsessive-compulsive disorder and some cases of schizophrenia.

Panic attacks: Anxiety attacks characterized by palpitations, a sense of imminent doom, fear of losing control, tightness in the chest, hyperventilation, lightheadedness, nausea, and peripheral paresthesias. There are no cardiopulmonary, endocrine, or other physical disorders that might account for the symptoms. Seen in a wide variety of psychotic and nonpsychotic disorders as well as in normal people subjected to sufficient stress.

Paranoia: A psychotic disorder characterized by delusions of grandeur and persecution, suspiciousness, hypersensitivity, hyperalertness, jealousy, guardedness, resentment, humorlessness, litigiousness, and sullenness. Paranoid schizophrenia is listed separately as a subtype of schizophrenia. Paranoid ideation is a consistent finding in paranoid patients, who are convinced that people are thinking "bad thoughts" about them, that they are being followed, that they are the object of evil conspiracies, etc. It includes ideas of reference, ideas of persecution, grandiose ideas, and ideas of jealousy. Paranoid ideation differs from paranoid delusions in that the ideas are held with less conviction. Paranoid style is a character style featuring hypervigilance, litigiousness, rigidity, humorlessness, jealousy, sullenness, suspiciousness, and hyperattention to evidence in the environment that corroborates paranoid suspicions.

Perseveration: Repetitive behavior or repetitive expression of a particular word, phrase, or concept during the course of speech. Seen in organic mental disorders, schizophrenia, and other psychotic disorders.

Phobia: (See Anxiety.) An admittedly irrational fear of a particular object or situation, to the extent that the person's life is dominated by avoidance behavior.

Posturing: The assumption of various abnormal bodily positions, often a feature of catatonia.

Poverty of content of speech: Speech that is persistently vague, overly concrete or abstract, repetitive, or stereotyped.

Poverty of speech: Speech that is decreased in amount and nonspontaneous, consisting mainly of brief and unelaborated responses to questions.

Pressure of speech: (See Flight of ideas.) Speech that is rapid and unstoppable, as if the speaker is driven to continue speaking. Speech is often loud and emphatic and hard to interrupt. It can dominate conversations or go on when no one is listening or responding. A feature of mania and seen also in other psychotic conditions, organic mental disorders, and nonpsychotic conditions associated with stress.

Psychomotor agitation: Motor restlessness and hyperactivity associated with tension, anxiety, and irritability.

Psychomotor retardation: Decreased motor activity, slowed speech, poverty of speech, delayed response to questions, and low, monotonous voice tones associated with feelings of fatigue.

Psychosis: A level of disordered thinking in which the person is unable to distinguish reality from fantasy because of impaired ability to test reality. Psychosis may be transient (hours or days) or persistent (months or years). The characteristic deficit in psychosis is not "loss of touch with reality" but loss of the ability to process experience appropriately, ie, the inability to differentiate data coming from the outside world from information originating in one's inner world of preconceptions, expectations, and emotions. Psychosis can be defined as an impairment of reality testing. Reality sense can be impaired in the absence of psychosis. One may have the "sense" of being followed when that is not the case and may experience hallucinations. One may have a quite distorted view of his or her strengths or weaknesses. If these hypotheses, no matter how bizarre, can be tested against objective evidence and as a result be rejected or at least doubted, psychosis can be ruled out. As reality testing—the capacity to challenge bizarre perceptions—becomes further impaired, the subject becomes less able or willing to look at or be swayed by external evidence. "Ideas" solidify as delusions, which progressively become more bizarre and complex. Thought becomes more and more preoccupied with fantasy and the subjective world as external cues are progressively ignored. The boundary between nonpsychotic and psychotic ideation and perception is not sharp. There is a spectrum from minimally distorted to grossly distorted nonpsychotic thinking, from mild impairment to severe impairment of reality testing, and from mild psychosis with circumscribed delusions to the extremely bizarre and disorganized psychotic state.

Reality sense: (See Psychosis.) Feelings, thoughts, and perceptions about the way things are.

Reality testing: (See Psychosis.) The process of testing thoughts or hypotheses against cues identified in the external world.

Schneiderian first-rank symptoms: Symptoms believed by Kurt Schneider, a German psychiatrist, to be pathognomonic of schizophrenia in the absence of organic disease: (1) Certain kinds of auditory hallucinations—hearing one's thoughts spoken aloud, hearing voices conversing with one another, or hearing voices keeping a running commentary on one's behavior. (2) Somatic hallucinations—frequently of a sexual nature, accompanied by delusional beliefs consistent with the sensations. The physical sensations are commonly attributed by the person to external causes, forces, energies, or hypnotic suggestion. (3) Thought withdrawal—the belief that other people are taking one's thoughts away. (4) Thought insertion—the belief that someone else is implanting thoughts into one's head. (5) Thought broadcasting—the belief that one's thoughts are known by others, as if everyone else could read one's mind. (6) Delusional perceptions—attaching abnormal significance, usually with self-reference, to a genuine perception. For example, the subject interprets a stop sign as an exhortation from another world to "stop being such a bad person." (7) Delusions of being controlled—the belief that one's actions, feelings, and impulses are really derived from, influenced by, or directed by external people or forces.

Stereotyping: An isolated, purposeless movement performed repetitively. A feature of catatonia and seen also in schizophrenia. Intoxication with amphetamine-like drugs will also produce stereotypical behavior.

Stupor: A particular level of diminished consciousness (ie, one stage more alert than coma) in which mental and physical activity is minimal as a result of organic impairment. Stupor can also refer to a functional state in which the patient appears to be unaware of the environment, unresponsive, and motionless but aware of the surroundings. A feature of catatonia and seen also in severe depression and schizophrenia.

Tangentiality: A disturbance of communication in which the subject "takes off on a tangent" away from a central idea or question and does not return. It may be a digression or an introduction of a new theme. It is related to loosening of associations and speech derailment in that there is a jump from one thought or topic to another. Tangentiality has been used synonymously with loosening of associations; however, the latter is characterized by repeated derailments with many associations that seem disconnected. Tangential thinking can be quite coherent as long as it successfully evades the central theme. A feature of a wide variety of pathological and normal states.

Thought broadcasting, thought insertion, thought withdrawal: See Schneiderian first-rank symptoms.

Thought disorder: Any disturbance of thinking that affects language, communication, thought content, or thought process. A disorder of thought content is characterized by delusions or marked illogicality. A formal thought disorder is a disorder in form or process of thinking, as distinguished from content of thought. Formal thought disorder is characterized by a failure to follow semantic, syntactic, or logical rules. It may range from simple blocking and mild circumstantiality to loosening of associations and loss of reality testing. Classically, formal thought disorder is the hallmark of schizophrenia.

Vegetative signs: In describing signs of depression, the term refers to disturbances of sleep, loss of appetite, weight loss, constipation, and loss of sexual interest. Vegetative functions refer to autonomic physiological functions related to growth, nutrition, or homeostasis of the organism.

REFERENCES & SUGGESTED READINGS

American Psychiatric Association: *Diagnostic and Statistical Manual of Mental Disorders,* 4th ed. American Psychiatric Association, 1994.

Campbell RJ: *Psychiatric Dictionary,* 7th ed. Oxford University Press, 1996.

Engel G: The need for a new medical model: A challenge for biomedicine. Science 1977;196:129.

Guest J: *Ordinary People.* Viking, 1976.

Smyth FS: The place of the humanities and social sciences in the education of physicians. J Med Educ 1962;37:495.

Section II.
Psychiatric Assessment

Introduction to Clinical Assessment: The Mayor of Wino Park

9

Howard H. Goldman, MD, MPH, PhD

Wino Park is an unoccupied rectangle of land "south of Market" in San Francisco. Open on two sides, this space has been somewhat crudely developed as a temporary haven for a shifting population of about 50 men and a few older women who lounge there out of the wind during the day. At night, these people are allowed to sleep in metal shelters if they have no better place to go. The police leave them alone if they remain quiet. There have been a few assaults and small-change robberies in Wino Park but no murders, no rapes, and no drug dealing that anyone knows of.

John Francis ("Red") Kimball, self-appointed Mayor of Wino Park, whose story is told in more detail in Chapter 14, has lived in the park for 4 or 5 months. After a night in jail, he is now in restraints in a police ambulance on his way to Memorial Hospital Emergency. As the ambulance backs to the unloading dock he shouts and struggles, complains loudly of brutal treatment, threatens legal action, and invokes retribution by powerful "friends downtown." With professional skill and no hard feelings, the attendants transfer the Mayor from the ambulance litter to a hospital gurney, strap him down, exchange paperwork and a few words of explanation with hospital intake personnel, and depart along a beam of revolving blue light in a crackle of radio code words.

In the reception area the Mayor alternately scowls and cajoles. He wants a cigarette. He wants to be liked and knows he won't be, a trashy drunk in a bored, intolerant time and place, a burden on the taxpayers, uncared for, welcome nowhere, all but homeless. He was married once but drank too much, was impotent, hit his wife, and lost her to California's smoothly functioning no-fault marital dissolution system. He lived for a while in a hotel in the Tenderloin district where the night manager agreed to receive and hold his monthly welfare and disability checks by arrangement with adult protective services workers. The Mayor now lives in Wino Park as his life slowly worsens. He drinks only wine, and not a lot of that by skid row standards—"up to 2 quarts a day" as described in Chapter 14. When not somnolent with drink he postures and harangues his fellows in the Park, turning away scorn with knowing glances. In occasional bursts of resolve he holds "news conferences" at downtown crosswalks, speaking into nonexistent microphones, raising an arm to take questions from the less favored correspondents in the back rows, fielding tough questions with quotable quips, expounding plans to extend ever grander services to his threadbare constituency if only the supervisors had the guts and the vision. Now there is talk of closing Wino Park. Nothing is so fierce as the functionary's loyalty to his function. Thinking about it the Mayor sometimes gets wild.

The Mayor has been to Memorial Hospital before, but he's worse this time. His assaults are more than bluster, and he is given three injections of diazepam that night. When he wakes he is nervy, somehow jaunty, and sexually aggressive with the female nurses. He is assigned to a senior medical student not yet at ease with psychiatric patients, whose job it is to deal with the Mayor until a decision can be made about what to do with him. Dealing with him means first recording vital signs and starting some tests for the Mayor's bulging file. With help from a technician, blood is drawn and sent for analysis. Urine and stool samples are taken. There is much vulgar comment and protest. The student has an ophthalmoscope; it's his favorite instrument but not an easy one to use. You have to get close, and this patient smells. You have to focus, and this patient jerks around. The medical student stands uncertainly with the instrument in his hand, wondering what to do, looking for all the world like a lost television reporter holding a field mike. Tomorrow is Father's Day and the student has been so busy that he hasn't even sent his father a card. Why is this rumball "mayor" sitting there as if he expects special treatment? Without thinking the student asks the most provocative question the Mayor has ever heard: "Mr Kimball, what brings you to the hospital at this time?"

THE MAYOR GRANTS AN INTERVIEW*

I'm the Mayor of Wino Park. They talk about closing me down. That's how I started drinking more and got real bad, turning yellow, blacking out. Next thing I know, I'm staring you in the face, like old times, we're buddies from way back, I remember last night, everything. You were scared, I could tell. I was a mess, right? But I walked in under my own steam, right? The Mayor don't need help. I see double, did you know that? I have pains in my belly, too.

I wasn't always like this. They didn't elect me Mayor for nothing. I have the gift. Sometimes I talk too much, give away my secrets. Like that cop, moving me along. I wasn't causing nobody any trouble. I was doing God's own work. "It's my secret fate to help people," I whispered that to the cop. I shouldn't have touched him. You can't touch cops these days. They overreact, like my old man. *He just couldn't stop hitting me! Sure I talked back to him! The way he yelled at Ma, then he was sorry. She couldn't have kids after me, something was wrong, she didn't come home with me from the hospital they said.* [Long pause.] He died in one of these places. Goddamn him. [Starting to cry.] Goddamn him.

INTRODUCTION TO CLINICAL ASSESSMENT

This was the first of many interviews with the Mayor. He stayed at the hospital for 3 weeks, undergoing extensive diagnostic evaluation, beginning treatment, and continuing in monitored rehabilitation after discharge. His evaluation included daily interviews, examinations and tests, and a personality assessment. These subjects are discussed in Chapters 10–13. Chapter 14 consists of the details of the assessment procedure and its results, presented in one commonly used case study format.

---

* Note that the Mayor's response to the medical student's query is somewhat at variance with the facts developed in Chapter 14.

The Psychiatric Interview

10

David E. Reiser, MD

Patient interviewing is a core skill in medicine. Despite technical advances, the bedrock of diagnosis and treatment continues to be communication. The doctor and patient must talk. Both, but particularly the doctor, must also know how to listen. No diagnostic test or apparatus can ever replace the human bond that forms the basis of medical practice, the doctor-patient relationship. The primary tool the physician utilizes to cement that relationship is a skillful and sensitive interview.

SIMILARITIES BETWEEN THE PSYCHIATRIC INTERVIEW & THE GENERAL MEDICAL INTERVIEW

The goal of all communication between doctor and patient is to facilitate *diagnosis and treatment* and further the aims of the *working alliance* between doctor and patient. Because of this, the psychiatric interview is similar in many ways to the general medical interview. It is useful to review the similarities before discussing important differences.

Diagnosis

Diagnosis and individualized assessment (formulation) are major goals of medical interviewing. An accurate diagnosis is the basis of every evaluation, and the diagnosis becomes the benchmark against which treatment success or failure is subsequently measured. This may seem obvious. What is not always appreciated, however, is the relationship between effective interviewing and accurate diagnosis.

Many patients withhold important medical information, fearing that it is too trivial or perhaps embarrassing to bring up. This is most apt to occur if the physician appears busy or impatient. For example, a modest girl in her teens presents to her family practitioner with complaints of fatigue. She has only recently entered puberty and is bashful about her sexuality. A brusque and hurried interview that focuses too quickly on a checklist of her symptoms may fail to elicit a symptom that embarrasses her—she has frequent urges to urinate. To the physician, this information is vital to a possible diagnosis of diabetes. To the patient, however, it is embarrassing, and it will be disclosed only in an atmosphere of openness and trust.

The interview also determines *what* is diagnosed. In a hurried, narrowly focused interview, for example, a physician might be able to elicit symptoms of congestive heart failure in a 60-year-old man. This information will do little good, however, if the physician notices nothing about the temperament and coping style of the patient. A skilled interviewer might go on to learn that for the past year this patient has been despondent over the death of his wife. Since her death, in fact, he has been noncompliant in the matter of taking medications, including digitalis. He says, "They gave my wife drugs toward the end, and that's what killed her." Bringing out these fears and attitudes is just as critical as eliciting a 10-day history of severe orthopnea.

Thus, good interviewing is essential both in establishing an accurate diagnosis and in gaining insight into the personality and coping style of the patient.

Treatment

Effective interviewing is also essential for effective treatment. For example, a physician makes a diagnosis of pneumococcal pneumonia in a 78-year-old widow living in a hotel for pensioners. He prescribes oral ampicillin, his receptionist schedules a return visit, and he considers his job done. Five days later, he learns that the patient has been admitted to the hospital in severe respiratory distress. What the physician failed to appreciate was the presence of Alzheimer's disease (discussed in Chapters 5 and 16). Not only had the patient failed to take her medication—she never had the prescription filled, forgetting all about it as soon as she left the physician's office.

Studies of patient compliance show that only 50–70% of patients comply with the therapeutic regimens prescribed by their physicians. Distrust, unexpressed anxiety, and confusion about physicians' instructions are the common reasons for noncompliance. *Most instances of noncompliance, in fact, seem to stem from breakdowns in the doctor-patient relationship.* Doctors think they communicate clearly to their patients, and patients think they understand what their physicians tell them—yet serious breakdowns in communication still occur.

The interview can be therapeutic in its own right. The prospect of help, the experience of being understood, and the impact of new insight offered by a trusted and respected physician can all have a therapeutic effect.

Effective interviewing must include, at a minimum, creation of an atmosphere conducive to a patient's expression of questions and concerns, opportunities for appropriate patient education, and meaningful follow-up. The doctor who walks out the door saying, "Call me if you have any questions," has not done enough. Patient education pamphlets, videotapes, and reprints can all be helpful. Yet there seems to be no substitute for an effective doctor-patient relationship, and the interview is the agent that cements it.

The Working Alliance

No treatment protocol is maximally effective if a good doctor-patient relationship has not been established. Regardless of our biotechnical skills, success depends to a great extent on the patient's compliance and trust. The working alliance can be defined as an agreement between physician and patient, based on mutual rapport and trust, to undertake treatment *together*. Steps in that process may entail discomfort and risk; they are deemed worth the risk when both believe that such steps may improve the patient's condition. In some treatments, this working alliance may simply be assumed. In others, it must not be taken for granted. A physician prescribing penicillin for streptococcal sore throat is not apt to read every paragraph of a pharmacology textbook concerning adverse drug reactions to the patient. At the other extreme, in the realm of "heroic medicine," there are dramatic instances of high technology being applied to medical conditions once thought to be unmanageable by any means. In such cases, patients may have to be given detailed information about all potential risks of treatment, and the working alliance obviously entails much communication between physician and patient regarding numerous critical details. Between such extremes lie most of medicine's daily challenges. In almost all cases, however, a physician's success with patients depends on the ability to establish an alliance based on trust and to communicate the necessary facts effectively.

As the foregoing is intended to suggest, there are many similarities between the psychiatric and the medical interview. This deserves to be emphasized, for the psychiatric interview is too often set apart in the clinician's mind as something abstract and specialized, based on knowledge and principles that need to be grasped only by psychiatrists. But as Harry Stack Sullivan (1962) has said, "Man is more simply human than otherwise." Psychiatric patients are not so different from other patients. Something has gone wrong, and they are seeking help. But like most patients, they are ambivalent about help, wanting it yet fearful of what might lie in the future—knowing that they need an expert to intervene yet unhappy with the realization that they cannot handle the problem themselves.

DIFFERENCES BETWEEN THE PSYCHIATRIC INTERVIEW & THE GENERAL MEDICAL INTERVIEW

The psychiatric interview differs from the medical interview in that the psychiatric patient must communicate personal concerns about disturbed mental functioning through language that can be formed only as a process of mentation. Depending on the psychiatric condition, this problem can be great or small; but in all cases, special tact and sensitivity are required of the psychiatric interviewer.

Diagnosis

The impediments to diagnosis posed by a psychiatric condition can vary considerably. A patient with a nonpsychotic disorder characterized by anxiety or depression may be able to communicate with no greater difficulty than any other patient. Many psychiatric conditions, however, affect the patient's ability to communicate and comprehend what is going on, as shown in the following examples:

1. A patient suffering from a psychotic disorder such as paranoid schizophrenia may be experiencing a flood of derogatory and frightening auditory hallucinations at the time of the interview. He may be convinced that someone is plotting to poison him and steal all of his possessions. The physician who walks into the room, extends a hand, and begins with a friendly introduction may be in for a rude surprise. Instead of smiling back obligingly, the patient may back into a corner, raise his fists in front of him, and say, "You're not coming near me with that poison!"

2. A manic patient may rush about the examination area uttering profanities, hardly able or willing to heed the doctor's reassurances. She may be busy testing all of the water faucets in the emergency area, convinced she has a magic formula for converting tap water into liquid uranium.

3. A demented patient may be outwardly cooperative. He will sit compliantly, nod when asked if he understands, and smile affably. Unfortunately, he thinks it is 1924 and is firmly convinced that the doctor interviewing him is his high school football coach.

4. A sociopathic patient may give a heart-wrenching story about the anguish of narcolepsy, leading the physician to miss the twinkle in her eyes as she asks for a prescription for 100 amphetamine tablets, "just like my doctor gives me back home."

The psychiatric interview may require multiple evaluations over time. A patient suffering from a psychiatric disorder, particularly in its acute stage, may be unable to tolerate a detailed, lengthy interview at the first meeting. At an early stage of illness a depressed patient may be too despondent and withdrawn to be helpful as a detailed informant. A manic patient may be more interested in reeling off profit projections from her latest scheme to establish a nationwide chain of boutiques than in reporting that she stopped taking her lithium. A paranoid patient may eye the clinician suspiciously, convinced that there are microphones strapped to his body. In all such cases, the clinician must be prepared to terminate the interview and resume it later when the patient's condition improves. Nothing is gained by attempting to force patients to endure the interviewing process beyond a comfortable limit.

The more acutely impaired a psychiatric patient is, the more the science of observation becomes critical. The science of observation will be elucidated further in the next section. It will suffice here to note that words are not the only source of information during an interview. Communication in a variety of other modes—including facial expressions and body language—conveys the underlying mood. If a clinician walks into the examining room and finds a disheveled, tense young man with clenched fists darting fearful glances around the room, the clinician has observed a great deal though the patient has not yet said anything.

The psychiatric interviewer must be prepared to seek out ancillary sources of data. People are usually part of a social network. Important members of this network will often be present in the emergency or acute care setting with the patient—friends, employers, spouses, ex-spouses, etc. When such people come with the patient to the acute care setting, it is usually worth spending some time talking with them, always with the patient's knowledge. Even when no one comes in with the patient, it is often good practice to seek such people out later for the help they can provide as informants. Stresses in a relationship often underlie psychiatric decompensation. The collateral information from people who know the patient is often invaluable.

Similarly, the physician should search old medical records, call prior treating physicians, and seek out other potential sources of data (school, military, employment records, etc) that may help in understanding the patient now. The patient's confidentiality, dignity, and trust must always be respected, but data obtained from collateral sources may be critical for effective diagnosis.

Treatment

There was a time when little other than communication was available to a psychiatrist treating patients. Antipsychotic drugs, effective antidepressants, and benzodiazepines are quite recent developments. The future holds prospects for effective somatic and pharmacological treatments, but communication will no doubt continue to play a central role.

The Working Alliance

Psychiatric patients, like many medical patients, are ambivalent about needing professional help. Even though they want help with problems they are unable to solve, they may feel humiliated and defeated by the mere fact of needing assistance. Wanting to change patterns of behavior, they nevertheless fear giving up familiar ways of coping. Patients who have great hopes for the results of treatment may also have great fear of failure. Cultural proscriptions and taboos about psychiatry and the "stigma" of psychiatric treatment reinforce such attitudes. A patient with a diseased heart or kidney usually does not feel shame to the same degree a patient with alcoholism or psychosis does. For these reasons, the interviewer must be sensitive to the importance of empathy, respect, and trust in order to develop a good working alliance with the patient. Regardless of what patients say or how they behave, the interviewer should assume that seeking psychiatric help is a distressing and conflict-laden event for all patients.

THE SCIENCE OF OBSERVATION

Illustrative Case

A group of medical students and their preceptor went to interview a 79-year-old woman in the orthopedics unit. She was in a semiprivate room and had a visitor, a woman in her mid-40s. Flowers, cards, and a framed photograph on the bedside table—of a handsome man in his late 50s wearing clothes styled in the late 1970s—showed that the patient was not alone in the world. She was in good spirits, with a hip that was only sprained and not more seriously injured. She asked her visitor to return another time—happy, she said, "to have some young people to talk to."

The preceptor was then unexpectedly called away to an emergency and urged the students to proceed with the interview for at most 20 minutes.

Later, the preceptor offered to anticipate the students' impressions of the old woman though he had been with her less than a minute before he was called away. The students were astonished at how much he had been able to observe in that time: that she was a widow, because she wore a wedding band and the picture would have been more recent—or there would have been none—if her husband were still alive; that she had grown children and maintained close ties with them, because a greeting to "the kids" (her grandchildren?) had gone with the visitor, who said, "Goodbye, Mom," and because the patient related so well to the young medical students; and that she belonged to several clubs and social groups, because there were so many flowers and cards—some with a great many signatures—in the room.

Most students think of the interview chiefly as something that they *do, perform,* and *conduct.* This is true, of course, but the interview is also a time to *ob-*

serve, perceive, and *take in.* The first concept of the interview is active and intrusive; the second is passive and receptive. In fact, the interview involves both, but most physicians err in the direction of being too active. One of the essential skills of observation is staying quiet so the patient can talk and so things can happen that need to be noted.

There are two phases to the observation component of the interview: active vigilance and what Freud (1912) called even-hovering attention.

Active vigilance is most appropriate during the first few minutes of the interaction. The "first few" minutes begin right away, as soon as the therapist and patient see each other, and not when they have settled down, with names exchanged and notes taken, so that the interview can formally "start." In the illustrative case above, the phase of active vigilance began the instant the group walked to the patient's bedside. During this phase of the interview, the student should take in as much as possible, actively and aggressively processing data that come in through all of the senses. How does the patient first greet the interviewer? Does he or she offer a hand or sit passively? Does the patient make eye contact? Is the handclasp firm and warm, or is it cold and clammy? Are there any books on the bed or table? What is the patient wearing? What are the first jokes and casual banter uttered by the patient? Are there any unusual sounds or smells in the room?

When the interview formally begins, the phase of active vigilance continues for the first few minutes of the dialogue. The student should make an effort to remember *everything* the patient says. What was the *very first* thing the patient said? What was the accompanying emotional tone? The following illustrate the importance of the patient's initial remarks:

1. "Whatever it is they're accusing me of, I didn't do it!" one patient "joked" at the start of an interview. It turned out that this man had been riddled with guilt since the suicide of his son 2 years previously. That is when his health began to fail.
2. "I wouldn't have nothin' to offer anyhow! Go away and leave me alone!" This patient turned out to be deeply tormented and embittered by her children's recent decision to place her in a nursing home.

After the phase of active vigilance, the student should shift to **even-hovering attention.** Students will discover, particularly if they have been vigilant in the first few minutes of the interaction, that they can remember the rest of the interview without resorting to detailed notes. Note taking is in fact discouraged except to jot down a few key facts, since a student with head lowered over a notepad is not looking at the patient and paying attention.

After the first few minutes, simply adopt a relaxed and receptive stance. *Listen!* Allow whatever the patient is saying to come into your mind freely. Allow yourself also to attend to the thoughts, ideas, and random associations that you are having while the patient is talking. There will be time for more focused and directive interviewing later.

Many students have conceptual difficulties that interfere with observation. One involves finding a balance between skeptical inquiry and jumping to conclusions. Another is an almost universal tendency to attribute what transpires in an interview to how well the interview was conducted. In the illustrative case, although most of the students were impressed by the preceptor's acumen, a few of them were angered by it and even felt the preceptor had jumped to conclusions. This does happen, and students are right to be cautious. Any conclusions drawn from limited data should be regarded as hypotheses, not certainties, and physicians should not hesitate to modify or expand their ideas about patients' problems as more data become available. At the same time, they should give the science of observation the benefit of the doubt before dismissing all hunches that can be extracted from small pieces of observable data. To be nonjudgmental and resist premature appraisal is laudable, but physicians cannot afford to ignore the clinical data the initial interaction so often provides.

The converse of this is that physicians should never assume that the data a patient provides are always perceived by them and the patient in the same way. Just as some interviewers ignore small yet important facts, others erroneously assume that they understand what the patient means even when the patient speaks in ambiguous terms. Patients talk about "not being myself lately" or being "out of sorts," "without get-up-and-go." The clinician should never assume that these and similar phrases are automatically clear. "Not being myself" could mean "I've been sexually impotent," or it could mean "I cry all night, and I've just bought a gun to kill myself with." It never hurts to ask, "What do you mean when you say you are not yourself?" "Out of sorts in what way, specifically?" "What do you mean by get-up-and-go?" The clarifying responses the patient then provides may startle the physician, who thought the patient meant something else entirely.

Regarding the concern that the student is always responsible for how an interview goes, only experience will teach that the interview is less influenced by what the examiner does than by the temperament and mood of the patient. It is primarily patients who shape the interview—and they do so with the same coping styles, wishes, fears, and conflicts with which they shape (or fail to shape) their lives. This is precisely why the interview provides such valuable data: it *replicates* the coping pattern and difficulties of the patient.

Students are always eager to learn how to correct what they did wrong and to understand what they could have done to make an interview go better. Interviewing technique is important, and students are right to ask for constructive criticism. But sooner or later they must also understand that how an interview goes usually says more about the patient than about the student. To assert this principle is not to deny responsibility for contemplating one's own limitations but to recognize an important diagnostic principle of psychiatry.

CONTENT & PROCESS

Illustrative Case

A 51-year-old construction foreman was being evaluated on a neuropsychiatry unit for symptoms of forgetfulness. He had had only a sixth-grade education but was highly regarded on the job and boasted of being a "self-made man." A medical student was conducting the initial evaluation interview. In responding to a question about the family, the patient began to speak derisively about his son, whom he had sent to college but who was now staying at home, collecting unemployment insurance, and playing a guitar and dreaming of riches on the rock scene. "He may have a college degree, but there's things I know that only life can teach!"

The medical student listened attentively and respectfully. Then he said, "It sounds like your son doesn't always respect what you know, what experience has taught you."

"That's right!"

The medical student then made an important intuitive connection. "I'm probably about the same age as your son," he said. "I hope I don't come across as a know-it-all with you. I'm a student—I told you that. Be sure to let me know if I'm not understanding something."

"No, doc, you're doing all right. You're all right."

All interpersonal communication has both a content and a process (Reiser and Schroder, 1980). Everyone is accustomed to focusing on the *content* of communication, but it is often the *process* that communicates what is most important. Music offers a good analogy: the content forms the basic notes of communication, while process comprises the rhythm, timing, chord structure, and harmony. Content is the literal *what* that is being said; process is the timing and flow, the all-important *way* in which something is said.

Although there is process communication in all interactions, its importance obviously varies. In asking a store clerk how much something costs, the process is hardly important unless local custom encourages bargaining. In the doctor-patient interaction, however, process is always important. Regardless of what the problem is, the patient will always have concerns about the doctor. "Can this person help me?" "Does he care about me?" "Does she find my problem dis-

gusting?" "Trivial?" "Has he ever seen anyone with my problem before?" The foreman in the illustrative case had an important concern: would the young "doctor" treat him with understanding and respect? Although the specifics may vary, the concerns are universal, and addressing them sympathetically will help establish a good working alliance. Because patients can rarely express these concerns directly, they almost always do so through process, though they are not always aware of it.

Mastering and understanding the process level of communication are exacting skills that take time and experience to acquire. The interviewer can usually detect the process level of a patient's communications by asking three questions: (1) What is the patient telling me about his or her concerns *right now?* (2) What is the patient telling me about his or her feelings *right now?* (3) What is the patient telling me about his or her feelings concerning what is going on between us *right now?*

This is how the student understood his patient's concerns in the illustrative case. *Right now,* the patient was saying he was concerned about whether the young student would patronize him. *Right now,* he was saying that he wanted to be treated with respect even though he was not an educated man.

Attention to process often answers another key question in the psychiatric interview: *why now?* A 46-year-old man with a 20-year history of manic-depressive illness comes to the emergency room markedly depressed. *Why now?* A young college senior develops a delusion that he is part of an international scheme. *Why now?*

What has been going on in the patient's life? The answer is always critical. It will frequently be found in the process of a patient's communication more than in the content. In the case of one very depressed man, for example, the process level of his communication dwelt extensively on themes of rejection and loss. He even told a sad joke about a man who was a cuckold. This process unfolded while the patient ostensibly disclosed only content. "I've been married 15 years to a good woman." This prompted the interviewer to inquire further about the patient's marriage and enabled him to learn that the patient suspected his wife had started an affair. This was the *why now?* for this patient's illness.

Finally, the concept of process is closely related to the phenomenon of **transference,** discussed in Chapter 31. In the psychiatric relationship, the intense feelings a patient has toward his or her therapist may be critical. Success in psychotherapy often depends on the skillful handling of these feelings. In certain forms of therapy, such as psychoanalysis and psychoanalytically oriented psychotherapy (see Chapter 31), an understanding of the patient's transference actually becomes an integral part of the process of treatment itself. With few exceptions, the nature and extent of the transference will also be communicated in process.

THE "A.R.T." OF INTERVIEWING

Every psychiatric interview may be conceptualized as having three phases: *A*ssessment, *R*anking, and *T*ransition (Reiser and Schroder, 1980).

Assessment

The assessment phase of the interview is the maximally open-ended, nondirective phase of the interaction. The setting should be a quiet and private place where doctor and patient can talk in an unhurried manner. Both should be seated and able to interact in normal tones at about the same eye level. If such a setting is not available, an empathic interview can go a long way toward overcoming the disadvantages of noise and lack of privacy. In all cases, the interviewer should try to ensure the best setting possible under the circumstances.

The interviewer should introduce and identify himself or herself, clearly explain the purpose of the meeting with the patient, and then invite the patient to begin in as open-ended a manner as possible. Some interviewers use a standard phrase, eg, "What sort of troubles have you been having?" or, "Tell me about the problem that brings you here." Some simply begin with a look of interest and an inviting gesture of the hand.

There are several reasons why it is important to start in an open-ended manner. First, an invitation to talk tells the patient, "You're important to me. I am interested in everything about you. Everything that concerns you is potentially of concern to me." Communicating this attitude is always important in medicine, but is even more important when working with patients who have problems that damage their sense of self-worth and their ability to trust others. Second, the clinician can often discern subtle but important clues to disturbances in thought processes. In response to the open-ended beginning of the interview, does the patient proceed to tell his or her story in a logical, goal-directed manner, ramble in a loose and incoherent way about seemingly unrelated concerns, or start to cry and seem unable to articulate any story at all? Is there inappropriate laughter? Is there a rush of language amounting to pressure of speech? These and similar incongruities of affect and cognitive disturbances (see Chapter 11) can be readily diagnosed if the interviewer is appropriately nondirective. If the examiner too quickly launches into a content-intensive, checklist style of interviewing, such data may be missed. A third reason for beginning in an open-ended manner is perhaps the most important. The physician may be wrong in assuming he or she knows what is most important in the patient's presentation. If a patient entering an emergency room appeared belligerent and paranoid and expressed fears of gangland revenge, the physician may have initially assumed that the person was suffering from a psy-chosis of the paranoid type, probably schizophrenia. Yet this conclusion would have to be reassessed if, in the course of an open-ended interview, the patient began to talk about his activities as a drug dealer and his recent heavy use of cocaine.

During the assessment phase, the patient will raise concerns, describe symptoms, and offer other clues the clinician will wish to investigate further. These will range from the patient's medical and past psychiatric history to family relations and vocational and financial difficulties. After a time—usually 3–10 minutes—the clinician will be ready to begin the second phase of the interview process.

Ranking

During the ranking phase of the interview, the physician makes decisions about the order in which different areas of inquiry should be examined. During the 3- to 10-minute assessment phase, the patient may introduce numerous areas of interest worth pursuing. What comes first? It is common practice to proceed first with the medical history, particularly the present illness, but this is seldom necessary (except, of course, in true emergencies) and may be ill-advised. It is best to postpone the medical history if it is suspected that the patient has apprehensions about the doctor-patient relationship itself. These concerns are usually expressed in process (as in the illustrative case described above). When these concerns are significant, they need to be dealt with before other data are obtained. Thus, the physician might rank a given patient's problems as follows: (1) concerns about whether I will understand that he is afraid to come to the hospital, (2) a 3-week history of depression and suicidal ideation, (3) the breakup of a marriage, and (4) the loss of a job after 20 years. The physician might then proceed by saying, "Before we talk further about your depression, Mr Smith, do I get the feeling you're afraid I'll insist you be hospitalized tonight?" Within each ranked area, the examiner should proceed from an open-ended, nondirective style to a progressively more focused and defined inquiry. Thus, the physician might say, "Tell me more about this feeling of hopelessness." After the patient has attempted to do so, the clinician's inquiry would become progressively more directive: "Have you lost any weight over the past few weeks?" "How many pounds would you say you've lost?" etc. Finally, questions that require the most specific type of responses may be asked: "Would you say you've lost a couple of pounds or 10 pounds in the last 2 weeks?" A good rule in ranking is to let the patient's priorities control whenever possible. The physician may be eager to elicit data concerning sleeplessness and euphoria or a 20-year drinking history. The patient may be much more troubled by concerns about being hospitalized or perhaps by something else altogether—something concerning the family or changes in employment or health.

Transition

Assessment and ranking are complex clinical skills that develop gradually as experience and knowledge increase; transitions are fairly easy from the first day. A transition consists of telling the patient when and why the subject of the interview is being changed. After the assessment phase, for example, the clinician may say, "It sounds like you're very concerned about the effect your drinking is having on your wife. But right now I'd like to hear more about why you think you want to end it all." In this instance, the clinician has properly given assessment of suicidal ideation a very high priority. The clinician ranked this consideration first after listening to many of the patient's concerns and then made a transition by telling the patient exactly what the focus of attention was and why.

Transitions may also be used to return to a more open-ended interview, after a specific line of inquiry has run its course. After a careful review of systems, the clinician might say, "Now that I've gotten the basics I need concerning your medical history, perhaps we could return to something you mentioned earlier—that your grandmother was hospitalized once for a psychiatric problem and things didn't go well. Could you tell me more about that?"

The line of questioning is usually clear in the clinician's mind, but the patient cannot be expected to understand what the clinician is up to. Great care must be taken to avoid confusion in changing the topic of inquiry.

"A.R.T." Sequence

Although assessment, ranking, and transition have been presented in sequence, all three actually go on simultaneously. For example, during a review of systems, the clinician may discover a new fact that should be assessed more thoroughly then and there, indicating a need to return to the assessment phase of the interview. As the doctor-patient relationship proceeds, new facts are always emerging that require reassessment and ranking.

SPECIFIC INTERVIEWING TECHNIQUES

The foundation of good psychiatric interviewing—indeed all medical interviewing—is a working alliance between doctor and patient in a spirit of growing mutual trust. No amount of skill in technique can compensate for basic defects in this alliance. Conversely, a patient will usually forgive the doctor any number of mistakes if basic trust is there. The most potent single interviewing technique, therefore, is *empathy*, an appreciation of what the patient is going through. It is far more important than any special technique, more meaningful to the patient than anything learned from this or any other book. With that understood, the remainder of this chapter can be given over to comments about "tricks of the trade" of interviewing adapted from Reiser and Rosen (1984).*

1. **Pay attention to the patient's comfort.** Too often, students see patients in crowded institutional settings where their dignity, privacy, and comfort are neglected. Doctors converge around the bedside in large groups and literally "talk down" to the supine patient. Introductions are mumbled or omitted altogether. Perhaps some of this is inevitable, but the psychiatric interviewer should be more meticulous in such matters. A quiet and private setting should be found if possible. Doctor and patient should both be comfortable and able to interact at eye level. Perhaps this sort of courtesy should not be called a technique at all. But its benefits for the patient and the interviewing process are so frequently overlooked that it must be underscored.

2. **Remember the basics.** As emphasized in previous sections, *understanding* the patient is more important than rigid adherence to classic technique. Nevertheless, a few of the standard interviewing rules and nostrums are helpful. (a) Don't ask two questions at the same time. ("Have you ever been bothered by voices or odd beliefs?") (b) An open-ended question is usually preferable to a closed-ended one. (c) Don't ask questions calling for negative answers. ("You haven't had any experience with 'voices,' have you?") (d) Avoid being judgmental. ("Have you had any disgusting or obscene thoughts?") (e) Make liberal use of facilitating remarks. ("I see. . . . Tell me more. . . . How was that for you? . . . Go on. . . .") (f) Ask for clarification. ("Can you explain what you meant by that? I'm not sure I exactly followed that.")

3. **Don't be afraid to be yourself.** The student should not try to imitate a portrait of Freud in a double-breasted suit. If a patient tells a joke and the joke is funny, go ahead and laugh. If the patient wants to know something about you—where you come from, whether you are married and have children—go ahead and answer. It is an unfortunate myth that the doctor-patient relationship should be totally unilateral, with the patient telling all and the doctor revealing nothing. In an unselfconscious way, always respecting the patient's dignity, you should feel free to tell who you are, both in the facts you disclose and the attitude you convey. There are times when it is appropriate—indeed indicated—to touch a patient on his or her hand or shoulder. That may be perceived as "phony" if you are naturally reserved, and so you may not be able to bring it off. If that is the case, don't force it. But you should never be afraid to reach out and be human. Physical contact is a potent "drug" that—like any drug—may have major side effects. It takes experience to know when to touch as well as when not to. Still, too much has been written about

---

* Adapted and reproduced with permission of the copyright holder, University Park Press.

the psychiatrist as an iceberg—silent, cold, and unbending. Remember also that a patient can be "touched" in many ways. An empathic expression of understanding or a sincere look of concern on your face can often touch a patient more deeply than your hand on his or her shoulder. Be yourself. When you communicate, whether through words or by laying on your hands, be guided by your answer to the question, "Am I doing this for my patient?"

4. Encourage the expression of feelings. Some patients are under strong cultural proscriptions against public displays of affect, particularly grief and rage. Physicians may have the same attitude and, if so, may believe that if a patient starts to cry, for example, something must have gone wrong with the interview. Most psychiatric patients are in emotional states they feel they cannot express—usually rage and sorrow. Almost without exception, they should be encouraged to let these feelings come out. ("There are tears in your eyes. His death has left you *very* sad, hasn't it?") The only case in which encouraging expression of affect is contraindicated is when a patient is in danger of total loss of control, signaled by escalating behavior—a louder and louder voice, tenser body habitus, etc. In such circumstances, the interviewer should demand that affect be controlled.

5. Consider the patient in developmental terms. As this textbook makes clear, growth and development do not cease at age 21. It is often useful to consider the patient's stage of development. Might this depressed 50-year-old woman be suffering from "empty nest syndrome" (depression because the children have all left home)? Might this agitated psychotic young man be struggling with emotional conflicts related to sexual intimacy and separation from his family? A developmental perspective can assist the interviewer in understanding the patient's concerns, particularly if the patient and interviewer are of widely disparate ages.

6. Remember that the patient is more scared than you are. A young man is nervous about meeting you and about the implications of having a psychiatric disturbance. Will you read his mind? Will you find him unlikable? Is he on a course leading to incurable insanity? Or do you find his problems laughably trivial, not worthy of serious attention or compassion? Inexperienced clinicians are often apprehensive in approaching a psychiatric patient, but not nearly so apprehensive as the patient usually is, and knowing this may enable you to be of help sooner than otherwise.

7. Tell the patient what you think he or she is feeling. Imagine that you are suffering from a psychiatric disorder—eg, that you have developed severe phobic symptoms. You have become afraid to travel by air, then by car, and now are afraid even to leave your home on foot. Which of the following would seem more empathic to you? "Can you describe your reaction to these events?" or "You must feel like a prisoner! How painful for you!" Some clinicians argue against what may seem to be putting words in a patient's mouth. That is a pitfall to be avoided, but the risk is exaggerated. If you are occasionally wrong about what a patient is feeling, the patient will tell you so. If you are consistently wrong, something has prevented you from forming an empathic bond with that patient. If you are not sure you know what the patient is feeling, it is easy enough to ask, "What is this like for you?" or "How was that for you?" in order to elicit a report of the patient's affective experience. Clinicians miss a good opportunity to interact therapeutically when they do know how the patient is feeling but fail to communicate their insight to the patient.

8. When an interview bogs down, try repeating the patient's last words. This technique was first popularized by the psychologist Carl Rogers (1951), who felt it was maximally nondirective and encouraged patients to proceed in the direction they preferred. Overreliance on this technique, however, is counterproductive. All psychiatric interviews have a purpose, which is not restricted to letting a patient go wherever he or she wants. The interview should follow the patient's lead, but sometimes the physician must be directive. Repeating the patient's last words is a technique that can be effective and should be used when needed. Encouraging nods of the head or supportive murmurs can accomplish the same thing. Periods of silence should be permitted also.

9. Go ahead and ask the "unaskable." If you are in touch with your own feelings as well as those of your patient, you may realize that a patient is very scared, angry, or depressed. It may even occur to you that the patient is thinking of committing suicide. Fortunately, most do not, but even if a patient does not act on suicidal thoughts, he or she may feel terribly isolated and alone. Many patients think about death but feel they cannot tell anyone. A similar burden is imposed by other intense affects patients dread sharing. If you think that a patient might be suicidal, ask the question, tactfully and respectfully. It is impossible to put such an idea into a patient's head, which is what interviewers sometimes fear; but it is quite possible and very dangerous to ignore a patient's nonverbal signals. Most people who attempt suicide have seen a physician recently, often without indicating their intent, and many go on to use medications prescribed by the physician in the attempt. Thus, in the case of suicide, clinicians must always ask the "unaskable."

The same principle applies to many other areas—if you suspect alcoholism, drug abuse, child battering, or some other socially "delicate" problem, you must not be afraid to inquire. Occasionally you may give offense, but less often than one might think. Special note should be made of the subject of sexuality. Despite our "liberated" times, it is surprising how often interviewers overlook inquiring about sexual concerns. Sex is part of being human and is frequently affected by illness, particularly psychiatric illness. Usually, however, the physician must inquire firmly and directly if he or she hopes to be of any help in this aspect of the patient's welfare. Ultimately, it is not just suicide and sex but all taboos to which the admonition *ask!* applies: fear of death, mutilation, sexual dysfunction, madness, suicide. A patient will let you know if you should back off. More often, the patient will open up with an outpouring of gratitude and relief.

10. **Learn to be quiet.** When patients come to a point in their story at which they are about to disclose something uncomfortable, they will often fall silent. Silence can be socially awkward, but as a psychiatric interviewer you must learn to take advantage of it. When a patient falls silent, be silent too. The pressure does build, and it may seem awkward for a time, but the patient usually goes on to tell the interviewer what is really bothering him or her. Most interviewers would do well to listen more and talk less. If silence becomes unduly protracted, it may be useful to say something neutral—"Go ahead. . . . Yes, go on. . . . I'm listening"—to relieve awkwardness and encourage the patient to continue.

11. **Pay attention to body language.** Body language is one of many ways in which patients try to communicate. This subject has received considerable attention in both medical and lay publications, perhaps more than it deserves. Yet body language is an important way in which both patients and doctors express themselves. And unlike the tongue, the body seldom lies.

Body language can be particularly revealing at the beginning of the interview. Observe how patients position themselves and move. Watch how they sit or stand, seek or avoid eye contact, etc. Body language is a reliable form of communication that everyone uses. The trick, as with other observational skills, lies in being *conscious* of what is observed.

12. **Start broadly and then focus in.** As the above discussion of the "A.R.T." of interviewing makes clear, it is rarely necessary to focus narrowly on any agenda at the outset of an interview. Allow the patient at least 3–10 minutes for assessment, the most open-ended phase of the interview. Books about interviewing list many techniques for staying broadly focused

or narrowing in. They speak of open-ended versus closed-ended questions, of compound versus simple sentences, of facilitating responses, etc. Although such labeling may be useful for some students, most do not find this kind of analysis helpful. Instead, as in cinematography, the interviewer should think of technique as involving a gradual focusing in, from wide-angle distance shots to narrow-angle close-ups. The interviewer's responses during the assessment phase are broadly focused wide-angle responses consisting of empathic silences, repeating the patient's last words, identifying the patient's affect ("That must have made you very sad!"), requesting clarification, etc. As the interviewer begins to focus in, questions become more directed: "Tell me more about this depression, Mr Jones." Or, "You mentioned that you and your wife have been fighting. Tell me more about what's going on there." As the camera angle narrows progressively, the questions naturally become more constricting: "How long have you been feeling that life was hopeless?" "How many pounds have you lost?" Now the emphasis is on specific data, chronology of symptoms and their nature and severity, their relations to other symptoms, etc. At this stage, the interviewer inquires about symptoms and signs directly related to the diagnostic criteria for specific mental disorders. Finally, the interviewer may focus on the most narrowly directed question of all—those that can only be answered yes or no: "Have you ever had blackouts?" "Have you found yourself thinking that everyone is against you?"

SUMMARY

The 12 interviewing techniques discussed above, coupled with an understanding of the content/process distinction and the "A.R.T." of interviewing, should enable the psychiatric interviewer to obtain a meaningful story from the patient. The interviewer should always remember, however, that technique is invariably secondary to the human dimension of interviewing—above all, establishing empathy, respect, and trust.

REFERENCES & SUGGESTED READINGS

Balint M: *The Doctor, His Patient, and the Illness.* International Universities Press, 1972.

Bernstein L, Bernstein R (editors): *Interviewing: A Guide for Health Professionals.* Appleton & Lange, 1985.

Davis M: Variations in patients' compliance with doctors' orders: Analysis of congruence between survey responses and results of empirical investigations. J Med Educ 1966;41:1037.

Freud S: Recommendations to physicians practicing psychoanalysis (1912). In: *Standard Edition of the Complete Psychological Works of Sigmund Freud.* Vol 12. Hogarth Press, 1958.

MacKinnon RA, Michels R: *The Psychiatric Interview in Clinical Practice.* W.B. Saunders, 1971.

Reiser DE, Rosen DH: *Medicine as a Human Experience.* University Park Press, 1984.

Reiser DE, Schroder AK: *Patient Interviewing: The Human Dimension.* Williams & Wilkins, 1980.

Rogers CL: *Client-Centered Therapy.* Houghton Mifflin, 1951.

Simons RC, Pardes H: *Understanding Human Behavior in Health and Illness.* Williams & Wilkins, 1985.

Stroudemire A (editor): *Clinical Psychiatry for Medical Students.* Lippincott, 1990.

Stroudemire A: *Human Behavior: An Introduction for Medical Students.* Lippincott, 1990.

Sullivan HS: *Schizophrenia as a Human Process.* Norton, 1962.

The Mental Status Examination

11

Jonathan Mueller, MD, Ralph J. Kiernan, PhD, & J.W. Langston, MD

The mental status examination is an instrument used by the clinician to assess a patient's orientation, attention, feeling states, speech, thought patterns, and specific cognitive skills. Like a lens or filter, it allows the clinician to perceive details and patterns whose nature might otherwise be only vaguely delineated. This examination, along with a careful history, physical examination, and laboratory examination, provides the foundation for psychiatric diagnosis and clinical assessment. Table 11–1 lists the major elements of the mental status examination organized in hierarchical format.

As Hughlings Jackson pointed out, functions most recently evolved (phylogenetically and ontogenetically) are the most vulnerable to disruption. Psychiatrists study disruption of thoughts, feelings, and behaviors that emerge from the organic functioning of the brain: The hierarchical structure of the mental status examination reflects the fact that higher cortical functions, such as abstract thought, may be distorted or disrupted by pathological processes at many levels. It is obvious that a stuporous patient's appreciation of abstract similarities cannot be tested, but it is often forgotten that other factors also constrain assessment of thought processes. For example, a patient who is unable to attend because of fever or metabolic disturbance cannot make new memories, although the neuronal substrate for "memory making" may be structurally intact. Among the factors that affect the interpretation and conduct of the mental status examination are disturbances of attention, vigilance, or concentration; emotional turmoil; perceptual disturbances (impaired vision or hearing); and receptive or expressive language disorders. A patient unwilling to cooperate with the examination will neither reveal intact functions nor disclose deficits. Failure to recognize limitations at any of these levels will lead to errors both in diagnostic formulation and in determination of appropriate treatment.

Although the mental status examination will be presented here as a separate part of the clinical examination (chief complaint; history of present illness; past medical, psychiatric, and social history, etc), it must be emphasized that the mental status examination is not simply an encapsulated or isolated part of the evaluation. Information noted throughout the interview will later be reported in the mental status examination, and information gained during formal mental status testing may prompt the physician to reevaluate the medical history or to seek confirmation of details by returning to specific items later in the examination. When a patient has a memory disorder, for example, the clinician should suspect omissions and inconsistencies in the history and investigate other sources if needed.

Physicians do not always have multiple opportunities to evaluate patients and may be called on for urgent decisions about a patient's capacity for self-care, potential for violence, suicidal risk, or hold on reality. Particularly in emergency room and consultation/liaison settings, there is a premium on prompt assessment. To maximize the yield of the mental status examination, the clinician must be ever mindful of the privileged nature of the relationship with the patient and of the impact specific questions may have on the patient. Initially, the examiner should explain the purpose of the mental status examination, indicating that it is part of every complete patient evaluation. It may help reduce the patient's anxiety and avoid offending the patient to add, "You may find some of the questions very easy and some quite difficult to answer." The clinician must be able to note subtle behavioral clues (a change in voice tone, averted gaze, a tear, a swallow, a sigh, or hesitancy to discuss a particular matter) without losing track of material that must be covered in order to complete the examination. Although the examiner should have a structured scheme for covering all aspects of the mental status examination, a "shopping list" approach is not appropriate. Nevertheless, certain complaints, signs, or symptoms do require that a mental checklist be consulted. For example, if a patient experiences hallucinations, it is essential to obtain a detailed description of the phenomenon.

1. Are hallucinations auditory, visual, tactile, olfactory, or gustatory?

Table 11–1. Organizing the mental status examination (hierarchical format).

1. Presentation
2. Motor behavior and affect
3. Cognitive status
4. Thought
5. Mood

2. Are they elementary (simple points or lines) or complex (formed figures)?
3. Do visual hallucinations occur only in one part of the visual field?
4. Are they disturbing or comforting?
5. Is the hallucinating patient commanded to perform certain acts (eg, do things harmful to self or others), and if so can the commands be resisted?
6. Do the hallucinations seem to emanate from a particular source?

GENERAL FORMAT OF THE MENTAL STATUS EXAMINATION

The goal of the mental status examination is to assess—both qualitatively and quantitatively—a range of mental functions at a specific time. A clear record of the data provides a baseline for future examinations. Quantification of elements of the mental status examination enables the clinician to assess deterioration or improvement in specific functions over time.

Assessment of cognitive strengths and weaknesses traditionally has been done by psychologists. Physicians who wish to benefit from precise measurement of cognitive function must either master the psychological literature on the subject or learn to make their own assessments. Quantitative assessment of higher cortical functions (cognitive status examination) is a process that is essential for proper diagnosis and management of organic mental disorders. Specifically, attention, language, constructional ability, recent memory, calculation, and reasoning abilities such as appreciation of similarities and practical judgment can all be assessed in a graded fashion.

One practical way to characterize cognitive dysfunction is systematically to probe areas of intellectual functioning with screening questions difficult enough that a right answer implies an adequate level of function in that area and renders further testing of that area unnecessary. If the patient fails the **screening** item, the examiner presents a very easy question followed by a series of increasingly difficult ones (the **metric**). This "screen/metric" approach provides a graded quantitative measure of the degree of functional impairment in specific areas. Such an approach is rapid and efficient, since time is not wasted examining areas in which the patient has obvious strengths.

Several standardized brief mental status examinations serve as cognitive screening devices but are insensitive to important aspects of mental status. Textbooks often provide very detailed "laundry list" approaches to mental status examinations that may exhaust both patient and examiner when used rigidly and in their entirety. Such mental status examination formats are rarely presented hierarchically and do not provide quantifiable results. The following approach

to the standardized and quantified mental status examination is recommended for routine use in single or serial assessments. Although its organization differs from that of standard examinations in current use, it contains the same elements. A detailed outline of this mental status examination is provided in Table 11–2. Many of the terms are defined in the Glossary of Psychiatric Signs & Symptoms (Chapter 8) or elsewhere in the text.

Table 11–2. Detailed elements of the mental status examination (hierarchical format).

1. Presentation
Level of consciousness; coma to alert wakefulness (Glasgow Coma Scale; see Table 11–3)
General appearance: body habitus; hygiene; cosmesis; dress
Attitude: degree of cooperation and effort

2. Motor behavior and affect
Motor behavior: akinesia; involuntary movements; mannerisms
Affect: facial expression; gestures; speech characteristics; pressure, volume, prosody

3. Cognitive status
Attention
  Attention span: digit span; number of trials required to learn four words
  Concentration and vigilance: serial subtraction; letter cancellation tasks; months of year backward
Orientation: for personal identity; place; time
Language
  Fluency: spontaneous speech; description of picture
  Comprehension: of spoken or written language performing commands of graded complexity; response to "yes/no" questions; pointing to named or described items
  Repetition: sentences of graded difficulty; isolated words; letters; numbers
  Naming: objects and parts of objects to visual confrontation (or on tactile presentation)
  Reading: aloud for comprehension; paragraph; sentence; words; letters; numbers
  Writing: written description of picture; write name and address; write from dictation; copy a written phrase, word, or letter
  Spelling: words of graded difficulty
Memory
  Verbal memory: four unrelated words recalled after 5 minutes; recall of short story or paired words
  Visual memory: reproduction of figures; recall of where examiner hides object
Constructional ability: reproducing figures from memory; copying figures; constructing blocks or token designs
Calculations: addition, subtraction, multiplication, and division
Reasoning
  Practical judgment
  Abstraction: similarities and proverb interpretation

4. Thought
Process: coherence; goal directedness; logicality
Content: hallucinations; delusions; preoccupations; suicidal or homicidal ideation
Insight: nature of illness and awareness of factors that affect the course of the illness

5. Mood
Relation to affect and congruence with thought content

PRESENTATION

Level of Consciousness

Fluctuations in degree of alertness should be documented as precisely as possible. (For example, "Patient yawning and drowsy but responds to verbal encouragement with cooperation that never lasts more than 20 seconds.") Level of consciousness can be described along a continuum from coma to full alertness. **Coma** is a state in which neither verbal nor motor responses can be elicited by noxious stimuli. (In moderate to light coma, motor reflexes but not psychological responses may be elicited.) **Stupor** is a state in which vigorous and repeated stimulation is required to rouse the patient. **Somnolence** and **lethargy** are less obtunded states in which drowsy, inactive, and indifferent patients respond to stimulation in delayed or incomplete fashion. **Drowsiness** is a sleeplike state from which the patient cannot be roused fully by minor stimuli. **Alert wakefulness** is a state in which responses to auditory, tactile, or visual stimuli are prompt and appropriate.

The Glasgow Coma Scale (Table 11–3) developed by Teasdale and Jennett (1974) is a graded approach to assessment of impaired consciousness on the basis of eye opening and verbal and motor responses to various stimuli. The scale ranges from 3 for deep coma to 15 for alert wakefulness. It has been demonstrated to have great value in predicting degree of recovery in traumatic brain injury.

General Appearance

The examiner notes clothing, personal hygiene, and any use of cosmetics, documenting details of fastidiousness or inattention (eg, "a 3-day growth of beard with food spilled on his nightshirt"). Is the patient robust in appearance? Does he or she appear physically ill, with signs of alcoholism (eg, palmar erythema, facial flushing, spider angiomas) or endocrine disease (eg, cushingoid)? Special attention is paid to idiosyncrasies of appearance. These details should be recorded carefully enough so that a third party would be able to recognize the patient from the description without having seen the patient.

Attitude

Is the patient cooperative, evasive, arrogant, bemused, or apathetic? The patient's attitude toward the examiner and the examination situation determines to a large extent how much and what kind of information will be derived.

MOTOR BEHAVIOR & AFFECT

Motor Behavior

Are the patient's movements rapid, abrupt, clumsy, graceful, or totally absent? Is the level of motor activity fairly constant, or do abrupt periods of fitful hyperactivity alternate with apathetic withdrawal? If the patient displays unusual responses, how are they provoked? Are movements coherent and goal-directed, or do they have no discernible purpose? Are there bizarre repetitive stereotyped movements? Does behavior include nail biting (anxiety), tapping the feet (anxiety or akathisia), or sticking the tongue out and licking the lips repetitively (buccolingual-masticatory syndrome of tardive dyskinesia)?

If the patient is mute, does he or she consistently avoid the examiner's gaze, closing eyes tightly and resisting efforts to lift the lids (catatonic negativism or malingering)? Do the patient's movements repeat those of the examiner (echopraxia)? Will the patient's limbs remain in unnatural positions if placed there (called catalepsy or "waxy flexibility")? Is a mute patient able to write if handed a pencil or to nod yes or no in response to certain questions (indicating either aphemia or hysterical mutism)? Is there any change in behavior depending on whether the examiner discusses nonpersonal events rather than more personal issues such as the health of either the patient or the patient's immediate family?

Affect

"Affect" may be considered the observable correlate of emotion, ie, the outer manifestation of inner states. It may be characterized as bright, sluggish, voluble, expansive, anguished, tearful, etc. The examiner pays particular attention to the range, intensity, lability, and appropriateness of affective behavior.

Affect has three components: facial expression, gestures, and speech. Although speech and language are often described together, there is a rationale for considering the flow, volume, pressure, rhythm, and intonation of speech as kinetic phenomena apart from language. The emotional coloring (prosody) of speech

Table 11–3. Glasgow Coma Scale.

	Coma Scale[a]
Eyes open (E)	
Spontaneously	4
To speech	3
To pain	2
None	1
Best verbal response (V)	
Oriented	5
Confused	4
Inappropriate words	3
Incomprehensible sounds	2
None	1
Best motor response (M)	
Obeys commands	6
Localizes pain	5
Withdrawal	4
Flexion to pain	3
Extension to pain	2
None	1

[a] Summed Glasgow Coma Scale = E + M + V; range from 3 for deep coma to 15 for alert wakefulness.

may be impaired in major depression, in dysfunction of the basal ganglia, in Broca's aphasia ("motor" aphasia), or secondary to damage of the right cerebral hemisphere (see Chapter 5).

The term "witzelsucht" refers to a facetious jocularity sometimes observed in association with frontal lobe lesions.

"Blunted" affect is grossly diminished in range of emotional expression.

Explosions of tears or anger ("catastrophic reactions") can occur in organically impaired individuals confronted with tasks once simple but now difficult or impossible to perform.

Cognitive Status

Arguments can be made for assessing the patient's cognition at either the outset or the conclusion of the mental status examination. The authors believe that a structured assessment of the patient's cognitive status is best performed immediately after the clinician has noted the patient's initial presentation, motor behavior, and affect, before an attempt is made to assess thought and mood. Impairments in cognitive ability may masquerade as either thought disorder (aphasia may appear as "concreteness of thought") or mood disturbance (an amnestic patient given the diagnosis of cancer 2 days previously may make no spontaneous mention of this and may therefore appear to deny or be indifferent to the diagnosis).

Attention

Is the patient so preoccupied or easily distracted that cooperation with the examiner is impossible? Is there a visual field cut, inattention to a visual hemifield in the absence of a field cut, or neglect of one side of the body?

A. Immediate Recall: Immediate recall refers to the retention of small amounts of information for up to 30 seconds. Material "in" immediate recall requires further processing before it can enter more permanent memory stores.

Proper assessment of attention is of great importance, since it may have implications for further evaluation and treatment. In the presence of an attentional deficit, the examiner must be wary of drawing inferences from further testing of higher cortical functions. Since inattention is a hallmark of acute confusional state, its presence should prompt a search for remediable (toxic, metabolic, or infectious) medical problems. However, inattention may also be seen in nonorganic mental disorders such as brief psychotic reaction and posttraumatic stress disorders. As a general rule, digit span (see below) is preserved in the early stages of dementia, and it is not until cortical degeneration is well advanced that impaired attention is found.

Attention span may be assessed by having the patient repeat a list of words or a digit sequence presented at the rate of one digit per second. It is impor-

tant that the digits not be grouped (by rhythmic clusters or intonation) and that they be somewhat random (eg, not all odd or all even). This should be practiced, since it is difficult to present a string of digits in this fashion without clustering. Intact forward repetition of six digits rules out major attentional disturbance. Inability to repeat at least five digits is considered abnormal.

Patients who fail the initial screening task of six-digit repetition are presented with a metric: digit sequences of increasing length, beginning with three-digit numbers. The examiner discontinues this task only after the patient has missed twice at a given level (eg, two mistakes at the five-digit level).

B. Concentration and Vigilance: The ability to sustain attention over a longer period may be referred to as "concentration" or "vigilance." Serial 7s (see later section on Calculations) or repetition backward of a digit sequence or the months of the year (or days of the week) may be used to assess concentration. Psychiatric disorders such as anxiety, depression, and schizophrenia may impair vigilance without disrupting digit repetition.

Orientation

Orientation is assessed with reference to person, place, and time. Orientation to **person** (ability to give one's own name when asked to do so) reflects "overlearned" information and is seldom if ever lost in organic brain disease. Failure to give one's own name occurs in hysterical dissociation and most often reflects negativism, confusion, distraction, hearing impairment, or receptive language disorder.

Orientation to **place** can be tested with reference to country, state, county, city, type of building, name of building, location of building, and location in the building. A patient may know he or she is in a hospital but not know the city or state.

Orientation to **time** may be tested with reference to year, season, month, day of week, and date. Because time changes more frequently than location, it is more vulnerable to disruption and thus is the most sensitive index of disorientation. (However, time of day cannot be used as a screen for orientation to time, since patients may know or guess the time of day from numerous cues but have no idea of the month or year.)

Language

Failure to assess language in a systematic fashion is a shortcoming of many mental status examinations and can lead to diagnostic confusion. Word-finding difficulty (anomia), for example, may be mistakenly thought to reflect a disorder of memory or judgment. Aphasia (see Chapter 5) is a language disorder often mistakenly attributed to confusion, dementia, hysteria, or psychosis.

Language proficiency is assessed by testing four parameters: fluency, comprehension, repetition, and naming. (Reading and writing will not be discussed here.)

A. Fluency: Fluency refers to the ability to produce sentences of normal length, rhythm, and melody. It is commonly assessed by listening to the patient's spontaneous speech. Is speech hesitant, stammering, or inarticulate? Are words mumbled or spoken too softly to be heard? Is the volume constant, or does it decrease toward the end of the sentence? Does the patient use bizarre syntax resulting in nonsense? What is the range of vocabulary? Is speech "empty," consisting of few substantive words and frequent circumlocutions? (The function or some particular attribute of an item may be offered as a substitute for its name—eg, "the thing that holds it on your shirt," rather than "the clip of the pen.") Patients may become adept at masking word-finding difficulty by skirting certain issues or using unobtrusive circumlocutions.

A helpful method for assessing fluency is to have the patient describe what he or she observes in a picture. Although this is not truly spontaneous speech, there are distinct advantages to presenting each patient with a uniform speech stimulus. The examiner quickly learns to note neglect of details and to recognize subtle word-finding difficulties. When the patient has completed the description, the examiner can return to specific details of the picture that have been omitted or incorrectly described. Verbatim recording of a patient's description of the picture is essential. Special attention is paid to paraphasic errors, which consist of distortions involving either individual letters ("brain clumor") or whole words (eg, "stick" for pencil). Speech is described for clinical purposes in an all-or-nothing fashion as either "fluent" or "nonfluent."

B. Comprehension: Just as intact auditory perception is essential for optimal interactions between geriatric patients and friends or hospital staff, language comprehension is also crucial. Since repetition and comprehension may be "dissociated" in language disorders that spare the perisylvian speech areas (see Chapter 5), it is dangerous to infer intact comprehension from a patient's ability to repeat what is said. Thus, any consistent tendency by the patient to echo or repeat should actually raise a question of comprehension deficit. It is as if these patients are trying to "run the tape by" one more time in order to extract as much information from it as possible.

There are many ways to assess comprehension at the bedside. The patient can be asked to point to objects the examiner names or whose function is described. This method is limited by objects that are at hand and by the examiner's skill in abstract description of common objects. Another approach is to present questions that can be answered yes or no. If this is done, the examiner must ask at least six questions, since the patient has a 50–50 chance of answering any one question correctly. (It should also be noted that some aphasic patients are unable to say yes or no even when they know the answer.)

A graded screening and metric approach to testing comprehension that has proved useful is as follows:

The screening item consists of obeying a three-step command. At least five objects are placed in front of the patient, who is told to "turn over the paper, hand me the pen, and point to your nose." A patient who fails this task is asked to perform the metric, which consists of three one-step commands, two two-step commands, and one three-step command. Success in performing each of the one-step commands rules out major apraxic problems. (See Chapter 5 for discussion of ideomotor apraxia.)

The metric is performed (for example) as follows:

One-step commands: (1) Pick up the pen. (2) Point to the floor. (3) Hand me the keys.

Two-step commands: (1) Point to the pen and pick up the keys. (2) Hand me the paper and point to the coin.

Three-step command: Point to the keys, hand me the pen, and pick up the coin.

A surprising number of patients are unable to perform a three-step command despite intact cooperation, attention, and auditory acuity. Careful documentation of inability to comprehend and comply with complex requests (ie, subclinical language disorder) is of great value to the nursing staff and others who manage the patient on the ward. Documentation of such deficits minimizes the risk that these patients will be wrongfully considered negativistic or uncooperative.

C. Repetition: Sentences that are short and contain high-frequency ("everyday") words are the easiest to repeat. Longer sentences that contain low-frequency words or short grammatical function words with no objective referents ("from," "and") are more difficult to repeat. An appropriate screening sentence for repetition might be "The beginning movement revealed the composer's intention." The patient who fails this is given a series of phrases or sentences of graded difficulty as the metric: "Out the window." "He swam across the lake." "The winding road led to the village." "He left the latch open." "The honeycomb drew a swarm of bees." "No ifs, ands, or buts." Because the bizarre speech of patients with Wernicke's aphasia is fluent, the physician may incorrectly conclude that these patients are psychotic or in a confusional state. Demonstration of paraphasic errors on repetition tasks provides elegant proof of primary language dysfunction. Repetition is impaired in all of the major perisylvian aphasic syndromes.

D. Naming: Naming parts of an object (eg, "tentacle") is even more difficult than naming the object itself ("octopus"). Thus, an appropriate screening question turns out to be naming a pen and its parts on visual confrontation: cap or cover, point or nib, and clip. (The patient who can name a pen and its parts has intact naming ability and does not have aphasia.)

Although an individual who names items correctly does not have aphasia, not every patient who manifests naming difficulties has aphasia. Otherwise healthy individuals who are physically exhausted or sleep-deprived often manifest dysnomia, which may be an early nonspecific sign of generalized cerebral dysfunction secondary to metabolic disturbance. Aphasic dysnomia may occur as an isolated and dramatic deficit with localized left hemispheric lesions, or it may exist as part of a larger aphasic syndrome.

Unless naming is carefully assessed, the clinician runs the risk of mistaking word-finding difficulty for "thought blocking," amnesia, or impaired judgment. Accordingly, language is assessed prior to memory.

Memory

A. Verbal Memory: A general impression of the patient's memory can be gained from the way in which he or she presents the history. Is there internal consistency, or are there gaps and contradictions? Does the patient remember the physician's name from a past encounter, or does the patient confabulate, claiming to have met an individual whom he or she has never seen before? Is there a period for which the patient has poor recall? If so, is the patient unable to recall either personal or general information from that period (organic amnesia), or is there selective inability to recall personally relevant information (psychogenic amnesia)?

1. Recent memory—The ability to recall events of the past minutes or days reflects recent memory. (Orientation to place and time also actually reflects memory.) Recent memory is assessed clinically by asking the patient to learn new information. This is commonly done by presenting four unrelated words. The patient is told that he or she will be asked for these words later in the examination. The examiner must be certain the patient can repeat all four words before going on with other parts of the examination, which constitute "interference material." (The number of trials required to learn four words is another measure of attention.) Failure to make sure that the patient can repeat all four words invalidates any conclusions about recent memory as a specific ability area—the patient may simply not have been attending to the task, and apparent failure to recall may really reflect initial failure to register material.

For each word a patient is unable to recall after 5 or 10 minutes, a category prompt (eg, "a color" or "an animal") is given. If the patient is still unable to recall the word, a list of three or four words—one of which is the test word—is presented. Points may be assigned on the basis of whether a word is recalled on command (3 points), following a prompt (2 points), or recognized from a list (1 point). Five to 10 minutes after either a depressed patient or a severely amnestic alcoholic has been given four words to learn, neither may be able to recall any of the words when asked to do so. The depressed patient, however,

will usually respond to category prompts or recognize the words from lists, whereas an alcoholic patient with Korsakoff's syndrome may not even recall having been given a list of words to learn. The examiner who simply records "none of four words recalled at 5 minutes" for both of these patients fails to distinguish two very different situations. Moreover, a maximum 12-point scoring system (four items, each rated 0–3) allows the clinician to monitor improvement or deterioration of memory following administration of agents such as thiamine, digitalis and diuretics, or tricyclic antidepressants. Clinicians who ask patients what they had for breakfast should verify the answer by asking the nursing staff. It is worth repeating that the distinction between attentional and amnestic deficits is crucial. *The diagnosis of amnestic syndrome cannot be made in the presence of an attentional deficit.*

2. Remote memory—The ability to recall the events of weeks or years ago is difficult to assess clinically, since the examiner seldom knows enough about the patient to ask pertinent or verifiable questions. Unless the examiner is prepared to seek corroboration (such as what schools the patient actually attended or the dates of military service), there is no point in asking such questions. Questions about past presidents, dates of wars, and events that affect everyone (such as President Kennedy's assassination) are helpful, but evaluation of responses remains problematic, since failure to recall may reflect increasing forgetfulness (as in senile dementia) or a period of time during which the patient was unable to lay down memories. With resolution of memory problems (eg, following traumatic amnesia secondary to head injury, or in response to thiamine treatment of Wernicke-Korsakoff syndrome), older memories tend to return before more recent ones (Ribot's law).

B. Visual Memory: Patients may be asked to reproduce designs or report details of pictures after delays of seconds or minutes. Alliteratively, the examiner may ask the patient to remember a series of items (eg, clock, window, chair) or where the examiner places or hides an item such as a dollar bill (eg, behind a picture).

Constructional Ability

Although testing of constructional ability is frequently omitted from the routine mental status examination, it may be helpful in the detection of organic brain disease. Patients may be asked to copy drawings, manipulate blocks, or reconstruct a figure using tokens. Before the examiner draws conclusions about a patient's constructional ability, it is essential to assess visual acuity, motor functions (strength, praxis, and coordination), and tactile sensation.

As a screening test for constructional ability, the patient is instructed to study two figures for 10 seconds and is then asked to reproduce them from memory. Successful completion of the screen requires intact immediate visual recall as well as significant visual-spatial ability.

Individuals who fail the screen are asked to copy a series of increasingly difficult figures.

Calculations

The patient's education and professional background should be considered before calculating ability is tested. The traditional "serial 7s" task, in which the patient is asked to "subtract 7 from 100 and then continue, subtracting 7 from each answer," is a difficult task for many high school graduates (ie, over two-thirds are unable to get into the 50s without an error in less than 30 seconds). In addition to calculating ability, the task requires sustained concentration and is easily disrupted by anxiety; for this reason, difficulty with serial 7s should not be taken as evidence of dyscalculia. Simple addition, subtraction, and multiplication often assess rote learning (a type of remote recall) rather than calculating. Thus, an appropriate assessment of calculations involves tasks that fall somewhere between the two examples. Some patients find it simpler to address problems in daily life, such as making change from a purchase, rather than solving formal math problems. As a screening device, the question "How much is 5 × 13?" is appropriate. The following are examples of metric items:

How much is 5 + 3?
How much is 15 + 7?
How much is 39 ÷ 3?
How much is 31 − 8?

Reasoning

Cognition can be subdivided into two areas: practical judgment and abstraction (similarities and proverb interpretation).

A. Practical Judgment: Assessing practical judgment is particularly important in the evaluation of thought disorders, character disorders, or dementia. This area is difficult to appraise because many judgment questions can be answered "correctly" by the aid of simple memory (remembering what one's parents or teachers said should be done in a given situation). Practical judgment also reflects the patient's social and financial background. (A prosperous physician who loses his wallet in the airport in Denver, Colorado, might call home to have money wired to him, whereas an adolescent runaway might turn to Traveler's Aid, go to a local church, or try to hitchhike.)

1. Screening question—The patient is asked, "What would you do if you were stranded in the airport in Denver, Colorado, with only a dollar in your pocket?" Acceptable answers are calling a friend or family member to wire money and going to Traveler's Aid. If the patient claims to know people in the Denver area, the examiner should say, "For the purposes

of this question, imagine you are in an airport far away from anyone you know." If the patient suggests using credit cards, the examiner should say, "For the purposes of this question, imagine you do not have credit cards." Patients should be asked to explain their answers further when vague or partially correct answers are given.

2. Metric—The patient is asked the following series of questions. A score of 2 points is given for a fully correct answer, 1 point for a partially correct or vague answer, and no points for an incorrect answer. Examples of 2-point, 1-point, and 0-point answers for each item are given below.

a. What would you do if you woke up at 1 minute before 8:00 AM and remembered an appointment downtown at 8:00 AM? *Answers:* 2 points—call the person; 1 point—dress as quickly as I can and rush downtown; 1 point (vague)—cancel the appointment; 0 points—go back to bed.

b. What would you do if while walking beside a lake you saw a 2-year-old child playing alone at the end of a pier? *Answers:* 2 points—remove the child from the pier and look for the parents; 1 point—tell the child to get away from the water; 1 point (vague)—make sure the child is not harmed; 0 points—yell for help, look for a lifeguard, go for help.

c. What would you do if you came home and found a broken pipe was flooding the kitchen? *Answers:* 2 points—shut off the main water valve; 1 point—call the plumber; 1 point (vague)—stop the water; 0 points—mop up the mess.

B. Abstraction: (Similarities and proverb interpretation.)

1. Similarities—The ability to appreciate the commonality between two objects is tested as part of the Wechsler Adult Intelligence Scale. Low native intelligence, psychosis, distraction, or dementia may produce impairment in abstracting ability.

a. Screening question—The patient is told, "I am going to ask you how some things are alike." A specific example is then given: "For example, a hat and a coat are alike because they are both clothing." As a screening item, the patient is asked, "In what way are painting and music alike?" Only the abstract responses "art" or "forms of art" are passing. Less specific abstract responses, such as both are "artistic" or "created," are not passing answers.

b. Metric—The patient is told, "I have some other pairs of items. Again, I want you to tell me how they are alike. In what way are a rose and a tulip alike?" Each item is similarly introduced. The first time a patient responds with a difference between the items, that response is recorded and the patient is told, "That is how they are different. I want you to tell me how they are alike." Regardless of whether the patient goes on to give a good answer, no credit is given. Subsequent "difference" responses are not corrected or credited with points.

1. Rose-tulip: 2 points—flowers; 1 point—grow, have petals, need water, smell nice; 0 points—pretty, same color, fresh, outdoors.
2. Bicycle-train: 2 points—vehicles, means of transportation; 1 point—ride them, wheels, toys; 0 points—go fast, have tracks.
3. Watch-ruler: 2 points—measuring instruments; 1 point—have numbers, tell how much; 0 points—are useful, have many parts.
4. Corkscrew-hammer: 2 points—tools; 1 point—used by humans, made of metal, do work; 0 points—cut into things, are strong.

2. Proverb interpretation—Another means of assessing a patient's capacity to abstract is to ask for the patient's interpretation of a proverb. Proverbs such as "There's no use crying over spilled milk" and "The grass is always greener on the other side of the street" are easier than "People who live in glass houses shouldn't throw stones" or "Every cloud has a silver lining." Proverb interpretation is strongly influenced by culture, educational level, and socioeconomic class.

THOUGHT

Assessment of thought may be divided into several areas: process, content, cognitive functions (abstraction and judgment), fund of knowledge, and insight. Each will be discussed briefly. (For more detail the reader is referred to the discussion of Psychopathology and to the Glossary of Psychiatric Signs & Symptoms in Chapter 8.)

Thought Process

Process of thought is assessed by noting coherence of speech and reflects the way in which mental associations are made. Thought process may be described as concrete, tangential (getting off the track of the subject and failing to return), circumstantial (digressive but able to return to the subject), perseverative (sticking to a single thought, phrase, or word), loose (absence of logical thought progression), or incoherent. "Thought blocking" refers to sudden cessation of thought or speech. It may occur in schizophrenia, and lesser degrees are seen in anxiety states such as obsessive-compulsive disorders. In rare instances, thought process may be so disrupted that the examiner has little or no idea of the content of a patient's thought.

Thought Content

In assessing the content of a patient's thought, the examiner notes preoccupations, ambitions, phobias, and perceptual disturbances (such as illusions and hallucinations). Patients may be asked, "Do you have the feeling that you control your own thoughts?" On careful questioning, patients may admit that they believe thoughts are inserted into or withdrawn from

their minds or broadcast to others, or that their thoughts are controlled by outside forces.

Specific fears or beliefs should not be taken at face value, but their origins should be explored. A statement such as "I don't want to go out of my house," for example, may have widely different meanings. A patient with a right parietal lobe tumor may no longer be able to find the way home after walking to a nearby store. One suffering from a major depressive disorder may feel too tired to go for a walk or may have lost all interest in former sources of pleasure. A schizophrenic patient may fear being overtaken by enemies and tortured. Yet another individual may fear open streets or becoming trapped in a crowd.

Patients who deny specific delusions may still claim to have a special relationship with God. It is often helpful to ask patients, "How do you think others feel about you?" (admired, shunned, unappreciated, etc).

Although visual and olfactory hallucinations may occur in "functional" psychoses such as schizophrenia or mania, they tend to occur more frequently in association with organic disease. Patients should be asked to describe how vivid and frequent their hallucinations are, in what circumstances they occur (on falling asleep or waking), and whether they are pleasant, comforting, or terrifying. They should be asked to identify the source of the hallucination (whether it originates within the patient or is projected from some outer source). If hallucinations consist of commands, patients should be asked whether they are able to resist the commands. Patients who are asked if they have special bodily feelings may respond that they feel dead or unreal inside.

Insight

The patient's degree of understanding of his or her medical or psychological problems is a measure of insight. The patient may be asked, "How do you understand your problems?" or "What has been most helpful to you in dealing with this problem in the past?" Although insight and understanding are often essential to working with patients, some patients are able to acquire insight only after their behavior has changed. It is always important to look for cognitive, perceptual, or informational explanations of "poor insight" before imputing to patients psychodynamic defenses against insight.

MOOD

Since patients with word-finding difficulty or memory disturbances may be unable to describe or recall their mood over the past few days or weeks, interpreting a patient's subjective report of mood requires knowledge of language skills and memory function. For this reason mood is not assessed or described until cognition has been assessed.

The term "mood" denotes a persisting subjective

state-of-feeling tone as reported by the patient. If the patient does not volunteer a description of his or her mood, the examiner may ask, "How are you feeling inside?" or "What are your spirits like?" Mood may be characterized (for example) as blue, despondent, anxious, fearful, bored, exuberant, irritable, or restless.

Are there dissociations between affect and reported mood? Does the patient with immobile facies say that he or she feels nothing inside or report that he or she feels sad but cannot cry? Does the facial expression of a schizophrenic patient who describes inner feelings of fear or emptiness reflect this, or does he or she wear a "silly" smile while describing inner turmoil? Patients with pseudobulbar palsy (which results from disruption of fibers connecting frontal motor cortex with brainstem nuclei subserving emotional expression) may report episodes of laughing or crying uncontrollably, breaking into laughter when they feel blackly depressed, or crying when amused.

MENTAL STATUS & INTELLIGENCE

Mental status examination and intelligence testing are often combined. Elements of the mental status examination are tested in formal tests of intelligence. Abnormalities in mental status (eg, attention or memory) clearly affect ability to complete tests of intelligence (see Chapter 13 for a detailed discussion of tests of intelligence). Conversely, some rough measures of intelligence, particularly fund of knowledge, often are included in mental status examinations. Our formal examination format does not include measurement of fund of knowledge, but it is briefly described here for the sake of completeness.

The patient's **fund of knowledge** may be assessed by asking questions about a wide range of subjects (politics, literature, art, history, geography, etc). In addition to reflecting educational level, the questioning may also help evaluate recent and remote memory. Although intelligence often manifests itself in a wide range of interests, some individuals with superior intelligence actually have very restricted interests. Vocabulary (noted under speech) represents a particular example of fund of knowledge and correlates highly with intelligence.

REFERENCES & SUGGESTED READINGS

Benson DF: *Aphasia, Alexia and Agraphia.* Churchill Livingstone, 1979.

Campbell RJ: *Psychiatric Dictionary,* 6th ed. Oxford University Press, 1989.

Cummings JL: *Clinical Neuropsychiatry.* Grune & Stratton, 1985.

Kiernan RJ, Mueller J, Langston JW, Van Dyke C: The neurobehavioral cognitive status assessment. Ann Intern Med 1987;107:481.

Schwamm LH, Van Dyke C, Kiernan RJ, Merrin EL, Mueller J: The neurobehavioral cognitive status examination: Comparison with the cognitive capacity screening examination and the mini-mental state examination in a neurosurgical population. Ann Intern Med 1987;107:486.

Taylor J (editor): *Selected Writings of John Hughlings Jackson.* Basic Books, 1958.

Teasdale G, Jennett B: Assessment of coma and impaired consciousness: A practical scale. Lancet 1974;2:81.

Van Dyke C, Mueller J, Kiernan RJ: The case for psychiatrists as authorities on cognition. Psychosomatics 1987; 28:87.

Walsh KW: *Neuropsychology.* Churchill Livingstone, 1977.

Physical Examination & Laboratory Evaluation

Frederick G. Flynn, DO, COL, MC, & Jonathan Mueller, MD

The ability to perform a physical examination is, like any other skill, acquired and maintained by frequent practice. Many psychiatrists who have completed their training—and particularly those whose practices are exclusively outpatient—often do not perform physical examinations. This is unfortunate, because internists and other specialists often perform abbreviated neurological examinations, but rarely perform a mental status examination, despite neuropsychiatric symptoms. As the role of the neurosciences and other branches of medicine becomes increasingly important in the practice of modern psychiatry, the ability of the psychiatrist to perform relevant physical examinations should become a central concern of psychiatric education. Since the purpose of the physical examination is to confirm or refute hypotheses that have been formulated on the basis of the patient's history and a review of systems, these areas will be considered first.

MEDICAL HISTORY & REVIEW OF SYSTEMS

Medical History

Detailed attention to the medical history reassures patients that they are being seen by a physician who recognizes the interplay between physical and mental distress. As an expression of concern for the patient's reactions to and feelings about illness, history taking helps to establish a working alliance between patient and therapist. The medical history obtained from a psychiatric patient may provide clues to the cause of changes in mental status and inevitably sheds light on the patient's biological limitations—to what existential psychotherapists term the patient's "being in the world."

The earliest events that influence central nervous system development are experienced in utero. These may include maternal illness, use of prescription medication, physical and emotional abuse, as well as abuse of alcohol, nicotine, narcotics, and other psychoactive drugs. Patients are often unaware of major prenatal events. Thus, documentation from previous medical records and history obtained from siblings, parents, or other relatives may be crucial.

Early childhood illnesses or developmental problems may be significant either because of enduring effects on major organ systems or because of suspicions they raise about immunological compromise. Major medical illnesses in a child or other members of the family may result in prolonged separation of the child from the parents or a significant decrease in time spent with—and interest shown in—a developing child's accomplishments or difficulties.

Surgical procedures, regardless of the age at which they are performed, have special importance as events during which control of the body is relinquished to a team of professionals. Hip fracture in an elderly patient may precipitate a series of physical and psychological events culminating in loss of autonomy. Any major surgical procedure exposes the patient to risks of hypotension and anesthesia. Cardiac surgery is particularly noted for having neurobehavioral sequela. "She has never been the same since her operation" is a frequent observation made by friends and family of elderly patients. Persistent confusion is common in elderly patients after surgical procedures or during minor illnesses, particularly when there is an underlying dementia. Changes in medications may also precipitate acute confusional states in the elderly. Often acute confusional states will last for days beyond the discovery of the cause and the initiation of treatment. All current medications and dosage schedules should be listed, along with past and present use of alcohol and other substances.

Special attention should be devoted to documenting the occurrence of neurological disturbances. Seizures, stroke, headaches, dizziness, gait disturbance, head trauma, blackouts, loss of consciousness, language problems, and memory problems all have great bearing on psychiatric assessment. A family history of any of the above neurological conditions can be very helpful in differentiating conditions that may present in similar fashion (eg, complex partial seizures and confusional migraine). Likewise, endocrine, metabolic, vascular, autoimmune, toxic, infectious, nutritional, neoplastic, degenerative, and focal and/or diffuse central nervous sytem lesions may all present initially as psychiatric illness.

Review of Systems

The following list is not exhaustive but provides examples of physical dysfunction with major implications for psychiatric assessment and management.

A. Nervous System and Sensory Organs:
Complaints of headache may arise from a wide range of causes, including stress, migraine, hypoxia, brain tumor, subarachnoid hemorrhage, cerebrovascular disease, and meningitis. Since binocular diplopia very rarely represents a conversion phenomenon, complaints of double vision should always trigger a search for disorders of neurological origin, such as Wernicke's encephalopathy, multiple sclerosis, cranial nerve palsies, brain tumor, and stroke. Visual hallucinations or illusions may arise from structural damage to any part of the visual system, eg, from anterior ocular disease (ie, cataract formation, or diseases of the macula, choroid, or retina), or injury to the optic nerve or tract, visual radiations, or the occipital cortex. Ocular damage that results in hallucinatory phenomena is known as the Charles Bonnet syndrome. Hallucinations confined to one visual hemifield or one visual quadrant suggest structural damage from disease or injury, focal seizure emanating from the visual cortex, or migraine. Older patients should be asked about changes in hearing or vision, since correction of these deficits (hearing aid or glasses) can improve the ability of patients to care for themselves and to lead independent social lives. Loss of hearing may lead to paranoid ideation or auditory hallucinations. Uncorrected end organ hearing loss may result in the spurious misinterpretation that a patient has a dementia or a receptive aphasia. Gait disturbance in the elderly may be due to a primary lesion in the brain (eg, cerebellum or frontal lobe), but is more often due to a combination of sensory input problems such as visual loss and diminished proprioception.

B. Cardiovascular System: Recurrent anxiety may reflect cardiac arrhythmia (particularly paroxysmal atrial tachycardia), angina, or mitral valve prolapse. Worsening of congestive heart failure with attendant drowsiness or hypoxemia may be easily mistaken for depression. Any history of angina, arrhythmia, or myocardial infarction should be noted. Heart disease may impose significant limitations on the patient's life-style, and cardiac medications may have psychoactive effects.

C. Respiratory System: Episodic shortness of breath or hyperventilation may occur secondary to panic attacks or may be seen in the context of general anxiety disorders. Conditions such as chronic obstructive pulmonary disease, emphysema, congestive heart failure, pulmonary embolism, and pneumonia must always be considered when anxiety is assessed. Excessive daytime hypersomnolence may be a symptom of obstructive sleep apnea (OSA). Fatigue, memory, and concentration problems as well as cognitive slowing are all complaints that may be associated with OSA.

D. Gastrointestinal System: Vague recurrent abdominal symptoms may be seen in patients with somatoform disorders (eg, conversion disorder and somatization disorder), but abdominal distress due to organic causes (eg, regional enteritis, ulcerative colitis, and porphyria) may be accompanied by prominent psychological distress. In the case of porphyria, frank psychosis may be experienced. Anorexia is a vegetative sign of depression, but loss of appetite may also arise from numerous organic causes, particularly cancer. Hyperphagia with weight gain may be a sign of diabetes mellitus (eating habits reflect rapidly changing blood glucose levels) or may occur in atypical cases of depression or rare cases of ventromedial hypothalamic disorders. Diarrhea may be due to irritable bowel syndrome or a malabsorption syndrome. Diarrhea accompanied by nausea, polyuria, and polydipsia may be a sign of lithium toxicity. Diarrhea associated with lymphadenopathy and dementia suggest Whipple's disease. Hypomotility or atony of the bowel, on the other hand, may be caused by use of psychiatric medications with anticholinergic properties (eg, tricyclic antidepressants, low-potency neuroleptics, and antiparkinsonism medications). Pernicious anemia or surgery of the stomach and/or proximal small intestine may result in cognitive and mood changes secondary to vitamin B_{12} malabsorption.

E. Genitourinary System: Frequency of urination is a cardinal symptom of diabetes mellitus, but may also reflect anxiety states, use of diuretics, or lithium toxicity. Inability to initiate urination should suggest anticholinergic toxicity in patients taking psychiatric medications and is a major concern in elderly men with prostatic hypertrophy. Episodes of incontinence, if accompanied by loss of consciousness, suggest either vasovagal phenomena or seizures. Spinal cord lesions (eg, secondary to trauma or multiple sclerosis) above the S1–2 level can produce a spastic bladder. The triad of dementia, ataxia, and incontinence in an elderly person should raise the question of normal-pressure hydrocephalus—a potentially reversible condition. Impotence may occur secondary to either medication or other forms of neurologic diseases, particularly spinal cord impairment.

PHYSICAL EXAMINATION

The patient's general appearance provides the clinician with much information about the severity and acuteness or chronicity of the illness. Failure to note subtle or obvious signs of physical illness may lead to prolonged, costly, and unnecessary or inappropriate treatment. Detection of a physical sign, on the other hand, may afford the physician unexpected leverage in treating an illness that was initially thought to be psychiatric. It is the rule rather than the exception that medical illnesses have behavioral manifestations and emotional consequences. In addition, some somatic illnesses present with psychiatric symptoms.

Vital Signs

With psychiatric patients it is essential to record vital signs early in therapy—if possible before medications are started or before they are changed. Orthostatic measurements (with the patient lying supine and then standing) of pulse and blood pressure are particularly valuable.

A. Pulse: Tachycardia may reflect anxiety, pain, or ingestion of adrenergic agonists or anticholinergic substances. Dehydration may result in compensatory tachycardia. Furthermore, some arrhythmias (particularly paroxysmal atrial tachycardia) produce marked anxiety. Tachycardia and anxiety are commonly associated with stimulants or illnesses such as hyperthyroidism. The liberal use of beverages containing caffeine may result in anxiety and tachycardia. Inquiry about caffeine use may result in significant cost savings. The reduction or discontinuation of caffeine intake with resultant normalization of pulse rate may save the patient a costly cardiac or autonomic evaluation. Bradycardia is common in patients with anorexia nervosa. Return of the pulse rate to the normal range in these patients is one means of monitoring protein ingestion. Bradycardia may also be seen in hypothyroidism or patients taking β-blockers.

B. Blood Pressure: Hypertension has multiple medical causes and places the patient at significant risk of cerebrovascular and cardiovascular accidents as well as renal complications. Situational stress may elevate blood pressure on a transient or chronic basis. Concurrent ingestion of monoamine oxidase inhibitors and wines or cheeses containing tyramine may lead to dangerous episodes of hypertension. Some antihypertensive drugs can produce episodes of major depression and may also cause impotence. In addition, psychotropic medications may produce postural hypotension via peripheral blockade of α-adrenergic receptors. The low potency neuroleptics, monoamine oxidase inhibitors, and tertiary tricyclic antidepressants commonly produce orthostatic hypotension. Dehydration, particularly in the elderly, may also cause orthostatic changes.

C. Temperature: Hypothermia is a potentially dangerous complication of antipsychotic medications in the elderly. Hyperpyrexia may reflect infection anywhere in the body (including the central nervous system), atropine poisoning, toxicity due to dopamine-blocking agents ("neuroleptic malignant syndrome"), or the hypermetabolic state of delirium tremens. Malignant catatonia, also associated with hyperpyrexia, has numerous causes. Malignant hyperthermia can also be seen after the use of certain inhalation anesthetics. Environmental exposure may result in hypothermia in cold climates or prolonged contact with water. Heat stroke results in hyperthermia with significant neuropsychiatric sequelae or death.

D. Respiratory Rate: While hyperventilation may arise in the context of stress disorders, anxiety states, or panic attacks, it may also reflect metabolic acidosis with a compensatory respiratory drive. Severe metabolic acidosis can be seen in certain toxic ingestions, most commonly in chronic alcoholics. The substances include methanol, ethylene glycol, and paraldehyde. Salicylate poisoning may also result in a severe metabolic acidosis with an increased anion gap. Central respiratory drive may be diminished by barbiturates, benzodiazepines, alcohol, or brainstem compression or lesions.

Head

Evidence of head trauma such as skull deformities or scars should be noted. Palpation of the skull may disclose skull deformities covered by hair that would otherwise not be noticed on observation alone. Patients may be amnestic for the actual event if the trauma was associated with loss of consciousness. An increase in cranial circumference or an unusual cranial shape suggests congenital abnormalities or long-standing hydrocephalus. Periocular ("raccoon eyes") as well as retroauricular ecchymosis may be seen in orbital and basilar skull fracture, respectively.

A. Face and Mouth: Hyper- or hypotelorism (wide- or narrow-set eyes) may suggest congenital central nervous system abnormalities. Adenoma sebaceum (multiple papules over the bridge of the nose and cheeks) occurs in tuberous sclerosis. A "port-wine" stain that involves the first division of the fifth cranial nerve, but may extend outside of its territory suggests Sturge-Weber syndrome. A heliotrope rash involving the upper eyelids suggests dermatomyositis. Vesicular lesions within the first division of the trigeminal nerve suggests herpes zoster ophthalmicus and may result in postherpetic neuralgia, an extremely painful condition. A "butterfly" rash over the nose and cheeks suggests the possibility of systemic lupus erythematosus. A round or moon-shaped face may reflect idiopathic Cushing's disease or ingestion of corticosteroids. Hair loss from the lateral eyebrows occurs in syphilis, leprosy, and hypothyroidism. A sore, raw tongue suggests vitamin deficiency, a large tongue suggests hypothyroidism, and greenish discoloration of the tongue suggests brominism. Repetitive tongue movements are common in edentulous patients, but may also be seen in patients with involuntary buccal, lingual, and masticatory movements (tardive dyskinesia), which may occur as a late complication of neuroleptic drug use. Regular tremor of the lips (an early parkinsonian complication of dopamine-blocking drugs) has been termed the "rabbit syndrome." Lack of facial expression may be a symptom of schizophrenia, major affective disorder, dementia, idiopathic Parkinson's disease, or right hemisphere, caudate, or medial frontal lesions, or may reflect drug-induced akinesia.

B. Eyes: Dilated pupils may reflect stress, anticholinergic toxicity, or hyperadrenergic states. Hyperadrenergic states, in turn, may reveal endogenous disease (hyperthyroidism, Addison's disease, pheochromocytoma, or carcinoid) or exogenous use of psychostimulants (amphetamine, PCP, cocaine, methylphenidate, and caffeine). Constricted pupils suggest ingestion of a narcotic, but brainstem lesions at the pontine level may also cause pinpoint pupils. Herniation of the uncus (a structure on the medial aspect of the temporal lobe) secondary to increased intracranial pressure compresses the pupilloconstrictor fibers of the third cranial nerve, causing the ipsilateral pupil to become fixed and dilated. Extraocular muscles may be affected in Wernicke's encephalopathy, progressive supranuclear palsy, ischemic disease, intracranial mass lesions, multiple sclerosis, diabetes, hyperthyroidism, autoimmune cranial neuropathies, myasthenia gravis, and myopathies, or following ingestion of phencyclidine, phenytoin, or barbiturates. Rust-colored rings in the cornea's deepest layer (Kayser-Fleischer rings) are a hallmark of Wilson's disease. Blink rate may be an indicator of central dopaminergic function. Diminished central dopamine usually results in decreased eye blink (eg, Parkinson's disease), whereas increased central dopamine results in increased blink rate (eg, schizophrenia, psychostimulants).

Neck

Thyroid enlargement or tenderness is significant, since symptoms of both hyper- and hypothyroidism can be mistaken for primary psychiatric disease. Carotid bruits suggest advanced atheromatous disease and have special significance if the individual has a history of transient ischemic attacks, reversible neurological deficits due to ischemia, or stroke. Neck stiffness with pain on flexion (meningismus) suggests meningeal irritation. Signs of trauma to the neck associated with headache and hemisensory, hemiparesis, or language disturbances should raise the suspicion of carotid artery dissection. Hyperextension of the neck followed by brainstem symptoms and signs should raise suspicion of a vertebral artery dissection. Involuntary torsion of the head and neck to one side (torticollis) may occur as drug-induced dystonia or in association with dystonia musculorum deformans, a rare neurological disorder.

Heart

Congestive heart failure (characterized by a third or fourth heart sound on auscultation) may be associated with hypoxia, anergy, and agitation. Unless the cardiac condition is recognized, "psychiatric signs" may be mistakenly treated with antianxiety, antipsychotic, or antidepressant medications. The midsystolic click of a prolapsed or "floppy" mitral valve is increasingly recognized in association with anxiety attacks. Paroxysmal atrial tachycardia may cause secondary anxiety or may arise from an anxious state. Tachycardia may also be due to the use of psychoactive medications or increased metabolic states, such as hyperthyroidism. Patients with a history of cardiac surgery may present with a host of neurobehavioral

symptoms, particularly memory problems, concentration difficulties, depression, and anhedonia.

Lungs

Hypoxia from any cause (including asthma, congestive heart failure, pneumonia, pneumothorax, or pulmonary embolism) may produce either quiet or agitated confusional states. Pneumonia is a reversible cause of dementia syndromes in the elderly. Patients presenting with confusion, dementia, or new onset of neurobehavioral symptoms, and who have a history of smoking, should be evaluated for central nervous system (CNS) metastatic disease, metabolic encephalopathy, or remote effects of cancer. Patients with a history of toxic fume exposure may have dyspnea and hypoxia associated with neurological and mental status changes.

Abdomen

The presence of multiple surgical scars may suggest a number of psychiatric illnesses (eg, conversion disorder, somatization disorder, chronic factitious illness, repeated ingestion of foreign bodies by schizophrenic individuals or by patients with borderline personality disorder) or may reveal the numerous abdominal crises seen in acute intermittent porphyria. Hepatomegaly and vascular spiders suggest chronic alcohol abuse. A bloated abdomen may suggest starvation, fecal impaction (one of the most common causes of acute confusion in a demented patient), ischemic bowel disease, malabsorption, or an abdominal tumor. A bloated abdomen may also be seen in patients with aerophagia, common in anxiety states.

Skeleton

Bony abnormalities may reflect congenital defects or may have arisen slowly in the context of collagen vascular disease. The cranioskeletal abnormalities of gigantism most frequently arise secondary to pituitary dysfunction. Bony lesions associated with neurological and neurobehavioral features include myeloma, Cushing's disease or syndrome, exogenous corticosteroids, Paget's disease, hyper- or hypoparathyroidism, metastatic disease, osteoporosis, soft tissue tumors, such as sarcomas and fibrosarcomas, meningiomas, osteomyelitis, rickets, neurofibromatosis (Von Recklinghausen's disease), and cranial dysplasia.

Extremities

Palmar erythema suggests collagen vascular disease, hepatic disease, alcoholism, or syphilis. Multiple laceration scars over the inner aspects of the forearms or wrists are stigmas of multiple suicidal gestures occasionally seen in severely ill patients with borderline personalities. Clubbing of the digits may reflect cardiac or pulmonary disease. Yellowish staining of the fingertips suggests a smoking habit. Nail fragility can be seen in conditions such as hypothyroidism. Mees lines (horizontal white lines across the nails) may be a reaction to arsenic or thallium toxicity. Periungual fibromas, classically seen in tuberous sclerosis, may be associated with a longitudinal groove through the nail. Significant trauma to the fingertips, including partial amputation, should raise the suspicion of a primary sensory deficit. Conditions that cause a lack of pain sensation, such as severe neuropathies (seen classically in leprosy), syringomyelia, and congenital absence of pain sensation, may all result in significant damage to the tips of digits. Loss of hair; thin, smooth, shining skin; and color change on temperature exposure can all be seen with autonomic disturbances in the extremities (eg, reflex sympathetic dystrophy—commonly referred to now as complex regional pain syndrome). The tremor of Parkinson's disease is initially a resting tremor of the hands and may be unilateral. Other forms of tremor may be seen with lithium use, in hyperadrenergic states (eg, anxiety, amphetamine abuse, alcohol withdrawal), or in benign familial (essential) tremor. The central obesity of Cushing's disease is accompanied by peripheral loss of fatty tissue, with the skin of the hands taking on the quality of parchment.

NEUROLOGICAL EXAMINATION

Cranial Nerves

A. Cranial Nerve I (Olfactory): Unilateral or bilateral anosmia may occur secondary to trauma and disruption of the olfactory nerves as they travel through the cribriform plate or a meningioma of the olfactory groove. Olfactory hallucinations may represent onset of a simple or complex partial seizure. Structural lesions of the medial temporal lobe may also cause olfactory hallucinations. Although olfactory hallucinations can occur in schizophrenia, they should always warrant an organic evaluation, because they are more often associated with central nervous system disease. Smokers, as well as patients with Parkinson's and Alzheimer's disease, often have diminished olfaction. Testing of the olfactory nerve should always be done with a nonnoxious substance (eg, coffee or wintergreen). Noxious substances such as ammonia may stimulate cranial nerve V and give spurious results in a hyposmic patient.

B. Cranial Nerve II (Optic): If visual acuity is poor, does it improve if the patient puts on glasses or looks through a pinhole (which corrects for refractive errors)? Is the patient taking anticholinergic drugs that impair accommodation required for near vision? Is there a homonymous visual field cut, suggesting a lesion of the optic chiasm or tract, visual radiations, or visual cortex, or is there monocular blindness, suggesting lesions anterior to the chiasm (ie, damage to the optic nerve or retina)? Constricted visual fields that fail to expand the field of vision when the distance between patient and target is increased should raise the suspicion of hysterical visual field constriction. Claims of blindness in the presence of intact optikinetic nystagmus should raise the suspicion of hysterical blindness, whereas claims of intact vision in the presence of objective evidence of severe visual loss (eg, failure to maneuver around furniture) suggest an occipital lobe lesion (Anton's syndrome—denial of blindness). Examination of the fundi may demonstrate blurring of the disk margins (associated with increased intracranial pressure) or arteriolar narrowing that suggests hypertension.

C. Cranial Nerves III (Oculomotor), IV (Trochlear), and VI (Abducens): If nystagmus is present, does it reflect therapeutic or toxic levels of drugs (eg, barbiturates or phenytoin) or alcohol intoxication or withdrawal? Is the nystagmus secondary to phencyclidine ingestion? If gaze paralysis is present, is it caused by thiamine deficiency associated with Wernicke's encephalopathy or by abducens palsy (often a nonspecific sign of increased intracranial pressure), or does it reflect the internuclear ophthalmoplegia seen in multiple sclerosis? Is there limitation of vertical gaze, as seen in progressive supranuclear palsy or with pineal tumors (Parinaud's syndrome)?

D. Cranial Nerve V (Trigeminal): Is facial sensation intact over all three branches of the trigeminal nerve? In cases of conversion (hysterical) anesthesia, sensory loss usually extends to the mandibular angle (innervated by the second cervical nerve). In conversion anesthesia, there may also be a dramatic change from the zone of anesthesia to a zone of acute perception at the midline of the face. Anatomically there is a midline overlap of terminal axons from both trigeminal nerves; therefore in true facial sensory loss, perceptual change should be noted before the midline is reached. The use of a tuning fork is also helpful in differentiating hysterical sensory loss from organic loss. Because the skull is a solid bony structure that can transmit vibratory sensation to the unaffected side, the patient with organic disease can perceive the tuning fork even if it is placed on the affected side of the forehead. The individual with hysterical sensory loss will often sharply demarcate perception of vibration at the midline of the forehead, between what cannot and what can be perceived.

E. Cranial Nerve VII (Facial): Is there facial asymmetry either at rest or on spontaneous motion? Is the entire hemiface involved (peripheral lesion), or is the forehead spared (central lesion)? Is a cortical lesion suggested by aphasia with right central facial paresis or by aprosody (loss of speech melody) with left central facial paresis? In upper motor neuron lesions affecting cortical bulbar fibers innervating the contralateral facial nucleus, there may be disassociation between a volitional and a mimetic smile. When asked to smile, the patient may demonstrate an obvious central facial paresis. If the patient is observed smiling spontaneously, however, in response to a humorous or flattering comment, the facial muscles may be seen to work symmetrically. Alternate supranuclear pathways from limbic structures to the facial nuclei most likely account for this discrepancy.

F. Cranial Nerve VIII (Acoustic and Vestibular Components): Is there sensorineural or conductive hearing loss? High-frequency hearing loss (presbycusis) is common in the elderly. Occasionally deficits mistakenly interpreted as a comprehension problem due to an aphasia or dementia may actually be secondary to a primary hearing deficit, correctable with a hearing aid. These patients should have hearing tests and brainstem auditory evoked potentials. A rare, but important condition the psychiatrist should recognize is pure word deafness. This is often mistaken for hysterical hearing loss or primary paranoia. It is due to a lesion that disconnects receptive language centers from association cortex. It does not, however, affect the patient's ability to write without error or accurately hear and interpret nonverbal auditory stimuli (eg, a doorbell, telephone, or barking dog). The quick and appropriate response to these latter stimuli often raises a false suspicion that the patient is hysterical or malingering. Perpetuating this spurious conclusion is the fact that many of these patients do appear paranoid when conversations occur around them and they do not understand what is said. Before diagnosing "hysterical" gait disorder, be certain the patient does not have position-induced vertigo secondary to labyrinthine dysfunction.

G. Cranial Nerves IX (Glossopharyngeal) and X (Vagus): Is the gag reflex intact, absent (patient at risk for aspiration), or overly brisk (associated with the "emotional incontinence" of pseudobulbar paralysis)? Swallowing is a complex act and may be grossly impaired despite an intact gag reflex.

H. Cranial Nerve XI (Accessory): Is there asymmetry of sternocleidomastoid muscle strength or diminished bulk of the trapezius muscle on palpation? Formerly, the prevailing view was that in cases of suspected conversion (hysterical) hemiparesis, patients would complain of an inability to turn the head toward the side of the weakness. Because turning the head in one direction is a function of the contralateral sternocleidomastoid muscle, the propensity to turn the head away from the hemiparesis would suggest an intact sternocleidomastoid muscle ipsilateral to the hemiparesis, and would, therefore, raise the suspicion of hysterical conversion. However, some patients may have ipsilateral supranuclear innervation of the accessory nucleus. Therefore, weakness of head-turning in a patient with hemiparesis should not be a criterion for differentiating a conversion disorder.

I. Cranial Nerve XII (Hypoglossal): Does the tongue deviate from the midline? If so, is this a sign of a brainstem lesion, or does it reflect a supranuclear lesion? Although the hypoglossal nucleus has bilateral supranuclear innervation, there is a greater number of contralateral fibers. Consequently, an upper motor neuron lesion may cause slight deviation of the tongue off midline to the side of the hemiparesis.

Motor System
A. Muscle Mass: Is there asymmetry of face, body, or limb muscle mass? Loss of muscle mass may be due to congenital disease, disuse atrophy, motor neuron, neuropathic, and myopathic disease. Enlarged, well-defined muscle mass may suggest anabolic steroid or growth hormone use. The absence of expected muscle mass loss in previously diagnosed states (eg, polio) should raise the suspicion of an inaccurate diagnosis or conversion disorder.

B. Muscle Tone: Is there parkinsonian cogwheel rigidity, lead pipe rigidity of an upper motor neuron disease, or the flaccidity of a lower motor neuron disease? Are muscles rigid secondary to dystonia? Is there the "waxy flexibility" of cataleptic catatonia or the rigid resistance of negativistic catatonia? Does the examiner encounter the ratchet-like gegenhalten (paratonia) of frontal lobe disease, characterized by increasing resistance in response to the examiner's attempts to passively move the patient's limbs at increasing speeds? Latent increased tone in an upper limb may be unmasked by passively moving the limb while asking the patient to perform an augmentation maneuver with the opposite limb. This may be accomplished by having the patient draw a "square in the air" with the limb opposite to the one being passively flexed and extended while simultaneously pronating and supinating the extremity. This may be a common finding in early Parkinson's disease.

C. Strength: Strength may be graded on a 6-point scale in which 5 = normal strength, 4 = movement against gravity and applied force, 3 = movement against gravity only, 2 = movement with gravity eliminated, 1 = trace movement, and 0 = no movement. Attention is paid to comparisons of left versus right, proximal versus distal, and upper versus lower motor strength.

D. Coordination: Is performance impaired on testing of finger-to-nose, heel-to-shin, and rapidly alternating (rhythmic) movements (all suggesting cerebellar hemispheric disorders), or does ataxia affect chiefly the lower limbs and trunk (suggesting midline cerebellar disorders)? Beware of inferring coordination deficits in the presence of weakness.

E. Reflexes:
1. Muscle stretch reflexes—Are tendon reflexes symmetrical or asymmetrical? Is there hyperreflexia consistent with upper motor neuron disease, or does areflexia accompany flaccid paralysis? A brisk jaw jerk suggests bilateral corticopontine involvement. Diffusely brisk reflexes may be seen in withdrawal from alcohol, benzodiazepine, or barbiturates; catatonic excitement; hyperthyroidism; magnesium or calcium deficiency; or CNS stimulants. Diffusely sluggish reflexes may be seen in barbiturate, alcohol, or benzodiazepine intoxication. Prolonged relaxation

time of the muscle stretch reflex suggests hypothyroidism.

2. Pathological reflexes—

a. Babinski's sign—Does stimulation of the plantar surface of the foot produce plantar flexion ("down-going" toe) or dorsiflexion (extension) of the great toe (Babinski's sign)? An "up-going toe" suggests pyramidal tract (upper motor neuron) lesions that may be at the level of the spinal cord, brainstem, or cerebral hemispheres.

b. Primitive reflexes—Can reflexive sucking, grasping, rooting, or snouting be elicited? Multiple primitive reflexes suggest diffuse frontal lobe disorders, but taken individually, these primitive reflexes are of questionable diagnostic significance. A unilateral grasping reflex may indicate involvement of the frontal lobes.

F. Gait and Station: Does the patient walk in a stooped fashion, with slow, shuffling steps and diminished arm swing? If so, is this parkinsonian picture drug induced or idiopathic? Is gait wide based and ataxic? Gait ataxia may be due to alcoholic intoxication, permanent ataxia secondary to alcoholic cerebellar degeneration, degenerative cerebellar disease, remote effects of carcinoma, primary or metastatic tumor, hypothyroidism, or intoxication with psychotropic or anticonvulsant agents such as phenobarbital. The gait ataxia associated with hypothyroidism is very similar to that of alcoholic cerebellar degeneration. Is one leg moved forward in circumduction and the arm on that side held in flexion over the chest? This occurs most commonly following stroke of the contralateral hemisphere. A very dramatic theatrical gait of lunging characteristically associated with the inability to stand and walk (astasia-abasia) is most often associated with conversion hysteria.

G. Movements: Is there asymmetry of movement (paralysis, neglect), poverty of movement, or excess of movement? Are there spontaneous dyskinetic movements (Huntington's chorea, tardive dyskinesia, levodopa-induced dyskinesia, Wilson's disease), tremors (resting parkinsonian tremor, benign familial tremor, cerebellar "intention" tremor), myoclonic jerks, or fasciculations?

Sensation

Sensory loss is characterized with reference to location and to the modalities involved. Does the patient fail to respond only to pinprick and changes of temperature (small fiber neuropathy, lateral spinal cord or brainstem lesion), or is there also diminished proprioceptive sensation (large fiber neuropathy, dorsal column, or ventral medullary lesion)? Is the deficit limited to one extremity, or are upper and lower extremities involved symmetrically (evidence of polyneuropathy)? Is the loss of sensation a crude inability to perceive the stimulus, or is it instead a specific inability to localize or recognize the stimulus? Tests of sensory extinction (failure to perceive sensation on one side of the body when bilateral areas are simultaneously stimulated), stereognosis (ability to recognize and name an object after feeling its shape), or graphesthesia (ability to recognize a number or letter "written" on the skin) allow the clinician to recognize syndromes of cortical sensory loss associated with parietal lesions.

LABORATORY EXAMINATIONS & OTHER DIAGNOSTIC TESTS

Just as the physical examination provides an opportunity to confirm or refute hypotheses formulated on the basis of the history and review of systems, the request for laboratory and other diagnostic tests should also derive from and be dictated by findings in the history, review of systems, and physical examination. If utilized in this way, the laboratory provides relevant diagnostic and prognostic data that benefit the patient and allow clinicians to sharpen their observational skills. Indiscriminate ordering of laboratory tests, on the other hand, is costly, short-circuits the traditional medical practice of careful examination leading to formulation of hypotheses, and can be detrimental to the patient-physician relationship. Laboratory tests are essential elements of the modern psychiatrist's diagnostic and therapeutic resources. Even as recently as a decade ago, this was not the case. Biological tests in psychiatry may be anatomic (magnetic resonance imaging [MRI], computed tomography [CT], angiography), functional (electroencephalography [EEG], evoked potentials, single-photon emission computed tomography [SPECT], positron emission tomography [PET]), or diagnostic (cerebrospinal fluid [CSF]/serum Venereal Disease Research Laboratories [VDRL], antinuclear antibody [ANA], tissue culture). Advances in psychopharmacology in the past two decades have led to a demand for refined quantitative measures of medication levels. Over the next decade, advances in research in psychiatry and neuroimmunology may make it necessary for psychiatrists to become conversant with biological probes of the immune system. The recent development of genetic probes has made testing for familial hereditodegenerative diseases readily accessible. The testing has improved accuracy of diagnosis and has assisted in genetic counseling of the family.

This section discusses the role of laboratory and other diagnostic studies in general psychiatric practice. Some of the laboratory tests described are used primarily as research tools and are not in routine use in clinical practice (eg, dexamethasone suppression test, PET scan). It cannot be emphasized too strongly that negative test results do not constitute proof that organic disease is not present. Normal findings on neurological examination, for example, do not rule out a demyelinating process that is in remission any more than negative findings on electroencephalography rule out a seizure disorder. Thus, test results must always be viewed as part of the larger clinical picture.

DIAGNOSTIC WORKUP

A. Acute Confusional State (Delirium):

The hallmark of the acute confusional state is a deficit of sustained attention. Delirium is sometimes used interchangeably with acute confusional state; however, the former usually implies the addition of agitated, hyperactive, or psychotic behavior. The workup of a confused patient is similar to that of a demented patient (see below). Special concern, however, is directed toward the toxicology screen. Among the substances for which psychiatrists most often screen are the following: heavy metals (mercury, lead, arsenic), hallucinogens (LSD, phencyclidine, tetrahydrocannabinol), atropinic substances (phenothiazines, antidepressants, sedatives, antiparkinsonism drugs), stimulants (amphetamines, cocaine, methylphenidate), central nervous system depressants (alcohol, phenobarbital, phenytoin), anxiolytics (benzodiazepines, meprobamate), and pain medications/street narcotics (morphine, heroin, hydromorphone, meperidine).

B. Dementia:

Alzheimer's disease is the most common form of dementia. Although definitive diagnosis can be made only by brain biopsy or autopsy, clinical correlation of the patient's history and examination with NINCDS/ADRDA or *DSM-IV* criteria can improve the probability of the diagnosis being correct. Recent serum and CSF tests for Alzheimer's disease, when used with the clinical assessment, may exceed a greater than 90% accuracy of diagnosis. Apolipoprotein E (Apo E) is a transporter of cholesterol. Alleles of Apo E include 2, 3, and 4. Individuals with the Apo E4 allele have the highest associated risk of developing Alzheimer's disease, whereas those with the Apo E2 allele have the lowest associated risk. Risk associated with the Apo E3 allele lies in between. CSF analysis for Tau protein and β-42 amyloid is also predictive. High CSF Tau and low amyloid β-42 is associated with the diagnosis of Alzheimer's disease. Despite the prevalence of Alzheimer's disease there are many other causes of dementia. These other causes of dementia should be ruled out, as many are treatable.

1. Blood, plasma, or serum values—Values for the following should be obtained: hemoglobin, hematocrit, white blood cell count, vitamin B_{12}, folic acid (red blood cell), sodium, calcium, magnesium, creatinine, urea nitrogen, glucose (fasting), bilirubin (direct and indirect), total protein, lactic acid, partial thromboplastin time, aspartate aminotransferase, thyroxine, erythrocyte sedimentation rate, arterial blood gases, and ceruloplasmin (in patients under 50 years of age).

2. Antigen and antibody tests—The following tests should be performed: ANA to rule out collagen vascular disease, CSF/serum VDRL, treponema pallidum hemagglutination (TPHA), and fluorescent treponemal antibody absorption (FTA-ABS) for syphilis. CSF immunoglobulin gamma (IgG), IgG synthesis rate, and oligoclonal bands for multiple sclerosis, cryptococcal antigen, and directigens against specific microbes when infectious meningitis is suspected may also be included in the evaluation. Additional serum antibody tests such as antiphospholipid antibody, anticardiolipin antibody, and lupus anticoagulant may also be performed, particularly in cases of stroke syndromes in patients without known risk factors.

3. HIV testing—HIV testing is an essential element in the workup, particularly for patients in high-risk groups.

4. Other studies—

a. Chest x-ray.

b. Electrocardiography (ECG)—A baseline ECG is important before starting treatment with drugs, because many psychotropic medications may produce tachycardia or other arrhythmias.

c. Electroencephalography (EEG)—The EEG may be helpful in documenting dysrhythmia or epileptic discharge. Provocative maneuvers such as sleep, sleep deprivation, and photic stimulation may be used to lower the seizure threshold.

Epilepsy is ultimately a clinical diagnosis, and findings on the EEG may or may not corroborate the diagnosis. Abnormal electroencephalographic tracings may be seen in patients who never have clinical seizures. Likewise, patients with frank clinical seizure disorders may have unremarkable electroencephalographic tracings. Many patients with hysterical seizures (pseudoseizures) also have a history of true seizures. Observation of a clinical seizure with concomitant electroencephalographic tracings that show no epileptic discharge makes possible a diagnosis of pseudoseizure. It does not exclude a coexisting true seizure disorder, however.

The EEG is extremely helpful in assessing toxic, metabolic, and infectious causes of confusion. In the vast majority of organically induced confusional states the EEG will show slowing. One important exception is barbiturate delirium, in which the EEG is characterized by excessive fast activity. Specific EEG patterns may be seen in certain diseases. Triphasic waves may be seen in hepatic or renal disease and periodic spike and high-amplitude slow waves can be seen in Creutzfeldt-Jakob disease. Periodic lateralizing epileptiform discharges (PLEDS) may be seen in diseases such as herpes encephalitis, and frontal epileptiform rhythmic delta activity (FERDA) in diffuse cerebral vascular disease or diencephalic mass lesions. Specialized EEG applications are often available at large teaching medical centers. Continuous video EEG telemetry is a helpful tool for identifying difficult-to-diagnose epilepsy and pseudoseizures. Electrocorticography allows electrodes to be applied to the surface of the brain and helps to identify functional brain areas in preparation for seizure surgery. Intraoperative EEG monitoring can be performed during major cardiac, vascular, or neurosurgical procedures. Continuous EEG monitoring can also help to diagnose nonconvulsive status epilepticus and to guide induced barbiturate coma to ensure burst suppression. The EEG may be used as an adjunct to clinical diagnosis of brain death but should never be used exclusively in making that diagnosis.

d. Computed tomography (CT)—CT scan of the brain is the test of choice for suspicion of an acute intracranial hemorrhage. Otherwise the MRI is the imaging procedure of choice for all other intracranial pathology.

e. Magnetic resonance imaging (MRI)— Imaging of the head is an essential tool in the investigation of dementia syndromes. Although generalized atrophy of the brain correlates poorly with the degree of cognitive dysfunction, focal atrophy of the frontal and temporal lobes may suggest a history of Pick's disease or significant closed head injury. Isolated infarction of strategic brain regions (eg, dominant inferior parietal lobe, hippocampus, or dorsomedial thalamus) may produce dementia or amnestic syndromes, whereas numerous infarctions can combine to produce the picture of multi-infarct dementia. Other structural abnormalities to be excluded in the workup of dementia include brain tumors (primary or metastatic), subdural hematomas, and normal-pressure hydrocephalus. Chronic abusers of alcohol, some schizophrenics, and a subpopulation of elderly patients with depression (but without dementia) have abnormal findings on MRI scan of the brain. Use of gadolinium further enhances the resolution of intracranial pathology seen with MRI. Findings such as these, along with possible applications in the treatment of patients with neurobehavioral disorders, indicate that brain imaging will become increasingly important in psychiatric assessment. Magnetic resonance angiography (MRA) can be utilized as a screen for aneurysms, vascular malformations, occlusion, and sometimes changes consistent with vasculitis. When CNS vasculitis is clinically suspected, and MRA is unrevealing, an angiogram is warranted.

f. Lumbar puncture (LP)—LP is usually performed to detect evidence of hemorrhage, infection, cancer, or primary vasculitis involving the central nervous system. In the presence of an unrecognized space-occupying lesion of the brain, a sudden drop in CSF pressure following lumbar puncture may result in herniation of the uncus through the tentorial notch. Although consequences of this may be catastrophic, the fear of herniation is often overstated. Imaging of the head is warranted to confirm or rule out a suspected intracranial hemorrhage. If meningitis is suspected, intravenous administration of broad

spectrum antibiotics should be begun immediately. An imaging study of the head should be performed to rule out a mass or other space-occupying lesion. If there is no space-occupying lesion then an LP should be performed. Despite increased intracranial pressure, fluid may be needed to confirm the diagnosis and establish sensitivity to antibiotics. In this case, a 22-gauge needle should be utilized with measurement of an opening pressure. If elevated, only a few milliliters of fluid should be removed for the purpose of diagnostic studies. For a nonemergent LP, the needle is inserted in the L4–5 interspace (as in the emergent LP), but 20 mL or more of fluid may be withdrawn. Opening and closing pressures, as well as gross appearance (color and turbidity) of the fluid, are noted. Samples are assayed for cell count, cell type, and protein and glucose levels (a simultaneous serum glucose should be drawn to avoid spurious results); submitted for VDRL and FTA-ABS tests for syphilis; and stained and cultured for bacterial and fungal organisms. For detection of specific fungal infections, such as *Cryptococcus neoformans,* latex agglutination testing may reveal positive results in over 90% of cases. Special studies, such as protein electrophoresis (autoimmune and inflammatory disease), oligoclonal bands (multiple sclerosis, inflammatory and infectious diseases, carcinoma and paraneoplastic processes), polymerase chain reaction (PCR) (herpes encephalitis, tuberculous meningitis), and antineuronal antibodies, including anti-Hu (encephalomyelitis), anti-Yo (cerebellar degeneration), and anti-Ri (brainstem encephalitis) antibodies all associated with paraneoplastic syndromes, may be necessary.

g. Positron emission tomography (PET)— The PET scan offers a means of monitoring local central nervous system metabolism, ie, examining brain function in vivo. A biological tracer labeled with a positron-emitting radionuclide is administered by parenteral injection or inhalation. The tomograph is formed by an external detector that determines the distribution of activity. Radioisotopes such as ^{15}O, ^{13}N, ^{11}C, and ^{18}F are commonly used. Measurements of local cerebral blood flow, extraction and metabolism of oxygen and glucose, protein synthesis, neurotransmitter storage, receptor distribution, and drug distribution can be made. [^{18}F]Fluorodeoxyglucose (FDG) is a common marker, used for glucose uptake and metabolism. Functional imaging can be made of the normal brain as well as, in a variety of neurological disorders including cerebrovascular disease, movement disorders, epilepsy, dementia, and psychiatric conditions. Psychiatric disorders being studied with PET include obsessive-compulsive disorder (OCD), depression, and schizophrenia. Common metabolic patterns on PET scanning include hypometabolism in bilateral posterior temporal-parietal areas (Alzheimer's disease), in medial-temporal areas (complex partial seizures-interictal), in bilateral caudate nuclei (Huntington's disease), and in bilateral frontal lobes (schizophrenia), and hypermetabolism of orbitofrontal cortex and caudate nuclei (OCD). An interesting pattern of hypometabolism can be seen in frontal stroke. Not only is hypometabolism evident in the infarct area, but also in remote regions known to be functionally associated, such as the contralateral cerebellum. This is known as diaschisis. Use of PET is restricted due to the requirement of an on-site or regional cyclotron. The introduction of mini-cyclotrons has enhanced accessibility to PET.

h. Single-photon emission computed tomography (SPECT)—SPECT is a sensitive test of blood flow perfusion. This procedure is a functional representation of perfusion at the time of a radionucleotide injection. It has more widespread use than PET because it does not require a cyclotron. SPECT can measure focal and diffuse hypoactivity or hyperactivity. Like PET, remote diaschisis can be detected in addition to the local region of injury or illness. This test serves as a functional adjunct to structural imaging studies such as MRI and CT. It has been utilized in cerebrovascular disease, epilepsy, degenerative disease, and neuropsychiatric disorders, particularly depression.

i. Evoked potentials—Visual, auditory, and somatosensory evoked potentials are useful in neurologic diagnosis when lesions either totally disrupt or prolong conduction along these respective pathways. Multiple sclerosis is the classic disease that often demonstrates abnormalities in all three types of evoked potentials. An event-related potential (ERP) such as the P-300 is a measure of attention to a target stimulus. The "300" refers to the number of milliseconds from the stimulus to positive wave deflection that occurs over sensory association cortex. This potential is often prolonged in conditions affecting attention.

j. Neurosonology—Intravascular blood flow can be studied utilizing carotid and vertebral artery duplex Doppler ultrasonography. Stenosis and ulcerative lesions may be detected in both symptomatic and nonsymptomatic individuals. Transcranial Doppler ultrasonography (TCD) is a noninvasive way of studying intracranial hemodynamics.

k. New neurodiagnostic tools—A host of new functional tests and imaging studies are rapidly assuming a role in the evaluation of normal brain function and disease.

Magnetic resonance spectroscopy (MRS). Unpaired protons and neutrons align themselves with the magnetic field. Radiofrequency pulsing causes nuclei to absorb and emit energy. The readout is in the form of a spectrum. MRS can measure a host of compounds in specific areas of the brain. Chemicals such as N-acetylaspartate (NAA), creatine, choline, and amino acid neurotransmitters are but a few. Specific spectrographic patterns are associated with certain disease. For example, Alzheimer's disease demonstrates decreased concentrations of NAA in the tem-

poral lobes and increased inositol in the occipital lobes. Decreased NAA has been demonstrated in the frontal and temporal lobes of schizophrenic patients. MRS is also being used to measure the concentration of psychotherapeutic drugs in the brain as well.

Perfusion, diffusion, and functional MRI. Echoplanar imaging (EPI) is a technique designed to produce ultrafast imaging. Utilizing paramagnetic contrast agents, perfusion imaging reveals perfusion failure in acute ischemic stroke. Diffusion MRI is highly sensitive for water diffusion, helping to identify ischemic injury within minutes after arterial occlusion. The severity and volume of injury may also be measured by this process. Diffusion MRI has also been shown to be valuable in the early detection and characterization of brain tumors. Functional MRI (fMRI) detects tissue perfusion based on blood flow and local quantity of oxygenated hemoglobin in response to neuronal activity. Detection of this local perfusion is made on the spin-spin or transverse relaxation time (T2) sequence of imaging. The benefit of this technique is the ability to localize specific functions (eg, lexical language processing) to specific anatomic brain regions. Drawbacks include the lengthy time of the study, which may require the patient to lie still for up to 3 hours.

Magnetoencephalography (MEG) and transcranial magnetic stimulation (TMS). Electrical fields of the brain have corresponding magnetic fields oriented at right angles. Changes in magnetic fields secondary to the functions of billions of cortical neurons can be detected with magnets placed on the scalp. MEG can detect activity deep within the brain because there is less attenuation by the skull and scalp seen in typical EEG. Drawbacks to MEG include the fact that recordings need careful shielding and extensive computational algorithms to maximally localize a signal, as well as the necessity to supercool magnets. This latter requirement utilizes superconducting quantum interference devices (SQUIDs), which operate at near absolute zero. Consequently MEG is not portable like EEG. TMS provides the opportunity to alter magnetic fields of the brain. Frequency, pulse duration, and intensity of the magnetic field all contribute to the amount of neuronal stimulation. Pulse rates below 5 Hz may decrease metabolism in underlying cortex. Rates between 15 and 25 Hz may increase local cerebral metabolism, but rates above 25 Hz may actually induce seizures. Regions of the brain subjected to trains of pulses may be transiently inhibited, but rebound and exhibit prolonged increased activity. TMS has been used to treat parkinsonian tremor and severe depression. In the latter, administration of TMS to the left frontal lobe has been reported to ameliorate depression. The frequency and duration of administration required to treat depression are limiting factors at this time.

l. Genetic testing—Some of the most exciting developments in diagnostic research are taking place in the field of molecular genetics. Advances in this area have resulted in identification of specific chromosomal sites of altered gene morphology contributing to the expression of pathology in a variety of neurodegenerative and psychiatric disorders. A detailed discussion of neurogenetics is beyond the scope of this chapter. However, just a few examples of how genetics has better defined some common neurodegenerative diseases are worth noting. Alzheimer's disease has been definitely linked to four chromosomes. The most common late-onset autosomal dominant and sporadic form has been linked to chromosome 19 and specifically genetic expression of apolipoprotein E (discussed in more detail in this chapter). The rare earlier-onset familial autosomal dominant forms include abnormalities on chromosomes 21, 14, and 1, with gene coding for amyloid precursor protein, and presenilin I and II, respectively. Other candidate genes may be found on chromosome 12 and possibly 17. The spinocerebellar degenerations once clinically characterized are now defined by the nature of trinucleotide repeat expansions (repetitive base pair triplets in DNA) at specific gene sites on chromosomes 3, 6, 11, 12, 14, 16, and 19. Molecular genetics has also shed light on immediate early gene expression, such as c-*fos* and c-*jun* in response to injury such as stroke. These genes are involved in promoting the synthesis of nerve growth factor (NGF) and free radical scavengers. These are involved in brain protection and repair. Another genetic research tool is the "knockout" gene. When a candidate gene felt to be responsible for a specific function or behavior is identified, techniques to knock out the gene in experimental animals affords scientists the opportunity to study the resultant behavior and disease. Subsequent studies could possibly lead to genetic manipulation of these identified genes in order to avoid later disease expression. Genetic testing of symptomatic patients with suspected neurodegenerative diseases may be warranted, however, testing of asymptomatic family members lends itself to ethical debate, and is too controversial to recommend in most cases.

C. Depression: The diagnosis of depression should be made on clinical grounds (*DSM-IV* criteria) as there is no laboratory test that provides a definitive diagnosis. There are chemical patterns of catecholamine and indolamine metabolites in blood and CSF, as well as hormonal variations of pituitary-adrenal and pituitary-thyroid axis responses in depression. These are not pathognomonic for depression, as stress due to many physical and emotional causes may also alter neurotransmitter and hormonal chemistry. The old concept of "exogenous" and "endogenous" depression should be abandoned. Whether depression is due to a medical illness, or significant personal psychosocial stressors, neurotransmitter systems of the brain are altered. Depression due to a medical illness (eg, hypothyroidism) may resolve after successful treatment of the under-

lying illness. Other medical illnesses in which depression is common (eg, Parkinson's disease, multiple sclerosis) may warrant treatment of the depression in addition to treatment of the underlying disease. There is increasing evidence that major depression probably impairs neuroimmunological responses rendering the depressed patient more susceptible to physical illness. This may underlie an increased incidence of common cold symptoms, chronic fatigue syndrome, fibromyalgia, and migraine among depressed patients.

As with all other neuropsychiatric conditions a thorough medication history is paramount in the effective treatment of depression. Depression may be directly related to medication the patient is taking (eg, β-blockers).

1. Catecholamines—The metabolite of norepinephrine (NE), 3-methoxy-4-hydroxyphenylglycol (MHPG), is decreased in patients with severe depressive disorders. This is particularly true in patients prone to suicide. Patients with 24-hour urine MHPG levels of less than 1000 μg are felt to be good candidates for treatment with antidepressants that predominantly block the reuptake of NE (eg, desipramine). Patients with depression may also demonstrate a lower urinary NE:E (epinephrine) ratio than those without depression.

2. Serotonin—Serotonin (5-hydroxytryptamine, 5-HT) is an indoleamine that plays a critical role in mood stability. Its metabolite, 5-hydroxyindoleacetic acid (5-HIAA), is low in the CSF of depressed patients. The degree of diminished 5-HIAA is directly proportional to violent behavior, including self-directed violence. Hence suicidal patients are often found to have very low CSF concentrations of this metabolite. The recent recognition of seven 5-HT receptor types and a host of subtypes has underscored the complexity of the role of serotonin in behavior. Some of these receptor types are antagonistic of other 5-HT receptors. For example, antidepressive effects are achieved with both $5-HT_{1A}$ agonists as well as $5-HT_2$ antagonists.

3. Other neurotransmitter systems—Down-regulation of β-adrenergic receptors occurs with chronic use of tricyclic antidepressants. The timing of this down-regulation correlates clinically with the delayed effect of antidepressants after the onset of their use. β-Blockers up-regulate these receptors. The propensity for β-blockers to cause depression can be understood. Selective cortical β-adrenergic receptor agonists may have a potential role in the treatment of depression if peripheral effects can be minimized. Acetylcholine may also up-regulate β-adrenergic receptors. Given this premise the anticholinergic effects of the tricyclics may serve an adjunctive role in treating depression. This effect is probably negligible however, as the efficacy of selective serotonin reuptake inhibitors (SSRIs) is well established, and they have essentially no anticholinergic properties. Plasma and CSF γ-aminobutyric acid (GABA) levels are low in anxious depression. Drugs that act on GABA receptors may serve to reduce the anxiety often associated with depression.

4. Dexamethasone suppression test—The development of the dexamethasone suppression test as a biological probe of the hypothalamic-pituitary-adrenal axis (eg, for diagnosis of Cushing's disease) was initially hailed as a landmark for biological psychiatry. Proceeding from the observation that some depressed patients have high serum cortisol levels, researchers soon discovered that these levels failed to be suppressed in response to exogenous corticosteroid administration, a response also found in patients with Cushing's disease.

The dexamethasone suppression test (as modified for psychiatric use) is performed by giving 1 mg of dexamethasone orally at 11 PM, obtaining serum cortisol levels at 8 AM, 4 PM, and 11 PM the following day. If any of these cortisol levels is 5 μg/dL or greater, the patient is described as "failing to suppress" and thus is said to have a positive, or abnormal, response.

Although at first the test was thought to have high specificity (few false-positive results), it is now known that many patients with dementia (without depression) or stress have abnormal dexamethasone suppression test results. Moreover, the test is only 45% sensitive, yielding a significant number of false-negative results.

Because of the increasing number of false-positive results (eg, in patients with dementia and schizophrenia), few indications exist at present for clinical diagnostic use of the dexamethasone suppression test. Nevertheless, because suppression of cortisol levels correlates with a good response to both electroconvulsive treatment and antidepressant agents, serial tests may be helpful in monitoring drug responses. Normalization of the dexamethasone suppression test should not be used as an indicator to stop antidepressant therapy.

a. Causes of false-positive results—These include pregnancy (high doses of estrogens), Cushing's disease or syndrome, major physical illness (as well as trauma, fever, dehydration, nausea), severe weight loss (malnutrition, anorexia nervosa), hepatic enzyme induction (eg, with use of phenytoin, barbiturates, meprobamate), uncontrolled diabetes mellitus, dementia, stroke, and epilepsy.

b. Causes of false-negative results—These include Addison's disease, corticosteroid therapy, hypopituitarism, and therapy with high doses of benzodiazepines, cyproheptadine, or indomethacin.

5. Thyrotropin-releasing hormone (TRH) stimulation test—TRH, a tripeptide released from the hypothalamus, stimulates secretion of thyroid-stimulating hormone (TSH) from the pituitary. In normal patients, injection of synthetic TRH (protirelin) produces an increase in TSH level of about 5–25

mIU/L above baseline. An increase of less than 7 mIU/L is considered a blunted response and may correlate with depression. The TRH stimulation test and the dexamethasone suppression test detect different subpopulations of depressed patients, since there is only a 30% overlap in results. The TRH stimulation test may be particularly helpful in detecting the depressed patient with subclinical hypothyroidism or lithium-induced hypothyroidism.

The protocol is as follows: The patient should be instructed to take nothing by mouth for 8 hours prior to the test. A baseline TSH level is obtained before administration of protirelin, 0.5 mg intravenously, infused over 1 minute. TSH levels are determined at 15, 30, 60, and 90 minutes. A major question about the test is whether it detects trait or state abnormalities, since blunted TSH responses persist following treatment.

Psychiatric conditions that may cause false-positive results (blunted response) include mania, alcohol withdrawal, and anorexia nervosa. Other conditions causing false-positive results include old age, starvation, chronic renal failure, Klinefelter's syndrome, and testing repeated too frequently (pituitary TSH levels may be depleted if the test is done more often than once a week).

6. Thyroid function tests—Thyroid function tests are an integral part of the assessment of both depression and mania as well as dementia syndromes. There is a 10% incidence of thyroid failure in depressed patients with fatigue. In overt hypothyroidism the T4 is decreased while the TSH is significantly increased. Elevated titers of thyroid autoantibodies to microsomes (anti-M) and thyroid globulin (anti-T) suggest autoimmune thyroiditis.

D. Sleep Disorders: Disturbances of sleep may be primary as in narcolepsy, parasomnias, and central sleep apnea, or may be secondary to medical, neurological, or psychiatric illness. The International Classification of Sleep Disorders (ICSD) lists over 90 causes of disturbed sleep. The two most common complaints associated with sleep are excessive daytime sleepiness and insomnia. These often coexist. The depressed patient who cannot fall asleep, or who awakens in the middle of the night and cannot get back to sleep, may demonstrate excessive sleepiness during the day. Diagnostic sleep testing should not be ordered as a "knee jerk" response to complaints of sleep disturbance. The medical history is key to whom should have formal diagnostic sleep testing. A cancer patient who is in pain and depressed may have insomnia. Treatment focus on the pain and depression will often ameliorate the insomnia. Sleep disturbances and shifts in sleep-wake cycles are the rule rather than the exception in dementia, and in patients with incapacitating neurological disease, such as multiple sclerosis, seizures, Parkinson's disease, or amyotrophic lateral sclerosis (ALS). Excessive sleep, as well as insomnia, may be seen in depressed patients, while patients in the manic phases of bipolar disorder may go for days with no sleep. Medication history for prescription and over-the-counter drugs is extremely important in considering their effects on sleep.

1. Polysomnography—This sleep study usually averages 8 hours in duration, and measures the time, number of cycles, and characteristics of rapid eye movement (REM) and the four stages of non-REM sleep. Monitoring utilizes an electrocardiogram (ECG), electroencephalogram (EEG), electrooculography (EOG), electromyography (EMG), and measures chest expansion, blood oxygen saturation, body movement, and body temperature. Optional measurements include penile tumescence, galvanic skin response, and gastric acid (with particular attention paid to gastroesophageal reflux [GER]). The most common sleep disorder for which polysomnography is performed is obstructive sleep apnea (OSA). Repetitive episodes of air movement obstruction last at least 10 seconds each and are associated with hypopneas (greater than 50% reduction in airflow) or apneas. This may result in a significant drop in O_2 saturation. The most common clinical scenario for OSA is an overweight male with excessive daytime sleepiness and a history of snoring, absence of breathing during sleep for greater than 10-second periods, and gasping for air during sleep with frequent awakenings. The consequences of untreated OSA are significant, including hypertension and cardiopulmonary disease. These patients will often have a host of neuropsychiatric complaints as well (eg, problems with memory, concentration, fatigue, irritability, and depression). Polysomnography is also helpful in diagnosing sleep cycle abnormalities, circadian rhythm disorders, periodic limb movement disorders, restless legs syndrome, and various parasomnias including REM behavior disorder, sleep walking, and night terrors.

2. Multiple sleep latency test (MSLT)—This has a similar monitoring setup to the polysomnogram, but consists of at least four daytime naps, rather than monitoring under continuous sleep. This is a helpful test in the evaluation of patients with unexplained excessive daytime sleepiness or with clinically suspected narcolepsy. In addition to excessive daytime sleepiness the narcoleptic patient may also clinically demonstrate cataplexy, hypnagogic (occurring while falling asleep) or hypnopompic (occurring while awakening) hallucinations, and sleep paralysis. All of these latter features are felt to clinically correlate with the physiologic aspects of REM sleep, namely dreaming and loss of motor tone. The mean sleep latency in a person with normal sleep is greater than 10 minutes. In narcolepsy the mean latency to sleep onset is less than 5 minutes. In normal sleep the first REM period occurs 80–90 minutes after sleep onset. In narcolepsy sleep may actually begin with REM. Hence the hallucinatory experiences occur as a

continuum of dreaming directly out of wakefulness. The sudden loss of tone (sleep paralysis) is also a sign of REM inception. This loss of tone may also occur during upright awake states, causing the individual to collapse to the ground or slump if sitting (cataplexy). It may be triggered by a sudden emotional experience (even hearing a humorous story or joke!). Stimulants such as methylphenidate and *d*-amphetamine still remain the treatment of choice for narcolepsy. Some drugs presently in Phase III trials promise to be as efficacious as the stimulants without the propensity to dependence or abuse.

Monitoring Therapeutic Drug Levels

A. Lithium: Careful monitoring of serum lithium levels is essential in the management of any patient receiving this medication. Patients should have a series of baseline serum and urine studies performed before going on lithium. Thyroid functions, electrolytes, blood urea nitrogen, creatinine, urine-specific gravity, and an ECG are warranted. Lithium can cause hypothyroidism, renal concentrating defects, and leukocytosis. Lithium competes with sodium for reabsorption in the proximal tubule. Therefore an increase in sodium intake may result in lithium diuresis and a drop in therapeutic level. Thiazide diuretics may enhance sodium diuresis and result in lithium toxicity. Lithium may also cause cardiac conduction defects. Different individuals tolerate or require different levels of lithium. While acutely manic patients may require and tolerate blood levels of 1–1.8 mEq/L, a therapeutic blood level for one individual may be a toxic blood level for another. Elderly individuals, for example, are occasionally maintained effectively at a blood level of 0.4 mEq/L and show signs of toxicity when levels rise to 0.6 or 0.7 mEq/L. Because lithium is cleared from the central nervous system more slowly than from the peripheral circulation, it may be prudent to discontinue (rather than simply lower the dosage of) lithium if toxicity occurs. There are well-documented reports of toxicity continuing for as long as 1 week after serum lithium levels have fallen well below the therapeutic range. Lithium levels should be drawn 12 hours after the bedtime dose. During the stabilization period of the patient they should be drawn twice weekly and every month thereafter.

B. Tricyclic Antidepressants: Before initiating tricyclic antidepressants an ECG is important. At therapeutic concentration these drugs have quinidine-like effects; however, if a patient has a cardiac conduction deficit, even therapeutic levels may produce complete heart block. Plasma concentrations may be tested when using both tertiary and secondary tricyclics. This may be done routinely, in high-risk patients, in patients who have a poor response, despite normal dose ranges, or in those whom toxicity is suspected. Some of the tricyclics have active metabolites. For example, desipramine is a metabolite of imipramine, and nortriptyline is a metabolite of mitriptyline. These metabolites should also be measured. Optimal therapeutic results on imipramine usually occur at concentrations between 200 and 250 ng/mL. There appears to be no further benefit above 250 ng/mL. Levels of 125 ng/mL, or higher, render the most favorable response to desipramine. Nortriptyline is unique among the tricyclics in that the drug has a therapeutic window between 50 and 150 ng/mL. Above 150 ng/mL the clinical efficacy is diminished. Blood levels should be drawn 12 hours after the nighttime dose. For the level to accurately reflect clinical efficacy the patient should be on the same daily dose for a minimum of 5 days.

Studies of tricyclic antidepressants have indicated that there may be as much as a 20-fold difference in blood levels among age-matched individuals receiving the same dosage. Thus, failure to respond to an antidepressant medication may reflect not only lack of patient compliance but also individual differences in absorption, metabolism, or excretion of the drug.

C. Nontricyclic Antidepressants: Although blood levels of these drugs can be measured, treatment ranges have not been as well established as for nortriptyline.

D. Anticonvulsants: Methods are available to evaluate blood levels for all of the well-known anticonvulsant medications. Monitoring of serum levels is important in the management of individuals with seizure disorders. Drug dosage, however, should be based on the patient's therapeutic response. If seizures persist, the physician should increase the anticonvulsant in small increments until the seizures are controlled or clinical toxicity ensues, rather than adjusting dosage on the basis of serum level alone. Commonly, patients are optimally managed either slightly below or above the recommended serum therapeutic range. Levels may fluctuate, depending on other drugs taken by the patient. The physician should determine patient compliance before evaluating whether seizures are refractory to certain medications. Monotherapy is always the desired management strategy in treating epilepsy, however, more than one anticonvulsant may be required in patients refractory to a single drug.

Some basic principles to be followed in the use of anticonvulsants include the following: (1) a complete blood count, liver function tests, blood urea nitrogen, and creatinine should be drawn as a baseline and followed periodically; (2) the majority of anticonvulsants should be titrated into a therapeutic range to avoid side effects; (3) accurate plasma drug levels can be made only after a steady state has been obtained (five times the half-life of the drug at a fixed daily dose); (4) for anticonvulsants with high protein binding a free level of drug should also be drawn in conditions that may alter protein binding (eg, anorexia, pregnancy) to avoid spurious results; (5) the clinician should be aware of drug-drug interactions, as anticonvulsant levels may vary high or low depending on what other drugs the patient is taking; gabapentin has essentially no protein binding, so addition of this drug has little effect on the levels of the other anticonvulsants; (6) the clinical state of the patient should be the primary guide in determining if drug dose should be adjusted, and not the plasma concentration, which should be more of a guide to avoiding toxicity.

REFERENCES & SUGGESTED READINGS

Adams, RD, Victor M, Ropper AH: *Principles of Neurology,* 6th ed. McGraw-Hill, 1997.

Ader R: Psychoneuroimmunology: Interactions between the brain and the immune system. In: *Neuropsychiatry.* Fogel BS, Schiffer RB (editors), Rao SM (assoc. editor). Williams & Wilkins, 1996.

American Psychiatric Association: *Diagnostic and Statistical Manual of Mental Disorders,* 4th ed. American Psychiatric Association, 1994.

Bailey H: *Demonstration of Physical Signs in Clinical Surgery,* 15th ed. J. Wright & Sons, 1973.

Bogousslavsky J, Fisher M: *Textbook of Neurology.* Butterworth-Heinemann, 1998.

Cummings JL, Benson DF: *Dementia: A Clinical Approach,* 2nd ed. Butterworth-Heinemann, 1992.

DeJong RN: *The Neurologic Examination,* 4th ed. Harper & Row, 1979.

DeMoranville BM, Jackson I: Psychoneuro-endocrinology. In: *Neuropsychiatry.* Fogel BS, Schiffer RB (editors), Rao SM (assoc. editor). Williams & Wilkins, 1996.

Enna SJ, Coyle JT: *Pharmacological Management of Neurological and Psychiatric Disorders.* McGraw-Hill, 1998.

Feinberg TE, Fara MJ: *Behavioral Neurology and Neuropsychology.* McGraw-Hill, 1997.

Galasko D et al: High cerebrospinal fluid Tau and low amyloid beta-42 levels in the clinical diagnosis of Alzheimer's disease and relation to apolipoprotein E genotype. Arch Neurol 1998;55:937.

Kaplan HI, Sadock BJ: *Pocket Handbook of Primary Care Psychiatry.* Williams & Wilkins, 1996.

Kaplan HI, Sadock BJ: *Pocket Handbook of Psychiatric Drug Treatment,* 2nd ed. Williams & Wilkins, 1996.

Kaplan HI, Sadock BJ: *Synopsis of Psychiatry-Behavioral Sciences/Clinical Psychiatry,* 8th ed. Williams & Wilkins, 1998.

Masters CL, Beyreuther K: Science, medicine and the future: Alzheimer's disease. Br Med J 1998;316:446.

Mayeux R et al: Utility of the apolipoprotein E genotype in the diagnosis of Alzheimer's disease. N Engl J Med 1998;338:506.

Mesulam MM: *Principles of Behavioral Neurology.* F.A. Davis, 1985.

Patten J: *Neurological Differential Diagnosis,* 2nd ed. Springer-Verlag, 1996.

Plum F, Posner JB: *The Diagnosis of Stupor and Coma,* 3rd ed. F.A. Davis, 1980.

Riggs JE (editor): *The Neurology of Aging—Neurologic Clinics.* W.B. Saunders, 1998.

Sandson TA, Price BH: Diagnostic testing and dementia. In: *Diagnostic Testing in Neurology—Neurologic Clinics.* Evans RW (editor). W.B. Saunders, 1996.

Wiebers DO et al: *Mayo Clinic Examinations in Neurology,* 7th ed. Mosby, 1998.

Psychological Testing

13

Daniel S. Weiss, PhD, & Ellen S. Krantz, PhD

Just as medicine has been advanced by the development of objective tests of a variety of different systems and functions, ie, cholesterol level, blood pressure, and cardiac function, so too has the understanding of psychological and intellectual functioning been advanced by the development of tests of functions in the domain of mind and brain. It is probably fair to say that a significant part of the knowledge base of psychology as a discipline is a result of the efforts of early investigators such as Binet and Cattell to quantify abilities and capacities of human behavior. A thorough history of this development is not needed to appreciate the extraordinary contribution that the testing of intellectual capacities has made to understanding human behavior and functioning. The attempt to apply scientific methods to human behavior, which gave rise to the modern discipline of psychology, began in the latter part of the nineteenth century.

At present, psychological testing may be divided into two broad domains: personality and vocational assessment and intellectual and neuropsychological assessment. Thus, the term psychological testing covers a broad range of activities and functions. In addition, in the past 10–15 years, the practice of neuropsychological assessment has become so specialized that the average psychologist can no longer perform competent neuropsychological testing without advanced postdoctoral training. As a consequence, depending on the question posed for psychological testing, the physician needs to be aware of the skills and training of the psychologist to whom the patient is referred.

This chapter is divided into two sections. The first describes intelligence and neuropsychological testing and the circumstances under which it typically occurs. The second concentrates only on personality assessment—psychological testing aimed at evaluating the typical attributes and psychological processes that characterize an individual, but omits coverage of vocational assessment.

INTELLIGENCE TESTING

The early psychologists received their first professional training in a variety of other disciplines. Many were educators with special interests in the applications of psychology to the problems of the mentally retarded or the intellectually gifted. They set out to define the criteria for intelligence and to standardize them on large samples of subjects, but controversies arose—still not entirely resolved (Sternberg and Kaufman, 1998)—concerning the nature of intelligence and how it might be measured. The most basic argument was whether intelligence consisted of a single general factor, designated g, which might manifest itself in a variety of ways, or whether what we call intelligence in fact consists of a number of correlated but distinct facets, in some form of a hierarchy.

However the controversy is theoretically resolved, in practice the most widely used individually administered intelligence tests measure performance in several different areas. The Wechsler intelligence scales serve as an example and are the most widely used and commonly accepted individual measures of intelligence.

The original Wechsler-Bellevue Intelligence Scale published in 1939 has gone through several revisions. The currently used tests are the **Wechsler Adult Intelligence Scale-III** (WAIS-III; Wechsler, 1997) and the **Wechsler Intelligence Scale for Children-III** (WISC-III; Wechsler, 1991). The scales for adults and children have the same structural design, but the material used is adapted to specific age levels.

The WAIS-III and the WISC-III comprise a series of subtests that are divided into a verbal and a performance group. The scoring of the Wechsler scales yields an estimate of **verbal IQ, performance IQ, full scale IQ, and a number of factor indices.** The subtests of the verbal section for the WAIS-III include vocabulary, similarities, arithmetic, digit span, information, and comprehension; the performance section comprises picture completion, digit symbol-coding, block design, matrix reasoning (newly added), and picture arrangement. Symbol search, letter-number sequencing, and object assembly can be substituted for other subtests under certain circumstances. The four index scores are verbal comprehension, perceptual organization, working memory, and processing speed.

The verbal subtests in the WISC-III are information, similarities, arithmetic, vocabulary, and comprehension; digit span is supplementary. The performance subtests of the WISC-III are picture completion, coding, picture arrangement, block design, and object assembly; symbol search can substitute for coding and mazes is supplementary. The WISC-III also yields four factor indices: verbal comprehension, perceptual organization, freedom from distractibility, and processing speed.

Administration of the WISC-III is appropriate for children aged 6 years to 16 years 11 months. Assessment of children using the WISC-III can assist in the diagnosis of childhood disorders including learning and developmental disabilities and contribute to formulating remedial or educational interventions.

The Wechsler scales yield a standardized IQ that is normalized separately for a variety of age groups. The concept of IQ was derived from the Stanford-Binet test. The intelligence quotient, hence IQ, was based on the ratio of mental age to chronological age. On the Wechsler scales, subjects' IQ scores are compared with those of other individuals in the same age group. This makes the WAIS-III particularly useful in measuring the intelligence of older people because it is not confounded by the procrustean ratio that was initially used, and the norming process included more older subjects than in previous editions.

Controversies regarding intelligence tests have not been limited to the question of whether what we call intelligence is a single factor or a function of many factors. Important social issues have been raised regarding the cultural bias of tests (in favor of certain ethnic or socioeconomic groups), different definitions of intelligence in different cultures, and the way in which test scores might be used in making decisions about access to educational opportunity (Sternberg and Kaufman, 1998).

The stratification of the sample used to normalize the 1997 edition of the WAIS-III represents an attempt to eliminate such bias. It was based on national standardization samples (from ages 16 to 89) using census data and stratifying on the basis of age, sex, race/ethnicity, educational level, and geographic region. The revision updated items, included new artwork, and made the content more culturally neutral. Similarly, the WISC-III has attempted to establish its normative samples more representatively and has modified some of the item content to make it more modern and culturally sensitive.

The distribution of IQ scores in the actual sample for the WAIS-III and WISC-III closely parallels that of a theoretical normal curve. The mean score is 100 with a standard deviation of 15. Scores from 90 to 109 are characterized as "average." Scores from 80 to 89 and from 110 to 119 are considered "low average" and "high average," respectively. Scores from 70 to 79 are "borderline," and scores from 120 to 129—the corresponding scores on the upper side—

are "superior." Finally, scores of 69 or below are categorized as "intellectually deficient," whereas at the upper end, scores of 130 and above are called "very superior." About 2.5% of the total sample falls in each of the latter two categories. In the Wechsler system each of the subtests has also been standardized, with a mean score of 10 and a standard deviation of three.

The most obvious misuse of an intelligence test such as the WAIS-III would be to reduce its findings to a single numerical result—the IQ. From what has been said about the standardization of each subtest, it is clear that a person might conceivably have a full scale IQ 100 but subtest scores almost entirely in the high average and the low average ranges.

It should be clear also that factors other than intelligence may influence performance on an IQ test. Consider the apathetic or rebellious adolescent who is required to take the test. Fatigue, illness, or medication may also adversely affect performance. These and other factors are taken into account by various indices of measurement error.

In practice, the WAIS-III or WISC-III is most frequently administered as one part of a battery of psychological tests. Just how the test results are used will depend on what the diagnostic question is. As with all other tests, the results are most meaningful in the context of a carefully elicited history.

Although almost everyone will do better on one section of the test than the other, scores for the verbal and the performance sections are usually in the same general range. When they are not, evaluation of the disparity follows two steps. The first is to determine if the difference is greater than would be expected because of the error inherent in measurement. If the difference is significant, it is nonetheless important to examine the base rate of such a difference. For example, about 24% of the normative sample of the WAIS-III had a VIQ-PIQ discrepancy of 15 or more points. There are a variety of explanations for such discrepancies other than error, including some form of organic brain damage. When such differences are found, the possible interpretations are by no means limited to that one explanation, and all information about the patient must be considered. Matarrazo (1990) made an important contribution by noting the difference between testing and assessment, particularly with respect to the proportions of the normative sample that have various degrees of disparity. His emphasis on the differences has called attention to the fact that there is more differential in performance that is more or less normal than many psychologists believed before these data were systematically collected.

Although the Wechsler scales are not expressly designed to detect organic deficits as such, they are generally included in the battery of tests used for assessing brain damage or other deficits in neurological functioning.

NEUROPSYCHOLOGICAL TESTING

Impairment of psychological functions such as perception, attention, concentration, reasoning, memory, or speech may occur at any age either suddenly or gradually, and may be transient or permanent. Impairment may be related to some event such as an injury or accident or may not be readily attributable to any apparent cause. Even when the cause is known, such as a head injury from a motor vehicle accident, it is not always clear what the degree of impairment is or what the functional outcome may be. A thorough neuropsychological assessment is very helpful in clarifying the type of deficits and the degree of impairment, even with information available from imaging studies. It may also be useful to establish, to the extent possible, the relative contributions of psychological and organic factors.

The purpose of neuropsychological assessment is to gather data that can assist in the diagnostic process, to provide data that inform rehabilitation therapies, to advise and counsel the patient and referring clinician directly, and to measure progress or decline in function over time. A comprehensive report is typically the product of a neuropsychological evaluation. The report should provide an interpretation of test results, behavioral observations about the patient in the context of the evaluation, a diagnostic summary and conclusions targeting the implications of the test data, and recommendations for future treatment and follow-up. A neuropsychological evaluation can be an important functional component in discharge planning following hospitalization or in an outpatient setting.

Many referrals to the neuropsychologist raise the question of differential diagnosis. Lezak (1995) explains that the most common referral questions have to do with the possibility that brain disease may underlie an emotional or personality disturbance, or that behavioral decline or cognitive complaints may have a psychological rather than an organic basis. In many complex cases in which the referral question is one of differential diagnosis, a precise determination may not be possible until an ongoing disease process overwhelms the patient's functioning, or unless "hard" neurological signs emerge. When the findings of a neuropsychological examination are unclear, repeated examinations over time may bring out performance inconsistencies or may reveal progressive deterioration that clarifies the diagnosis.

An organic brain disorder can also complicate or imitate severe functional behavioral disturbances. The primary symptoms may involve marked mood or character change, confusion or disorientation, disordered thinking, delusions, hallucinations, bizarre ideation, ideas of reference or persecution, or any other of the thought and behavior disturbances typically associated with schizophrenia or affective psychoses. The neuropsychologist's task is to evaluate the patient for evidence of typical left- or right-hemisphere problems. Identification of such lateralizing signs makes a strong case for organicity. Similarly, specific patterns on memory tests, such as recent memory being more severely affected than remote memory, point to an organic problem. In addition, a pattern of low scores on tests involving attentional ability and new learning compared to higher scores on tests of knowledge and skill suggests an organic presentation. Lezak indicates that when attempting to determine whether a psychotically disturbed patient is brain damaged, the examiner will require a clear-cut pattern of lateralized dysfunction or organic memory impairment, a number of signs, or a pattern of considerably lowered test scores before concluding that brain damage is likely present. Goldstein and Watson (1989) indicate that inconsistent or erratic expression of cognitive defects is more suggestive of a psychiatric disturbance alone. The subtle behavioral expression of many brain diseases, particularly in the early stages, and the overlap of symptoms of organic brain diseases and functional disturbances make differential diagnosis difficult.

Patients may require specific modifications if English is not their native language. Poor English skills or lack of English ability may invalidate the test procedures. Both verbal and nonverbal tests that involve complex instructions may be problematic. Whenever possible, a non–English-speaking patient should be referred to a psychologist who is fully fluent in the patient's native tongue. When this is not possible, an interpreter can assist with translation, though this is far from ideal. Spreen and Strauss (1998) note that simple translation of English-language tests may distort the results, particularly in the case of verbal tests that may be much more difficult or much easier in translation, thus invalidating the available norms.

Tests explicitly intended to assess neuropsychological impairment in great detail are available, but are time intensive for both the patient and the professional administering the test. They are not ordinarily requested or performed unless there is clear evidence of an organic deficit that requires more detailed examination.

Neuropsychological evaluation developed using a fixed battery of tests, the best known of which is the Halstead-Reitan battery (Reitan and Wolfson, 1993a), an elaborate and complicated series of tests that requires extensive training in its administration and interpretation. The original battery included the Minnesota Multiphasic Personality Inventory (MMPI) (see section later in chapter), the Wechsler-Bellevue Intelligence Scale, as well as a variety of other tests. Since Reitan's original work, the MMPI is no longer a required part of the battery and the Wechsler-Bellevue has gone through three revisions (the Wechsler Adult Intelligence Scale [WAIS], the WAIS-R, and the WAIS-III). Consequently, contemporary use of the Halstead-Reitan battery has included some modifications that Reitan may not endorse. Reitan and Wolfson have also published a battery for younger (1993b) and older children (1992). Reitan and Wolfson (1988) have also developed a general neuropsychological deficit scale.

The full battery currently includes the following tests: Category Test, Trail-Making Test, Tactual Performance Test, Rhythm Test, Speech-Sounds Perception Test, Finger Oscillation Test, Grip Strength, Reitan-Klöve Sensory-Perceptual Examination, Aphasia Screening Test, Tactile Finger Recognition, and Finger-Tip Number Writing. The interpretation of test battery results is a complex procedure that cannot be described briefly. The basic procedures involve determining when an individual's performance is outside the range of normal performance, if the performance implies problems on one or the other side of the brain, and whether the deficits in performance appear to fit a pattern of rapid onset or a slower, more gradual deterioration.

An alternative to and extension of the fully fixed battery is the Boston Process approach. It originated in the efforts of Edith Kaplan (1983). This approach is based on an analysis of the qualitative nature of behavior as it is observed during the administration of various neuropsychological tests as well as the overall performance. Thus, in addition to recording whether a patient passes or fails an item, specific observations about how the item is passed or failed are also recorded by the clinician. Such observations can be very helpful in making differential diagnostic decisions that could not be made only with knowledge of actual level of performance. For example, a patient who uses strategies randomly and inconsistently but who performs quickly may earn a normal score that would appear to suggest no difficulties, but observing the strategies reveals that there is some pathological process at work.

An alternative approach to the evaluation of lesions to the brain has been developed by Luria (1966) of the Soviet Union. In Luria's opinion, current psychological tests are too complex and provide no more than gross evaluations of cognitive processes.

He has assumed that complex behavioral processes are, in fact, not localized but distributed in broad areas of the brain and that the contribution of each cortical zone to the organization of the whole functional system is quite specific. He has accordingly undertaken a careful analysis of specific disturbances in the neuropsychological examination for diagnosis of focal brain injury. Luria's approach has been gaining adherents, but his methods are not yet widely used in the United States.

On the basis of Luria's approach and techniques, Christensen (1979) developed a battery to test 10 neuropsychological functions. Many common tests are incorporated into this battery, including elements of the mental status examination such as digit span, certain memory tests, and serial 7s (see Chapter 11). De-

tailing the variety of tests in Christensen's adaptation of Luria's neuropsychological investigation is beyond the scope of this text. The reader is referred to the writings of Christensen (1979) and Lezak (1995).

Christensen's battery adapts its tests to the needs of each patient (as does Luria's "experimental" approach); thus, the results are difficult to interpret. The battery is not comprehensive, and most patients will require further testing—eg, of intelligence and some memory functions not already covered in the battery.

Golden and his colleagues (1981) at the University of Nebraska developed a standardized battery from the many tests used by Luria and Christensen. The battery, called the **Luria-Nebraska Neuropsychological Battery,** tests the 10 functions referred to previously. The scales for scoring correspond to the 10 functions, but with reading and writing placed on separate scales and with motor and tactile functions scored on right-hemisphere, left-hemisphere, and pathognomonic scales. Although standardized, this battery suffers from some of the same limitations as Christensen's battery. The Luria-Nebraska battery distinguishes between normal controls and neurologically impaired patients, but its reliability and usefulness have been questioned (Lezak, 1995). Though its use has continued to grow somewhat since its publication, the Luria-Nebraska still is not as widely accepted as the Halstead-Reitan battery, and is seen by many as having significant limitations.

Other Approaches

In *Neuropsychological Assessment,* Lezak (1995) describes several other batteries and composite tests for brain damage, including one of her own design. In addition, she describes many other neuropsychological tests. Of interest and relevance are the aphasia tests developed by Kaplan and associates (Goodglass and Kaplan, 1972; Kaplan et al, 1983). The reader is referred to these works and to the discussions on aphasia testing in Chapters 5 and 11. Similarly, Spreen and Strauss (1998) clearly describe an eclectic approach to neuropsychological assessment that selects appropriate standardized tests from the literally hundreds available and uses them to focus on the key questions under study.

PERSONALITY ASSESSMENT

When Sir William Osler suggested that the patient was more important than the disease, he was emphasizing the importance of understanding the life circumstances and personality of the individual patient. When physicians make diagnoses, whether of somatic or psychiatric disorders, they must also consider the nature of the person who has the disorder. Concern with the psychological context in which the symptoms appear helps the clinician understand the meaning and implications of the presenting complaint and the particular symptom pattern. What the current episode of illness means to the patient and what coping resources and personal strengths and weaknesses the patient possesses will influence the clinician's approach to evaluation, setting of treatment objectives, and choice of treatment plans.

Personality is the composite of enduring attributes of an individual's psychological makeup. Today, despite agreement on the importance of a patient's personality in understanding the presentation of symptoms and the choice of treatment for virtually any mental disorder, there are still fundamental questions about what personality is and how it should be defined.

DEFINITIONS OF PERSONALITY

There are probably as many definitions of personality as there are authors who have written about the subject. Allport's (1937) definition is as apt as any: "Personality is the dynamic organization within the individual of those psychophysical systems that determine his unique adjustments to his environment." Two German terms, representing two views of personality, further explain the concept. *Persönlichkeit* denotes the distinctive impression that someone makes on another. This word derives from the Latin *persona* and connotes the sense we get about how individuals choose and perform their social roles. Behind the mask, however, is a complex player donning various roles. The term *personalität* denotes this more fundamental or basic concept of personality used in psychiatric clinical situations. This definition of personality, which goes beyond exhibited behaviors to reach the core of identity, is considered by some to be synonymous with the term *self* and is a key concern in psychodynamics.

DIAGNOSTIC AND STATISTICAL MANUAL OF MENTAL DISORDERS, 4TH EDITION (DSM-IV) CLINICAL EVALUATION OF PERSONALITY TRAITS & DISORDERS

In *DSM-IV,* axis II is used to record observations about personality, including personality traits and, when appropriate, personality disorders. *Personality traits* are defined as "enduring patterns of perceiving, relating to, and thinking about the environment and oneself and are exhibited in a wide range of social and personal contexts." The diagnosis of *personality disorder* is made "only when personality traits are inflexible and maladaptive and cause either significant functional impairment or subjective distress." In addition, a person may meet diagnostic criteria for a personality disorder (eg, borderline personality disorder) and also demonstrate histrionic or avoidant personality traits. All of this information is recorded on

axis II in a complete clinical evaluation according to *DSM-IV* (see Chapter 24).

The major clinical and diagnostic dilemma is determining when (at what point or under what circumstances) a set of personality traits (or the patient's "personality") becomes "maladaptive" or is "overly rigid." Personality assessment is one tool the clinician employs in making decisions about the nature and range of a patient's personality.

The major use of personality assessment, however, is in the context of an overall request for diagnostic psychological testing. In these circumstances personality measures are the central measures employed, but an IQ test may also be used. The most frequent use of this type of assessment is to evaluate the patient with a myriad of problems that have many possible causes. Psychological testing is often used to rule in or rule out some potential diagnoses. For example, some personality disorder may occur along with moderate brain dysfunction and a profound learning disability. A second typical occasion for personality assessment is in the forensic arena for custody evaluations, parole decisions, or criminal responsibility evaluations.

PERSONALITY ASSESSMENT PROCEDURES

The goals of assessment usually consist of one or more of the following: (1) to assess psychological processes, (2) to assess personality traits, (3) to assess psychological structures, (4) to aid in diagnosis, and (5) to formulate treatment plans.

FEATURES OF PSYCHOLOGICAL TESTS FOR PERSONALITY ASSESSMENT

Standardization

The greatest advantage of using psychological tests for personality assessment is that both the stimuli used to elicit information and the conditions under which the stimuli are administered are standardized. This means that differences in response may be attributed to differences in the respondents.

Another important feature of standardization is the use of "fixed-choice" responses. This limitation on how responses may be made—for example, answering only "true" or "false" to the questions on the Minnesota Multiphasic Personality Inventory-2 (MMPI-2)—facilitates comparison of personality assessments by one individual with that of others. Because another source of information that might vary is held constant, other types of information about personality are made clearer.

In personality assessment tools with fixed-response formats, the scoring or keying of responses is also fixed. For example, the patient may respond only "true" or "false" to item 169 on the MMPI-2: "When I get bored, I like to stir up some excitement." The manner in which the choice affects the score is also standardized: if the patient responds "true," this scores a point on the basic clinical scale measuring hypomania. If the patient answers "false," the score on this and all other scales is not affected. The meaning of this single response in terms of personality assessment is not subject to interpretation by the examiner or by the clinician. With the MMPI-2, the clinician's contribution lies in interpreting the pattern of scale scores (see "Interpretation" section later in this chapter).

Although stimuli (eg, the 10 inkblot cards of the Rorschach test) are standardized, each card is not just one more of the same thing, ie, the stimuli are not interchangeable. In the Rorschach inkblots, there is a range of variation in certain dimensions (color, clarity, and form). Used as a set, they are standardized, but certain stimuli tap certain personality processes. Similarly, in the MMPI-2, some items are scored on more than one scale (eg, on scales of depression and schizophrenia), whereas others are scored only on one scale or only on the other. In personality assessment, this explains the usual clinical practice of using a battery of psychological tests that vary in types of procedures, stimuli, response formats, and scoring methods. The result is a test battery that evokes a wide range of responses that elucidate and inform different aspects of personality.

Reliability & Validity

It is essential that psychological tests of all kinds, not just those of personality, be both reliable and valid. If a measure is **reliable,** its results are stable or consistent across subsequent testing assuming that nothing about the patient's personality has changed. Without reliability, a psychological test is useless.

A measure or set of measures is said to be **valid** if it actually measures what the authors claim it does. For example, a measure of defensiveness should be related to other indices of being defensive, such as being reluctant to acknowledge failings or presenting an exaggerated, socially desirable self-description. At the same time, to be valid a measure should not be related to indices that are conceptually independent. The measure of defensiveness, for example, should not be related to intelligence or degree of depression.

Careful research is required to establish the reliability and validity of measures of personality and other psychological constructs, so that their use can assist in diagnostic assessment and treatment planning. Caution is required in the use of any but the most established and well-researched measures.

CLASSIFICATION OF PSYCHOLOGICAL TESTS FOR PERSONALITY ASSESSMENT

Psychological tests are most easily classified as either objective or projective. A clever explanation of

the distinction is offered by the psychologist George Kelly (1958): "When the subject is asked to guess what the examiner is thinking, we call it an objective test; when the examiner tries to guess what the subject is thinking, we call it a projective device." There are, of course, psychological tests and assessment devices that do not neatly fit into these categories, but most are predominantly one or the other.

Objective Tests

Objective tests are tests whose scoring (numerical results) can be produced mechanically. This generally implies that the response format is standardized. Examples of such tests in personality assessment are the MMPI-2, the California Psychological Inventory (CPI), and the Millon Clinical Multiaxial Inventory-II. Another objective test familiar to medical students is the Medical College Admission Test. What is not objective in such tests is the meaning of the results or scores. As shown in the clinical example in Chapter 15, the training, experience, and skill of the psychologist come into play in the interpretation and synthesis of the results of the various tests.

Projective Tests

Projective tests are less structured than objective tests in response format and in scoring. The term projective was coined by Frank (1939), based on the following assumption: Because of the unstructured and ambiguous nature of the stimuli and response options available to the respondent, the responses must be *projections* of the patient's "way of seeing life, his meanings, significances (sic), patterns, and particularly his feelings." In projective methods, the kinds of responses are not fixed, scoring is usually time consuming, several scoring systems often exist for each technique, scoring may differ from clinician to clinician, and the interpretation of the results of projective methods frequently requires integrative thinking on the part of the clinician. The best known example of a projective test is the set of inkblots developed by Rorschach.

MINNESOTA MULTIPHASIC PERSONALITY INVENTORY-2 (MMPI-2)

The MMPI was the most thoroughly researched objective personality assessment instrument. Item development and testing began in the late 1930s. The test authors, Hathaway and McKinley (a psychologist and a physician), undertook the mammoth task of test construction, recognizing the acute need for an objective measure of various dimensions of psychopathological disorders to aid clinicians in diagnosis and treatment planning. The MMPI was designed to provide for multiphasic assessment of psychopathological changes in much the same way that medical checkups are multiphasic.

In 1989, the MMPI-2 was introduced, an updated version designed to preserve the best of the original measure but to address some of the dated item phrases and mechanics of administration and to add some new items so that assessment would be in accord with current diagnostic conceptions. Many psychologists have applauded the appearance of MMPI-2, but others have been more cautious in adopting it without more empirical evidence about the comparability of results from the original. This is because the scoring and some of the normative data are different enough from the original version so that some of the configural results from the profiles are not comparable.

Administration

The MMPI-2 comprises 567 "true" or "false" items. In the most popular version of the MMPI-2, the items are arranged in booklet form so that the first 370 are all that are needed for the basic scales. Nonetheless, typical administration uses all the items. The patient is instructed to read each item and decide "if it is true as applied to you or false as applied to you." Typically, test subjects use a computer-scannable answer sheet.

Scoring & Scales

Items comprising the various scales were selected by empirically determining which distinguished between groups of interest. In this way, the authors of the MMPI and the MMPI-2 did not decide at the outset how paranoid patients would respond to different items. Scoring is based on data that indicate how paranoid patients respond to the items as compared to controls.

The results from either the MMPI or the MMPI-2 are scores on 3 validity scales and 10 clinical scales. These scores are expressed in T-scores and typically are plotted on a profile. T-scores have a mean of 50 and a standard deviation of 10. One major difference between the original MMPI and the MMPI-2 is how the T-scores are calculated; this difference in the distribution of scores is a major reason why some are still cautious in using the MMPI-2. For an individual patient tested with both the old and the new versions, the same scores may not mean the same thing.

The validity scales of both versions indicate how likely it is that the patient responded truthfully and accurately. Some patients respond in a pattern indicating a wish to appear healthy; others respond as if they want to appear disturbed. The validity scales can also pick up random responding—eg, when patients lose their place on the answer sheet so that the marks are off by one or two items for the last hundred. One useful feature of the MMPI-2 is the addition of a similar scale (F-Back) that addresses this issue for the latter set of items. Finally, problems in reading and comprehension may be spotted by the validity scales. The MMPI-2 added additional scales (VRIN and TRIN) targeted at identifying inconsistent response patterns.

The clinical scales of the MMPI and MMPI-2 index a variety of useful personality dimensions. The hope that they would be truly multiphasic has now been abandoned. Nonetheless, it would be very rare for a personality assessment to be conducted without the MMPI or MMPI-2. The clinical scales are Hypochondriasis, Depression, Hysteria, Psychopathic Deviate, Masculinity-Femininity, Paranoia, Psychasthenia, Schizophrenia, Hypomania, and Social Introversion. The scale names are only broad labels and detailed information about exactly what they measure is beyond the scope of this chapter.

In addition to the standard scales, there are scales for Alcoholism, Posttraumatic Stress Disorder, and a whole set of Personality Disorder scales. For these additional scales as well as for the standard scales, it should be emphasized that they are not like a medical diagnostic test. There is no instance in which a certain score establishes a specific diagnosis. Rather, the scales assemble a pattern of tendencies that probably characterizes the individual patient and may help a clinician or judge make a decision about management or disposition in a particular case.

Interpretation

It is probable that about 90–95% of MMPI and MMPI-2 tests scored are also interpreted with the aid of some type of computerized formula. These are an outgrowth of the early use of MMPI code types on the profiles in the 1950s and 1960s. Some of the current programs can be used on a personal computer; others are commercially and centrally operated and generate a four- or five-page single-spaced report. These computerized interpretive reports have the advantage of being done blind to everything about the subject except age, sex, and perhaps educational level and marital status. Thus, the conclusions cannot be influenced by other clinical information. Nevertheless, they also have the disadvantage of being uninformed about certain trends that could modify conclusions. In any case, almost all reports rightly emphasize that the results are not specific but are based on statistical trends observed in other patients with very similar score profiles. In this respect, such results need to be viewed in the context of the complete diagnostic evaluation and to be synthesized with other data rather than be seen as "facts" about the patient.

RORSCHACH PSYCHODIAGNOSTICS

The set of 10 published Rorschach inkblots is part of a series developed and used by the Swiss psychiatrist Hermann Rorschach in his clinical research. Rorschach was interested in fantasy, and he noticed that specific kinds of blots evoked fairly consistent responses from certain groups of patients. These findings were published in his monograph, *Psychodiagnostics* (1942), but his work was cut short by his death at the age of 38.

The Rorschach technique is probably the best known personality assessment measure. This is due not only to the extremely widespread use of the technique but also to early claims and hopes that it could and would provide an "x-ray" of the mind. Despite its mystique, the Rorschach technique is actually among the most thoroughly researched measures used in all of psychological testing, and today there is good documentation of its range of usefulness as well as its limitations. Much of the credit for this work is due to the psychologist John Exner, whose system of administration and scoring is now the standard in the field (Exner, 1996).

Administration

The 10 inkblots are ambiguous stimuli that provoke associations. The standard series is reproduced on cards that are 18×24 cm ($7 \times 9\frac{1}{2}$ inches) and numbered from I to X. Card I is shown in Figure 13–1. Five of the blots (I, IV, V, VI, and VII) are in black and white; the others include colors. The examiner gives the patient a statement of directions explaining that a series of inkblots will be shown and that the patient will be asked to tell what they look like. When the first card is offered, the patient is asked, "What might this be?"

During the first phase of the test, the **free association phase,** the examiner records each response as nearly verbatim as possible, notes the orientation of the blot for each response (eg, upside down), and interferes as little as possible.

After all 10 blots have been presented, there is usually an **inquiry phase.** Each blot is given back to the patient, and the examiner reads back the patient's response and asks what about the blot prompted that response. During this phase of the procedure, patients may give additional responses. These are noted, and the same inquiry procedure is followed for these additional responses. In the Exner system, even though new responses may be made during the inquiry phase, *only free association responses are scored.*

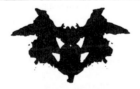

Figure 13–1. Card I of the Rorschach Psychodiagnostics, reduced to one-sixth of actual size. (Reproduced, with permission of the copyright holder, Hans Huber AG Buchhandlung Verlag.)

Scoring

The great bulk of the work in an assessment using the Rorschach is devoted to scoring the responses. There is no one "official" scoring procedure, as there is for the MMPI-2 or the WAIS-III. Major scoring systems were developed in the late 1930s and early 1940s. More recently, Exner proposed an integrative scoring system with more detailed normative data, and this system has become the standard for scoring.

All of the major scoring systems follow Rorschach's original scheme in noting four categories: (1) location, (2) determinants, (3) contents, and (4) popularity. Exner uses two other categories: organizational activity and form quality. Exner's scoring system is presented below.

A. Location: Scoring of location is based on the part of the inkblot used as the basis for the response. The common categories of location are (1) the whole blot, (2) a common detail, (3) an unusual detail, and (4) the white space around or in the middle of the blot. (All of the scoring categories use abbreviated symbols, such as W for whole, but the full set is of interest only to advanced examiners.)

B. Determinant: Scoring of determinants is based on the qualities of the blot that were used in forming the precept, ie, what made it look like the object described by the patient. The major categories of determinants are (1) form, (2) movement, (3) color (chromatic), (4) color (achromatic), (5) texture (shading-derived), (6) dimensionality (shading-derived), (7) shading (general or diffuse), (8) dimensionality (form-derived), and (9) pairs and reflections.

C. Content: There are 27 content categories. Examples with Exner's numbers are (1) whole human, (7) animal detail, (14) blood, (19) fire, (25) sex, and (26) x-ray.

D. Popularity: There are specific responses given frequently to specific cards. Exner has tabulated 13 popular responses; several are listed here, with popularity number shown in parentheses and Rorschach card number shown in brackets: (1) [I] bat or butterfly; (6) [IV] animal skin or human figure dressed in fur; (10) [VII] human heads or faces, usually those of women or children; and (13) [X] crab, lobster, or spider.

E. Organizational Activity: The scoring of organizational activity is indexed by the symbol Z. It is a complex feature to score and it deals with the patient's process of integrating the various features of the inkblot to form an organized and coherent percept.

F. Form Quality: Most scoring systems evaluate how well the percept "fits" the actual blot. Exner uses a four-level system for scoring quality of fit: superior (+), ordinary (o), weak (w), and minus (−). The minus response is defined as "the distorted, arbitrary, unrealistic use of form as related to the content offered, where an answer is imposed on the blot area with total, or near total, disregard for the structure of the area."

Interpretation

Despite the heavy and involved emphasis on scoring, conclusions about personality structure and functioning have come less from formal scoring and more from a movement back and forth between what theory suggests about psychopathological disorders and what the responses to the Rorschach inkblots suggest about the patient's style of processing information. Although Exner's scoring system is quite detailed and empirically based, his instructions for interpretation are much less mechanical. They emphasize a two-stage process of (1) initially generating many hypotheses about defenses, contact with reality, intelligence, fantasy life, and sexuality, based on the formal scoring of the whole record, the specific scoring of each response, the sequence of responses, and the content of the verbalization; and (2) integrating the hypotheses and modifying or ruling out the contradictory ones. After this process, a coherent personality description is written.

Although some writers have argued that interpretation of the Rorschach record should be blind, without reference to any other information about the patient, this method is not recommended. The Rorschach technique is not a parlor game; it is an aid to understanding personality functioning. As such, all available information about the person's functioning is useful. If several psychological tests have been used, on the other hand, Exner recommends that the Rorschach record be examined first, so that some hypotheses are not prematurely ruled out by non-Rorschach information.

Issues in the Use of the Rorschach Technique

Despite the great strides made by Exner in standardizing scoring, the value of the Rorschach technique in personality assessment continues to depend almost exclusively on the clinician's write-up of the record, which involves some degree of subjectivity. This makes it difficult to evaluate the technique, but some conclusions are possible.

First, by itself, the Rorschach record cannot provide a diagnosis. Hypotheses about personality styles or defenses can be entertained, but it is inappropriate to use the Rorschach record to validate these hypotheses. Second, Exner's work amply demonstrates that there are no universal meanings for any card. There is no "father card," "mother card," or "sex card," as many writers have argued. Third, the administration process is as ambiguous as the blots are. The record of responses may be influenced by characteristics of the examiner or by the context in which the examination takes place. Fourth, like psychodynamic formulations of conflict and defense, the yield from a Rorschach record must be viewed as a working formulation to be modified on the basis of other information as it becomes available.

Another projective test commonly used in psychological assessment is the Thematic Apperception Test (TAT). The respondent creates a story to a series of fixed cards. The available evidence about the reliability and validity of the TAT is such that it is difficult to reconcile its continuing use and popularity with the meager evidence that important additional information can be gleaned from it. Unlike the Rorschach, which has benefited substantially from Exner's systematic attention to scoring, the TAT has no such champion.

BROAD ISSUES IN PERSONALITY ASSESSMENT BY PSYCHOLOGICAL TESTING

Three themes have run through the discussion of psychological tests in this chapter.

1. Despite the search for standardization and uniformity in the use of psychological tests for personality assessment or neuropsychological evaluation, different clinicians have different systems and choose different tests. Thus, the interpretation of a battery of psychological tests depends on who does the interpreting. In an analogous fashion, the test results depend on who the patient is; results may be accurate indicators, or they may reflect *individual differences in responses that are not primarily indicative of the attributes being assessed.* This is why tests do not have perfect predictability and why it is difficult to determine with high accuracy a complete picture of a patient's functioning.

2. The research evidence about the utility of testing has been disappointingly mixed. It is not clear how much more information is gained after using the MMPI-2, by also administering the Rorschach and the TAT. In this area, clinicians have been somewhat resistant to take seriously the research evidence, viewing it as simplistic, naive, and not in touch with clinical realities. There are clinical examples in which results of the battery of tests have suggested a personality assessment that is not what any one test would have suggested. The issue here is one of cost and time effectiveness. Like laboratory tests in clinical medicine, psychological tests must be evaluated for redundancy, cost, and possibility of yielding incrementally useful and new information. This concern is less true of neuropsychology evaluation, however.

3. The major area requiring more careful scrutiny is the area of agreement among clinicians—not in scoring of psychological tests but in interpreting the results. If trained clinicians cannot reach an acceptable level of agreement about interpretation, then more structured formats for interpretation must be developed to aid in standardizing the kinds of categories used and inferences made from the testing results.

REFERENCES & SUGGESTED READINGS

Allport GW: *Personality: A Psychological Interpretation.* Holt, 1937.

Butcher JN et al: *Minnesota Multiphasic Inventory (MMPI2). Manual for Administration and Scoring.* University of Minnesota Press, 1989.

Christensen AL: *Luria's Neuropsychological Investigation,* 2nd ed. Wiley, 1979.

Exner JE: *The Rorschach: A Comprehensive System,* 3rd ed. 3 Vol set. Wiley, 1996.

Frank LK: Projective methods for the study of personality. J Psychol 1939;8:839.

Golden CJ et al: A standardized version of Luria's neuropsychological tests. In: *Handbook of Clinical Neuropsychology.* Filskov S, Boll TJ (editors). Wiley, 1981.

Goldstein G, Watson JR: Test-retest reliability of the Halstead-Reitan Battery and the WAIS in a neuropsychiatric population. Clin Neuropsychol 1989;3:265.

Goodglass H, Kaplan E: *Assessment of Aphasia and Related Disorders.* Lea & Febiger, 1972.

Kaplan EF, Goodglass H, Weintraub S: *The Boston Naming Test,* 2nd ed. Lea & Febiger, 1983.

Kelly GA: Man's construction of his alternatives. In: *The Assessment of Human Motives.* Lindzey G (editor). Rinehart, 1958.

Lezak MD: *Neuropsychological Assessment,* 3rd ed. Oxford University Press, 1995.

Luria AR: *Higher Cortical Functions in Man* (translated by B Haigh). Basic, 1966.

Matarazzo JD: Psychological assessment versus psychological testing: Validation from Binet to the school to the courtrooms. Am Psychol 1990;45:999.

Reitan RM, Wolfson D: *Traumatic Brain Injury: Recovery and Rehabilitation.* Vol 2. Neuropsychology Press, 1988.

Reitan RM, Wolfson D: *Neuropsychological Evaluation of Older Children.* Neuropsychology Press, 1992.

Reitan RM, Wolfson D: *The Halstead-Reitan Neuropsychological Test Battery: Theory and Clinical Interpretation,* 2nd ed. Neuropsychology Press, 1993a.

Reitan RM, Wolfson D: *Neuropsychological Evaluation of Young Children.* Neuropsychology Press, 1993b.

Rorschach H: *Psychodiagnostics.* Huber, 1942 (Grune & Stratton, 1951).

Spreen O, Strauss E: *A Compendium of Neuropsychological Tests,* 2nd ed. Oxford University Press, 1998.

Sternberg RJ, Kaufman JC: Human abilities. Annu Rev Psychol 1998;49:479.

Wechsler D: *The Measurement of Adult Intelligence.* Williams & Wilkins, 1939.

Wechsler D: *Wechsler Intelligence Scale for Children–Third Edition.* The Psychological Corporation, 1991.

Wechsler D: *Wechsler Adult Intelligence Scale–Third Edition.* The Psychological Corporation, 1997.

The Clinical Case Summary: The Mayor of Wino Park & His Uncle

14

Howard H. Goldman, MD, MPH, PhD, & David Anderson, MD

The following is a case study of the Mayor of Wino Park, briefly introduced as a character sketch in Chapter 9. The standard sequence for presenting clinical psychiatric cases is set forth in Table 14–1. The hypothetical data needed to complete this clinical case summary would have been collected during the Mayor's 3-week hospitalization, during which he underwent an extensive evaluation, including all of the elements presented in Chapters 10–13. Although the case is presented here primarily to demonstrate the form and content of a case summary, the details of the case also illustrate the complex interaction of biological, psychological, and social factors in medicine and psychiatry. Following the case study of the Mayor is a case study of his uncle, written by an internist in general medical practice.

CASE SUMMARY 1

A. Identifying Data: John F. ("Red") Kimball is 54 years old, divorced, unemployed, currently subsisting on Social Security Disability Insurance (SSDI) benefits, and living on the streets or in Wino Park, a protected urban camping ground in San Fran-

cisco. The night manager of the Billings Hotel on Pine Street receives and holds the patient's monthly check. The patient prefers to be addressed as Mayor and referred to as the Mayor.

B. Informant: The patient is a poor historian. Throughout his hospital stay, his responses to inquiries have been marked by inconsistencies, gaps, and confabulation. His ability to give a useful past history has improved as his attention span increases with treatment, but his history of the present illness continues to be marred by deficits in short-term memory.

To supplement the history, we obtained medical records from previous hospitalizations, outpatient clinic records, and school and military records. No work history documentation could be obtained, nor could any family member be located to verify the history. During an earlier admission, a lifelong acquaintance corroborated much of the patient's early life history as presented in this case study.

C. Chief Complaint: "They closed Wino Park—and I'm yellow, have the shakes, and somebody's trying to poison me."

D. History of the Present Illness: While living in Wino Park off and on for the past 5 years, the Mayor had been in good health except for a few episodes of depression treated with tricyclic antidepressants and supportive psychotherapy. During the past year, he appointed himself mayor of all the homeless alcoholics and other unemployed and mentally ill people who slept in the park. He considered himself their spokesman, and during the past 3 months, following the announcement that the park was to be closed, he felt constant pressure to "save" their haven. He began giving impromptu "news conferences" to anyone who would listen at downtown intersections during rush hour or before groups of tourists waiting for cable cars. He also began to drink more heavily, consuming several quarts of wine daily.

About 10 weeks prior to the present admission, the Mayor was arrested for threatening an officer who attempted to take him into custody when he was found drunk, wandering the streets. He was released the next morning, but the desk sergeant thought he seemed depressed and perhaps in need of medical evaluation, so he was sent to the hospital in a police

Table 14–1. Suggested format for a clinical case summary.

Identifying data
Informant (sources of information) and assessment of
   reliability
Chief complaint
History of the present illness
Past medical and psychiatric history
Review of systems
Habits
Family history
Social history
Developmental history
Physical examination
Neurological examination
Mental status examination
Diagnostic tests
Differential diagnosis
Provisional psychosocial formulation
Hospital course
Multiaxial diagnosis
Psychosocial formulation
Continuing treatment plan and disposition

ambulance. He admitted he had been in a "black mood" for the past couple of weeks, with no appetite, and had been losing weight, waking up at night, and then unable to get back to sleep. He was obviously agitated, said he could not concentrate, and thought a lot about death when he wasn't casting about for some magical solution to the Wino Park "crisis," as he saw it. His preoccupation with death and veiled threats of suicide ("Maybe I'll end it") led to his admission to a psychiatric inpatient unit for observation and protective detention. He signed himself out after 72 hours, proclaiming, "There's nothing wrong with me!" His discharge diagnosis was recurrent unipolar depression. He refused to stay in the hospital for a trial of treatment with antidepressant medication. He could not be committed because he denied suicidal intentions and had not developed delirium tremens. He also refused referral to an outpatient clinic.

The Mayor continued to be depressed and drank "to kill the pain of going insane" and to stop the "shakes." There was no apparent change in his condition until 2 weeks before the present admission, when he became jaundiced, more agitated, confused, and paranoid. He was afraid that someone had contaminated the wine with some kind of poison or "Yellow Dye Number Nine," and he was organizing people to march to the liquor stores to pull the wine off the shelves. At that point he was sleeping only a few hours a night. He became extremely irritable (euphoric one moment, angry the next), and his scheming, grandiosity, and paranoid ideation increased. His speech was pressured, tangential, and at times almost incomprehensible. The "people's press conferences" at downtown intersections became disruptive, and the police were called on several occasions, but there were no arrests or contacts with the health care system until the day of admission.

On the day of admission, Wino Park was closed, and all the homeless men and women were being turned out or relocated. The Mayor refused to go. When the police said they would have to arrest him if he did not leave, he became agitated, running around furiously and talking loudly. All of the pathological thought, affect, and behavior of the previous 2 weeks intensified. He threatened loudly that he would kill anyone who touched him and then kill himself. When he seemed close to collapse from exhaustion, the police grabbed him, handcuffed him, called for an ambulance, and drove him to the hospital again.

E. Past Medical and Psychiatric History: Medical records indicate that the patient was the 35-week product of a difficult pregnancy and labor complicated by abnormal maternal bleeding secondary to multiple small uterine fibroid tumors. The patient's mother had a hysterectomy following delivery; she was separated from her baby for 4 weeks, was unable to nurse him, and then was hospitalized for depression for 4 months postpartum.

During childhood, the patient had measles, mumps, and chicken pox but no other infectious diseases except for an occasional cold. A fractured clavicle at age 8 years was inflicted by his alcoholic father. He had an appendectomy at age 13, shortly after his mother died. (The appendix was normal, according to the pathology report.)

At age 20, the patient received a medical discharge from the Navy for a "character disorder" and was noted to be an alcoholic and occasional binge drinker. Between the ages of 20 and 35, he was working, married, and in excellent health. He was divorced at age 35, and his drinking increased. (For details, see Social History.) For the next 5–10 years, his work history was interrupted by several admissions to alcohol treatment centers, outpatient alcohol counseling, and periods of ambulatory psychiatric treatment for depression. Once, while depressed, he was treated with thyroid hormone; he became acutely psychotic and agitated and was thought to have bipolar affective disorder (manic-depressive illness).

At age 45, the patient became severely depressed and suicidal. He was committed to a state mental hospital because he had refused treatment in a voluntary general hospital psychiatric unit. On admission, he was heavily sedated with antipsychotic medication because of agitation and auditory hallucinations consisting of voices commanding him to kill himself. Because of the imminent danger of suicide, he underwent a course of 12 electroconvulsive treatments, which dramatically improved his mental status, especially his agitation and suicidal ideation. He remained somewhat depressed and stayed in the hospital for 3 months. A trial of tricyclic antidepressants and supportive psychotherapy was successful in further reducing his symptoms, and he was discharged with a prescription for amitriptyline, 200 mg daily at bedtime. He went to live in a single-room-occupancy hotel in the "Tenderloin district" of San Francisco. He was seen as an outpatient for several years in a clinic operated by the county, but his drinking was not controlled, and he stopped his medication. He was readmitted to various hospitals several times. As noted earlier, his sole source of support was SSDI funds. The night manager at the hotel serves as his conservator.

The patient became so mentally disorganized, paranoid, and unmanageable that he could no longer stay at the hotel. He was accepted at a board and care home for alcoholic men but would not agree to the restrictions. He could not be committed to a hospital, because he was not dangerous to himself or others, and so he began his life on the streets and in Wino Park 5 years prior to the current admission.

The Mayor has no documented history of endocrine disorders, including thyroid disease and Cushing syndrome. He has no history of acute liver disease, gastritis, or other gastrointestinal disorders, although his liver enzyme levels have been elevated in the past. There is no record of jaundice prior to this illness. He has never had delirium tremens or any seizure disorder, and he has no known allergies.

F. Review of Systems: In addition to having the symptoms and signs mentioned in the history of the present illness, the patient admits to seeing double from time to time and losing his footing occasionally. Pertinent negative findings include the absence of focal neurological and endocrinological signs and symptoms (other than those mentioned above, eg, diplopia, tremor) and no abnormalities in stool color. He also denies dizziness with changes in posture and denies difficulty initiating his urine stream.

G. Habits: The Mayor drinks up to 2 quarts of wine daily. He has been drinking since he was 12 years old; he admits to having been a binge drinker as a teenager and an alcoholic since his 20s. There is no other history of drug abuse. He has smoked one pack of cigarettes daily since age 15, plus occasional cigars.

H. Family History: The patient is the only child of Francis Kimball and Jean-Marie Thibodeau Kimball. Francis Kimball died at age 55, when the patient was 35, of injuries sustained in an accident at the state mental hospital where he had been a patient for nearly 5 years. Mr Kimball had been away without leave from the hospital, had gotten drunk, started a fight with another patient, was pushed over a wall, and fell 10 feet and struck his head. He had been hospitalized for bipolar affective disorder (manic-depressive illness) and alcoholism. He had no other known disorders. Jean-Marie Kimball died at age 32 of breast cancer. She had no known illnesses other than postpartum depression and uterine fibromyomas. All of the grandparents died before they reached age 50: one by suicide, one from "heart disease," one from influenza, and one from tuberculosis.

I. Social History: As a child, John F. Kimball lived with both parents, although their occasional extended absences from home (caused by parents' illnesses and father's alcoholism) necessitated informal foster care with neighbors and with "aunts and uncles" for up to 3 months at a stretch. John attended parochial school for 6 years, completed junior high, and attended high school in the public schools in San Francisco. His performance was uneven; he did well with some subjects and teachers and poorly with others. He was good in dramatics, athletics, and public speaking, had many friends, and was elected class treasurer as a sophomore. He became depressed as a senior, did poorly, and dropped out before graduation. He entered the Navy and served for 3 years. He spent time in the "brig" for insubordination, drunkenness, and being AWOL. He was never promoted above the rank of Seaman First-Class and was discharged for medical reasons with a diagnosis of "character disorder and alcoholism."

Building on some skills he learned in the Navy and on his persuasive manner, the patient got a union card and a job as a machinist. He worked in a dry dock, repairing ships. He was liked by his workmates; they drank and caroused together, and Kimball became union shop steward. For a time he was involved in union politics and attended local election rallies.

"Red" Kimball married a girl from his old neighborhood shortly after discharge from the Navy. They lived in a flat and "got along fine," but he insisted they have no children. She acquiesced reluctantly until she turned 30. At that time, she began to complain about "feeling empty" and wanting a family. He began to spend less time at home and more time with "the boys," and his drinking increased. He became impotent, and they stopped having sexual relations altogether. Their marriage slowly deteriorated as he became more depressed and his alcoholism worsened. They began to fight, and he abused her physically on two occasions. She filed for dissolution of the marriage; the patient has not seen his wife since the decree became final.

The remainder of the social history is conveyed along with the past history, discussed earlier. As noted, the patient is homeless, unemployed, and supported by SSDI.

J. Developmental History: The Mayor's life began with a 5-month separation from his mother, who was hospitalized with postpartum complications, including a hysterectomy and postpartum depression. As a newborn, he was raised by a neighbor and supported by his father, whose alcoholism made him an undependable caretaker. Mrs Kimball returned home and took up the child-rearing responsibility with renewed energy, but she never seemed able to get emotionally close to her son. The same was true of Mr Kimball, although when he was sober, he was a great "pal" to his son, teaching him to box and play games.

Little is known of the Mayor's childhood from age 2 to 6 years. In spite of never feeling emotionally close to her son, his mother tended to "spoil him" with small favors and took him with her everywhere. As his father's absences became more frequent and longer in duration, "Red" Kimball became protective of his mother. The Mayor's earliest traumatic memories are of his father's physical assaults on his mother. He was terrified and felt guilty that he couldn't help her. Once he did step in the way of his father's blows and sustained a fractured clavicle. He began to "hate" his "old man" and felt confused when his father confessed to him in tears—drunk and begging forgiveness. The image of the "pal" was incongruent with the hated "old man." As a child, "Red" thought almost everything was his fault because he had been "bad."

Ages 7–12 were marked by minor school difficulties and further troubles at home. "Red" took his first drink at age 12 and became drunk easily at first but soon developed tolerance to large quantities of alcohol. His mother died when he was 13 years old, and he was extremely quiet, withdrawn, and guilty. He had no one to talk to, and his sadness turned to anger and resentment toward his parents, who had neglected him. And the anger turned quickly to guilt for having hateful feelings toward his parents. A few months later, he complained of intense stomach cramps and was operated on for suspected appendicitis, but the surgical specimen was normal.

The patient reached puberty at about age 14, engaged in homosexual horseplay (group masturbation) with some friends at age 15, and had his first heterosexual experience at age 16. He related no history of sexual dysfunction other than episodes of impotence during his marriage (described above) and while drunk. Other details of social and sexual relationships are discussed in the social history.

K. Physical Examination: On admission the patient was a plethoric man who seemed older than his stated age, with a barrel chest, thin limbs, and protruding abdomen. He was in apparent distress, shouting and waving his arms. His sclerae were yellow and his skin jaundiced where it was not tanned from prolonged exposure.

1. Vital signs—Pulse 120 and regular, respiration 24, labored; blood pressure 169/90 left arm, sitting; temperature 100° F. At the time of admission, only a limited examination could be performed because of the patient's lack of cooperation. A cursory examination of the lungs, heart, and abdomen revealed no acute disease. The examination was completed the following morning, when pulse was 88 and regular, respiration 12 and regular, blood pressure 110/60 in both arms with no significant orthostatic drop in blood pressure, and temperature 99° F.

2. Head, eyes, ears, nose, and throat—Several scars on the face and scalp healed by secondary intention, marked scleral icterus, spider angiomas and injected veins on the nose, nasopharyngeal congestion.

3. Neck—Supple, no thyromegaly, no lymphadenopathy.

4. Thorax and lungs—Increased anteroposterior diameter, lungs clear to percussion and auscultation, although breath sounds were distant, and the chest was slightly hyperresonant. No gynecomastia.

5. Heart and great vessels—The point of maximum impulse was felt in the fifth intercostal space two fingerbreadths to the left of the midclavicular line; the impulse was hyperdynamic. Heart sounds were all within normal limits, with no murmurs, rubs, or clicks. All peripheral pulses were felt; no bruits.

6. Abdomen—Icteric skin, appendectomy scar. Abdomen distended with ascites fluid wave. Tenderness in the right upper quadrant, with an enlarged liver felt 4 cm below the costal margin. No splenomegaly, no masses, no costovertebral angle tenderness. Bowel sounds were normal.

7. Rectum—Prostatic hypertrophy (2/4) with no discrete mass. Stool test for occult blood was negative.

8. Genitourinary tract—Normal adult male with slight testicular atrophy. Normal pattern of pubic hair.

9. Extremities—No bony abnormalities, full range of motion.

L. Neurological Examination:

1. Mental status—(See below.)

a. Cranial nerves—I, II, V, VII–XII tested and all within normal limits; III, IV, VI, pupils equal, round, and reacting to light and accommodation, but abduction and conjugate gaze were paralyzed; diplopia was evident.

2. Motor system—

a. Muscle mass and tone—Normal.

b. Strength—Full strength (5/5).

c. Coordination—Slight asterixis and dysdiadochokinesia, demonstrated in difficulties with finger-to-nose and heel-to-shin tests.

d. Reflexes—All 3/4 without clonus, except that ankle jerks were absent; Babinski, Hoffmann absent.

e. Gait and station—Wide-based gait.

f. Movements—Normal fluidity without tics, chorea, or dyskinesia; mild resting tremor in both hands (1/4).

g. Sensation—Diminished pain and vibration sense in the extremities, feet worse than hands; no extinction on simultaneous stimulation.

M. Mental Status Examination:

1. Overview—Exaggerated alertness and easy distractibility; disheveled, with poor personal hygiene but a certain flair to his carriage and disarray; unco-operative at times but with perseverance able to complete the examination; hyperactive, unable to sit for more than 3–4 minutes at a time.

2. Emotion—Labile, expansive, irritable, with rapid shifts from tearful sadness to red-faced anger. Affect was appropriate. (Thoughts were consistent with affect.)

3. Attention—Failed the seven-digit screening test, only able to recall three digits on second try. Unable to perform serial 7s or 3s.

4. Orientation—To person, place (that it was a hospital only), and time (only to year, not month or day).

5. Memory—Attention deficit made memory assessment difficult. With effort and repetition, the patient was able to immediately recall three items, but he could not remember any of them at 5 minutes even with prompting and reinforcement. Visual memory was similarly impaired. The patient confabulated to fill in the gaps in recent memory. Long-term memory was adequate for a period prior to 4 or 5 years ago. He knew the United States presidents and current events of the period.

6. Speech and language—Pressured and incessant, but fluent, with normal comprehension; repetition and naming both intact. Two- and three-step commands could not be assessed because of memory deficits.

7. Constructional ability—Unable to perform tests requiring memory. The patient was able to copy test figures when they were in front of him.

8. Calculations—Able to pass the screening test (5 × 13).

9. Thought—

a. Thought process—Thought process markedly disturbed, occasionally incoherent. When coherent, the patient had flight of ideas, was tangential, but did not demonstrate looseness of association.

b. Thought content—Content marked by mood-congruent auditory hallucinations saying "you are to blame" or laughing derisively. The patient was preoccupied by guilt and images of death alternating with "grandeur." He had paranoid delusions that someone was trying to poison the wine in the liquor stores—"Yellow Dye Number Nine is making me yellow all over!" He denied ideas of reference, thought broadcasting, or other delusions of control. He also denied complex hallucinations of several voices conversing and had no visual, tactile, or gustatory hallucinations, illusions, or other preoccupations.

c. Cognitive functions—Refused to interpret proverbs or answer screening questions: "Don't bother me with that nonsense. . . . My time is too valuable." Judgment grossly impaired. Did demonstrate some ability to abstract when he tried to take over a nurse's responsibility of explaining to a patient why he should take his medication. He implored the patient, "Take that stuff and your mood might get to be like mine. Besides, it'll help you get out of here quicker if you do like they say!"

d. Fund of knowledge—Knew the presidents and current events up to 4–5 years ago.

e. Insight—Aware of the reasons for hospitalization but expended considerable energy denying problems and displacing them onto the politics of the demise of Wino Park.

N. Diagnostic Tests:

1. Laboratory tests—Serum electrolytes and blood urea nitrogen were normal. Blood ammonia was trivially elevated to 120 μg/dL on admission but fell into the normal range within 3 days. Thyroid studies were normal. Serum aspartate aminotransferase, alkaline phosphatase, and bilirubin were all elevated on admission and returned toward normal by discharge. Bilirubin fell from 4.1 mg/dL to 1.8 mg/dL (mostly direct). Serum albumin was depressed; gamma globulin was elevated. Prothrombin time was in the high normal range. Hematological evaluation showed a mild macrocytic anemia and moderate leukocytosis with a shift to the left. Erythrocyte sedimentation rate was mildly elevated. Serum iron was normal; serum folate was low. Urinalysis and electrocardiography were normal. Blood glucose was normal. Hepatitis B and C profiles were negative.

2. X-rays—Chest films showed slight cardiomegaly and evidence of mild emphysema; there was no evidence of congestive heart failure. A CT scan of the head was normal, with no evidence of tumor, infarct, or subdural hematoma.

3. Neuropsychological tests—Full-scale Wechsler Adult Intelligence Scale had been 110 on a previous evaluation. On this admission, the patient's concentration and memory were so impaired that a complete reexamination was impossible. All tests requiring short-term memory were failed. Results of the screening Bender Gestalt Test, however, were normal. The examiner noted that when the patient was tested near the end of his manic episode, he copied the test figures flamboyantly and large in size.

4. Personality assessment—No testing was done on this admission. Previous tests included a Minnesota Multiphasic Personality Inventory; results showed high scores on psychasthenia, masculinity, paranoia, and hysteria. On one administration, he also showed an elevation on the depression scale; at another time, the hypomania scale was elevated.

O. Differential Diagnosis: The differential diagnosis on admission was not complicated because of the well-established prior diagnoses of affective disorder and alcohol dependence, the recurrence of classical symptoms and signs during this episode of illness, and a strong family history of affective illness. For the sake of completeness, other diagnoses were considered: organic affective syndrome, delirium tremens, and especially the nonaffective psychotic disorders (eg, schizophrenia, acute paranoid disorder). No organic cause could be identified, although it is possible that encephalopathy associated with the patient's alcoholic hepatitis may have exacerbated or precipitated his psychosis. The same may be said of his alcohol intoxication. On alcohol withdrawal, there was no worsening of his mental status, no increase in tremor, and no seizures—effectively eliminating delirium tremens from the diagnosis. The pattern of the Mayor's illness without persistent psychosis and with prolonged intervals free of illness precluded a diagnosis of schizophrenia; delusional disorder and the other psychotic illnesses were ruled out only by the presence of the full-blown manic episodes and depressive episodes in the Mayor's history and by current findings on mental status examination. On admission, he demonstrated most of the symptoms and signs of manic episode (see Table 20–1); shortly after admission, he developed a major depressive episode (see Table 20–1). This pattern replicated at least one earlier cycle of bipolar affective disorder.

A diagnosis of alcohol dependence could also be made unequivocally (see Table 17–2). The diagnosis of alcohol amnestic syndrome was straightforward (see Chapter 17 and Table 17–2), having been made in the presence of a gaze palsy characteristic of Wernicke's encephalopathy often associated with Korsakoff's psychosis (amnestic syndrome). The diagnosis of alcoholic hepatitis was based on the acute onset of jaundice in an alcoholic and marked abnormalities in hepatic function. Alcoholic cirrhosis was suggested by the presence of ascites; however, *definitive* diagnosis can be based only on liver biopsy, which was not performed, because it was considered too dangerous and because the Mayor was uncooperative. Hematological evaluation revealed a macrocytic anemia, also probably caused by chronic alcoholism and folate deficiency.

P. Provisional Psychosocial Formulation: Too little information was available on admission to develop a formulation, although the initial psychological themes centered on losses and self-esteem.

Q. Hospital Course:

1. Week 1—The first week was devoted to a thorough evaluation, reported in this case summary, and to initial treatment of the patient's many problems. Treatment of agitation and insomnia began with oxazepam, 30 mg four times daily, reduced to 15 mg three times daily by the end of the week. When baseline renal and endocrine studies were completed, the patient was started on lithium carbonate, 600 mg orally three times daily for 5 days until a therapeutic level of 1.1 mEq/L was achieved, and a maintenance dose of 300 mg three times daily was established. In evaluative and supportive psychotherapy, the patient revealed many important losses and separations in his life. The psychological themes are discussed in the psychosocial formulation below. The Mayor appeared to become depressed by the end of the first week, as his manic signs and symptoms abated with aggressive treatment. During this period, he was confined to the ward. Attempts to contact family and friends were unsuccessful. Social service personnel set about finding the patient a place to live after discharge.

Oxazepam was initially selected to control agitation for two reasons: it is less toxic to the liver than the antipsychotic medications and it would help control alcohol withdrawal symptoms and seizure activity associated with delirium tremens if any of these should occur. The patient was observed closely for delirium tremens, but this did not develop. He was also given thiamine, 50 mg intravenously on admission, followed by 50 mg intramuscularly daily thereafter to reverse the Wernicke-Korsakoff syndrome (gaze paralysis and memory disturbance). The gaze paralysis cleared rapidly, but the patient was left with an impairment in memory. Folic acid was given orally, 1 mg daily, for the anemia.

The hope was that abstinence and improved nutrition would permit the patient's liver to heal and that laboratory values would return toward normal and the jaundice would subside. A definitive diagnosis could not be made; a biopsy was not advisable because of poor patient cooperation and the risk of excessive bleeding (prothrombin time was in the high normal range).

2. Week 2—The Mayor's affect deteriorated into a depressive episode. He complained of a return of agitation, loss of appetite, thoughts (but no plans) of death and suicide, and difficulty concentrating. Feelings of guilt and failure dominated his individual therapy sessions and his comments in ward group therapy meetings. At the beginning of the week, he was involved in ward activities; by the end of the week, he had lost interest in everything and seldom left his room. He was watched closely to prevent a suicide attempt. In spite of only 1 week of symptoms and signs of depression, he was started on paroxetine, 20 mg in the morning. Oxazepam was tapered to 15 mg at bedtime.

3. Week 3—The third week was characterized by slow improvement in mental status. Concentration and attention improved. There was no psychosis. Affect lightened slightly. The patient's sleep improved, and he was taking two meals daily by the end of the week. He still felt guilty and was negative, but he stopped ruminating about death and suicide. Arrangements were made for him to go to a board and care home for alcoholics, but he could not obtain a bed for 2 weeks. Plans to keep him until his depression had completely resolved had to be dropped because he insisted on discharge, as did the utilization management team at the hospital. He was not suicidal and could not be committed involuntarily to a state mental hospital for further care. His conservator at the single-room-occupancy hotel agreed to look after him and let him stay there again. The Mayor also agreed to take his medication and continue in treatment in the hospital's outpatient department. He was making progress in treatment and was beginning to see that he needed to forgive himself for his imagined wrongdoings and to develop a less intense and extreme style in dealing with other people.

By the time of discharge, the patient still had signs of impaired memory and depressed affect, but he was free of psychosis, and his attention span was normal. His jaundice was clearing, and his liver function was returning toward normal.

R. Multiaxial Discharge Diagnosis:

1. Axis I—

Bipolar disorder (see Table 20–1).

Manic episode on admission.

Depressive episode by discharge.

Alcohol dependence (see Table 17–2).

Alcohol amnestic disorder (Korsakoff's psychosis) (see Chapter 17 and Table 17–2).

2. Axis II—Histrionic and passive-aggressive traits are probably secondary to affective disorder.

3. Axis III—

Alcoholic hepatitis with jaundice.

Wernicke's syndrome.

Congestive heart failure and chronic obstructive pulmonary disease.

Alcoholic cirrhosis (suspected clinically).

Peripheral neuropathy.

Macrocytic anemia.

4. Axis IV—

Psychosocial and environmental problems.
Loss of "home" and status as "Mayor."
Acute physical illness perceived as threat.

5. Axis V—

Global assessment of function.
Current: 20 (in danger of harm).
Past year: 35 (inability to function).

S. Psychosocial Formulation: The Mayor is an angry, guilt-ridden man with bipolar affective disorder complicated by alcoholism and its psychological and physiological concomitants. His life story represents a cyclic struggle to achieve a sense of self-worth and self-forgiveness in the face of hardships, losses, separations, and failures. One can only speculate on the interplay of heredity and environment in the evolution of this man's psychopathology; he has a strong family history of affective disorder and alcoholism. In many ways he has repeated the history of his father—in his illness and in his personal life.

The Mayor's depression may be viewed as a response to his losses and separations, beginning at birth: his mother's hospitalizations and depression, his father's repeated absences and ultimate institutionalization and death, and his mother's death all provoked sadness, anger, and a feeling that perhaps he was unloved, unlovable, or perhaps even so "bad" that he made these terrible events and problems happen. The anger fed his guilt, and when it became too intense, it triggered a morbid retreat into depression and alcohol abuse or an angry flight into mania. Manic euphoria, grandiosity, and the projection of his anger onto others in paranoid fantasies briefly protected him from pain and guilt. (For example, it was *others* who were trying to poison him with Yellow Dye Number Nine, not *he* who was intoxicating himself and his liver with wine.)

The Mayor's sense of guilt and inadequacy appears to stem from the confusion, terror, and helplessness he felt while witnessing his mother's abuse at the hands of his father. He also fell victim to his father's wrath, which hurt him and confused him further. His alliance with his mother may be viewed as overdetermined (ie, having many causes). His failure to develop a bond with his mother during infancy and her resentment at the loss of her ability to have more children following his birth set up a cycle of reaction formations leading to a studied closeness between them. They tried to overcome their own unconscious resentments toward each other and to compensate for the bond that did not develop in infancy.

The father, too, worked at being a "pal" when he wasn't drunk, depressed, or "away." During childhood, the patient felt doubly guilty about his mother (causing her unhappiness and not protecting her from attack)—a pain he says he felt in his "gut." In retrospect, his symptoms of appendicitis shortly following his mother's death may be seen as a manifestation of this pain. In spite of anger toward his father, he emulated him—all the way to the hospital.

The patient's marriage was also in many respects patterned after that of his parents. It was a hostile dependent relationship that lasted 15 years. However, the Mayor's marriage ended not with the death of his wife but in divorce following injury and abuse. In this case, the abusiveness stemmed from his wife's wish to have children and the Mayor's adamant opposition. One can speculate that his violent opposition derived from a fear that were he to be a father, he might abuse his "son" (he could only imagine a boy child) and disappoint him ("as my father disappointed me").

The Mayor wants everyone to love him but is unable to get close to anyone. He lacks the capacity for intimacy. His charm, dramatic style, and engaging personality have brought him no closeness and no increase in self-esteem. These he has manufactured in flights into mania—an escape from his severe depression. He projects his disappointments, failures, and anger onto others who he believes are out to get him, especially authority figures, teachers, superiors in the Navy, his bosses at work, the police, alcohol manufacturers, his wife, and his doctors.

Bipolar affective disorder and alcoholism have isolated the Mayor from the things he wanted most but were denied him by fate, circumstance, and heredity. A biological predisposition to affective disorder coupled with environmental circumstances and emotional deprivation and trauma combine to explain the man and his illness.

The patient's sensitivity to loss and stress and the loss of his "home" in the park and his status as Mayor precipitated this episode of illness. He says, "I *was* the Mayor of Wino Park!" The park had been an asylum for a homeless man who needed his expansive fantasies to feel a sense of worth. The Mayor will soon be 55, the age at which his father died in a mental hospital. Whether the Mayor survives will depend in part on the ability of health care professionals to control his disorder biomedically, understand his illness and his defenses psychologically, help him find a new home and social support, and capitalize on his strengths, such as his wit, charm, and capacity for leadership.

T. Continuing Treatment Plan and Disposition:

1. Biomedical treatment plan—

Lithium carbonate, 300 mg orally three times daily.
Paroxetine, 20 mg in the morning.
Thiamine, 100 mg orally three times daily.
Folic acid, 1 mg orally daily.
General internal medicine follow-up in 2 weeks.
Psychotropic medications to be monitored by psychiatrist.
Lithium levels to be determined weekly or until stabilized.

2. Psychological treatment plan—
Continue in weekly individual supportive treatment focusing on interpersonal skills; sessions limited to 30 minutes, as tolerated.
Referral to Alcoholics Anonymous.
Visit from nurse if patient fails to comply with his appointments.

3. Social treatment plan—The patient was transferred to an alcoholism board and care home from his discharge residence at the hotel in San Francisco. Alcoholics Anonymous will help him to build a new social network as well as reinforce his abstinence. SSDI checks will be transferred from the hotel to the board and care home after a 1-month trial. Conservatorship might also be transferred to the board and care home operator.

CASE SUMMARY 2

A. Identifying Data: This is a 74-year-old white male, retired school teacher.

B. Chief Complaint: "The pain in my arm is driving me crazy."

C. History of the Present Illness: The patient, who is well known to this physician, had an episode of herpes zoster of the right C-7 dermatome approximately 4 years ago. Following the initial episode, he developed pain in his right arm, which had been well controlled with nonsteroidal anti-inflammatory drugs and capsaicin ointment. Although there was some residual pain while on these medications, it was quite tolerable and did not interfere with his daily activities. Over the past 8 weeks or so he has noticed that the pain is bothering him more, although he says it really is not more severe. He wants something done about it. There has been no recurrence of rash in the area, no injury, nor any new neurological symptoms such as weakness, numbness, or tingling. The patient simply states that the pain bothers him more.

On further discussion, he also complains of feeling more tired than usual for the past 2 months. His activity level has not increased but, in fact, has decreased because he has not felt like doing very much. He has been getting his usual 6–7 hours of sleep but has had to go to bed earlier because he has been waking up early in the morning and then is unable to return to sleep. The pain does not wake him up; he just wakes up. He denies that shortness of breath or any other physical symptom awakens him. There has been a 5-lb weight loss over the past couple of months as a result of decreased appetite; however, he denies nausea, vomiting, diarrhea, constipation, hematochezia, melena, emesis, or hematemesis. He also reveals that he has been more irritable lately and that his wife has been "on his nerves," though he is not sure why he has felt this way.

The patient says that he has been worrying a lot recently. When asked what he is worrying about, he states, "I worry about my health a lot, and I worry about my nephew." His nephew has a history of mental illness and had recently been evicted from the residential hotel he had been living in; he is now homeless and on the street. (The Mayor of Wino Park is the son of the patient's wife's brother.) Although he felt guilty about not offering to take this nephew into his home, his wife being firmly against it, he knew that the nephew would probably not agree to come live with him anyway. He also has been worried about money, although he knows objectively that he and his wife are comfortable on their current retirement income. He no longer has the desire to do much of anything and, in fact, is not even going to church anymore. This used to be his primary social activity. He says that he hasn't been enjoying it lately and "just doesn't have the energy." He denies any heat or cold intolerance, change in his skin or hair, or palpitation or tremor.

There is no suicidal plan, but when questioned about suicide he said, "Sometimes I think it wouldn't be too bad if a truck ran me over."

About 20 years ago he had an episode of depression that was not treated with medication and resolved after approximately 1 year. There is no history of manic episodes. He feels very similar now and states, "I don't want to get that low again."

He has no other complaints at this time.

D. Past Medical History:

1. Herpes zoster 4 years ago, which resulted in postherpetic pain in the right C-7 dermatome.
2. Hypertension for approximately 34 years, which has been well controlled on medication.
3. Coronary artery disease with stable angina. The patient has less than one episode of exertional chest pain per month, which is easily relieved with rest and/or one sublingual nitroglycerin tablet. He has no history of myocardial infarction.
4. He has a history of hypercholesterolemia.
5. There is a history of degenerative joint disease with chronic aching in both knees.

He denies any history of diabetes, liver disease, renal disease, lung disease, tuberculosis, or rheumatic fever. He denies any allergies. He denies any history of blood transfusions. He denies any history of ever having had surgery.

He drinks alcohol rarely, that is, less than one drink per week, and he has never been a heavy drinker. He smoked one pack of cigarettes per day for 20 years but quit 30 years ago.

His current medications include long-acting propranolol, 160 mg every day; isosorbide dinitrate, 20 mg orally three times a day; ibuprofen, 800 mg orally three times a day; capsaicin ointment to his right arm four times a day; and nitroglycerin sublingual, as needed.

E. Family History: The patient's father died at the age of 80 of congestive heart failure, which followed a myocardial infarction. He had had long-standing hypertension and a history of alcohol abuse. His mother died at the age of 90 of "natural causes." He has four brothers, three of whom have hypertension and one of whom has coronary artery disease. The other brother is healthy as far as he knows. His siblings are otherwise well. He is married and has two healthy sons. His maternal grandfather died of colon cancer. His family history is otherwise negative.

F. Social History: The patient is a retired school teacher who is married and lives with his wife of 52 years. They have lived in South San Francisco since they were married and have many friends. One of their children lives in town and is very supportive. His main hobbies are being involved in church group activities, bowling, and reading. The patient has a bachelor's degree. He has no grave financial concerns at this time.

G. Review of Systems: He has occasional headaches. He wears bifocals. He has corns, which are sometimes painful. He has occasional mild constipation. Otherwise, the review of systems is negative except as mentioned in the history of present illness.

H. Physical Examination: This is a well-developed white male who appears to have a sad affect. Vital signs: blood pressure is 140/80, right arm sitting; pulse is 66; respirations are 12. The skin is without lesions. The head, ears, eyes, nose, and throat examination shows that he is normalocephalic; the skull shows no evidence of trauma. Extraocular movements are intact. Pupils are equal, round, and reactive to light. The fundi are benign except for mild arteriolar narrowing. His nose, mouth, and throat examination is completely within normal limits. The neck is supple without jugular venous distention, thyromegaly, or bruit. The chest is clear to auscultation and percussion. A coronary examination reveals S1, S2, and S4 without S3 or murmur. The abdomen is benign with normal bowel sounds and no tenderness, guarding, rebound, rigidity, organomegaly, or mass. The extremities are without edema or cyanosis. A rectal examination reveals normal tone and mucosa without mass, and brown guaiac-negative stool is present. A neurological examination reveals normal mental status—the patient is alert and oriented to name, place, date, and time. His long-term and short-term memory are intact. Concentration is decreased by test of serial 7s. Interpretation of proverbs and the ability to identify similarities between two objects are appropriate. There is no evidence of excessively concrete thinking. Judgment appears to be intact. He is able to follow complex commands and to copy a drawing of a house without difficulty. Cranial nerves II–XII are intact. Motor strength is 5 out of 5 throughout. Sensory examination is intact to light touch, pinprick, and position. There is hyperesthesia along the C-7 dermatome on the right arm. The reflexes are 2+ and symmetrical. There is no Babinski. Finger-to-nose and heel-to-shin testing are normal. Gait is normal. Romberg test is negative.

I. Assessment:

1. The constellation of symptoms—anhedonia, depressed mood, sleep and appetite disturbance, fatigue, and irritability—strongly suggests a diagnosis of major depression, particularly in this patient who has a history of a past depressive episode. Hypothyroidism or hyperthyroidism may present with nonspecific symptoms in elderly patients, but this patient has no history of thyroid disease and no physical examination finding to suggest either disorder. Occult malignancy may occasionally present in this fashion, but again, there is no corroborating historical or physical examination evidence to support this diagnosis.

2. Arm pain. Most likely the patient's increased distress with his arm pain is related to his depression. As noted in the history of present illness, the pain is not more severe. There is nothing on physical examination to suggest a change in his neurological status.

3. Hypertension, well controlled.

4. Coronary artery disease appears to be stable.

5. Hypercholesterolemia was stable at last check 3 months ago.

6. Degenerative joint disease has been stable and well controlled on current medications.

J. Plan: The diagnosis of probable major depression was discussed with the patient, and various therapeutic options including psychotherapy and/or pharmacotherapy were offered. The patient agreed that he had been feeling depressed and felt that he needed treatment; however, he felt that he would prefer not to have psychotherapy at this point in his life. He agreed to begin therapy with desipramine in low dose. In addition to its antidepressant properties, desipramine was chosen because it has been demonstrated to be helpful in treating neuritic pain. The possible side effects of the medication, including dry mouth, sedation, urinary retention, and postural dizziness, were discussed. The patient was warned about these and told that should he develop postural dizziness or urinary retention, he should call or come to the emergency room. Desipramine was begun at 10 mg orally at bedtime. The patient was also told that he should not expect a response from this medication immediately and that the dosage would need to be increased gradually as tolerated. He agreed to return in 1 week for follow-up.

Thyroid-stimulating hormone, complete blood count, and biochemical profile were ordered.

All other medical problems are stable, and current treatments were to be continued.

K. Course of Treatment: The results of all diagnostic tests were normal. The patient began desipramine, 10 mg orally at bedtime, as instructed the evening it was prescribed. Over the next 2 days he began to notice increasing episodes of chest pain and went to the emergency room. He was evaluated and admitted for possible unstable angina. When seen the following day by his primary physician it became clear that the patient had been experiencing chest pains only when standing up and had spent 1½ days in bed because of fear of standing up. From supine to standing position, the patient's blood pressure fell from 140/70 to 80/50, his heart rate increased from 80 to 110, and he developed chest pain that could be relieved by lying down. The chest pain was caused by coronary ischemia secondary to decreased perfusion and increased oxygen demand brought about by hypotension and tachycardia, respectively. The desipramine was then stopped, since it was felt to be the cause of his orthostasis and tachycardia. Within 2 days his orthostatic symptoms had completely abated, and he was able to return to his prior activity level. The patient's depressive symptoms continued, and he was started later on fluoxetine, initially at 10 mg per day followed by an increase to 20 mg per day, given in the morning. In the 2 weeks after his dose reached 20 mg per day the patient began to feel much better. He noticed an increase in his energy level and an improvement in his sleep patterns. He began to enjoy things, and his appetite improved. His mood brightened. His arm pain, though no less intense, bothered him much less than it had prior to treatment. The patient was continued on fluoxetine for 12 months, after which it was stopped with no recurrence of the patient's depressive symptoms.

Section III.
Mental Disorders

Classifying Mental Disorders: *Diagnostic and Statistical Manual of Mental Disorders,* Fourth Edition (*DSM-IV*)

15

Harold A. Pincus, MD, Michael B. First, MD, Allen Frances, MD, & Laurie E. McQueen, MSSW

Note to Reader on Use of *DSM-IV* in This Text

By arrangement with the American Psychiatric Association, the authors of *Review of General Psychiatry* have borrowed freely from *DSM-IV.* Most of what we have taken from *DSM-IV* is identified as such in the tabular matter, eg, "Table 20–1. *DSM-IV* diagnostic criteria for mood disorders." Language from the diagnostic criteria of *DSM-IV* reproduced in this text otherwise than in the tables is in quotes. The quoted passages are reproduced exactly as they appear in *DSM-IV.* The tables have been normalized to the style of the book in small matters of punctuation and spelling.—HHG.

The *Diagnostic and Statistical Manual of Mental Disorders,* 4th edition (*DSM-IV*), represents the standard classification of mental disorders used in the United States and internationally. The fourth edition was developed over a 5-year period, involving hundreds of psychiatrists and other mental health professionals from the United States and 40 other countries. Revisions from the *DSM-III-R* were the result of a systematic, empirically based methodology that documented in detail the basis for decisions made.

The DSM system was originally developed to provide a single coding reference for mental disorders. In addition to its usefulness for medical record keeping, the system has evolved to serve a number of other important functions in clinical practice, research, and education. By providing categories of disorders, the classification provides a succinct communication tool for clinicians and researchers and allows information collected in each milieu to be read-

ily translatable and valuable for the other. For researchers, explicit criterion sets defining homogeneous populations have allowed great advances in refining diagnostic assessment, investigating the etiology of mental disorders, and developing more effective treatments. Categorizing disorders aids the clinician's predictive power, allowing him or her to estimate more accurately, for example, symptoms or features that might be expected, the typical course of the disorder, and optimal treatments. The organizing principle of the DSM system also facilitates differential diagnosis by grouping disorders by shared phenomenology. Additionally, the classification system serves as an educational tool, providing an organized method to learn a great deal of complex information.

Although the classification system has advanced psychiatric diagnosis, it should be recognized as one tool among several in patient diagnosis and care, and it should be understood that no classification system can be applied without adequate clinical training and judgment.

HISTORY OF CLASSIFICATIONS OF MENTAL DISORDERS

Efforts to classify mental illness have existed for thousands of years. Egyptian and Sumerian references to senile dementia, melancholia, and hysteria date back to 3000 BC. Ancient Greeks and Romans described five categories of disorders, including phrenitis, mania, melancholia, hysteria, and epilepsy.

Throughout the struggle to classify mental disorders adequately and accurately, several challenging issues have persisted. For example, whereas some systems favored a large number of narrowly defined conditions (eg, a system proposed by Boissier de

Sauvages in the sixteenth century identified over 2400 conditions, each of which was essentially a symptom), others were based on more inclusive, broad conceptualizations (eg, Phillippe Pinel in the eighteenth century proposed a system of only four clinical types, including mania, melancholia, dementia, and idiotism). Classification systems have also varied in the extent to which categorization of disorders could be based on etiology (eg, in the early nineteenth century William Griesinger predicted that all mental disorders would be classified according to their underlying brain lesion), the course of the illness (eg, Benedict-Augustin Morel depicted schizophrenia solely in terms of the course of the illness in the early nineteenth century), or the description of symptom patterns.

Emil Kraepelin, in the latter half of the nineteenth century, developed a system that drew from these various approaches. Kraepelin studied groups of patients whose disorders had the same course in order to determine their shared clinical features. This overall approach was largely retained in the development of the current DSM system.

DSM & ICD

Several systems developed in the United States prior to DSM had been devised primarily to collect statistical information and included manuals developed by the U.S. Army (and Veterans Administration), the World Health Organization (WHO), and earlier attempts of the American Psychiatric Association in conjunction with the New York Academy of Medicine.

DSM-I, published in 1952 by the American Psychiatric Association, presented short glossary definitions of 106 mental disorders and was the first classification to emphasize clinical utility. *DSM-I* was a variant of the WHO's *International Classification of Disease*, 6th edition (ICD-6). The sixth edition of the ICD was the first to include a section of mental disorders. The term "reaction" was used throughout the *DSM-I*, largely on the basis of Adolf Meyer's psychobiological view that mental disorders embodied reactions of the personality to psychological, social, and biological factors.

The relationship between the ICD system and the DSM system would continue. In 1968, ICD-8 and *DSM-II* were published. Seventy-six new categories had been added from *DSM-I* to *DSM-II*, representing advances in the field that allowed greater specificity. Additionally, the DSM no longer included the term "reaction," which had been used throughout *DSM-I*.

DSM-III, published in 1979, represented a major shift in the approach to psychiatric diagnosis and included many important innovations. Explicit criteria, suggested earlier by the British psychiatrist Stengel, were incorporated in the definition of each disorder. Multiaxial assessment was added, guiding the clinician in comprehensive case assessment using multiple domains of information. The system also established a descriptive approach that was neutral in regard to etiology. The development of *DSM-III* was also the first to include field trials, which involved more than 500 clinicians, to test the utility of the system in clinical practice. The ICD-9 did not incorporate explicit criteria or multiaxial assessment, mainly because its primary use was statistical collection, whereas *DSM-III* had been developed specifically for researchers and clinicians as well as for standard coding purposes. Because of problems in compatibility of medical terminology across the United States, a clinical modification (CM) of ICD-9 for use in the United States (ICD-9-CM) was developed that allowed the specific *DSM-III* terms to be incorporated in the ICD coding system. *DSM-III-R* was developed to correct some factual errors and inconsistencies revealed by the use of *DSM-III;* it was published in 1987.

The Development of *DSM-IV*

Work on the revision of *DSM-III-R* began in 1988 and was prompted by the desire to achieve greater compatibility with the ICD-10, which had begun to be developed at that time. The process of developing the *DSM-IV* was remarkable in that it involved an unprecedented number of individuals and established a systematic methodology for considering changes to the system via a three-step empirical process. In part this reflected the rapidly expanded research base that was available. The process also addressed the concern of the field that arbitrary changes in the system would disrupt research, education, and clinical practice.

Work began with the appointment of a 27-member *DSM-IV* Task Force. Thirteen work groups, each with 5–10 members, were established, and each was responsible for a major section of the manual. Members were chosen for the diversity of their expertise and perspectives. Each work group chair was also a Task Force member to facilitate communication across the work groups. The Task Force and each work group also worked with advisory committees of 50–100 people. Advisors representing a variety of professions and specialties helped outline major issues and contributed research and clinical expertise. Many international advisors were also members of the WHO ICD-10 team. Those developing *DSM-IV* and ICD-10 held several meetings in addition to ongoing communications to reconcile significant differences in the systems.

The three-step empirical process included (1) 150 systematic, comprehensive literature reviews addressing nosological issues of most concern and relevance to the field, (2) reanalysis of existing but previously unanalyzed data sets to provide additional data relevant to *DSM-IV* issues, and (3) field trials assessing the reliability of several suggested criteria sets, including *DSM-III, DSM-III-R*, ICD-10, and *DSM-IV*. Evaluation of this empirical evidence, compatibility with ICD-10, conservativeness to *DSM-III-R,* and clinical utility were all important factors in considering changes to the existing system. Interaction and input from the field were also sought through numerous presentations and publications.

The *DSM-IV* was specifically developed to be compatible not only with the ICD-9-CM, but also with ICD-10 and ICD-10-CM, which the U.S. government plans to implement sometime after 2001. With the implementation of ICD-10-CM, a greater level of correspondence between the United States and other countries will have been achieved. In addition, the ICD-10-CM provides the *DSM-IV* diagnostic name for disorders and greater coding specificity for *DSM-IV* disorders than ICD-9-CM, which contained many antiquated names and required use of the same codes for several *DSM-IV* disorders.

CENTRAL CONCEPTS OF THE *DSM-IV*

Definition of a Mental Disorder

As for many concepts in science and medicine, it is inherently difficult to provide a definition for mental disorder that accurately accounts for all situations. Even the use of the term "mental disorder" has the unfortunate consequence of implying that there is a fundamental difference between mental disorders and "physical" disorders.

Although difficult, it is useful and necessary to provide some guidelines on what is meant by a mental disorder for use in the DSM system. *DSM-IV* notes:

> Each of the mental disorders is conceptualized as a clinically significant behavioral or psychological syndrome or pattern that occurs in an individual and that is associated with present distress (a painful symptom) or disability (impairment in one or more important areas of functioning) or with a significantly increased risk of suffering death, pain, or disability or an important loss of freedom. It is also noted that an expectable or culturally sanctioned response to a particular event (eg, bereavement for loss of a loved one) should not be considered a disorder. Nor should circumstances of deviant behavior or conflict with society be considered mental disorders unless the conflict represents individual dysfunction as detailed above.

Descriptive, Categorical Approach to Diagnosis

DSM-IV disorders are categorized according to a description of symptoms that emerge in a certain pattern or cluster. In most cases, this descriptive system attempts to be neutral in regard to underlying pathology. For example, Major Depressive Disorder is categorized by the presence of depressed mood or loss of interest coupled with symptoms such as insomnia and loss of appetite. There is no implication that all whose symptom pattern meets this description will be alike in regard to etiology. There are some exceptions to this general approach. Mental Disorders Due

to a General Medical Condition (eg, Major Depressive Disorder Due to Hypothyroidism) or Substance-Induced Disorders (eg, Cocaine-Induced Anxiety Disorder) do specify an etiology and are distinguished from the more common primary mental disorders for which no specific etiology has been determined. As more is learned about the underlying causes of mental disorders, the system will undoubtedly move toward a one-to-one correspondence of disorder to cause.

Although the categorical approach is useful in organizing and conveying information, important limits in its use should be recognized. Categorical systems are most useful in situations in which there are distinct boundaries among groups, groups are mutually exclusive, and groups are homogeneous. Unfortunately, these conditions are imperfectly met, given limitations in the current state of knowledge. However, alternative approaches, for example, dimensional systems, have their own limitations. The dimensional approach describes variables distributed on a continuum, as opposed to having the distinct boundaries that are assumed in a categorical system. Dimensional models have received some support in recent research, particularly for the personality disorders, but at present data are not complete enough to justify changing the format of psychiatric diagnosis in clinical use.

Multiple Diagnosis & Differential Diagnosis

DSM-IV allows for multiple diagnoses in most situations in which an individual's symptom presentation meets the criteria for more than one disorder. Although some diagnostic hierarchies exist for situations in which a more pervasive mental disorder encompasses a less pervasive condition (eg, the diagnosis of Dementia, which is characterized by impaired memory, subsumes the diagnosis of Amnestic Disorder), many hierarchies have been eliminated, however, through the revisions of the DSM. There was little empirical evidence to justify the importance of diagnosing certain disorders to the exclusion of others. Allowing multiple diagnoses also improves reliability and retains more information. However, it should not be assumed that an individual whose symptom pattern meets the criteria for more than one diagnosis has multiple independent conditions; it is plausible that co-occurring conditions that have been given separate labels in DSM are actually part of a single complex syndrome. Alternatively, multiple diagnoses may result because some symptoms are part of the conceptualization of more than one diagnostic category.

Reliability & Validity of *DSM-IV* Criteria

The reliability of psychiatric disorders refers to the degree to which different users of the classification concur on a diagnosis across different cases. Reliability is a necessary but not sufficient aspect of validity, a term referring to the extent to which the criterion set identifies a group of individuals that shares important characteristics beyond the criteria themselves (eg, course or outcome, treatment response, biological or psychological parameters, or etiology). The reliability of psychiatric diagnoses has increased with the use of operational criterion sets. Empirical data demonstrating improved reliability have been used to revise items in a criterion set or even the entire conceptualization of a disorder. The development of the *DSM-IV* benefited from the expanded research base available and from the rigorous application of that data base in considering the validity of proposed changes in the system. For example, it was determined that consideration of adding a new diagnostic category to the system would be contingent, in part, on empirical evidence of antecedent validators (eg, precipitating factors, family history), concurrent validators (eg, biological, physiological, and psychological variables), and predictive validators (eg, treatment response).

MAJOR CHARACTERISTICS OF *DSM-IV*

The *DSM-IV* is organized according to the 16 major diagnostic classes (Table 15–1). An additional section is included for conditions that may be a focus of clinical attention but are not considered mental disorders. Except for the Disorders Usually First Diagnosed in Childhood or Adolescence (grouped together based on typical age of onset) and Mental Disorders Due to a General Medical Condition, Substance-Induced Mental Disorders, and Adjustment Disorders (grouped together based on common etiology), classes of disorders are grouped according to common presenting symptoms to facilitate differential diagnosis.

Diagnostic Criteria

Each disorder within the *DSM-IV* is described by a criterion set. Most criterion sets are a mixture of

Table 15–1. Sixteen major diagnostic classes.

Disorders Usually First Diagnosed in Infancy, Childhood, or Adolescence
Delirium, Dementia, and Amnestic and Other Cognitive Disorders
Mental Disorders Due to a General Medical Condition Not Elsewhere Classified
Substance-Related Disorders
Schizophrenia and Other Psychotic Disorders
Mood Disorders
Anxiety Disorders
Somatoform Disorders
Factitious Disorders
Dissociative Disorders
Sexual and Gender Identity Disorders
Eating Disorders
Sleep Disorders
Impulse-Control Disorders Not Elsewhere Classified
Adjustment Disorders
Personality Disorders

polythetic (ie, a certain proportion of symptoms from a set needs to be present for the criterion to be met) and monothetic (ie, all conditions of the particular criterion must be met) criteria. Although polythetic approaches may allow for more heterogeneity in the diagnosis than is desirable (eg, two individuals diagnosed with the same disorder may not share a single symptom), they are useful because for most disorders, there are symptoms that are often but not invariably present, and these symptoms would be excluded by a purely monothetic criterion set.

Criterion sets are provided as clinical guidelines and because it has been shown that use of such criterion sets enhances agreement among clinicians and researchers. However, clinical judgment plays a critical part in the application of the criteria to the evaluation of any individual.

Descriptive Text

Detailed text is included for each diagnosis. Information is presented in nine sections. The *Diagnostic Features* section includes illustrative examples of criteria and definitions of terms used in the criterion set. *Subtypes and/or Specifiers* provides definitions concerning applicable subtypes or specifiers. *Recording Procedures* provides guidelines for reporting the name of the disorder and for selecting the appropriate code. *Associated Features and Disorders* describes symptoms that often are related to the disorder but are not essential to the diagnosis. Other mental disorders that have been found to be commonly comorbid with the disorder are also listed. Laboratory findings, physical examination findings, and general medical conditions that may be associated with the disorder are also included in this section.

The *Specific Age, Culture or Gender Features* section includes information on particular symptom presentations that may occur across the life span, between the different sexes, or among different cultural groups. *Prevalence* notes data on point and lifetime prevalence when known (eg, data from national epidemiological studies are included). *Course* describes the typical age of onset, duration of the disturbance, and progression (ie, if the disorder usually worsens or improves with age). Also noted is whether the disorder is characterized by a single episode, recurrent episodes, or an unremitting course.

The *Familial Pattern* section notes whether the disorder is more frequent among first-degree biological relatives than among the general population. Guidelines on how to distinguish the disorder from others with similar symptoms are described in the *Differential Diagnosis* section.

Multiaxial Assessment

DSM-IV retains the multiaxial system first incorporated in *DSM-III* (Table 15–2). The purpose of the system is to facilitate comprehensive evaluation by requiring that five categories of information, or

Table 15–2. Summary of the five *DSM-IV* axes.

Diagnostic axes

Axis I	Clinical Disorders	
	Other Conditions That May Be a Focus of Clinical Attention	
Axis II	Personality Disorders and Mental Retardation	
Axis III	General Medical Conditions	

Other domains for assessment

Axis IV	Psychosocial and Environmental Problems
Axis V	Global Assessment of Functioning

"axes," be collected for each individual being assessed.

Axes I, II, and III are diagnostic axes. Axis I is used to note the presence of all mental disorders in *DSM-IV* except for the Personality Disorders and Mental Retardation, which are noted on Axis II. Axis I can also be used to record "Other Conditions That May Be a Focus of Clinical Attention" (eg, bereavement, relational problems, problems related to abuse or neglect). Axis II can also be used to report maladaptive personality features or defense mechanisms. General medical conditions are recorded on Axis III. The term "general medical condition" refers to conditions and disorders that are listed outside of the Mental Disorders section of the *International Classification of Disease*. Ideally, more specific terminology should be used to identify a class of disorders (eg, neurological conditions) or a specific disorder (eg, multiple sclerosis). Although a separate axis is provided to note these conditions, there should be no inference that there are fundamental or conceptual differences among the three axes; rather, the purpose of delineating Axis III is to encourage a comprehensive clinical assessment and to highlight the possible interaction between a general medical condition and the diagnosis or treatment of a mental disorder.

General medical conditions noted on Axis III can be related to Axis I disorders in one of the following ways. (1) The clinician has ascertained that a psychiatric disorder is caused by the pathophysiological consequences of a general medical condition. In these situations, a Mental Disorder Due to a General Medical Condition is noted on Axis I, and the general medical condition is noted on both Axis I and Axis III (eg, an anxiety disturbance caused by the effects of hyperthyroidism would be noted as Anxiety Disorder Due to Hyperthyroidism on Axis I, and hyperthyroidism would be noted on Axis III). (2) The clinician judges that a general medical condition is affecting the course, severity, or treatment of a mental disorder (but is not etiologically related to the mental disorder). In these situations, the general medical condition is coded solely on Axis III, and the mental disorder is noted on Axis I or II (eg, an individual with liver disorder may have difficulty metabolizing certain medications used to treat the mental disorder). (3) The clinician feels that there is no specific relationship between an existing mental disorder and a general medical condition but chooses to note the general medical condition on Axis III to ensure a comprehensive record.

Axis IV is available to note psychosocial or environmental problems that may affect the diagnosis or care of an individual. These may include problems at work, homelessness, poverty, and problems related to access to health care (Table 15–3). In some situations, the psychosocial or environmental condition is the primary focus of clinical attention and should therefore be recorded on Axis I.

The clinician's assessment of the individual's level of occupational, social, and psychosocial functioning is recorded on Axis V, using the Global Assessment of Functioning (GAF) Scale (Table 15–4). This information is helpful in planning a treatment regimen and in predicting likely treatment outcome. Ratings on the GAF scale are usually for the current period (ie, at the time of evaluation) and assist the clinician in monitoring the individual's progress in global terms. Three additional scales—the Social and Occupational Functioning Assessment Scale (SOFAS), Global Assessment of Relational Functioning (GARF), and the Axis for Defensive Mechanisms—have been added to an appendix of the *DSM-IV* as additional references.

Appendices to *DSM-IV*

DSM-IV includes 10 appendices. *Diagnostic Decision Trees* provide a diagnostic algorithm organized by presenting symptom that is useful in differential diagnosis. The *Criteria Sets and Axes Provided for Further Study* appendix contains proposed criterion sets for use in research settings. The *DSM-IV* Task Force determined that there was insufficient empirical evidence to include these conditions as official diagnostic categories but hoped that inclusion of proposed criterion sets would facilitate further research.

An additional appendix, *Outline for Cultural Formulation and Glossary of Culture-Bound Syndromes*, contains glossary definitions of culture-bound syndromes and an outline for assessing the potential impact of an individual's cultural context on psychiatric evaluation. Culture-bound syndromes are most commonly found in, or are unique to, particular societies or cultural areas (eg, *amok*, an outburst of aggressive or homicidal behavior followed by exhaustion and

Table 15–3. Axis IV, Psychosocial and Environmental Problems.

Problems with primary support group (childhood, adult, parent-child)
Problems related to the social environment
Educational problems
Occupational problems
Housing problems
Economic problems
Problems with access to health care services
Problems related to interaction with the legal system/crime
Other psychosocial problems

Table 15–4. Axis V, Global Assessment of Functioning (GAF) Scale.[a]

Code	Assessment
100 | 91	Superior functioning in a wide range of activities, life's problems never seem to get out of hand, is sought out by others because of his or her many positive qualities; no symptoms
90 | 81	Absent or minimal symptoms (eg, mild anxiety before an exam), good functioning in all areas, interested and involved in a wide range of activities, socially effective, generally satisfied with life, no more than everyday problems or concerns (eg, an occasional argument with family members)
80 | 71	If symptoms are present, they are transient and expectable reactions to psychosocial stressors (eg, difficulty concentrating after family argument); no more than slight impairment in social, occupational, or school functioning (eg, temporarily falling behind in schoolwork)
70 | 61	Some mild symptoms (eg, depressed mood and mild insomnia) *or* some difficulty in social, occupational, or school functioning (eg, occasional truancy, or theft within the household), but generally functioning pretty well, has some meaningful interpersonal relationships
60 | 51	Moderate symptoms (eg, flat affect and circumstantial speech, occasional panic attacks) *or* moderate difficulty in social, occupational, or school functioning (eg, few friends, conflicts with peers or co-workers)
50 | 41	Serious symptoms (eg, suicidal ideation, severe obsessional rituals, frequent shoplifting) *or* any serious impairment in social, occupational, or school functioning (eg, no friends, unable to keep a job)
40 | 31	Some impairment in reality testing or communication (eg, speech is at times illogical, obscure, or irrelevant) *or* major impairment in several areas, such as work or school, family relations, judgment, thinking, or mood (eg, depressed man avoids friends, neglects family, and is unable to work; child frequently beats up younger children, is defiant at home, and is failing at school)
30 | 21	Behavior is considerably influenced by delusions or hallucinations *or* serious impairment in communication or judgment (eg, sometimes incoherent, acts grossly inappropriately, suicidal preoccupation) *or* inability to function in almost all areas (eg, stays in bed all day; no job, home, or friends)
20 | 11	Some danger of hurting self or others (eg, suicide attempts without clear expectation of death; frequently violent; manic excitement) *or* occasionally fails to maintain minimal personal hygiene (eg, smears feces) *or* gross impairment in communication (eg, largely incoherent or mute)
10 | 1	Persistent danger of severely hurting self or others (eg, recurrent violence) *or* persistent inability to maintain minimal personal hygiene *or* serious suicidal act with clear expectation of death
0	Inadequate information

[a] Consider psychological, social, and occupational functioning on a hypothetical continuum of mental health–illness. Do not include impairment in functioning due to physical (or environmental) limitations. (*Note:* Use intermediate codes when appropriate, eg, 45, 68, 72.)

amnesia for the episode, most commonly seen in southeastern Asian countries).

Other appendices include ICD-9-CM and ICD-10 coding aids, numerical and alphabetical lists of the disorders, a glossary of technical terms, and an annotated listing, by disorder, of differences from the *DSM-III-R* to the *DSM-IV.*

USE OF THE DSM-IV

Coding & Reporting

Numerical codes for each disorder or condition listed in the manual are provided and are derived from the *International Classification of Disease,* 9th revision, Clinical Modification (ICD-9-CM). Use of these codes facilitates medical record keeping and statistical comparison both in the United States and

internationally. Although the ICD-10 has been released in the United States and elsewhere, use of the ICD-9-CM codes has been retained in the United States at least until the year 2001. An appendix to the *DSM-IV* provides a listing of *DSM-IV* Classification using ICD-10 codes for future reference.

However, similar to what had been done for ICD-9-CM, a "clinical modification" to the ICD-10 (ie, ICD-10-CM) has been developed for use in the United States to allow for greater coding specificity. Within the next few years, this new coding classification system will replace the antiquated ICD-9-CM with an alpha-numeric coding structure (ie, F32.0 Major Depressive Disorder, Single Episode, Mild replaces 296.21) that will allow for greater coding specificity reflecting current knowledge and more flexibility for coding in the future as medical knowledge increases.

Indicating Severity

Specific definitions of severity are provided for some disorders (eg, Major Depressive Disorder, Bipolar Disorder, Conduct Disorder). For the other disorders in which specific definitions of severity are not provided, generic definitions of "mild," "moderate," and "severe" can be utilized. "Mild" indicates that there are few symptoms in excess of what is necessary to make the diagnosis and that impairment in social, occupational, or important areas of functioning is not more than mild. "Severe" indicates that many symptoms in excess of those needed to make the diagnosis are present and that symptoms are so severe that functioning is greatly impaired. "Moderate" is used for cases with severity between mild and severe.

Course Modifiers

Course modifiers are provided to note circumstances in which full criteria for a disorder were met in the past but are not currently met: "In partial remission" may be indicated when the symptoms no longer meet full criteria for the disorder but some symptoms are still present. "In full remission" is used when symptoms are no longer present but the clinician judges that it is clinically relevant to note the history of the diagnosis. "Prior history" may also be used to indicate that an individual's symptoms at one time met the criteria for a disorder but the individual considered completely recovered. The distinction between "in full remission" and "prior history (recovered)" involves a number of issues, for example, length of time since the symptoms were present and the duration of disturbance. Some groups of disorders have specific sets of course modifiers (eg, Substance Dependence, Major Depressive Disorder).

Ways of Indicating Diagnostic Uncertainty

DSM-IV includes a number of conventions useful in indicating diagnostic uncertainty. A clinician can defer a more precise diagnosis until more information can be gathered while at the same time indicating what is known. Terms useful in this regard are detailed in Table 15–5.

Caveats in the Use of *DSM-IV*

The introduction to the *DSM-IV* notes several caveats in the use of the system, including the limitations of the categorical approach and need for clinical judgment as previously detailed. It is essential to note these limitations, as DSM is often used outside of the clinical and research venues. For example, although the DSM may be of value in forensic settings (eg, by facilitating understanding of the typical characteristics of a particular disorder), several cautions should underscore its use. Rarely does clinical diagnosis in itself answer questions of primary concern to the law, such as competence, criminal responsibility, or disability. Individual case assessment beyond the DSM diagnosis is critical in all forensic situations. Impairments and disabilities vary across and within the diagnostic categories, and the existence of a mental disorder does not necessarily imply that an individual has impaired control over his or her actions. Further, although the DSM reflects the consensus of the field when it is published, new information is constantly generated and may be pertinent as well.

Special care must also be urged when a clinician is unfamiliar with the cultural referents of the individual being evaluated. A clinician unaware of the individual's culture may mistake thoughts or actions that are an accepted and typical part of that person's milieu (eg, seeing a deceased relative during grieving)

Table 15–5. Terms useful for indicating diagnostic uncertainty.

Term	Examples of clinical situations
V Codes (for other conditions that may be a focus of clinical attention)	Insufficient information to know whether or not a presenting problem is attributable to a mental disorder, eg, academic problem; adult antisocial behavior
799.9 Diagnosis or condition deferred on Axis I	Information inadequate to make any diagnostic judgment about an Axis I diagnosis or condition
799.9 Diagnosis deferred on Axis II	Information inadequate to make any diagnostic judgment about an Axis II diagnosis
300.90 Unspecified mental disorder (nonpsychotic)	Enough information available to rule out a psychotic disorder, but further specification is not possible
298.90 Psychotic disorder not otherwise specified	Enough information available to determine the presence of a psychotic disorder, but further specification is not possible
[Class of disorder] not otherwise specified	Enough information available to indicate the class of disorder that is present, but further specification is not possible, because either there is not sufficient information to make a more specific diagnosis or the clinical features of the disorder do not meet the criteria for any of the specific categories in that class, eg, depressive disorder not otherwise specified
Specific diagnosis (provisional)	Enough information available to make a "working" diagnosis, but the clinician wishes to indicate a significant degree of diagnostic uncertainty, eg, schizophreniform disorder (provisional)

as symptoms of a mental disorder. Evaluation of personality syndromes and disorders may be particularly difficult as the concept of self varies tremendously across cultural reference groups. Several innovations in the *DSM-IV* have been added to assist clinicians in these situations. As previously described, a text section for each disorder describes variations in symptom presentations that may be expected across cultural groups. Additionally, an outline guideline for cultural formulation and list of culture-bound syndromes have also been added.

It is also noted that the use of *DSM-IV* in determining an appropriate diagnosis is just one step in the proper treatment of the individual. Additional information beyond that needed to make a diagnosis is necessary for the formulation of an appropriate treatment plan.

Future Directions

The descriptive text in the *DSM-IV* (eg, Associated Features, Prevalence, Course, Differential Diagnosis) has undergone revision to maintain its accuracy and currency. The revision process includes comprehensive systematic literature reviews to identify the evidence base, development of evidence-based rationales for each update, and multidisciplinary peer review of the proposed revisions. The text revision will be published in the year 2000.

In addition, there are a number of nosological questions that continue to be the focus of discussion within the psychiatric community. It is hoped that the ongoing dialogue about these issues will inform the *DSM-V* process and stimulate further research. Among the issues that will need to be addressed are the following:

Strategies for subthreshold disorders— Certain subthreshold conditions have been proposed to constitute psychiatric disorders and were added to the *DSM-IV* Appendix (Mixed Anxiety/Depression, Minor Depression, Brief Recurrent Depressive Disorder, Mild Neurocognitive Disorder). From the standpoint of financial coverage for treatment, it might be desirable to include these and certain other subthreshold conditions as psychiatric disorders, particularly in primary care settings, but do they have adequate reliability and validity? Furthermore, the conceptual basis and specific criteria have not yet been well established for how boundaries should be drawn between normality, subthreshold conditions, and "threshold" conditions. Should subthreshold conditions be added if there are no clear treatment implications?

The role of laboratory tests in psychiatric diagnosis—Although laboratory tests are mentioned as an associated feature in the text for certain *DSM-IV* disorders, they are not part of the criteria sets (except for mental retardation and learning disorders). The question of whether such tests should be added to criteria sets was debated during the *DSM-IV* process and it is likely to be raised during the *DSM-V* process

for other disorders as well (eg, Alzheimer's). Such laboratory testing is already included in many neurological and general medical diagnoses.

Personality disorders—The classification of personality disorders remains controversial. The issue of whether personality disorders should be classified using a dimensional approach rather than a categorical system was debated for *DSM-IV* and was discussed in the *DSM-IV* Options Book. A dimensional approach has some practical and conceptual advantages but may be difficult to apply in clinical settings. The current categorical system has also been criticized as not being adequately useful to clinicians. Another controversial issue involves the Axis I/Axis II dichotomy. Although many felt that putting the personality disorders on a separate axis in *DSM-III* ensured specific attention to long-standing characterological issues, questions have arisen regarding the wisdom of maintaining them on a separate axis.

Rethinking the multiaxial system—Although *DSM*'s multiaxial system is widely considered useful because it allows evaluation of patients across several different domains, this system is thought to have some limitations. Alternatives were considered for *DSM-IV*, such as not having separate axes for Personality Disorders and medical conditions, making Axes IV and V optional, and adding ratings of defense and coping styles. Is the current system optimal? How many axes and which axes should be included? Should new axes, such as a family history axis, be added? Are there domains of information that would be most useful in the future for the individual clinician and the health care system?

Beyond diagnosis, the assessment of psychiatric patients faces a number of challenges presented by health care reform and managed care and the needs of patient care. New methods for measuring and reviewing psychiatric care that may not reflect good research or the perspective of clinicians are rapidly being developed by public and private entities. Mental health providers and their patients are being held to "criteria" for the determination of access to services or evaluation for inclusion in care networks. A wide range of clinical and policy issues is affected by the selection and application of psychiatric measures: eligibility determinations, outcomes assessment, pricing, risk adjustment, disability assessment, as well as quality assurance/utilization-related activities.

The American Psychiatric Association has developed the *Handbook of Psychiatric Measures,* which is envisioned as a "toolbox with instructions" that evaluates for clinicians and health administrators available psychiatric measures. Measures in a range of domains of assessment including symptoms, functioning, and outcomes are evaluated for their components, reliability, validity, strengths, and weaknesses.

The *Handbook of Psychiatric Measures* consists of three main sections. The first provides a general discussion of the selection, application, and uses of measures in clinical settings, and in health care evaluation, and discusses the various properties of measures and how their clinical utility is evaluated. Psychiatric measures that are non-disorder specific (ie, diagnostic interviews, measures of severity and functioning, patient satisfaction) comprise the second section, and measures specific to psychiatric disorders (eg, mood disorders, schizophrenia) are presented in the third section.

The main purpose of the *Handbook of Psychiatric Measures* is to provide clinicians working in mental health or primary care settings with a compendium of the available rating scales and tests that may be useful in the clinical care of their patients or to assist them in interpreting treatment and services research studies. The manual is also designed to provide guid-ance to clinicians, policy makers, and planners on how to select, use, and interpret clinical measures.

The development of the *DSM-IV* has been based on a careful three-step process of collecting, examining, and contributing to the creation of the most recent research available via literature review, data re-analysis, and field trials. Future revisions of the system will benefit from the ever-evolving data base of psychiatric research and will no doubt result in the classification becoming more reliable, useful, and based on a more profound understanding of etiology and pathogenesis of mental disorders.

Efforts are underway to expand the scientific base in psychiatry so there are more data responsive to issues in the development of *DSM-V* after the turn of the century.

REFERENCES & SUGGESTED READINGS

American Psychiatric Association: *Diagnostic and Statistical Manual of Mental Disorders.* American Psychiatric Association, 1952.

American Psychiatric Association: *Diagnostic and Statistical Manual of Mental Disorders,* 2nd ed. American Psychiatric Association, 1968.

American Psychiatric Association: *Diagnostic and Statistical Manual of Mental Disorders,* 3rd ed. American Psychiatric Association, 1979.

American Psychiatric Association: *Diagnostic and Statistical Manual of Mental Disorders,* 3rd ed, revised. American Psychiatric Association, 1987.

American Psychiatric Association: *Diagnostic and Statistical Manual of Mental Disorders,* 4th ed. American Psychiatric Association, 1994.

American Psychiatric Association: *Handbook of Psychiatric Measures.* American Psychiatric Association (in press).

Frances A et al: DSM-IV work in progress. Am J Psychiatry 1990;147:1439.

Frances A, Widiger TA, Pincus HA: The development of DSM-IV. Arch Gen Psychiatry 1989;46:373.

Pincus HA et al: DSM-IV and new diagnostic categories: Holding the line on proliferation. Am J Psychiatry 1992;149:112.

APPENDIX: *DSM-IV* CLASSIFICATION

NOS = Not Otherwise Specified.

An *x* appearing in a diagnostic code indicates that a specific code number is required.

An ellipsis (. . .) is used in the names of certain disorders to indicate that the name of a specific mental disorder or general medical condition should be inserted when recording the name (eg, 293.0 Delirium Due to Hypothyroidism).

Numbers in parentheses are page numbers.

The current severity of a disorder may be specified after the diagnosis as

Mild	currently meets
Moderate	diagnostic
Severe	criteria

In Partial Remission
In Full Remission
Prior History

DISORDERS USUALLY FIRST DIAGNOSED IN INFANCY, CHILDHOOD, OR ADOLESCENCE

Mental Retardation
Note: These are coded on Axis II.
317	Mild mental retardation
318.0	Moderate mental retardation
318.1	Severe mental retardation
318.2	Profound mental retardation
319	Mental retardation, severity unspecified

Learning Disorders
315.00	Reading disorder
315.1	Mathematics disorder
315.2	Disorder of written expression
315.9	Learning disorder NOS

Motor Skills Disorder
315.4	Developmental coordination disorder

Communication Disorders
315.31	Expressive language disorder
315.32	Mixed receptive-expressive language disorder
315.39	Phonological disorder
307.0	Stuttering
307.9	Communication disorder NOS

Pervasive Developmental Disorders
299.00	Autistic disorder
299.80	Rett's disorder
299.10	Childhood disintegrative disorder
299.80	Asperger's disorder
299.80	Pervasive developmental disorder NOS

Attention-Deficit and Disruptive Behavior Disorders
314.xx	Attention-deficit/hyperactivity disorder
.01	Combined type
.00	Predominantly inattentive type
.01	Predominantly hyperactive-impulse type
314.9	Attention-deficit/hyperactivity disorder NOS
312.xx	Conduct disorder
.81	Childhood-onset type
.82	Adolescent-onset type
.89	Unspecified type
313.81	Oppositional defiant disorder
312.9	Disruptive behavior disorder NOS

Feeding and Eating Disorders of Infancy or Early Childhood
307.52	Pica
307.53	Rumination disorder
307.59	Feeding disorder of infancy or early childhood

Tic Disorders
307.23	Tourette's disorder
307.22	Chronic motor or vocal tic disorder
307.21	Transient tic disorder
	Specify if: Single episode/recurrent
307.20	Tic disorder NOS

Elimination Disorders
—.—	Encopresis
787.6	With constipation and overflow incontinence
307.7	Without constipation and overflow incontinence
307.6	Enuresis (not due to a general medical condition)
	Specify type: Nocturnal only/diurnal only/nocturnal and diurnal

Other Disorders of Infancy, Childhood, or Adolescence
309.21	Separation anxiety disorder
	Specify if: Early onset
313.23	Selective mutism

313.89   Reactive attachment disorder of infancy or early childhood
      Specify type: Inhibited type/disinhibited type

307.3   Stereotypic movement disorder
      Specify if: With self-injurious behavior

313.9   Disorder of infancy, childhood, or adolescence NOS

DELIRIUM, DEMENTIA, AND AMNESTIC AND OTHER COGNITIVE DISORDERS

Delirium

293.0   Delirium due to . . . *[Indicate the general medical condition]*

——.—   Substance intoxication delirium (*refer to substance-related disorders for substance-specific codes*)

——.—   Substance withdrawal delirium (*refer to substance-related disorders for substance-specific codes*)

——.—   Delirium due to multiple etiologies (*code each of the specific etiologies*)

780.09   Delirium NOS

Dementia

294.xx   Dementia of the Alzheimer's type, with early onset (*also code 331.0 Alzheimer's disease on Axis III*)
   .10   Without behavioral disturbance
   .11   With behavioral distrubance

294.xx   Dementia of the Alzheimer's type, with late onset (*also code 331.0 Alzheimer's disease on Axis III*)
   .10   Without behavioral disturbance
   .11   With behavioral disturbance

290.xx   Vascular dementia
   .40   Uncomplicated
   .41   With delirium
   .42   With delusions
   .43   With depressed mood
      Specify if: With behavioral disturbance

Code presence or absence of behavioral disturbance in the fifth digit for dementia due to a GMC.

294.1x   Dementia due to HIV disease (*also code 042 HIV on Axis III*)

294.1x   Dementia due to head trauma (*also code 854.00 head injury on Axis III*)

294.1x   Dementia due to Parkinson's disease (*also code 332.0 Parkinson's disease on Axis III*)

294.1x   Dementia due to Huntington's disease (*also code 333.4 Huntington's disease on Axis III*)

294.1x   Dementia due to Pick's disease (*also code 331.1 Pick's disease on Axis III*)

294.1x   Dementia due to Creutzfeldt-Jakob disease (*also code 046.1 Creutzfeldt-Jakob disease on Axis III*)

294.1   Dementia due to . . . *[indicate the general medical condition not listed above] (also code the general medical condition on Axis III)*

——.—   Substance-induced persisting dementia (*refer to substance-related disorders for substance-specific codes*)

——.—   Dementia due to multiple etiologies (*code each of the specific etiologies*)

294.8   Dementia NOS

Amnestic Disorders

294.0   Amnestic disorder due to . . . *[Indicate the general medical condition]*
      Specify if: Transient/chronic

——.—   Substance-induced persisting amnestic disorder (*refer to substance-related disorders for substance-specific codes*)

294.8   Amnestic disorder NOS

Other Cognitive Disorders

294.9   Cognitive disorder NOS

MENTAL DISORDERS DUE TO A GENERAL MEDICAL CONDITION NOT ELSEWHERE CLASSIFIED

293.89   Catatonic disorder due to . . . *[Indicate the general medical condition]*

310.1   Personality change due to . . . *[Indicate the general medical condition]*
      Specify type: labile type/disinhibited type/aggressive type/apathetic type/paranoid type/other type/combined type/unspecified type

293.9   Mental disorder NOS due to . . . *[Indicate the general medical condition]*

SUBSTANCE-RELATED DISORDERS

a *The following specifiers may be applied to substance dependence:*
   With physiological dependence/without physiological dependence
   Early full remission/early partial remission
   Sustained full remission/sustained partial remission
   Remission on agonist therapy/in a controlled environment

The following specifiers apply to substance-induced disorders as noted:
[I] With onset during intoxication
[W]With onset during withdrawal

Alcohol-Related Disorders
Alcohol Use Disorders
303.90   Alcohol dependence[a]
305.00   Alcohol abuse

Alcohol-Induced Disorders
303.00   Alcohol intoxication
291.81   Alcohol withdrawal
    Specify if: With perceptual disturbances
291.0   Alcohol intoxication delirium
291.0   Alcohol withdrawal delirium
291.2   Alcohol-induced persisting dementia
291.1   Alcohol-induced persisting amnestic disorder
291.x   Alcohol-induced psychotic disorder
  .5   With delusions[I,W]
  .3   With hallucinations[I,W]
291.89   Alcohol-induced mood disorder[I,W]
291.89   Alcohol-induced anxiety disorder[I,W]
291.89   Alcohol-induced sexual dysfunction[I]
291.89   Alcohol-induced sleep disorder[I,W]
291.9   Alcohol-related disorder NOS

Amphetamine (or Amphetamine-Like)-Related Disorders
Amphetamine Use Disorders
304.40   Amphetamine dependence[a]
305.70   Amphetamine abuse

Amphetamine-Induced Disorders
292.89   Amphetamine intoxication
    Specify if: With perceptual disturbances
292.0   Amphetamine withdrawal
292.81   Amphetamine intoxication delirium
292.xx   Amphetamine-induced psychotic disorder
  .11   With delusions[I]
  .12   With hallucinations[I]
292.84   Amphetamine-induced mood disorder[I,W]
292.89   Amphetamine-induced anxiety disorder[I]
292.89   Amphetamine-induced sexual dysfunction[I]
292.89   Amphetamine-induced sleep disorder[I,W]
292.9   Amphetamine-related disorder NOS

Caffeine-Related Disorders
Caffeine-Induced Disorders
305.90   Caffeine intoxication
292.89   Caffeine-induced anxiety disorder[I]
292.89   Caffeine-induced sleep disorder[I]
292.9   Caffeine-related disorder NOS

Cannabis-Related Disorders
Cannabis Use Disorders
304.30   Cannabis dependence[a]
305.20   Cannabis abuse

Cannabis-Induced Disorders
292.89   Cannabis intoxication
    Specify if: With perceptual disturbances
292.81   Cannabis intoxication delirium
292.xx   Cannabis-induced psychotic disorder
  .11   With delusions[I]
  .12   With hallucinations[I]
292.89   Cannabis-induced anxiety disorder[I]
292.9   Cannabis-related disorder NOS

Cocaine-Related Disorders
Cocaine Use Disorders
304.20   Cocaine dependence[a]
305.60   Cocaine abuse

Cocaine-Induced Disorders
292.89   Cocaine intoxication
    Specify if: With perceptual disturbances
292.0   Cocaine withdrawal
292.81   Cocaine intoxication delirium
292.xx   Cocaine-induced psychotic disorder
  .11   With delusions[I]
  .12   With hallucinations[I]
292.84   Cocaine-induced mood disorder[I,W]
292.89   Cocaine-induced anxiety disorder[I,W]
292.89   Cocaine-induced sexual dysfunction[I]
292.89   Cocaine-induced sleep disorder[I,W]
292.9   Cocaine-related disorder NOS

Hallucinogen-Related Disorders
Hallucinogen Use Disorders
304.50   Hallucinogen dependence[a]
305.30   Hallucinogen abuse

Hallucinogen-Induced Disorders
292.89   Hallucinogen intoxication
292.89   Hallucinogen persisting perception disorder (flashbacks)
292.81   Hallucinogen intoxication delirium
292.xx   Hallucinogen-induced psychotic disorder
  .11   With delusions[I]
  .12   With hallucinations[I]

292.84	Hallucinogen-induced mood disorder[I]
292.89	Hallucinogen-induced anxiety disorder[I]
292.9	Hallucinogen-related disorder NOS

Inhalant-Related Disorders
Inhalant Use Disorders

304.60	Inhalant dependence[a]
305.90	Inhalant abuse

Inhalant-Induced Disorders

292.89	Inhalant intoxication
292.81	Inhalant intoxication delirium
292.82	Inhalant-induced persisting dementia
292.xx	Inhalant-induced psychotic disorder
.11	With delusions[I]
.12	With hallucinations[I]
292.84	Inhalant-induced mood disorder[I]
292.89	Inhalant-induced anxiety disorder[I]
292.9	Inhalant-related disorder NOS

Nicotine-Related Disorders
Nicotine Use Disorder

305.10	Nicotine dependence[a]

Nicotine-Induced Disorders

292.0	Nicotine withdrawal
292.9	Nicotine-related disorder NOS

Opioid-Related Disorders
Opioid Use Disorders

304.00	Opioid dependence[a]
305.50	Opioid abuse

Opioid-Induced Disorders

292.89	Opioid intoxication
	Specify if: With perceptual disturbances
292.0	Opioid withdrawal
292.81	Opioid intoxication delirium
292.xx	Opioid-induced psychotic disorder
.11	With delusions[I]
.12	With hallucinations[I]
292.84	Opioid-induced mood disorder[I]
292.89	Opioid-induced sexual dysfunction[I]
292.89	Opioid-induced sleep disorder[I,W]
292.9	Opioid-related disorder NOS

Phencyclidine (or Phencyclidine-Like)-Related Disorders
Phencyclidine Use Disorders

304.90	Phencyclidine dependence[a]
305.90	Phencyclidine abuse

Phencyclidine-Induced Disorders

292.89	Phencyclidine intoxication
	Specify if: With perceptual disturbances
292.81	Phencyclidine intoxication delirium
292.xx	Phencyclidine-induced psychotic disorder
.11	With delusions[I]
.12	With hallucinations[I]
292.84	Phencyclidine-induced mood disorder[I]
292.89	Phencyclidine-induced anxiety disorder[I]
292.9	Phencyclidine-related disorder NOS

Sedative-, Hypnotic-, or Anxiolytic-Related Disorders
Sedative, Hypnotic, or Anxiolytic Use Disorders

304.10	Sedative, hypnotic, or anxiolytic dependence[a]
305.40	Sedative, hypnotic, or anxiolytic abuse

Sedative-, Hypnotic-, or Anxiolytic-Induced Disorders

292.89	Sedative, hypnotic, or anxiolytic intoxication
292.0	Sedative, hypnotic, or anxiolytic withdrawal
	Specify if: With perceptual disturbances
292.81	Sedative, hypnotic, or anxiolytic intoxication delirium
292.81	Sedative, hypnotic, or anxiolytic withdrawal delirium
292.82	Sedative-, hypnotic-, or anxiolytic-induced persisting dementia
292.83	Sedative-, hypnotic-, or anxiolytic-induced persisting amnestic disorder
292.xx	Sedative-, hypnotic-, or anxiolytic-induced psychotic disorder
.11	With delusions[I,W]
.12	With hallucinations[I,W]
292.84	Sedative-, hypnotic-, or anxiolytic-induced mood disorder[I,W]
292.89	Sedative-, hypnotic-, or anxiolytic-induced anxiety disorder[W]
292.89	Sedative-, hypnotic-, or anxiolytic-induced sexual dysfunction[I]
292.89	Sedative-, hypnotic-, or anxiolytic-induced sleep disorder[I,W]
292.9	Sedative-, hypnotic-, or anxiolytic-related disorder NOS

Polysubstance-Related Disorder

304.80	*Polysubstance dependence[a]*

Other (or Unknown) Substance-Related Disorders

Other (or Unknown) Substance Use Disorders

304.90 Other (or unknown) substance dependence[a]

305.90 Other (or unknown) substance abuse

Other (or Unknown) Substance-Induced Disorders

292.89 Other (or unknown) substance intoxication
   Specify if: With perceptual disturbances

292.0 Other (or unknown) substance withdrawal
   Specify if: With perceptual disturbances

292.81 Other (or unknown) substance-induced delirium

292.82 Other (or unknown) substance-induced persisting dementia

292.83 Other (or unknown) substance-induced persisting amnestic disorder

292.xx Other (or unknown) substance-induced psychotic disorder
  .11 With delusions[l,W]
  .12 With hallucinations[l,W]

292.84 Other (or unknown) substance-induced mood disorder[l,W]

292.89 Other (or unknown) substance-induced anxiety disorder[l,W]

292.89 Other (or unknown) substance-induced sexual dysfunction[l]

292.89 Other (or unknown) substance-induced sleep disorder[l,W]

292.9 Other (or unknown) substance-related disorder NOS

SCHIZOPHRENIA AND OTHER PSYCHOTIC DISORDERS

295.xx Schizophrenia

The following classification of longitudinal course applies to all subtypes of schizophrenia:

Episodic with interepisode residual symptoms (*specify if:* With prominent negative symptoms) episodic with no interepisode residual symptoms/continuous (*specify if:* With prominent negative symptoms)

Single episode in partial remission (*specify if:* With prominent negative symptoms)/single episode in full remission

Other or unspecified pattern

  .30 Paranoid type
  .10 Disorganized type

  .20 Catatonic type
  .90 Undifferentiated type
  .60 Residual type

295.40 Schizophreniform disorder
   Specify if: Without good prognostic features/with good prognostic features

295.70 Schizoaffective disorder
   Specify type: Bipolar type/depressive type

297.1 Delusional disorder
   Specify type: Erotomanic type/grandiose type/jealous type/persecutory type/somatic type/mixed type/unspecified type

298.8 Brief psychotic disorder
   Specify if: With marked stressor(s)/without marked stressor(s)/with postpartum onset

297.3 Shared psychotic disorder

293.xx Psychotic disorder due to . . . *[indicate the general medical condition]*
  .81 With delusions
  .82 With hallucinations

——.— Substance-induced psychotic disorder (*refer to substance-related disorders for substance-specific codes*)
   Specify if: With onset during intoxication/with onset during withdrawal

298.9 Psychotic disorder NOS

MOOD DISORDERS

Code current state of major depressive disorder or bipolar I disorder in fifth digit:

 1 = Mild
 2 = Moderate
 3 = Severe without psychotic features
 4 = Severe with psychotic features
   Specify: Mood-congruent psychotic features/mood-incongruent psychotic features
 5 = In partial remission
 6 = In full remission
 0 = Unspecified

The following specifiers apply (for current or most recent episode) to mood disorders as noted:
 [a]Severity/psychotic/remission specifiers/[b]chronic/[c]with catatonic features/[d]with melancholic features/[e]with atypical features/[f]with postpartum onset
The following specifiers apply to mood disorders as noted:
 [g]With or without full interepisode recovery/[h]with seasonal pattern/[i]with rapid cycling

Depressive Disorders

296.xx   Major depressive disorder
.2x   Single episode[a,b,c,d,e,f]
.3x   Recurrent[a,b,c,d,e,f,g,h]
300.4   Dysthymic disorder
      Specify if: Early onset/late onset
      Specify: With atypical features
311   Depressive disorder NOS

Bipolar Disorders

296.xx   Bipolar I disorder
.0x   Single manic episode[a,c,f]
      Specify if: Mixed
.40   Most recent episode hypomanic[g,h,i]
.4x   Most recent episode manic[a,c,f,g,h,i]
.6x   Most recent episode mixed[a,c,f,g,h,i]
.5x   Most recent episode depressed[a,b,c,d,e,f,g,h,i]
.7   Most recent episode unspecified[g,h,i]
296.89   Bipolar II disorder[a,b,c,d,e,f,g,h,i]
      Specify (current or most recent episode): hypomanic/depressed
301.13   Cyclothymic disorder
296.80   Bipolar disorder NOS
293.83   Mood disorder due to . . . *[indicate the general medical condition]*
      Specify type: With depressive features/with major depressive-like episode/with manic features/ with mixed features
——.—   Substance-induced mood disorder (*refer to substance-related disorders for substance-specific codes*)
      Specify type: With depressive features/with manic features/with mixed features
      Specify if: With onset during intoxication/with onset during withdrawal
296.90   Mood disorder NOS

ANXIETY DISORDERS

300.01   Panic disorder without agoraphobia
300.21   Panic disorder with agoraphobia
300.22   Agoraphobia without history of panic disorder
300.29   Specific phobia
      Specify type: Animal type/natural environment type/blood-injection-injury type/situational type/other type
300.23   Social phobia
      Specify if: Generalized

300.3   Obsessive-compulsive disorder
      Specify if: With poor insight
309.81   Posttraumatic stress disorder
      Specify if: Acute/chronic
      Specify if: With delayed onset
308.3   Acute stress disorder
300.02   Generalized anxiety disorder
293.83   Anxiety disorder due to . . . *[indicate the general medical condition]*
      Specify if: With generalized anxiety/with panic attacks/with obsessive-compulsive symptoms
——.—   Substance-induced anxiety disorder (*refer to substance-related disorders for substance-specific codes*)
      Specify if: With generalized anxiety/with panic attacks/with obsessive-compulsive symptoms/with phobic symptoms
      Specify if: With onset during intoxication/with onset during withdrawal
300.00   Anxiety disorder NOS

SOMATOFORM DISORDERS

300.81   Somatization disorder
300.82   Undifferentiated somatoform disorder
300.11   Conversion disorder
      Specify type: With motor symptom or deficit/with sensory symptom or deficit/with seizures or convulsions/with mixed presentation
307.xx   Pain disorder
.80   Associated with psychological factors
.89   Associated with both psychological factors and a general medical condition
      Specify if: Acute/chronic
300.7   Hypochondriasis
      Specify if: With poor insight
300.7   Body dysmorphic disorder
300.82   Somatoform disorder NOS

FACTITIOUS DISORDERS

300.xx   Factitious disorder
.16   With predominantly psychological signs and symptoms
.19   With predominantly physical signs and symptoms
.19   With combined psychological and physical signs and symptoms
300.19   Factitious disorder NOS

DISSOCIATIVE DISORDERS

300.12	Dissociative amnesia
300.13	Dissociative fugue
300.14	Dissociative identity disorder
300.6	Depersonalization disorder
300.15	Dissociative disorder NOS

SEXUAL AND GENDER IDENTITY DISORDERS

Sexual Dysfunctions
The following specifiers apply to all primary sexual dysfunctions:
Lifelong type/acquired type/generalized type/situational type/due to psychological factors/due to combined factors

Sexual Desire Disorders
302.71	Hypoactive sexual desire disorder
302.79	Sexual aversion disorder

Sexual Arousal Disorders
302.72	Female sexual arousal disorder
302.72	Male erectile disorder

Orgasmic Disorders
302.73	Female orgasmic disorder
302.74	Male orgasmic disorder
302.75	Premature ejaculation

Sexual Pain Disorders
302.76	Dyspareunia (not due to a general medical condition)
306.51	Vaginismus (not due to a general medical condition)

Sexual Dysfunction Due to a General Medical Condition
625.8	Female hypoactive sexual desire disorder due to . . . *[indicate the general medical condition]*
608.89	Male hypoactive sexual desire disorder due to . . . *[indicate the general medical condition]*
607.84	Male erectile disorder due to . . . *[indicate the general medical condition]*
625.0	Female dyspareunia due to . . . *[indicate the general medical condition]*
608.89	Male dyspareunia due to . . . *[indicate the general medical condition]*
625.8	Other female sexual dysfunction due to . . . *[indicate the general medical condition]*
608.89	Other male sexual dysfunction due to . . . *[indicate the general medical condition]*

—.—	Substance-induced sexual dysfunction (*refer to substance-related disorders for substance-specific codes*) *Specify if:* With impaired desire/with impaired arousal/with impaired orgasm/with sexual pain *Specify if:* With onset during intoxication
302.70	Sexual dysfunction NOS

Paraphilias
302.4	Exhibitionism
302.81	Fetishism
302.89	Frotteurism
302.2	Pedophilia *Specify if:* Sexually attracted to males/sexually attracted to females/sexually attracted to both *Specify if:* Limited to incest *Specify type:* Exclusive type/nonexclusive type
302.83	Sexual masochism
302.84	Sexual sadism
302.3	Transvestic fetishism *Specify if:* With gender dysphoria
302.82	Voyeurism
302.9	Paraphilia NOS

Gender Identity Disorders
302.xx	Gender identity disorder
.6	In children
.85	In adolescents or adults *Specify if:* Sexually attracted to males/sexually attracted to females/sexually attracted to both/sexually attracted to neither
302.6	Gender identity disorder NOS
302.9	Sexual disorder NOS

EATING DISORDERS

307.1	Anorexia nervosa *Specify type:* Restricting type; binge-eating/purging type
307.51	Bulimia nervosa *Specify type:* Purging type/nonpurging type
307.50	Eating disorder NOS

SLEEP DISORDERS

Primary Sleep Disorders
Dyssomnias
307.42	Primary insomnia
307.44	Primary hypersomnia *Specify if:* Recurrent

347	Narcolepsy	
780.59	Breathing-related sleep disorder	
307.45	Circadian rhythm sleep disorder	

307.45 Circadian rhythm sleep disorder
Specify type: Delayed sleep phase type/jet lag type/shift work type/unspecified type

307.47 Dyssomnia NOS

Parasomnias
307.47 Nightmare disorder
307.46 Sleep terror disorder
307.46 Sleepwalking disorder
307.47 Parasomnia NOS

Sleep Disorders Related to Another Mental Disorder
307.42 Insomnia related to . . . [indicate the Axis I or Axis II disorder]
307.44 Hypersomnia related to . . . [indicate the Axis I or Axis II disorder]

Other Sleep Disorders
780.xx Sleep disorder due to . . . [indicate the general medical condition]
.52 Insomnia type
.54 Hypersomnia type
.59 Parasomnia type
.59 Mixed type
——.— Substance-induced sleep disorder (*refer to substance-related disorders for substance-specific codes*)
Specify type: Insomnia type/hypersomnia type/parasomnia type/mixed type
Specify if: With onset during intoxication/with onset during withdrawal

IMPULSE-CONTROL DISORDERS NOT ELSEWHERE CLASSIFIED
312.34 Intermittent explosive disorder
312.32 Kleptomania
312.33 Pyromania
312.31 Pathological gambling
312.39 Trichotillomania
312.30 Impulse-control disorder NOS

ADJUSTMENT DISORDERS
309.xx Adjustment disorder
.0 With depressed mood
.24 With anxiety
.28 With mixed anxiety and depressed mood
.3 With disturbance of conduct

.4 With mixed disturbance of emotions and conduct
.9 Unspecified
Specify if: Acute/chronic

PERSONALITY DISORDERS

Note: These are coded on Axis II.
301.0 Paranoid personality disorder
301.20 Schizoid personality disorder
301.22 Schizotypal personality disorder
301.7 Antisocial personality disorder
301.83 Borderline personality disorder
301.50 Histrionic personality disorder
301.81 Narcissistic personality disorder
301.82 Avoidant personality disorder
301.6 Dependent personality disorder
301.4 Obsessive-compulsive personality disorder
301.9 Personality disorder NOS

OTHER CONDITIONS THAT MAY BE A FOCUS OF CLINICAL ATTENTION

Psychological Factors Affecting Medical Condition
316 . . . [Specified psychological factor] affecting . . . [indicate the general medical condition]
Choose name based on nature of factors:
Mental disorder affecting medical condition
Psychological symptoms affecting medical condition
Personality traits or coping style affecting medical condition
Maladaptive health behaviors affecting medical condition
Stress-related physiological response affecting medical condition
Other or unspecified psychological factors affecting medical condition

Medication-Induced Movement Disorders
332.1 Neuroleptic-induced parkinsonism
333.92 Neuroleptic malignant syndrome
333.7 Neuroleptic-induced acute dystonia
333.99 Neuroleptic-induced acute akathisia
333.82 Neuroleptic-induced tardive dyskinesia
333.1 Medication-induced postural tremor
333.90 Medication-induced movement disorder NOS

Other Medication-Induced Disorder
995.2   Adverse effects of medication NOS

Relational Problems
V61.9   Relational problem related to a mental disorder or general medical condition
V61.20   Parent-child relational problem
V61.10   Partner relational problem
V61.8   Sibling relational problem
V62.81   Relational problem NOS

Problems Related to Abuse or Neglect
V61.21   Physical abuse of child
           (*code 995.54 if focus of attention is on victim*)
V61.21   Sexual abuse of child
           (*code 995.53 if focus of attention is on victim*)
V61.21   Neglect of child
           (*code 955.52 if focus of attention is on victim*)
—.—   Physical abuse of adult
V61.12   (if by partner)
V62.83   (if by person other than partner)
—.—   Sexual abuse of adult
V61.12   (if by partner)
V62.83   (if by person other than partner)

Additional Conditions That May Be a Focus of Clinical Attention
V15.81   Noncompliance with treatment
V65.2   Malingering

V71.01   Adult antisocial behavior
V71.02   Child or adolescent antisocial behavior
V62.89   Borderline intellectual functioning
780.9   Age-related cognitive decline
V62.82   Bereavement
V62.3   Academic problem
V62.2   Occupational problem
313.82   Identity problem
V62.89   Religious or spiritual problem
V62.4   Acculturation problem
V62.89   Phase of life problem

ADDITIONAL CODES

300.9   Unspecified mental disorder (nonpsychotic)
V71.09   No diagnosis or condition on Axis I
799.9   Diagnosis or condition deferred on Axis I
V71.09   No diagnosis on Axis II
799.9   Diagnosis deferred on Axis II

Multiaxial System
Axis I   Clinical Disorders
           Other Conditions That May Be a Focus of Clinical Attention
Axis II   Personality Disorders
           Mental Retardation
Axis III   General Medical Conditions
Axis IV   Psychosocial and Environmental Problems
Axis V   Global Assessment of Functioning

Dementia, Delirium, & Amnestic Disorders

16

Phillip Grob, MD, David Lorreck, MD, Renée Binder, MD, & Ellen Haller, MD

Prior editions of this book discussed delirium, dementia, and amnestic disorders in a broader chapter entitled Organic Mental Disorders (following the convention in the *Diagnostic and Statistical Manual of Mental Disorders* [*DSM*]). This category encompassed psychological and behavioral disorders whose abnormalities resulted from known biological causes and pathophysiological mechanisms. In contrast to these organic disorders, psychiatric illnesses such as schizophrenia or bipolar disorder were categorized as "functional disorders" with no identifiable organic etiology. This organic/functional dichotomy became increasingly problematic as evidence grew for central nervous system dysfunction in the major "functional" mental disorders. In addition, this dichotomy left clinicians with no satisfactory alternative term for conditions that were not "organic mental disorders." Finally, the organic versus nonorganic distinction encouraged the continued stigmatization of mentally ill individuals by suggesting that "functional" disorders such as schizophrenia were not true medical disorders.

In the *Diagnostic and Statistical Manual of Mental Disorders,* 4th edition (*DSM-IV*), the section on organic mental disorder is completely reorganized, and the term "organic" is eliminated. The disorders of delirium, dementia, and amnesia are classified as **cognitive disorders** and will be presented in this chapter. Other diagnoses previously classified within the Organic Mental Disorder section of *DSM-III-R* are now called **secondary** if caused by a specific medical disorder (eg, mood disorder resulting from hypothyroidism or personality change resulting from stroke) or **substance induced** if substance intoxication or withdrawal is judged to be etiologically related to the disturbance (eg, cocaine psychotic disorder with delusions). The secondary disorders are now classified phenomenologically with related disorders. For example, secondary mood disorders are in the Mood Disorder section of *DSM-IV* and are discussed in Chapter 20 of this book. The substance-induced disorders are all classified together in *DSM-IV* under the title Substance-Related Disorders. If a patient presents with depression, for example, the clinician can readily use *DSM-IV* criteria to assess whether the depression (1) is secondary to an underlying condition such as hypothyroidism, (2) is caused by withdrawal from a substance such as cocaine or by intoxication with a substance such as a barbiturate, or (3) is a primary psychiatric condition.

SYMPTOMS & SIGNS OF COGNITIVE DISORDERS

A. Common Symptoms and Signs: In evaluating a patient with a psychological or behavioral disturbance, certain signs and symptoms suggest that the disorder is a cognitive disorder, as described in this chapter. These signs and symptoms include the following:

1. Fluctuating performance on serial mental status examinations.
2. Memory impairment.
3. Disorientation.
4. Cognitive impairment, eg, dyscalculia, or reduced fund of information.
5. Visual hallucinations or illusions.
6. Tactile hallucinations or illusions.
7. Motor restlessness.
8. Impaired judgment and poor impulse control.
9. Autonomic symptoms (tachycardia, fever, sweating, hypertension).
10. Sudden onset without any previous personal or family psychiatric history—at any age, but particularly in a patient over 40.
11. Lack of expected response to traditional treatment.
12. Prior physical illness or current physical symptoms.
13. History of recent drug or medication intake.

Although any of these symptoms and signs may be present in any psychiatric disorder, when they are elicited, it is important first to consider cognitive disorders or secondary or substance-induced disorders in the differential diagnosis.

B. Etiology: A single psychiatric syndrome may have many organic causes, and a single cause can result in different syndromes. For example, neurosyphilis can cause delirium, dementia, secondary psychotic disorder, secondary mood disorder, or secondary personality change. Even in the same patient, a given cause may lead first to one syndrome and then to another. For example, neurosyphilis may first present as a secondary mood disorder or a secondary personality change, but then may progress to dementia. Similarly, infection with the human immunodeficiency virus (HIV) may cause a variety of disorders, including delirium, dementia, secondary psychotic disorder, and secondary mood disorder.

C. Factors Affecting Symptoms and Signs:
Even if a specific, identifiable cause is present, the course of illness for a given individual depends on physical, psychological, and social factors:

1. Physical factors affecting symptoms and signs include the following:
   a. The degree of insult sustained by the central nervous system (CNS). For example, brain tumor is manifested differently depending on the size and location of the tumor and whether intracranial pressure is increased. Pernicious anemia is manifested differently depending on the serum level of vitamin B_{12}.
   b. The rate at which whole-brain involvement occurs. For example, the sequelae of a brain tumor depend on whether the tumor grows slowly or rapidly. In the case of heavy metal poisoning, effects depend on whether intoxication is gradual or acute.
   c. The physical condition of the patient. For example, an elderly patient with several concurrent medical diagnoses is more prone to developing a substance-induced delirium when prescribed a CNS-active medication than is a younger, healthier patient.
2. Psychological factors affecting symptoms and signs include the following:
   a. The patient's personality and psychological defense mechanisms. For example, in response to the same specific brain insult, a patient with a paranoid personality may become more paranoid, and a patient with an obsessive personality may become more obsessive.
   b. The patient's intelligence and education. For example, the signs of dementia are often quite subtle in a well-educated patient with above average intelligence who can still do very well on a cognitive examination.
   c. The patient's level of premorbid psychological adjustment. For example, a patient who was relatively well adjusted before dementia may be better able to tolerate a mild deficit than a patient with preexisting psychological difficulties.
   d. The patient's level of current psychological stress and conflict. For example, a patient who has recently lost a spouse or has been forced to retire may have more difficulty tolerating even mild deficits in cognitive functioning than a patient without current stress.
3. Social factors affecting symptoms and signs include the following:
   a. The degree of social isolation versus support. For example, a patient with dementia of the Alzheimer's type may function well while living with a healthy spouse, but may then deteriorate if the spouse becomes ill and needs hospitalization.
   b. The degree of familiarity patients have with their environment. For example, patients with dementia often function poorly and become easily confused in an unfamiliar hospital environment (a phenomenon known as "sundowning" because it tends to worsen at night), although they may be able to take care of themselves fairly well in their own home.
   c. The level of sensory input. Either insufficient or excessive sensory input (eg, being in a darkened room in a nursing home without a calendar or attempting to rest in an Intensive Care Unit surrounded by lights, noise, and constant activity) may cause increased confusion in a patient with delirium and/or dementia.

DEMENTIA

Definition

Dementia is a syndrome manifested by several cognitive deficits that include memory impairment involving at least one of the following: aphasia, agnosia, apraxia, or a disturbance in executive functioning (the ability to plan, sequence, abstract, and organize) that interferes with social, occupational, or interpersonal skills. Tables 16–1, 16–2, 16–3, and 16–4 list the *DSM-IV* criteria for dementias. The most commonly used brief test for cognitive function is the Folstein Mini-Mental Status Examination (MMSE) (Table 16–5).

The patient with dementia is forgetful, has difficulty learning new information, and will often try to minimize or deny deficits. Typically, recent memory is worse than remote memory. A patient may be un-

---

Table 16–1. Diagnostic criteria for dementia (all types).

The development of multiple cognitive deficits manifested by both of the following:
1. Memory impairment (inability to learn new information and to recall previously learned information)
2. At least one of the following cognitive disturbances:
   a. Aphasia (language disturbance)
   b. Apraxia (inability to carry out motor activities despite intact motor function)
   c. Agnosia (failure to recognize or identify objects despite intact sensory function)
   d. Disturbance in executive functioning (ie, planning, organizing, sequencing, abstracting)

Table 16–2. *DSM-IV* diagnostic criteria for dementia of the Alzheimer's type.

A. See Table 16–1

B. The course is characterized by gradual onset and continuing cognitive decline

C. The cognitive deficits cause significant impairment in social or occupational functioning and represent a significant decline from a previous level of functioning

D. The cognitive deficits in A are not caused by any of the following:

1. Central nervous system conditions that cause progressive deficits in memory and cognition (eg, cerebrovascular disease, Parkinson's disease, Huntington's disease, subdural hematoma, normal-pressure hydrocephalus)

2. Systemic conditions that are known to cause dementia (eg, hypothyroidism, vitamin B_{12} or folic acid deficiency, niacin deficiency, hypercalcemia, neurosyphilis, HIV infection)

3. Substance-induced conditions

E. The deficits do not occur exclusively during the course of delirium

F. Not better accounted for by another Axis I disorder (eg, major depressive disorder, schizophrenia)

Table 16–4. *DSM-IV* diagnostic criteria for dementia other than Alzheimer's or vascular.

A. See Table 16–1

B. The cognitive deficits cause significant impairment in social or occupational functioning and represent a significant decline from a previous level of functioning

C. The deficits do not occur exclusively during the course of delirium

D. There is evidence from the history, physical examination, or laboratory findings of a medical condition (for dementia from other general medical conditions) or substance use (for substance-induced persisting dementia) judged to be etiologically related to the disturbance, or (for dementia of multiple etiologies) there is evidence of multiple etiologies (eg, head trauma plus chronic alcohol use, dementia of the Alzheimer's type with the subsequent development of vascular dementia)

---

able to recall names of three objects after 5 minutes, but may have excellent recall of events that occurred in childhood.

In addition to defects in memory, language skills and constructional abilities are also frequently impaired. Patients may have difficulty repeating a phrase or naming objects pointed to by the examiner. Constructional ability may be tested by having the patient draw intersecting pentagons or a clock face with the hands set at a certain time.

Patients with dementia also develop difficulty with abstract thinking. For instance, they may be unable to state how a chair and a desk are similar. Interpretations of proverbs are usually concrete.

It is not unusual, as the dementia progresses, for patients to develop accentuation of their premorbid character traits; for example, a normally suspicious patient may develop frank paranoia. With frontal lobe

Table 16–3. *DSM-IV* diagnostic criteria for vascular dementia.

A. See Table 16–1

B. Focal neurological signs and symptoms (eg, exaggeration of deep tendon reflexes, extensor plantar response, pseudobulbar palsy, gait abnormalities, weakness of an extremity) or laboratory evidence indicative of cerebrovascular disease (eg, multiple infarctions involving cortex and underlying white matter) that are judged to be etiologically related to the disturbance

C. The cognitive deficits cause significant impairment in social or occupational functioning and represent a significant decline from a previous level of functioning

D. The deficits do not occur exclusively during the course of delirium

---

disease patients may lose normal social inhibitions and consequently may demonstrate inappropriate sexual behaviors.

Patients with dementia will often have abnormalities other than cognitive ones. Their grooming and hygiene may be impaired. Their affect may be labile or shallow. Mood may be depressed, particularly early in the course of the illness when patients are more aware of their cognitive deficits. The thought process is often remarkable for perserveration. Delusional thinking or hallucinations may develop, with paranoid delusions being particularly common. Confabulation may occur. Insight and judgment become progressively more impaired.

The *DSM-IV* allows clinicians to characterize the nature of an individual's dementia, such as Alzheimer's type or vascular type. Different codes exist for an uncomplicated dementia and for dementias with delirium, delusions, hallucinations, affective disturbances, behavioral disturbances, or communication disturbances. The diagnosis is made on the basis of the predominant features of the patient's presentation.

Dementia of the Alzheimer's type is further characterized by age of onset; a patient is diagnosed with early onset if symptoms develop at age 65 or younger, or with late onset if symptoms develop after 65 years of age.

Epidemiology

Dementia is found predominantly in elderly persons, although certain etiological factors may cause dementia at any age. The diagnosis of dementia may be made at any time after the IQ is fairly stable (usually by age four). Chronic neurological disorders are the cause of such early dementias.

Dementia of the Alzheimer's type is by far the most common form of dementia, accounting for approximately 40–65% of all cases. Prevalence is 1% at 65 years of age, and doubles every 5 years. Alzheimer's dementia (AD) affects as many as four million citizens of the United States. This number is likely to

Table 16–5. Folstein Mini-Mental Status Examination.[a]

	Patient ....
	Examiner ....
	Date ....

Maximum
Score   Score

ORIENTATION

5   ( )   What is the (year) (season) (date) (day) (month)?
5   ( )   Where are we: (state) (county) (town) (hospital) (floor).

REGISTRATION

3   ( )   Name 3 objects: 1 second to say each. Then ask the patient all 3 after you have said them.
Give 1 point for each correct answer. Then repeat them until he learns all 3.
Count trials and record.
Trials

ATTENTION AND CALCULATION

5   ( )   Serial 7's. 1 point for each correct. Stop after 5 answers. Alternatively spell "world" backwards.

RECALL

3   ( )   Ask for the 3 objects repeated above. Give 1 point for each correct.

LANGUAGE

9   ( )   Name a pencil, and watch (2 points)
Repeat the following "No ifs, and, or buts." (1 point)
Follow a 3-stage command:
      "Take a paper in your right hand, fold it in half, and put it on the floor" (3 points)
Read and obey the following:

CLOSE YOUR EYES (1 point)

Write a sentence (1 point)
Copy design (1 point)
_____ Total score
ASSESS level of consciousness along a continuum _____

                                    Alert   Drowsy   Stupor   Coma

INSTRUCTIONS FOR ADMINISTRATION
OF MINI-MENTAL STATUS EXAMINATION

ORIENTATION

1. Ask for the date. Then ask specifically for parts omitted, eg, "Can you also tell me what season it is?" One point for each correct.
2. Ask in turn "Can you tell me the name of this hospital?" (town, county, etc). One point for each correct.

REGISTRATION

Ask the patient if you may test his memory. Then say the names of 3 unrelated objects, clearly and slowly, about one second for each. After you have said 3, ask him to repeat them. This first repetition determines his score (0–3) but keep saying them until he can repeat all 3, up to 6 trials. If he does not eventually learn all 3, recall can not be meaningfully tested.

ATTENTION AND CALCULATION

Ask the patient to begin with 100 and count backwards by 7. Stop after 5 subtractions (93, 86, 79, 72, 65). Score the total number of correct answers.

If the patient cannot or will not perform this task, ask him to spell the word "world" backwards. The score is the number of letters in correct order, eg dlrow = 5, dlorw = 3.

RECALL

Ask the patient if he can recall the 3 words you previously asked him to remember. Score 0–3.

LANGUAGE

Naming: Show the patient a wrist watch and ask him what it is. Repeat for pencil. Score 0–2.

Repetition: Ask the patient to repeat the sentence after you. Allow only one trial. Score 0 or 1.

3-Stage command: Give the patient a piece of plain blank paper and repeat the command. Score 1 point for each part correctly executed.

Reading: On a blank piece of paper print the sentence "Close your eyes" in letters large enough for the patient to see clearly. Ask him to read it and do what it says. Score 1 point only if he actually closes his eyes.

Writing: Give the patient a blank piece of paper and ask him to write a sentence for you. Do not dictate a sentence, it is to be written spontaneously. It must contain a subject and verb and be sensible. Correct grammar and punctuation are not necessary.

Copying: On a clean piece of paper, draw intersecting pentagons, each side about 1 in., and ask him to copy it exactly as it is. All 10 angles must be present and 2 must intersect to score 1 point. Tremor and rotation are ignored.

Estimate the patient's level of sensorium along a continuum, from alert on the left to coma on the right.

[a] From Folstein et al (1975).

double over the next 30 years. The annual economic toll of AD in the United States in terms of health care expenses and lost wages of both patients and their caregivers is estimated at 80–100 billion dollars.

Of the remaining types of dementia, the second most common type is vascular dementia (10–40%) followed by mixed Alzheimer's–vascular dementia and less common forms of dementia.

Etiology & Pathogenesis

The pathogenesis of dementia depends largely on the etiology. Approximately 5–15% of all dementias are reversible, and if their cause is identified and treated the prognosis is good. On the other hand, neurodegenerative dementias such as AD are progressive and incurable and ultimately end in death.

A. Dementia of the Alzheimer's Type: AD is a neurodegenerative disease of the brain with an average duration of 8–10 years between onset and death, and a variable course of progression that ranges from 4 to 20 years. AD has an insidious onset, most commonly after the age of 60 years, although in rare instances as early as 40 years of age, followed by progressive deterioration.

AD is divided into three stages based on functional and cognitive capacity. Although variable, the MMSE can be used to track the course of cognitive impairment. Typically, early AD MMSE is equal to or greater than 18, moderate AD MMSE is between 12 and 18, and severe AD MMSE is less than 12. On average the MMSE score declines by 3 points per year.

In terms of functional capacity, with early AD, judgment is typically intact as are activities of daily living (ADL). With moderate AD, judgment is severely impaired and patients generally require assistance with ADLs and some form of supervised care. With severe AD, judgment is essentially lost and patients are completely dependent on others for ADL and self-care. They may not be oriented to family members or to self, may become bed bound, and may consequently develop decubiti, infection, or other illness, which ultimately may lead to death.

Short-term memory loss is usually the earliest manifestation of AD. This is typically associated with mild aphasia and impaired visuospatial ability, which evolve into fluent aphasia and constructional apraxia. Other cognitive functions such as calculations, reasoning, judgment, and executive functioning also become impaired. Typically behavioral aggression, psychomotor agitation, frank psychosis, and affective or personality changes, although not an early consequence of AD, may ensue as the illness progresses.

The major neuropathological features of AD are neuritic plaques, amyloid deposition in plaques, and neurofibrillary tangles spread diffusely through the cerebral cortex and hippocampus. These features remain the pathognomic findings for diagnosis, which can be made histologically only definitively at au-

topsy. Hence the clinical diagnosis of AD is based on clinical presentation and on exclusion of other causes of dementia.

In AD degeneration in the cortical neurons and the associated reduction in the number of cortical synapses have been correlated with the severity of dementia. The most common distribution is in the hippocampus, a structure deep in the brain involved with encoding memory, and in the temporal and parietal lobes. In general, the greater the involvement of the frontal lobe, the more likely the development of mood and behavioral symptoms.

As noted, the two key abnormal findings in the brain of individuals with AD are amyloid plaques and neurofibrillary tangles. Plaques are dense deposits of an amyloid protein (called β-amyloid) and other associated proteins and nonnerve cells (glial cells and microglia) that gradually build up outside and around neurons, forming insoluble deposits that interrupt synaptic transmission, resulting in neuronal cell death.

β-Amyloid is a protein fragment snipped from a larger protein, called the amyloid precursor protein (APP), during metabolism. APPs are normally associated with nerve cell membranes (transmembrane). For reasons that are not clear, β-amyloid may develop when APP is abnormally cleaved by proteases. The abnormally large β-amyloid peptide (40–42 amino acids) rapidly forms insoluble "sticky" aggregates that are key to the development of plaques and consequent cell death. Theories regarding the toxicity of β-amyloid to neuronal cells include formation of free radicals, local inflammatory response, depletion of intracellular choline, and disruption of potassium channels.

Neurofibrillary tangles are abnormal collections of intracellular phosphorylated proteins. The primary component of tangles is one form of the protein, tau, which is involved in microtubule stability in normal neurons. Abnormal tau proteins of AD result in microtubule disintegration and the consequent development of neurofibrillary tangles, which consist primarily of paired helical abnormal tau proteins.

Although AD is a generalized neurodegenerative disorder, the cholinergic (acetylcholine) pathways are the neurotransmitter system most aggressively affected early in the disease. Ninety percent of cholinergic neurons arise from the nucleus basalis of Meynert in the basal forebrain, with projections to frontal, parietal, temporal, and subcortical structures. This is consistent with short-term memory loss as the presenting symptom of AD, as the temporal lobe projections to the hippocampus are part of the core circuit that encodes new memories. There are also decreased levels of choline acetyltransferase (CAT), the enzyme involved in the synthesis of acetylcholine, and decreased concentrations of acetylcholine in the cerebrospinal fluid. The depletion of acetylcholine concentrations has been correlated with memory and cognitive impairment in AD and restoration of cholinergic function is a primary goal in current pharmacological treatment strategies.

In addition to its effects on the cholinergic system, AD also results in the loss of noradrenergic neurons in the locus ceruleus and of serotonergic neurons in the dorsal raphe nuclei. In addition, researchers have found decreased levels of γ-aminobutyric acid (GABA), substance P, somatostatin, and corticotropin-releasing factor.

The two most significant risk factors for AD are advanced age and positive family history. As noted previously, the prevalence of AD doubles every 5 years after the age of 65. The prevalence of dementia is 25–30% in the 85- to 90-year-old population. The prevalence trend in the very old (greater than 90) is unclear due to the limitations of study size and data in this population.

Genetic familial risk factors can be seen in the effect of positive family history in sporadic cases (90% of AD) as well as in the 10% of AD that appears to be familial. Having one affected sibling or parent doubles the risk of AD; having two affected parents or one parent and one sibling increases the risk three- to fourfold.

Mutations on chromosomes 1, 14, and 21 are associated with some forms of early familial AD (FAD). The defective gene on chromosome 1 has been named presenilin 2, which is involved in the development of β-amyloid plaques. The presenilin 2 gene has been linked to the abnormally high prevalence of AD among families descended from a group of Germans (called Volga Germans). Only a very small fraction of early-onset FAD is caused by this presenilin 2 gene mutation. The defective gene on chromosome 14 has been named presenilin 1, which is more commonly implicated in the development of β-amyloid plaques. The defective gene on chromosome 21 results in the abnormal processing of APP, resulting in the accumulation of neuritic plaques. Furthermore, patients with Down syndrome (trisomy 21) who survive the fifth decade of life show the neuropathological brain changes of AD and may suffer significant cognitive decline.

Together, presenilins 1 and 2 and mutations in the APP gene account for nearly 50% of early-onset FAD. The gene(s) for the remaining 50% has yet to be identified.

Another important risk factor in late-onset familial and sporadic AD may be the inheritance of the E4 allele of apolipoprotein E (Apo E), a cholesterol carrier protein whose gene is located on chromosome 19. Every person has two Apo E genes, one inherited from each parent. Of the three common alleles of Apo E, E2 may be protective against AD, E3 appears neutral, and E4 appears linked to an increased risk for developing AD, both in late-onset familial AD and in sporadic AD. The greatest risk is in individuals with two copies of Apo E E4, with studies suggesting up to

90% developing AD by age 85. How Apo E E4 increases a person's susceptibility to AD is not known.

Currently genetic testing is not part of routine clinical practice. Since 90% of AD is sporadic, Apo E testing would have no negative or positive predictive value, assuming individuals live to age 85.

Age and positive family history are the only clear risk factors for AD. Head injury, gender, education, diet, occupational exposures, and thyroid disease have shown to be possible risk factors in AD. However, these other risk factors have not been found to be very significant consistently and appear to be sensitive to sampling methodology. Recent studies have made clear that there is a long preclinical phase of AD, with disease expression occurring when a critical threshold of neuronal compromise is reached. This would suggest that many vectors of neuronal injury, particularly cerebrovascular disease, would enhance and hasten the expression of AD.

The etiology of AD is likely multifactorial in which genetic and environmental factors combine with aging to overcome the ability of neurons to maintain homeostasis. This impaired neuronal metabolism results in damaged mitochondria, damaged cytoskeleton, increased release of excitotoxic neurotransmitter glutamate, activation of local inflammatory mechanisms, aberrant phosphorylation of membrane proteins, and, ultimately, premature dysfunction and neuronal cell death.

B. Vascular Dementia: Vascular dementia accounts for approximately 15% of all dementias. Typically, patients have risk factors such as hypertension, cardiac disease, diabetes, and strokes. Vascular dementia was classically characterized by an abrupt onset and stepwise deterioration of dementia, as opposed to the insidious onset and gradual progression seen more commonly in AD. However, it is possible for vascular dementia to resemble AD in its onset and course. The pattern of cognitive impairment is often patchy, depending on the location of vascular compromise, and there are often focal upper motor neuron signs (eg, reflex or tone asymmetry).

There are two forms of vascular dementia. Classical multi-infarct dementia involves multiple completed strokes in cortical and possibly subcortical areas. The other form is associated with the small vessel disease and microangiopathy of chronic vascular risk factors (eg, hypertension, diabetes mellitus, smoking, hypercholesteremia), and was classically described as Binswanger's disease. The classic presentation of this type of primarily subcortical vascular dementia is diminished attention and concentration and prolonged response latency. Due to the extensive subcortical-frontal connections, frontal lobe behavioral syndromes (eg, apathy, disinhibition) can be frequently seen. The decrement in verbal fluency and the ablation of short-term memory are less prominent than in AD. Behavioral manifestations are variable depending on the vascular region involved.

Brain imaging studies usually show multiple vascular lesions of cortical and subcortical regions. Functional imaging scans with positron emission tomography (PET) or single-photon emission computed tomography (SPECT) will usually show a patchy reduction in cerebral blood flow.

Although hypertension, cerebrovascular disease, diabetes, and AD are all common diseases of aging, the prevalence of mixed (AD and vascular) dementia has been underreported, due to unrealistic efforts to define dementia distinctly as either of the Alzheimer or vascular type. Previous studies suggesting higher prevalences of vascular dementia probably included mixed disease. AD, vascular dementia, and mixed AD/vascular dementia comprise 80–90% of clinical dementia.

C. Alcohol-Related Dementia: Chronic alcohol use has long been considered an etiology of dementia. This has been subject to debate as a neuropathological entity, has been hard to identify, and there has been no clear dose relationship between alcohol use and cognitive functioning. However, the heavy neurological comorbidity due to nutritional compromise, increased cerebrovascular disease, head injuries, Wernicke's encephalopathy, and Korsakoff's syndrome may be the de facto etiology for alcohol-related dementia, or at least heavy risk factors for developing dementia.

D. Dementia due to Parkinson's Disease: Parkinson's disease (PD)-induced dementia accounts for 5–10% of all dementias. Parkinson's disease is a slowly progressive neurologic condition associated with dopamine deficiency and characterized by the triad of resting tremor, bradykinesia, and rigidity. Its onset is usually in middle to late life. Approximately 40–50% of patients with PD develop dementia. The dementia of PD is insidious in onset and develops late in the disease course. Subcortical patterns of cognitive deficits (eg, diminished attention and concentration, slowing of response, and apathy) are common. Histopathologically, there is neuronal loss and gliosis primarily in the lateral substantia nigra.

E. Dementia due to Lewy Body Disease: Lewy body disease (LBD) typically has a more rapid onset with a fluctuating course. Visual hallucinations, parkinsonian symptoms, and susceptibility to delirium are common early in the course. Patients with LBD are remarkably sensitive to extrapyramidal side effects of antipsychotic medications. The pathognomonic histopathologic feature of LBD is the presence of Lewy inclusion bodies in the cerebral cortex.

F. Frontal Lobe Dementias: Pick's disease and other forms of frontotemporal dementias are noteworthy for the early presentation of impaired executive functioning and personality and behavioral changes, including disinhibition, affective blunting, and deterioration of social skills. Memory deficits become more apparent as the disease progresses. In Pick's disease, there is profound atrophy of the frontal and/or temporal lobes, with characteristic Pick inclusion bodies found on autopsy. It typically presents between the ages of 50 and 60 years, though it may begin later. There is also a non-Pick body form of frontotemporal dementia.

G. Other Progressive Dementing Disorders: Other progressive neurodegenerative diseases cause irreversible dementias. Creutzfeldt-Jakob disease is a rapidly progressive spongiform encephalopathy associated with a slow virus or prion. Individuals with Creutzfeldt-Jakob disease frequently demonstrate a heightened startle response. Huntington's disease is an autosomal dominant neurodegenerative disorder that affects the basal ganglia and other subcortical structures. Onset is usually before age 50, is associated with a clear autosomal dominant transmission family history, and presents with involuntary movements and behavioral changes, with dementia being a later complication. Progressive supranuclear palsy is another dementia presenting with more rapid course and extrapyramidal symptoms. A distinguishing feature may be the prominence of vertical voluntary gaze paresis while retaining involuntary vertical gaze reflexes.

H. Dementia due to Other Causes: Many other medical conditions can present as a dementia and are important to consider in the differential diagnosis because they are potentially reversible. These reversible dementias account for approximately 10% of dementias. Reversible causes of dementia, listed in Table 16–6, include endocrine disturbances (eg, hypothyroidism, hypoglycemia), nutritional deficiencies (eg, thiamine, niacin, or vitamin B_{12} deficiency), structural abnormalities (eg, brain tumor, subdural

Table 16–6. Causes of dementia from medical conditions.

Intracranial	Infections
Tumor	Neurosyphilis
Chronic subdural	AIDS
hematoma	Chronic meningitis (TB,
Normal-pressure	fungal, parasitic)
hydrocephalus	Cerebral abscess
Head trauma	Heavy metal poisoning
Metabolic	Mercury
Hypoxemia	Lead
Electrolyte disturbance	Arsenic
Dehydration	Thallium
Renal or hepatic failure	Collagen-vascular disease
Wilson's disease	Systemic lupus
Porphyria	erythematosus
Endocrinopathies	Temporal arteritis
Thyroid disease	Sarcoidosis
(myxedema,	Drug toxicity
hyperthyroidism)	Chronic alcoholism
Adrenal disease	Chronic substance abuse
Parathyroid disease	Anticholinergic agents
Pituitary disease	Antihypertensive agents
Deficiency states	Anticonvulsants
Vitamin B_{12}	Miscellaneous
Folate	Disulfiram
Thiamine	Cimetidine
Niacin (pellagra)	Antineoplastic agents

hematoma, normal-pressure hydrocephalus), infectious conditions (eg, neurosyphilis, HIV), renal and hepatic disorders, the toxic effect of long standing substance abuse (eg, ethanol abuse), and iatrogenic, ie, pharmocological toxicity due to undiagnosed CNS side effects, toxicity, or polypharmacy interactions.

The extent of the reversibility is contingent on the nature of the disorder and the timeliness of diagnosis and treatment. For instance, dementia secondary to HIV, although not fully reversible, may be improved by antiviral medications. On the other hand, dementia secondary to normal-pressure hydrocephalus, which may present as dementia, ataxia, and urinary incontinence, may be fully or partially reversed if the diagnosis is made and treatment (shunt placement) is initiated promptly.

Differential Diagnosis

Distinguishing dementia from other cognitive disorders and from both primary and secondary psychiatric disorders is critical. Common clinical dilemmas in geriatric care are distinguishing dementia from depression, delirium, or the cognitive changes of normal aging. Chronically mentally ill patients may also be incorrectly diagnosed with dementia. There is also debate whether chronic schizophrenia can be a primary etiology of dementia. A chronic schizophrenic patient with profound social regression and severe negative symptoms may be difficult to distinguish from a patient with dementia.

A. Major Depression and Related Affective Disorders: Depression in older individuals frequently presents with atypical features such as predominant cognitive deficits. Some older individuals with depression may even deny feeling sad. The cognitive dulling associated with depression in older people has been described as pseudodementia or the dementia syndrome of depression. The cognitive impairment in these patients is temporary and improves as the depression resolves. Table 16–7 contrasts the clinical features of cognitive consequences of depression (pseudodementia) and dementia. Clinical features that suggest an underlying depressive disorder include a more sudden onset of cognitive decline. This may or may not be preceded by depressive symptoms. These individuals may have a prior history of affective disorders, may present with neurovegeta-

tive signs such as appetite, sleep, and energy disturbances, and may have various somatic complaints. In addition, depressed patients tend to exaggerate their cognitive deficits and display poor effort on cognitive examination, frequently answering with the words "I don't know." In contrast, patients with dementia frequently minimize, rationalize, and attempt to conceal and compensate for their deficits. Depressed patients often show inconsistent deficits of both recent and remote memory, whereas patients with early dementia tend to have a more intact remote memory, with severe short-term deficits. Depressed patients' memory deficits are more responsive to prompting and encouragement than patients with AD. In content, the responses of depressed patients are characterized more by "near misses" and poor effort than the gross errors of truly demented patients.

Even with these clues to differentiating between cognitive changes due to depression and dementia, it may be difficult to make the distinction. In addition, patients with dementia may become secondarily depressed. In a patient in whom the distinction is quite unclear, a reasonable approach would be to treat a suspected depression and then see if the patient continues to show signs of dementia well after the depressive episode has resolved.

B. Delirium: Although cognitive impairment exists in both delirium and dementia, the clinical course of each is quite distinct. Delirium has a widely fluctuating clinical course with an acute onset, whereas dementia typically has a more insidious progressive course with less acute onset. Table 16–8 contrasts the clinical features of delirium and dementia. Critical in the distinction is assessing the level of consciousness and measuring cognitive capacity serially. It should be stressed that for patients with dementia (as well as any neurologically vulnerable patient) the risk of developing a superimposed delirium is great.

C. Normal Aging: In normal aging memory losses are slight and do not interfere with activities of daily living. The speed of mental processing may slow with aging, but aging is not synonymous with dementia. Cognitive changes associated with normal aging include prolonged latency of response, slower set shift, decreased attention and concentration, slower acquisition and processing, and less efficient memory. However, with normal aging, language, ac-

Table 16–7. Differentiation of pseudodementia and dementia.

The Dementia Syndrome of Depression	Dementia
Sudden onset	Gradual onset
Vegetative signs common	Vegetative signs less common
Patients expose cognitive deficits	Patients conceal cognitive deficits
Patients often respond "I don't know"	Patients attempt to answer questions
Variability in cognitive performance	Consistently poor cognitive performance
Inconsistent effort	Consistent effort
Recent and remote memory may be equally poor	Recent memory worse than remote memory
Sundowning uncommon	Sundowning common

Table 16–8. Clinical features of delirium and dementia.

Delirium	Dementia
Abrupt onset	Insidious onset
Fluctuating course over 24 hours with nocturnal exacerbation	Stable course over 24 hours
May have asterixis or coarse tremor	Often have no abnormal involuntary movements
Often incoherent speech with fluctuating rate	Often normal speech except for word-finding difficulties, perseveration
Visual hallucinations most common; occasionally, patients have both auditory and visual hallucinations	Often have no hallucinations
Fleeting, poorly organized delusions	Often have no delusions, sometimes paranoid
Reduced consciousness	Clear consciousness
Impaired orientation	Impaired orientation
Globally impaired attention	Normal attention except in severe cases
Globally impaired cognition	Globally impaired cognition

quired skills, judgment, personality, and social or occupational functioning remain intact.

D. Schizophrenia: Both schizophrenia and dementia cause a deterioration from a previous level of functioning, impaired abstract thinking, and poor judgment. However, although schizophrenia can be of late onset, it typically manifests during adolescence or young adulthood. In addition, patients with schizophrenia have prominent thought disorganization or psychotic symptoms that may fluctuate over time, with cognitive capacity frequently changing with exacerbation of level of illness.

E. Factitious Illness: In factitious disorders, patients present with psychological symptoms in a conscious attempt to mimic psychiatric illness. In these individuals, symptoms are worse when the patient is aware of being observed, and the symptoms are not consistent with what is observed in true dementia. For example, a patient simulating memory impairment will often show equal difficulty with both recent and remote memory, whereas in true dementia recent memory is usually more impaired than remote memory. Also, in true dementia a patient will often be oriented to his or her name but not to time or place; patients with factitious illness often state they do not know their own name, a finding seen only in the very late stages of true dementia.

Diagnosis

In diagnosing a dementia the clinician must first aggressively rule out any potential reversible causes of the disorder. Ideally, a complete history should be obtained from someone who knows the patient well, as well as from the patient. Attention should be paid to medications, drug and alcohol use, onset and course of impairment, as well as psychosocial and medical antecedents. A physical examination should be performed with full neurological evaluation. A comprehensive mental status examination should be performed, as should a standardized cognitive measure such as the MMSE.

The following laboratory tests should be obtained as part of the dementia workup: complete blood count, complete chemistry profile, urinalysis, thyroid function tests, folate and vitamin B_{12} levels, and

VDRL/RPR

syphilis serology. Additional studies are obtained based on history and examination. These may include toxicology screen, sedimentation rate, HIV and Lyme disease serology, heavy metal screen, antinuclear antibody, neuropsychological testing, chest x-ray, lumbar puncture, and neuroimaging. A chest x-ray may assist in determining the presence of pneumonia, congestive heart failure, and chronic obstructive pulmonary disease. Cerebrospinal fluid (CSF) is not routinely evaluated. A lumbar puncture may be performed for cases with unusual presentation (ie, early onset, rapid progression), suspicion of neurosyphilis, neuroborreliosis, or metastatic carcinoma. Recently developed CSF diagnostic markers for Alzheimer's disease include decreased amyloid precursor protein or tau-related markers (eg, Alzheimer 50 antigen). However, the sensitivity and specificity of these tests do not supersede the diagnostic accuracy of a good clinical history and examination. Neuroimaging is not routinely obtained as part of a dementia workup but is often useful. Structural neuroimaging such as computed tomography (CT) or magnetic resonance imaging (MRI) can demonstrate atrophy, white matter ischemic changes, infarcts, space occupying lesions, and normal-pressure hydrocephalus. Quantitative studies of hippocampal atrophy may have some predictive diagnostic value in dementia. Functional imaging such as SPECT or PET provide information on metabolic function by measuring cerebral blood flow or cell uptake of glucose. In Alzheimer's dementia parietotemporal deficits are typically seen earlier than frontal deficits. Parietotemporal hypometabolism and right-left asymmetry are the most consistent findings in functional imaging of Alzheimer's disease. Vascular dementias, on the other hand, show asymmetric cortical and subcortical focal deficits often with a patchy distribution. Functional imaging may also be useful in attempting to differentiate between cognitive deficits due to depression and dementia.

Illustrative Case

The patient was a 65-year-old married and recently retired dentist whose chief complaint was depression. He had experienced a series of professional difficulties over the years, including a prosecution for fraud after billing two insurance companies for the same service. He had never done anything like this in the past, and at a pretrial hearing he claimed he had been confused, and the charges were dropped. The patient later decided to retire and sold his practice impulsively and, as his family thought, improvidently. In retirement, the patient became depressed and suicidal and decided to seek psychiatric help.

The mental status examination showed depressed affect. However, the patient had no vegetative signs and no history of mental illness. He had difficulty finding the psychiatrist's office and went to the wrong part of the building several times. He had problems in recent memory and calculation and could not remember where his daughter lived. A complete medical history revealed that the patient had minor problems with urinary incontinence as well as ataxia. A CT scan revealed ventricular dilatation consistent with normal-pressure hydrocephalus. He was diagnosed with dementia secondary to normal-pressure hydrocephalus. A neurosurgical shunt to divert cerebrospinal fluid from the cerebral ventricular space to the atrium of the heart reversed his dementia as well as his secondary depression.

In the above case, the incident of billing two insurance companies was probably an early sign of deterioration of previously good judgment.

Treatment

A multitiered approach to management of dementia includes psychosocial support to the patient and caregivers and psychopharmacological support to the patient for cognitive, behavioral dysfunction and psychotic or affective symptoms. The main goals of treatment are to optimize function, slow the progression of the dementia, and improve the quality of life. By maximizing functional capacity and improving cognition, mood, and behavior, institutionalization may be prevented or delayed.

A. Psychosocial Treatment of Dementia: There is a wide range of psychosocial strategies used to improve the quality of life and maximize function. These can be classified as cognitive, behavioral, environmental, integration of self, and socialization-enhancing interventions.

Early in dementia, using mnemonic cues, color codes, and other strategies can improve concentration and memory.

Behavioral-oriented approaches include general measures such as structured daytime activity, toileting and exercise schedule, and specific interventions for problem behaviors. Addressing specific behavioral problems can be done by keeping an ABC log: antecedent, behavior, consequence. Using a behavioral diary, an individual may be able to then manipulate the environment so as to prevent the antecedent from occurring. Environmental interventions include music, white noise, natural lighting, low stimulus areas, use of objects with sharp contrasts, and picture cues.

Integration of self-interventions include reminiscence groups, validation therapy (ie, affirm rather than correct patients' false statements), and simulated presence (ie, a care provider, prior to going away, can make a video talking about past shared events with pauses to let the patient respond). Socialization and pleasure-enhancing interventions include art therapy, recreational therapy, intergenerational encounters, and animal therapy.

For a patient with insomnia, a multifaceted psychosocial intervention might include exclusion of daytime napping, exposure to natural lighting or light therapy, regular daytime exercise, a warm bath prior to bedtime, and provision of a dark quiet environment at night.

Caregiver intervention is a critical component of treating dementia. This can include individual and family counseling, education, support groups, and respite services such as an adult day program for the patient. The treating physician should be observant of potential caregiver burnout and depression, which occur frequently.

B. Pharmacological Treatment of Dementia: Pharmacological treatment of dementia can be classified into two types: treatment for slowing the rate of cognitive decline and treatment for psychiatric conditions secondary to dementia, such as depression, psychosis, and agitation.

1. Pharmacological treatment for slowing the rate of cognitive decline—Various mechanisms have been proposed for slowing neuronal cell death or improving the cholinergic deficits associated with AD. These include enhancing neurotransmission with acetylcholinesterase inhibitors, reducing the formation of free radicals with antioxidants, and decreasing the possible inflammatory component of AD with anti-inflammatory drugs. Of these, evidence suggests that the mechanism of enhancing neurotransmission is most effective, and this is currently the primary method used by clinicians.

a. Acetylcholinesterase inhibitors—The cholinergic hypothesis for AD is based on the association between cholinergic cell loss and cognitive decline. Enhancing the cholinergic system has, in fact, been shown to have a mild to moderate positive effect on cognition in 30–50% of patients with AD. Not clear yet is the duration of this effect or whether it affects the rate of cognitive decline.

There are two acetylcholinesterase inhibitors approved for the treatment of mild to moderate AD. These medications inhibit the ability of acetylcholinesterase to degrade acetylcholine in the synapse, thereby increasing concentrations of acetylcholine at muscarinic and nicotinic receptors, both peripherally and in the brain. The first approved acetylcholinesterase inhibitor, tacrine, is currently not readily used because of its potential for liver toxicity, need for blood monitoring, and short inhibitory action resulting in the need for dosing three times per day.

Arcep

Donepezil, a second-generation acetylcholinesterase inhibitor, is the drug of choice: it has fewer risks and side effects than tacrine, as well as a greater ability to cross the blood-brain barrier and longer duration of inhibitory action, with a consequent dosing schedule of one time per day. The recommended starting dose is 5 mg daily, which may be increased to 10 mg daily after 1 month if further improvement is desired. Side effects, which are primarily related to parasympathetic stimulation, include nausea, diarrhea, gastritis, insomnia, muscle cramps, and anorexia. Relative contraindications include reactive airway disease, first-degree heart block, sick sinus syndrome, and peptic ulcer disease. Although both tacrine and donepezil may produce mild but measurable improvement in cognition, they provide symptomatic improvement but do not prevent the inevitable course of neurodegeneration.

Other acetylcholinesterase inhibitors are in clinical trials and may become available in the near future. In addition to enhancing acetylcholine levels, acetylcholinesterase inhibitors may impede disease progression and impede neuronal cell death by enhancing neurotrophic regeneration and slowing the formation of β-amyloid plaques.

b. Antioxidants—It is believed that an excess of oxygen-based free radicals contributes to the development and progression of AD, and taking antioxidants may slow the rate of cognitive decline by impeding neuronal death. Vitamin E, given in an average maintenance dose of 800–1000 units twice a day, is well tolerated and frequently used. Estrogen also appears effective in lowering the likelihood of developing AD, possibly by having neuroprotective properties. Studies have indicated that postmenopausal women who used estrogen had a one-third lower risk of developing AD than nonusers. Women with a history of long-term use had the lowest risk. The use of estrogen is contraindicated in individuals with a history or family history of breast cancer.

c. Anti-inflammatory drugs—Recent research suggests that inflammatory and immune systems are linked to neuronal death in AD. Reactive microglia may induce an immune reaction resulting in the formation of inflammatory cytokines such as interleukin-1 and interleukin-6, which are known to promote the synthesis of β-amyloid protein. Anti-inflammatory agents are currently in clinical trials.

d. Other agents—Additional agents that are being studied for possible neuroprotective effects include nicotine, melatonin, gingko biloba, nerve growth factor, and antiamyloid agents.

2. Pharmacological treatment for related psychiatric conditions—

a. Depression—Major depression is a common comorbid illness of AD, vascular dementia, dementia secondary to Parkinson's disease, and other less common dementias. Based on the severity of dementia, presenting signs and symptoms of depression will vary. The clinician should monitor for change in mood, affective blunting or lability, irritability, neurovegetative signs, change in self-attitude, suicidal thoughts, and abrupt cognitive changes. Depression may be the presenting symptom of a dementia and individuals with cognitive deficits secondary to depression are at increased risk for developing a dementia.

The choice of antidepressants is based on patient medical and psychiatric history and status. Common first-line antidepressants, because of their safety and side effect profile, include the selective serotonergic reuptake inhibitors (SSRIs) such as sertraline, paroxetine, fluoxetine, and citalopram. Alternative first-line antidepressants include bupropion, venlafaxine, and mirtazapine. Tricyclic antidepressants such as nortriptyline, although effective, are less often recommended as first-line drugs because of their anticholinergic property, potential for causing orthostatic hypotension, delayed cardiac conduction, and lethality in overdose. Similarly, monoamine oxidase inhibitors such as phenelzine are not drugs of first choice because of their drug and food interaction risks, including the need to avoid tyramine-containing foods. Stimulants are sometimes used to treat severe apathy or depression, particularly in medically compromised individuals.

b. Psychosis—Psychotic manifestations associated with dementia are delusions and hallucinations. Delusions are frequently of a persecutory nature and tend to address core environmental issues, for instance, accusing a family member of stealing. This is in contrast to the more bizarre delusions commonly seen in schizophrenia. Visual hallucinations occur more frequently than auditory hallucinations, but may be difficult to distinguish from illusions, eg, reflections on windows interpreted as strangers in the house.

When psychotic symptoms cause distress or potentially dangerous behaviors antipsychotic medication is indicated. Historically haloperidol and other high-potency antipsychotics have been used in treating psychosis in dementia. Although usually effective, they frequently cause untoward effects such as akathisia, parkinsonism, and tardive dyskinesia. Because of their anticholinergic properties, lower-potency antipsychotics such as thioridazine are best avoided in treating patients with dementia. The new-generation antipsychotics such as risperidone, quetiapine, and olanzapine are usually effective in diminishing psychotic symptoms and are less likely to cause the side effects seen with high- and low-potency older antipsychotics.

c. Agitation—About 60% of all patients with dementia experience agitation, particularly in the middle and late stages of the disease. Agitation is most commonly associated with frontal, right parietal, and limbic pathology. Agitation implies a wide array of behavioral disturbances including psychomotor activation, restlessness, combativeness, aggression, screaming, cursing, sundowning, and disinhibition. These behaviors, along with incontinence, are often critical factors in leading to placement in a nursing home.

Before addressing agitation pharmacologically, it is imperative to rule out other causes for such behaviors including pain, constipation, insomnia, depression, anxiety, infection or other underlying medical problems, delirium, and side effects from medications such as akathisia. It is also essential to attempt nonpharmacologic intervention prior to resorting to medication.

Although antipsychotics have shown to be effective in treating dementia with behavioral disturbances, they are to be used only if other interventions are ineffective. This is explicitly expressed in the Omnibus Budget Reconciliation Act of 1987 (COBRA, 1987) in terms of treatment of patients in federally financed nursing homes.

Perhaps the safest and most effective drugs for treating agitation and other behavioral disturbances in dementia are those not approved by the Food and Drug Administration for such specific use. Frequently used first-line medications include the anxiolytic buspirone, the antidepressant trazodone (at low doses), and antiepileptic drugs such as valproic acid and gabapentin. Depression may present atypically in dementia as agitation, and will often respond well to an SSRI antidepressant. Benzodiazepines are frequently used in patients with dementia who exhibit agitation or anxiety. However, because of frequent side effects (eg, increased confusion, disinhibition, falls, delirium) they should be used sparingly, in a time-limited fashion, and as a last resort, while attempting to stabilize the patient on other medications.

DELIRIUM

Definition

Delirium is a transient, potentially reversible dysfunction in cerebral metabolism, etiologically related to metabolic derangements, that has an acute or subacute onset and is typically manifested by alterations of levels of consciousness and change in cognition. It is the most common psychiatric syndrome found in a general medical hospital, particularly among older patients.

Numerous physiological insults are potential putative agents for inducing the delirium syndrome. Whether the syndrome develops depends on the vulnerability of the patient's brain and the intensity of the putative agent. Hence, individuals with dementia may develop a delirium when confronted with what otherwise might be a minor insult, such as a urinary tract infection, or the addition of a medication with anticholinergic side effects.

The delirium syndrome may manifest itself in numerous ways, but key to the presentation is a change in the level of consciousness, from a hyperactive

state (ie, increased arousal and psychomotor activity), a hypoactive state (ie, decreased arousal and psychomotor activity), or a mixed form with fluctuations between states.

The *Diagnostic and Statistical Manual of Mental Disorders* (*DSM*) is the key reference regarding the criteria for the diagnosis of delirium. Since its inception in 1952, different editions have contained different criteria (see Table 16–9). The diagnostic features of delirium in the current *DSM* (*DSM-IV*) are as follows:

1. Disturbance of consciousness (ie, reduced clarity of awareness of the environment), with reduced ability to focus, sustain, or shift attention.
2. Change in cognition (such as memory deficit, disorientation, language disturbance) or the development of a perceptual disturbance that is not better accounted for by a preexisting or evolving dementia.
3. The disturbance that develops over a short period of time (usually hours to days) and tends to fluctuate during the course of the day.
4. Evidence from the history, physical examination, or laboratory findings of a general medical condition, substance intoxication or withdrawal and/or medication side effect judged to be etiologically related to the disturbance.

Epidemiology

There are few definitive data on the epidemiology of delirium. Past research has been confounded in part by variability of diagnostic criteria.

Current data indicate that delirium occurs in 10–20% of patients on acute medical/surgical wards. Some authors report that the incidence of delirium in elderly patients presenting to the emergency room is as high as 80%. Delirium is infrequent in the young and middle-aged and, when present, is often associated with alcohol or illicit drug use. The incidence of delirium increases progressively with each decade past the age of 40.

Certain groups are most at risk for developing delirium: (1) elderly patients, (2) patients with preexisting brain damage (eg, dementia, strokes), (3) patients on polypharmacy or withdrawing from addictive substances, and (4) medically compromised patients (eg, individuals with AIDS, burn patients).

Table 16–9. *DSM-IV* diagnostic criteria for delirium.

A. Disturbance of consciousness (ie, reduced clarity of awareness of the environment) with reduced ability to focus, sustain, or shift attention

B. Change in cognition (such as memory deficit, disorientation, language disturbance) or development of a perceptual disturbance that is not better accounted for by a preexisting, established, or evolving dementia

C. The disturbance develops over a short period of time (usually hours to days) and tends to fluctuate during the course of the day

Delirium can be triggered in sick or medically stable patients by environmental changes and psychological stressors. Commonly associated triggers include sensory deprivation, high noise levels, lack of normal diurnal cycles, sleep deprivation, and depression.

The syndrome of delirium is associated with increased morbidity, mortality, rate of institutionalization and length of stay, and cost of hospitalization. As the population ages, with the associated increase in polypharmacy and comorbid diseases, the prevalence of delirium will likely increase. Although classically defined as an acute event, the frail and cognitively impaired may subacutely develop a delirium. Polypharmacy, disruption of sleep-wake cycle, sensory compromise, or other myriad risk factors may have a cumulative effect.

Etiology & Pathogenesis

The etiology of delirium is usually multifactorial, involving both baseline patient vulnerability and the number and severity of insults. Risk factors tend to have multiplicative effects.

As noted, advanced age is one of the most important risk factors for developing delirium. Physiological changes that occur with aging make the elderly person less resistant to stress and acute disease and more susceptible to pharmacological side effects because of impairment of drug distribution, metabolism, and excretion. Albumin levels in elderly adults are decreased, and allow more unbound drug to circulate. Age-related decreases in liver blood flow and hepatic enzyme function lower drug metabolism. Renal blood flow, number of functional glomeruli, and creatinine clearance are decreased, decreasing renal excretion. The normal age-related changes in the brain that increase vulnerability to delirium include loss of neurons, with associated lowering of neurotransmitter levels, particularly dopamine and acetylcholine.

The physiological basis of delirium is poorly understood. Several theories exist including failure of cerebral oxidative metabolism with a subsequent decrease in neurotransmitter production. By reversing cerebral hypoxia, clinical manifestations of delirium, such as

confusion, and diffuse background electroencephalogram slowing (alpha activity) can be reversed. There are also data to support cholinergic dysfunction as an etiology of delirium. Anticholinergic drugs and AD, both associated with low levels of cerebral acetylcholine, place patients at increased risk for delirium. Currently, cholinergic medications such as donepezil are being examined in clinical trials in delirium.

Lymphokines have been shown to influence delirium in individuals with inflammation and infection. Cancer patients treated with interleukin-2 and lymphokine-activated killer cells have a 50% chance of developing delirium. Symptoms are dose related and cease after discontinuing therapy.

The diagnosis of delirium is all the more difficult because of the variability of presentation in a frail individual with preexisting physiological and neuropsychiatric vulnerabilities. For instance, an elderly individual with agitated behavior may be found to have a low hematocrit, cardiac failure, pulmonary insufficiency, and chronic pain from arthritis. Each clinical finding may be a potential contributor to an apparent delirium. If this individual had a preexisting dementia and was on multiple medications, the presentation, which is not uncommon, becomes more complicated.

It is imperative that the clinician organize the potential causes of delirium into a usable diagnostic hierarchy. Some of the numerous causative factors for delirium will be reviewed using the mnemonic "I WATCH DEATH" (see Table 16–10).

A. Infections: Infections are a common cause of delirium. The extent of the neuropsychiatric effect of an infection is largely contingent on the preexisting neurological vulnerability of the individual. Sepsis may cause a delirium in any individual, whereas a urinary tract infection is more likely to induce a delirium in a frail elderly individual.

In addition to extracranial sources of infection such as pneumonia or urinary tract infection, less common intracranial infections such as meningitis or encephalitis need also be considered in the differential diagnosis. Meningitis and encephalitis are typically acute febrile illnesses often associated with nonspecific neurological signs such as a stiff neck.

Table 16–10. Causative factors for delirium.

Causative Factor	Examples
Infection	Meningitis, encephalitis, systemic infection
Withdrawal	Alcohol, benzodiazepines, barbiturates
Acute metabolic	Electrolyte and acid-base abnormalities, renal disease, hepatic disease, postoperative state
Trauma	Concussion, heat stroke, severe burns
CNS pathology	Cerebrovascular accident, seizure, subdural or subarachnoid hemorrhage, neoplasms, infections
Hypoxia	Anemia, cardiac failure, respiratory failure, hypotension, pulmonary embolus, carbon monoxide poisoning
Deficiencies	Vitamin B_{12}, folate, thiamine
Endocrinopathies	Hyper- or hypothyroidism, hyper- or hypocortisolism, hypoglycemia
Acute vascular	Septic shock, hypertensive encephalopathy
Toxins or drugs	Amphetamines, anticholinergics, anticonvulsants, antihistamines, clonidine, digitalis, hallucinogenics, levodopa, narcotics
Heavy metals	Arsenic, lead, manganese, mercury

B. Withdrawal: Withdrawal from alcohol as well as other potentially physiologically addicting drugs such as benzodiazepines and barbiturates can cause delirium. A chronic elderly alcoholic with poor social support and nutritional status is at risk for developing Wernicke's encephalopathy, which may manifest as confusion, ataxia, and ophthalmoplegia (eg, lateral gaze paresis). As Wernicke's encephalopathy is the result of thiamine deficiency, prompt treatment with thiamine is critical. Korsakoff's syndrome, a potentially permanent amnestic disorder, may be a sequelae of Wernicke's encephalopathy.

The following information can be of help in evaluating whether an individual is withdrawing from ethanol:

1. History of ethanol use, including average use and last drink. History of blackouts, delirium tremens, or seizures.
2. Medical complications associated with alcohol use such as elevated liver function enzymes (with aspartate aminotransferase typically greater than alanine aminotransferase), elevated mean corpuscular volume (MCV) and related macrocytic anemia, cirrhosis or evidence of chronic liver failure such as ascites, decreased albumin, or increased coagulation time.
3. Physical examination indicative of a hyperadrenergic state such as hypertension, tachycardia, tremor, diaphoresis, pupillary constriction, and hyperreflexia.

With regard to withdrawal from other drugs (such as benzodiazepines), delirium is commonly an unintended iatrogenic epiphenomenon that warrants regular review of drug intake and appropriate toxicology screen.

C. Acute Metabolic: Electrolyte disturbances are most commonly associated with dehydration due to impaired thirst mechanisms, mobility, and access to water. Particularly vulnerable are medically compromised individuals with possible dehydration, renal or hepatic failure, or nutritional deficiencies.

D. Trauma: Individuals who have sustained focal neurological trauma such as a concussion, or those with systemic trauma such as heat stroke, severe burns, or invasive surgery, are at increased risk for developing delirium.

E. CNS Pathology: Less than 10% of all cases of delirium are due to acute CNS lesions. Examples of CNS insults that can lead to delirium are stroke, subdural hemorrhage, subarachnoid hemorrhage, neoplasms (both primary and metastatic), aneurysms, abscesses, parasitic cysts, seizures, postelectroconvulsive therapy, vasculitis, hydrocephalus, and infections. For example, consider the possibility of a subarachnoid hemorrhage in a delirious individual who had a brief period of unconsciousness followed by a headache. Stroke patients are at higher risk for developing delirium if the stroke occurred in the inferior temporooc-

cipital, right parietal, or right prefrontal regions as these areas are involved with attention capacity.

F. Hypoxia: Cerebral hypoxia predisposes individuals to developing delirium. Patients should be assessed for anemia, cardiac failure, hypotension, respiratory failure, pulmonary embolism, and carbon monoxide poisoning. Vital signs, physical examination, hematocrit, and arterial blood gas can assist with the determination of cerebral hypoxia.

G. Deficiencies: Nutritional deficiencies are particularly common among the very young and old as well as with alcoholics and medically compromised patients.

H. Endocrinopathies: Examples of endocrinopathies that can induce delirium include diabetes mellitus (hyper- or hypoglycemia), Graves' disease (hyperthyroidism), and Addison's disease (hypoadrenocortisolism).

I. Acute Vascular: Examples of acute vascular events that can cause delirium are shock and hypertensive encephalopathy.

J. Toxins or Drugs: Medications are one of the most common causes of delirium, particularly in elderly individuals. Table 16–11 lists some of the classes of medication that most commonly cause delirium. The most regularly associated classes of drugs are anticholinergics, sedative hypnotics, and narcotics. Commonly used medications with anticholinergic properties include antiparkinsonian medications, such as trihexiphenidyl; tricyclic antidepressants, such as amitriptyline; low-potency antipsychotics, such as chlorpromazine; antihistamines, such as diphenhydramine; over-the-counter sleep aids, which frequently contain diphenhydramine; and bladder antispasmodics, such as oxybutynin. Classical anticholinergic effects include peripheral vasodilation (red), anhidrosis and dry mucous membranes (dry), delirium (mad), and impaired visual accommodation (blind). Thus the saying: "red as a beet, dry as a bone, mad as a hatter, and blind as a bat." Unfortunately for the clinician, the presentation of an anticholinergic-induced delirium is typically more subtle, often with only a change in behavior or mild confusion. It cannot be stressed enough that diphenhydramine is not a benign sleep aid, despite being available over the counter, and is a potent precipitant of delirium.

K. Heavy Metals: Last in the "I WATCH DEATH" mnemonic are the heavy metals, such as ar-

Table 16–11. Classes of medication that cause delirium.

Anticholinergics *benadryl, anti psychotic, atropine, Parkinson's*
Benzodiazepines
Cimetidine
Alcohol
Nonsteroidal anti-inflammatories
Cardiac drugs: digoxin, β-blockers, diuretics
Centrally acting antihypertensives
Narcotics
Other central nervous system depressants

senic, lead, manganese, and mercury. If clinical suspicion arises, heavy metal analysis should be performed.

Differential Diagnosis

Other brain disorders and some psychiatric disorders can present with signs and symptoms resembling delirium. Examples of organic brain disorders that may mimic delirium are Charles Bonnet syndrome (isolated visual hallucinosis), partial complex seizures, and absence seizures. Psychiatric conditions that may mimic delirium include dementia, major depression, schizophrenia, and delusional disorder. Of these, the hardest differential diagnosis is often between delirium and dementia. This is complicated by the fact that over 50% of hospitalized patients with dementia may also have delirium. Table 16–12 lists some important distinctions between the two disorders.

Diagnosis

The diagnosis of delirium is purely clinical. Delirium often goes unrecognized as the symptoms can be subtle and fluctuate through the course of the day. As many as 19 of 20 delirious patients are not accurately diagnosed.

A detailed history should always be obtained, when possible from collateral sources. This should include baseline cognitive capacity and recent cognitive and behavioral changes. A full medical and psychiatric history should also be obtained. Attention should be given to recent trauma, exposure to infections, medication use, including over-the-counter drugs, and alcohol and illicit drug use.

Mental status testing is essential, including a test of cognitive ability such as the Folstein Mini-Mental Status Examination (MMSE). This is a brief structured test of cognitive function used as a screening tool for cognitive impairment and organic mental disorders. It has a sensitivity of 82% and a specificity of 87%, but does not differentiate between delirium and dementia. In addition, baseline measures are influenced by level of education and cultural background. To follow the fluctuating course of delirium, serial MMSEs can be instructive. Another test, the Delirium Rating Scale, can be used to assist in differentiating delirium from dementia.

A diagnostic physical examination should include vital signs, cardiac and respiratory status, and upper motor neuron and other focal neurological functioning.

Diagnostic tests should be ordered to screen for common causes of delirium. General tests include toxicology screening, complete blood count with differential, chemistry profile including magnesium, phosphorus, and calcium, liver function studies, urinalysis, blood culture, electrocardiogram, chest x-ray, and either arterial blood gas or pulse oximetry.

Other studies such as thyroid function tests, syphilis serology, HIV serology, lumbar puncture, electroencephalogram, and neuroimaging are not routinely performed, but are carried out when clinically indicated.

Illustrative Case

A 43-year-old woman brought to the hospital by members of her family reported that during the few days just prior to admission she had become increasingly frightened and suspicious. The patient felt that her upstairs neighbors were threatening her and that it was unsafe to be at home. She said she had seen babies being lowered from the window of the upstairs apartment. Her family stated that these ideas had no basis in reality.

On initial mental status examination, the patient was agitated and frightened, had pressured speech, and was preoccupied with persecutory ideas. She was fully oriented to time and place, and her memory was intact. The admitting third-year medical student and resident diagnosed her with a psychotic disorder, not otherwise specified, and did not (at the time of admission) suspect a delirium.

On the first day of hospitalization, the patient's mental status changed markedly. It appeared first to improve but then worsened. She became more agitated and disoriented. She developed visual hallucinations (she saw her mother in her hospital room), illusions (shadows on the wall were misinterpreted as a person), and problems in memory (she could not recall three objects). In addition, she became tremulous, tachycardiac, diaphoretic, and hypertensive.

Urine screen showed high barbiturate levels; however, the patient denied drug use. A diagnosis of barbiturate withdrawal delirium was made, and the pa-

Table 16–12. Delirium versus dementia.

	Delirium	Dementia
Onset	Rapid	Slow and progressive
Reversibility	Potentially reversible	Usually not reversible
Deficits	Focal cognitive	Global cognitive
	Affects attention primarily	Affects memory primarily in early stages
	Fluctuating level of awareness	Level of awareness usually intact in early stages
	Fluctuating level of attention	Level of attention usually intact in early stages
Course	Fluctuating and variable over course of day	Typically no acute daytime fluctuations
Urgency	Needs immediate medical workup	Nonurgent

tient was successfully treated with gradually decreasing doses of barbiturates to prevent seizures.

Treatment

The treatment of delirium involves treating the primary causative condition, providing supportive care, and preventing injurious behaviors.

General principles of managing delirium are used for all patients. These include providing fluids and nutrition, providing a calm quiet environment, and establishing appropriate sleep cycles. The patient needs to be frequently reoriented and explanations should be given for almost all activity involving the patient.

It is preferable to avoid restraining a delirious patient who is agitated. However, either physical or pharmacological restraints may be necessary when behavioral and supportive measures are ineffective. The risks of physical restraints include increased agitation, increased risk for decubiti, and strangulation. Frequently, around the clock sitters (including friends and family) may reduce the need for restraints by reorienting and reassuring the patient. Although the hospital may balk at the cost of a 24-hour sitter, it can be advocated as cost effective if it decreases the patient's length of stay and comorbidity.

Pharmacological intervention is sometimes necessary. There is no ideal drug for delirium and some drugs used to treat delirium, such as benzodiazepines, can exacerbate rather than alleviate the symptoms being addressed. However, for delirium secondary to alcohol or sedative hypnotic withdrawal, benzodiazepines are the drug of choice. Haloperidol, a high-potency antipsychotic, is commonly used to treat agitation due to delirium. Haldoperidol, although effective, may have untoward effects including extrapyramidal symptoms and neuroleptic malignant syndrome. For severe agitation, a dose of up to 5 mg haloperidol intramuscularly or intravenously can be given every 6–8 hours and may be doubled every 30 minutes until behavioral control is achieved, up to a maximum bolus of 40 mg. Once the patient is sleepy but arousable the dose can be halved and given every 12 hours. The drug can then be tapered as clinically indicated. Dosing is typically much lower in elderly patients. Newer antipsychotics such as quetiapine, olanzapine, and risperidone can be used to treat agitation and carry fewer risks and side effects than haloperidol, but can be administered only orally.

Prognosis

Delirium carries a high risk of morbidity and mortality, long-term institutional placement, and cognitive decline. Many cases of subclinical dementia are unmasked by delirium. Consequences of the immobility and confusion associated with delirium include dehydration, malnutrition, and decubiti. Among delirious hospitalized medical patients mortality is as high as 20–40%.

Many delirious patients recover their premorbid cognitive functioning completely when the delirium is reversed. Those most likely to fully recover are patients with identifiable and completely treated medical conditions such as an infection and those with drug-induced delirium.

AMNESTIC DISORDERS

Definition

In the *DSM-IV* amnestic disorders are characterized by the development of memory impairment, as manifested by a decrease in the ability to learn new information or the inability to recall previously learned information, in the absence of other significant cognitive impairment (see Table 16–13). This memory disturbance must cause a significant decline in social or occupational functioning. The diagnosis of amnestic disorder cannot be made when a patient has dementia or delirium. Amnestic disorders are differentiated from dissociative disorders such as dissociative identity disorder by the presence of a causally related medical condition, such as head trauma or carbon monoxide poisoning. Table 16–14 lists some medical conditions known to cause amnestic disorder. Substance-induced persisting amnestic disorder is an additional *DSM-IV* diagnosis, and it has the same criteria except that the disorder is caused by substance use (eg, alcohol, drugs of abuse, medications). These disorders are classified as transient, if the memory impairment lasts for 1 month or less, or chronic, if the duration is for more than 1 month.

Epidemiology

Amnestic disorder is relatively uncommon. No adequate studies exist on the incidence or prevalence of amnestic disorders. Amnesia is most commonly found in alcohol use disorders and in head injury. Recent trends suggest a decrease in the frequency of amnesia related to chronic alcohol use and an increase in the frequency of amnesia secondary to head trauma.

Table 16–13. *DSM-IV* diagnostic criteria for amnestic disorder related to a general medical condition.

A. The development of memory impairment as manifested by the inability to learn new information or the inability to recall previously learned information

B. The memory disturbance causes significant impairment in social or occupational functioning and represents a significant decline from a previous level of functioning

C. The memory disturbance does not occur exclusively during the course of delirium or dementia

D. There is evidence from the history, physical examination, or laboratory findings of a general medical condition (including physical trauma) judged to be etiologically related to the memory impairment

Table 16–14. Causes of amnestic disorder.

Korsakoff's syndrome (thiamine deficiency)
Brain trauma
Cerebral anoxia
   Cardiac arrest
   Acute respiratory failure
   Anesthetic accident
   Carbon monoxide poisoning
   Drowning
   Strangulation
Space-occupying lesions
   Neoplasms
   Abscess
   Subarachnoid hemorrhage
Cerebrovascular accident
   Infarction of posterior cerebral artery distribution
   Bilateral hippocampal infarction
Infection
   Herpes simplex virus encephalitis
   Tuberculous meningitis
Electroconvulsive therapy (ECT)
Temporal lobe epilepsy
Transient global amnesia
Acute hypoglycemia
Substance induced
   Anticholinergic agents
   Benzodiazepines
   Heavy metal poisoning

Etiology & Pathogenesis

The major neuroanatomical structures involved in memory and in the development of amnestic disorders are diencephalic structures such as the thalamus (dorsomedial and midline nuclei) and medial temporal lobe structures, such as the hippocampus, mamillary bodies, and amygdala. Although amnesia usually results from bilateral injury to these structures, unilateral damage, particularly of the left hemisphere, may also result in amnesia. Other anatomical regions may also be involved in the symptoms seen in amnesia, eg, confabulation and apathy are often seen with frontal lobe damage.

Among alcoholics, the most common cause of amnestic disorder is thiamine deficiency. The nutritional deficiency causes Wernicke's encephalopathy and Korsakoff's syndrome. Other causes of thiamine deficiency include starvation, carcinoma of the stomach, hemodialysis, prolonged intravenous hyperalimentation, hyperemesis gravidarum, and gastric plication. Neuroanatomical lesions seen in Korsakoff's syndrome involve the mamillary bodies, thalamic nuclei (dorsomedial, anteroventral, and pulvinar nuclei), and often the terminal portions of the formix. Histopathological findings include small blood vessel hyperplasia and hemorrhages, hypertrophy of astrocytes, and axonal changes. Korsakoff's syndrome is often preceded by Wernicke's encephalopathy, a syndrome manifested by confusion, ataxia, and ophthalmoplegia. Although the confusion of Wernicke's encephalopathy typically resolves within a month, Korsakoff's amnestic syndrome accompanies or follows untreated Wernicke's encephalopathy in 85% of all cases. The onset of Korsakoff's syndrome is often gradual, with recent memory affected more than remote memory. Individuals often appear passive or apathetic and may confabulate. One-third to one-fourth of patients with Korsakoff's syndrome gradually recover completely within a year if thiamine is promptly administered. One-fourth have no improvement in their symptoms.

Other causes of amnestic syndromes include head trauma (both closed and penetrating), cerebrovascular disease, multiple sclerosis, hypoxia (including carbon monoxide poisoning), hypoglycemia, herpes simplex encephalitis, space-occupying lesions, medications (particularly benzodiazepines), seizures, and electroconvulsive therapy.

Amnesia secondary to electroconvulsive therapy is typically retrograde for approximately 5 minutes before treatment and antegrade for about 5 hours following treatment. Mild memory deficit may continue for up to 9 months following termination of electroconvulsive therapy, but these deficits are usually subtle and there are no data to support the claim of permanent amnesia.

Transient global amnesia is a variant of amnestic disorder. It is characterized by the acute onset of retrograde and antegrade amnesia, which typically resolves within 6–24 hours. Often individuals with transient global amnesia have a clear sensorium and lack insight into their condition. Transient global amnesia is presumed to be a cerebrovascular disorder involving transient impairment in blood flow through the vertebrobasilar arteries resulting in ischemia to the temporal lobe and diencephalic regions. Some cases of transient global amnesia are associated with epilepsy, migraine headache, and hypertension. Although patients with transient global amnesia tend to improve completely, approximately 20% will have a recurrence.

Differential Diagnosis

Before diagnosing amnestic disorder clinicians should rule out more common causes of memory impairment such as normal aging, dementia, and delirium.

With normal aging memory impairment may occur, but with no accompanying impairment in social or occupational functioning. With dementia, memory loss occurs alongside other cognitive deficits. In delirium, memory loss is accompanied by impairment in attention and concentration.

Other disorders that may resemble an amnestic disorder include the dissociative disorders, factitious disorder, and malingering. Unlike amnestic disorder, these disorders often present with selective or inconsistent memory deficits. For instance, individuals with dissociative disorder may lose orientation to self, which is uncommon with amnestic syndromes. In addition, individuals with these conditions typically do not have an underlying medical condition and usually do have underlying intrapsychic and psychosocial stressors.

Diagnosis

To be diagnosed with amnestic disorder an individual must have impairment in memory and new learning with otherwise preserved intellectual functioning. Memory loss is antegrade or retrograde. In antegrade amnesia memory impairment is of events following neurologic insult. In retrograde amnesia memory impairment is of events preceding the insult. The amnestic period may start from the point of trauma or may include memory preceding the trauma.

Typically short-term and recent memory are impaired, whereas long-term and immediate memory tend to remain intact. Recent memory involves the ability to retain new material after attention is distracted, eg, recalling three objects after 3 minutes. Immediate memory involves the ability to retain new information without disturbing attention, eg, repeating five digits backward. Whereas orientation to place and time may be impaired in severe amnesia, orientation to person is rarely lost. The more remote the memory the less likely it will be impaired.

The onset of symptoms may be sudden, as in head trauma, or gradual, as in thiamine deficiency. Patients may also appear bewildered and may attempt to hide their confusion by confabulating or making up memories. Insight is usually poor and there may be subtle or gross changes in personality.

The course and prognosis of an amnestic disorder are variable and contingent on the specific cause. The onset may be sudden or gradual, the symptoms may be transient or persistent, and the outcome can range from complete recovery to permanent amnesia.

Transient amnestic disorder with full recovery can be seen in electroconvulsive therapy, benzodiazepine use, and epilepsy. Cases in which permanent amnesia often follows include head trauma, carbon monoxide poisoning, and herpes simplex encephalitis.

Illustrative Case

The patient was a 28-year-old married construction worker who was transferred to the psychiatric hospital from a medical ward. Ten days before admission, after learning that his wife was having an affair, he went to the basement and hanged himself with a rope looped over a water pipe. His wife saw him hanging and became confused about what to do. She tried unsuccessfully to burn the rope with a match and then ran to a neighbor for help. By the time the patient was cut down, he had suffered pulmonary and cardiac arrest and had dilated pupils. He had been hanging by the neck for about 10 minutes. He was resuscitated and was having spontaneous respirations within 24 hours of the anoxic episode. Ten days later, he was transferred to the psychiatric unit. Initial mental status examination revealed a patient who was conscious, alert, and feeding himself. He was oriented to self but disoriented as to place and time. Reading, writing, and spelling were not affected.

The patient was able to repeat six digits forward. However, his recent memory was impaired, and he was unable to recall any of three objects after 5 minutes. Remote memory was also impaired; he did not know he was married and remembered nothing about the suicide attempt. He did not remember past presidents or details of his work history. His distant memory was better, in that he remembered his birthplace and some details of his early life, eg, physical punishment by his stepfather. He was also able to abstract proverbs.

Physical and neurological examinations were within normal limits except for an elevated right hemidiaphragm and right upper extremity weakness from the traction injury of the patient's upper brachial plexus, primarily the C5 root. This weakness improved during the course of his 2-week hospitalization, although the memory impairment remained. The patient was transferred to a long-term rehabilitation hospital. When evaluated 3 months later, he was able to learn new material but had no memory for the period during which he was not storing new information. Remote memory had also improved, and he was able to remember more details of his past life.

This patient met criteria for a diagnosis of amnestic disorder caused by anoxia.

Treatment

Treatment of an amnestic disorder must begin, whenever possible, with identifying and treating the underlying cause, for instance, giving thiamine to an individual with chronic alcohol use who is at risk for Wernicke's encephalopathy and Korsakoff's syndrome. Typically, in such a case, 100 mg of thiamine per day is given intramuscularly for the first 3 days, followed by 100 mg of thiamine per day given orally until nutritional status improves.

Otherwise, treatment is typically supportive, including psychodynamic and cognitive-behavioral therapy, and educating patients and their families.

SUMMARY

Important points relevant to the diagnosis and treatment of the disorders discussed in this chapter compared to primary psychiatric disorders can be summarized as follows:

1. It is often difficult by clinical presentation to determine whether psychiatric symptoms are caused by dementia, delirium, amnesia, or another cognitive disorder, are secondary to a general medical condition or are substance induced, or are part of a primary psychiatric disorder. Symptoms and signs that point toward a diagno-

sis of a cognitive or secondary psychiatric disorder are reviewed at the beginning of this chapter.

2. A vigorous search for an underlying cause for the presenting psychiatric symptoms is important in any case in which a diagnosis other than a primary psychiatric disorder is suspected. If a specific cause is identified and is treatable,

some or all of the psychiatric symptoms may be reversible.

3. In addition to identifying and treating any underlying cause, important aspects of treatment include supportive care, education of patients and their families, and the judicious use of psychoactive medications to control psychiatric symptoms.

REFERENCES & SUGGESTED READINGS

Arnold SE, Kumar A: Reversible dementias. Med Clin North Am 1993;77:215.

Bender KJ: Treating behavioral and cognitive symptoms of Alzheimer's disease. Psychiatric Times (Supplement) 1–4, August 1998.

Bennett DA, Knopman DS: Alzheimer's disease: A comprehensive approach to patient management. Geriatrics 1994;49:20.

Blass JP, Wisniewski HM: Pathology of Alzheimer's disease. Psychiatr Clin North Am 1991;14:397.

Cantillon M, De La Puente AM, Palmer BW: Psychosis in Alzheimer's disease. Sem Clin Neuropsychiatry 1998; 3:34.

Cooper JK: Drug treatment of Alzheimer's disease. Arch Intern Med 1991;151:245.

Erickson KR: Amnestic disorders: Pathophysiology and patterns of memory dysfunction. West J Med 1990;152:159.

Erkinjuntti T, Sulkava R: Diagnosis of multi-infarct dementia. Alzheimer Dis Assoc Dis 1991;5:112.

Fish DN: Treatment of delirium in the critically ill patient. Clin Pharmacol 1991;10:456.

Folstein MF, Folstein SE, McHugh PR: Mini-Mental State: A practical method for grading the cognitive state for the clinician. J Psychiatr Res 1975;12:189.

Gambert SR: Alzheimer's disease: When to initiate treatment and what to expect. Clin Geriatr 1998;6:42.

Hales RE, Yudofsky SC, Silver JM: Treatment of aggression and agitation in the elderly. Clin Geriatr 1995;3:49.

Lipowski ZJ: Update on delirium. Psychiatr Clin North Am 1992;15:335.

McDonald WM, Nemeroff CB: Neurotransmitters and neuropeptides in Alzheimer's disease. Psychiatr Clin North Am 1991;14:421.

Mirski DF, Brawman-Mintzer O, Mintzer JE: Pharmacological treatment of aggressive agitation in patients with AD. Clin Geriatr 1998;6:47.

Musselman DL, Hawthorne CN, Stoudemire A: Screening for delirium: A means to improved outcome in hospitalized elderly patients. Rev Clin Gerontol 1997;7:235.

Progress Report on Alzheimer's Disease. Alzheimer's Disease Education and Referral (ADEAR) Center. NIA, NIH Pub. No. 99-3616, 1998.

Reuter JB, Girard DE, Cooney TG: Wernicke's encephalopathy. New Engl J Med 1985;312:1035.

Shua-Haim JR, Sabo MR, Ross JS: Delirium in the elderly. Clin Geriatr 1999;7:47.

Siu AL: Screening for dementia and investigating its causes. Ann Intern Med 1991;115:122.

Small GW, Rabins PV, Barry PP et al: Diagnosis and treatment of Alzheimer's disease and related disorders. JAMA 1997;278:1363.

Webster J: Recognition and treatment of dementing disorders in the elderly. Clin Geriatr 1999;7:61.

17 Substance-Related Disorders: Alcohol & Drugs

H. Westley Clark, MD, JD, MPH, Terry Michael McClanahan, MA, Nick Kanas, MD,
David Smith, MD, & Mim J. Landry

of drinkers 30% binge
10% heavy drinkers

Alcoholism and drug abuse are major problems in the United States. Clinically, the correct terminology for alcoholism and drug abuse is "psychoactive substance use disorders" or, more recently, "substance-related disorders." The epidemiology of substance-related disorders varies. Approximately 111 million Americans age 12 and older used alcohol in 1997. Of that number, 32 million were binge drinkers and 11 million were heavy drinkers (Substance Abuse and Mental Health Services Administration [SAMHSA], 1998). At the same time nearly 24.2 million Americans used illicit substances. These included heroin, cocaine, marijuana, phencyclidine (PCP), LSD, methamphetamine, and other drugs. This number does not include those who smoke cigarettes or drink caffeine-based products excessively.

The *Diagnostic and Statistical Manual of Mental Disorders,* 4th edition (*DSM-IV*) defines substance-related disorders in broad and functional terms, encompassing both alcoholism and drug abuse. This approach allows the clinician to ask similar questions about any substance in deciding whether the patient shows evidence of dependence or abuse. Specific measures are designed to address alcoholism as a separate diagnostic entity, of course, while other measures are designed to address different drugs of abuse.

No single cause exists for the development of substance-related disorders: biomedical, psychological, and social factors all play a role (Figure 17–1). Stressful events sometimes serve as catalysts for drinking and drug-using behavior. For many drugs, increased use can lead to both psychological and physical dependence, which results in a number of important biomedical, psychological, and social sequelae. For alcoholism, these may be cirrhosis, depression, and marital and occupational problems; for other drugs, such as cocaine dependency, these may be myocardial infarction, depression, and marital, legal, and occupational problems.

Alcoholism has been characterized as a primary chronic disease with genetic, psychosocial, and environmental factors influencing its development and manifestations. It is often progressive and fatal. Alcoholism is characterized by impaired control over drinking, preoccupation with the drug (alcohol), use of alcohol despite adverse consequences, distortion in

thinking, and denial of either excessive drinking or its sequelae. Each of these symptoms may be continuous or periodic. Drug abuse can also be characterized in genetic, psychosocial, and environmental terms. The disease process is progressive, although not as often fatal, if cigarette smoking is excluded. Substance abuse can simply be defined as using a psychoactive substance drug to such an extent that it interferes with health, occupational, or social function.

DIAGNOSIS

Alcoholism and drug abuse or dependence must be distinguished from mere use, although some have described any use of illicit psychoactive substances as drug abuse. Without the psychosocial dysfunction associated with the more narrow view of drug abuse, however, the clinician may get caught in a struggle with the patient over the larger social view of the appropriateness of certain behaviors. The sequelae of alcohol and drug abuse are stressful and lead to more alcohol or drug abuse, further dependence, and additional sequelae—and the cycle continues. Treatment for alcohol and drug abuse follows a similar pattern: target the stage of dependence on the psychoactive substance, target the important sequelae, and, finally, explore and modify predisposing causes. The exception to this strategy occurs in maintenance therapies, such as methadone maintenance for people dependent on opioids or nicotine maintenance for people dependent on nicotine. In the case of maintenance therapies, the use of approved pharmacological agents occurs in conjunction with psychosocial interventions. The clinician needs to remember that many patients, if not the majority, use multiple psychoactive substances. Therefore, a patient who presents with one substance, such as cocaine abuse, may actually need urgent intervention for alcohol withdrawal prior to continuing treatment for cocaine.

DIAGNOSTIC WORKUP

Some of the effects of alcohol and drug abuse are encompassed in the *DSM-IV* criteria for substance de-

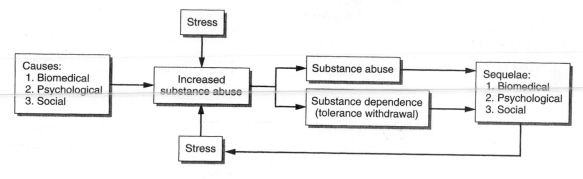

Figure 17–1. A conceptual model of substance abuse.

pendence and abuse (see Table 17–1). Table 17–2 lists several biomedical, psychological, and social complications of alcoholism, which are quite similar to those of drug abuse. There are, however, sequelae specific to a given drug or route of administration. Hyperthermia may occur with cocaine abuse, but not with benzodiazepine abuse; abscesses may occur with injection drug use (eg, heroin, cocaine, or methamphetamine), but not with drugs that are smoked; seizures may occur with cocaine intoxication and with benzodiazepine withdrawal. The clinician should be aware that with psychoactive substances, signs and symptoms may occur that are characteristic of the intoxication state, the withdrawal states, and chronic use. These signs and symptoms vary according to the state in which the patient presents. The *DSM-IV* lists intoxication states for all major substances except nicotine (Table 17–3). It lists no withdrawal states for caffeine, cannabis, hallucinogens, inhalants, or phencyclidine. Clinically, however, a withdrawal state is associated with caffeine.

History

A complete history and a mental status examination are essential to the workup (Clark and McClanahan, 1998). While obtaining the history the possibility of substance abuse is explored by inquiring, in a nonjudgmental manner, about the consumption of alcohol and other drugs of abuse. The setting in which the patient presents can inform the practitioner about an approach to the alcohol or drug question. A patient presenting in an emergency situation may respond to questions differently than one presenting for nonemergency treatment. Patients often understate their use of psychoactive substances and may deny any relationship between these substances and their presenting problems. Other patients seeking more powerful drugs or hospitalization, conversely may overstate their use of psychoactive substances. Consequently, knowledge of which substance produces which psychological symptoms enables the clinician to focus questions about the psychoactive substance. A history of blackouts, morning tremor, and marital

or job problems, for example, should alert the clinician to the possibility of alcoholism. Alternatively, a history of hyperactivity, paranoia, or psychosis may suggest the use of amphetamines or cocaine. How the question about substance abuse is posed to the patient is important: the inquiry should initially be in general terms, then, gradually, become more specific. Indirect questions such as "How much alcohol do you drink daily?" or "Have you ever used cocaine?" are less threatening initially than direct questions such as, "Is alcohol or is cocaine a problem for you?" If alcoholism or other drug abuse is suspected, an interview with a spouse, family members, or friends is indicated.

Type of Substance or Substances Used

Patients may readily acknowledge using licit substances, such as products containing alcohol or nicotine, or taking prescription medications, but may be reluctant to acknowledge misuse. The clinician must inquire about the following:

- alcohol, cigarettes, or other products containing nicotine;
- sedative-hypnotics, particularly benzodiazepines and barbiturates;
- opiates and opioids;
- stimulants, such as amphetamines and cocaine;
- and hallucinogens, including substances as diverse as LSD, PCP, and cannabis.

Table 17–1 outlines the *DSM-IV* criteria for abuse of (and dependence on) these substances in general, including polysubstance abuse. Because polysubstance abuse is increasing among substance abusers, asking about the use of multiple substances is critical when confronted by a patient in whom the use of psychoactive substances must be assessed.

Level of Psychoactive Substance Consumption

In 1995, beer accounted for 57.4% of the per capita alcohol consumed, liquor for 29.6%, and wine

Table 17–1. *DSM-IV* diagnostic criteria for substance-related disorders.

DEPENDENCE AND ABUSE
Substance Dependence

A maladaptive pattern of substance use, leading to clinically significant impairment or distress, as manifested by three or more of the following occurring at any time in the same 12-month period:
(1) tolerance, as defined by either of the following:
    (a) need for markedly increased amounts of the substance to achieve intoxication or desired effect
    (b) markedly diminished effect with continued use of the same amount of the substance
(2) withdrawal, as manifested by either of the following:
    (a) the characteristic withdrawal syndrome for the substance (refer to criteria A and B of the Criteria sets for withdrawal from the specific substances)
    (b) the same (or closely related) substance is taken to relieve or avoid withdrawal symptoms
(3) the substance is often taken in larger amounts or over a longer period than was intended
(4) a persistent desire or unsuccessful efforts to cut down or control substance use
(5) a great deal of time is spent in activities necessary to obtain the substance (eg, visiting multiple doctors or driving long distances), use the substance (eg, chain smoking), or recover from its effects
(6) important social, occupational, or recreational activities given up or reduced because of substance use
(7) continued substance use despite knowledge of having had a persistent or recurrent physical or psychological problem that was likely to have been caused or exacerbated by the substance (eg, current cocaine use despite recognition of cocaine-induced depression, or continued drinking despite recognition that an ulcer was made worse by alcohol consumption)

Specify if:
With Physiological Dependence: Evidence of tolerance or withdrawal (ie, either item (1) or (2) is present).
Without Physiological Dependence: No evidence of tolerance or withdrawal (ie, neither item (1) nor (2) is present).
There are modifiers that address the issue of course. First, it is most important to recognize that once a person has ever had a pattern of substance use that meets criteria for dependence, the person can no longer qualify for a diagnosis of abuse for that substance. However, the patient may meet criteria for early remission, full or partial, or sustained remission, full or partial. There is a modifier that applies to a patient who is **on agonist therapy,** such as methadone maintenance or nicotine replacement, when the agonist medication is not being abused. There is also a modifier that applies to a patient who is **in a controlled environment** for 1 month or longer where no criteria for dependence or abuse are met, but the person is in an environment where controlled substances are highly restricted, such as locked hospitals, therapeutic communities, or substance-free jails.

Substance Abuse

A. A maladaptive pattern of substance use leading to clinically significant impairment or distress, as manifested by one or more of the following occurring at any time during the same 12-month period:
    (1) recurrent substance use resulting in a failure to fulfill major role obligations at work, school, or home (eg, repeated absences or poor work performance related to substance use; substance-related absences, suspensions, or expulsions from school; neglect of children or household)
    (2) recurrent substance use in situations in which it is physically hazardous (eg, driving an automobile or operating a machine when impaired by substance use)
    (3) recurrent substance-related legal problems (eg, arrests for substance-related disorderly conduct)
    (4) continued substance use despite having persistent or recurrent social or interpersonal problems caused or exacerbated by the effects of the substance (eg, arguments with spouse about consequences of intoxication, physical fights)
B. Has never met the criteria for Substance Dependence for this class of substance.

SUBSTANCE INTOXICATION AND SUBSTANCE WITHDRAWAL
Substance Intoxication

The development of a reversible substance-specific syndrome due to recent ingestion of (or exposure to) a substance. (Note: different substances may produce similar or identical syndromes.)

Substance Withdrawal

The development of a substance-specific syndrome due to the cessation of, or reduction in, substance use that has been heavy and prolonged.
The substance-specific syndrome causes clinically significant distress or impairment in social, occupational, or other important areas of functioning.
Not due to a general medical condition and not better accounted for by another mental disorder.

for 13% (National Institute on Alcohol Abuse and Alcoholism [NIAAA], 1997). Daily alcohol consumption can be estimated using the following conversion: one 12-ounce can of beer (4% ethanol) = one 1.5-ounce shot of hard liquor (40% ethanol) = one 5-ounce glass of wine (12% ethanol); each contains approximately 0.5 ounces or 12 grams of ethanol.

Alcoholics with a high tolerance of alcohol may consume the equivalent of a liter or more of hard liquor per day. A high daily consumption rate is just one indication that an alcohol problem exists, and this observation should be used in conjunction with other symptoms and signs in making the diagnosis.

When assessing the use of cigarettes, obtaining a current and past use pattern such as a pack-per-day assessment is helpful (Ziendonis et al, 1998). Depending on the smoker, nicotine dependence may occur with as few as 10 cigarettes per day or as many as several packs per day. When assessing the use of illicit substances, the bias of the clinician may result in embracing a zero tolerance view, which dictates that any use of illicit substances is abuse.

Table 17–2. Sequelae of alcoholism.

Biomedical
Birth defects
Blackouts
Bone fractures
Cardiomyopathy
Cerebellar degeneration
Cirrhosis
Delirium tremens
Dementia
Esophageal varices
Esophagitis
Fatty liver
Gastritis
Hepatitis
Hypertension
Hypothyroidism
Increased risk of cancer
   (mouth, pharynx, larynx, esophagus,
   liver, pancreas)
Intoxication
Korsakoff's syndrome
Myopathy
Nutritional deficiency, especially vitamin
   (thiamine, folate) deficiency
Pancreatitis
Peripheral neuropathy
Pneumonia
Portal hypertension
Seizures
Sexual dysfunction
   (impotence, amenorrhea)
Subdural hematoma
Tuberculosis
Wernicke's syndrome
Psychological
Angry outbursts
Anxiety
Craving for alcohol
Denial
Dependency
Depression
Guilt
Hallucinosis
Loneliness
Paranoia
Suicidal ideation
Use of other drugs
Social
Automobile accidents
Family problems (marital, child abuse,
   domestic violence)
Financial problems
Inadequate shelter
Legal problems
Social isolation
Vocational problems

The National Commission on Marijuana and Drug Abuse uses a five-tier approach to illicit and nonprescription psychoactive substances: (1) experimental use or short-term, nonpatterned trials of the drug; (2) social-recreational use, or use in social settings among friends; (3) circumstantial-situational or self-limited use of variable pattern, frequency, intensity, and duration; (4) intensified or long-term patterned use at least once a day; and (5) compulsive or frequent and intense use of relatively long duration. In an attempt to quantify the use of illicit substances, the pattern is quite important; in fact, the pattern of use may be more informative than the quantity of substance used. The user of nonpharmaceutical psychoactive substances often does not know how much of the purported psychoactive substance is consumed or received from the substance peddler.

An alternative to quantifying drug use in terms of grams or ounces is to ask the patient how much money is routinely spent on the purchase of the substances. Knowing the price may not be helpful in determining the quantity of consumption, but it can be helpful in determining the level of dysfunction associated with the use of the substance. A patient who earns $100 a day, but spends $75 on drugs, has very little left for living expenses; hence, this patient's use of illicit substances is clearly dysfunctional.

Denial of Problems Associated with Psychoactive Substance Use

Many people who suffer from the effects of psychoactive substance use disorders deny either the presence or the extent of their problem. In some cases, denial is characteristic of the individual's defense mechanism in other contexts. Extreme forms of denial may represent reactions to stress from past traumatic events, sequelae of alcoholism or other drugs, or even stress associated with the treatment process itself. The intensity of denial may vary, and a patient may deny problems previously acknowledged. If denial is confronted too vigorously, increased anxiety and anger may result, producing more denial or a flight from treatment. Alternatively, the patient may confront the clinicians in an angry or threatening manner, particularly if the patient feels threatened by being identified as a substance abuser. Clinician-initiated confrontation should be modified according to the therapist's assessment of the patient's ability to face the problem.

Major Psychiatric Sequelae of Psychoactive Substance Use

The clinician should determine if the patient is currently under the influence of a psychoactive substance. The use of psychoactive substances follows a basic three-part pattern: (1) intoxication, (2) withdrawal, and (3) residual effects. A patient smelling of alcohol who has a staggering gait is usually under the influence of alcohol. Patients who are tolerant of alcohol may be intoxicated, however, without any gross evidence of dysfunction, eg, no slurring of speech or staggering gait. The patient may mask the odor of alcohol by the use of mouthwash, chewing gum, or mints. An example of a residual effect is a blackout.

Alcohol-Induced Blackouts

Blackouts are a form of anterograde amnesia, in which the patient is unable to recall events that occurred during a bout of drinking even though he or she was conscious and active during this time. Black-

Table 17–3. Major effects of substance-related diagnoses from *DSM-IV*.

Substance	Intoxication	Withdrawal	Abuse	Dependence
Alcohol	X	X	X	X
Amphetamine	X	X	X	X
Caffeine	X		X	X
Cannabis	X	X	X	X
Cocaine	X	X	X	X
Hallucinogen	X	X	X	X
Inhalant	X		X	X
Nicotine	X	X	X	X
Opioid	X	X	X	X
Phencyclidine	X	X	X	X
Sedative-hypnotic-anxiolytic	X	X	X	X

outs can last for several minutes or for days; their frequency is an index of the severity and duration of alcoholism. Blackouts occur in 64–94% of alcoholics; predisposing factors include gulping drinks on an empty stomach and not sleeping. Blackouts are generally unrelated to organic disturbances as measured by neuropsychological testing. The differential diagnosis of alcoholic blackouts includes head trauma, carbon monoxide poisoning, hysteria, and malingering.

Drug-Induced Psychosis

Psychosis is a frequent complaint of patients presenting for psychiatric care. Psychoactive substances are notorious for producing undesirable side effects, such as psychosis. The *DSM-IV* states that psychosis can be associated with intoxication and withdrawal. Drugs such as alcohol, amphetamines, marijuana, hallucinogens, inhalants, opioids, PCP, and sedative-hypnotics may produce psychosis. In many situations, the presentation is that of an acute emergency; in other situations, the patient presents with a more stable psychosis that does not attain emergency level. In either situation the clinician, not knowing the obvious cause of the psychosis, must make a differential diagnosis. Diagnoses include (1) paranoid schizophrenia, (2) bipolar mood disorder during the manic phase, (3) anxiety disorders, particularly with panic attacks, (4) amphetamine- or cocaine-induced psychotic reactions, (5) drug intoxication with psychedelics, PCP, or other sympathomimetic drugs (eg, ephedrine, cocaine), (6) hyperthyroid crisis, including ingestion of thyroid preparations, and (7) pheochromocytoma.

Stimulant Psychosis

Numerous difficulties exist in diagnosing acute amphetamine toxicity. Amphetamine use is concealed in some cases, and the clinician encounters an acutely agitated, anxious, paranoid, or belligerent patient whose abnormal behavior is not due to any obvious cause. A history from friends or relatives may provide important clues; a history of recurrent episodes of hyperactivity and paranoia treated for long periods with antipsychotic medication suggests paranoid schizophrenia. Chronic amphetamine use may produce a similar pattern, however, and should

be considered. Urine tests are usually quite helpful in revealing the presence of amphetamines.

Amphetamine psychosis results from prolonged high-dose amphetamine abuse, often in association with sleep deprivation. The clinical manifestations of full-blown amphetamine psychosis resemble those of a functional paranoid psychosis, but they are dose related and have a much shorter course. Unless the individual suffers from a persistent psychotic disorder such as schizophrenia, the psychotic reaction will resolve as the amphetamine or methylphenidate is excreted from the body.

Cocaine psychosis, which is more commonly found with either free-base cocaine, such as "crack" cocaine, or with injection cocaine, may be more transient than the psychosis of amphetamine use. Psychosis, of course, can be found with any form of cocaine or amphetamine taken in sufficiently high doses over sufficiently long periods of time. Toxicology screens may reveal the presence of cocaine or its major metabolite, benzoylecgonine, assisting in the diagnosis. The absence of a positive toxicology screen, however, does not rule out the possibility of a cocaine psychosis.

When either amphetamine or cocaine is withdrawn, a residual depression may occur. This depression may abate with the passage of time or it may require hospitalization. Patients presenting with suicidal ideation, which often occurs with cocaine or amphetamine use, should be assessed for hospitalization. Naturally, then, the patient using cocaine or amphetamine may present as a medical emergency. Discussion of the emergency response to drug abuse occurs in Chapter 41.

Phencyclidine Psychosis

The phencyclidines (PCP) may cause an acute psychosis; this is a medical emergency and should be treated promptly. In some people, PCP may also produce a prolonged psychosis unrelated to toxic blood levels; in others, it may precipitate a psychotic reaction that lasts a month or more and appears clinically similar to functional psychosis. The clinician must recognize the need to inquire about the use of PCP. PCP is not used as commonly as it once was, however; its use has been reported in St. Louis and

Philadelphia (called "love boat" or "wet") and in Texas, where it is combined with embalming fluid (National Institute on Drug Abuse [NIDA], 1996).

Summarizing all the major conditions associated with the use of psychoactive substances is impossible. Naturally, the psychiatric presentation of a patient may be affected by the use of a specific substance. A general spectrum of psychiatric symptoms includes acting out, angry outbursts, anxiety, depression, denial, flashbacks, paranoia, personality changes, sleep dysfunction, and suicidal ideation. This list is neither complete nor exhaustive. The clinician needs to understand that patients presenting with psychological or biomedical symptoms may be users of psychoactive substances.

MENTAL STATUS EXAMINATION

The general psychiatric mental status examination is described in Chapter 11. A clinician interviewing a patient about his or her substance abuse problems may begin with the mental status examination and then explore substance abuse issues if they surface early. If a patient presents with a chief complaint of substance abuse the mental status examination can augment the history by capturing current evidence of elements such as the patient's presentation, motor behavior, cognitive status, thought, and mood. The mental status examination can reveal clinical data that may be either consistent or inconsistent with the history. Thus, a patient who describes alcohol as a primary drug and appears pressured, agitated, diaphoretic, and paranoid, but who describes drinking alcohol recently, may either be intoxicated, in withdrawal, or manifesting symptoms from a second substance of abuse (eg, cocaine).

Another element of the mental status examination is memory, specifically the loss of short-term memory in the withdrawal state. A mild memory deficit may be obscured by the retention of verbal skills, which would appear to suggest the patient is tracking new information that is provided. Memory deficits may also be accompanied by attention deficits, particularly in alcoholics in early stages of sobriety. Cognitively based programs use lectures and videos for psychoeducation: as a result of memory and attention deficits their messages may not be assimilated. Of course, the mental status examination, which assesses thought and mood elements, is critical, as these elements are affected by a broad spectrum of agents.

PHYSICAL EXAMINATION

A complete physical examination should be performed after the history and mental status examination. In the early stages of alcoholism, pertinent physical findings may be limited to evidence of

hepatomegaly, tremor, or mild peripheral neuropathy. In more advanced stages, a number of physical signs may exist that are consistent with the sequelae listed in Table 17–2. With other drugs of abuse, pertinent physical findings may be limited, eg, in patients injecting drugs, track marks, abscesses (healed or active), or evidence of subcutaneous injections (skin popping) may be present. Pupillary changes may also be apparent on physical examination. Opioid intoxication may produce pupillary constriction, whereas opioid withdrawal may produce pupillary dilation. Pupillary dilation also may occur with cocaine and hallucinogen intoxication. A patient who "snorts" (intranasal insufflation) cocaine may show a perforated nasal septum, whereas a patient who only smokes cocaine ("crack") would not. A patient who smokes cocaine may, however, show signs of burns or singes of facial hair. Although peripheral neuropathies occur with chronic alcohol consumption, they can also occur with chronic low-level exposure to solvents.

LABORATORY & X-RAY FINDINGS

It is possible to collect important information about the substance abuse status of a patient using screening techniques and laboratory measurements. Urine toxicology screens are helpful in determining the presence of metabolites from drug use, particularly unsuspected polysubstance abuse. Many hospitals and clinics have the ability to screen for substances such as cocaine, amphetamines, opioids, marijuana, and PCP. Furthermore, a number of spot-screening tests are readily available for the same purpose. Screening tests are set to a certain point called a cut-off: specimens testing "positive" have quantities of metabolites above the cut-off; specimens testing negative have quantities of metabolites below the cut-off. Clinicians must also be aware that because of technical limitations, screening tests may result in false negatives. A patient may have recently used a psychoactive substance but still test negative. Screening tests may also result in false positives. A patient taking over-the-counter cold medications containing pseudoephedrine may screen positive for amphetamine, but on confirmatory testing with gas chromatography/mass spectroscopy will test negative. As a result, confirmatory tests are recommended for forensic purposes; for situations that could result in legal, economic, or psychological injury to a patient; and for any situation in which a definitive answer is needed.

Alcohol testing can be accomplished by using a breathalyzer, or by testing urine, blood, or saliva. Unlike drug testing, which will test positive for a substance at the nanogram per milliliter level, alcohol levels are measured at a higher level of milligrams per deciliter. Alcohol levels are more closely associated with intoxication than the more minute levels of drug toxicology. Thus, a cocaine level of 300 ng/mL is not necessarily associated with intoxication, whereas an alcohol level of 200 mg/dL is. For the purpose of driving a motor vehicle state laws usually define alcohol intoxication at either 80 or 100 mg/dL or 0.08 or 0.100 mg%. Table 17–4 summarizes the signs of alcohol intoxication correlated with progressive blood alcohol levels. The relationships between ingestion of alcohol, the blood ethanol concentration, and the signs of intoxication vary; they depend on the history of use, rate of ingestion, and alterations in absorption, metabolism, and excretion. Alcohol is usually fully absorbed from within 30 minutes to 2 hours, depending on both the beverage ingested and food intake.

In addition to toxicology screens, screens for serum levels of aspartate aminotransferase (AST, SGOT), alkaline phosphatase, γ-glutamyltranspeptidase, and bilirubin (increased levels indicate liver damage) should be performed. An abnormal erythrocyte and a mean corpuscular volume (macrocytosis) indicate possible liver disease, folate deficiency, or the toxic effect of alcohol on the developing erythroblast. A serum creatinine should be done for evidence of renal damage; hepatitis B and C screens also should be done, because both are associated with injecting drug use and polydrug abuse. Given the incidence of venereal diseases associated with the use of drugs and alcohol, a Venereal Disease Research Laboratories or rapid plasma reagin test should be done. Urinalysis and chest x-ray should be performed in all cases. Fractures, subdural hematomas, pneumonia, tuberculosis, and lung cancer may be associated conditions in patients abusing substances. Tuberculin skin tests

Table 17–4. Signs of intoxication correlated with blood alcohol levels.[a]

Blood Alcohol Level (mg/dL)[b]	Signs of Intoxication
20–99	Muscular incoordination Impaired sensory function Changes in mood, personality, and behavior
100–199	Marked mental impairment Incoordination Prolonged reaction time Ataxia
200–299	Nausea and vomiting Diplopia Marked ataxia
300–399	Hypothermia Severe dysarthria Amnesia Stage 1 anesthesia
400–700	Coma Respiratory failure Death

[a] Reproduced, with permission, from Becker CE, Roe RL, Scott RA: *Alcohol as a Drug.* Medcom Press, 1974. Copyright 1974 by Williams & Wilkins.
[b] Lethal dose varies. For adults, it is 5–8 g/kg; for children, 3 g/kg. If there is no food intake, lethal dose occurs before above doses are absorbed. Signs of intoxication are more apparent when blood alcohol level is rising than when it is falling.

should be routinely administered to any patient suspected of being a substance abuser. Because the use of psychoactive substances is associated with unprotected sexual activities or with the transmission of infected body fluids through shared drug paraphernalia, serious consideration should be given to asking the patient to agree to a human immunodeficiency virus (HIV) test. Naturally, the HIV test should be done with appropriate pre- and posttest counseling.

SPECIFIC SUBSTANCES OF ABUSE

STIMULANTS

General nervous system stimulants are widely used in the United States: The two most prevalent are nicotine in tobacco products and caffeine in coffee, tea, sodas, and other products. (Although tobacco and caffeine abuse are given diagnostic codes and diagnostic criteria in *DSM-IV,* they are not discussed separately in this text because of space limitations.) Stimulant abuse has become a serious problem: SAMHSA (1998) reports that in 1997 approximately 111 million Americans age 12 and older were current alcohol users; 32 million engaged in binge drinking; about 11.2 million were heavy drinkers; and an estimated 64 million were current smokers. Major stimulants of abuse are cocaine (a derivative of the coca plant), synthetic stimulants such as amphetamine and amphetamine-like drugs (eg, methylphenidate) (Table 17–5), and methamphetamine. Most of these substances have legitimate medicinal value: cocaine is approved for topical anesthesia; amphetamines and amphetamine-like drugs are approved for narcolepsy, hyperkinesia, and short-term diet control; and amphetamines are approved for the short-term treatment of depression, particularly in the elderly.

The management of stimulant abuse is complicated by the availability of cocaine "look-a-likes" (eg, ephedrine, lidocaine) that resemble cocaine in appearance, contain no controlled substance, and may themselves be toxic. The potent central nervous system stimulants have a high potential for abuse. In the drug culture, the primary routes of cocaine administration are nasal insufflation, smoking free-base "crack" cocaine or "ice" (a potent form of smokable methamphetamine), and injection. For instance, methamphetamine use is highest in San Francisco (69.2 per 100,000) where the preferred route of administration (NIDA, 1996) varies with ethnicities; Asian-Americans and Pacific Islanders prefer to smoke methamphetamines whereas African-Americans prefer intranasal use. Administration of amphetamines is either oral or by injection. Dependence on stimulants can develop, but this is primarily psychological, with no well-defined abstinence symptoms other than de-

Table 17–5. Drugs.

Anabolic steroids
Nicotine
Sedatives
  Barbiturates
    Butabarbital
    Butalbital
    Pentobarbital
    Secobarbital
  Barbiturate-like
    Glutethimide
    Meprobamate
  Chloral hydrate
  Methaqualone[a]
  Benzodiazepines[b]
    Alprazolam
    Chlordiazepoxide
    Diazepam
    Lorazepam
    Triazolam
Stimulants
  Amphetamines
  Cocaine
  Methylphenidate
  Phenmetrazine
  Caffeine
Opiates and Opioids
  Codeine
  Heroin
  L-Acetylmethadol
  Methadone
  Morphine
  Opium
  Fentanyl analogues
  Hydromorphone
  Meperidine
  Hydrocodone
  Propoxyphene hydrochloride
Phencyclidine (PCP)
Inhalants
  Glue
  Gasoline
  Solvents
  Correction fluids
  Anesthetics
  Thinners
Hallucinogens[c]
  LSD
  DET, DMT
  Psilocin, psilocybin
  Mescaline
  MDMA "Ecstasy"
    DOB, DOM, MDA, MMDA, MDE

[a] Withdrawn in 1983. Not legally available after 1984.
[b] Short list, see reference text for more complete list.
[c] LSD, lysergic acid diethylamide; DET, diethyltryptamine; DMT, dimethyltryptamine; MDMA, N-methyl-3,4-methylenedioxymethamphetamine; DOB, 4-bromo-2,5-dimethoxyamphetamine; DOM, 4-methyl-2,5-dimethoxyamphetamine; MDA, 3,4-methylenedioxyamphetamine; MMDA, methylenedioxyamphetamine; MMDA, 3-methoxy-4,5-methylenedioxyamphetamine; MDE, N-ethyl-3,4,-methylenedioxyamphetamine.

pression or lethargy. These stimulants can, however, lend themselves to compulsive use and high-dose abuse. Because high-dose abuse of short-acting stimulants, such as cocaine, lends itself to compulsion, loss of control, and continued use despite adverse consequences, it represents a form of addictive disease.

Because "crack" cocaine is prepared by a simplified basification technique that yields free-base cocaine in small, proportionately less expensive dosage units, fewer obstacles are involved with this rapid delivery form of cocaine. Free-base cocaine vaporizes at approximately 100 °C; it can be easily smoked. The pulmonary route enhances rapid and thorough plasma cocaine concentration. Euphoria is swift and marked, followed by severe depression, which is typically self-medicated with additional cocaine; this, in turn, leads to a progression and worsening of symptoms.

Amphetamine may be taken orally in low doses to enhance physical or emotional performance, or it may be taken in high doses, either orally or intravenously, to produce euphoria and a "rush" (ie, a burst of energy accompanied by a physical sensation in the head and neck). High-dose oral use can also produce psychotic reactions. Even moderate doses of amphetamine in conjunction with physical exertion at high environmental temperatures may contribute to heat stroke through interference with regulation of body temperature. Several deaths of bicyclists have been attributed to this phenomenon.

Many people are occasional amphetamine users, taking low oral doses while studying for an examination or for "treatment" of obesity. Although obese patients are often under medical care, they are not always carefully supervised and some may abuse the drug. Amphetamine is at times used orally or intravenously to counteract the effects of other drugs. Once a pattern of amphetamine use is established, the drug is frequently used to counteract the effects of amphetamine abstinence.

Clinical Features

In addition to euphoria, stimulation, relief of fatigue, and suppression of appetite, other possible effects of stimulant use include excitation, increased pulse rate and blood pressure, and insomnia. Massive overdoses of amphetamine occasionally occur in suicide attempts, in intravenous users who obtain unusually potent preparations, and in children who inadvertently ingest the drug. Patients may be unconscious following seizures, with hypertensive crises or even cerebrovascular accidents.

PHENCYCLIDINE (PCP) ABUSE

The phencyclidines are "dissociative anesthetics" that have a mechanism of action quite different from other hallucinogens; in the drug culture, they are used for "mind-altering" experiences. These substances have a high potential for chronic toxicity.

PCP and its analogs, including ketamine, can be produced cheaply and easily with readily accessible ingredients. Their use has increased among minority groups and less affluent young people, but is rare among "substance-sophisticated" populations. About

95% of users experience no crisis, but the 5% who become seriously intoxicated present a difficult management problem; without warning, the user may alternate between coma and violence.

PCP produces its effects by binding to high-affinity PCP receptors in the brain. PCP receptors also appear to be responsive to substances called σ-opioids, which produce psychotomimetic effects in humans. Research shows that PCP receptors are most dense in the hippocampus, frontal cortex, and superior colliculus. By binding to PCP receptors, a substance will block the N-methyl-D-aspartic acid (NMDA)-type glutamate receptor, which is linked to the excitation of the central nervous system. Thus, a PCP agonist will have an antiexcitatory effect on the nervous system.

Clinical Features

The term "PCP syndrome" has been used to describe the pattern of PCP toxicity. The PCP syndrome is manifested in the following four stages, which may or may not be successive:

A. Stage 1 (Acute PCP Toxicity): Reactions of acute PCP toxicity are a direct result of PCP intoxication; these may include coma, hypertension, seizures, respiratory depression, and psychosis and agitation. Patients with acute toxicity may report to psychiatric emergency units with symptoms of paranoia, thought disorder, negativism, hostility, and grossly altered body image, or they may be referred for treatment as a result of their assaultive and antisocial behavior.

B. Stage 2 (PCP Toxic Psychosis): The development of prolonged toxic psychosis is apparently not related to toxic blood levels of PCP and does not inevitably follow Stage 1.

C. Stage 3 (PCP-Precipitated Psychotic Episodes): In some individuals, PCP may precipitate a psychotic reaction that lasts a month or more and appears clinically similar to functional psychosis. Characteristics of PCP-precipitated psychotic episodes are of the schizoaffective type, with paranoid features and a waxing and waning thought disorder. Most individuals in Stage 3 have odd or eccentric personality disorders, which is the major prognostic indicator.

D. Stage 4 (PCP-Induced Depression): PCP frequently produces a depressive reaction with severe cognitive impairment. Depression may follow any of the previous stages, but the diagnosis is missed by many clinicians, particularly when depression follows Stage 3. The condition lasts from a day to several months, but it is usually completely reversible after withdrawal and abstinence from PCP.

PSYCHOTOMIMETIC AMPHETAMINE ABUSE

Some of the amphetamines have characteristics similar to "psychedelic" drugs. 3,4-Methylenedioxyamphetamine (MDA), N-methyl-3,4-methylenedi-

oxymethamphetamine (MDMA), and N-ethyl-3,4-methylenedioxyamphetamine (MDE) are several of the more popular psychotomimetic drugs. MDA is known in some areas as the "love drug," MDMA is referred to as "Ecstasy," and MDE is called "Eve." These "designer" drugs have two basic qualities: they enhance insight and empathy, and they stimulate the central nervous system.

At low doses, MDMA and MDE can produce a state of well-being and self-insight, heightened empathy, and lowered psychological defenses leading to open communication. Because of these effects some psychotherapists and psychiatrists have used MDMA and MDE in therapy. At higher doses, however, the stimulant properties of these drugs emerge.

Research has revealed acute MDMA toxicity syndromes (at low, medium, and high doses), prolonged toxicity syndromes, and MDMA-induced anxiety syndromes. The acute and prolonged toxicity syndromes are dose related and can be treated like stimulant toxicity. The MDMA-induced anxiety syndromes, however, which emerge some time after MDMA ingestion or persist in the absence of MDMA in the bodily fluids, should be treated as anxiety disorders. Patients with these anxiety syndromes typically respond to psychotherapy and protocols for nonpsychoactive anxiety. At the upper dosage limits, or in people with underlying cardiac problems, MDMA, MDE, and MDA can result in death from hypothermia, cardiac fibrillation, or other complications.

Clinical Features

Reports indicate that users of MDMA also have nausea, jaw clenching and teeth grinding, increased muscle tension, blurred vision, and a postuse dysphoria. Animal studies suggest the possibility of degeneration of serotonergic nerve cells and serotonin depletion with chronic use; what import this has for humans is unclear.

BARBITURATE & OTHER SEDATIVE-HYPNOTIC ABUSE

The category of depressant drugs includes a wide variety of substances that differ markedly in their physical and chemical properties, but share the common characteristic of causing generalized depression of the central nervous system. This drug group includes sedative-hypnotics (eg, barbiturates) and antianxiety agents (eg, benzodiazepines), which are widely prescribed in the United States. Some drugs, such as the barbiturates, are diffuse depressants of the central nervous system with no specific receptors. Others, such as the benzodiazepines, have a specific receptor in the brain and, thus, have a more specific action.

Depressant drugs listed in Table 17–5 include the barbiturates, barbiturate-like substances, benzodiazepines, carbamates, and chloral hydrate. In addition to euphoria and reduction of aggressive or sexual drives, other possible effects of these drugs include drowsiness, respiratory depression, and nausea. Although drugs classified as central nervous system depressants differ in their pharmacological actions and the onset and duration of their effects, all exhibit some degree of cross-tolerance and cross-dependence. These depressant drugs are also cross-tolerant to alcohol; their concomitant use with alcohol increases the risk of abuse and overdose.

BARBITURATES

The barbiturates are the oldest of the sedative-hypnotics and can be classified as ultrashort-, short-, intermediate-, and long-acting. Ultrashort-acting barbiturates, such as thiopental, are used for anesthesia because of their rapid onset and brief duration. As a consequence, the ultrashort-acting barbiturates are rarely abused. The short- and intermediate-acting barbiturates include secobarbital and pentobarbital; they are used primarily for insomnia. Their short duration of action and short-to-intermediate duration of disinhibition make them the most commonly abused drugs in the barbiturate class. The long-acting barbiturates have a very low abuse potential. The onset of effects can take up to 1 hour and can last up to 16 hours, making these drugs useful as anticonvulsant agents.

Clinical Features

Patients who have taken an overdose of barbiturates or other sedative-hypnotics arrive at the emergency room with a variety of signs and symptoms that must be interpreted quickly and accurately. A sedative-hypnotic overdose is a life-threatening emergency that cannot be treated definitively by nonmedical personnel. Signs and symptoms of sedative-hypnotic overdose include slurred speech, staggering gait, sustained vertical or horizontal nystagmus, slowed reactions, lethargy, and progressive respiratory depression, which is characterized by shallow and irregular breathing, leading to coma and possibly death.

Most patients treated for an overdose of sedative-hypnotics are acutely intoxicated or in a coma following ingestion of a single large dose, but they usually are not physically dependent on the drug. Unless the sedative-hypnotic has been used daily for more than a month in an amount equivalent to 400–600 mg of a short-acting barbiturate, a severe withdrawal syndrome will not develop.

BENZODIAZEPINES

Benzodiazepines are one of the most widely used drug groups in the United States. The indications for their use are anxiety, muscle spasm, seizures,

and treatment of acute alcohol withdrawal symptoms. Benzodiazepines are representative of the broad sedative-hypnotic class. Often inappropriately called "minor tranquilizers" (in contrast to the neuroleptics or "major tranquilizers," such as chlorpromazine or haloperidol), the benzodiazepines have varying duration of action, including short-acting (alprazolam) and long-acting (diazepam) benzodiazepines. All, however, have approximately equal abuse potential.

One of the major reasons for the popularity of benzodiazepines is they have a much wider therapeutic index than the barbiturates. Death from an overdose of benzodiazepines is very unlikely, although the therapeutic index and danger from overdose are greatly increased when benzodiazepines are taken in combination with alcohol. Most cases of benzodiazepine-related overdose seen in emergency rooms are associated with alcohol ingestion.

Substantial variations exist in individual reactions to the use of benzodiazepines. Most individuals who take benzodiazepines within the therapeutic range over long periods experience no significant withdrawal. People with a psychobiological predisposition to addiction (often with a past history or family history of alcoholism), however, who take benzodiazepines in dosages within the therapeutic range for over 3 months, may manifest severe withdrawal psychosis and seizure on abrupt cessation of this drug.

Some physicians switch from a medium- or longer-acting benzodiazepine, such as diazepam, to a shorter-acting benzodiazepine, such as alprazolam, in the mistaken belief that the shorter-acting drug has less potential for abuse. They may lower the equivalent dose as well, prompting the emergence of a sedative-hypnotic abstinence syndrome (eg, anxiety and insomnia). All benzodiazepines have the same potential for abuse; the use of shorter-acting benzodiazepines should be limited to their intended therapeutic purpose (eg, relief of panic). Patients with benzodiazepine dependence should enroll in a formal program of gradual detoxification. Alternatives to psychoactive medications should be sought for patients with both a dependence on benzodiazepines and a diagnosis of anxiety disorder. Therapeutically effective medications with a lower potential for dependence (eg, imipramine rather than alprazolam in a drug-dependent patient with a history of panic disorder) should also be sought. If these alternatives, coupled with stress reduction education, relaxation training and exercise, and biofeedback fail, and if major dysfunction is present, then a benzodiazepine is the drug of choice.

Clinical Features

If a benzodiazepine is taken at a dosage several times the therapeutic dosage for approximately 1 month, physical dependence can develop and abrupt cessation can produce sedative-hypnotic withdrawal symptoms, such as withdrawal psychosis and seizures.

Treatment   *Flumazenil*

A. Overdose: The ways in which an acute sedative-hypnotic overdose can be managed in an emergency situation are described in Chapter 41.

B. Withdrawal: Both the barbiturate and non-barbiturate sedative-hypnotics can produce physical dependence for the duration of withdrawal sequelae, determined in part by the differing metabolic properties and duration of action of the primary drug dose. Physical dependence on large doses of a short-acting barbiturate may be produced, for example, when the drug is abruptly stopped. The peak risk of seizure occurs at about the second day. Conversely, with a longer acting nonbarbiturate sedative-hypnotic such as diazepam, a large or even standard therapeutic dose over a long period of time produces physical dependence. Abrupt cessation, particularly by the fifth or sixth day, can cause withdrawal seizures as well as withdrawal psychosis. All of these withdrawal syndromes from sedative-hypnotics can be managed by detoxification with phenobarbital, a long-acting barbiturate. A "phenobarbital stabilization period" should continue for 2 days, followed by graded reduction of phenobarbital dosage over 7–20 days.

If the history of barbiturate abuse is variable, or if the patient is using multiple sedative-hypnotics, a challenge of short-acting pentobarbital (100–200 mg) or long-acting phenobarbital (100–200 mg) can be used to test the individual's tolerance before starting the detoxification schedule. A person who does not have sedative-hypnotic tolerance will respond to the challenge with signs of sedation, ataxia, and mild intoxication; a person with developed tolerance will show minimal effect.

Addiction to a wide variety of other nonbarbiturate sedative-hypnotic substances—prescribed primarily for insomnia—with high-abuse potential can occur if the individual takes 5–10 times the therapeutic dose for approximately 1 month. This group includes glutethimide, ethchlorvynol, and methaqualone*. Physical dependence on barbiturates and barbiturate-like substances can cause an extremely severe withdrawal syndrome with features of psychosis, seizure, and amnestic disorder. If these medications have been taken for longer than 1 month or have been self-administered in high doses, they should not be abruptly stopped; the medication should either be gradually reduced or the phenobarbital substitution and withdrawal technique (detoxification) should be initiated.

Illusonogen

HALLUCINOGEN DRUG ABUSE

Hallucinogen abuse escalated in the 1960s and continues to be a significant problem. In 1996 there were

an estimated 1.1 million new hallucinogen users. This is approximately twice the average annual number of users during the 1980s (SAMHSA, 1998). A list of common hallucinogens is found in Table 17–5. Although LSD is the most widely known hallucinogen, marijuana and PCP also belong in this category. Hallucinogens characteristically result in euphoria and an altered perception of visual and auditory stimuli; other effects include poor judgment, impaired perception of time and space, altered consciousness without delirium, sedation, overstimulation, and intellectual impairment. Hallucinogens produce perceptual distortions of an actual phenomenon in the environment (illusions) more commonly than they produce a nonexistent phenomenon (hallucinations).

Clinical Features

A. Acute Toxicity: In acute hallucinogenic drug toxicity, individuals are aware of having taken a drug (eg, LSD), but they are in a state of severe anxiety and panic. They feel they cannot control the drug's effects, and they want to be rescued immediately. The diagnosis depends on a thorough understanding of the phases of the hallucinogenic experience. The course of the hallucinogenic "trip" (based on ingestion of 100–250 mg of LSD) can be described in three overlapping phases. The precise duration of each phase depends on dosage, individual idiosyncrasies, and the setting in which the drug is taken.

1. Phase 1 (sensory phase)—This phase, which lasts from ingestion to hour 5, is characterized by sensory changes—visual, auditory, tactile, olfactory, gustatory, and kinesthetic effects—and awareness of internal bodily functions.

2. Phase 2 (symbolic, recollective, and analytic phase)—From hours 2 to 8, manifestations include visual imagery characterized by vivid colors, hallucinations or illusions, altered visual perceptions, mood and affect changes, and altered communication.

3. Phase 3 (heightened sensibility phase)—From hours 2 to 10, insight, integration, and transformation of perceptions are heightened. Manifestations include (1) concern with philosophy, religion, and cosmology; (2) exaggeration of character traits and psychodynamic conflicts; (3) exaggerated emotion; and (4) feelings of heightened psychological perception and insight.

B. Chronic Toxicity: Four recognized chronic reactions to hallucinogens or psychedelics occur: (1) prolonged psychotic reactions, (2) flashbacks, (3) depression severe enough to be life-threatening, and (4) exacerbation of preexisting psychiatric illness.

Treatment

External stimuli such as bright lights, loud music, and strangers coming or going may be interpreted as

---

* Withdrawn in 1983 and not legally available after 1984.

hostile by the patient having a "bad trip." A quiet room in a supportive environment (with trusted individuals) is a good place to "talk down" a frightened patient. Sitting on pillows on the floor is recommended for both patient and clinician. A nonthreatening physical setting also allows the clinician to avoid adopting an overly authoritative or threatening style.

Empathy and self-confidence are essential attributes of physicians or others dealing with people undergoing hallucinogenic crises. Anxiety or fear is almost certainly communicated to the patient, who may perceive the fear in an amplified manner. Physical contact is often reassuring but may be misinterpreted. When approaching patients who have been "tripping," the clinician must be guided by judgment and previous experience.

Psychotic reactions usually occur in patients with preexisting psychological problems. These reactions are similar to functional psychotic states; they can be severe and prolonged. Appropriate treatment often requires residential care and then outpatient counseling.

"Flashbacks" are transient, spontaneous recurrences of drug effects long after the hallucinogenic intoxication has dissipated. These episodes cease with time but, in extreme cases, the patient should be referred for antipsychotic medication and outpatient therapy.

INHALANTS

Inhalation to produce an altered state of consciousness is an ancient practice. Inhalants generally refer to volatile substances such as glue, gasoline, solvents, cleaners, hair sprays, correction fluids, amyl nitrite, and degreasers. Nitrous oxide, "laughing gas," is also considered an inhalant. The inhalants, then, are made up of different substances that have different effects and different toxicities. Most of these substances, however, are products that can be found nearly anywhere. As a group they are cheap, legal, and easily accessible, particularly the organic solvents. The use of inhalants, generally favored by those under 20 years of age, has increased in the 1990s. For instance, there were an estimated 382,000 new inhalant users in 1991; by 1996 the number of new inhalant users increased to an estimated 805,000 (SAMHSA, 1998). The age group with the most significant increase of use of inhalants were youths aged 12–17.

It is unusual for a solvent abuser to appear at a hospital or outpatient clinic for treatment. An inexperienced user may suffer from anoxia or ventricular fibrillation, which progresses to death. The history given by the patient or relative will be the most important source of information about the inhalant. The *DSM-IV* describes inhalant intoxication, listing 13 possible symptoms, including euphoria, lack of coordination, slurred speech, and unsteady gait. The inhalant-intoxicated individual may clearly resemble the alcoholic "drunk" without the odor of al-

cohol. The *DSM-IV* recognizes an inhalant delirium, persisting dementia, psychotic disorder with delusions, and psychotic disorder with hallucinations; dependence and abuse are also recognized.

Most of the inhalants do not produce chronic or irreversible changes. Some, such as toluene, however, can cause irreversible dementia, cerebellar ataxia, and spasticity if inhaled chronically.

No specific treatment exists for inhalant abuse. Clinical treatment is symptomatic; psychiatric treatment is nonspecific.

MARIJUANA ABUSE

Marijuana, hashish, and other cannabis preparations have hallucinogenic and sedative properties. The primary active constituent is tetrahydrocannabinol (THC). At low to moderate doses, marijuana usually produces a sense of well-being, relaxation, and emotional disinhibition. A range of sensory and perceptual distortions, milder than those associated with LSD, may occur. Increased heart and pulse rates and a small decrease in blood pressure are common. At high doses, marijuana produces LSD-like effects, such as hallucinations, disorganized thought, panic, paranoia, agitation, and rare psychotic reactions sometimes accompanied by rage and violence.

Clinical Features

DSM-IV describes cannabis intoxication, cannabis delirium, cannabis psychotic disorder with delusions, and cannabis anxiety disorder. Tolerance to cannabis can develop, and a mild withdrawal syndrome of insomnia, anxiety, restlessness, perspiration, loss of appetite, and upset stomach is also seen. Chronic, heavy use compromises pulmonary functioning and suppresses testosterone (a particular problem for adolescents) and the immune system.

Perez-Reyes (1988) reported that the effects of marijuana and alcohol appear additive in that marijuana enhances the effects of alcohol on psychomotor skills. Lukas (1992) found marijuana may also alter the bioavailability of alcohol, reducing the peak plasma level.

A small subgroup of chronic marijuana users fulfills the *DSM-IV* diagnostic criteria for marijuana dependence. These users typically smoke marijuana daily, and they have family and personal histories of psychoactive substance dependence. Sometimes a person who is dependent on another drug (eg, alcohol or cocaine) may perceive marijuana as benign and attempt to use it in a controlled manner while abstaining from the primary drug. Invariably, this person returns to the use of the primary drug after using marijuana. It is important to help people dependent on psychoactive substances understand that abstinence from all mood-altering drugs is the most critical aspect of recovery.

OPIATE & OPIOID ABUSE

An opiate is a remedy containing or derived from opium and an ~~opioid is any synth~~etic narcotic that has opiate-like activities, but is <u>not derived from opium</u>.

Drugs in the opiate and opioid class include the natural substances derived from the opium poppy, such as opium, morphine, and codeine; semisynthetics, such as diacetylmorphine (heroin); and synthetic narcotic analgesics (opioids), such as meperidine, methadone, and fentanyl (Table 17–5). Opiates have been used as analgesics since ancient times, and some of them are still the analgesics of choice for severe pain. These opiates, whose adverse effects are drowsiness, respiratory depression, constricted pupils, and nausea, are also prescribed for reduction of aggressive or sexual drives. The effects for which these drugs are used illicitly include euphoria and "escape."

Clinicians must recognize that patients who receive opioids for the treatment of pain are often subsumed under the category of addicts. Many physicians undermedicate patients suffering from intractable pain, whether from cancer or from a benign condition. Thus, patients often appear preoccupied with medications, demanding increased dosages. Weissman (1989) has applied the term "pseudoaddiction" to this situation. Prescribing and administering inadequate amounts of opioids for the appropriate relief of pain makes "pseudoaddiction" more a reflection of the attitudes and knowledge of the clinician than an accurate assessment of the patient.

Clinical Features

The combination of pinpoint pupils and a declining level of consciousness is presumptive evidence of overdose of an opiate (eg, heroin or morphine) or an opioid. Although pinpoint pupils are an important diagnostic sign, the pupils <u>may be dilated as a consequence of hypoxia in cases of advanced coma.</u>

Medical complications associated with the direct pharmacological effects of opiates and opioids are relatively rare. They include constipation, decrease in sexual desire, and impairment of sexual functioning. In the "drug culture," however, opiates such as heroin are usually administered intravenously, producing a broad range of "needle diseases," including abscesses, hepatitis, and endocarditis. Addicts (eg, physicians and nurses) who inject meperidine or other pharmaceutical opioids, rather than heroin, and who use sterile needles have a much lower incidence of "needle disease."

Treatment

A. Overdose: Fortunately, overdose with either an opiate or an opioid can be reversed by administration of the narcotic antagonist naloxone (Narcan). This is usually done in the emergency unit. The intravenous route is preferred with 2–3 mg given initially. If the patient is in shock and has low blood pressure, 1 mg can be injected sublingually initially, and the injection repeated sublingually or intravenously to gain a response. The sublingual injection site must be carefully watched for oozing blood, which may be aspirated and cause serious consequences.

In opiate or opioid overdose, pupillary dilation and an elevation in the level of consciousness will occur within 20 seconds to 1 minute following intravenous administration of naloxone. If this response is obtained, a second injection of naloxone, 2 mg intravenously, should follow for prolonged effect. For overdose by methadone or propoxyphene napsylate, both long-acting preparations, repeated doses of naloxone will be required every 1–2 hours. *Note:* Naloxone is a short-acting narcotic antagonist and an ultrarapid opiate detoxicant and the opiate effect will outlast the antagonist effect of a single dose. Thus, the antagonist must often be repeated to maintain adequate respirations (Allen, 1997). The availability of a specific reversal agent does not mean that general supportive measures such as clearing the airway, maintaining respiration, keeping the patient warm, and elevating the feet can be neglected.

B. Dependence: Detoxification from opiate dependence can be accomplished on either an inpatient or an outpatient basis, depending on the severity of the situation and the time available to accomplish the treatment. A long-acting narcotic, such as methadone, is substituted for the opiate to which the patient is addicted. The methadone dosage during the first 2 days is usually 10–40 mg; this is followed by a gradual dosage reduction over a 3- to 21-day period, until the patient is drug free. Methadone itself can produce dependence; it is a long-acting narcotic and can be abused.

Nonnarcotic medication may be used on an outpatient basis to relieve symptoms of narcotic withdrawal. This includes the use of a sedative, a hypnotic, and an antispasmodic for relief of anxiety, insomnia, and gastrointestinal upset, respectively. Drugs such as clonidine (α_2-adrenergic agonists) can be used to suppress autonomic hyperactivity (eg, nausea, vomiting, intestinal cramps, and diarrhea); other medications are used to suppress pain and insomnia. Some outpatient detoxification centers use a less potent narcotic medication, such as propoxyphene. Acupuncture and other nondrug approaches have also been used on an outpatient basis for detoxification.

C. Maintenance: Long-acting opioids, such as methadone and L-acetylmethadol (LAM), are used to treat opioid-dependent individuals. By substituting an oral medication, such as methadone or LAM, the individual dependent on illicit opioids should not need to consume those substances. Buprenorphine, a partial μ-opioid agonist, is currently being investigated for both opioid detoxication and maintenance purposes. The use of oral medications removes the risk of sharing contaminated needles and syringes, which put the user at risk for HIV disease.

EPIDEMIOLOGY

ALCOHOL

Data from SAMHSA (1998) indicate that 51% of the total population age 12 and older currently use alcohol; the usage rate is over 60% for the age group from 21 to 39. Young Americans aged 18–25 are the most likely to engage in binge drinking or to drink heavily; of this group 46% are binge drinkers and one in five is a heavy drinker.

Alcohol use is also highly correlated with the use of illicit drugs. Of the 11.2 million heavy drinkers, 30% are current illicit drug users; of the binge drinkers, 18% are.

Alcohol consumption can be assessed based on age, gender, ethnicity, religious affiliation, socioeconomic status, geographic region, and social class. Fifty-eight percent of males are current alcohol users, compared with 45% of females. Males (23%) are significantly more likely to engage in binge drinking than females (8.1%) or to be heavy drinkers (8.9% for males versus 2.1% for females). Whites continue to represent the highest group of drinkers at 55%, followed by Latinos (42%) and African-Americans (40%).

Bucholz (1992) cites data from the Epidemiologic Catchment Area (ECA) study indicating that approximately 23.8% of men have a lifetime prevalence of alcoholism compared to 4.6% of women. Lifetime prevalence for Hispanic-Americans is higher (16.7%) than for whites (13.6%) and African-Americans (13.8%), although for Hispanic-American women it is lower. Overall, the ECA data show a male-to-female ratio of about 5.5:1. However, Grant et al (1991) report data from the National Health Interview survey, conducted by the National Center for Health Statistics, that show a male-to-female ratio of 3:1.

When income is used as a variable, the ECA data show an inverse relationship. Men with incomes greater than $50,000 show a much lower proportion of alcoholism than either the 1-year or lifetime prevalence. However, remission rates were higher in the higher income brackets than in the lower income brackets. ECA data also demonstrate a high frequency of comorbidity; approximately 47% of all alcoholics meet the criteria for a second lifetime psychiatric disorder. Although at first it may seem somewhat dated, the ECA study continues to represent the most comprehensive and empirically sound study to date.

DRUGS

The use of illicit drugs is a function of age. For most drugs, a higher lifetime prevalence exists for older age groups, which is not surprising: older cohorts have had more time to experiment with drugs than younger cohorts. Experiences such as marriage appear to facilitate the reduction of marijuana and other illicit drug use. Data from the National Institute of Drug Abuse Monitoring the Future Study, 1975–1992 (Johnson et al, 1993) indicate that among young adults 80% of 31- to 32-year-olds have used illicit drugs, compared to 41% of 1992 high school seniors. The annual prevalence rates are higher, however, among high school seniors: 27% compared to 22% of the 31- to 32-year-olds. This pattern of a higher lifetime prevalence as a function of age, but a lower annual prevalence during the later twenties, holds true for all illicit drugs except marijuana and cocaine. Data from SAMHSA (1998) corroborate these findings: comparing lifetime illicit drug use, the prevalence rate is 58.6% among 35- to 39-year-olds and 37.8% among 16- to 17-year-olds.

Unlike other illicit drugs, the lifetime, annual, and current use of cocaine is higher among the older age groups. Cocaine, in general, appears to be used more frequently among people in their twenties than those in their late teens. In 1997, lifetime prevalence for "crack" cocaine reached about 10.5% for those in their late twenties and early thirties (SAMHSA, 1998) compared to 3.3% (Johnston et al, 1997) for high school seniors. SAMHSA data report a lifetime cocaine usage rate of 24.5% for 35- to 39-year-olds, the highest of any age group, 6.9% for 16- to 17-year-olds, and 8.9% for 18- to 25-year-olds.

When looking at the annual and current use of LSD, the data from Johnston et al (1997) reveal that 8.8% of the respondents in the 18-year-old age group reported annual experience, which has increased every year since 1991. Furthermore, 2.5% of the 18-year-olds reported current use. SAMHSA data indicate that the number of past-month heroin use increased from 68,000 in 1993 to 325,000 in 1997, but as a percentage of the total population this remains negligible.

SUBSTANCE-RELATED DISORDERS IN PHYSICIANS

Substance-related disorders that occur in physicians, residents, or medical students are no less a major problem than when they occur in any other group. Physicians appear to have experimented with illicit substances consistent with their contemporaries; furthermore, the rate of alcoholism and other substance use disorders appears similar to that of others within their socioeconomic class. In the National Household Survey on Drug Abuse, Hughes et al (1992a) reported that physicians were less likely to have used cigarettes, marijuana, cocaine, and heroin in the past year than their age and gender counterparts. Based on a mailed, anonymous, self-report survey of 9600 physicians, with a 59% response rate, Hughes et al observed that physicians were more likely to have used alcohol, prescription minor opiates, and benzodiazepines than the comparison group. The use of alcohol, however, was attributed more to socioeconomic class than to profession, whereas the use of minor opiates and benzodiazepines was attributed more to access. Thus, although physicians may not drink more than other members of their socioeconomic class, they still drink more than the average population. The risk of alcoholism, then, is real, although not disproportionate. Others contradict these findings. For instance, O'Connor and Spickard (1997) state that the prevalence of alcohol and illicit drug abuse among physicians probably approximates the general population, and that abuse of prescriptive medications may be more prevalent. In a review of disciplinary acts taken by the Medical Board of California, Morrison and Wickersham (1998) report that 14% of sanctions were due to the abuse of alcohol or other drugs.

In an attempt to study resident physicians 3 years removed from medical school, Hughes et al (1991) mailed an anonymous survey to 3000 young physicians in 1987; they reported data on the 60% who responded. Alcohol was found to be the most widely used substance among residents, with 87% reporting use in the past month, but only 5% reporting use daily. Slightly less than 10% of the residents smoked cigarettes in the past month, with 5% smoking at least one cigarette on a daily basis. Seven percent of the respondents smoked marijuana in the past month, but only 0.3% were daily users. Almost 4% of the residents used benzodiazepines in the past month, although none reported daily use. Nevertheless, this particular finding suggests some residents are using controlled substances for self-medication, which is a potential problem. Only 1.4% of the residents acknowledged an experience with cocaine in the past month. Less than 1% of the respondents reported past-month experiences with amphetamines, psychedelics, LSD, barbiturates, heroin, or other opiates. When Hughes et al (1992b) analyzed their data by specialty, they found that residents in psychiatry and emergency medicine showed higher rates of substance use and residents in anesthesiology showed lower rates of substance use than residents in other specialties.

Physicians, nurses, and other health care professionals who develop substance abuse problems usually require some form of intervention. Those who become substance dependent are likely to require formal treatment. Substance dependence can interfere with the ability to practice medicine and can increase the likelihood that either patient care or professional misconduct may result. This may become evident in the diversion of medications such as opioids and benzodiazepines.

Specialized treatment programs have been designed to meet the needs of health professionals who suffer from substance abuse or substance dependence. Furthermore, Ikeda and Pelton (1990) noted that several state licensing boards and state medical societies sponsor diversion programs for physicians. In fact, Missouri has created a program (the Missouri Physicians' Health Program) in which confidential voluntary referrals are given treatment. Bohigian (1996) reports that the program has achieved a recovery rate of 94%. Finally, self-help groups such as Alcoholics Anonymous (AA), Narcotics Anonymous (NA), Cocaine Anonymous (CA), Rational Recovery, or Secular Organizations for Sobriety may offer assistance to the professional who needs community support for recovery. Consequently, the prognosis for substance-using physicians is improved if the problem is identified early and they receive prompt, comprehensive treatment.

ETIOLOGY, PATHOGENESIS, & NATURAL HISTORY OF SUBSTANCE-RELATED DISORDERS

Numerous factors have been identified as potential causes for substance-related disorders. In some patients, one factor may predominate; in others, several factors may interact, while in many, no clear-cut cause can be found. In addition, a stressful event may be the final precipitant that initiates the addictive cycle.

A. Biomedical Factors: Evidence supporting a role of biomedical factors in substance-related disorders comes from genetic, physiological, biochemical, and prenatal data.

1. Genetic factors—A number of twin, genetic marker, and adoption studies support the conclusion that susceptibility to adverse effects of alcohol and predilection for uncontrollable drinking are hereditary. Similar evidence applies to other substances of abuse, particularly the opioids and cocaine. Particularly intriguing are the studies showing alcoholism is more likely to occur in adopted children whose biological parents were alcoholics than in those whose biological parents were nonalcoholics. Two types of alcoholism emerge from these adoption studies. In Type 1, or milieu-limited alcoholism, both genetic predisposition and environmental factors play a role. This form of alcoholism, found more often among female alcoholics than in their male relatives, presents after the age of 25 and is not associated with criminality. In Type 2, or male-limited alcoholism, genetic factors appear stronger; there is more criminal behavior and an earlier age of onset. Cloninger (1987) has related Type 1 alcoholism to passive-dependent personality traits and Type 2 alcoholism to sociopathic personality traits. Schuckit (1994) noted that the sons of alcoholics tended to display a low level of response to alcohol well before they subsequently developed alcoholism a decade later. This low-level response is posited to represent the absence of the normal warning signs that inform other drinkers it is time to stop drinking. Alternatively, this low-level response might motivate the hyporesponder to consume more alcohol to generate an effect.

An explosion of scientific activity has occurred in research into the alleles of the dopamine D_2 receptor. Noble (1993) notes that an association exists with alcoholism of the A1 allele of the D_2 dopamine receptor gene. Other data indicate the dopamine receptor gene is also associated with other substance use disorders. Using the technique of restriction fragment length polymorphism (RFLP), researchers continue to pursue the link between specific genes and substance abuse.

In contrast, research on a genetic relationship to drug abuse is in an early developmental stage. Uhl et al (1993) observed that no study has identified substance abusers or controls by sampling randomly from the general population. Controlled studies, however, have produced data that support the notion that DRD2 variants contribute to interindividual differences in vulnerability to drug abuse.

2. Physiological factors—Physiological studies have correlated alcoholism with hypofunction of the adrenal cortex or the thyroid gland. In these studies, it is unclear whether endocrine hypofunction leads to alcoholism or vice versa; thus, a clear causal relationship is still unproved. Many Asians have a physiological response to alcohol characterized by facial flushing, headaches, tachycardia, and itching, which may account for the low rate of drinking in this population. This response, which occurs in 30–50% of Asians, is the result of the genetic lack of one form of aldehyde dehydrogenase (ALDH), the primary enzyme in the liver that breaks down acetaldehyde, the first metabolite of alcohol.

3. Biochemical factors—Because of the association of alcoholism and depression, numerous studies have attempted to relate alcoholism to levels of monoamine oxidase, also thought to be related to alcoholism. These studies have generally measured monoamine oxidase levels in platelets and have found levels are lower in alcoholics than in controls. Because platelet levels of monoamine oxidase are strongly affected by genetic factors, some have speculated this may be an important biochemical link between hereditary influences and the affective state of alcoholics. Other brain proteins have been implicated in alcoholism, primarily neurotransmitters (such as γ-aminobutyric acid, glycine, and glutamate), proteins that control the opening and closing of ion channels, and second messenger systems. Data are still being accumulated in these promising areas of research.

Dopamine has been implicated in the activity of the psychostimulants, such as cocaine and amphetamine. A receptor for cocaine has been identified that appears to be a site on the dopamine transporter of dopamine nerve terminals. Di Chiara and Imperato (1988) asserted that dopaminergic mechanisms may be a final common pathway for many substances that produce addictive behavior. Sora et al (1998) believe that rather than a single neurotransmitter system multiple neurotransmitter systems or the entire neurotransmitter system itself may be more important for the pathway to addiction.

Disturbances in the endogenous opioid system have been suggested as either a cause of opioid dependence or as a consequence of chronic opioid dependence. Altered opioid receptor proteins may give rise to a chronic addiction.

4. Prenatal factors—Infants whose mothers drink heavily during pregnancy often show biological defects such as decreased size and weight. Fetal alcohol syndrome, a neonatal condition characterized by neurophysiological dysfunction and various anatomic malformations, has been described. In infants whose mothers use drugs during pregnancy, there may be residual effects that affect the infant. Certainly a withdrawal syndrome is associated with opioids, benzodiazepines, nicotine, and possibly cocaine. Whether there are long-term sequelae to these syndromes awaits longer term studies. Clark and Weinstein (1993) noted, however, that the literature on prenatal substance exposure has expanded dramatically in the past 7 years.

B. Psychological Factors: Data supporting psychological causes of alcoholism and drug abuse are from three sources: (1) psychoanalytic case studies, (2) personality assessments using psychological testing, and (3) theories of learning.

1. Emotional conflicts—Psychoanalytic theory holds that early developmental deprivations and trauma may result in painful conflicts that are repressed. Symptoms such as anxiety and depression may occur when these conflicts begin to enter conscious awareness. Reactivation of conflicts may be triggered later in life by stress or by events that are reminiscent of the original deprivations and trauma (see section on "Role of Stress"). Alcohol and drugs are seen as releasing inhibitions, thus allowing expression of these repressed conflicts. More recently, substance abuse has been seen as an attempt to return to normal or to relieve emotional suffering. Brehm and Khantzian (1992) note that with this more modern view, the "self-medication" hypothesis has been developed; the substance user chooses an appropriate substance to titrate negative emotions. Thus, opiates help the addict control feelings of rage that erupt from earlier traumas in his or her life, cocaine is used to cope with feelings of anergy and fatigue that come from depression or low self-esteem, and alcohol can be used to help emotionally restricted individuals experience affect and to surmount fears of intimacy and closeness. Khantzian (1988) believes these factors have treatment implications, as they assist the clinician in understanding the patient's need for "control, containment, contact, and comfort."

2. Personality traits—Psychological testing has been used to explore common personality characteristics found in alcoholics. Several studies using the Minnesota Multiphasic Personality Inventory (MMPI) have shown that alcoholics demonstrate an abnormal elevation on the D (depression) and Pd (psychopathic deviance) scales. Some of these data on personality traits support the notion that alcoholics exhibit oral-dependent and depressive character traits, which is consistent with the psychoanalytic position previously mentioned. Because psychological tests often are administered to adults who are already identified as alcoholics, it is possible that years of drinking may encourage the emergence of clinically abnormal character traits later in life. For example, Vaillant (1980) has presented prospective data supporting the notion that oral-dependent traits may result from, rather than cause, alcoholism. Stabenau (1992) contends that antisocial personality disorder (ASP) is a strong predictor for alcohol abuse and dependence. Other studies have found a relationship between alcoholism and ASP.

As with alcoholism, psychological testing has been used to explore the dimensions of drug abusers. Craig and Weinberg (1992) report on studies that have used the Millon Clinical Multiaxial Inventory (MCMI) to characterize drug addicts. It was noted that antisocial character traits were prominent among those addicted to opiates and cocaine. Brooner et al (1992) note, however, that although both are associated with chronic drug use, ASP must be distinguished from antisocial behavior, as the former is associated with behavior that is more problematic.

3. Learned behavior—Learning theory has also been used to develop a causal model of substance use. Many alcoholics report that being intoxicated reduces anxiety and replaces it with a feeling of well-being. On the other hand, many drug abusers find cues in their environment facilitating their relapse by "reminding" them of their substance of abuse. The concept of "reminders" belongs to a line of research into substance abuse by Childress et al (1993) called "cue reactivity." Because people are drawn toward pleasurable states, drinking behavior, for example, is reinforced and gradually becomes a learned behavior (a habit). The same can be said for other substances of abuse.

C. Social Factors: The importance of social factors as a cause of alcoholism or drug abuse is supported by data from surveys and field studies that show relationships between the particular social variable under study and the rates of substance use. Some of the most important variables, such as sex, age, and ethnicity, are discussed in the previous section on "Epidemiology."

Family structure also plays an important role in both alcoholism and drug abuse. Using general systems theory, the substance abuser's family may be conceptualized as a maladaptive system whose stability depends on one member fulfilling a sick role. Although the family is dysfunctional, it is in a homeostatic state. Any attempt on the part of the physician or therapist to change the behavior of one family member will disturb the other family members; this will result in an increase in their anxiety and their attempt to resist the disturbing influence. This "systems" view has important implications for treatment because the entire family should be considered in the treatment plan.

D. Role of Stress: An interaction of biomedical, psychological, and social factors may lead to the gradual development of alcoholism or drug dependence. In some substance abusers, however, an acute traumatic life event (eg, the death of a spouse, physical illness, or even delayed posttraumatic stress disorder) leads to increased drinking or drug use as a coping mechanism in dealing with resultant anxiety and depression. In the diagnostic workup of substance abusing patients, making specific inquiries into a history of drinking or drug escalations after stressful events is useful.

TREATMENT & PROGNOSIS

A. Effect of the Physician's Attitude on Treatment: The physician's attitude affects the treatment of alcoholics and drug abusers. Attitudinal barriers include moralistic views that substance abusers are "bad" people; frustration over substance abusers being difficult, time-consuming patients who often leave treatment prematurely or offer little financial or ego reward; and pessimism over the "revolving-door syndrome," whereby, despite a great expenditure of time and energy on the part of the physician, the patient may later return for treatment in an inebriated or postintoxicated state. It is also true that physicians tend to treat those problems that interest them, for example, internists focus on biomedical issues and psychiatrists focus on psychosocial issues. To treat substance abusers properly, equal attention must be given to biomedical, psychological, and social issues; this is a difficult conceptual stance for many physicians.

Attitudinal barriers begin in the medical school and house staff years. Fisher et al (1975) found a general tendency for the expression of pessimism and negative moral views as students and physicians ascended the ladder of medical training: house staff members were more negative than second-year medical students and they, in turn, were more negative than first-year medical students. Chappel et al (1977) found that a course in substance abuse taught to second-year medical students significantly improved their attitudes; they took a less moralistic and more therapeutic view of the problem. Because the prognosis for curing alcoholism is better than the prognosis for curing many other conditions, it is important to educate physicians about alcoholism and its treatment so they will know how to deal with this problem.

B. Abstinence Versus Controlled Consumption: A key question in the treatment of individuals suffering from substance-related disorders is whether the goal should be permanent abstinence or moderate controlled use. For no substance is the debate about use more poignant than alcohol. Alcoholism has been conceptualized as a loss of ability to control consumption, perhaps because of a neurophysiological feedback dysfunction affecting the ability to regulate alcohol intake based on interoceptive cues. According to the theory, alcoholics must, therefore, be regarded as inherently unable to control their drinking behavior, so attempts at controlled drinking are doomed to failure. Furthermore, strict abstinence in the treatment of alcoholics has a long tradition and is a basic philosophic stance of AA, one of the oldest and most successful treatment programs. Because clinical experience has shown that most alcoholics who attempt controlled drinking ultimately fail, most workers in the field are skeptical about controlled drinking as a basic treatment goal. Nevertheless, because of the positive health effects of light to moderate alcohol consumption, moderation training has been recommended for those problem drinkers who are not alcohol dependent (Sitharthan et al, 1997).

For drugs of abuse, caffeine is perhaps the only substance with support for moderate consumption. Most of the other drugs of abuse are illicit and, thus, have negative consequences associated with them, which clearly suggest that if abuse becomes an issue, a return to moderate use is not practical. Clinically, marijuana is a drug about which many patients do not complain and support for moderate consumption may occur. Just as the abstinence model is articulated by AA, however, NA and CA discourage the use of psychoactive substances. These two organizations, parallel to AA, are available for community support of patients whether or not they are in formal treatment programs.

C. Disulfiram (Antabuse): Disulfiram produces an unpleasant reaction in the presence of alcohol and is used as a deterrent to drinking; its primary action is in blocking aldehyde dehydrogenase in the liver. When a patient taking disulfiram drinks ethyl alcohol, acetaldehyde cannot be converted to acetate, and the level of acetaldehyde in the blood may increase 5- to 10-fold. The alcohol-disulfiram reaction is thought to be a result of this increased level of acetaldehyde.

Nausea and flushing usually occur within 30 minutes and the full-blown reaction, which may include anxiety, dyspnea, headaches, tachycardia, and hypertension, usually lasts 30–90 minutes. More serious reactions may occur in individuals who are unusually sensitive or who have consumed large amounts of alcohol. For this reason, patients undergoing an alcohol-disulfiram reaction should be carefully monitored in an emergency room, and appropriate treatment for possible convulsions, myocardial infarction, or cardiovascular collapse should be available.

Disulfiram has a number of potential side effects, most of which are rare. The most common of these are drowsiness, metallic or garlic taste in the mouth, fatigue, and headaches. Disulfiram has synergistic effects with commonly prescribed medications (eg, benzodiazepines, barbiturates, monoamine oxidase inhibitors), and its use in pregnant women has been associated with fetal abnormalities. It has also been shown to produce psychotic reactions in patients with a history of major depression, mania, borderline personality, or schizophrenia.

The usual dose of disulfiram is 250 mg/day, generally taken in the evening because it causes drowsiness. Sensitivity to alcohol develops within 12 hours after taking the first dose, although antacids and iron decrease its absorption and may prolong this timeframe. Disulfiram is eliminated from the body slowly, and patients should be warned that they cannot drink for 1–2 weeks after medication is stopped. Disulfiram should seldom be prescribed continuously for more than 3–6 months, because side effects are time related. Because many of the side effects are also dose related, the dose should rarely exceed 500 mg/day. Alcoholics taking disulfiram should be carefully cautioned about side effects, the risks of the alcohol-disulfiram reaction, and unrecognized sources of alcohol, such as wine vinegar sauces, and medications containing alcohol (eg, cough syrup). Occasionally, patients are sensitive to the alcohol in aftershave lotion or aerosol deodorants; therefore, use of talcum powder and alcohol-free deodorants may be advisable. Banys (1988) contends that disulfiram is most useful in patients who (1) can tolerate a treatment relationship, (2) are relapse prone, but are in treatment, (3) have failed with less structured approaches, (4) are in early abstinence and are in crisis or under severe stress, (5) are in established recovery, but are not in individual or group psychotherapy because of relapse risk, or (6) specifically request it.

Hughes and Cook (1997) report that there is no reasonable evidence that disulfiram increases patients' abstinence rates. However, in a review of 38 outcome studies, they conclude that disulfiram may be helpful in reducing the quantity of alcohol consumed and the number of days of drinking.

D. Naltrexone: Naltrexone is an opiate antagonist approved for use in the treatment of opiate addiction and in the treatment of alcohol dependence. For the opioid-dependent patient who has been detoxified, the idea is to maintain the patient on this agent. Naltrexone has a high affinity for opiate receptors, is well absorbed orally, and has antagonist activity up to 72 hours. Maintenance naltrexone blocks the effects of opioids and is administered after a naloxone challenge test has determined whether the patient is still physically dependent on opiate agonists, such as heroin. Because naloxone is short acting, a positive response (ie, evidence of withdrawal) would last only about 1 hour, whereas the precipitation of withdrawal by naltrexone might last 24 hours.

For the patient suffering from alcoholism, naltrexone may be used as an adjunct to social and psychotherapeutic techniques. Volpicelli et al (1995) and others have reported that clinical trials have shown that naltrexone increases abstinence rates, decreases drinking days, decreases craving, and delays relapse. It should be noted, however, that naltrexone is not a "magic bullet"; in fact it is only modestly effective.

Naltrexone may have side effects, such as abdominal pain, headache, and mild increases of blood pressure. If evidence of moderate hepatic disease exists, naltrexone should not be administered. The major problem with naltrexone therapy is the high dropout rate. Normally, 40% of those who start naltrexone quit in the first month; only 10–20% take it for 6 months or longer. Recovering health professionals and parolees operating under the direction of the criminal justice system have a much higher continuation rate than other people.

E. Treatment Settings and Effectiveness:
Substance abuse treatment is provided in a spectrum of public and private facilities whose programs are also more flexible in terms of the type of problems they are willing to treat. In the 1980s, many programs were restricted to the treatment of alcoholism. The effectiveness of alcohol and drug abuse treatment, however, has been called into question. Although short-term abstinence rates of 40–60% are achievable in the first year, the evidence does not support an abstinence effect for longer term treatment of alcohol abuse. On the other hand, methadone maintenance and therapeutic communities appear to achieve significant program goals of both reduced drug use and crime. Marsha Lilli-Blanton (1998) notes that major studies (SAMHSA, 1997; RAND, 1994), which have evaluated the progress of thousands of people, conclude that drug abuse treatment was effective when outcomes were assessed 1 year after treatment.

Three types of treatment settings are available for alcoholics and drug abusers: (1) specialized substance abuse treatment programs, (2) AA, NA, and CA, and (3) treatment by the individual physician.

Specialized Substance Abuse Treatment Programs

The number of specialized treatment programs serving the substance abuse population increased in the 1980s. Because of budget considerations and poor reimbursement policies by insurance companies, however, this trend has weakened in recent years. Patients are either self-referred to these programs or they are referred by community agencies, physicians, and other professionals. Many of these programs include detoxification facilities, an inpatient rehabilitation unit, and an outpatient clinic.

A. Detoxification Facilities: The settings in which detoxification occurs will depend on the nature of the substance on which the patient is dependent and on the unique condition of the patient. Alcohol is a good representative substance in the discussion of detoxification facilities. Detoxification from alcohol may be done in one of three settings. To prevent late withdrawal reactions, patients should be carefully observed for at least 5 days. Severely ill patients should be hospitalized and treated in a general medical ward or specialized unit capable of dealing with potential complications. Indications for admission include impending or frank delirium tremens, medical problems that might be aggravated by the stress of withdrawal, and severe functional problems, such as suicidal or homicidal ideation or a psychotic condition. Patients with a history of medical complications or delirium tremens during previous withdrawals should also be considered for hospitalization.

Because only 5% of alcoholics require hospitalization for detoxification, most are managed in a social model detoxification setting. These centers provide a nonthreatening environment in which the patient is kept active and is provided with support and attention. The centers are usually staffed by nonprofessionals and are not licensed or staffed to handle severe illness or to dispense medications, therefore, patients referred to such settings should be both ambulatory and physically well.

Finally, some alcoholics may be managed in an outpatient clinic, and withdrawal symptoms can be aided by benzodiazepines. This type of withdrawal program should be reserved for physically and psychologically stable patients who are well motivated and have friends or relatives who can give them support and monitor their use of benzodiazepines.

These three settings are representative for all substances of abuse. A general discussion of intervention for other substances occurred earlier in this chapter. Thus, although cocaine dependence does not generally require hospitalization for detoxification, medical sequelae, such as chest pain or suicidal ideation, may necessitate hospitalization. Patients dependent on cocaine may want to be isolated from the substance of abuse; they may enter a social model detoxification facility for a week or more to remove themselves from the environment in which the drugs are being sold. Finally, outpatient clinics offering supportive care and pharmacotherapy in the form of antidepressants, such as fluoxetine, may be of assistance to the cocaine-using patient.

B. Inpatient Rehabilitation Units: Inpatient rehabilitation units were once very important settings for dealing with the sequelae of alcoholism and other drugs. These facilities are becoming more scarce primarily due to cost of treatment. However, federal grants are commonly funding private facilities to develop short-term (less than 6 months) therapeutic communities. Rehabilitation units offer a variety of services, including general medical workups; disulfiram treatment; naltrexone treatment; individual, group, and family therapy; recreational therapy; educational films and discussions; vocational testing and counseling; AA, NA, and CA groups; and careful attention to discharge planning, eg, help in finding a place to live and a temporary source of financial aid. Individuals referred to these units include patients who cannot remain abstinent outside a controlled setting, patients who need a period of hospitalization to stabilize their social situation, and patients who might benefit from an intensive therapeutic experience that may involve up to 10 hours a day of therapeutic work. Substance abusers with severe psychiatric or medical disorders do not generally do well in these intense, demanding programs. Programs are available, however, that can accommodate or that are devoted to the special needs of dual-diagnosis patients. Increasingly, insurance companies require inpatient rehabilitation programs to justify the presence of patients within the program. As a result, instead of the fixed length of stay popular in the 1980s, variable lengths of stay are becoming the norm.

C. Outpatient Substance Abuse Clinics: Many of the treatment services offered by outpatient substance abuse clinics parallel those previously described. Patients often spend years enrolled in outpatient programs, however, the focus is on long-term management and the uncovering of predisposing causes. Substance abusers in outpatient programs must be able to function outside a controlled environment.

D. Effectiveness of Programs: The measurement of the effectiveness of substance abuse treatment is complicated by the myriad of substances abused, the variations in populations studied, and the comorbidities present. Furthermore, a lack of consistency has developed in deciding what outcome variables are critical and what constitutes success. Finally, the consensus in the substance abuse treatment community is that substance abuse as a phenomenon is a chronic relapsing process; hence substance abusers may have recurrent episodes of treatment during the course of their lives. This, of course, is no different from other psychiatric conditions or, for that matter, many medical conditions.

In several reviews of specialized treatment programs, 30–40% of alcoholics were found to be significantly improved after 1–2 years. These results were adjusted statistically to account for program dropouts and patients whose improvement was "spontaneous" (ie, it could not be attributed to the treatment program). Success was measured as continuous abstinence or improved biomedical or psychosocial status. Outpatient programs are slightly

more successful than inpatient programs, although combined programs give the best results. Treatment programs vary greatly, depending on patient motivation and treatment setting. Poorly motivated alcoholics who are ordered by a judge to participate in a program, usually as a way of retaining a driver's license or staying out of jail, improve at a rate of about 10%, whereas improvement rates approaching 70% have been reported in highly motivated patients who are enrolled in multifaceted programs and who receive support from family and employers.

1. Alcoholics Anonymous—Alcoholics Anonymous (AA) was founded in 1935 by two recovering alcoholics. In 1989, there were nearly 48,000 AA groups in the United States and Canada; members now total over 500,000. AA is a self-help organization of nonprofessionals that emphasizes group support and surrender to a "higher power" to achieve permanent total abstinence. Sponsors and program members are available to help alcoholics 24 hours a day and sober interactions are encouraged through frequent meetings and club activities.

Although AA surveys usually report a 1-year continuous abstinence rate of nearly 60%, dropout rates are high, approaching 50% in the first 3 months (Chappel, 1997). When these data are considered in the analysis, the 1-year improvement rate approximates that of specialized alcoholism treatment programs. Nevertheless, for those who accept the AA model and remain in treatment, the program offers an important and often lifesaving source of support and abstinence. About one-half of those who participate for 3 months will be abstinent and continue to participate throughout the next year; a member who has been abstinent for 1–5 years has a good chance (86%) of completing the following year without drinking. Spin-offs of AA—Al-Anon and Alateen for adults and teenagers living with alcoholics—have been helpful in providing support.

NA and CA, self-help groups that focus either on narcotics or cocaine, are other spin-offs of AA. Although each group pursues its mission of self-help in much the same way as AA does, each has developed its own steps and traditions. NA and CA groups are available in many communities.

There are other self-help groups: Rational Recovery, whose principles are based on Albert Ellis, and Secular Organizations for Sobriety (SOS). These organizations offer self-help for those who object to those components of AA, NA, and CA that are considered religious. Galanter et al (1993) presented data that suggest a positive impact for Rational Recovery.

2. Treatment by an individual physician—Individual physicians in private, clinic, or hospital-based settings are an important treatment source for alcoholics and substance abusers. Although most physicians concern themselves with aspects of treatment of substance abuse that represent their area of expertise, a growing number are taking an eclectic view that integrates biomedical, psychological, and social factors in the treatment plan. It is critical that physicians familiarize themselves with community resources and establish channels for referral to other professionals who may have more expertise in some aspects of treatment. Therapeutic approaches should be flexible, supportive, and nonjudgmental. Physicians should remember that substance abuse is a disorder characterized by loss of control over drinking behavior or drug use, frequent relapses, a chronic course, and a variety of causes and effects. The physician who takes responsibility for constructing and coordinating all aspects of the patient's care (emotional and physical) will be more likely to have a successful treatment plan. Galanter (1993) offers a network therapy model for the individual therapist in office practice; this addresses many of the issues raised above by using psychodynamic and behavioral therapy while engaging the patient in a network composed of family members and friends.

E. Phases of Treatment for Substance Abuse: In planning treatment for the substance abuser, the physician should base priorities on each patient's biomedical, psychological, and social needs. The following discussion approaches treatment in terms of four sequential phases, each with typical problems and possible solutions (Table 17–5). Not all

patients enter treatment in Phase 1 or 2, however, and some patients may skip a phase depending on individual needs.

1. Phase 1 (acute crisis)—In evaluating a substance abuser, the first consideration is whether the patient is experiencing a life-threatening crisis (Table 17–6). The possibility of an acute medical or psychiatric emergency should be considered in every alcoholic or drug addict. Although the specific details of treatment are beyond the scope of this chapter, measures usually include immediate hospitalization and vigorous medical or psychiatric intervention (eg, administration of intravenous fluids, precautions against suicide attempts, and one-on-one nursing care). If family violence has occurred, family therapy and even a home visit by the staff may be useful. Substance-abusing patients hospitalized for another problem must be observed for the appearance of withdrawal symptoms, particularly if they were dependent on alcohol, benzodiazepines, or opioids.

2. Phase 2 (withdrawal from alcohol or drugs)—After acute crisis is ruled out, safe withdrawal from the effects of alcohol or drugs can be started (Table 17–6). Patients admitted to the hospital with delirium tremens should be placed in a well-lit room; they will require frequent observation (and possible restraints). The principles of care include re-

Table 17–6. Phases of treatment of alcoholism and drug abuse.

Phase of Treatment	Typical Problems	Possible Solutions
Phase 1 (acute crisis)	Biomedical: gastrointestinal bleeding (eg, alcohol); angina (eg, cocaine); coma (eg, opioids)	Appropriate medical intervention, which may include hospitalization
	Psychological: hallucinosis (eg, alcohol, LSD, or stimulants); paranoia (eg, PCP, marijuana, stimulants, alcohol); suicidal ideation (eg, stimulants, alcohol, LSD)	Appropriate psychiatric intervention, which may include hospitalization
	Social: family violence (eg, alcohol, stimulants, PCP)	Appropriate psychiatric intervention, which may include hospitalization; family therapy; home visit; domestic violence counseling
Phase 2 (withdrawal from substance abuse)	Biomedical: impending delirium tremens (eg, alcohol); impending seizures (eg, benzodiazepines); impending gastric distress (eg, opioids)	Medical or social model detoxification; outpatient detoxification; appropriate medical intervention
	Psychological: denial; worry about health; stressful life events	Counseling; brief individual or group therapy; AA/NA/CA
	Social: inadequate food and shelter; financial problems	Counseling; social services referral
Phase 3 (sequelae of substance abuse)	Biomedical: chronic medical problems; malnutrition	Appropriate medical intervention; vitamin supplements, proper diet, and exercise; disulfiram (alcohol); methadone (opioid); naltrexone (opioid)
	Psychological: denial; depression; guilt; stressful life events; craving for alcohol or drugs	Counseling; brief individual or group therapy; antidepressants; behavior modification techniques
	Social: family, housing, vocational, and legal problems; loneliness; unfilled leisure time	Counseling; social services referral; family therapy; recreational therapy; AA/NA/CA, Al-Anon or Alateen; halfway house
Phase 4 (focus on predisposing causes)	Biomedical: genetic factors	Counseling
	Psychological: neurotic and personality disorders; major affective disorders; schizophrenia	Long-term group therapy; antidepressants, major tranquilizers; therapeutic communities; individual therapy
	Social: sociocultural and familial influences	Counseling

assurance, careful monitoring of vital signs, and intravenous fluids with electrolytes and vitamins. Most alcoholics have low thiamine stores, and glucose solutions may cause further depletion of thiamine; therefore, thiamine should be added to intravenous fluids to prevent Wernicke's syndrome. Intravenous benzodiazepines are generally used, often in high doses, for delirium tremens. The physician must be alert to complications associated with delirium tremens (eg, seizures and marked autonomic hyperactivity), as well as the possibility of associated medical problems (eg, pneumonia or subdural hematoma). With treatment, most alcoholics recover from delirium tremens, although the mortality rate may reach 15%. Opioid-dependent patients admitted for rapid detoxification protocols need appropriate supportive care.

The detoxification from benzodiazepines must be carefully instituted to avoid seizures. Sees (1991) reviewed pharmacological adjuncts for treatment of withdrawal syndromes and offers practical recommendations.

In addition to biomedical problems during the withdrawal period, psychosocial issues should also be addressed. Many substance abusers deny or minimize the extent of psychological or social problems. Others are legitimately worried about their health or they are recovering from a stressful life event, such as a death in the family or a divorce, which served as the reason for the latest drinking or drug-using spree. Supportive counseling or brief individual or group therapy may be instituted as soon as the patient's sensorium clears and his or her medical status improves. Because compliance with treatment may be affected by problems, such as having no money and nowhere else to go, the physician may wish to either offer advice or make referrals to appropriate social service agencies.

3. Phase 3 (sequelae of alcoholism or drugs)—After dealing with acute problems and withdrawal, concern should focus on the sequelae of alcoholism or drugs. Some patients in this phase of treatment may be admitted directly to an outpatient clinic; others with more tenuous biomedical and psychosocial status should first be admitted to an inpatient rehabilitation unit. Chronic medical problems such as peripheral neuropathy, cirrhosis, or dementia should be managed appropriately. Vitamins and suitable instructions on the importance of diet and exercise will improve physical status. Disulfiram (Antabuse) should be prescribed for patients who need this added incentive to avoid alcohol. Naltrexone may be given to decrease cravings and to delay relapse. Patients dependent on opioids, and who are eligible for methadone maintenance, should be referred for this treatment. Alternatively, if the patient prefers to remain opioid free, naltrexone may be given.

Psychologically, many substance abusers experience depression, guilt, or the impact of stressful life events during this phase, particularly as the denial defense begins to crumble. Counseling or brief individual or group therapy may help. Antidepressants or lithium carbonate may be useful for substance abusers with major mood disorders. Newly abstinent substance abusers, particularly alcoholics, cocaine addicts, or opioid addicts, are particularly prone to experience a psychological craving for their substance of abuse. The intensity of the craving is correlated with anxiety or environmental factors, such as seeing an advertisement for alcohol, cues in their neighborhood, or experiencing a stressful life event. Behavior modification techniques that use aversive conditioning have been used to reduce craving in some alcoholics. Mild electric shock or emetics such as apomorphine or emetine are given while the patient drinks in a controlled setting, usually an inpatient or rehabilitation unit. The goal of such treatment is to create an aversion to alcohol that will persist after treatment. Aversive and other behavioral techniques are not effective as the sole form of treatment, but they have been used with success in multifaceted programs that address both drinking behavior and associated psychosocial problems. Covert sensitization (aversion therapy) and other newer behavioral techniques that use fantasy and imagination to develop conditioned aversion to alcohol have also shown promise, although not all patients can be successfully trained to use these techniques (see Chapter 33). Onken et al (1993) edited a NIDA Monograph that reviewed behavioral treatments for drug abuse.

Years of substance abuse may lead to family difficulties, inadequate shelter, a poor job history, legal and financial problems, loneliness, and trouble filling leisure time in a nonalcoholic context. The physician may wish to counsel the patient on these matters or to refer the patient to appropriate social agencies for food stamps, vocational counseling, and so forth. Family therapy may be helpful, because patterns of family interaction become more rigid when substance abusers are using than when they are clean or sober. Recreational activities and hobbies may help the alcoholic fill leisure time. Community self-help groups, such as AA, NA, and Rational Recovery are useful in giving support as well as encouraging and reinforcing abstinence.

In some communities, another referral source is the substance abuse halfway house, which Rubington (1977) defines as "a transitional place of indefinite residence of a community of persons who live together under the rule and discipline of abstinence from alcohol and other drugs." This setting provides the abstinent substance abuser with a clean and sober environment in the company of other recovering substance abusers who are able to offer support and advice. Food and shelter are provided, and many halfway houses have their own therapeutic programs, which may include vocational counseling *and informal "rap" groups.* Although the stay is usually limited to a few months, many alcoholics are functioning at a higher level by this time and are ready to live independently.

4. Phase 4 (focus on predisposing causes)—After the sequelae of alcoholism and drugs have been managed, focusing on predisposing causes of the problem is appropriate (Table 17–6). The physician should be sensitive to the patient's concerns involving genetic and sociocultural factors. Some substance abusers feel that genetic factors doom them to a life of alcoholism or drug abuse; for this reason, they approach treatment pessimistically. Others blame their religious and cultural background, age, or gender, or are reluctant to seek treatment from physicians of different ethnic backgrounds. Counseling that emphasizes support and reassurance may be effective in alleviating concern, exploring stereotypes, and breaking cultural barriers.

For many substance abusers, psychological issues are important predisposing causes of drinking or drug use. Diagnostically, these may include dysthymic and generalized anxiety or posttraumatic stress disorder; personality problems such as antisocial, dependent, or borderline disorder; major affective problems such as bipolar or major depressive disorder; and schizophrenia. For substance abusers with neurotic problems and borderline personality disorders, long-term individual therapy may be useful. Substance abusers with other personality disorders do best in group therapy. Therapy emphasizing insight and interpersonal learning tends to be stressful for substance abusers, so they need additional group experiences providing support and emphasizing abstinence, such as offered by AA, NA, and CA or a "rap" group. Assertiveness training groups have also been useful for many substance abusers. Finally, for substance abusers with major affective disorders or schizophrenia, treatment with antidepressants, lithium carbonate, or major tranquilizers may be helpful. Minor tranquilizers, such as the benzodiazepines, have addictive potential and should not be used for long periods, if at all. Treatment matching, ie, finding the most appropriate treatment for the specific needs of the patient, may be the most critical variable in determining the outcome of the care given to the patient.

SUBSTANCE ABUSE & HUMAN IMMUNODEFICIENCY VIRUS DISEASE

As of December 1997 (the most recent complete reporting period), 641,086 cases of acquired immunodeficiency syndrome (AIDS) in the United States had been reported to the Centers for Disease Control and Prevention, of which 202,406 (31.5%) were associated with illicit drug use. Of these, 161,872 (80%) were in both women and heterosexual men reported to be injecting drug users (IDUs) and 40,534 (20%) were in men who had sex with men who were

also IDUs; in addition, there were 7335 pediatric AIDS cases in which the mothers were either IDUs or sex partners of IDUs. The substance abuser risks various health complications ranging from drug-related violence and automobile accidents to liver disease. The sharing of needles by addicts carries the risk of direct transmission of hepatitis and AIDS.

Unfortunately, psychoactive drug use increases a person's risk-taking behavior, including unsafe sexual practices. The use of intravenous amphetamines, for example, is often associated with sexual activity, particularly in some homosexual men who use stimulants to sustain erections for many hours. It is critical that such high-risk individuals receive access to both AIDS education and substance abuse education and treatment. AIDS and AIDS-related complex (ARC) add another dimension to differential diagnosis of chemical dependence and psychiatric disorders. The astute clinician must assess whether psychiatric symptoms (particularly anxiety or depression) are (1) symptoms of drug use (or withdrawal), (2) symptoms of an endogenous disorder, (3) a psychological reaction to, or fear of, AIDS, or (4) an indication of the effects (eg, depression and delirium) of HIV on the central nervous system. The psychiatrist who has no experience with psychoactive substance use disorders or with AIDS-related psychological disorders should engage in multidisciplinary cooperation with other health care professionals, including paraprofessional substance abuse and AIDS counselors, when treating psychoactive substance abusers in this high-risk category. Multiple drug-resistant tuberculosis is also a great concern among the providers of treatment to substance abusers, particularly those who are HIV positive and those who have AIDS or ARC.

SUMMARY

Substance-related disorders are serious disorders characterized by loss of control over alcohol consumption or drug use; a chronic, relapsing course; and a number of biomedical, psychological, and social causes and effects. In the diagnostic workup, a complete history, mental status examination, and physical examination, along with appropriate laboratory tests, are essential. Because substance abuse affects both sexes and people of all ages, races, and socioeconomic classes, the physician should be alert to its possibility when evaluating any patient. Case finding is made difficult by denial of alcoholism or drug abuse by patients, negative physician attitudes, and the presence of alcoholism or drug abuse among physicians.

Permanent abstinence is the major treatment goal for alcoholics and drug abusers. Therapeutic approaches should be flexible, supportive, and nonjudgmental. Important treatment settings include inpatient and social model detoxification units, inpatient rehabilitation wards, outpatient substance abuse clinics, and substance abuse halfway houses. Disulfiram (Antabuse), methadone maintenance, or community self-help groups (such as AA) are important adjuncts to treatment. By addressing issues involving acute crises, withdrawal, and sequelae and causes of substance abuse, the physician may play a key role in coordinating the treatment of substance-abusing patients.

REFERENCES & SUGGESTED READINGS

Allen LN: Drugs of abuse. In: *Psychotropic Drugs.* Keltner, Folks (editors). Mosby, 1997.

Banys P: The clinical use of disulfiram (Antabuse): A review. J Psychoactive Drugs 1988;20:243.

Becker CE, Roe RL, Scott RA: *Alcohol as a Drug.* Medcom Press, 1974.

Bohigian GM et al: Substance abuse and dependence in physicians: The Missouri Physicians' Health Program. South Med J 1996;89:1078.

Brehm NM, Khantzian EJ: A psychodynamic perspective. In: *Substance Abuse, A Comprehensive Textbook,* 2nd ed. Lowinson JH, Ruiz P, Millman RB (editors). Williams & Wilkins, 1992.

Brooner RK et al: Antisocial behavior of intravenous drug abusers: Implications for diagnosis of antisocial personality disorder. Am J Psychiatry 1992;149:482.

Bucholz KK: Alcohol abuse and dependence from a psychiatric epidemiologic perspective. Alcohol Health Res World 1992;16:197.

Chappel JN et al: Substance abuse attitude changes in medical students. Am J Psychiatry 1977;134:379.

Chappel JN: Long-term recovery from alcoholism. Psychiatr Clin North Am 1993;16:177.

Childress AR et al: Cue reactivity and cue reactivity interventions in drug dependence. NIDA Research Monograph 1993;137:73.

Clark HW, McClanahan TM: Contemporary issues in dual diagnosis. In: *New Treatments for Chemical Addictions.* McCance-Katz E, Kosten TR (editors). American Psychiatric Press, 1998.

Clark HW, Weinstein M: Chemical dependency. In: *Occupational and Environmental Reproductive Hazards: A Guide for Clinicians.* Paul M (editor). Williams & Wilkins, 1993.

Cloninger CR: Neurogenetic adaptive mechanisms in alcoholism. Science 1987;236:410.

Craig RJ, Weinberg D: Assessing drug abusers with the Millon Clinical Multiaxial Inventory: A review. J Subst Abuse Treat 1992;9:249.

Di Chiara G, Imperato A: Drugs abused by humans preferentially increase synaptic dopamine concentrations in the mesolimbic system of freely moving rats. Proc Natl Acad Sci USA 1988;85:1207.

Fisher JC et al: Physicians and alcoholics: The effect of medical training on attitudes toward alcoholics. J Stud Alcohol 1975;36:949.

Galanter M: Network therapy for addiction: A model for office practice. Am J Psychiatry 1993;150:28.

Galanter M, Egelko S, Edwards H: Rational recovery: Alternative to AA for addiction? Am J Drug Alcohol Abuse 1993;19:499.

Hayner GN, McKinney HE: MDMA: The dark side of Ecstasy. J Psychoactive Drugs 1986;18:341.

Hughes PH et al: Resident physician substance use in the United States. JAMA 1991;265:2069.

Hughes PH, Cook CC: The efficacy of disulfiram: A review of outcome studies. Addiction 1997;92;381.

Hughes PH et al: Prevalence of substance use among U.S. physicians. JAMA 1992a;267:2333.

Hughes PH et al: Resident physician substance use, by specialty. Am J Psychiatry 1992b;149:1348.

Ikeda R, Pelton C: Diversion programs for impaired physicians. West J Med 1990;152:617.

Johnston LD, O'Malley PM, Bachman JG: National survey results on drug abuse from the Monitoring the Future Study, 1975–1992. Vol II. NIDA. NIH Publication No. 93-3598, 1993.

Kaufman E: Family therapy: A treatment approach with substance abusers. In: *Substance Abuse, A Comprehensive Textbook,* 2nd ed. Lowinson JH, Ruiz P, Millman RB (editors). Williams & Wilkins, 1992.

Khantzian EJ: The primary care therapist and patient needs in substance abuse treatment. Am J Drug Alcohol Abuse 1988;14:159.

Lillie-Blanton M: Drug abuse—Studies show treatment is effective, but benefits may be overstated. (Testimony, 07/22/98, GAO/T-HEHS-98-185.)

Lowinson JH, Ruiz P, Millman RB (editors): *Substance Abuse, A Comprehensive Textbook,* 2nd ed. Williams & Wilkins, 1992.

Lukas SE et al: Marihuana attenuates the rise in plasma ethanol levels in human subjects. Neuropsychopharmacology 1992;7:77.

Morrison J, Wickersham P: Physicians disciplined by a state medical board. JAMA 1998;279:1889.

National Institute on Drug Abuse (NIDA): Epidemiologic trends in drug abuse: Volume I, highlights and executive summary, Community Epidemiology Work Group. NIH Publication No. 96-4126, 1996.

National Institute on Alcohol Abuse and Alcoholism (NIAAA): Surveillance report #43: Apparent per capita alcohol consumption: National, state, and regional trends, 1977–95. USDHHS, 1997.

Noble EP: The D2 dopamine receptor gene: A review of association studies in alcoholism. Behav Genet 1993;23:119.

O'Connor PG, Spickard A: Physician impairment by substance abuse. Med Clin North Am 1997;81:1037.

O'Farrell TJ: Marital and family therapy in alcoholism treatment. J Subst Abuse Treat 1989;6:23.

Onken LS et al: Behavioral treatments for drug abuse and dependence. NIDA Research Monograph 1993;137.

Perez-Reyes M et al: Interaction between marihuana and ethanol: Effects on psychomotor performance. Alcoholism Clin Exp Res 1988;12:268.

RAND: Controlling cocaine: Supply versus demand. Rand Doc No. MR-331. RAND Corporation, 1994.

Rubington E: The role of the halfway house in the rehabilitation of alcoholics. In: *The Biology of Alcoholism. Vol 5: Treatment and Rehabilitation of the Chronic Alcoholic.* Kissin B, Begleiter H (editors). Plenum Press, 1977.

Schuckit MA: Low level of response to alcohol as a predictor of future alcoholism. Am J Psychiatry 1994;151:184.

Sees KL: Pharmacological adjuncts for the treatment of withdrawal syndromes. J Psychoactive Drugs 1991;23:371.

Sharp CW, Beauvais F, Spence R (editors): Inhalant abuse: A volatile research agenda. NIDA Research Monograph 129, 1992.

Sitharthan T et al: Cue exposure in moderation drinking: A comparison with cognitive-behavior therapy. J Consult Clin Psychol 1997;65:878.

Smith DE: Cocaine-alcohol abuse: Epidemiological, diagnostic and treatment considerations. J Psychoactive Drugs 1986;18:117.

Sora I et al: Cocaine reward models: Conditioned place preference can be established in dopamine- and in serotonin-transporter knockout mice. Proc Natl Acad Sci USA 1998;95:7699.

Stabenau JR: Is risk for substance abuse unitary? J Nerv Ment Dis 1992;180:583.

Substance Abuse and Mental Health Services Administration (SAMHSA): National Treatment Improvement Evaluation Study. DHHS Publication No. (SMA) 97-3154. Center for Substance Abuse Treatment, 1997.

Substance Abuse and Mental Health Services Administration (SAMHSA): Preliminary results from the 1997 National Household Survey on Drug Abuse. DHHS Publication No. (SMA) 98-3251. Office of Applied Studies, 1998.

Uhl G et al: Substance abuse vulnerability and D2 receptor genes. Trends Neurosci 1993;16:83.

Vaillant GE: Natural history of male psychological health: VIII. Antecedents of alcoholism and orality. Am J Psychiatry 1980;137:181.

Volpicelli JR et al: Medical management of alcohol dependence: Clinical use and limitations of naltrexone treatment. Alcohol Alcoholism 1995;30:789.

Weissman DE, Haddox JD: Opioid pseudoaddiction: An iatrogenic syndrome. Pain 1989;36:363.

Wesson DR, Smith DE, Steffen SC: Crack and ice. Treating smokable stimulant abuse. Hazelden Foundation, 1992.

Ziedonis DM, Wyatt SA, George TP: Current issues in nicotine dependence and treatment. In: *New Treatments for Chemical Addictions*. McCance-Katz E, Kosten TR (editors). American Psychiatric Press, 1998.

Schizophrenic Disorders 18

Bruce Africa, MD, PhD, Oliver Freudenreich, MD, & Stuart R. Schwartz, MD

The term "schizophrenia" denotes a severe and prolonged mental disturbance manifested as a wide range of disturbed thought, speech, and behavior. Though discussed as one disease, schizophrenia may be more appropriately considered a group of disorders of uncertain cause with similar clinical presentations, invariably including thought disturbances in a clear sensorium, often with characteristic symptoms such as hallucinations, delusions, bizarre behavior, and deterioration in the general level of functioning. Schizophrenia is a disorder that is found in all countries and societies of the world; about 1 in every 100 persons will develop schizophrenia in their lifetime.

CONCEPTS OF SCHIZOPHRENIA

Descriptions of illness consistent with the concept of schizophrenia date back 3400 years to 1400 BC and are found throughout history; they become frequent only after the social and industrial revolutions of the eighteenth century when physicians were given control of asylums. Emil Kraepelin, a German psychiatrist attempting to classify all subsequently described psychoses of the nineteenth century, introduced the term "dementia praecox" in 1896. He classified psychotic disorders "without known organic etiology" into three groups based on clinical presentation and course. Kraepelin used the term **manic-depressive insanity** for the group of disorders characterized primarily by exacerbations and remissions in disturbances of affect rather than cognition. He linked a second syndrome, **paranoia,** with this group because the psychosis was limited and did not produce severe deterioration of affect or function. **Dementia praecox** was the term Kraepelin used for his third group, which featured severe disturbances in functioning that began in adolescence and progressively worsened and in which "failure of volition" was a prominent feature. Kraepelin did note that there were variations in course, and he considered **paraphrenia** to be a less severe development of dementia praecox (Kraepelin, 1909/1919).

In 1911, Eugen Bleuler, a Swiss psychiatrist, classified the functional psychoses into just two groups by introducing the term **schizophrenia.** Schizophrenia, literally translated as "splitting of the mind," remained the dominant term worldwide for the psychoses described below. Bleuler believed that four psychological processes were central to the illness: **autism** (a turning inward, away from the world), **ambivalence** (the condition of having two strong but opposite feelings at the same time), and primary disturbances in **affect** and **associations.** Like Kraepelin, Bleuler assumed that the schizophrenia syndrome was separate from manic-depressive illness and that underlying biological determinants eventually would be discovered for each (Bleuler, 1911/1950). Modern studies of manic-depressive and schizophrenic psychoses actually began after 1911, when serology had provided a means of identifying patients with tertiary syphilis, who accounted for about one-third of those considered severely mentally ill, and later when public health measures had reduced the nutritional avitaminoses.

Eugen Bleuler's criteria were used broadly to designate a group of patients about twice as large as Kraepelin's group. Kasanin conceptualized a "schizoaffective" grouping of those who exhibited signs and symptoms that resembled a combination of the signs and symptoms found in parts of the two Bleulerian psychoses. These additional patients were identified by Langfeldt as "schizophreniform," ie, "other than true schizophrenia." His work in the 1930s had established that those who remitted, either spontaneously or after treatment, were mostly from this group.

The controversy about the definition of "schizophrenia" has led to many different conclusions about its natural course and treatment outcome. The varied conclusions have, in turn, confused the student as much as have the varied symptomatic behaviors of patients with schizophrenia with whom they interact. No matter how narrow the initial diagnostic criteria, there are marked variabilities in both the final outcome and the clinical presentations seen at different times over any individual patient's lifetime. Different observers, even within a single diagnostic system, seeing the patient at different times, attain contradictory impressions and gain a dissimilar perspective.

The currently accepted concept of the schizophrenic disorders recognizes (Table 18–1) deterioration from a previous level of functioning, characteristic symptoms involving multiple psychological processes, clear-cut psychotic features during the active phase of the illness, and a tendency toward chronicity. Thus, the diagnosis of schizophrenia is

Table 18–1. *DSM-IV* diagnostic criteria for schizophrenia.

A. *Characteristic symptoms:* Two (or more) of the following, each present for a significant portion of time during a 1-month period (or less if successfully treated):
(1) delusions, (2) hallucinations, (3) disorganized speech (eg, frequent derailment or incoherence), (4) grossly disorganized or catatonic behavior, (5) negative symptoms (ie, affective flattening, alogia, or avolition).
Note: Only one Criterion A symptom is required if delusions are bizarre or hallucinations consist of a voice keeping up a running commentary on the person's behavior or thoughts, or two or more voices conversing with each other.

B. *Social/occupational dysfunction:* For a significant portion of the time since the onset of the disturbance, one or more major areas of functioning such as work, interpersonal relations, or self-care are markedly below the level achieved prior to the onset (or when the onset is in childhood or adolescence, failure to achieve expected level of interpersonal, academic, or occupational achievement).

C. *Duration:* Continuous signs of the disturbance persist for at least 6 months. This 6-month period must include at least 1 month of symptoms (or less if successfully treated) that meet Criterion A (ie, active-phase symptoms) and may include periods of prodromal or residual symptoms. During these prodromal or residual periods, the signs of the disturbance may be manifested by only negative symptoms or two or more symptoms listed in Criterion A present in an attenuated form (eg, odd beliefs, unusual perceptual experiences).

D. *Schizoaffective and mood disorder exclusion:* Schizoaffective disorder and mood disorder with psychotic features have been ruled out because either (1) no major depressive, manic, or mixed episodes have occurred concurrently with the active-phase symptoms or (2) if mood episodes have occurred during active-phase symptoms, their total duration has been brief relative to the duration of the active and residual periods.

E. *Substance/general medical condition exclusion:* The disturbance is not due to the direct physiological effects of a substance (eg, a drug of abuse, a medication) or a general medical condition.

F. *Relationship to a pervasive developmental disorder:* If there is a history of autistic disorder or another pervasive developmental disorder, the additional diagnosis of schizophrenia is made only if prominent delusions or hallucinations are also present for at least a month (or less if successfully treated).

Classification of longitudinal course (can be applied only after at least 1 year has elapsed since the initial onset of active-phase symptoms):

Episodic With Interepisode Residual Symptoms (episodes are defined by the reemergence of prominent psychotic symptoms); *also specify if:* **With Prominent Negative Symptoms**
Episodic With No Interepisode Residual Symptoms
Continuous (prominent psychotic symptoms are present throughout the period of observation); *also specify if:* **With Prominent Negative Symptoms**
Single Episode In Partial Remission; *also specify if:* **With Prominent Negative Symptoms**
Single Episode In Full Remission
Other or Unspecified Pattern

---

made only after careful examination of the cross-sectional signs and symptoms at presentation and an appraisal of the longitudinal course of the illness.

ONSET OF SCHIZOPHRENIA

Although schizophrenia usually has its onset when the person is in the teens or early 20s, there clearly is a continuum of onset with cases occurring early (before puberty) and late (after age 45). Schizophrenia beginning in childhood often indicates a more severe disease process that is more difficult to treat. Autism and childhood schizophrenia are no longer considered to be the same disorder. Schizophrenia can begin later in life and is sometimes called late paraphrenia; clinically the typical patient is a suspicious person with delusions of persecution and hallucinations but with little formal thought disorder and affective flattening. The onset of adult schizophrenia is noted when family and friends observe that the person has changed and is no longer the same. The individual functions poorly in significant areas of routine daily living, such as work or school, and in social relations. There is often a notable lack of concern for self-care in an individual who has previously been capable of it. As they lose their grip on reality, patients experience the following feelings:

A. Perplexity: At the onset of illness, patients report a sense of strangeness about the experience as well as confusion about where the symptoms are coming from and why their own everyday experience is so markedly changed.

B. Isolation: The schizophrenic person experiences an overwhelming sense of being different and separate from other people. They experience intense loneliness.

C. Anxiety and Terror: A general sense of discomfort and anxiety often pervades the experience. This may be made more acute by periods of intense terror caused by a "world within" that is experienced as dangerous or uncontrollable and is often attributed to external sources.

SYMPTOMS & SIGNS

In schizophrenia, severe disturbances occur in several of the following areas: language and communication, content of thought, perception, affect, sense of self, volition, relationship to the external world, and motor behavior. Any of these symptoms may be seen in other mental disorders, and none, by itself, is pathognomonic of schizophrenia. Furthermore, individuals who are well adapted and who have no evidence of any underlying psychopathological disorder may, when under stress, exhibit a syndrome that is similar to that seen in schizophrenic persons. It is the character of symptoms involved and the degree of impairment over time that establish the diagnosis of schizophrenia. Disabling symptoms characteristic of schizophrenia do not preclude development of other psychiatric disorders, nor are schizophrenic patients devoid of ordinary human characteristics—feelings, thoughts, and actions.

Disturbances in Language & Communication

The schizophrenic individual thinks and reasons according to private, and often idiosyncratic, rules of logic. The form of thinking is disordered (formal thought disorder). The individual cannot maintain a consistent train of thought; ideas slip from one track to another, and communication is severely impaired (so-called **derailment** or **looseness of associations**). **Circumstantiality** (irrelevant detours in speech) or **tangentiality** (continuing digressions in speech, so that the conversation fails to reach the anticipated goal) may also occur. There may be **poverty of content of speech,** in which little information is communicated because many words are vague, overabstract, overconcrete, repetitive, or stereotyped. A more severe symptom is the formation of **neologisms:** the schizophrenic individual's speech is filled with "new words" formed by condensing and combining several known words in a manner unique to the individual, who may often be able to provide a precise definition of the word used that may have personal, magical, or wish-fulfilling properties. Complete incoherence of speech (**word salad**) may occur, with a mixture of words lacking meaning and logical coherence.

The disorder in thought permeates many areas of the patient's life and may be shown not only in language but also in work and personal creative efforts (eg, arts, crafts). The following is a typical example of the thought disorder of the schizophrenic patient:

> If things turn by rotation of agriculture or levels in regards and timed to everything: I am referring to a previous document when I made some remarks that were facts also tested and there is another that concerns my daughter she has a lobed bottom right ear, her name being Mary Lou. . . . Much of abstraction has been left unsaid and undone in this product/milk syrup, and others due to economics, differentials, subsidies, bankruptcy, tools, buildings, bonds, national stocks, foundation craps, weather trades, government in levels of breakages, and fuses in electronics to all formerly "stated" not necessarily factuated.

Clinicians must recognize that this disturbance in language and communication cannot be attributed to lack of education, low intelligence, or a particular cultural background.

Disturbances in Content of Thought

Things go on in the mind of a schizophrenic patient that do not go on in the minds of other people. Distor-

tions of perception and idiosyncratic, illogical associations lead to incorrect conclusions; these are usually defended with emotion and may cause socially inappropriate behavior. A **delusion** is a false belief that may be fixed (ie, maintained over an extended period) or temporary. Certain delusions are particularly characteristic of schizophrenia patients, such as the notion that their thoughts are being broadcast into the external world so that others can hear them, or that thoughts are being inserted into their minds by another individual or superior force, or that an individual or machine is dominating and controlling their lives (**delusion of influence**). Events that are not related to the patient are commonly invested with a personal significance by the patient alone and are called **ideas of reference,** eg, a newspaper article or television program may be experienced by the patient as having a special personal message that relates directly to them. Delusions are commonly persecutory (belief that they are being watched, followed, or plotted against), grandiose (belief that they have special powers, influence, or wealth), or somatic in a nonmedical and often bizarre way (belief that something is rotting inside their bodies).

In normal adolescence, people often experience a sensation of heightened self-consciousness and believe that others are aware of their private thoughts and feelings. The schizophrenic patient experiences similar feelings with far greater distress, intensity, and conviction. A psychiatric nurse describes her own thought disturbances as follows:

> Not knowing that I was ill, I made no attempt to understand what was happening, but felt that there was some overwhelming significance in all of this, produced either by God or Satan. . . . The walk of a stranger on the street could be a "sign" to me which I must interpret. Every face in the windows of a passing streetcar would be engraved on my mind, all of them concentrating on me and trying to pass me some sort of message.

Disturbances in Perception

False perceptions in the absence of an external stimulus are called **hallucinations.** In schizophrenia, these are usually auditory. Visual, tactile, and olfactory hallucinations can occur in schizophrenia, but more often reflect delirium, dementia, or some other disorder. In auditory hallucinations, voices seem to speak directly to the patient or make comments (frequently negative) on the patient's behavior. "**Command hallucinations**" can be a compelling force working against the patient's own wishes, best interests, or safety. Hallucinations must be distinguished from **illusions,** which are false interpretations of a real stimulus.

Disturbances in Affect

Affect, or "feeling tone," refers to the outward expression of emotion, as opposed to mood, which is inferred from the combined data of affect and the patient's own communications. In schizophrenia, affect may be inappropriate, ie, inconsistent with the topic or context of communication. Affect may be extremely labile, showing rapid shifts from tears to joy for no obvious reason, or may be flattened, showing virtually no signs of emotional expression, with the voice monotonous and the face immobile. Patients may state that they no longer respond to life with normal intensity or that they are "losing their feelings." Physicians must be cautious in evaluating the affect of a patient, because use of antipsychotic drugs may produce a state that is nearly identical to the flattening of affect described above.

Disturbances in Sense of Self

Schizophrenic patients have lost touch with who they are. They may have doubts, concerns, and worries about the very nature of their identity. They may feel that the very core of their identity is dead, vulnerable, or changing in some mysterious way. The overwhelming sense of perplexity about this feeling is then translated into concerns about the meaning of existence. Two patients have described how they feel:

> I have experienced this process chiefly as a condition in which the integrating mental picture in my personality was taken away and smashed to bits, leaving me like agitated hamburger, distributed evenly throughout the universe.

> I am like a zombie living behind a glass wall. I can see all that goes on in the world, but I can't touch it. I can't reach it. I can't be in contact with it. I am outside. They are inside, and when I get inside, they aren't there. There is nothing there, absolutely nothing.

Disturbances in Volition

In schizophrenia, disturbance in self-initiated, goal-directed activity is very common and may grossly impair work performance or functioning in other roles. The disruption takes the form of inadequate interest, drive, or ability to complete a course of action successfully. Overwhelming ambivalence, which directs the individual toward two diametrically opposed courses of action, may lead to a stalemate with no goal-directed activity. In contrast, there may be a sense of mission, particularly in the early stages of schizophrenia, with a resulting outpouring of energy to complete a particular task while floridly exhibiting symptoms. These activities are perceived as bizarre by most of those in contact with the patient, and they also bring the patient into conflict with the authority figures within the consensual reality of the dominant culture.

Disturbances in Relationship to the External World

The individual with schizophrenia tends to withdraw from involvement with other people and to direct attention inward toward egocentric and illogical ideas and fantasies. The word "autistic" (not to be confused with autism, a different condition) has been used to describe the overwhelming, self-centered concerns of the patient with a schizophrenic disorder.

Disturbances in Motor Behavior

Motor disturbances range through both extremes. Decreased reaction to the environment can progress to an almost total reduction of spontaneous movements and activity (catatonic stupor) in which the individual acts like a zombie or assumes strange postures (waxy flexibility). Motion may also become constant, bizarre, or wildly aggressive (agitated catatonia), continuing until exhaustion, treatment, or death intervenes.

SUBTYPES OF SCHIZOPHRENIA

Schizophrenic disorders in the *Diagnostic and Statistical Manual of Mental Disorders,* 3rd and 4th editions (*DSM-III* and *DSM-IV*) were divided into four active and one residual subtypes on the basis of distinctive symptom clusters. Descriptions of these subtypes have evolved, since the time of Kraepelin and Bleuler, as attempts to identify different natural courses and/or responses to treatment within the spectrum of schizophrenia.

Disorganized Type

(Formerly called hebephrenia.) Features include incoherence and the lack of systematized delusions, disorganized behavior that is not catatonic, and blunted, inappropriate, or silly affect. The clinical picture is usually associated with a history of poor functioning and poor adaptation even before the illness, an early and insidious onset, and a chronic course without significant remissions. Social impairment is usually extreme.

Catatonic Type

Features include either excitement or stupor and mutism, negativism, rigidity, and posturing. The presence of catatonic symptoms alone, without other features of schizophrenic development, can indicate either a major mood disorder or a mental syndrome secondary to a general medical condition.

Paranoid Type

DSM-IV has simplified the criteria defining this subtype, requiring only a preoccupation with one or more fixed delusions and exclusion of the regressive symptoms (prominent disorganization of speech and behavior or inappropriate affect) seen in the other subtypes. Given the usual later age of onset and the limited number of symptoms, patients with this subtype tend to have a more stable clinical picture, with less deterioration and better prognosis than those with other subtypes. Patients in this subgroup may be quite intelligent and well informed.

Residual Type

Features include current lack of active-phase symptoms (Criterion A, Table 18–1) but definite experience of at least one schizophrenic episode in the past, with the continued presence of either negative symptoms or attenuated forms of two or more of the active-phase symptoms, eg, odd beliefs, unusual behavior, or marked eccentricity. The person is "burned out" and is not immersed in the fresh turmoil of the florid, active phase. These people often function as long-term outpatients, but find it very difficult to maintain gainful employment in settings without special support services or accommodations (eg, flexible hours).

Undifferentiated Type

Features include grossly disorganized behavior, hallucinations, incoherence, or prominent delusions, but the criteria for disorganized, catatonic, or paranoid types are not met.

POSITIVE, NEGATIVE, & COGNITIVE SYMPTOM DIMENSIONS

Around 1980, both researchers and clinicians recognized the limitations of the traditional system of subtyping schizophrenia based on phenomenology alone. Attempts were made to define meaningful subtypes by incorporating into the definition anatomical disturbances, treatment responses, and time courses, in addition to phenomenology. In 1980, Crow proffered his two-syndrome concept of schizophrenia, in which he suggested that there are two types of schizophrenia, each associated with a specific pathological process or dimension of pathology: type I with acute symptoms, potentially reversible, and due to a disturbance of dopamine regulation; and type II as a "defect state" with negative symptoms and brain abnormalities on computed tomographic (CT) studies. Although this was an oversimplification of a very complex problem, the model has had heuristic value in that it allows us to conceptualize (and study) schizophrenia as a disorder with separable disease processes that have different physiological processes and treatment responses. These dimensions are thought to be independent but can occur in the same patient. Subsequent elaborations and modifications (eg, Carpenter et al, 1988) led to the following useful three dimensions of pathology: positive symptoms (include hallucinations and delusions), degree of disorganization (in speech and behavior), and primary negative symptoms, or the deficit syndrome.

The positive symptoms are clearly nonspecific as they can occur in many other psychotic disorders; it is the positive symptoms that often respond best to neuroleptics. The primary negative symptoms are proba-

bly closest to Kraepelin's "weakening of the will and deterioration of the personality" and could represent the core of the disorder. They are deficit symptoms and include blunted affect, decreased interests and curiosity, diminished sense of purpose, and decreased social drive. Special care must be taken not to confuse these negative symptoms with secondary negative symptoms that are the result of treatments (neuroleptic-induced parkinsonism) or depression.

A fourth important illness dimension is the neurocognitive dimension. Although it has long been known that on careful testing, all patients with schizophrenia display neurocognitive deficits, it is surprising that we have begun to investigate their importance in rehabilitation only recently. Key for a successful outcome seems to be minimal deficits in verbal memory and attention (Green, 1996). It is often the patients' cognitive deficits in conjunction with their negative symptoms rather than their more dramatic positive symptoms that are most important in their daily lives and their rehabilitation.

DIFFERENTIAL DIAGNOSIS

The differential diagnosis must consider **Mental Disorders Due to General Medical Conditions,** which often present with bizarre delusions and hallucinations similar to those of acute schizophrenia. Disorientation and memory impairment strongly suggest a general medical disorder, whether acute or chronic. Toxic psychoses associated with use of stimulants, hallucinogens, or phencyclidine (PCP) may include symptoms identical to those found in schizophrenia. Any history of drug use provided by such a patient is notoriously unreliable, but the diagnosis is suggested when a psychotic condition clears up dramatically after only a few days of close supervision. Medical disorders associated with alcohol use may mimic schizophrenia, particularly a chronic paranoid type. Metabolic and circulatory disorders, such as those from (1) acute anoxia or chronic arteriosclerosis, (2) hyperthyroidism or iatrogenic high-dose steroids, or (3) many other general medical conditions, specifically including central nervous system diseases of acute onset, must be ruled out.

The diagnostician must distinguish schizophrenia from the severe mood disorders (particularly bipolar or manic-depressive illness), since the appropriate treatment for and course of these disorders are markedly different. Until 20 years ago, it was not widely appreciated that patients with mood disorders, when acutely psychotic, could present with the signs and symptoms of schizophrenia. The course of disease in a patient with a mood disorder is generally intermittent, with symptom-free intervals between episodes of illness. The course in schizophrenia, particularly without treatment, is persistent and often downhill. The schizophrenic patient is always markedly vulnerable to stress, and some thought disorder can usually be found on formal evaluation. A family history of schizophrenia suggests a diagnosis other than a psychotic mood disorder. A family history of mood disorder is so common that it should not be used to argue against the diagnosis of schizophrenia in the patient.

Conditions such as schizophreniform or atypical psychosis may resemble schizophrenia at one point in the clinical picture, but the psychoses are short lived and have a different course. Individuals with severe personality disorders may have transient psychotic symptoms similar to those of schizophrenia, but, in contrast to schizophrenia, these are very brief, and there are long periods of much better social functioning. The low level of functioning and odd behavior with impoverished affect of mental retardation may be confused with schizophrenia.

Individuals who are members of subcultural or religious groups may have beliefs or experiences that are difficult to distinguish from pathological delusions or hallucinations. When such experiences can be explained by the patient's known association with such subcultural groups or values, they should not be considered evidence of schizophrenia. The developmental struggles of normal adolescence may resemble the onset of a pattern of abnormal thinking. Even an experienced observer may have difficulty making the correct clinical diagnosis of schizophrenia.

NATURAL HISTORY

The onset of schizophrenia usually occurs in the second and third decades of life, although paranoid schizophrenia may appear later. In some patients the onset of illness appears to be sudden, but an accurate history will usually reveal that prodromal symptoms were present for weeks or months before the clear-cut schizophrenic symptoms appeared. Depression, anxiety, suspiciousness, hypochondriasis, marked difficulty in concentrating, and restlessness are among the usual prodromal symptoms. The patient often presents initially to a family physician and emphasizes hypochondriacal concerns or bizarre somatic delusions. There is commonly some event in the person's life that is reported to have triggered the development or worsening of schizophrenia. In other patients, it is impossible to define a clear-cut precipitating event; psychosocial stressors may be understated, as the individual retreats from a painful reality.

The characteristic presentation of schizophrenia is a gradual withdrawal from people, activities, and social contacts, with increasing concern for abstract and sometimes idiosyncratic ideas. The acute stage of psychosis may be florid, with prominent hallucinations, delusions, and severe disorders in thinking. After the active psychotic period, there is often a stage of postpsychotic depression that may last many

months, even when treated. Gradually, symptoms may disappear, and the person may recover with no apparent residual deficits; a long remission may follow. Some patients experience only a single episode and remain symptom free for most of their lives. Although the course of the illness can fluctuate over several decades following its onset in early adulthood, a characteristic expression of illness is established in 75% of patients within the first 5 years, and few changes in course occur after 15 years (Bleuler, 1978).

Each recurrence of illness leads to increasing impairment. Patients who are severely affected are able to function only marginally in the community and usually have periodic relapses requiring rehospitalization. Those patients whose illnesses are chronic, progressive, and deteriorating may require prolonged hospitalization or continuous supervision. Zubin and Spring (1977) have emphasized that the one feature all schizophrenic patients have in common is persistent vulnerability rather than persistent illness. Some patients are highly vulnerable and have repeated or almost continual episodes of illness, whereas others are less vulnerable and have few episodes. When episodes develop in this latter group, they are not lifelong. Eventually the illness may remit, with or without treatment. A majority of schizophrenic patients today spend most of their lives in the community and are superficially indistinguishable from the rest of the population.

After the active phase of illness, impairment may vary widely. During the acute stage, psychotic symptoms are always associated with significant impairment. The individual may require hospitalization to ensure that basic needs are met and that poor judgment does not lead to complications such as marked failure in social relations, work, and education, gross personal neglect, or suicide or violent behavior. Although there are many sensationalized accounts of violent acts committed by psychotic individuals, people with schizophrenia are generally no more dangerous than other people living in the community. There are two exceptions: patients who are symptomatic from their illness (which translates into shortly before, during, and after hospitalizations) and patients with concomitant substance use. Even then, the targets of violence are often family members, not strangers. The suicide rate among schizophrenics is 10%, and the average life expectancy is 10 years lower than the general population.

Prognosis When Treated

Kraepelin's original cohort proved to have only 4% lasting remissions, and a grim prognosis for schizophrenia was presumed—recovery usually led to a revised diagnosis. Diagnosis of a disease by its own outcome is logically unsound, and using a period of prolonged illness as a criterion for diagnosis selects for chronicity and poor outcome in schizophrenia. For the first half of this century, outcome was usually measured by discharge from hospital and the absence of readmission. Since 1970, measurements of residual thought disorder, social function, and work function have been included as more adequate descriptors of the patient's quality of life. Cognitive criteria have recently gained prominence and all of these criteria have been found to vary semiindependently, suggesting that they measure different aspects of the individual's adaptation to illness.

The clinician attempting to provide a prognosis for a schizophrenic patient must consider not only the symptoms but also the total picture of that individual: abilities as well as disabilities and assets as well as liabilities. The clinician must evaluate the stresses and demands made on the patient, the world in which the patient lives, and the world the patient creates for himself or herself, often with internal distortion of external reality.

DSM-IV includes an estimate of the prognosis. The prognosis is good if the onset of illness is sudden and a precipitating stress is clearly identifiable and if the patient's social functioning was adequate before illness developed or if the patient performed successfully in a work situation outside the family environment. The prognosis is poor if the onset of illness is insidious, with slowly emerging symptoms and no clearly identifiable precipitating stress, and if the individual was not functioning adequately (socially, economically, or intellectually) before the onset of illness.

Data from a 15-year retrospective study of treatment-resistant patients indicate that as the chronic illness progresses, the significance of certain prognostic factors (predictors) changes. For example, previous work and social accomplishments are the major predictors of outcome in the first decade of illness. In the second decade, the presence of affective symptoms (particularly depression) is a positive predictor, whereas symptoms of paranoia or assaultiveness and the presence of family overinvolvement are negative predictors. Beyond the second decade, a family history of schizophrenia is the most important negative prognostic factor.

The diagnosis and prognosis become more certain the longer the follow-up. Studies of treatment effects on acute episodes of schizophrenia are usually 2–24 months long (short term), and 5-year studies (mid term) are adequate for determining the effects of most interventions. Long-term studies of the complete course of illness require about 15 years, and six such comparable studies have appeared in the English literature (Table 18–2). A seventh, very long-term study primarily describes patients with schizophrenia who survived into their senium (Ciompi, 1980).

The combined data indicate that patients as a group have diverse outcomes under all treatment conditions and that the somatic therapies, previously accepted as interrupting the acute exacerbation and improving short-term prognosis, also improve long-term outcome in both the broad and the narrow schizophrenia spectra.

EPIDEMIOLOGY

The major difficulties in epidemiologic studies of schizophrenia have been the differences in diagnostic criteria, the absence of a definitive conceptual framework, and the lack of a clearly associated factor that can be quantified, eg, a single pathognomonic symptom, sign, biochemical phenotype, or genetic marker.

The 1968 New York/London study showed that differences in diagnostic criteria led to schizophrenia being diagnosed twice as frequently in New York than in London. Each city was subsequently found to hold an extreme position within its respective culture. The World Health Organization's International Pilot Project for Schizophrenia (WHO IPPS) demonstrated that investigators in nine widely different world cultures could achieve high reliability among themselves (80–90%) when they used agreed-on diagnostic criteria both within their own cultures and in each of the other cultures studied. Prospective follow-up data at 10 years have been published and are consistent with those summarized in Table 18–2, but show better social outcome in the less industrialized countries (Jablensky et al, 1992).

Table 18–2. Studies of long-term outcome in schizophrenia.

| Author[a] | Diagnostic Criteria | At Follow-Up | | Treatment | Outcome (%)[b] | | |
		Years (avg)	N		Good	Fair	Poor
Bleuler	Bleuler	22	176	Social	22	33	47
Huber	Bleuler-Schneider	22	213	Social	15	45	40
		22	287	Social plus ECT[c]	28	41	31
Ogawa	*ICD-9*	24	130	Social plus neuroleptics	31	46	23
Tsuang	*DSM-III*	35	186	Social	20	26	54
McGlashan	*DSM-III*	15	163	Psychosocial	14	23	64
Harding	*DSM-III*	32	82	Psychosocial plus neuroleptics	34	34	32

[a] Information in table extracted in part from references in Hegarty et al (1994).
[b] Outcomes are in terms of overt psychopathology; social functioning outcomes are better in all studies.
[c] ECT, electroconvulsive therapy.

The current standard base for psychiatric epidemiology in the United States is the National Institutes of Mental Health (NIMH)-sponsored Epidemiologic Catchment Area (ECA) Program, which followed over 18,000 persons in four urban centers and one area of towns from 1980 to 1985. Data include sufficient elderly, black, and Hispanic probands to allow extrapolation to the U.S. population of that era. The ECA "lifetime prevalence rate" of 1.4% for *DSM-III* schizophrenia is consistent with the 1% figure reported in most other studies. Although lifetime rates between 0.1% and 10% have been reported in some areas, these probably reflect cultural and genetic isolation as well as the known differences in study design and disease definition. Rates of 40% within large, multigenerational families or 0% in an isolated area of Micronesia with over 1000 adults have been reported from well-designed studies.

The incidence of both onset of illness and treatment is highest for men between 15 and 24 years of age and for women, between 25 and 34 years of age. Both sexes have an average prodrome of over a year, when psychosocial changes are noted by others but treatment is avoided. Perhaps the most striking feature of schizophrenia documented by the ECA is the history of treatment in only half of the affected population in spite of the severity of the disorder. The later age of onset and better outcome of schizophrenic women than men is the single most consistent finding since Kraepelin, and the difference is more pronounced since neuroleptic agents and community socialization have become the foundations of treatment. For both sexes, however, the number of those in treatment peaks between the ages of 35 and 44. Symptoms do attenuate after the age of 50 and less active treatment is required in the elderly after a life-long struggle with the disease.

Patients with schizophrenia account for about 40% of hospital beds occupied. The chronicity of the disease and the often profound impairment experienced by schizophrenic patients have made it the most serious and disabling mental illness known worldwide. Mania may be just as severe, but the impairment is shorter lived and more amenable to treatment. Dementia is extremely disabling, but its onset is typically in later life. The appearance of schizophrenia during the early adult years and its persistence throughout decades heighten the loss to society of productive human beings and emphasize the personal tragedy for affected patients and their families.

ETIOLOGY & PATHOGENESIS

Intensive research has led to many hypotheses concerning the "etiology of schizophrenia"; many different single causative factors for these schizophrenic syndromes have been discovered and proposed, but none has been replicated or confirmed. If schizophre-

nia is not a unitary disorder, however, but a syndrome of multiple causes and discrete subtypes, then research attempting to arrive at a "unitary hypothesis" of the disorder will continue to be unproductive. Comparing "schizophrenic patients" with controls in pursuit of a single causative agent may be as fruitless as comparing "the retarded" with controls or comparing febrile with afebrile patients.

Many specific findings, however, seem to be different in subgroups of schizophrenic patients as opposed to "normal controls," particularly during acute illness. The relationships of these associated findings to the causes and effects of schizophrenia serve as the basis for our current biopsychosocial model of the illness. Studies from the following four areas have improved our understanding of schizophrenia and have led to major innovations in treatment: (1) genetics, (2) the influence of family, (3) the influence of social and environmental factors, and (4) neurobiology. Although information from each of these areas is important, none can exclusively explain the development of schizophrenia. Most studies indicate that the disorder is best understood as a heterogeneous "spectrum of schizophrenia."

Genetics

Until recently, genetic investigations have focused on the elements of consanguinity, adoption, and monozygotic multiple births. In studies in consanguinity the incidence of schizophrenia in the relatives of an index case is compared with the incidence in control families. Closer consanguinity correlates with a higher incidence of schizophrenia (Table 18–3), whereas patients with schizophreniform, schizoaffective, or delusional disorder have similar patterns of consanguinity with relation to schizophrenia as do controls.

The two variables of genetics and cultural environment were isolated by studying children who had been adopted shortly after birth and who had subsequently developed schizophrenia. These studies confirmed the existence of a genetic component in the predisposition to schizophrenia. Nine percent of the members of schizophrenic children's biological families were themselves schizophrenic, whereas only 2% were schizophrenic in the biological families of non-schizophrenic children; the incidence of schizophre-

Table 18–3. Genetic relationship correlated with incidence of schizophrenia.[a]

Relationship	Incidence (%)
General population	1
Sibling schizophrenic	8
One parent schizophrenic	12
Dizygotic twin schizophrenic	14
Both parents schizophrenic	39
Monozygotic twin schizophrenic	47

[a] Data from Kety and Matthysse (1988).

nia in the adopting families of these two groups of children was the same. Whether the schizophrenic parent was the father or the mother made no difference.

Independent analyses of these data have confirmed the original findings, suggesting that the genetic expression can manifest itself in the "schizophrenia spectrum" of paranoid, schizoid, and schizotypal personality disorders. A later follow-up showed that in some cases one of the adopting parents manifested schizophrenia for the first time after the adoption had taken place. In these cases, most of the children with at least one schizophrenic biological parent developed schizophrenia, but none of those with nonschizophrenic biological patients did. Although traditional linkage studies have shown linkage to many chromosomes, none of these linkages has been replicated. The search for a single disease gene has been disappointing. Because of recent advances in molecular biology, the entire genome can be systematically screened for genes that might influence a person's risk for schizophrenia. The largest genome-wide scan to date, examining 43 schizophrenia pedigrees, suggests that there is no single gene that causes a large increase in the risk of schizophrenia. It should be noted that the failure to identify a single disease locus strongly supports our conceptualization of schizophrenia as a complex genetic-developmental-environmental disease. It does not discredit the idea that schizophrenia is a disease with a genetic contribution.

A different approach, the candidate gene method, examines putative disease genes at the molecular level using cloning and sequencing techniques. In this way, genotypes of the dopamine receptor, for example, are being compared between normal and schizophrenic patients.

Although a genetic factor is involved in the predisposition to schizophrenia, it is not sufficient to ensure development of the disorder, as is shown by the considerable discordance in incidence and outcome in monozygotic twins.

In summary, only 20% of those who become schizophrenic have a first-degree relative with the overt illness, and most data are inconsistent with a single-major-locus model for a "schizophrenic gene." The best current models involve polygenic (multiloci) and epigenetic contributions. Put differently, schizophrenia is a complex genetic disease like, for example, hypertension. Although a rare gene might eventually be found to be responsible for some cases of schizophrenia around the world, in the vast majority of cases, multiple genes, perhaps in interaction, will be found to be responsible (Moldin and Gottesman, 1997).

Influences of Family

Early studies of the influence of family and culture focused on patterns of deviance in communication such as the "double bind," in which there is a contradiction between the overt linguistic content of speech and the emotional tone or nonverbal actions that are inherent parts of face-to-face human communication.

These studies resulted in considerable emotional pain for families trying to cope with disturbed family members. Therapists often blamed the family for the patient's illness, further disrupting family relationships. Fortunately, particularly for families that remain involved with relatives who have schizophrenia, this assignment of blame has been discredited.

Another variable in family communication, "expressed emotion," defined as high when the family consistently directs intrusive, hostile, and overtly critical comments toward the patient, has been studied. It has been established that reducing high levels of expressed emotion in the families of those who suffer from schizophrenia has a beneficial effect on outcome. A 15-year prospective study indicates that high levels of deviance in communication and high levels of expressed emotion are predictors of schizophrenia in persons at high risk, eg, children of a schizophrenic patient. Fortunately, family education can affect these interactional patterns and the longitudinal course of illness in a favorable manner. These observations also may lead to feelings of "blame" among family members, who need to learn better patterns of involvement. It is clear today that family members do not cause schizophrenia. It is, however, also clear that the degree of expressed emotions in a given family can influence the rate of relapse of the affected family member (Butzlaff and Hooley, 1998).

Influences of Society

It is clear that the onset of schizophrenia in young adults coincides with a developmental stage during which an individual separates from the family of origin and finds new roles in society, including new peer relationships and a new work role. The onset of schizophrenia is often associated with failure to adapt successfully to the changes required by these new social roles. The following studies identify several societal factors that clearly have a strong association with schizophrenia. These factors appear to have a major impact on the emergence of schizophrenia in those who are constitutionally susceptible to its development.

A. Population Density: Population density has been correlated with prevalence, although in a manner that seems applicable only to urban settings. Specifically, there is a strong correlation between the prevalence of schizophrenia and the local population density within districts of cities that have a total population greater than 1 million. In smaller cities of 100,000–500,000 people, the correlation is weaker, and it disappears altogether in smaller towns. These data probably reflect differences in (1) those who migrate to cities through choice or necessity, (2) the environmental stresses and social support patterns found in cities, (3) the tolerance for deviant behavior, which determines case finding, and (4) the availability of treatment. A recent study has supported, but reinterpreted, these findings (Torrey and Bowler, 1990).

B. Socioeconomic Class: A second factor consistently confirmed by many studies is the association of schizophrenia and lower socioeconomic class. One theory states that the conditions of life in lower socioeconomic classes are causal factors in the development of schizophrenia. The alternative theory states that patients who develop schizophrenia tend to drift into the lower social classes because of their inability to perform adequately in many life functions. They have difficulty engaging in productive work and in forming social networks. This "drift hypothesis" is supported by the finding that schizophrenic individuals are more likely to be of a lower social class than their parents.

C. Date of Birth: A third factor affecting the incidence of schizophrenia is a birth date in the winter months. In both Europe and the United States, incidence of schizophrenia is significantly increased in those born between January and April; a complementary peak in incidence is found in South Africa during the months corresponding to winter in the Southern Hemisphere (July, August, and September). This finding has led to many intriguing hypotheses, of which the occurrence of prenatal infections in the mother during the second trimester seems best supported by current data.

D. Industrialization: Industrialization is another factor that seems to affect the incidence of schizophrenia. In developing countries the incidence of schizophrenia has risen, and the outcome has worsened, as the countries have increased their contact with industrialized nations. One explanation suggested for the putative "increase in insanity since 1800" is that this is the specific result of industrialization on the general social order and human beings. As industrial development proceeds, an even more definite difference in the presenting symptoms of schizophrenia occurs; hebephrenic and catatonic schizophrenias become less common, whereas paranoid schizophrenia becomes more common. This pattern is consistent with the shift that has occurred in the United States over the past 60 years; the number of people presenting with catatonic symptoms has dramatically decreased, whereas the number of those showing paranoid symptoms has increased.

E. Other Factors: Several other factors have been proposed as possible influences on the development of schizophrenia. The data are not as consistent and well established as those for the factors previously mentioned. One element is **stress,** as subjectively perceived by the patient and reported after the development of illness. The idea is not that stress causes schizophrenia but that the number of identifiable stressful events (particularly loss of a meaningful person or relationship) clearly increases during the time just before the recognized onset of schizophrenia. The causal relationship between events and the decreased coping skills of the person in the disease prodrome is unclear. The effects of **emigration** and the resulting obvious **cultural dislocation** have also been proposed and extensively studied as risk factors likely to increase the incidence of schizophrenia, but they have not been uniformly confirmed. Many other environmental influences, from allergy to xenophobia, have been explored, but none has proven to be a major etiological factor in the pathogenesis of the schizophrenic disorders.

Specific Neurobiological Findings in Identified Patients

A. Anatomic: Schizophrenia is an illness in which thoughts and behavior are disordered without the gross dysfunction in cognition or sensorium that is usually associated with delirium or dementia. Through the 1970s, individuals with schizophrenia were considered not to have abnormalities in the gross anatomy of their brains. The higher structural resolutions of CT and magnetic resonance imaging (MRI) scans have shown that a subgroup of schizophrenic individuals had enlarged lateral and third ventricles (which imply changes in the periventricular limbic-striatal area) and decreased size of the frontal and temporal lobes. An MRI study of 15 sets of monozygotic twins discordant for schizophrenia found small anterior hippocampi and enlarged ventricles only in the afflicted twin, on the left in 14 cases and on the right and in the third ventricle in 13 cases, a difference not seen in monozygotic twin controls without schizophrenia. The finding of enlarged lateral ventricles has been one of the most replicated findings in biological psychiatry, although the molecular basis for this process remains enigmatic since no glial scarring suggestive of neuronal degeneration is found. It appears to antecede the clinical expression of the disease, has been correlated with a poorer outcome, and might be progressive in a "Kraepelinian" subgroup of patients with a severe form of the disease (Davis et al, 1998). Brain imaging studies implicate at least the prefrontal cortex, the cingulate cortex, the temporal cortex, and the hippocampal formation as areas with abnormalities. However, abnormalities in other areas, including the thalamus and the cerebellum, have been described.

Recent studies of abnormalities in the brains of individuals with schizophrenia have moved from the macroscopic level to the cellular and the molecular level with no clear picture emerging quite yet. Probably the most intriguing hypothesis has been Weinberger's neurodevelopmental hypothesis of schizophrenia (Weickert and Weinberger, 1998). His hypothesis postulates a lesion during early brain development that remains clinically silent until early adulthood, when unnecessary interneuronal dendrites are "pruned" to establish the neuropsychiatric brain structure of adulthood. This hypothesis can be examined by studying cortical cytoarchitecture. It is based on the fact that the mammalian cortex evolves from the embryonic neural crest "from the inside out," ie, earlier migrating cells travel a shorter distance, and cerebral growth is achieved by the migration of later cells through the cortical layers established by the earlier migrating cells. Once it arrives at a final location ("normal" or not) the cell rapidly connects to most adjacent cells rather nonspecifically.

Only in two periods, one beginning in gestation and continuing through 2 years of age and the other in adolescence, are unnecessary interneuronal dendrites "pruned" to establish the neuropsychiatric brain structure of adulthood. Cytoarchitectonic studies have found a variety of disturbances in the layering of the cortex in some schizophrenic patients; a decrease of specific cells in the topmost cortical layer (I) has been described, and an increased number of the "missing cells" are found "stuck" in the two lower layers (II and III). The layers studied develop normally during the second trimester of pregnancy, dating this disturbance of neuronal migration to events in utero. Possible candidates for faulty brain development are molecules that regulate neuron growth, neuronal migration, and cortical development. Moreover, it makes it plausible that certain environmental events, such as an infection during the second trimester of pregnancy, or, later, obstetric complications, both of which have been implicated in the etiology of schizophrenia, could cause a disturbance in brain development that is not progressive.

B. Biochemical: Biochemical studies have provided an understanding of the workings of both the normal human synapse and the altered ones found in schizophrenia. Most studies have concentrated on the synaptic junction, ie, from presynaptic controls of neurotransmitter release through intercellular metabolism and postsynaptic receptor blockade. The focus has shifted from this initiation phase of drug action (drug-receptor interaction and on the cell surface) to the adaptation phase of drug action (events occurring "downstream," involving cytoplasmic second messenger gene activation and gene regulation). Newer imaging techniques such as positron emission tomography (PET) and magnetic resonance spectroscopy (MRS) are applied to study receptors and drug effects in the living brain (eg, Farde et al, 1992).

After it was recognized that lysergic acid diethylamide (LSD) interacted preferentially with serotonergic cells in the brainstem raphe, serotonin (5-hydroxytryptamine, 5-HT) was considered to be "the most likely of the known neurotransmitters" to be involved in schizophrenia. In 1964, however, Carlsson showed that dopamine (3-hydroxytyramine) was selectively affected by conventional neuroleptics. He was awarded the Nobel Prize for this discovery and most subsequent biochemical studies of schizophrenia have focused on the brain's dopamine system.

Five subtypes of dopamine receptors (D_1 through D_5) have been biochemically characterized; they all are G-protein coupled, either stimulating or inhibiting cyclic adenosine monophosphate (cAMP) production. Neuroanatomically, the dopaminergic system consists of only 1% of the neurons in the brain, and most of them are found in four well-defined tracts: the nigrostriatal tract, originating in the mid-brain and terminating in the basal ganglia; the mesolimbic and mesocortical tracts, both originating in an overlapping area of the mid-brain but projecting to the limbic system and to the frontal cortex, respectively; and the tuberoinfundibular tract, with cell bodies in the hypothalamus projecting to the infundibulum and the anterior pituitary. Typical, high-potency neuroleptics that have dominated the treatment of schizophrenia from 1970 to the mid-1990s are highly selective for the D_2 receptor. This D_2 receptor blocking effect explains many of the typical actions and side effects of neuroleptics: D_2 receptor blockade of the nigrostriatal tract results in extrapyramidal symptoms (EPS), the suppression of positive symptoms seems to be related to blocking excess dopamine in the mesolimbic tract, and inhibition of the tuberoinfundibular leads to hyperprolactinemia since dopamine is the "prolactin inhibiting factor" (PIF). A putative dopamine deficiency in the mesocortical system might be responsible for negative symptoms, and a better understanding of cortical D_1 and D_3 receptors could lead to better treatments, since blocking D_2 receptors in this pathway exacerbates negative symptoms (Lidow et al, 1998).

There are linear correlations between the established clinical potencies of the individual "typical neuroleptic" and the binding of these drugs to D_2 receptors. Studies using PET have shown that the D_2 receptors of the basal ganglia are highly blocked by conventional doses of typical neuroleptics in living humans, and that the D_2 receptor density of the basal ganglia among schizophrenic patients prior to neuroleptic treatment is similar to that in nonschizophrenic controls.

Four so-called "atypical" neuroleptics are available in the United States: clozapine, risperidone, olanzapine, and quetiapine (Kane, 1997). Clozapine was released in 1990 despite its significant risk of agranulocytosis, since it can be effective even in patients who show no response to conventional treatments. All atypical neuroleptics share one property: they produce few if any EPS at typical clinical doses. They also appear to provide a better outcome in schizophrenia, not only in the reduction in positive, negative, and possibly cognitive symptoms but also in the reduced risk for tardive dyskinesia and neuroleptic malignant syndrome. The biochemical basis for this clinical difference probably has to do with the extent to which atypical neuroleptics interact with the serotonergic, adrenergic, and cholinergic neurotransmitter receptors, while maintaining sufficient effects on both the D_1, D_2 and possibly the D_3 dopaminergic receptors. Since neurotransmitter systems are interdependent and often form feedback loops, multiple systems are involved in the production of efficacy as well as the production of side effects. Risperidone, for example, combines potent D_2 receptor blockade with potent 5-HT$_2$ blockade. The effect of risperidone on the serotonin system clearly has a modifying effect on the dopamine system in the basal ganglia, since risperidone produces few EPS despite potent D_2 receptor blockade (Kapur and Remington, 1996).

To briefly summarize, dopamine continues to play a major role in our theories of schizophrenia, but more attention is being paid to (1) regional differences in dopamine transmission and receptor subtypes, including the possibility that there is a lack of dopamine in some areas and an excess in others; (2) the modifying influences of other neurotransmitter systems, such as the serotonin system or the *N*-methyl-D-aspartate receptor on dopamine release; and (3) changes occurring in the cells at the level of gene activation and gene regulation.

C. Physiological: Another investigational approach compares physiological measures of brain function among patients with schizophrenia, their relatives, and normal controls. Using measures such as reaction time, event-related potentials, continuous performance task, ocular motor movement abnormalities, and sensorimotor gating, it is clear that patients with schizophrenia show deficits in the elementary areas of information processing and attention: patients might have difficulties filtering out unimportant stimuli from their environment; it has been suggested that gating failures lead to misinterpretation of the environment and to delusions. The same deficits can often be found in relatives of individuals with schizophrenia or premorbidly in children at high risk for schizophrenia. This supports the view that information-processing abnormalities are a trait-linked marker of vulnerability to schizophrenia

An example of one of these physiological markers is a sensorimotor gating abnormality in which patients with schizophrenia fail to suppress the so-called P50 wave that can be measured after they hear a click; interestingly, this abnormality can be seen in about 50% of clinically asymptomatic relatives of patients with schizophrenia (suggesting autosomal dominant transmission), it does not improve with neuroleptics (suggesting a nondopaminergic mechanism), and it has been linked to an abnormality in the nicotinic receptor (Adler et al, 1998).

Various **abnormalities in eye movements** are highly associated with schizophrenia. Saccadic eye movements are abnormally jerky in 80% of schizophrenic patients who are not taking medication, in 45% of nonschizophrenic relatives of schizophrenic patients, and in only 7% of controls. The concordance of abnormalities between twins is 71% for monozygotic twins and 54% for dizygotic twins; both rates are higher than the concordance for the actual development of schizophrenia.

Changes in cerebral metabolism have been found using the increased sensitivities of PET and studies in cortical regional blood flow (cRBF). Decreased metabolism of the medial-frontal areas, when the schizophrenic patient is challenged with tests that utilize these areas in normal individuals, and an associated increase in medial temporal activity have been demonstrated. Differential activation of the auditory cortex has been shown in actively hallucinating paranoid schizophrenics, and this abnormal activity normalizes after combined pharmacological and psychosocial treatment.

The anatomic, biochemical, and physiological findings summarized above are highly consistent and, taken together, form the "scientific basis" for current studies of schizophrenia. The student must understand, however, that altered activities of neuronal systems are not considered to be the "cause" of schizophrenia, but they are implicated in the manifestation of symptoms. In fact, all typical neuroleptics are equally effective in reducing acute positive symptoms, regardless of whether these are manifested in schizophrenia, mania, or the psychoses developing in medical-surgical patients, such as those treated with corticosteroids or experiencing the complex metabolic derangements found on the intensive care units (ICU).

Some students become discouraged by our inability to understand schizophrenia given the often seemingly disconnected facts that at present do not lend themselves to one theory. However, currently available imaging studies such as single-photon emission computed tomography (SPECT) or PET have already provided a refined understanding of, for example, the interplay between dopamine and serotonin. New techniques such as MRS or functional MRI (fMRI) will allow us to describe the neurobiology and circuitry that underlie psychiatric signs and symptoms. Although we still do not understand the etiology of schizophrenia, an understanding of the pathophysiology of schizophrenia, just like an understanding of the pathophysiology of diabetes mellitus, is often sufficient to treat the syndrome.

TREATMENT

The consequences of schizophrenia are painful and unacceptable both to the patient and to the surrounding community. The magnitude of these consequences has led to a wide range of treatments and protective strategies. Even before the development of a conceptual framework to explain schizophrenia, physical methods were used to protect society and to help families and caretakers minimize the disruption caused by schizophrenia. Treatments in the nineteenth and early twentieth centuries involved sedation, restraint, and confinement. Hospital treatment often resulted in continuous institutionalization until death, usually hastened by nutritional and infectious diseases. Occasionally, a combination of psychological, social, and biological treatments was followed by remission sufficient for discharge. These cases served as the bases of both hope and clinical reports throughout much of this century.

The probability of eventual discharge from hospitals for patients who have developed schizophrenia for the first time has increased over each decade of this century. The psychosocial therapies developed since the 1920s have played a major role in this process. Until the 1950s patients were removed from society to an institution; there they could be observed and treated, and society could avoid contact with people they considered to be frightening and disturbed. The dramatic increase in release rates since the late 1950s could not have occurred without the introduction of neuroleptics earlier in the decade. **Neuroleptic treatment** controls acute symptoms, allows the reduction of hospitalization from years to days, prolongs remission, and helps make the current outcome for patients treated for schizophrenia much better than the untreated natural course.

Until the 1930s the only somatic treatments that were actually beneficial involved either the induction of prolonged coma/sleep by chemical means or forced, very prolonged immobilization using restraints, jackets, and sheet packs. Convulsive treatments, originally induced by chemicals but electrically induced (electroconvulsive treatment or ECT) since the 1940s, became the treatment of choice for acute schizophrenia until being displaced by the neuroleptics in the 1960s. At present, the use of ECT in the treatment of schizophrenia is limited to the occasional patient. It is typically used after pharmacotherapy has failed to treat a patient's severe psychosis or if there is severe suicidality or presentation of life-threatening catatonia. The response to ECT is often rapid and dramatic. It should be noted that ECT was supplanted by pharmacotherapy not because ECT is inferior or involves risks but for a variety of other factors including ease of administration of drugs and stigma attached to ECT. In recent years, there has been renewed interest in ECT as a treatment for schizophrenia based on the concern that prolonged psychosis might be neurotoxic and the belief that aggressive treatment could prevent deterioration (Fink and Sackeim, 1996).

Contemporary treatment of schizophrenia always involves a combination of biological, psychological, and social methods called **combined treatment.** The psychiatrist usually works as part of a treatment team, and in many cases the family is actively incorporated into the treatment plan.

Psychosocial Treatment

It is useful conceptually to divide the treatment of schizophrenia into three phases since their respective goals and treatment strategies vary: an acute phase, a stabilization phase, and a stable phase.

In the acute phase, the aim is to reduce acute symptoms, prevent harm, and improve role function. This is the beginning of an attempt to engage patients and develop a treatment alliance with them. Consideration needs to be given to the appropriate (ie, least restrictive) setting in which patients can be treated in a way that is safe for both them and for their environment. This can range from supervision by a family member at home to a day hospital admission to involuntary commitment to a state facility. The acute phase is often the easiest phase in which to engage family members because their motivation is high.

During the stabilization phase it is important to continue to minimize stress, to enhance patients' adaptation to life, and to educate patients and their families about early signs of relapse.

During the stable phase treatment is designed to minimize risk of relapse on the one hand and to optimize functioning on the other. Knowledge about patients' neurocognitive status becomes important now as it will guide cognitive and vocational rehabilitation efforts. Training in social skills that uses behavioral techniques to teach skills useful in everyday life can be very helpful to patients with negative symptoms. Since the patient's long-term course will be affected by the family's understanding of the illness, psychoeducational work with the family is very important in this phase of treatment. Some patients with no social support and difficulties accessing different community agencies might benefit from so-called case management, in which a designated person helps them steer through the bureaucracies. A successful but very intensive case management model with active treatment interventions has been developed (assertive community treatment); it enables marginally functioning individuals to live in the community. Key principles are support, emphasis on compliance, and assertive outreach if indicated to keep the patient in treatment.

Two points in the treatment of a patient with schizophrenia need to be emphasized: the sine qua non for successful treatment is a good therapeutic alliance with the patient and a good working alliance with the family. Many patients lack insight into the nature of their illness, attribute their symptoms to anything but a mental illness, and often do not acknowledge the need for treatment (David and Kemp, 1997). Often patients are noncompliant with treatment. Awareness of this allows the doctor to determine what made the patient decide not to follow treatment recommendations: was it side effects that were not explained, lack of understanding because of cognitive deficits, or the uninformed advice of a family member (Weiden and Zygmunt, 1997)? A good alliance with the patient, in which the patient trusts the physician, will allow the physician to treat the patient successfully. A good alliance with the family can prevent hospitalizations if family members help with medication or recognition of prodromal symptoms.

The overall therapeutic stance is usually supportive with a focus on the present and on problem solving. The psychiatrist listens carefully but interactively and attempts to understand each patient in a way that fosters development of a more adaptive, mature personality. In effect, the psychiatrist takes the role of a concerned but not overbearing parent who uses understanding and skill to promote the maximum possible development in a vulnerable individual. Although the diagnosis of schizophrenia carries a guarded prognosis, the situation is rarely hopeless, and usually much can be improved. The psychiatrist must communicate this understanding to the patient, the treatment team, and the family. Focusing on "recovery" promotes hope. Almost all patients can be better even if not completely well. Expectation, however, must be realistic: for some patients a return to college is within the range of possibility; for others even supported employment might be illusory.

Pharmacological Treatment

Initially, phenothiazines were the major type of drug used in both acute hospital treatment of psychosis and in the long-term stabilization of schizophrenic patients after their subsequent return to the community. Controlled prospective studies confirmed that use of phenothiazines achieved remission of symptoms in weeks rather than years in 90% of those experiencing an acute psychotic episode, that recovery was sufficient to enable patients to return to the community, and that the likelihood of rehospitalization could be reduced by half in patients who had been treated with phenothiazines in the hospital, regardless of the type of treatment received following discharge. The sooner neuroleptics can be employed to abort and contain the patient's psychosis, the better the long-term outcome. After the brief period required to clarify the diagnosis and rule out one of the psychoses caused by a general medical condition (2–3 days) it is unwise to defer medications in hopes that the patient will learn a lesson, be grateful for, or otherwise benefit from, the ongoing experience of a psychotic state. The typical antipsychotic drugs now employed include several classes of drugs in addition to the phenothiazines originally used (see Chapter 30).

A. Choice of Neuroleptic: All typical neuroleptics have been found to be equally effective among large groups of patients. Among typical neuroleptics the effective therapeutic dose required to treat a patient varies in relation to that drug's ability to block the dopamine receptor and the relative potencies reflect the drug's ability to block the various dopamine receptors; similarly, the side effects reflect the relative binding at other known neurotransmitter receptors. Individual patients may respond to one drug better than another, and a history of a favorable response to treatment with a given drug in either the patient or a family member should lead to use of that particular drug as the drug of first choice. If the initial choice is not effective in 2–4 weeks, it is reasonable to try another neuroleptic drug with a different chemical spectrum of neurotransmitter interactions. Today, most clinicians consider using an atypical neuroleptic such as risperidone or olanzapine initially in the treatment algorithm. Aside from milligram potencies, the primary differences among the neuroleptic agents involve side effects, which may affect compliance by conferring an advantage to the patient, eg, producing nighttime sedation with chlorpromazine or avoiding appetite stimulation with molindone. Clinically, risperidone, olanzapine, and quetiapine are often well tolerated because of fewer extrapyramidal symptoms (EPS), which can be a major factor for compliance with treatment; unfortunately, they often produce weight gain. Clozapine requires weekly monitoring of blood to detect developing agranulocytosis, increases the risk of seizure, and has many side effects that limit its use.

Useful generalizations may be made about the differences between the low- and high-potency neuroleptics. The low-potency drugs have much greater sedative and hypotensive properties, to which the patient often becomes more tolerant within a few weeks, but the greater risk of malignant hyperthermia and obesity associated with this group of drugs continues throughout the period of active drug use. Low-potency drugs also are inherently anticholinergic, so that the use of additional anticholinergic drugs to prevent EPS may be unnecessary.

The high-potency typical neuroleptics have little inherent anticholinergic activity and frequently produce EPS or dystonia, so that anticholinergic drugs are usually required, at least in the initial months of treatment. They may be more likely to produce **neuroleptic malignant syndrome,** a devastating acute illness characterized by fever, delirium, autonomic dysfunction, muscle rigidity, and a 20% mortality when untreated. The incidence of this iatrogenic disease may be as high as 1%, but, as with schizophrenia, the "disease" may be a grouping of various medical conditions.

The only long-acting (depot) neuroleptics available in the United States are the esters of fluphenazine and haloperidol, which may be given intramuscularly as infrequently as every 4 weeks to establish adequate drug levels. This type of drug treatment decreases relapse rates for outpatients who have been previously stabilized but does not produce the same relative benefit following inpatient treatment of an acute psychotic episode.

Conventional (typical) neuroleptics are still used for emergency treatment and for monthly injections, since no depot preparation exists for any of the atypical drugs, and for patients who cannot afford one of the newer medications.

B. Dosage of Neuroleptic: The proved efficacy of typical neuroleptics in reducing relapse rates and improving outcome led to some untoward consequences: patients who had been treated with high doses of antipsychotic drugs to control acute psychotic symptoms continued to receive high doses as maintenance levels in the absence of known contraindications to long-term use and in the belief that this would better prevent relapse. This mistaken idea was widely "noted for correction" by 1975, but some chronic patients cannot be removed from high doses without relapse. Many patients suffered from unacceptable side effects of high doses of neuroleptics, such as tardive dyskinesia (TD), an often irreversible, disfiguring movement disorder, and the psychiatric community recognized that it was essential to determine the minimum effective dose of antipsychotic medications. Fortunately, it was found that except during acute exacerbations of psychosis, lower doses of antipsychotic medications are consistent with excellent long-term control of symptoms in schizophrenia. Studies with both low-potency and high-potency (typical) neuroleptics established that acute psychotic symptoms respond more quickly to moderate doses (600–1000 mg of chlorpromazine or equivalent drug) than to low doses (below 300 mg of chlorpromazine or equivalent).

TD is characterized by repetitive, involuntary movements, usually of the mouth and tongue, but often of the thumb and fingers, and occasionally of a limb or the whole trunk. Although movement disorders occasionally occur spontaneously in later life, the major risk factors for the development of TD are older age and total cumulative exposure to dopamine antagonists, of which typical neuroleptics and the "bowel sedatives" (eg, diphenoxylate and metoclopramide) are the most widely used.

TD is thought to result from dopamine receptor supersensitivity following chronic receptor blockade by the typical neuroleptics. It appears to be a later manifestation of changes initially expressed as EPS. Anticholinergic drugs do not improve TD and may make it worse. The recommended treatment of TD has been to lower the dosage of any typical neuroleptic and hope for gradual remission of the choreoathetoid movements. Increasing the dosage of a typical neuroleptic briefly masks the symptoms of TD, but symptoms may reappear later as a reflection of the progression of receptor supersensitivity. The atypical neuroleptics clearly have a much lower risk of producing TD, with clozapine being completely devoid of this serious side effect.

Dosage strategies have been developed to balance the need for levels of neuroleptics adequate to treat psychotic symptoms and the risk of total lifetime dosage often required during chronic drug treatment. Three strategies—**low dose, targeted symptom,** and **drug holidays**—have been used to lower the maintenance doses in the years of illness following acute psychosis and hospitalization. The low-dose approach, which is the approach recommended for most patients, attempts to find the minimum, constant dose effective in preventing relapse. Studies have shown

that the minimum parenteral dose of fluphenazine or haloperidol decanoate is 5–10 mg intramuscularly every 2 weeks, and the minimum oral dose is about 5 mg every day; both dosages may have to be tripled at times of symptom exacerbation to prevent full relapse. The **targeted symptom** strategy calls for close monitoring of the patient by a treatment team and the use of medications only for specific symptoms. This might be a feasible strategy for occasional patients who can clearly identify their prodrome; it is, however, a strategy with a higher risk for relapse and TD. The use of **drug holidays,** in which a neuroleptic is not taken for 1–2 days each week, has fallen into disfavor, because it seems to decrease patient compliance and because it may exacerbate TD.

C. Duration of Drug Treatment: The most important principle to remember is that it takes time for a psychotic episode to resolve and that continuously increasing the dose does not hasten recovery. The psychosis gradually resolves only after 2–6 weeks on a neuroleptic in the range of 10–20 mg of haloperidol. Major reductions in this dosage should be avoided for at least 6 weeks and are best attempted 6 months after the episode. The patient should be alerted to note any signs of returning symptoms so that modest increases in dosage may be made, if necessary, to minimize recurrent symptoms and potential relapse. Gradual reduction in dosage should approach a minimum that enables the patient to function as well as possible at a level that is in accord with the patient's wishes and is also socially acceptable. It has been found that a large majority of patients cannot reduce dosage below a certain daily minimum (usually equivalent to 200–400 mg of chlorpromazine or 5 mg haloperidol orally per day) without permitting the return of psychotic symptoms within months. For most patients with recurrent episodes, lifelong maintenance treatment with neuroleptic medications is a necessary part of existence, permitting relative freedom from symptoms and a life in the community.

Thankfully, the newer antipsychotics have had a tremendous impact on many patients' quality of life, making it easier to take a medication lifelong. Risperidone, olanzapine, and quetiapine clearly have a much better side effect profile than conventional antipsychotics, particularly with respect to EPS. They also drastically minimize the risk of TD.

D. Adjunctive Drugs: Neuroleptics are the primary drugs used in the treatment of schizophrenic symptoms, but adjunctive drugs are often also used. The first, and most common, reason is to treat a side effect produced by a neuroleptic. EPS are decreased by anticholinergic agents, dystonias are relaxed by diphenhydramine, and akathisia may be reduced by propranolol. The second reason is to add another psychoactive drug to treat neuroleptic-resistant symptoms: lithium, carbamazepine, or valproate may stabilize moods, the benzodiazepines may calm anxiety or induce sleep, and antidepressants may ease depression in some patients with schizophrenia spectrum disorder.

Combined Treatment

Although neuroleptic medication may effectively normalize a patient's overt behavior, thought processes, and ability to communicate coherently, it does little to help a patient achieve those factors considered to be essential for enhancing the quality of life: the ability to relate to friends and loved ones, the ability to obtain adequate food, clothing, and shelter by performing work for recompense and social role, and the ability to evidence adult self-control of one's own life. The true task of the long-term treatment of schizophrenia is twofold: (1) to establish a psychologically stable baseline free from repeat psychotic episodes and (2) to help the patient build on this baseline to lead a life that is qualitatively enriched by reasonable personal, social, and vocational achievements. This allows the patient to resume human development without relapse into psychosis.

During initial hospitalization, patients have an involuntarily imposed social structure, constant companionship of trained personnel, and supervised medication. On return to the community, patients become responsible for complying with the medication requirements, although that task involves at least some association with a prescribing physician. Patients who cooperate with treatment remain in contact with a physician or a treatment institution over many years. The availability of the essential psychosocial therapies are dependent on either preexisting family resources and insurance or on the variable whims of the government controlling health policy. During this time, patients should assume increasing responsibility for their own well-being and understanding of their illness and life situation.

A major goal in the treatment of patients after discharge from the hospital is to help them recognize the stressful external situations or internal stimuli that indicate the start of a relapse. When patients become aware of these early signs of psychosis, they can often regain control of their lives by increasing the dosage of antipsychotic medication for a few weeks and by increasing their contact with the professionals treating them. This self-help is of major therapeutic benefit to patients, who find that they can exercise some measure of control over their illness and hope for a life that is not interrupted by recurrent hospitalization.

Most schizophrenic patients benefit from prudent use of antipsychotic medication in combination with supportive psychotherapy and work with the patient's family or significant others. Physicians may restrict their involvement to adjusting the dosage of medication, but a psychotherapist may find that increased therapy makes additional medications unnecessary. A long-term companion or a psychotherapist's time is always expensive; medicines may or may not be. Institutions are rarely able to provide the needed constancy of continuing interaction with the same therapist. For many chronically ill schizophrenic patients, one way of obtaining this desired constancy is to maintain a relationship with a family physician who understands the patient's vulnerability and needs and can monitor neuroleptic effects. The psychiatrist can be available to consult with the family doctor when required. The clinician hopes to observe and facilitate the following improvements in a schizophrenic person who is vulnerable to future psychotic episodes:

• Improvement in thought disorder, ranging from marked diminution to outright absence of symptoms.
• Greatly improved modulation of affect.
• Decreased susceptibility to transient psychotic symptoms.
• Realistic setting of personal ambitions.
• Ability to take credit for personal accomplishments.
• Improvements in social judgment.

SOCIAL SUPPORT SERVICES

All clinicians must be aware of the social context in which the patient with schizophrenia is being treated. As management has moved from long periods of institutionalization to brief hospital stays followed by treatment in community settings, there has been a change in the patient's needs. Discharge from institutional settings has meant greater personal responsibility for those who not only are impaired but also are typically impoverished and alone. At one time patients were provided with food, clothing, shelter, and medical care in controlled "total institutions," but patients with schizophrenia now find themselves exposed to the rigors of life in unsupportive communities. The patients' basic needs are no longer met, since meeting these needs requires funding by the government, charities, or the individual families, from all of whom the patient is often estranged. Services are provided in a number of different settings, and resources are scarce. Many patients with schizophrenia are now struggling to survive in the community. They are at greatly increased risk for homelessness, drug abuse, exploitation, suicide, AIDS, and a variety of other illnesses that give them a higher-than-normal mortality. A recent study provided the disturbing fact that 1 in 10 schizophrenic patients was homeless even before initial hospitalization and not only after a long, deteriorating course of illness (Herman et al, 1998). With deinstitutionalization now an accomplished fact, we will have to address the problem of how to provide treatment for a clearly identifiable minority of patients who need highly structured, 24-hour care. Currently, patients who do not live in the streets often find themselves housed but not treated in the criminal justice system, a phenomenon that has been termed "transinstitutionalization" (Lamb, 1998). To some observers the answer is to return these people to long-term hospitals; to others the answer is to improve their access to resources and health personnel within the community. Finally, we as a society need to decide what we consider adequate care for people with mental illnesses and how much we are willing to pay for it.

SUMMARY

Schizophrenic disorders are a complex syndrome characterized by a disturbance in reality testing, marked impairment of social functioning, and severe personality disorganization involving disturbances in thought, affect, and behavior. There is no single cause, although in many cases there do appear to be medical and biological bases present within early childhood. Psychosocial factors play an important part in the development and in the treatment of the schizophrenic disorders. Treatment should consist of various combined biopsychosocial methods and should include the formation of a therapeutic alliance with the schizophrenic person, as well as contact with friends and family, if needed and available. Although schizophrenia has remained the most serious psychiatric illness known for the past 200 years, a comprehensive approach to the care and treatment of schizophrenic disorders has improved the quality of life for patients and their families and also greatly improved the treated outcome as compared to the natural course.

Moreover, we might have reached the point at which early intervention to arrest the deterioration that comes from successive psychotic episodes has become a possibility and a goal. If efforts at prevention are to be successful for the next generation of young people with schizophrenia, we have to begin treatment as early as possible and keep the psychotic episodes as brief as possible. This means that families and society need to be better informed about signs and symptoms of psychosis in order to recognize the need for treatment in a young adult rather than blaming the psychotic person for being lazy or explaining his or her symptoms away as "adolescent turmoil." New medications hold promise for better treatment with fewer side effects, particularly when coupled with effective psychosocial treatments and support.

REFERENCES & SUGGESTED READINGS

Adler LE et al: Schizophrenia, sensory gating, and nicotinic receptors. Schizophr Bull 1998;24:189.

American Psychiatric Association: *Diagnostic and Statistical Manual of Mental Disorders*, 4th ed. American Psychiatric Association, 1994.

American Psychiatric Association: Practice guideline for the treatment of patients with schizophrenia. Am J Psychiatry 1997;154(April Suppl):1.

Andreasen NC, Carpenter WT Jr: Diagnosis and classification of schizophrenia. Schizophr Bull 1993;19:199.

Bleuler E: *Dementia Praecox, or the Group of Schizophrenias* (1911). Translated by Zinkin JJ. International Universities Press, 1950.

Bleuler M: *The Schizophrenic Disorders: Long-term Patient and Family Studies.* Translated by Clemens SM. Yale University Press, 1978.

Butzlaff RL, Hooley JM: Expressed emotion and psychiatric relapse. A meta-analysis. Arch Gen Psychiatry 1998; 55:547.

Carpenter WT Jr, Heinrichs DW, Wagman AMI: Deficit and nondeficit forms of schizophrenia: The concept. Am J Psychiatry 1988;145:578.

Ciompi L: Catamnestic long-term study on the course of life and aging of schizophrenics. Schizophr Bull 1980;6:606.

Crow TJ: Molecular pathology of schizophrenia: More than one disease process? Br Med J 1980;280:66.

David A, Kemp R: Five perspectives on the phenomenon of insight in psychosis. Psychiatric Annals 1997;27:791.

Davidson L, McGlashan TH: The varied outcomes of schizophrenia. Can J Psychiatry 1997;42:34.

Davis KL et al: Ventricular enlargement in poor-outcome schizophrenia. Biol Psychiatry 1998;43:783.

Farde L et al: Positron emission tomographic analysis of central D1 and D2 dopamine receptor occupancy in patients treated with classical neuroleptics and clozapine. Relation to extrapyramidal side effects. Arch Gen Psychiatry 1992;49:538.

Fink M, Sackeim HA: Convulsive therapy in schizophrenia? Schizophr Bull 1996;22:27.

Glass LL et al: Psychotherapy of schizophrenia: An empirical investigation of the relationship of process to outcome. Am J Psychiatry 1989;146:603.

Green MF: What are the functional consequences of neurocognitive deficits in schizophrenia? Am J Psychiatry 1996;153:321.

Harding CM, Zahniser JH: Empirical correction of seven myths about schizophrenia with implications for treatment. Acta Psychiatr Scand 1994;90(Suppl 384):140.

Hegarty et al: One hundred years of schizophrenia: A meta-analysis of the outcome literature. Am J Psychiatry 1994; 151:1409.

Herman DB et al: Homelessness among individuals with psychotic disorders hospitalized for the first time: Findings from the Suffolk County Mental Health Project. Am J Psychiatry 1998;155:109.

Jablensky A et al: Schizophrenia: Manifestations, incidence, and course in different cultures. A World Health Organization Ten-Country Study. Psychol Med 1992; Monograph (Suppl 20).

Kane JM: The new antipsychotics. J Pract Psychiatry Behav Health 1997;3:343.

Kapur S, Remington G: Serotonin-dopamine interaction and its relevance to schizophrenia. Am J Psychiatry 1996; 153:466.

Kendler KS, Karkowski LM, Walsh D: The structure of psychosis. Latent class analysis of probands from the Roscommon Family Study. Arch Gen Psychiatry 1998; 55:492.

Kety SS, Matthysse S: Genetic and biochemical aspects of schizophrenia. In: *The New Harvard Guide to Psychiatry.* Nicholi AM (editor). Belknap Press of Harvard University Press, 1988.

Kraepelin E: *Dementia Praecox and Paraphrenia.* Translated by Barclay RM. Livingstone, 1919.

Lamb HR: Deinstitutionalization at the beginning of the new millennium. Harvard Rev Psychiatry 1998;6:1.

Lehman AF, Steinwachs DM, and the Co-Investigators of the PORT Project: At issue: Translating research into practice: The Schizophrenia Patient Outcomes Research Team (PORT) Treatment Recommendations. Schizophr Bull 1998;24:1.

Lidow MS, Williams GV, Goldman-Rakic PS: The cerebral cortex: A case for a common site of action of antipsychotics. TiPS 1998;19:136.

Moldin SO, Gottesman II: At issue: Genes, experience, and chance in schizophrenia—positioning for the 21st century. Schizophr Bull 1997;23:547.

Olney JW, Farber NB: Glutamate receptor dysfunction and schizophrenia. Arch Gen Psychiatry 1995;52:998.

Robins E, Guze SB: Establishment of diagnostic validity in psychiatric illness: Its application to schizophrenia. Am J Psychiatry 1970;126:983.

Steadman HJ et al: Violence by people discharged from acute psychiatric inpatient facilities and by others in the same neighborhoods. Arch Gen Psychiatry 1998;55:393.

Torrey EF, Bowler A: Geographical distribution of insanity in America: Evidence for an urban factor. Schizophr Bull 1990;16:591.

Weickert CS, Weinberger DR: A candidate molecule approach to defining developmental pathology in schizophrenia. Schizophr Bull 1998;24:303.

Weiden PJ, Zygmunt A: Medication noncompliance in schizophrenia: Part I. Assessment. J Pract Psychiatry Behav Health 1997;3:106.

Wyatt RJ, Damiani LM, Henter ID: First-episode schizophrenia. Early intervention and medication discontinuation in the context of course and treatment. Br J Psychiatry 1998;172(Suppl 33):77.

Zubin J, Spring B: Vulnerability—a new view of schizophrenia. J Abnorm Psychol 1977;86:103.

Delusional & Other Psychotic Disorders

19

Edward L. Merrin, MD

Although classic psychotic symptoms (delusions, hallucinations, disorganized speech and behavior, inappropriate or blunted affect) are popularly associated with the diagnosis of schizophrenia, they are by no means pathognomonic of that or any other disorder. Accurate identification of the primary psychiatric condition underlying these symptoms is important for selecting treatment and predicting outcome. For many patients, the diagnosis of schizophrenia or mood disorder with psychotic features will be appropriate (see Chapters 18 and 20). This chapter reviews a group of less commonly diagnosed disorders: schizophreniform disorder, schizoaffective disorder, delusional disorder, brief psychotic disorder, and shared psychotic disorder.

An accurate diagnosis of psychosis based on the *Diagnostic and Statistical Manual of Mental Disorders,* 4th edition (*DSM-IV*), like all medical diagnoses, depends on obtaining a detailed history and performing a careful clinical examination. The physician should always be alert to the possibility that the psychotic symptoms are caused by a primary medical or neurological disorder (see Chapter 16) or by the effects of intoxication with or withdrawal from substances of abuse or prescribed medications (see Chapter 17). When these etiological factors have been ruled out it is then important to consider the longitudinal pattern of symptoms rather than limiting the evaluation to a cross-sectional look at the patient's current clinical state only. The following issues are particularly important in the differential diagnosis of the psychotic disorders discussed in this chapter: (1) the presence or absence of specific psychotic symptoms, (2) the degree of recovery from episodes of illness, (3) the duration of symptoms, (4) the presence or absence of prominent mood symptoms and when they occur in relationship to psychotic symptoms, and (5) the presence or absence of specific medical or substance-induced etiological factors.

These five areas are built into the *DSM-IV* criteria for schizophrenia, and allow each of the disorders discussed in this chapter to be distinguishable from schizophrenia and from each other. Table 19–1 has been constructed to facilitate this differential diagnosis. The five columns (A–E) correspond to the *DSM-IV* criteria for schizophrenia. As each disorder is de-

scribed it should be possible to refer to Table 19–1 to understand how the disorder being discussed is distinguished from the other disorders.

SCHIZOPHRENIFORM DISORDER

Symptoms & Signs

Schizophreniform disorder is a psychotic illness with symptoms typical of schizophrenia but without the chronic course of that disorder. To satisfy the diagnostic criteria for schizophreniform disorder, patients must display psychotic symptoms sufficient to meet *DSM-IV* criteria for the active phase of schizophrenia, but they must return to their previous level of functioning within 6 months. Criteria for schizophreniform disorder are listed in Table 19–2.

Natural History & Prognosis

The long-term course of schizophreniform disorder is variable. In some patients, there is only a single psychotic episode, whereas in others there are repeated episodes separated by varying lengths of time. First episodes usually occur in late adolescence or early adulthood, often in association with a specific precipitating crisis. A better prognosis is associated with good social and occupational functioning before the onset of illness, an abrupt rather than insidious onset, and confusion or disorientation during the most acute phase of the episode. Blunted or flat affect is a poor prognostic sign.

The diagnosis of schizophreniform disorder is often provisional and may have to be changed as the patient is followed over a period of months or years. About half of patients with schizophreniform disorder will either improve or recover, whereas only one-third of schizophrenic patients will substantially improve. Those who do less well are often eventually rediagnosed as schizophrenic. However, follow-up studies indicate that in a substantial number of patients, later episodes take the form of depression or mania.

Differential Diagnosis

Schizophreniform disorder is differentiated from psychotic disorder associated with a general medical condition and from substance-induced psychotic dis-

Table 19–1. Differential diagnosis of schizophrenic-like psychotic symptoms keyed to *DSM-IV* criteria for schizophrenia.

	A. Psychotic Symptoms[a]	B. Decline in Functioning	C. Duration	D. Mood Changes	E. "Organic" Etiology
Schizophrenia (see Chapter 18)	Full schizophrenic syndrome	Yes	At least 6 months	Not prominent	No
Mood disorder with psychotic features (see Chapter 20)	Any positive symptoms	Variable	At least 2 weeks	Always present during illness	No
Schizophreniform disorder	Full schizophrenic syndrome	No	1–6 months	Not prominent	No
Schizoaffective disorder	Full schizophrenic syndrome	Variable	Delusions or hallucinations for 2 weeks without mood symptoms	Present during a substantial portion (but not all) of the illness	No
Delusional disorder	Nonbizarre delusions only	No	At least 1 month	Not prominent	No
Brief psychotic disorder	Any positive symptoms[b]	No	1 day to 1 month	Not prominent	No
Shared psychotic disorder	Any shared delusion	Unspecified	Unspecified	Not prominent	No
Psychosis due to general medical condition (see Chapter 16)	Any hallucinations or delusions	Unspecified	Unspecified	Unspecified	Yes
Substance-induced psychotic disorder (see Chapter 17)	Any hallucinations or delusions	Unspecified	Unspecified	Unspecified	Yes

[a] The "full schizophrenic syndrome" is defined as meeting Criterion A of the *DSM-IV* criteria for schizophrenia.
[b] "Positive symptoms" include delusions, hallucinations, disorganized speech, or grossly disorganized or catatonic behavior.

order by the lack of evidence from history, physical and mental status examination, and laboratory tests of specific medical (encephalitis, neoplasm, endocrine disorders, etc) or substance-induced (psychostimulant or hallucinogenic drug intoxication, drug withdrawal, etc) etiological factors. Schizophreniform disorder is distinguished from schizophrenia by its shorter course (less than 6 months for prodromal, active, and residual symptoms combined) and by the absence of deterioration from previous

Table 19–2. *DSM-IV* criteria for schizophreniform disorder.

A. Meets Criteria A, D, and E of schizophrenia.

B. An episode of the disorder (including prodromal, active, and residual phases) lasts at least 1 month but less than 6 months (When the diagnosis must be made without waiting for recovery, it should be qualified as "provisional")

Specify if

Without good prognostic features

With good prognosis features as evidenced by at least two of the following:

(1) onset of prominent psychotic symptoms within 4 weeks of the first noticeable change in unusual behavior or functioning
(2) confusion or perplexity at the height of the psychotic episode
(3) good premorbid social and occupational functioning
(4) absence of blunted or flat affect

levels of functioning. The diagnosis of brief psychotic disorder is suggested rather than schizophreniform disorder when the illness has been present for less than 1 month. There may also be fewer psychotic symptoms than necessary to meet the symptom Criterion A for schizophrenia in brief psychotic disorder. The mood disturbances in schizophreniform disorder, unlike those in major depression, bipolar disorder, or schizoaffective disorder, are brief in duration relative to the total length of the episode. Psychotic symptoms in delusional disorder are limited to understandable, plausible-sounding (although unlikely) delusions and do not include prominent hallucinations, loose associations, or bizarre delusions.

Illustrative Case

A 31-year-old male vocational nurse was hospitalized for his third episode of psychosis. He complained of the recent onset of difficulty focusing his thoughts, intrusive ideas of a bizarre nature ("there's a telepath in my old lady's body"), and auditory hallucinations of the voices of so-called telepaths who controlled his body movements. These symptoms had so impaired his functioning that he lost his job. Mental status examination revealed pressured speech, loose associations, and occasional idiosyncratic word usage. Various tics and twitches occurred that the patient attributed to the influence of the "telepaths." His symptoms gradually cleared after several weeks of treatment with antipsychotic drugs, and he was able to return to living with his girlfriend and active employment. There were no residual psychotic symptoms.

As a child the patient had always formed friendships and seemed well adjusted despite frequent family moves. His father was a salesman who was interested in the occult. A younger brother and sister had both suffered from psychotic disorders of an unknown type. The patient's first episode of psychosis occurred at age 25 after a romantic disappointment. A second episode occurred 3 years later during a period of unemployment and economic distress. In each case the disturbance remitted completely within a few months.

Epidemiology

Schizophreniform disorder is less common than schizophrenia and occurs with equal frequency in men and women. Some studies have indicated that schizophreniform disorder is genetically related to schizophrenia, but other recent reports (Kendler and Walsh, 1995) refute this.

Etiology & Pathogenesis

The specific causes of schizophreniform disorder are unknown. Neurodevelopmental, traumatic, and genetic models are among those proposed as explanations for these findings, but none points to any currently identified specific pathological mechanism.

Treatment

Acute episodes of schizophreniform disorder are best treated in a hospital setting, where a structured supportive environment is provided. Exceptions to this may be made if adequate support is present in the home or an alternate facility such as a day hospital is available. Patients who present for treatment in early stages of decompensation may also be treatable on an outpatient basis. Although a few patients improve spontaneously after hospital admission, most will require medication. The neuroleptic drugs are the usual indicated treatment. Supplementation by benzodiazepines such as lorazepam during the most acute period of treatment may reduce the dose of neuroleptics required and thereby reduce the risk of side effects such as parkinsonism and tardive dyskinesia. Treatment itself proceeds in a fashion identical to that used for schizophrenia, with doses of antipsychotic drugs being gradually increased over a period of days or weeks until maximum benefit is achieved (see Chapter 30). Symptoms such as insomnia, agitation, suspiciousness, and disorganized thoughts may recede dramatically during the first few days of treatment, but auditory hallucinations and delusions may clear more gradually. The newer "atypical" neuroleptics, such as risperidone, olanzapine, and quetiapine, offer less risk of long-term neurologic side effects as well as less drug-induced parkinsonism. The newer drugs, however, are expensive. Clozapine should probably not be used to treat schizophreniform disorder because of its potential side effects. It is most indicated in treatment of refractory cases of schizophrenia and similar disorders, which by definition are probably excluded from the diagnosis of schizophreniform disorder. When patients fail to respond to traditional treatment in a reasonable period of time, alternate treatments such as lithium carbonate, carbamazepine, and electroconvulsive therapy have been employed, although their efficacy is less well established.

After clinical stabilization, neuroleptic drugs are gradually withdrawn unless symptoms recur. It is useful to teach patients to recognize early signs of decompensation. Maintenance drugs as well as a diagnostic reassessment may be required if relapse occurs.

Suicide is of critical concern in the treatment of patients with schizophreniform disorder, particularly after psychotic symptoms have subsided. Many patients enter into a prolonged depression, which may be part of the natural history of the disorder or represent a psychological reaction to the realization that one has been mentally ill. These postpsychotic depressions respond poorly to antidepressant treatment, and the risk of suicide is high. Patients should be monitored closely after discharge from the hospital and rehospitalized if suicidal ideation becomes apparent.

SCHIZOAFFECTIVE DISORDER

Symptoms & Signs

For decades there has been controversy about whether patients with admixtures of schizophrenic and mood symptoms were suffering from schizophrenia, an atypical variety of bipolar disorder, or a separate disorder entirely. A number of diagnostic labels have been applied to this group of patients, including (but not limited to) cycloid psychosis, atypical schizophrenia, good-prognosis schizophrenia, and remitting schizophrenia. The term "schizoaffective disorder," originated by Jacob S. Kasanin in 1933, has prevailed, although the boundaries with other disorders are still debated. In modern diagnostic practice, many of these patients are diagnosed as having psychotic mood disorders.

Patients with schizoaffective disorder display psychotic symptoms consistent with the acute phase of schizophrenia, but these symptoms are frequently accompanied by prominent manic or depressive symptomatology. At other times, schizophrenic symptoms unaccompanied by mood symptoms are present. Schizoaffective disorder is further divided into bipolar (history of manic episodes) and depressive types. The *DSM-IV* criteria for this disorder are shown in Table 19–3.

Natural History & Prognosis

Schizoaffective disorder can present at any age, but it is most commonly first seen in young adulthood. Prognosis can be estimated from the relative promi-

Table 19–3. *DSM-IV* criteria for schizoaffective disorder.

A. An uninterrupted period of illness during which, at some time, there is either a major depressive episode or manic episode concurrent with symptoms that meet Criterion A for schizophrenia (see Table 19–1)

B. During the same period of illness, there have been delusions or hallucinations for at least 2 weeks in the absence of prominent mood symptoms

C. Symptoms meeting criteria for a mood episode are present for a substantial portion of the total duration of the active and residual periods of the illness

D. Not due to the direct physiological effects of a substance (eg, drugs of abuse, medication) or a general medical condition

Specify if

Bipolar type: If disturbance includes a manic or a mixed episode (or manic or a mixed episode and major depressive episodes)

Depressive type: If major depressive episode only

nence of schizophrenic and mood symptoms; more prominent and persistent schizophrenic symptoms are associated with poorer outcome, whereas more frequent and persistent mood symptoms predict more positive outcome. The presence of mood-congruent delusions and hallucinations (eg, the belief by a depressed woman that she has sinned or a manic individual's belief that he or she is the Messiah) predicts better outcome than mood-incongruent psychotic symptoms. Age of onset may also be a factor, as the functional status of adolescents diagnosed with schizoaffective disorder resembles that of schizophrenia more than it does mood disorders.

Differential Diagnosis

A longitudinal rather than cross-sectional approach is essential for the differential diagnosis of schizoaffective disorder, since it is the temporal relationship between psychotic and mood symptoms that distinguishes it from schizophrenic and mood disorders. Both psychotic disorder associated with a general medical condition and psychotic disorder that is substance induced may cause the symptoms of schizoaffective disorder directly or modify the manifestations of another psychotic disorder. For example, recent use of cocaine or amphetamines may produce a variety of manic, delusional, or hallucinatory symptoms. Withdrawal from cocaine may induce profound depressive symptoms accompanied by delusions or hallucinations. Schizoaffective disorder differs from major depression or bipolar disorder with psychotic symptoms in that although a full mood syndrome (manic or major depressive episode) is accompanied by psychotic symptoms, delusions or hallucinations have been present without them for at least 2 weeks. It differs from schizophrenia or schizophreniform disorder in that the total duration of any mood symptoms present is not brief in relation to the total duration of the illness. In

more descriptive terms, patients with a predominantly schizophrenic clinical picture who suffer from occasional periods of depression or elation are diagnosed as schizophrenic. For patients whose psychotic symptoms occur only during mood disturbances, the most appropriate diagnosis is major depression or bipolar mood disorder with psychotic features. The remaining patients have schizoaffective disorder.

In delusional disorder mood symptoms are also relatively brief in duration, and psychotic symptoms are limited to nonbizarre delusional systems. Brief psychotic disorder differs from schizoaffective disorder in that a full mood syndrome is not present, and psychotic symptoms may not be sufficient to satisfy criteria for schizophrenia.

Illustrative Case 1

A 65-year-old man of German descent had been hospitalized frequently since his 30s for an illness characterized in part by auditory hallucinations and paranoid delusions. After each hospitalization, he recovered enough to return to his full-time job. On retiring, he took up residence in a downtown hotel while receiving injections of depot fluphenazine. Within a few months he became markedly depressed. A trial of tricyclic antidepressant drugs resulted in a euphoric mood accompanied by pressured speech, insomnia, and poor judgment. The antidepressant medication was discontinued, but the depression returned within a few months, and the patient was hospitalized.

On admission to the hospital, the patient was severely slowed in his movements and speech and walked with a stooped gait. He slept poorly and had little appetite. He insisted that therapeutic efforts were best spent on other patients, because he was a worthless person for whom there was no hope. He wanted to be dead but lacked the initiative or "courage" to commit suicide. There were no delusions or hallucinations apparent, and his speech was well organized and logical. He responded dramatically within 10 days after resumption of the antidepressant drug in a lower dosage. A diagnosis of bipolar disorder was made, and prophylactic lithium treatment was begun. The fluphenazine was discontinued.

Several months later the patient discontinued lithium because of a tremor and began to pace around his hotel, sleeping poorly and eating only one meal daily. He also stopped bathing and shaving. He presented himself again to the hospital in a filthy, disheveled state; he was lice ridden and had lost 20 pounds. He was not visibly depressed or elated but was negativistic and turned his head and glared frequently as if responding to a voice. After several days of treatment with moderate doses of haloperidol, he began to respond to questioning by his physician. He denied having been depressed and insisted that nothing was wrong with him. He admitted hearing women singing happy German children's songs and often sang along with them. He also discussed his belief that Jews were attempting to harm him and his grandchildren as retaliation for what the Germans had done to them during World War II. He claimed that he had felt this way for years but often avoided discussing it with his doctors. He described a series of seemingly ordinary incidents that had happened through the years that he felt proved his point.

Illustrative Case 2

A 44-year-old divorced black male presented with a 20-year history of traveling about the country, almost annual psychiatric hospitalizations, and alcohol abuse. The usual diagnosis had been paranoid schizophrenia. Two months before his latest request for inpatient care he had been started on lithium treatment for the first time but discontinued it because of increased urination and dysuria. He also stopped taking the chlorpromazine that had been prescribed. He complained of sleeplessness and weight loss and became loud and belligerent when his need for hospitalization was questioned.

Mental status examination revealed a guarded, somewhat sarcastic, physically thin man who spoke in increasingly loud tones with a considerable degree of pressure and circumstantiality. His behavior on the ward was intrusive and loud, and he slept little. His mood was irritable, and he was frequently pacing, talking, or otherwise active. When questioned about auditory hallucinations, he became extremely defensive and denied hearing voices. He did say, however, that he sometimes picked up information from "the wrong channel" but ignored it. He had gotten "into trouble" in the past when he paid attention to what he had heard.

Treatment was started with lithium. Small doses of haloperidol had to be added temporarily because his pressured, irritable manner caused conflicts with other patients. After 1 week his behavior was considerably subdued, but it became apparent that he was hallucinating. He spent most of the day off the ward in animated conversation with nonexistent persons. At that point serum lithium levels were within the therapeutic range. Addition of haloperidol in standard doses eliminated the hallucinations, but withdrawal of lithium resulted in a return of manic behavior.

Epidemiology

Estimates of the prevalence of schizoaffective disorder vary widely, but schizoaffective manic patients appear to comprise 3–5% of psychiatric admissions to typical clinical centers. At one point it was widely believed that schizoaffective disorder was associated with increased risk of mood disorders in relatives. This may have been because of the number of patients with psychotic mood disorders who were included in schizoaffective study populations. The current diagnostic criteria define a group of patients with a mixed genetic picture. They are more likely to have schizophrenic relatives than patients with mood dis-

orders but more likely to have relatives with mood disorders than schizophrenic patients.

Etiology & Pathogenesis

Although the causes of schizoaffective disorder are unknown, it is suspected that this diagnosis represents a heterogeneous group of patients, some with atypical forms of schizophrenia and some with very severe forms of mood disorders. There is little evidence for a distinct variety of psychotic illness. It follows then that the etiology is probably identical to that of schizophrenia in some cases or to mood disorders in others.

Treatment

Most schizoaffective patients require neuroleptic medication, often on a long-term basis, to control psychotic symptoms, as well as treatment for mood symptoms.

Combining lithium, carbamazepine, or valproate with a neuroleptic has been shown to be superior to neuroleptics alone in schizoaffective patients with manic symptoms. The degree of benefit for an individual patient should be considered carefully, as each of these agents carries an additional set of risks (see Chapter 30). Lithium–neuroleptic combinations may produce severe extrapyramidal reactions or confusion in some patients. Carbamazepine or valproate are frequently employed when lithium is not effective or well tolerated. Granulocytopenia can occur during the first few weeks of carbamazepine treatment, and neuroleptic blood levels may be increased substantially due to hepatic enzyme induction. Valproate can cause liver toxicity and platelet dysfunction, although those problems are uncommon. More recently, the anticonvulsants lamotrigine and gabapentin have shown promise in the treatment of manic symptoms, although there have been no systematic studies of their use in schizoaffective disorder at this time. Calcium channel blockers such as verapamil may also be an effective treatment for manic symptoms but are seldom prescribed for that purpose. Benzodiazepines such as lorazepam and clonazepam are effective adjunctive treatment agents for acute manic symptoms, but long-term use may result in dependency.

Treatment of the schizoaffective depressed patient has not been studied as well as the schizoaffective patient with mania. Administration of a neuroleptic drug is required, but it is not clear whether adding an antidepressant is beneficial. Preliminary evidence suggests that atypical neuroleptics have antidepressant properties. If so, they would become the preferred choice in these patients. Continued depressive symptoms might necessitate the addition of antidepressant medication. Although the utility of lithium, carbamazepine, or valproate in the treatment of schizoaffective depression has not been clearly established, patients who have histories of manic episodes in the past will need to be on mood stabilizers to minimize the risk of antidepressant-induced switches into mania. Polypharmacy of this type requires monitoring for drug interactions. Manic symptoms can occur when antidepressants are administered, particularly in patients with a prior history of those symptoms, even when a mood stabilizer is being used. Tricyclics are the worst offenders, whereas selective serotonin reuptake inhibitors (SSRIs) and bupropion are less likely to induce mania. Administration of multiple drugs with anticholinergic properties can create toxicity, including delirium. Lower-potency standard neuroleptics such as chlorpromazine and thioridizine, most tricyclic antidepressants and monoamine oxidase (MAO) inhibitors, and agents such as benztropin used to treat drug-induced parkinsonism are common offenders. Of the newer medications, clozapine, the SSRI paroxetine, and the atypical neuroleptic olanzapine also have anticholinergic activity. Carbamazepine induces hepatic enzymes and may result in increased serum levels of other medications, and some antidepressants, particularly fluoxetine, inhibit metabolism of many drugs through action on the cytochrome P450 system. Thus, dosages of medications may have to be adjusted downward when they are added. Many clinicians are choosing to minimize the drawbacks of polytherapy by using atypical neuroleptics for psychotic symptoms and by choosing newer antidepressants rather than tricyclics. Newer antidepressants are also much safer in overdose, an important consideration in depressed psychotic patients. They may be indicated when there is a history of previous positive response, when other drugs have failed, or when there is a history of manic episodes. Both lithium and heterocyclic antidepressants are effective prophylactic agents in recurrent unipolar depression. Newer drugs are still under study, and their effectiveness in preventing recurrences of schizoaffective depression has not been demonstrated.

DELUSIONAL DISORDERS

Symptoms & Signs

Delusional disorders are characterized by prominent well-organized delusions and by the relative absence of hallucinations, disorganized thought and behavior, and abnormal affect. Although not as common as schizophrenia or psychotic mood disorders, they are consistently encountered in psychiatric settings. The older name for this disorder, paranoia, was first used by Kahlbaum in 1863 and incorporated as a category of illness in Kraepelin's 1912 textbook. Since it is the delusional beliefs of a persecutory nature that are most commonly described, the term "paranoia" has become associated with suspiciousness or persecutory beliefs. To avoid confusion, the term "delusional disorder" is used in *DSM-IV*. The criteria for its diagnosis are shown in Table 19–4.

The disorder is usually marked by the onset of delusional ideas that become the focus of the pa-

Table 19–4. *DSM-IV* criteria for delusional disorder.

A. Nonbizarre delusions (ie, involving situations that occur in real life, such as being followed, poisoned, infected, loved at a distance, having a disease, or being deceived by one's spouse or lover) of at least 1 month's duration

B. Has never met Criterion A for schizophrenia (*Note:* Tactile and olfactory hallucinations are not excluded if related to the delusional theme)

C. Apart from the impact of the delusion(s) or its ramifications, functioning is not markedly impaired and behavior is not obviously odd or bizarre

D. If mood episodes have occurred concurrently with delusions, their total duration has been brief relative to the duration of the delusional periods

E. Not due to the direct physiological effects of a substance (eg, drugs of abuse, medication) or a general medical condition

tient's life. The delusional beliefs themselves are internally consistent; in fact, the clinician may have difficulty deciding where legitimate grievances or misfortunes end and psychotic fantasies begin. What begins as a frustrating experience with a government agency or employer may become a complex conspiracy that involves everyone in the patient's surroundings. These patients may resort to litigation or appeal to public authorities for assistance; as these efforts are frustrated, those agencies and individuals are viewed as having joined the ranks of the enemy. A sense of self-importance and of messianic mission may develop over time as patients see themselves standing alone against injustice. Remarkably, outside of their delusional concerns, these patients behave and communicate in a normal fashion. Their emotional responses conform to our expectations of a normal person facing the same threat or danger. They may feel strongly motivated to discuss their beliefs and try to engage the clinician as an ally. They rarely have insight into the fact that they are ill, and their attendance in a psychiatric setting is often the result of pressure from family or courts. Comorbid psychiatric disorders such as mood disorders or alcohol dependence may be present as well. Depression, perhaps with suicidal ideation, is not unusual when a patient has exhausted all personal resources coping with a life that has become a nightmare.

Delusional disorders are further classified according to the type of delusion that is most prominent:

Patients with **erotomanic** delusional disorder mistakenly believe that a particular person, usually of higher social status than the patient (eg, a film star, politician, or college professor), is deeply in love with them. The patient may attempt to communicate with this person by letter, by telephone, or even by forced intrusion into the person's home. The patient may provide idiosyncratic interpretations of the public statements or gestures of the target person as evidence of attempts by this person to respond.

Patients with delusional disorder of the **grandiose**

type believe that they are special or have very important talents or abilities. Such patients may spend much of their time working on ideas for great inventions, which they may represent as having important potential benefits for humanity but which will seem lacking in substance to the listener. They may believe they are persecuted by those who envy their talents; in such cases the boundary between delusional disorder of the persecutory type and of the grandiose type may become blurred.

Patients with delusional disorder of the **jealous** type mistakenly believe that their spouse or lover is unfaithful, often based on mysterious clues that seem to appear everywhere. They may gather evidence based on random events, bits of conversation, or misplaced household items to support their suspicions.

Patients with delusional disorder of the **persecutory** type believe that they are victims of an organized plot. They may feel that they are being pursued, that their telephone is tapped, or that their reputation is being purposely maligned.

Patients with prominent **somatic** delusions may believe that they have some dread disease or are dying. In one particular manifestation, patients complain of infestation with insects or parasites; such patients are likely to present for treatment at a dermatologist's office rather than in a psychiatric setting. They frequently offer jars or bottles with "specimens" they have saved for laboratory analysis; often these appear to be pieces of skin or other nonspecific material.

In **mixed delusional disorder** more than one type of delusion is present, without any one clearly predominating. In some cases grandiose, jealous, and persecutory delusions may co-occur.

Patients with **unspecified delusional disorder** have delusions that do not clearly fit other categories (eg, the delusion of doubles [Capgras's syndrome], in which patients believe that a loved one is a double or imposter and is not to be trusted).

Table 19–5 shows *DSM-IV* criteria for subtypes of delusional disorder.

Table 19–5. *DSM-IV* criteria for delusional disorder subtypes.

Erotomanic: Delusions that another person, usually of higher status, is in love with the individual

Grandiose: Delusions of inflated worth, power, knowledge, identity, or special relationship to a deity or famous person

Jealous: Delusions that one's sexual partner is unfaithful

Persecutory: Delusions that one (or someone to whom one is close) is being malevolently treated in some way

Somatic: Delusions that the person has some physical defect or general medical condition

Mixed: Delusions characteristic of more than one of the above types but no one theme predominates

Unspecified

Differential Diagnosis

The presence of nonbizarre, superficially plausible delusions for at least 1 month and the absence of history of both more pervasive psychotic symptoms and significant deterioration in social functioning are required for a diagnosis of delusional disorder. The content of the delusions forms the basis for classification into erotomanic, grandiose, jealous, persecutory, somatic, and unspecified types.

Delusional disorder must be distinguished from psychotic disorder associated with a general medical condition and from substance-induced psychotic disorder, both of which can present with prominent delusions. Schizophrenia, schizophreniform disorder, and schizoaffective disorder differ from delusional disorder in that delusions are accompanied by additional psychotic symptoms such as prominent auditory hallucinations, loosening of associations, poverty of speech, markedly illogical thinking, delusional content of a bizarre or absurd nature, or bizarre behavior. Delusional disorder differs from brief psychotic disorder in having a duration of 1 month or greater.

Delusional disorder accompanied by depression differs from major depression with psychotic features in that the total duration of the mood symptoms is brief compared to the total duration of the illness. Although depressed patients may experience virtually any type of delusion, persecutory beliefs associated with depression are often thematically related to an exaggerated feeling of guilt—they feel they are being punished for their crimes or otherwise deserve the treatment they are receiving. Both manic and delusional disorders can present with exaggerated feelings of self-importance and belligerence, but manic symptoms such as increased motor activity, excessive plans, hypersexuality, racing thoughts, or decreased need for sleep are not prominent or persistent in delusional disorder.

A more subtle distinction is between delusional disorder of the persecutory type and paranoid personality. In the latter, the patient may be generally suspicious of the motives of others but does not have actual delusions. In practice, however, it may be difficult to extract delusional ideas from paranoid patients, since they may conceal the extent of their suspiciousness when they do not trust the examiner.

Natural History & Prognosis

Most cases of delusional disorder are characterized by a gradual onset and chronic course, although more acute forms have been described. Onset is typically in middle life or later, with few first hospitalizations before age 35. Age of onset is oldest for the persecutory type and youngest for the somatic type, with the others falling in between. The prognosis of delusional disorder is variable. Many patients retain some of their delusional beliefs, and engaging them in treatment can be difficult. A satisfactory outcome is achieved if they can function in the community without feeling the need to act on or discuss their abnormal beliefs.

Illustrative Case 1 (Persecutory Type)

A 59-year-old divorced power company engineer became convinced that the design for a new nuclear power plant was faulty and unsafe. Despite 11 years with the company, he was fired, by his account, after repeatedly annoying his superiors with these concerns. Acting as his own attorney, he filed suits against the company, some protesting his firing, some to stop construction of the power plant, and even some to stop utility rate increases. He became well known to company and public officials, who saw him as a comic figure who was also somewhat tragic.

Meanwhile, the patient came to believe that because he had filed so many suits on his own behalf, a "grandfather" clause in the state law entitled him to be considered an attorney. He also began to believe that his efforts had made him unpopular with certain powerful groups, including the Mafia, the Bank of America, the FBI, and even the Vatican. He squandered his savings on a trip to Europe, where he attempted to pursue his investigations, until he was deported from England. Whenever local authorities would intervene, he assumed they were involved in the conspiracy and were helping to keep track of his whereabouts.

After his personal resources were exhausted and after an unsuccessful attempt to convince police that a "contract" was out on his life, he requested hospitalization for "protection." At the time of admission, the patient was well groomed and articulate. He rambled on about his delusions and fears unless interrupted firmly. There was no evidence of hyperactivity, hallucinations, or other delusional thinking. During his hospital stay he was neither overtalkative nor socially intrusive. He slept peacefully, believing that he was safe in the hospital. After treatment with moderate doses of a neuroleptic drug, he was able to leave the safety of the hospital for a halfway house. Careful questioning revealed that he continued to believe that there was a conspiracy against him, but felt less of a compulsion to discuss it or act on it.

Illustrative Case 2 (Somatic Type)

A 65-year-old former prizefighter had been making the rounds of local hospitals for 2 years with the complaint that his nose was shrinking. He feared that if this process progressed too far, he would not be able to breathe and would subsequently die. Although at times this depressed him, the depression was transient, whereas his frantic concerns about his nose continued unabated. Attempts by otolaryngolo-

gists to reassure him were unsuccessful and attempts on psychiatric units to treat him with trials of neuroleptics and antidepressants failed. He subsequently refused any psychiatric referral. At no time had there been evidence of hallucinations, other delusions, or disorganized thought. His behavior and level of self-care were totally appropriate. Multiple mental status examinations, neurological studies, and laboratory screenings failed to disclose evidence of underlying medical disease.

Epidemiology

Delusional disorder is relatively uncommon, representing 1–4% of all psychiatric hospital admissions. The incidence of the disorder is 1–3/100,000 population annually, and the prevalence is between 0.02% and 0.03%. The persecutory type is the most common form. Women are affected more often than men but not as predominantly as in mood disorders. Patients are more likely to have been married than schizophrenic patients. Low socioeconomic status and recent immigrant status are common associated factors. Additional populations at risk include elderly patients with impaired hearing, cognitive deficits, or other disabilities that limit social contacts. Genetic studies indicate a lack of familial relationships with either schizophrenia or mood disorder.

Etiology & Pathogenesis

The cause of delusional disorder is unknown, but a number of contributory psychological mechanisms have been proposed, particularly for the persecutory type. Kraepelin and Kretschmer postulated that the disorder resulted from overwhelming stress in a premorbid personality characterized by distrustfulness and hypersensitivity to slights. Later writers have postulated a developmental deficit in the ability to trust others. Cameron (1974) stressed that individuals with delusional disorder are unable to compare the perspectives of others with their own. They thus seem to be isolated, asocial people who must be vigilant lest something potentially threatening happen. Freud attributed paranoid thinking to **projection,** a psychological mechanism whereby ideas or feelings unacceptable to conscious awareness are disowned and attributed to (projected on) others. Salzman (1960) and Cameron (1974) believed that delusional symptoms developed from underlying feelings of vulnerability and worthlessness.

These psychological formulations have significant shortcomings. They lack diagnostic specificity; similar psychological themes are identifiable in patients with a variety of psychiatric disorders who happen to have persecutory delusions. Many patients with hypersensitive, asocial personalities develop other disorders (such as schizophrenia). In addition, similar phenomena may occur in otherwise normal individuals, sometimes under conditions of vulnerability such as drug intoxication or fatigue or in social or religious groups whose values isolate them from the larger community. In some circumstances, hypervigilant scanning of the environment for danger or treachery may be adaptive. Nonetheless, social isolation, whether a result of maladaptive personality functioning, physical limitations, or cultural dislocation, seems to be an important factor in the pathogenesis of persecutory symptoms and delusional disorders in general. Additional contributory causes obviously are present but are beyond our current understanding.

Treatment

The treatment of delusional disorder usually involves the use of neuroleptic medication. In cases of delusions of infestation some psychiatrists have claimed that pimozide, a butyrophenone similar to haloperidol, has specific efficacy. There are also anecdotal reports of delusional disorder responding to antidepressants after neuroleptic treatment has failed.

Delusional patients are unlikely to participate willingly in any treatment program unless there is some basis for trust in the physician. Patients with this disorder are wary of any situation in which they are not in control, and often suspect that medication may be designed to harm them or lower their resistance to outside influences. The very act of accepting medication may be viewed as an admission that their beliefs are false. Any side effect, however trivial, may frighten them into refusing further treatment. For this reason many psychiatrists are selecting atypical antipsychotics such as risperidone, olanzapine, or quetiapine because of their more favorable side effect profiles.

Paranoid patients feel that they have been disappointed by people who at first seem to be on their side but later betray them, and therefore they approach new relationships in guarded fashion. At the same time, they desire human contact and may wish to find someone to trust who can help them. A professional and respectful attitude is necessary to take advantage of this. A paternalistic approach will be perceived as insulting; an informal manner may imply that the physician does not take their concerns seriously. Complete frankness is called for—pretending to give credence to the patient's delusional ideas leads to an appearance of betrayal when the clinician's true feelings emerge. Clinicians should make clear that they do not accept what the patient asserts as true, *but that disagreement implies no disrespect.* It is pointless and counterproductive to use logical reasoning to argue or try to talk patients out of their delusions. As trust develops, evidence for and against the validity of the delusional beliefs can be mutually explored in the hope that the patient will spontaneously begin to question their truth. In many cases, the best result that can be achieved is to help these patients understand and accept that they have beliefs most others view as illogical and fallacious.

BRIEF PSYCHOTIC DISORDER

Symptoms & Signs

It is a common clinical observation that otherwise well-functioning people may develop psychotic symptoms in response to stress. In certain cultures, symptoms conform to certain patterns that are recognized by the individual's group as a valid and legitimate signal of distress. Psychiatrists in Europe have long recognized the existence of a "nonendogenous" or "psychogenic" form of psychotic illness that is distinct from schizophrenia or manic-depressive illness. Psychiatrists in the United States have been less interested in this phenomenon, although they have described cases of "hysterical psychosis" or acute reactions to combat such as the "3-day schizophrenias" of World War II.

Brief psychotic disorders may be preceded by a stressful event or series of events such as automobile accidents, divorces or separations, and financial setbacks. They may also be associated with the postpartum period. However, stressors may also be absent or seemingly mild in severity. The onset of symptoms is abrupt, without the gradually developing prodrome often seen in schizophreniform disorder or schizophrenia. Symptoms are often dramatic and florid and are often thematically related to precipitating circumstances. There may be emotional turmoil or confusion as well as psychotic symptoms of various types. Delusions, hallucinations (auditory hallucinations are common, but visual hallucinations occur occasionally), loose associations or disorganized speech, and bizarre and disorganized behavior are all common. Personality disorders are often noted after recovery from the psychotic symptoms and may become the clinical focus. The *DSM-IV* criteria for brief psychotic disorder are shown in Table 19-6.

Natural History & Prognosis

The disorder is marked by good premorbid functioning and short duration (no longer than 1 month). Onset is usually during young adulthood. There is always a full recovery, although patients may have repeat episodes, particularly if a basic personality defect is present that provides a window of vulnerability to stress. On follow-up, the diagnosis of brief psychotic disorder is still appropriate for about half of these patients. The rest are rediagnosed at some point as suffering from other psychotic disorders.

Differential Diagnosis

The diagnostic criteria for brief psychotic disorder distinguish it from various other mental disorders. The effects of a substance (such as withdrawal or intoxication from alcohol or drugs) or of a general medical condition should be ruled out by appropriate history taking, physical examination, and laboratory tests. The symptoms of brief psychotic disorder may resemble those of schizophrenia, schizophreniform

Table 19–6. *DSM-IV* criteria for brief psychotic disorder.

A. Presence of at least one of the following symptoms:

    (1) delusions
    (2) hallucinations
    (3) disorganized speech (eg, frequent derailment or incoherence)
    (4) grossly disorganized *or* catatonic behavior

    Note: Do not include a symptom if it is a culturally sanctioned response pattern

B. Duration of an episode of the disturbance is at least 1 day and no more than 1 month, with eventual full return to premorbid level of functioning

C. Not better accounted for by a mood disorder with psychotic features, schizoaffective disorder, or schizophrenia, and not due to the direct effects of a physiological substance (eg, drugs of abuse, medication) or a general medical condition

Specify if

    With marked stressor(s) (brief reactive psychosis): if symptoms occur shortly after and apparently in response to events that, singly or together, would be markedly stressful to almost anyone in similar circumstances in the person's culture

    Without marked stressor(s): if psychotic symptoms do *not* occur shortly after, or are not apparently in response to events that, singly or together, would be markedly stressful to almost anyone in similar circumstances in the person's culture

    With postpartum onset: if onset is within 4 weeks postpartum

disorder, or delusional disorder, but these disorders last longer than 1 month. Unlike mood disorders with psychotic features and schizoaffective disorder, a full manic or depressive syndrome is not present in brief psychotic disorder. The clinician should also be alert to the possibility of factitious disorder with psychological symptoms; evasive responses to questions or apparent inconsistencies in the history may suggest this possibility.

Illustrative Case

A 60-year-old widower was admitted to the urology service for evaluation of acute onset of inability to void. While a physician was explaining the nature of a planned diagnostic procedure, bright red blood appeared in the catheter bag in full view of the patient. He became extremely frightened and was convinced that he would not survive the upcoming procedure. When a psychiatric consultant visited him several hours later, he was sobbing uncontrollably and was unable to lie still. He overheard messengers from God telling him he would soon be dead, and he saw visions of his deceased wife, who promised him a reunion.

The patient's psychiatric history dated from World War II, when he had experienced two episodes of psychogenic amnesia and had traveled long distances before finding himself in strange cities. Since then, he had had periods of anxiety, particularly in crowded public situations, and he had finally stopped working at age 50. He had never been psychotic.

After 2 days of pharmacological treatment and frequent reassurance from the medical staff, his symptoms disappeared almost as dramatically as they had begun.

Epidemiology

Although the incidence of brief psychotic disorder is difficult to estimate, family studies suggest that relatives of these patients are prone to develop brief psychoses but not schizophrenia or mood disorders. The majority of patients diagnosed with this disorder are female.

Etiology & Pathogenesis

Psychological factors may be more important in brief psychotic disorder than in schizophreniform or schizoaffective disorders. When a person is confronted with a stressful situation, the natural response is to use familiar problem-solving behavior patterns either to achieve a resolution or to maintain psychological equilibrium until external events change. Psychotic symptoms may emerge when the patient's psychological defenses are completely overwhelmed. For some patients, only chaotic events such as natural disasters or combat experiences are severe enough to upset the equilibrium; other people may be overwhelmed by divorce, physical illness, or financial disaster. Some patients with character defects (ie, personality disorder) may be unable to cope with transitions or disappointments that most people would be able to tolerate, even though they might find them unsettling. Postpartum cases may be influenced by endocrine changes as well as psychological stress. In cases without associated stressors, there may be as yet undetermined biological causes.

Treatment

Patients should be assessed carefully for suicidal or homicidal ideation and appropriate steps should be taken to contain acute symptoms. Psychotropic medications are usually necessary to control agitation and insomnia. Neuroleptic medications should be limited to short-term use only, and symptomatic treatment with benzodiazepines such as lorazepam will often make the use of large amounts of neuroleptics unnecessary. Medication should be tapered off fairly soon after resolution of the acute disturbance. There is ordinarily no indication for maintenance therapy.

Psychological treatment may take several forms. Simply being removed from the crisis and being cared for by the hospital staff may allay the patient's anxiety enough to permit constructive discussion and problem solving. Enlisting the aid of family members may also be important for the same reason. Encouraging the patient to recount the events that led to the breakdown and to discuss their impact and meaning will facilitate recovery. Such discussion offers the patient a model for dealing with crises in the future. Longer-term psychotherapy directed at more fundamental psychological conflicts may be indicated for some patients.

SHARED PSYCHOTIC DISORDER

Symptoms & Signs

Shared psychotic disorder is an uncommon condition characterized by uncritical acceptance by one person of the delusional beliefs of another. Although two people are most commonly involved (folie à deux), cases have been reported involving three or more and in some instances an entire family. The patients are usually relatives or persons who have lived in intimate contact for a long time.

A characteristic feature of shared psychotic disorder is a pattern of dominance and submission. The dominant partner (primary case) is more seriously ill and suffers from a delusional psychosis—usually schizophrenia or delusional disorder. This individual is the originator of the delusions, passing them on to the passive partner. The submissive recipient is not otherwise psychotic prior to acquiring his or her partner's delusional beliefs. The content of the delusions is often persecutory or hypochondriacal and underscores the perceived hostility of the outside world, reinforcing social isolation and interdependence of the parties. This marked isolation becomes a strong motivation to maintain the close relationship at all costs. Hallucinations are also common, as are comorbid conditions such as dementia or mental deficiency. Table 19–7 lists the *DSM-IV* criteria for shared psychotic disorder.

Table 19–7. *DSM-IV* criteria for shared psychotic disorder.

A. A delusion develops in an individual in the context of a close relationship with another person(s), who has an already established delusion

B. The delusion is similar in content to that of the person who already has the established delusion

C. Not better accounted for by another psychotic disorder (eg, schizophrenia or a mood disorder with psychotic features), and not due to the direct physiological effects of a substance (eg, drugs of abuse, medication) or a general medical condition

Differential Diagnosis

The primary issue in differential diagnosis of shared psychotic disorder is ruling out the presence of schizophrenia or other psychosis in the submissive partner.

Natural History & Prognosis

Shared psychotic disorder occurs in older and younger patients with equal frequency. The prognosis for the submissive "recipient" is quite good if separation from the dominant partner is possible. In approximately 40% of reported cases, the recipient patient has responded to separation from the dominant partner alone. Treatment specific for the underlying illness is necessary for the primary case, with the final outcome depending on the diagnosis.

Illustrative Case

A hotel manager in a small town called the police because a guest family had stopped paying its bills and had been acting strangely. A 48-year-old man, his 25-year-old wife, and their infant son had registered 2 weeks previously and had not left the room except for the wife's trips to the grocery store. These forays had ceased the week before. The rent for the second week had not been paid despite frequent demands. Other guests complained of chanting and yelling during the night.

The husband was an unemployed laborer with a history of psychiatric hospitalizations and arrests for drunkenness and assault. He professed to be receiving messages from God directing him and his family to await the destruction of the world and the beginning of "the new order." His family would be among the few survivors and would play a leading role in the future of mankind. He heard the voice of God and of various angels, who gave him instructions.

His wife was an extremely introverted, socially awkward woman who had never dated before meeting her husband. She rarely had contacts with other adults without her husband being present; on those occasions, he would invariably speak for her.

The husband had to be forcibly removed from the hotel room by the police and was eventually committed to a state hospital. His wife initially resisted offers of help, fearing that if she left the hotel she would not be saved from the impending Armageddon. She gradually gave up these beliefs in response to simple reassurance. The child was placed in a foster home. The wife and husband were reunited after his release from the hospital and were lost to follow-up.

Epidemiology

There are no data on incidence or prevalence of shared psychotic disorder, but it is thought to be quite rare. Over 90% of cases involve members of a single family. The most common cases involve two sisters. Mother and child are next in frequency of occurrence, followed by father-child and husband-wife combinations. Pairings between friends and fellow mental patients are infrequent but have occurred.

Approximately 25% of the submissive (recipient) partners suffer from a physical disability such as hearing loss or stroke, which may increase their susceptibility to domination by their partners.

Etiology & Pathogenesis

Shared psychotic disorder is believed to arise as a result of interdependency between the partners and serves to preserve their relationship. For the mechanism to work, several conditions must be met. The primary case, already mentally ill, must be dominant in the relationship and be able to influence the submissive partner. There must be a distinct advantage for both partners in sharing the delusions. For the inducing partner, maintaining at least one human contact represents a chance to avoid complete isolation. The delusions represent a mode of communication providing a tie with their partner that partially offsets the alienation from outside reality. For the submissive partner, the delusions become a compromise, allowing a continuation of a dependent relationship.

Treatment

Treatment for the recipient generally consists of separation from the dominant partner. In many cases, the patient then becomes accessible to rational discussion and gives up the delusional system. However, because many patients will return to the same relationship, other steps may be indicated. These might include family or conjoint therapy as well as assistance in developing activities and interests outside the relationship.

REFERENCES & SUGGESTED READINGS

Schizophreniform Disorder

Benazzi F: *DSM-III-R* schizophreniform disorder with good prognostic features: A six-year follow-up. Can J Psychiatry 1998;43:180.

Casacchia M et al: Schizophreniform disorder: A 1-year follow-up study. Psychopathology 1996;29:104.

Kendler KS, Walsh D: Schizophreniform disorder, delusional disorder and psychotic disorder not otherwise specified: Clinical features, outcome and familial psychopathology. Acta Psychiatr Scand 1995;91:370.

Zhang-Wong J et al: Five-year course of schizophreniform disorder. Psychiatry Res 1995;59:109.

Schizoaffective Disorder

Doering S et al: Predictors of relapse and rehospitalization in schizophrenia and schizoaffective disorder. Schizophr Bull 1998;24:87.

Greil W et al: Lithium vs carbamazepine in the maintenance treatment of schizoaffective disorder: A randomised study. Eur Arch Psychiatry Clin Neurosci 1997;247:42.

Keck PE Jr et al: New developments in the pharmacologic treatment of schizoaffective disorder. J Clin Psychiatry 1996;57(Suppl 9):41.

Kendler KS et al: Examining the validity of *DSM-III-R* schizoaffective disorder and its putative subtypes in the Roscommon Family Study. Am J Psychiatry 1995; 152:755.

Marengo JT, Harrow M: Longitudinal courses of thought disorder in schizophrenia and schizoaffective disorder. Schizophr Bull 1997;23:273.

Delusional Disorder

Cameron NA: Paranoid conditions and paranoia. In: *American Handbook of Psychiatry.* Vol 3. Arieti S, Brady EB (editors). Basic Books, 1974.

Copeland JR et al: Schizophrenia and delusional disorder in older age: Community prevalence, incidence, comorbidity, and outcome. Schizophr Bull 1998;24:153.

Eastham JH, Jeste DV: Treatment of schizophrenia and delusional disorder in the elderly. Eur Arch Psychiatry Clin Neurosci 1997;247:209.

Evans JD et al: A clinical and neuropsychological comparison of delusional disorder and schizophrenia. J Neuropsychiatry Clin Neurosci 1996;8:281.

Fennig S et al: The consistency of *DSM-III-R* delusional disorder in a first-admission sample. Psychopathology 1996;29:315.

Fricchione GL et al: Psychotic disorder caused by a general medical condition, with delusions. Secondary "organic" delusional syndromes. Psychiatr Clin North Am 1995;18:363.

Herlitz A, Forsell Y: Episodic memory deficit in elderly adults with suspected delusional disorder. Acta Psychiatr Scand 1996;93:355.

Howard R: Drug treatment of schizophrenia and delusional disorder in late life. Int Psychogeriatr 1996;8:597.

Lo Y et al: Organic delusional disorder in psychiatric inpatients: Comparison with delusional disorder. Acta Psychiatr Scand 1997;95:161.

Manschreck TC: Delusional disorder: The recognition and management of paranoia. J Clin Psychiatry 1996; 57(Suppl 3):32.

Munro A, Mok H: An overview of treatment in paranoia/delusional disorder. Can J Psychiatry 1995; 40:616.

Salzman L: Paranoid state: Theory and therapy. Arch Gen Psychiatry 1960;2:679.

Yamada N et al: Age at onset of delusional disorder is dependent on the delusional theme. Acta Psychiatr Scand 1998;97:122.

Brief Psychotic Disorder

Jorgensen P et al: Acute and transient psychotic disorder: Comorbidity with personality disorder. Acta Psychiatr Scand 1996;94:460.

Pitta JC, Blay SL: Psychogenic (reactive) and hysterical psychoses: A cross-system reliability study. Acta Psychiatr Scand 1997;95:112.

Susser E et al: Epidemiology, diagnosis, and course of brief psychoses. Am J Psychiatry 1995;152:1743.

Shared Psychotic Disorder

Kraya NA, Patrick C: Folie à deux in forensic setting. Aust N Z J Psychiatry 1997;31:883.

Silveira JM, Seeman MV: Shared psychotic disorder: A critical review of the literature. Can J Psychiatry 1995; 40:389.

Mood Disorders

20

Victor I. Reus, MD

The British physician Aubrey Lewis once noted that the history of the diagnosis and treatment of melancholia could serve as a history of psychiatry itself. That observation seems particularly relevant today, since advances in the diagnosis and treatment of mood disorders have led to a dramatic increase in their perceived prevalence and to more rigorous criteria for placement in competing nosological categories.

The distinguishing characteristic of these disorders is a primary pervasive disturbance in mood. In this context, the term "mood" denotes an emotional state that may affect all aspects of the individual's life. The syndromes are characterized by pathologically elevated or depressed mood and should be regarded as existing on a continuum with normal mood. A diagnosis is appropriate when the mood disturbance is "primary" and central to the illness and not secondary to some other physical or psychological state. In the latter instance, the diagnosis would be incomplete without a reference to the precipitating cause. Although historically a precipitating stressful event was thought to be a critical element in the differential diagnosis of mood disorders, current opinion is that data of this sort lack diagnostic specificity and prognostic validity. Even so, when a mood disturbance following a stressful life event is a mild one that does not meet the criteria for any of the disorders discussed in this chapter, a diagnosis of **adjustment disorder with depressed mood** is warranted (see Chapter 23).

In this chapter, the class of mood disorders is divided into disorders in which there is a full major mood syndrome, disorders in which there is only a partial but persistent mood syndrome, and disorders that cannot be classified in either of these two ways (Table 20–1). Major mood disorders are further classified according to whether the patient has a history of a manic episode (Figures 20–1 and 20–2). A past or present history of a manic episode justifies a diagnosis of **bipolar I disorder,** which may be further subdivided on the basis of the presenting or most recent mood state (manic, depressed, or mixed). Some investigators have suggested that the spectrum of bipolar illness contains distinct subtypes characterized by the prominence of either mania or depres-

sion. If there is no history of a manic episode, and if the criteria of severity are met, a diagnosis of **major depressive disorder** is warranted. Major depression is further subclassified according to whether it is a first episode or a recurrence. Additional clinical features such as the presence of psychotic ideation or vegetative signs should also be specifically recorded. Although not authorized by the *Diagnostic and Statistical Manual of Mental Disorders,* 4th edition (*DSM-IV*), the term "unipolar" is sometimes used to describe this group of disorders.

Other specific mood disorders include cyclothymic disorder and dysthymic disorder. The term **cyclothymic disorder** encompasses individuals whose symptoms resemble those of bipolar disorder but are neither severe enough nor of sufficient duration to meet the criteria for diagnosis of bipolar or major depressive disorder. The term **dysthymic disorder** partially encompasses the group of individuals historically classified as suffering from depressive neurosis. These individuals have chronic depression that is not of sufficient severity or duration to meet the criteria for major depressive episode.

The terms **bipolar disorder NOS** ("not otherwise specified") and **depressive disorder NOS** are reserved for individuals who do not precisely meet any of the criteria just described. One example would be patients with a history of mood change occurring regularly during the premenstrual period.

BIPOLAR DISORDER

Symptoms & Signs

One essential criterion for a diagnosis of bipolar I disorder is a past or present history of a manic episode. Manic episodes are characterized by a predominantly elevated, expansive, or irritable mood that presents as a prominent or persistent part of the illness. Manic patients classically have abundant resources of energy and engage in multiple activities and ventures. At baseline and between episodes, the bipolar manic patient may indeed function at a high level of productivity, particularly in areas requiring creative talent. In the initial stages of an episode—and sometimes in attenuated episodes—the ventures

Table 20–1. *DSM-IV* criteria for mood disorders.

Manic episode

A. A distinct period of abnormally and persistently elevated, expansive, or irritable mood, lasting at least 1 week (or any duration if hospitalization is necessary).

B. During the period of mood disturbance, three (or more) of the following symptoms have persisted (four if the mood is only irritable) and have been present to a significant degree: (1) inflated self-esteem or grandiosity, (2) decreased need for sleep (eg, feels rested after only 3 hours of sleep), (3) more talkative than usual or pressure to keep talking, (4) flight of ideas or subjective experience that thoughts are racing, (5) distractibility (ie, attention too easily drawn to unimportant or irrelevant external stimuli), (6) increase in goal-directed activity (either socially, at work or school, or sexually) or psychomotor agitation, (7) excessive involvement in pleasurable activities that have a high potential for painful consequences (eg, engaging in unrestrained buying sprees, sexual indiscretions, or foolish business investments).

C. The symptoms do not meet criteria for a mixed episode.

D. The mood disturbance is sufficiently severe to cause marked impairment in occupational functioning or in usual social activities or relationships with others or to necessitate hospitalization to prevent harm to self or others or there are psychotic features.

E. The symptoms are not due to the direct physiological effects of a substance (eg, a drug of abuse, a medication, or other treatment) or a general medical condition (eg, hyperthyroidism).

Note: Manic-like episodes that are clearly caused by somatic antidepressant treatment (eg, medication, electroconvulsive therapy, light therapy) should not count toward a diagnosis of bipolar disorder.

Bipolar I disorder, single manic episode

A. Presence of only one manic episode and no past major depressive episodes.

Note: Recurrence is defined as either a change in polarity from depression or an interval of at least 2 months without manic symptoms.

B. The manic episode is not better accounted for by schizoaffective disorder and is not superimposed on schizophrenia, schizophreniform disorder, delusional disorder, or psychotic disorder not otherwise specified.

Specify if:
  Mixed: if symptoms meet criteria for a mixed episode

Specify (for current or most recent episode):
  Severity/Psychotic/Remission Specifiers
  With Catatonic Features
  With Postpartum Onset

Bipolar I disorder, most recent episode hypomanic

A. Currently (or most recently) in a hypomanic episode.

B. There has previously been at least one manic episode or mixed episode.

C. The mood symptoms cause clinically significant distress or impairment in social, occupational, or other important areas of functioning.

D. The mood episodes in Criteria A and B are not better accounted for by schizoaffective disorder and are not superimposed on schizophrenia, schizophreniform disorder, delusional disorder, or psychotic disorder not otherwise specified.

Specify:
  Longitudinal Course Specifiers (With and Without Interepisode Recovery)
  With Seasonal Pattern (applies only to the pattern of major depressive episodes)
  With Rapid Cycling

Bipolar I disorder, most recent episode manic

A. Currently (or most recently) in a manic episode.

B. There has previously been at least one major depressive episode, manic episode, or mixed episode.

C. The mood episodes in Criteria A and B are not better accounted for by schizoaffective disorder and are not superimposed on schizophrenia, schizophreniform disorder, delusional disorder, or psychotic disorder not otherwise specified.

Specify (for current or most recent episode):
  Severity/Psychotic/Remission Specifiers
  With Catatonic Features
  With Postpartum Onset

Specify:
  Longitudinal Course Specifiers (With and Without Interepisode Recovery)
  With Seasonal Pattern (applies only to the pattern of major depressive episodes)
  With Rapid Cycling

Bipolar I disorder, most recent episode mixed

A. Currently (or most recently) in a mixed episode.

B. There has previously been at least one major depressive episode, manic episode, or mixed episode.

C. The mood episodes in Criteria A and B are not better accounted for by schizoaffective disorder and are not superimposed on schizophrenia, schizophreniform disorder, delusional disorder, or psychotic disorder not otherwise specified.

Specify (for current or most recent episode):
Severity/Psychotic/Remission Specifiers
With Catatonic Features
With Postpartum Onset

Specify:
Longitudinal Course Specifiers (With and Without Interepisode Recovery)
With Seasonal Pattern (applies only to the pattern of major depressive episodes)
With Rapid Cycling

Bipolar I disorder, most recent episode depressed

A. Currently (or most recently) in a major depressive episode.

B. There has previously been at least one manic episode or mixed episode.

C. The mood episodes in Criteria A and B are not better accounted for by schizoaffective disorder and are not superimposed on schizophrenia, schizophreniform disorder, delusional disorder, or psychotic disorder not otherwise specified.

Specify (for current or most recent episode):
Severity/Psychotic/Remission Specifiers
Chronic
With Catatonic Features
With Melancholic Features
With Atypical Features
With Postpartum Onset

Specify:
Longitudinal Course Specifiers (With and Without Interepisode Recovery)
With Seasonal Pattern (applies only to the pattern of major depressive episodes)
With Rapid Cycling

Bipolar I disorder, most recent episode unspecified

A. Criteria, except for duration, are currently (or most recently) met for a manic, a hypomanic, a mixed, or a major depressive episode.

B. There has previously been at least one manic episode or mixed episode.

C. The mood symptoms cause clinically significant distress or impairment in social, occupational, or other important areas of functioning.

D. The mood symptoms in Criteria A and B are not better accounted for by schizoaffective disorder and are not superimposed on schizophrenia, schizophreniform disorder, delusional disorder, or psychotic disorder not otherwise specified.

E. The mood symptoms in Criteria A and B are not due to the direct physiological effects of a substance (eg, a drug of abuse, a medication, or other treatment) or a general medical condition (eg, hyperthyroidism).

Specify:
Longitudinal Course Specifiers (With and Without Interepisode Recovery)
With Seasonal Pattern (applies only to the pattern of major depressive episodes)
With Rapid Cycling

Bipolar II disorder

A. Presence (or history) of one or more major depressive episodes.

B. Presence (or history) of at least one hypomanic episode.

C. There has never been a manic episode or a mixed episode.

D. The mood symptoms in Criteria A and B are not better accounted for by schizoaffective disorder and are not superimposed on schizophrenia, schizophreniform disorder, delusional disorder, or psychotic disorder not otherwise specified.

E. The symptoms cause clinically significant distress or impairment in social, occupational, or other important areas of functioning.

Specify (for current or most recent episode):
Hypomanic: if currently (or most recently) in a hypomanic episode
Depressed: if currently (or most recently) in a major depressive episode

Specify (for current or most recent major depressive episode only if it is the most recent type of mood episode):
Severity/Psychotic/Remission Specifiers
Chronic
With Catatonic Features
With Melancholic Features
With Atypical Features
With Postpartum Onset

Specify:
Longitudinal Course Specifiers (With and Without Interepisode Recovery)

(continued)

Table 20–1. *(continued)*

With Seasonal Pattern (applies only to the pattern of major depressive episodes)
With Rapid Cycling

Hypomanic episode

A. A distinct period of persistently elevated, expansive, or irritable mood, lasting throughout at least 4 days, that is clearly different from the usual nondepressed mood.

B. During the period of mood disturbance, three (or more) of the following symptoms have persisted (four if the mood is only irritable) and have been present to a significant degree: (1) inflated self-esteem or grandiosity, (2) decreased need for sleep (eg, feels rested after only 3 hours of sleep), (3) more talkative than usual or pressure to keep talking, (4) flight of ideas or subjective experience that thoughts are racing, (5) distractibility (ie, attention too easily drawn to unimportant or irrelevant external stimuli), (6) increase in goal-directed activity (either socially, at work or school, or sexually) or psycho-motor agitation, (7) excessive involvement in pleasurable activities that have a high potential for painful consequences (eg, the person engages in unrestrained buying sprees, sexual indiscretions, or foolish business investments).

C. The episode is associated with an unequivocal change in functioning that is uncharacteristic of the person when not symptomatic.

D. The disturbance in mood and the change in functioning are observable by others.

E. The episode is not severe enough to cause marked impairment in social or occupational functioning, or to necessitate hospitalization, and there are no psychotic features.

F. The symptoms are not due to the direct physiological effects of a substance (eg, a drug of abuse, a medication, or other treatment) or a general medical condition (eg, hyperthyroidism).

Note: Hypomanic-like episodes that are clearly caused by somatic antidepressant treatment (eg, medication, electroconvulsive therapy, light therapy) should not count toward a diagnosis of bipolar II disorder.

Cyclothymic disorder

A. For at least 2 years, the presence of numerous periods with hypomanic symptoms and numerous periods with depressive symptoms that do not meet criteria for a major depressive episode. **Note:** In children and adolescents, the duration must be at least 1 year.

B. During the above 2-year period (1 year in children and adolescents), the person has not been without the symptoms in Criterion A for more than 2 months at a time.

C. No major depressive episode, manic episode, or mixed episode has been present during the first 2 years of the disturbance.

D. The symptoms in Criteria A are not better accounted for by schizoaffective disorder and are not superimposed on schizophrenia, schizophreniform disorder, delusional disorder, or psychotic disorder not otherwise specified.

E. The symptoms are not due to the direct physiological effects of a substance (eg, a drug of abuse, a medication) or a general medical condition (eg, hyperthyroidism).

F. The symptoms cause clinically significant distress or impairment in social, occupational, or other important areas of functioning.

Note: After the usual 2 years (1 year in children and adolescents) of cyclothymic disorder, there may be superimposed manic or mixed episodes (in which case both bipolar I disorder and cyclothymic disorder may be diagnosed) or manic depressive episodes (in which case both bipolar II disorder and cyclothymic disorder may be diagnosed).

Major depressive episode

A. Five (or more) of the following symptoms have been present during the same 2-week period and represent a change from previous functioning; at least one of the symptoms is either (1) depressed mood or (2) loss of interest or pleasure. **Note:** Do not include symptoms that are clearly due to a general medical condition, or mood-incongruent delusions or hallucinations. (1) depressed mood most of the day, nearly every day, as indicated by either subjective report (eg, feels sad or empty) or observation made by others (eg, appears tearful). **Note:** In children and adolescents, can be irritable mood, (2) markedly diminished interest or pleasure in all, or almost all, activities most of the day, nearly every day (as indicated by either subjective account or observation made by others), (3) significant weight loss when not dieting or weight gain (eg, a change of more than 5% of body weight in a month), or decrease or increase in appetite nearly every day. **Note:** In children, consider failure to make expected weight gains, (4) insomnia or hypersomnia nearly every day, (5) psychomotor agitation or retardation nearly every day (observable by others, not merely subjective feelings of restlessness or being slowed down), (6) fatigue or loss of energy nearly every day, (7) feelings of worthlessness or excessive or inappropriate guilt (which may be delusional) nearly every day (not merely self-reproach or guilt about being sick), (8) diminished ability to think or concentrate, or indecisiveness, nearly every day (either by subjective account or as observed by others), (9) recurrent thoughts of death (not just fear of dying), recurrent suicidal ideation without a specific plan, or a suicide attempt or a specific plan for committing suicide.

B. The symptoms do not meet criteria for a mixed episode.

C. The symptoms cause clinically significant distress or impairment in social, occupational, or other important areas of functioning.

D. The symptoms are not due to the direct physiological effects of a substance (eg, a drug of abuse, a medication) or a general medical condition (eg, hypothyroidism).

E. The symptoms are not better accounted for by bereavement, ie, after the loss of a loved one, the symptoms persist for longer than 2 months or are characterized by marked functional impairment, morbid preoccupation with worthlessness, suicidal ideation, psychotic symptoms, or psychomotor retardation.

Major depressive disorder, single episode

A. Presence of a single major depressive episode.

B. The major depressive episode is not better accounted for by schizoaffective disorder and is not superimposed on schizophrenia, schizophreniform disorder, delusional disorder, or psychotic disorder not otherwise specified.

C. There has never been a manic episode, a mixed episode, or a hypomanic episode. **Note:** This exclusion does not apply if all of the manic-like, mixed-like, or hypomanic-like episodes are substance or treatment induced or are due to the direct physiological effects of a general medical condition.

Specify (for current or most recent episode):
Severity/Psychotic/Remission Specifiers
Chronic
With Catatonic Features
With Melancholic Features
With Atypical Features
With Postpartum Onset

Major depressive disorder, recurrent

A. Presence of two or more major depressive episodes.

Note: To be considered separate episodes, there must be an interval of at least 2 consecutive months in which criteria are not met for a major depressive episode.

B. The major depressive episodes are not better accounted for by schizoaffective disorder and are not superimposed on schizophrenia, schizophreniform disorder, delusional disorder, or psychotic disorder not otherwise specified.

C. There has never been a manic episode, a mixed episode, or a hypomanic episode. **Note:** This exclusion does not apply if all of the manic-like, mixed-like, or hypomanic-like episodes are substance or treatment induced or are due to the direct physiological effects of a general medical condition.

Specify (for current or most recent episode):
Severity/Psychotic/Remission Specifiers
Chronic
With Catatonic Features
With Melancholic Features
With Atypical Features
With Postpartum Onset

Specify:
Longitudinal Course Specifiers (With and Without Interepisode Recovery)
With Seasonal Pattern

Dysthymic disorder

A. Depressed mood for most of the day, for more days than not, as indicated either by subjective account or observation by others, for at least 2 years. **Note:** In children and adolescents, mood can be irritable and duration must be at least 1 year.

B. Presence, while depressed, of two (or more) of the following: (1) poor appetite or overeating, (2) insomnia or hypersomnia, (3) low energy or fatigue, (4) low self-esteem, (5) poor concentration or difficulty making decisions, (6) feelings of hopelessness.

C. During the 2-year period (1 year for children or adolescents) of the disturbance, the person has never been without the symptoms in Criteria A and B for more than 2 months at a time.

D. No major depressive episode has been present during the first 2 years of the disturbance (1 year for children and adolescents); ie, the disturbance is not better accounted for by chronic major depressive disorder, or major depressive disorder, in partial remission.

Note: There may have been a previous major depressive episode provided there was a full remission (no significant signs or symptoms for 2 months) before development of the dysthymic disorder. In addition, after the initial 2 years (1 year in children or adolescents) of dysthymic disorder, there may be superimposed episodes of major depressive disorder, in which case both diagnoses may be given when the criteria are met for a major depressive episode.

E. There has never been a manic episode, a mixed episode, or a hypomanic episode, and criteria have never been met for cyclothymic disorder.

F. The disturbance does not occur exclusively during the course of a chronic psychotic disorder, such as schizophrenia or delusional disorder.

G. The symptoms are not due to the direct physiological effects of a substance (eg, a drug of abuse, a medication) or a general medical condition (eg, hypothyroidism).

H. The symptoms cause clinically significant distress or impairment in social, occupational, or other important areas of functioning.

Specify if:
Early Onset: If onset is before age 21 years
Late Onset: If onset is age 21 years or older

Specify (for most recent 2 years of dysthymic disorder):
With Atypical Features

(continued)

Table 20–1. *(continued)*

Seasonal Pattern Specifier

Specify if:

With Seasonal Pattern (can be applied to the pattern of major depressive episodes in bipolar I disorder, bipolar II disorder, or major depressive disorder, recurrent)

A. There has been a regular temporal relationship between the onset of major depressive episodes in bipolar I or bipolar II disorder or major depressive disorder, recurrent, and a particular time of the year (eg, regular appearance of the major depressive episode in the fall or winter).

Note: Do not include cases in which there is an obvious effect of seasonal-related psychosocial stressors (eg, regularly being unemployed every winter).

B. Full remissions (or a change from depression to mania or hypomania) also occur at a characteristic time of the year (eg, depression disappears in the spring).

C. In the last 2 years, two major depressive episodes have occurred that demonstrate the temporal seasonal relationships defined in Criteria A and B, and no nonseasonal major depressive episodes have occurred during that same period.

D. Seasonal major depressive episodes (as described above) substantially outnumber the nonseasonal major depressive episodes that may have occurred over the individual's lifetime.

Mood disorder due to . . . [*indicate the general medical condition*]

A. A prominent and persistent disturbance in mood predominates in the clinical picture and is characterized in either (or both) of the following: (1) depressed mood or markedly diminished interest or pleasure in all, or almost all, activities or (2) elevated, expansive, or irritable mood.

B. There is evidence from the history, physical examination, or laboratory findings that the disturbance is the direct physiological consequence of a general medical condition.

C. The disturbance is not better accounted for by another mental disorder (eg, adjustment disorder with depressed mood in response to the stress of having a general medical condition).

D. The disturbance does not occur exclusively during the course of a delirium.

E. The symptoms cause clinically significant distress or impairment in social, occupational, or other important areas of functioning.

Specify type:

With Depressive Features: if the predominant mood is depressed but the full criteria are not met for a major depressive episode

With Major Depressive-Like Episode: if the full criteria are met (except Criterion D) for a major depressive episode

With Manic Features: if the predominant mood is elevated, euphoric, or irritable

With Mixed Features: if the symptoms of both mania and depression are present but neither predominates

Substance-induced mood disorder

A. A prominent and persistent disturbance in mood predominates in the clinical picture and is characterized by either (or both) of the following: (1) depressed mood or markedly diminished interest or pleasure in all, or almost all, activities or (2) elevated, expansive, or irritable mood.

B. There is evidence from the history, physical examination, or laboratory findings of either (1) or (2): (1) the symptoms in Criterion A developed during, or within a month of, substance intoxication or withdrawal or (2) medication use is etiologically related to the disturbance.

C. The disturbance is not better accounted for by a mood disorder that is not substance induced. Evidence that the symptoms are better accounted for by a mood disorder that is not substance induced might include the following: the symptoms precede the onset of the substance use (or medication use); the symptoms persist for a substantial period of time (eg, about a month) after the cessation of acute withdrawal or severe intoxication or are substantially in excess of what would be expected given the type or amount of the substance used or the duration of use; or there is other evidence that suggests the existence of an independent non–substance-induced mood disorder (eg, a history of recurrent major depressive episodes).

D. The disturbance does not occur exclusively during the course of a delirium.

E. The symptoms cause clinically significant distress or impairment in social, occupational, or other important areas of functioning.

Note: This diagnosis should be made instead of a diagnosis of substance intoxication or substance withdrawal only when the mood symptoms are in excess of those usually associated with the intoxication or withdrawal syndrome and when the symptoms are sufficiently severe to warrant independent clinical attention.

Specific type:

With Depressive Features: if the predominant mood is depressed

With Manic Features: if the predominant mood is elevated, euphoric, or irritable

With Mixed Features: if symptoms of both mania and depression are present and neither predominates

Specify if:

With Onset During Intoxication: if the criteria are met for intoxication with the substance and the symptoms develop during the intoxication syndrome

With Onset During Withdrawal: if criteria are met for withdrawal from the substance and the symptoms develop during, or shortly after, a withdrawal syndrome

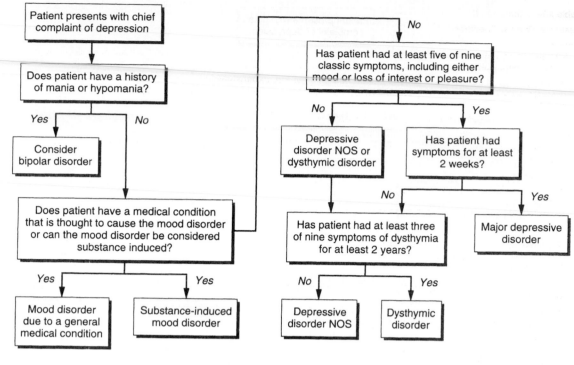

Figure 20–1. Differential diagnosis of depressive disorders.

may appear genuinely creative and perhaps only mildly eccentric. In time, however, as the investment in these activities becomes excessive, the individual loses the capacity to behave with reasonable caution and judgment and to conform to social expectations and norms. When the mood elevation is of a milder nature, either in severity or in duration, and is unassociated with a marked impairment in function, an assessment of hypomania rather than mania is made, resulting in a bipolar II disorder rather than a bipolar I diagnosis. It is not known whether these disorders are distinct in their etiology or exist on a continuum. In many manic episodes, particularly in the initial stages, the predominant mood is euphoria, although dysphoric mania is not as rare a condition as previously thought. The mood is often accompanied by a sense of absolute conviction or certitude, usually involving a self-perceived talent or perception but occasionally centering around more metaphysical and cosmic matters. A newly discovered or dramatically enhanced interest in religious or sexual experiences is a common feature. The euphoria experienced by the manic patient has an infectious quality and may mislead some people—even close associates—into accepting types of behavior that otherwise might not be tolerated. Manic patients can be quite engaging, and their well-known proclivity for buying sprees and improvident business ventures is often accompanied, at least for a time, by a remarkable ability to

obtain loans or gifts of money and encouragement from people whose judgment is usually better.

One of the primary early symptoms of a manic episode is a decreased need for sleep, so that in many cases the individual may not sleep for 3 or 4 days at a time. A "hunger" for social interchange may be manifested by frequent and inappropriate phone calls to distant acquaintances, particularly during late-night periods when social stimulation is minimal. Hypergraphia (excessive writing) and a fascination with music and playing musical instruments are frequently noted. Manic patients may also have a tendency to wear bright colors and unusual combinations of eccentric attire or may exhibit an attitude of carelessness about clothes or makeup. Public disrobing is also common.

Manic speech is characteristically rapid and discursive. Manic patients are difficult to interrupt and have difficulty not interrupting others who are speaking. The speech itself may involve rhyming, punning, and bizarre associations, but there are no pathognomonic elements. Manic patients are readily distractible and respond to both internal and external stimuli in a self-referential manner. Manic episodes that are more severe or that are observed later in the natural history of the disorder may be characterized by paranoia and irritability rather than euphoria and grandiosity. Anxiety and feelings of suspicion can cause the verbal output of such individuals to be markedly decreased, leading

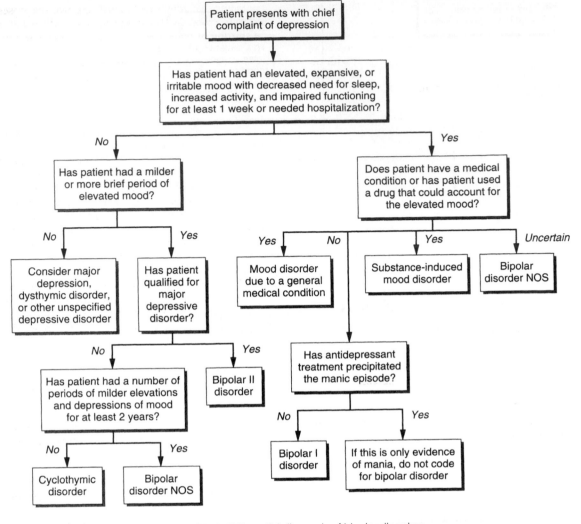

Figure 20–2. Differential diagnosis of bipolar disorders.

to erroneous diagnostic conclusions. Significant social aggression is rare, although acute mania and hypomania are common diagnoses in individuals with a history of psychiatric treatment who commit violent crimes. In some cases, severe depression may occur concomitantly with the manic state ("mixed state") or in abrupt alternation with the manic state. Suicidal risk is significantly elevated over the base rate for bipolar disorders in such individuals. True delusions and auditory hallucinations may be present, giving rise to difficult problems of differential diagnosis. The content of the delusions or hallucinations is often consistent with the predominant mood (mood-congruent).

In severe cases, mania can present as a state of catatonia. In such cases, the individual appears "willfully" unresponsive, often assuming a fixed posture and appearing mute except for occasional shouts or guttural sounds. Less severe states may be character-

ized by primitive delusions, fecal smearing, and extremes of tearfulness and emotional lability.

Natural History

A. Manic Disorder: Now that pharmacological treatment has become widespread, the complete natural history of a manic episode is seldom observed. Speed of onset, severity, and duration of the manic episode vary greatly in different individuals, depending, apparently, in part on genetic and other factors not clearly understood. Descriptions of past manic episodes are the best source of information about future episodes. Predictions about the future course of a patient experiencing a first manic episode are necessarily vague. In many individuals, the onset of the manic episode will be abrupt, occurring over a period of days or in some cases hours, and classically occurring in the early morning hours, first noted either as early morning awakening or inability to fall asleep. Other individuals experience a more protracted onset over a period of weeks. Increases in psychomotor activity, increased energy, and elevated mood are the most common early signs, with manic speech and thought disorder occurring later if at all. Not all individuals pass through the classical sequence of events or progress to the same level of severity. There have been reports of manic individuals who have no complaints of sleep disturbance or obvious euphoria but who appear not to differ either in the natural course of the illness or in response to treatment.

In some cases manic episodes appear to be self-limiting within days, weeks, or months. The variables that account for the wide reported ranges make assessments based on anything other than the individual's own past history unreliable. Chronic mania has been described and may remain stable at different levels of severity. Although lithium carbonate and the anticonvulsant agents carbamazepine, valproate, lamotrigine, gabapentin, and topiramate represent a dramatic advance in the treatment of bipolar disorders, 15–20% of manic patients respond inadequately to the medication and continue to present either episodically or chronically with classical signs of the disorder. Even with appropriate treatment, patients who present with rapidly alternating episodes of mania and depression or mixed states are more likely to remain ill for an extended period of time than are patients who are purely manic. Bipolar patients experiencing their first episode of depression have an approximately 20% chance of remaining depressed for at least 1 year, a rate comparable to that of individuals with pure depression. In subsequent episodes, the cumulative risk for development of chronic refractory depression rises to 30%.

B. Bipolar Disorder: Although bipolar illness has traditionally been associated with a relatively late age at onset, current evidence indicates a peak age of onset of between 20 and 25 years. Some surveys have indicated that premorbid symptomatology may start even earlier in adolescence and, more rarely, in early childhood. Onset after age 60 is rare and may reflect causation by an undiagnosed medical condition. Bipolar illness with onset during childhood or adolescence is commonly misdiagnosed, a fact that may reflect historical diagnostic bias or diagnostic confusion arising from normal physical and psychological developmental changes during this period. Differentiation of childhood bipolar disorder from attention-deficit disorder is particularly difficult.

Differential Diagnosis

Manic symptoms can occur in association with known organic disorders, but in such cases should be diagnosed as a mood disorder due to a general medical condition (ie, "secondary mania") rather than as bipolar disorder. There appear to be no clinical char-acteristics that might distinguish the two diagnoses, and it is probable that future research will result in the shifting of many manic diagnoses from a primary to a secondary category. The list of known causal agents is long and includes drugs (eg, corticosteroids, levodopa, stimulants), metabolic disturbances (such as those associated with hemodialysis), infections, neoplastic diseases, and epilepsy (particularly partial complex seizures).

In manic patients presenting with prominent delusions and hallucinations, the differential diagnosis is likely to include schizophrenia, paranoid type. Both syndromes can present with identical clinical symptoms, which means that the diagnosis can be based only on the clinical course or on secondary features such as the presence of a family history of mood disorder, the level of premorbid adjustment, a history of manic symptoms, or a prior response to treatment. The diagnosis of schizoaffective disorder is available for cases in which the clinician is unable to choose between manic episode and schizophrenia. Unfortunately, there is at present no agreement on how this category should be defined or on its etiological or prognostic relationship to schizophrenia or mood disorder (see Chapter 19).

Prognosis

Emil Kraepelin, the German psychiatrist who coined the phrase "manic depression," wrote that bipolar illness, in contrast to schizophrenia, usually has a good prognosis. In Kraepelin's original sample of 459 patients, 45% had only one attack, and very few had more than four episodes. The average duration of a pharmacologically untreated manic episode was 7 months, but a wide range was reported. Although most later studies have validated Kraepelin's findings, particularly when the disorder is compared to schizophrenia, it appears that the prognosis of bipolar illness is less favorable than originally reported. Up to 20% of patients respond inadequately to medication and must endure chronic or recurrent symptoms.

The phases of bipolar illness may differ in their responsiveness to treatment and in their effect on ultimate outcome. Some individuals, for example, experience complete remission of acute manic symptoms and benefit from prophylactic medication but continue to have unmodified or attenuated depressive episodes, with suicide being a significant risk. The best predictor of cycle frequency and treatment response is the personal and family psychiatric history. Once the episode has resolved, the duration of the symptom-free interval varies greatly in different individuals. In contrast to Kraepelin's original impression, it is now clear that most patients who satisfy the criteria for bipolar disorder will experience another episode within 2–4 years. The complete cycle—ie, from manic to depressed to manic state—may be as short as 48 hours or so long that the concept of cyclicity becomes meaningless. Patients with bipolar disorder who experience rapid cycles—three or more a year—respond less well to lithium than to anticonvulsants as compared to individuals with longer symptom-free intervals. The few available prospective studies of the course of bipolar illness indicate that for any given individual, the cycles become shorter as time goes on.

The prognosis thus depends on the frequency and duration of individual episodes and the response to medication. Because lithium is effective in moderating the severity of symptoms in most cases, there is always a strong possibility that recurrences represent failure of compliance with the drug regimen. Perhaps because of the quality of the mood experience, manic patients often utilize the psychological defense mechanism of denial, admitting that problems may exist but attributing them to overwork or to job or family stress. Patients with mild bipolar episodes may be able to function adequately during a period in which they demonstrate most of the symptoms of a manic episode. In such cases, factors such as psychological coping mechanisms, social supports, and socioeconomic status influence the outcome as much as response to medication.

Illustrative Case

A 27-year-old male graduate student in molecular biology was brought to the emergency room by his fiancée, who explained that over the preceding 2 weeks he had become increasingly irritable and suspicious and had undergone a "personality change." She noted that he had not slept at all for the past 3 nights and had become preoccupied by the belief that his research thesis would be regarded as the "new bible of the computer age." Fearing that his ideas might be stolen by government agents, he had constructed an elaborate mathematical code that would allow only him and his appointed "prophets" to understand the documented work. The patient was dressed in a mismatched three-piece suit he claimed was a disguise that would enable him to elude agents assigned to follow him. Although during the initial stages of the interview the patient refused to speak, he suddenly observed that since the interviewing physician was on the faculty of the university, he might be better able to understand the meaning of his research than the resident physician who screened him at the admission desk. He also remarked that the interviewing physician's name contained a syllable similar in sound and spelling to the Latin word for "trust" and suggested that their meeting must have been preordained. Throughout the remainder of the interview, the patient paced around the room, interrupting his responses to questions with associations to the interviewer's style of dress, a paperweight on the desk, and a book whose title he misread.

The history obtained from the fiancée revealed that the patient had never had any symptoms similar to these, but that for about 3 months during the past 12-month period he had felt too tired to go to class and had spent much of the day sleeping. She recalled that the patient had an aunt who was hospitalized twice following the birth of her two children and that an older brother had been married four times and was "quite moody."

After some urging by his fiancée, the patient agreed to enter the hospital and began taking medication, which he called "thought pills." Neuroleptic medication resulted in marked amelioration of symptoms within 5 days. After 2 weeks of treatment with lithium, his suspiciousness and grandiose beliefs diminished significantly. With partial recovery, the patient was mildly depressed and embarrassed about his recent behavior, but still seemed excessively concerned about the possible need to protect his research from industrial spies in the future.

Epidemiology

Multinational studies indicate that the lifetime risk of bipolar disorder is approximately 1–2%. Depending on how the phenotype is defined, the concordance rate for bipolar illness ranges from 65% to 85% in monozygotic twins and is 20% in dizygotic twins. Bipolar illness occurs in relatives of patients with bipolar disorder much more frequently than in relatives of patients with major depression; the rates for depression alone are approximately the same. Adoption studies show that rates of illness clearly depend on the risk associated with the biological rather than the adoptive parents. In general, bipolar probands have more relatives with bipolar disorder and mood disorder than unipolar probands.

Etiology & Pathogenesis

A. Biochemical Factors: Although many differences in biochemical indices have been described when patients with bipolar disorder are compared to normal control subjects, there is no agreement about which alterations have etiological significance and which are secondary effects or epiphenomena. Since the "switch" from depression into mania (and vice versa) can occur in minutes, attempts have been made to identify biochemical changes that might be associated with the switch. Specific changes in brain monoamine neurotransmitter metabolism and receptor function appear to be the most likely mechanisms. Although now regarded as too simplistic, the catecholamine hypothesis suggested that catecholamine (most specifically norepinephrine) deficiency was associated with motor retardation and depression, whereas catecholamine excess could result in excitement and euphoria. Since all of the major neurotransmitter systems are functionally linked, it is not surprising that changes in other major neurotransmitter systems have also been documented. Changes in dopaminergic function, GABAergic regulation, and adrenergic-cholinergic system imbalance have been reported during manic episodes. Trait-dependent alterations in platelet serotonin uptake, in cerebrospinal fluid levels of serotonin metabolites, and in endocrine response to serotonergic agonists have also been found in patients with bipolar illness. Neuroimaging studies have documented a number of abnormalities, including changes in amygdala, thalamus, hippocampus, and prefrontal cortex volume and increased white matter lesions in subcortical areas. Overall, however, there have been few biological studies of mania, since the nature of the syndrome makes compliance with research procedures difficult. Studies of the mechanism of action of lithium have pointed to the important regulatory functions of second messenger systems, particularly the phosphatidylinositol cycle, as well as modulation of glutamate activity.

Electrolyte disturbances have also been found in patients with bipolar disorders and may represent a defect of cellular membrane function. In general, sodium retention and potassium and water excretion increase during depression and decrease during manic intervals. Abnormal calcium homeostasis has also been reported. A variety of neuroendocrine changes have also been reported for patients with bipolar disorder who are in the depressed phase. About half of both bipolar and unipolar depressed patients show evidence of any or all of the following during a severe depressive episode: increased adrenal glucocorticoid function, decreased thyroid-stimulating hormone response to thyrotropin-releasing hormone, decreased basal prolactin levels, and decreased growth hormone response to insulin challenge.

Because of pharmacological parallels to temporal lobe epilepsy and beneficial responses to several anticonvulsant agents, some investigators have hypothesized that recurrent bipolar mood episodes derive from an endogenous "kindling" of electrical discharges in limbic areas of the brain. Others have emphasized patterns in alteration of circadian rhythmicity.

Thus far, the results of studies in molecular genetics have been inconclusive. Regions on chromosome 18p and 18q and on chromosomes 4 and 21 have received the strongest support, although no specific gene has thus far been isolated for what is most certainly a complex multigenic disorder.

B. Psychosocial Factors: There is no reliable evidence that psychosocial factors cause bipolar disorder, although life stresses may precipitate manic or depressed bipolar states and may in fact be necessary for the expression of symptomatology in milder bipolar syndromes. The lifetime prevalence of comorbid substance abuse exceeds 60%. Recent research in biological circadian rhythmicity suggests that subtle changes in the light-dark cycle (eg, seasonal variations) are an additional predictor of risk.

Treatment

A. Biomedical Therapies: Treatment of bipolar disorder depends on the specific form of behavioral disorder at presentation. Lithium carbonate or divalproex represents the preferred initial intervention for the acute manic state, even though 10–14 days may be required before full effect is achieved. A favorable response is reported in 65–75% of bipolar manic patients. Complications are relatively infrequent, but a transient "rebound" depression following resolution of a manic state is not uncommon. Overall response to lithium appears to improve as duration of treatment continues, resulting in a dramatic decrease in morbidity and mortality over the lifetime of the individual. (For a detailed discussion of the pharmacology of lithium, see Chapter 30.) The degree of psychomotor activation and the fragile structure of the treatment alliance in acute mania require that supplemental treatment with faster-acting neuroleptics or benzodiazepines be instituted in most cases. Chronic treatment with neuroleptics is to be avoided, as the risk of tardive dyskinesia is increased in mood disorders. For patients who do not respond satisfactorily to lithium or divalproex, the anticonvulsant drugs carbamazepine, lamotrigine, or gabapentin may be tried; studies show that these drugs have acute antimanic and possibly antidepressant effects in bipolar illness. Clonazepam and the calcium channel antagonist verapamil have emerged as other empirical alternatives, but these should not be considered agents of first choice. Treatment resistance may require combination therapy. Treatment of the depressive phase of bipolar illness is particularly problematic, as antidepressants may precipitate mania or result in more rapid cycling.

B. Psychosocial Therapies: Some form of psychosocial intervention is almost always indicated in the treatment of bipolar disorder, although its nature and extent will necessarily depend on the degree of disruption of family and financial situations, the baseline character of the individual, and the response to somatic treatment. The nature of the biological contribution to the disorder (see also Chapter 6) makes it almost impossible to ascertain in advance what the individual's ongoing psychosocial needs might be after acute symptoms subside. Some patients with bipolar disorder have infrequent recurrences, experience long symptom-free intervals, and are able to lead productive lives. Others may have a particularly malignant form of the syndrome or may exhibit pathological degrees of denial and lead turbulent lives calling for active psychosocial involvement by the therapist. Manual-based psychoeducational treatments specific to bipolar disorder and employing cognitive-behavioral strategies have recently been developed. Patients with bipolar disorder may also benefit from interventions that help to establish life-style regularity.

CYCLOTHYMIC DISORDER

Symptoms & Signs

Cyclothymic disorder is characterized by manic and depressive states not of sufficient severity or duration to meet the criteria for either bipolar disorder or major depression (Table 20–1). Symptoms must persist for at least 2 years (1 year in children and adolescents) and have no psychotic component. Individuals meeting the criteria for this diagnosis may experience an exacerbation of depression or mania sufficient to warrant a change in diagnosis. Most clinicians presently consider cyclothymic disorder to be an attenuated form of bipolar disorder rather than a personality disorder, as originally thought. Cyclothymic disorder is common in outpatient psychiatric practice and may be the diagnosis for as much as 3–4% of an unselected clinic population.

Cyclothymic patients suffer from short cycles of depression and hypomania that can at times be as severe as those observed in other disorders but that usually fail to meet the criteria for duration. It is often difficult to ascertain any regular pattern of mood switching, and patients will commonly describe mood changes that come and go spontaneously over the course of hours or days. Studies of behavioral characteristics of these patients show that they are extroverted sociable individuals who appear self-assured, energetic, and often impulsive. At times this cheerful exuberance turns into irritability and extreme sensitivity to rejection or loss. Cyclothymic patients are frequently described as "stimulus-seeking," a characteristic that leads them to become involved in daring hobbies and results in checkered work and school careers. Promiscuity and drug abuse are also noted, as is a history of repeated romantic disasters. Although many of these characteristics are likely to lead to a socially maladaptive life-style, cyclothymic individuals often achieve substantial success and status in society. This may in part reflect a cultural bias that values "outgoing" personality characteristics, but it is also an outcome of a periodic increase in energies and enthusiasms that leads to accomplishments beyond the reach of more placid individuals.

Natural History

Close examination of the cyclothymic patient's personal history will usually reveal an age at onset of symptoms of early to late adolescence. About a third of patients with this diagnosis will experience an intensification of symptoms during a 2-year follow-up, sufficient to meet the criteria for mania, hypomania, or major depression. The close relationship of cyclothymia to bipolar disorder is supported by the finding that treatment of the depressed phase with tricyclic antidepressants can result in pharmacologically induced hypomania in 40–50% of patients. There seems to be a higher risk for the natural development of formal depressive as opposed to manic episodes.

Differential Diagnosis

As mentioned previously, the main task in differential diagnosis is to determine the severity and duration of the altered mood state. A chaotic life history with poor interpersonal relationships often suggests a diagnosis of borderline personality. Many cyclothymic individuals experience difficulties in ego development and in achieving an integrated sense of self. These issues may come up more frequently in cyclothymic disorder than in formal bipolar disorder, since the milder and more evanescent quality of cyclothymia will make it more difficult for patient and family, friends, and therapist to recognize the constitutional contribution. The deleterious effects on personality development of a constantly changing and autonomous mood state that colors, in random fashion, the critical developmental experiences of childhood and adolescence should be obvious.

Prognosis

Since the syndrome is more broadly defined than either bipolar disorder or major depression, estimates of prognosis depend on assessments of the quality, quantity, and frequency of mood change and the effect of such changes both on the patient and on his or her social and professional world. The lifetime prediction of risk is unknown. Approximately 60% of these patients improve when treated with a mood stabilizer.

Illustrative Case

A 34-year-old divorced secretary sought psychotherapy because of her long history of unsatisfactory relationships with men. She was currently employed by an agency that provided temporary secretarial help and admitted that she had quit or been fired from several jobs because of her inability to keep regular working hours. She stated that she did not really like secretarial work and hoped to return to fashion modeling, an occupation she had pursued several years previously with modest success. She reported that she encountered difficulties even then from failing to show up for assignments and, on two occasions, from going to an appointment after having had several drinks. Further questioning revealed sporadic recreational use of marijuana, cocaine, and amphetamines. She attributed her difficulty in relationships with men to the fact that most of the men she had been attracted to were too career oriented and "homebody" types. She acknowledged that several individuals with whom she had been close described her as "moody." She described her life as alternating between times when she felt "buzzed, like on speed" and times when she felt "blank" and wanted to sleep most of the day. During these latter periods, she stated she felt somewhat better after drinking a bottle of wine but felt particularly guilty about the fact that her life was "not going anywhere." The family history revealed a turbulent family environment created principally by an abusive father with a history of binge drinking. Clinical and laboratory evaluation disclosed no organic cause of the mood disorder. The patient was started in psychotherapy and was given a trial of lithium carbonate. Over the succeeding year, she obtained permanent employment and reported an increased sense of emotional stability.

Epidemiology

This disorder seems to be more prevalent than previously acknowledged. It is more common in women, and there is apt to be a family history of mood disorder and "mood spectrum" problems such as alcohol abuse and antisocial personality.

Etiology & Pathogenesis

A. Biochemical Factors: Very little is known about biochemical changes in cyclothymic disorder. Most of the evidence has come from genetic studies linking the disorder to the major mood syndromes and from studies documenting a response to antimanic or antidepressant drug treatment.

B. Psychosocial Factors: Although the primary process responsible for sudden and recurrent mood change in cyclothymic individuals is thought to be biological and genetically transmitted, the psychosocial sequelae of such changes may emerge over time as the most significant aspect of the patient's discontent. This is particularly true for individuals with an early onset of the disorder. Persons who suffer recurrent unpredictable and intense mood upsets, seemingly unrelated to circumstance, develop major themes of loss and low self-esteem. A history of interpersonal conflicts and generalized anger is common, because the character of presentation is often subtle enough to escape the awareness of clinicians and the sympathy of friends.

Treatment

Biomedical treatment of cyclothymic disorder should be empirically derived and should be offered only if the individual's functioning is significantly adversely affected. A trial of a mood stabilizer may ameliorate manic symptoms and reduce the frequency of most cycles. Antidepressant medication may relieve symptoms of depression (see Chapter 30). Even with successful drug treatment, many patients with this disorder will benefit from psychotherapy that focuses on interpersonal relationships and self-image.

MAJOR DEPRESSION

Depression is one of the most prevalent medical disorders and has been recognized as a distinct pathological entity from early Egyptian times. In spite of this, the disorder is commonly undiagnosed and undertreated. Common usage of the word "depression" stems principally from the attempts of the nineteenth-century psychiatrist Emil Kraepelin to introduce a term that would have greater diagnostic specificity than "melancholia." Currently, the term melancholia denotes major depressive disorder with changes in endogenous or vegetative function, eg, disturbances of sleep, appetite, and libido.

Although clinicians, throughout most of this century, have attempted to subclassify the syndrome on the basis of symptoms and causes, many of the subclassifications proved to be invalid or unreliable. For example, the distinction between depressions that were "reactive" and those that were nonreactive or endogenous—ie, not precipitated by psychosocial stress—has not proved to be of predictive value. Such judgments in any case are highly subjective and depend on how detailed a history is obtained and how much weight is assigned by the patient or clinician to the changes that routinely occur in life. Distinctions on the basis of age have likewise proved suspect, with recent research indicating that depression during the involutional period is qualitatively no different from that experienced during any other stage.

Symptoms & Signs

A variety of studies have distinguished depressed individuals with prominent psychomotor retardation and anhedonia from those who evidence psychomotor activation, guilt, anxiety, and, occasionally, delusional thinking. The number and severity of somatic symptoms generally increase along with the severity of depression. Separating major depressions according to whether they are endogenous or autonomous has not been found to be useful, either in predicting drug response or in improving assessments of general risk. Individuals may in fact show endogenous features in one episode and not in another.

The character of depressive symptoms depends to a large extent on the severity of the disorder. In the most severe cases (10–15%), patients may present with an extensive paranoid or nihilistic delusional system and the experience of hallucinations, usually self-deprecatory in content and consonant with the underlying mood state. Mood-incongruent psychotic features are less frequently present. Because such individuals have more psychomotor disturbance and generally respond poorly to antidepressant medication, some investigators have considered psychotic depression as a separate entity and not simply a severe variant of major depression.

Depression occurs at any age and can present with primary symptoms that do not involve obvious mood change. Depression in children may be difficult to diagnose. Because of cognitive and linguistic developmental changes that occur in childhood, emotional states are experienced and projected differently. In older people, the most significant symptom may be a change in cognitive function. The term "pseudodementia" has been applied to a state clinically identical to irreversible senile dementia but that resolves with antidepressant treatment. Recent research questions the utility of this distinction, since an unremitting course and lack of pharmacological response of senile dementia are far from confirmed. In "masked depression," a condition in which there is no apparent mood change, the course of illness, prognosis, and response to treatment are the same as those associated with classical major depression. Depression is one of the most common missed diagnoses in the general medical clinic. It may be associated with a primary disorder such as an endocrinopathy, neoplasm, or viral infection, but it more commonly occurs independently in the context of a panoply of multisystemic somatic complaints. When the disease state is thought to be causal, a diagnosis of mood disorder due to a general medical condition should be given, rather than major depression.

Natural History

There is great variation in the clinical presentation and course of major depression. As the individual patient's history accumulates, recurrent episodes tend to develop a cyclic pattern of presentation, so that better judgments about the probable future course can be made.

Depression can occur at any age, but the average age at onset is between 30 and 40 years. In general, the earlier the age at onset, the more likely it is that there will be a recurrence. Symptoms develop either gradually over a period of many months or more dramatically over a shorter period, in many cases following a significant loss or episode of stress, although this is not necessary. If untreated, the depressive episode may resolve spontaneously over a period of weeks to months or may become chronic and remain essentially unchanged over a period of years. The mean duration for treated episodes is approximately 20 weeks. Although most patients with major depression respond well to somatic treatment, uncontrolled studies have revealed that recovery from major depressive disorder is not as good as once thought. Only about 50% of patients are completely recovered at 1-year follow-up. The prognosis worsens with increased severity of symptoms at onset, less acute onset, and occurrence of the acute episode superimposed on an underlying state of chronic depression. The risk of relapse after recovery from major depressive disorder is high for a short period—about 25% relapse within 12 weeks. For individuals with recurrent episodes, it is difficult to predict how soon another episode can be expected. The presence of a chronic underlying depression or a history of three or more depressive episodes significantly increases the risk of early relapse. In addition, there is evidence that the interval between episodes becomes

shorter as the individual ages. Chronic depression is associated with major decrements in functional abilities and results in significant societal burden. The total annual costs of depression have been estimated at 44 billion dollars. Depression has also been shown to be a major risk factor for the development of cardiovascular disease and death after a myocardial infarction.

At least 20–30% of patients with major depression and no history of mania will experience a manic or hypomanic episode later in life. Factors positively correlated with eventual bipolar outcome include pharmacological induction of mania, a history of postpartum depression, early onset (less than 25 years of age), and symptoms of hypersomnia and psychomotor retardation.

Differential Diagnosis

Depression occurs concomitantly with a number of different disease states, such as pancreatic and bronchogenic carcinoma, hypothyroidism, Cushing's syndrome, and cerebrovascular disease. When the mood state is felt to be etiologically related to the medical condition, the diagnosis of major depression should not be given. As noted, depression and dementia, particularly in the elderly, may be confused. However, patients with dementia may develop major depression as well. In some individuals, depression occurs in association with seasonal change, giving rise to the term "seasonal mood disorder." Such individuals have experienced improvement in mood through "phase advance" alteration of their sleep-wake cycle and through the administration of several hours daily of high-intensity light, usually during morning hours. A regulatory disturbance of pineal gland function and melatonin secretion has been hypothesized in these patients, and the syndrome itself has been conceptualized as an evolutionary remnant of the mammalian hibernation cycle. In *DSM-IV*, a seasonal pattern may be a specific diagnostic feature of either bipolar disorder or recurrent major depression.

Schizophrenia commonly presents with significant depressive symptoms, either during the acute phase or shortly following resolution of psychotic symptoms. In such cases the diagnosis of depressive disorder not otherwise specified is added to the primary diagnosis. The differential diagnosis between major depression with psychosis and schizophrenia with depressive signs is exceedingly difficult and can best be made by considering aspects of the patient's premorbid history and a family history of psychiatric disorder. Because a diagnosis of schizophrenia requires a duration of at least 6 months, the date of onset is important.

In dysthymic and cyclothymic disorders, aspects of the depressive syndrome may occur but are not of sufficient intensity or duration to meet the criteria for major depression. It should be remembered, however, that major depression can occur in these or other disorders as an independent, superimposed entity and should be recorded as such. The diagnosis of dysthymic disorder should not be given if an episode of major depression emerges in the first 2 years, however.

Patients with bipolar disorder, mixed type, may likewise exhibit features of severe depression but will also present manic symptoms.

Grief syndromes often present with behavioral and physiological changes identical to those observed in major depression. Major depression should not be diagnosed until it is determined that the reaction is either too severe or too prolonged to be explained as simple bereavement. Comorbidity with anxiety disorders and substance abuse is common.

Prognosis

In individual cases, estimates of the degree of recovery and the likelihood of staying well depend mostly on the patient's age at onset, the number of previous episodes, and the response to somatic and psychosocial treatment. Many individuals have only one depressive episode in a lifetime. The likelihood of recurrence is dramatically increased with the onset of a second episode and continues to rise slightly with each additional episode, eventually reaching a statistical plateau. In cases in which suicidal preoccupation is recurrently noted in successive episodes and in which profound delusional content is noted, the prognosis for recovery is generally poor.

Illustrative Case

The patient was a surgeon referred by an internist for evaluation of complaints of fatigue and hand tremor. During outpatient evaluation, the patient said that 4 months previously he began noticing a significant worsening of manual dexterity during surgery. He attributed his difficulties to a fine tremor that he demonstrated for the examiner. He felt guilty about several patients who had put their faith in him and had suffered for it. He was sure that people in the hospital were making disparaging comments about his condition, though he could offer no specific examples. He had become reluctant to schedule operations but at the same time said that his decreased income was mainly attributable to fewer referrals from colleagues and "the word getting out." Although this was the first occurrence of this kind, he felt that his whole career had been a sham and that his previous accomplishments were undeserved. He could see no medical or psychiatric solution to his difficulties and expressed an intention to retire, although he was only 47 years old and not financially able to do so.

Although the patient had full health and disability insurance coverage, he expressed great concern about the impending hardship to his family from medical expenses and his failure to earn a good income. This concern magnified even trivial expenditures; eg, he felt he could no longer buy a morning paper without jeopardizing his son's college education. He reported poor appetite and a weight loss of 15 lb in less than 2 months. He reluctantly acknowledged that he and his wife had not had sexual relations in 4 months because of his impotence. He was unable to read professional journals or popular reading matter. Direct questioning revealed early morning awakening, but he said this was not a problem. Despite a strong feeling that all of his troubles were related to the hand tremor, he agreed to enter the hospital for a trial of antidepressant medication. On the ward, he received a combination of drug treatment and individual and group therapy. After 10 days of drug treatment (imipramine, 200 mg orally daily), he began sleeping better and eating regularly. He continued to complain of depression but admitted to an increase in energy level, a decrease in tremulousness, and an ability to maintain an erection. A week later, he began to express an interest in returning to work and initiated plans for discharge.

Epidemiology

Although mood disorders are widely acknowledged to be common, their prevalence is difficult to determine because of differences in diagnostic procedures and criteria. Assessments of depressive symptoms—ie, intense, pervasive, and almost daily feelings of sadness or disappointment that affect normal functioning—show lifetime prevalence rates of 9–20%. (The relationship of such subjective assessments to the objective diagnosis of major depression is not known.) When more stringent criteria for major depression are used, prevalence of major depression is 3% for men and 4–9% for women. The lifetime risk is 8–12% for men and 20–26% for women. These figures also may be high, since they are largely dependent on subjective evaluations of individuals who have not sought treatment. There has been a progressive increase in rates of depression in successive birth cohorts throughout this century as well as a progressively earlier age of onset.

About 12–20% of persons experiencing an acute episode develop a chronic depressive syndrome, and up to 15% of patients who have depression for more than 1 month commit suicide.

Etiology & Pathogenesis

A. Biochemical Factors: Genetic studies and studies on the effect of specific antidepressant drugs have led to the conclusion that most cases of recurrent major depression have some biological basis. This does not mean, however, that psychological factors have no role in symptom formation or in precipitation of episodes of depression of lesser severity.

Family and genetic studies indicate that the risk rate among first-degree relatives of individuals suffering from major depression (unipolar) is approximately two to three times the risk in the general population. This, it should be noted, is approximately half the rate reported among first-degree relatives of individuals suffering from bipolar illness. The concordance rate is about 11% for dizygotic twins and approaches 40% for monozygotic twins. Biological parents of adopted probands have a much greater prevalence of mood disorder than adoptive parents.

The most prominent hypotheses generated to account for the actual mechanism of the mood disorder focus on regulatory disturbances in the monoamine neurotransmitter systems, particularly those involving norepinephrine and serotonin (5-hydroxytryptamine). It has also been hypothesized that depression is associated with an alteration in the acetylcholine-adrenergic balance and characterized by a relative cholinergic dominance. In addition, there are suggestions that dopamine is functionally decreased in some cases of major depression. Because the central nervous system monoamine neurotransmitter systems are widely distributed and involved in tonic regulation of autonomic functions, arousal, movement, sleep, aggression, and other vegetative functions, they are particularly well suited for their hypothesized role. Original reports suggesting that patients with endogenous depression experienced either decreased noradrenergic or serotonergic activity now appear to be overly simplistic. All the monoamine neurotransmitter systems are interrelated and subject to compensatory adaptation to perturbation over time. In addition, the discovery that many neuropeptides and hormones may serve as neurotransmitters and neuromodulators in certain contexts has underscored the complexity of the neural regulation of mood (see Chapter 6).

A significant number of patients have evidence of either increased or decreased noradrenergic function, as reflected by urinary levels of 3-methoxy-4-hydroxyphenylglycol (MHPG), the primary metabolite of central nervous system nonadrenergic function. Other major studies have pointed to a decrease in serotonergic activity in certain subgroups, as measured by levels of 5-hydroxyindoleacetic acid (5-HIAA), the principal metabolite of serotonergic activity in the brain, and 5-hydroxytryptamine (5-HT_{2A}) receptor binding. Depletion of tyrosine or tryptophan has also been shown to cause depression in vulnerable individuals. Most current hypotheses of neurotransmitter function in altered mood states have focused on changes in receptor sensitivity and second messenger systems. With a few exceptions long-term antidepressant treatment has been found to be associated with reduced postsynaptic β-adrenergic receptor sensitivity and enhanced postsynaptic serotonergic and cyclic adenosine monophosphate activity. In an effort to integrate these data, investigators have recently focused more on genomic regulation, specifically the role of transcription factors as causal agents.

Several specific abnormalities in neuroendocrine regulation may represent evidence of either primary disturbance in hypothalamic-pituitary control or secondary alteration in neurotransmitter function in limbic sites. The most consistent finding is that many patients with severe depressive disorder have an excess secretion of cortisol from the adrenal cortex stimulated by increased release of corticotropin-releasing factor from the hypothalamus. This is not simply a stress-related phenomenon, because the actual number of secretory episodes is increased, principally in the early morning hours when the system is normally quiescent. Many cortisol hypersecretors also have levels of norepinephrine, MHPG, and epinephrine in plasma and urine that are several times higher than normal. In addition to alterations in the pituitary-adrenal axis, elevation in serum triiodothyronine and thyroxine have been reported, as has a significant blunting of the response of thyroid-stimulating hormone to an infusion of thyrotropin-releasing hormone. Reports of changes in growth hormone, prolactin, luteinizing hormone, and testosterone regulation in major depressive disorder are contradictory.

From a neurophysiological perspective, the most replicable finding is that sleep in severe depression is characterized by decreased total sleep, decreased rapid eye movement (REM) latency (ie, sleep time from onset of sleep until the first epoch of REM sleep), increased REM density (ie, ratio of REM activity to REM time), and decreased stage 4 Δ sleep. Sleep electroencephalography does not differentiate subgroups of depressed patients but may help predict a positive response to antidepressant medication.

Immunological studies have identified a variety of subtle alterations in depression, including change in lymphocyte subsets, response to mitogen, natural killer cell activity, and cytokine regulation. Neuroimaging studies have found a variety of abnormalities in prefrontal cortex and cingulate gyrus and in periventricular white matter in geriatric patients suffering from depression.

B. Psychosocial Factors: Although psychosocial stress may play a role in the precipitation of a major depressive episode and shape the particular constellation of symptoms noted, current research indicates that environmental factors as such do not cause severe depressive episodes. However, depressed individuals are often unable to accept the concept of biological vulnerability and remain convinced that they themselves or changes in their environment are principally responsible for their mood state. Self-doubt, guilt, and an overriding sense of worthlessness will often lead to disruption in relationships with friends and family and to a withdrawal from work—actions that have understandable long-term effects on mood. Chronic depression and depressive personality traits may thus emerge as the psychological and social concomitants, and sequelae of recurrent biological depressive states. Histrionic and hostile character traits are often noted, as is a long history of difficulty in maintaining stable interpersonal relations. The presence of a personality disorder does not affect the symptom profile but does presage a worse outcome.

The observation that many patients with depression have similar distinctive personality traits led Freud and other psychoanalytic writers to see clinical depression as a psychologically reparative mechanism. The loss of a love object and the consequent psychic injury could be overcome only by self-punishment in which the internalized object was devalued. Freud maintained that ego development depended on successful resolution of object loss. Through a process of narcissistic identification, the ego became the target of revengeful aggressive treatment intended for the original object. Depression thus emerges as the construct of guilt over anger toward an ambivalently perceived (loved, hated) object. Other psychoanalytic writers have elaborated and adapted Freud's views, focusing on depression as an ego response to helplessness rather than internalized anger. Such formulations are undoubtedly useful for conceptualizing the origin of milder depressive episodes in individuals who are still socially functional and for understanding symptom formation in more severe depressive states. However, biological vulnerability is probably an essential prerequisite to the expression of major depressive disorder.

More recently, investigators have stressed the cognitive distortions that dramatically prolong the morbid mood state. The most common cognitive distortions involve negative interpretation of experience, a negative evaluation of the self, and pessimism about the future. Thus, a reverberating loop is established in which a dysphoric affect can give rise to distorted perceptions that in turn exacerbate the dysphoria. This formulation is helpful in understanding the tenacity with which depressed patients seem to cling to the depressive experience even in the face of apparent reward, success, and support.

One cognitive theory based on animal studies is called "learned helplessness." In this formulation, individuals in stressful situations in which they are unable to prevent or alter an aversive stimulus (ie, physical or psychic pain) withdraw and make no further attempts to escape even when opportunities to improve the situation become available. Another theory postulates that a reduction in the rate of positive reinforcement is the principal cause of depression. Low self-esteem is a consequence of the inability of depressed patients to engage in successful goal-seeking behaviors and a resultant low rate of positive reinforcement.

Cognitive and behavioral approaches to the depressive syndrome seem to be more useful for conceptually understanding the psychosocial effects of the depressive state and for planning psychotherapy than for explaining the origin of such episodes. An individual carrying a biological predisposition for recurrent depressive episodes may, for example, successfully negotiate biologically "vulnerable" periods during times of little conflict or stress.

Treatment

A. Biomedical Therapies: A trial of antidepressant medication is indicated for most individuals with major depression, particularly if melancholic features are present (Table 20–1). Most patients with depression are either undertreated or inappropriately treated. Benzodiazepines, which may exacerbate the problem, are prescribed much more often than tricyclic agents. Premature withdrawal of antidepressant medication and symptomatic relapse are also unfortunately common.

Drug selection should be based on the patient's general medical condition, the drug's side effects, and a personal or family history of therapeutic response to a specific agent. About 70% of patients with major depression respond favorably to antidepressant medication. Most cases of poor response result either from the patient's failure to take the medication as prescribed or from inadequate dosage. Selective serotonin reuptake inhibitors (SSRIs) have largely displaced tricyclic antidepressants as the initial treatment choice because of their better tolerated side effect profile. However, because the blood level from a given dosage varies as much as 30-fold in different individuals, in cases of nonresponse to certain antidepressant drugs it is useful to measure plasma drug levels, even in patients receiving maximal doses. The value of plasma levels is most clear with nortriptyline and desipramine. Although useful for titrating dosage into a general range, variations in blood levels within that range do not correlate well with clinical response.

Clear therapeutic benefit usually is noticed 14–21 days after starting treatment, although earlier and later responses are not uncommon. In general, objective signs of improvement (increased appetite, weight gain, improved sleep and affect, reduced agitation, increased purposeful activity) are noted before subjective improvement. A drug of a different class should be considered for patients whose symptoms do not improve after 6 weeks of medication with adequate blood levels. Alternatively, another drug may be added, such as liothyronine, lithium, buspirone, or a monoamine oxidase (MAO) inhibitor. A trial either of an MAO inhibitor alone or of lithium carbonate might be considered at this point.

MAO inhibitors—phenelzine or tranylcypromine—can be drugs of first choice for individuals who present with prominent anxiety associated with depression or who complain specifically of fatigue, hypersomnia, and weight gain rather than weight loss. Although lithium does not have as specific an antidepressant effect as more traditional antidepressant agents, it may help patients with clear periodicity of depressive recurrences and is a better prophylactic agent than traditional antidepressant agents.

How long maintenance treatment should be continued after acute symptoms have subsided is not always clear; current opinion indicates that indefinite treatment at the acute dosage is warranted if relapse is to be avoided.

Patients with very severe depressions and prominent delusional features are relatively refractory to traditional antidepressant treatment. The response often can be enhanced by addition of an antipsychotic agent. Electroconvulsive therapy should be considered in such cases and in cases of nondelusional major depression resistant to drug therapy. Most controlled studies have shown that electroconvulsive therapy is at least as effective as antidepressant medication in the treatment of major depression and often produces a much faster recovery. There are few contraindications to the use of electroconvulsive therapy, and side effects are limited to memory loss for the period just before and after treatment (see Chapter 30). In the past several years a series of studies have shown that transcranial magnetic stimulation, a procedure used originally in neurological diagnosis, can have an antidepressant effect. This intervention is currently being evaluated further.

B. Psychosocial Therapies: Psychotherapy is often indicated for major depression, particularly to improve social functioning following remission of acute symptoms. Controlled studies have indicated that the combination of psychotherapy and antidepressant medication is more effective than either used alone. It should be noted, however, that in most moderate to severe cases of major depression, drug therapy alone is significantly better than psychotherapy alone. Many psychotherapeutic approaches have been utilized, but therapies that focus on the depressed patient's interpersonal functioning and cognitive distortions appear to be the most productive. Insight therapy is made difficult by the depressed patient's tendency to interpret therapeutic suggestions as criticism. Cognitive therapy is often didactic in nature and may profitably include "homework assignments" in which the patient is asked to examine critically and test erroneous assumptions deriving from the depressive experience. For example, a patient may say, "I fail at everything I try to do." Asking that patient to keep a log of daily tasks and document the outcome of each effort affords the therapist an effective means of challenging the patient's derogatory self-image. Testimony from others who are able to state that the tasks were performed satisfactorily can be sought if necessary (see Chapter 33).

The involvement of family and spouse should not be neglected in treatment planning. This may take several forms, including education about the illness, emotional support, and consideration of interpersonal issues. Although prepubertal children with major depression who receive drug treatment usually show a return to normal functioning in areas such as school performance, ongoing deficits in peer and family relationships frequently continue and require specific intervention.

DYSTHYMIC DISORDER

Symptoms & Signs

The term "dysthymic disorder" was coined to denote in a specific operational way a group of patients formerly described as having "neurotic" or characterological depressions. Clinicians have long observed that these individuals experience chronic feelings of inadequacy and self-denigration and express these feelings in a dramatic manner that defies all attempts at treatment. Such patients describe a loss of interest or pleasure in most activities of daily life but do not have symptoms severe enough to meet the criteria for major depressive episode. Depressed mood may be unremitting or may alternate with short periods of normal mood lasting no longer than a few weeks. Dysthymic patients have a tendency to overreact to the normal stresses of life with depressive mood. They have low self-confidence but can be quite demanding and complaining, blaming others for their failures as much as they blame themselves. Obsessional traits are common. As a result of such attitudes, dysthymic patients tend to lead limited social lives and have unstable relationships with others. Abuse of alcohol and other drugs is common in this group of patients.

Natural History

Dysthymic patients often complain of having felt depressed throughout life. A specific time of onset usually cannot be identified or is described as having occurred very early in childhood or adolescence, with a subsequent history of many therapeutic interventions.

Individuals with a characterological predisposition to depressive experience may also be subject to recurrences of major depressive episodes and thus have "double depression" at certain points in their lives. Poor self-esteem, hopelessness, and chronic anhedonia can be viewed as learned phenomena initiated and reinforced at critical junctures by the major depressive event. Since depressive symptoms are usually mild or moderate in severity, morbidity associated with major depression, such as suicide, is less common. Dysthymic patients are frequent consumers of medical and mental health care resources, and a history of participation in self-help organizations can also often be obtained.

Differential Diagnosis

Dysthymic disorder is easily distinguished from major depression on the basis of severity and chronicity. Occasionally, individuals with dysthymic disorder experience periods of superimposed major depression, and both diagnoses are warranted during such periods. The personality characteristics of individuals with dysthymic disorder are such that an additional diagnosis of personality disorder may be warranted. Again, both diagnoses should be recorded regardless of the hypothesized causal relationship between the two diagnoses.

The essential feature of this diagnosis is the chronic nature of the depressed mood. Although normal individuals experience mood states similar to what is noted in dysthymic disorder, their depressions are not as persistent or generally as severe, and there is no ongoing interference with personal or social functioning.

Prognosis

A broad range of impairment is associated with dysthymic disorder. In some cases, social function and job performance are only mildly affected, but others are characterized by recurrent suicidal preoccupation and inability to sustain adequate performance at school or at work. Since the disorder undoubtedly encompasses a heterogeneous group of individuals, the prognosis depends on the response to psychotherapy, antidepressant medication, or both together.

Illustrative Case

A 34-year-old unmarried computer programmer was referred for evaluation of chronic depression. He stated that he had felt depressed his "whole life" and that previous psychiatric treatment had been of no benefit. The past history revealed that the patient, who had no siblings, had been socially isolated and shy and had avoided participation in athletics and social events during high school. He had a dependent relationship with his mother following the divorce of his parents when he was 4 years old. His college career was uneventful. When asked how he came to choose computer science as a major, the patient replied that it was more "logical" and "real" and did not require participation in small seminar sections, in which he felt he performed poorly.

The patient's primary complaint was that "life is meaningless." He complained of hypersomnia but admitted he often went to sleep a few hours after returning from work because "there is nothing else to do and television is bad." He had no hobbies and stated that he did not like to try things where "I'll look bad." He had been involved in two therapeutic relationships, one lasting 4 months and the other 2 years. He stated that he enjoyed the experience, particularly the longer relationship, but did not feel treatment "really changed anything." He denied ever having experienced any periods of increased energy but did admit that he could "think of being suicidal" if his life did not improve soon.

Epidemiology

The lifetime prevalence of dysthymic disorder is approximately 6%. Although defined more specifically than the older term "depressive neurosis," the disorder is common in the practice of most clinicians. Dysthymia is somewhat more prevalent in women. Information regarding genetic transmission or familial occurrence of the disorder is lacking, although it is believed that there may be a subgroup of individuals with dysthymia that experiences an attenuated form of a biologically based major depressive disorder.

Etiology & Pathogenesis

Biological and psychosocial theories of the causes of dysthymic disorder are similar to those discussed in the section on major depression, the primary distinction being that dysthymic disorder presents as a less severe but more chronic syndrome.

Treatment

Psychotherapy is the principal treatment resource for patients with dysthymic disorder, although a significant number of patients may benefit from a trial of an antidepressant drug. The guidelines for assessing the potential utility of drug therapy are a contributory family history and a past history of poor response to other forms of treatment.

Although individual psychotherapy is the most common psychosocial treatment offered, many individuals will benefit from group therapy and from active investigation and restructuring of maladaptive social functioning.

Psychotherapy with chronically depressed individuals is an emotionally draining process for the therapist, and recurrent examination of the therapist's own feelings toward the patient is required. Analysis of one's own anger, boredom, or frustration about some aspect of the patient's behavior can help to isolate the key issue in therapy and lead to symptomatic improvement. The patient's unrealistic and idealistic expectations of himself or herself may, for example, be transmitted to the therapist and give rise to overly optimistic expectations of progress in therapy. If the patient shows no subjective improvement over time, the therapist may inadvertently respond somewhat in the way significant individuals in the patient's life have responded. Interpretation of such personal experiences by the therapist can, in the proper context, be therapeutic.

Short-term focused psychotherapy and therapeutic programs that stress changes in interpersonal relationships and cognitive self-awareness are becoming more popular, in part because long-term analytic approaches to personality change are economically unfeasible. Family-centered approaches differ from individual methods in their direct focus on the "role of the sick member" in the family system rather than on the symptoms of the identified patient.

OTHER MOOD DISORDERS

Bipolar Disorder NOS

Some individuals with bipolar disorder not otherwise specified experience hypomanic episodes without intermittent depressive symptoms. Recurrent hypomania is often socially acceptable and adaptive for the individual. Hypomanic individuals usually experience benefits from increased energy, decreased need for sleep, increased gregariousness, and greater creativity without the disabling consequences of grossly inappropriate social behavior or delusional preoccupation. Most hypomanic episodes do not call for pharmacological treatment; however, in specific cases a trial of lithium carbonate may be advisable. The subtle nature of many hypomanic episodes results in frequent misdiagnosis. Patients and clinicians alike may see such episodes as "normal" and view only the depressive episodes as pathological. Rarely, bipolar disorder not otherwise specified is used to refer to patients in whom a manic episode is superimposed on schizophrenia or delusional disorder.

Depressive Disorder NOS

Depressive disorder not otherwise specified is a diagnosis given to individuals whose depressive symptoms do not meet the criteria for severity or duration noted in the previously described categories. Individuals may experience occasional brief and mild episodes of depression not associated with psychosocial stress or may have dysthymia with periods of normal mood that last longer than several months. The point prevalence of minor, "brief," and subsyndromal depressive disorders is estimated to be 7–8%. Recent clinical and biological studies suggest that these conditions exist on a continuum with melancholia and may respond to antidepressant treatment.

Diagnostic problems may arise with depressed individuals whose mood change is either associated with or follows a psychotic process. The rationale for putting patients in this category rather than some other such as schizoaffective disorder (also poorly defined) is unclear (see Chapter 19).

Historically, the diagnosis of "atypical" depressive disorder has been most often used to denote individuals with mood disorder with prominent phobic and anxious features, weight gain, hypersomnia, and marked interpersonal rejection sensitivity. In *DSM-IV* such atypical features may be coded under any of the other major mood disorders. Such individuals may respond to MAO inhibitor medication preferentially.

SUMMARY

It is difficult to conceive of an area in psychiatry in which the clinician's attitude, knowledge, and skills are more severely tested than in the diagnosis and treatment of mood disorders. Knowledge in this area has been accumulating at such a rate that even the most diligent physician would be hard pressed to keep up with all of the new developments in the field. As reviewed in this chapter, there is considerable evidence for a biological basis for most mood disorders. Data supporting this hypothesis have come from genetic, biochemical, psychopharmacological, and neuroendocrinological investigations, and the hope is that psychiatric diagnosis in this area will become a more objective process as these research efforts continue.

Although subgroups of mood disorders seem relatively distinct from one another as described, in clinical practice there is often considerable overlap between symptoms of different disorders as well as ambiguity about the class in which a given individual belongs. With the present state of knowledge, predictions about course of illness and response to treatment for patients with mood disorders remain as much an art as a science. Use of the biopsychosocial model in the understanding of mood disorders illustrates the awesome complexity of central nervous system regulation of affect but holds out promise of successful methods of treatment on many different levels.

REFERENCES & SUGGESTED READINGS

Alexopoulos GS: "Vascular depression" hypothesis. Arch Gen Psychiatry 1997;54:915.

Bauer MS et al: Manual-based group psychotherapy for bipolar disorder: A feasibility study. J Clin Psychiatry 1998;59:448\9.

Bauer MS et al: Clinical practice guidelines for bipolar disorder from the Department of Veteran Affairs. J Clin Psychiatry 1999;60:9.

Cassidy F et al: A factor analysis of the signs and symptoms of mania. Arch Gen Psychiatry 1998;55:27.

Dilsaver SC et al: Phenomenology of mania: Evidence for distinct depressed, dysphoric, and euphoric presentations. Am J Psychiatry 1999;156:426.

Dixon JF, Hokin LL: Lithium acutely inhibits and chronically up-regulates and stabilizes glutamate uptake by presynaptic nerve endings in mouse cerebral cortex. Proc Natl Acad Sci 1998;95:8363.

Drevets WC et al: Subgenual prefrontal cortex abnormalities in mood disorders. Nature 1997;386:824.

Druss BG, Rohrbaugh RM, Rosenheck RA: Depressive symptoms and health costs in older medical patients. Am J Psychiatry 1999;156:477.

Eaton WW et al: Natural history of diagnostic interview schedule/DSM-IV major depression. Arch Gen Psychiatry 1997;54:993.

Ebert D, Ebmeier K: The role of the cingulate gyrus in depression: From functional anatomy to neurochemistry. Biol Psychiatry 1996;39:1044.

Fawcett J: Bipolar II disorder. Psychiatr Ann 1996;26:S440.

Ghaemi SN, Boiman EE, Goodwin FK: Kindling and second messengers: An approach to the neurobiology of recurrence in bipolar disorder. Biol Psychiatry 1999;45:137.

Gullion CM, Rush AJ: Toward a generalizable model of symptoms in major depressive disorder. Biol Psychiatry 1998;44:959.

Judd LL et al: A prospective 12-year study of subsyndromal and syndromal depressive symptoms in unipolar major depressive disorders. Arch Gen Psychiatry 1998;55:694.

Kendler KS, Gardner CO: Boundaries of major depression: An evaluation of DSM-IV criteria. Am J Psychiatry 1998;155:172.

Kendler KS, Prescott GA: A population-based twin study of lifetime major depression in men and women. Arch Gen Psychiatry 1999;56:39.

Kessler RC et al: Lifetime panic-depression comorbidity in the national comorbidity survey. Arch Gen Psychiatry 1998;55:801.

Kovacs M et al: A controlled family history study of childhood-onset depressive disorder. Arch Gen Psychiatry 1997;54:613.

Kroeze WK, Roth BL: The molecular biology of serotonin receptors: Therapeutic implications for the interface of mood and psychosis. Biol Psychiatry 1998;44:1128.

Lave JR et al: Cost-effectiveness of treatments for major depression in primary care practice. Arch Gen Psychiatry 1998;55:645.

Levitan RD et al: Major depression in individuals with a history of childhood physical or sexual abuse: Relationship to neurovegetative features, mania, and gender. Am J Psychiatry 1998;155:1746.

Mann JJ: The neurobiology of suicide. Nature Med 1998;4:25.

Mann JJ et al: Toward a clinical model of suicide behavior in psychiatric patients. Am J Psychiatry 1999;156:181.

Musselman D, Evans DL, Nemeroff CB: The relationship of depression to cardiovascular disease. Arch Gen Psychiatry 1998;55:580.

Nonacs R, Cohen LS: Postpartum mood disorders: Diagnosis and treatment guidelines. J Clin Psychiatry 1998;59(Suppl 2):34.

Palsson S, Skog I: The epidemiology of affective disorders in the elderly: A review. Int Clin Psychopharmacol 1997;12(Suppl 7):S3.

Persons JB, Thase ME, Crits-Christoph P: The role of psychotherapy in the treatment of depression. Arch Gen Psychiatry 1996;53:283.

Phillips KA et al: Reliability and validity of depressive personality disorder. Am J Psychiatry 1998;155:1044.

Rush AJ, Thase ME: Strategies and tactics in the treatment of chronic depression. J Clin Psychiatry 1997;58(Suppl 13):14.

Shea MT et al: Does major depression result in lasting personality change? Am J Psychiatry 1996;153:1404.

Sobin C, Sackeim HA: Psychomotor symptoms of depression. Am J Psychiatry 1997;154:4.

Steffens DC, Krishnan KRR: Structural neuroimaging and mood disorders: Recent findings, implications for classification and future directions. Biol Psychiatry 1998;43:705.

Tohen M, Gannon KS: Pharmacologic approaches for treatment-resistant mania. Psychiatr Ann 1998;28:629.

Tondo L, Baldessarini RJ: Rapid cycling in women and men with bipolar manic-depressive disorders. Am J Psychiatry 1998;155:1434.

Tondo L et al: Lithium maintenance treatment of depression and mania in bipolar I and bipolar II disorders. Am J Psychiatry 1998;155:638.

Vaillant GE: Natural history of male psychological health, XIV: Relationship of mood disorder vulnerability to physical health. Am J Psychiatry 1998;155:184.

Weissman MM et al: Offspring of depressed parents. Arch Gen Psychiatry 1997;54:932.

21

Anxiety Disorders

John H. Greist, MD, & James W. Jefferson, MD

Anxiety and fear are ubiquitous emotions. The terms anxiety and fear have specific scientific meanings, but common usage has made them interchangeable. For example, a phobia is a kind of anxiety that is also defined in the *Diagnostic and Statistical Manual of Mental Disorders,* 4th edition (*DSM-IV*) as a "persistent or irrational fear." **Fear** is defined as an emotional and physiological response to a recognized external threat (eg, a runaway car or an impending crash in an airplane). **Anxiety** is an unpleasant emotional state, the sources of which are less readily identified. It is frequently accompanied by physiological symptoms that may lead to fatigue or even exhaustion. Because fear of recognized threats causes similar unpleasant mental and physical changes, patients use the terms fear and anxiety interchangeably. Thus, there is little need to strive to differentiate anxiety from fear. However, distinguishing among different anxiety disorders is important, since accurate diagnosis is more likely to result in effective treatment and a better prognosis.

The intensity of anxiety has many gradations ranging from minor qualms to noticeable trembling and even complete panic, the most extreme form of anxiety.

The course of anxiety also varies, with peak severity being reached within a few seconds or more gradually over minutes, hours, or days. Duration also varies from a few seconds to hours or even days or months, although episodes of panic usually abate within 10 minutes and seldom last more than 30 minutes.

The signs and symptoms of anxiety are detailed in the diagnostic criteria for the anxiety disorders (Tables 21–1 to 21–8).

If anxiety arises unexpectedly ("out of the blue"), it is called **uncued** or **spontaneous anxiety** (or if very intense, **spontaneous panic**). When anxiety occurs predictably in response to specific situations, it is called **cued, phobic,** or **situational anxiety** (or when extreme, **phobic** or **situational panic**). **Anticipatory anxiety** (or **anticipatory panic**) is the term used to describe anxiety triggered by the mere thought of particular situations.

The boundary between normal and pathological anxiety cannot be drawn with great precision or confidence. People sometimes seek treatment for anxiety only to find that the anxiety has disappeared before treatment begins. Physicians sometimes delay treatment until disruption of functioning is obvious or suffering is severe. These differences are understandable in the context of present knowledge regarding anxiety, attitudinal differences of both patients and doctors about seeking and giving help, and the effectiveness of various treatments. When anxiety substantially impairs work or social adjustment, most authorities agree that careful assessment is indicated and that treatment is likely to be worthwhile. Suffering itself is often justification for treatment, even if the person with anxiety can continue to function.

Anxiety commonly occurs as a manifestation of appropriate concern about medical and psychiatric disorders. Medical problems involving any body system can produce anxiety as a symptom. Drugs and dietary factors—particularly caffeine and alcohol—may also provoke anxiety.

ANXIETY & DEPRESSION

At least three-fourths of patients with primary depression complain of feeling anxious, worried, or fearful. Extreme anxiety may occur in agitated depression in the form of anguished facial expressions; lip biting; picking at fingers, nails, or clothing; handwringing; constant pacing; and inability to sit quietly. Conversely, primary anxiety can be depressing in its own right. If anxiety persists, particularly if it interferes with functioning, secondary depression is the rule rather than the exception. Some patients have both primary anxiety and primary depressive disorders. Although most patients with anxiety or depression fall clearly into the respective *DSM-IV* categories, differential diagnosis of anxiety and depression can be challenging and require several interviews, further evaluation, and trials of treatment.

THEORIES OF ANXIETY

A. Genetic: Isaac Marks (1986) has provided an elegant summary of the genetics of fear and anxiety disorders:

From protozoa to mammals, organisms have been selectively bred for genetic differences in defensive behaviour which are accompanied by differences in brain and other biological functions. Studies of twins indicate some genetic control of normal human fear from infancy onwards, of anxiety as a symptom and as a syndrome, and of phobic and obsessive-compulsive phenomena. Anxiety disorders are more common among the relatives of affected probands than of controls, especially among female and first-degree relatives; alcoholism and secondary depression may also be overrepresented. Familial influences have been found for panic disorder, agoraphobia, and obsessive-compulsive problems. Panic disorder in depressed probands increases the risk to their relatives of phobia as well as of panic disorder, major depression, and alcoholism. The strongest family history of all anxiety disorders is seen in blood-injury phobia; even though it can be successfully treated by exposure, its roots may lie in a genetically determined specific autonomic susceptibility. Some genetic effects can be modified by environmental means.

B. Psychodynamic: Although Freud at first proposed a physiological basis for anxiety, he later concluded that anxiety serves as a signal to the ego of the emergence of an unconscious conflict or impulse. His theory led to the development of psychoanalysis, used to study and treat emotional disorders. According to psychoanalytic theory, anxiety is seen as an emotion of the ego (the part of our mental apparatus that balances the impulses and demands of our childlike id, the stern and punitive controls of our parent-like superego, and external reality). Anxiety is also seen as the key indication of hidden psychological conflict.

C. Learned: Behavioral therapists hold that anxiety is a learned response to some noxious situation or stimulus. When a situation or stimulus provokes anxiety in a person, the person learns to reduce the anxiety by avoiding the situations that provoke it. Generalized anxiety disorder may result from the unpredictability of positive and negative reinforcement—the person is uncertain when and if avoidance behaviors will be effective in reducing anxiety.

It is also possible to develop anxiety in response to generally positive or neutral stimuli if these are associated with a noxious or aversive stimulus. This conditioning process is held to be responsible for the avoidance of neutral or benign situations in which distressing anxiety (such as panic) has occurred. Pairing of a recurrent anxiety-inducing thought (such as "contamination") with a compulsive behavior (such as hand washing) that reduces anxiety is thought to explain the development of obsessive-compulsive disorder.

D. Biochemical: When compared with normal controls, patients with anxiety disorders have significantly different physiological functioning (eg, higher heart rate, higher blood lactate levels, and greater oxygen debt during moderate exercise). Patients with panic disorders are more sensitive to a number of substances (eg, caffeine, lactate, isoproterenol, epinephrine, yohimbine, and piperoxan). Many of these substances increase activity of the locus ceruleus, the midbrain nucleus that supplies about 70% of the norepinephrine-releasing neurons in the central nervous system. Given these substances human subjects report increased anxiety and monkeys demonstrate fear behaviors similar to those they show when placed in a confrontational setting. Electrical stimulation of the locus ceruleus in monkeys produces a similar fear response, whereas its ablation reduces fear behaviors. Medications that inhibit functioning of the locus ceruleus also reduce fear responses in monkeys and anxiety in humans with anxiety disorders as well as in controls. Although α_2-agonists and β-adrenergic receptor blockers have been shown to have some antianxiety properties, the selective serotonin reuptake inhibitors, monoamine oxidase inhibitor antidepressants, and benzodiazepine drugs, which down-regulate function of the locus ceruleus (norepinephrine), are the most useful clinically.

The benzodiazepines have a second putative mode of action in that they potentiate γ-aminobutyric acid (GABA), a widely distributed inhibitory neurotransmitter. Discovery of benzodiazepine receptors in the central nervous system led to a search for endogenous benzodiazepines, and these have now been found (see Chapter 5).

Abnormal neurotransmission of serotonin is thought to explain part of the pathophysiology of obsessive-compulsive disorder, and potent serotonin uptake inhibitors are the most predictably effective medications for this disorder.

The apparent biochemical basis of every behavior, thought, and feeling does not dictate that biochemical abnormalities must be treated with chemicals—brain chemistry can also be changed by behavioral, psychological, and surgical interventions.

Epidemiology

In the National Institute of Mental Health Epidemiologic Catchment Area (NIMH-ECA) study (Myers et al, 1984), anxiety disorders were more prevalent over the preceding 6 months than any other mental disorder (8.3% of the populations surveyed in their homes). Of those with anxiety disorders, only 23% were receiving treatment. Other studies have found similar rates of anxiety disorders. The lifetime prevalence of anxiety disorders found in the National Comorbidity Survey (Kessler et al, 1994) was 24.9%.

PANIC DISORDER

DSM-IV identifies the common occurrence of panic attacks and the relative rarity of panic disorder. About 35% of the population experiences a panic attack in the course of a year and *DSM-IV* formally recognizes that panic attacks occur in a "variety of anxiety disorders." There is still substantial debate about the etiological importance of panic episodes or attacks in the development of agoraphobia. The NIMH-ECA study found a 6-month prevalence of panic disorder of only 0.7%; the prevalence of agoraphobia was 2.8%.

Symptoms & Signs

Table 21–1 lists criteria for panic attack (*DSM-IV*). The distressing constellation of sudden episodes involving pronounced alteration of physiological functions frequently leads to fears of death, "going crazy," or "doing something uncontrolled." Commonly, patients will experience 8 or 9 of the 13 symptoms. Panic attacks begin suddenly and usually abate within 10 minutes, rarely lasting 30 minutes or more. Patients may confuse panic with anticipatory anxiety early in the course of the disorder, although most, with experience, become expert at distinguishing between the two. Moving about during a panic attack makes many individuals feel somewhat better, but avoidance of situations in which panic has occurred leads to the development of phobias.

Criteria for panic disorder are listed in Tables 21–2 and 21–3. Basically, several unexpected (spontaneous or uncued) panic attacks must evoke fear of subsequent attacks or the effects of attacks or change behavior significantly. Panic disorder may occur with agoraphobia (Table 21–3) or without agoraphobia (Table 21–2). Agoraphobia occurs more often without than with panic disorder. Some individuals develop panic attacks after the onset of agoraphobia, and the diagnosis should then be changed from agoraphobia without panic disorder to panic disorder with agoraphobia, even though the more correct sequential description would be agoraphobia with panic disorder.

Differential Diagnosis

Somatic conditions should not be overlooked as causes of anxiety, nor should anxiety disorders be over-investigated or treated as somatic disorders. Most somatic causes of symptoms of anxiety are readily recognized if a careful history is taken and physical examination and indicated laboratory tests are performed.

Somatic conditions that may produce anxiety include those affecting the cardiovascular system (angina

Table 21–1. *DSM-IV* criteria for panic attack.

Note: A panic attack is not a codable disorder. Code the specific diagnosis in which the panic attack occurs.
A discrete period of intense fear or discomfort, in which four (or more) of the following symptoms developed abruptly and reached a peak within 10 minutes: (1) palpitations, pounding heart, or accelerated heart rate, (2) sweating, (3) trembling or shaking, (4) sensations of shortness of breath or smothering, (5) feeling of choking, (6) chest pain or discomfort, (7) nausea or abdominal distress, (8) feeling dizzy, unsteady, light-headed, or faint, (9) derealization (feelings of unreality) or depersonalization (*being detached from oneself*), (10) fear of losing control or going crazy, (11) fear of dying, (12) paresthesias (numbness or tingling sensations), (13) chills or hot flashes.

Table 21–2. *DSM-IV* diagnostic criteria for panic disorder without agoraphobia.

A. Both (1) and (2):
  (1) Recurrent unexpected panic attacks.
  (2) At least one of the attacks has been followed by 1 month (or more) of one (or more) of the following:
    (a) Persistent concern about having additional attacks.
    (b) Worry about the implications of the attack or its consequences (eg, losing control, having a heart attack, "going crazy").
    (c) A significant change in behavior related to the attacks.

B. Absence of agoraphobia.

C. The panic attacks are not due to the direct physiological effects of a substance (eg, a drug of abuse, a medication) or a general medical condition (eg, hyperthyroidism).

D. The panic attacks are not better accounted for by another mental disorder, such as social phobia (eg, occurring on exposure to feared social situations), specific phobia (eg, on exposure to a specific phobic situation), obsessive-compulsive disorder (eg, on exposure to dirt in someone with an obsession about contamination), posttraumatic stress disorder (eg, in response to stimuli associated with a severe stressor),
or separation anxiety disorder (eg, in response to being away from home or close relatives).

Table 21–3. *DSM-IV* diagnostic criteria for panic disorder with agoraphobia.

A. Both (1) and (2):
  (1) Recurrent unexpected panic attacks.
  (2) At least one of the attacks has been followed by 1 month (or more) of one (or more) of the following:
    (a) Persistent concern about having additional attacks.
    (b) Worry about the implications of the attack or its consequences (eg, losing control, having a heart attack, "going crazy").
    (c) A significant change in behavior related to the attacks.

B. Presence of agoraphobia.

C. The panic attacks are not due to the direct physiological effects of a substance (eg, a drug of abuse, a medication) or a general medical condition (eg, hyperthyroidism).

D. The panic attacks are not better accounted for by another mental disorder, such as social phobia (eg, occurring on exposure to feared social situations), specific phobia (eg, on exposure to a specific phobic situation), obsessive-compulsive disorder (eg, on exposure to dirt in someone with an obsession about contamination), posttraumatic stress disorder (eg, in response to stimuli associated with a severe stressor), or separation anxiety disorder (eg, in response to being away from home or close relatives).

pectoris, acute myocardial infarction, arrhythmias, congestive heart failure, shock), respiratory problems (asthma, emphysema, pulmonary embolism), neurological disorders (encephalopathy, seizure disorder, benign essential tremor, vertigo), hematological and immunological disorders (anemia, anaphylactic shock), and endocrine dysfunction (diabetes, hypothyroidism, hyperthyroidism, parathyroid disease, Cushing's disease, pheochromocytoma).

Medications may also provoke symptoms of anxiety. Antispasmodics, cold medicines, thyroid supplements, digitalis, stimulants, and—paradoxically—antianxiety and antidepressant medicines used to treat panic may all induce anxiety. Discontinuation of certain medications (eg, some blood pressure medicines, sleeping pills, and antianxiety drugs) may lead to withdrawal syndromes in which anxiety may be prominent. Caffeine, alcohol, and marijuana are frequent causes of symptoms of anxiety, including panic.

Illustrative Case

A 30-year-old woman had experienced panic episodes since age 20. They usually began spontaneously, "out of the blue," although they often appeared in the context of anger or other emotional extremes of sadness or disappointment. She had awakened from sleep experiencing a feeling of panic on several occasions. Although she worried initially that the settings or circumstances in which panic occurred might be causing the episodes, she later concluded that no reliable pattern could be detected. She neither smoked nor used alcohol and had discontinued use of caffeine because it made her feel jittery.

Attacks were characterized by rapid heart rate, sweating, nausea, chills, trembling, and a fear of doing something uncontrolled. Early severe episodes had included symptoms associated with hyperventilation, including "smothering," choking, chest discomfort, faintness, and paresthesias, but once she recognized their association with overbreathing, she was able to control them by learning to breathe "slow and shallow."

The patient reported increased frequency but not severity of panic attacks in the premenstruum. Family history was positive for similar episodes in her mother from ages 25 through 45 and for depression on both sides of her family.

After each of her first few attacks, the patient sought treatment in an emergency room or from her primary care physician, who had carefully examined her and, finding "nothing wrong," attempted to reassure her that her symptoms were a manifestation of anxiety. She had briefly used a benzodiazepine prescribed by her physician but objected to the "drugged" feeling it produced. Panic ceased for one 3-year period and occurred less than once per month for another 3 years. She remained, however, worried that panic could recur at any time. For the 2 years before she sought treatment, panic attacks had occurred at least twice per month. Imipramine in gradually increasing doses (see below) was prescribed, and at levels of 100 mg/d, panic attacks ceased for 6 months. They resumed when the dose was decreased to 75 mg/d.

Epidemiology

The NIMH-ECA study found a 6-month prevalence of panic disorder of only 0.7%, whereas the 12-month prevalence in the National Comorbidity Survey was 2.3%—a large discrepancy partly explained by the difference in measurement interval and partly by the difference in populations and questions in the assessment instruments.

More than one-third of individuals may experience a single episode of panic in any given year, a much smaller proportion will have repeated panic attacks, and less than 1% will develop panic disorder. The peak age at onset of spontaneous panic is between 15 and 25 years, and panic beginning after age 40 would suggest depression or a possible somatic cause. There is some genetic basis for panic disorder, although many who experience panic attacks come from families with no history of anxiety. Women have been thought to have panic disorder twice as commonly as men, but some of this difference may be related to cultural factors that permit women, more than men, to complain about and seek treatment for symptoms of panic or anxiety.

Etiology & Pathogenesis

The underlying pathophysiology of panic disorder is far from clear. It is commonly believed that panic disorder has a biochemical basis, but its precise characteristics have not been elucidated. Many authorities suspect that noradrenergic dysfunction, perhaps mediated through the locus ceruleus (Nutt et al, 1992), is involved, and drug treatments that alter this system have been shown to be of benefit. Panic appears pathogenetic for phobic complications of anticipatory anxiety and avoidance in some individuals, which may persist after panic has abated.

There may be an association between early separation anxiety manifested by school avoidance and the later development of agoraphobia.

Treatment

Treatment is largely empirical, since etiological factors have not been clearly established.

A. Psychological Treatment: Many case reports and personal testimonials claim positive benefits from the many varieties of psychotherapy, although no one type of psychotherapy is clearly any more or less effective than another. With psychotherapeutic approaches to anxiety disorders, as well as with behavioral therapy and drug therapy, nonspecific factors common to any good patient-clinician relationship (eg, expectation of success, belief in the treatment, reassurance, encouragement, empathy) probably account for much of the improvement achieved.

Cognitive therapy (see Chapter 33), which attempts to modify catastrophic negative thoughts that may accompany panic attacks, has been shown in controlled investigations to be an effective treatment for panic disorder (Barlow, 1998). Thus, an attempt can be made to help a patient with the following train of thought, "My heart just skipped a beat and my chest feels tight, so I must be having a heart attack and will surely die," to reinterpret these physiological symptoms to achieve a new train of thought, such as, "My heart just skipped a beat and my chest feels tight. These are familiar symptoms of panic. I can expect several other 'old friends' such as numbness and tingling of my fingers, feeling faint, shortness of breath, and trembling to appear soon. These are all symptoms of panic, which I have been through many times before. Panic is unpleasant but not dangerous, and I know this attack will end soon." This reassignment of the physiological components of panic from life-threatening to familiar and manageable may help a larger proportion of patients than other psychotherapies. It also includes elements of exposure therapy (see below).

B. Behavioral Therapy: There is growing evidence that exposure therapy can substantially reduce the frequency and severity of panic attacks (see Chapter 33). Agoraphobic patients who experience spontaneous panic attacks report marked reduction in the frequency and severity of panic when they carry out exposure therapy without medication. In some studies, panic attacks have stopped completely in two-thirds of patients. When hyperventilation is a substantial component of panic, teaching patients techniques to control it is often helpful. The voluntary induction of hyperventilation can be coupled with both education linking overbreathing with symptoms and instruction in diaphragmatic breathing.

Patients who experience only panic without anticipatory anxiety and avoidance can be exposed, in imagination, to the physiological aberrations associated with panic. Thus, they would be asked to imagine that the full constellation of symptoms of panic is emerging just as it does during a panic attack and to continue that fantasy until the anxiety associated with the panic attack dies down.

When panic attacks are accompanied by anticipatory anxiety and avoidance, exposure therapy is the treatment of choice. Exposure can be simply taught in an office setting in as little as 5 minutes. The patient is instructed to "find and face the things you fear and remain in contact with them until your anxiety subsides." The therapist must reiterate the instruction as treatment progresses and monitor compliance with written records kept by the patient for mutually agreed-on exposure tasks. Homework assignments constitute the bulk of exposure tasks, and enlistment of a family member or friend who can serve as cotherapist is often helpful. A self-help chapter in a book by Greist et al (1986) has been shown to be as effective as sessions with a behavioral therapist in treating individuals with agoraphobia.

C. Drug Therapy: Many consider medications to be the cornerstone of treatment of panic disorder (see Chapter 30). Most antidepressants (tricyclics, selective serotonin reuptake inhibitors, monoamine oxidase inhibitors, and others) substantially reduce the frequency and severity of panic attacks and often completely prevent them. They work even if depression is not present. Benzodiazepine anxiolytics are also effective antipanic drugs (alprazolam and clonazepam are the best-studied examples, but do not appear to be unique) and work more quickly than the antidepressants, although they carry a risk of dependence. All antipanic drugs should be started at low dosages and increased gradually until an effective dosage level is achieved. Relapse is common when antipanic drugs are discontinued; fortunately, their long-term use appears to be safe in most cases.

Although sometimes of ancillary benefit, β-adrenergic blocking agents (eg, propranolol) are not as effective as the above-mentioned drugs. Antipsychotics, barbiturates, meprobamate, and antihistamines are not recommended for treatment of panic attacks.

A combination of medication and cognitive-behavioral therapy is most beneficial for many patients. When the two therapies are combined, relapse rates following withdrawal from medication may be substantially lower.

AGORAPHOBIA

Symptoms & Signs

Agoraphobia is a fear of being caught in a situation from which a graceful and speedy escape to safety would be difficult or embarrassing if the patient felt discomfort (often in the form of panic). Situations likely to induce fear and avoidance include attendance at auditoriums, eating out (especially at formal sit-down restaurants), shopping in supermarkets, standing in lines, using public transportation, and driving under conditions in which opportunities to pull over, stop, or get off the highway quickly may be restricted. Being accompanied by a trusted family member or friend permits many agoraphobic individuals to increase the number of possibly uncomfortable situations they can endure and to extend the range of their excursions.

For those who panic, fear of fainting during an attack is the most common fear after fear of panic itself. Hyperventilation with its attendant decreases in blood carbon dioxide, ionized calcium, and phosphorus produces paresthesias, light-headedness, visual changes, and feelings of unreality that contribute to the fear of fainting. Actual fainting, although reportedly caused by hyperventilation, must be exceedingly rare, since none of the patients seen by the authors has fainted during a panic attack.

By definition, phobias are irrational fears involving avoidance of objects or situations that are extremely unlikely to cause harm and that most people approach without discomfort. Agoraphobic patients lament their inability to face everyday situations and often become discouraged, depressed, and demoralized by the constriction in their lives caused by agoraphobia.

Differential Diagnosis

Avoidance or withdrawal can occur in depression, schizophrenic and paranoid disorders, some organic mental disorders, other anxiety disorders (eg, social or specific phobia, obsessive-compulsive disorder, and PTSD), and certain personality disorders. This avoidance occurs in the context of other symptoms and signs that usually clarify the underlying diagnosis. Answers to a few simple questions (also useful with other anxiety disorders) are likely to point to or away from a diagnosis of agoraphobia:

1. Are there situations or things you avoid? What are they? (Agoraphobic patients are likely to describe situations in which they would feel caught or trapped.)
2. What do you feel will happen if you cannot avoid (the situations described in question 1)? (Expect agoraphobic patients to describe fears of panic, fainting, "going crazy," or dying.)
3. Do your fears seem exaggerated or out of proportion? (Most agoraphobic patients clearly recognize the unreasonableness of their fears and frequently describe them with words such as dumb, stupid, crazy, goofy, irrational.)
4. If you must face avoided situations, how do you bring yourself to do it? (Agoraphobic patients usually describe anticipatory anxiety that leads to excuses to avoid the situation or frank refusal to proceed, frequent requests that others accompany them, or use of alcohol or other sedatives to decrease anxiety.)
5. Have you ever experienced a decrease in anxiety if you could not leave the uncomfortable situation for a long time? (Most agoraphobic patients have found themselves in such situations from time to time, and most report a reduction in anxiety with this fortuitous exposure therapy.)

Prognosis

Agoraphobia may remit spontaneously, particularly if panic attacks abate or if life circumstances force or encourage patients to go about their business, producing a naturalistic behavior therapy. Typically, untreated agoraphobia runs a chronic and un-

dulating course with periods of relative exacerbation and remission and with major incapacity associated with anticipatory anxiety and avoidance. Abuse of alcohol and other substances becomes a problem for a small proportion of agoraphobic patients who derive initial antianxiety effects from these substances, rely on them increasingly, and develop both psychological and physiological dependence.

Agoraphobia can have devastating effects on both sufferers and their families. Roles within the family often change dramatically. For example, because of increased family responsibilities, spouses work fewer hours after their partners develop the disorder. Agoraphobia frequently leads to discouragement and complaints of tension, fatigue, obsessions, and depression.

With treatment, some individuals are cured, and most make substantial gains and resume their previous occupational and social roles with minor residual anxiety. A very small number of agoraphobic patients fail to respond to behavioral and drug treatments.

Illustrative Case

A 23-year-old woman who had experienced panic while driving on an expressway on three separate occasions became worried about driving on the expressway again; worrying about it brought on another panic attack. She stopped driving on the expressway but still experienced extreme anxiety in other situations in which means of egress were not readily available, such as standing in a supermarket checkout line, sitting in church, or sitting under a hair dryer at the beauty parlor. She became increasingly worried about panic attacks and avoided more and more settings in which they might occur, resulting in a feeling of helplessness. She was able to continue working only because a trusted friend conveyed her to and from work.

After reading about agoraphobia in a magazine, she recognized her disorder and sought treatment. Careful history taking revealed that she had last experienced a panic attack 3 months before coming to the clinic, but worried about attacks almost constantly (anticipatory anxiety). Treatment was begun with exposure therapy, and she made rapid gains in the range of her activities while experiencing progressively less discomfort. Panic attacks did not recur either in the treatment setting or spontaneously, and at 1-year follow-up she had regained her full range of activities, although she still worried somewhat that panic attacks might recur.

Epidemiology

The NIMH-ECA study reported a 6-month prevalence of agoraphobia of 3.8% for women and 1.8% for men. Some of the higher prevalence rates in females may be culturally determined. The age at onset peaks in the early 20s, and onset after age 40 is uncommon.

People who develop agoraphobia, although previously similar to others in social or marital status, marital and sexual adjustment, separation anxiety, dependency, and other personality characteristics, now, in terms of many of these attributes, experience a change for the worse.

Etiology & Pathogenesis

There is growing evidence that an agoraphobic trait disorder may be inherited. In two studies, specific severe trauma preceded the onset of agoraphobia in only 3% and 8% of people, respectively. However, less severe life stress events were reportedly twice as common in agoraphobic patients as in controls.

Commonly, panic leads to anticipatory anxiety of experiencing another panic attack in the same situation, which, in turn, leads to avoidance of that situation. Many patients report this sequence (and would therefore be diagnosed as having panic disorder), but others develop classical agoraphobic avoidance without ever experiencing panic. In some, panic occurs after entering agoraphobic situations (situational or phobic panic). The exact role of panic in the etiology of agoraphobia remains unresolved and is the subject of continuing study.

Treatment

A. Psychological Treatment: The effectiveness of specific psychotherapies for treatment of agoraphobia has not been established. All therapies (including medications and behavioral therapy) should include nonspecific but important elements of education and support; this may partly explain the improvement sometimes seen with psychotherapy.

B. Behavioral Therapy: Exposure therapy is the single most effective treatment for agoraphobia with and without panic attacks. Panic, anticipatory anxiety, and avoidance are all reduced by this straightforward approach when it is applied systematically according to simple instructions that many patients can put into practice by themselves or with the help of a family member or friend. Patients are also given suggestions for "coping tactics" to be used when anxiety rises to disturbing levels. Over the past decade, the average number of contact hours spent with an experienced behavioral therapist in the successful treatment of agoraphobia has declined from nearly 20 to less than 4. One controlled study (Swinson et al, 1992) demonstrated a substantial and sustained beneficial effect for specific exposure instructions given during a single encounter in or shortly after a patient presented at an emergency room with a panic attack. Avoidance, frequency of panic attacks, and depression all improved significantly; patients who received reassurance did not improve. The results of this study support both the cost effectiveness of this treatment technique and its self-help nature. Patients using exposure therapy develop a new improved attitude toward the fears they experience and the risks they are willing to take regarding those fears. This change in attitude often spreads to other areas of functioning, with beneficial results.

C. Drug Treatment: When panic is present, drug treatment is often employed (see Panic Disorder, above). In the absence of panic, exposure therapy alone is usually sufficient. Some patients have pronounced anticipatory anxiety when they begin exposure therapy; such patients may be given antianxiety medications. The lowest effective dose should be used, since some individuals may fail to learn how to deal effectively with anxiety-causing stimuli when no longer under the influence of anxiolytics. This is a phenomenon known as state-dependent learning: what is learned in a state in which medication is taken does not generalize to a state in which the medication is not taken. There is also a risk of dependence with most anxiolytics.

SOCIAL PHOBIA

Symptoms & Signs

The *DSM-IV* diagnostic criteria for social phobia (also called social anxiety disorder) are listed in Table 21–4. Individuals with social phobia have a persistent and recognizably irrational fear of performing in social situations, believing that their performance will be found wanting in some way and lead to embarrassment or humiliation.

Whereas some anxiety can provide people with a performance-enhancing "edge," social phobia produces anxiety of such great proportions that it interferes with performance. Social phobia can be quite specific (eg, public speaking) or may be generalized to many social aspects of the individual's life and, in its most extreme form, may merge into avoidant personality disorder.

Individuals asked to face their particular type of social phobia describe anticipatory anxiety and may experience situational panic attacks. Avoidance is a common complication of social phobia.

Differential Diagnosis

Marked anxiety and avoidance of social situations may occur in schizophrenia, major depression, obsessive-compulsive disorder, and paranoid and avoidant personality disorders. However, the reasons given for such avoidance and anxiety are closely tied to content appropriate for those specific disorders and seldom involve embarrassment or humiliation. For example, a patient who is paranoid may avoid social situations because of a delusional fear of being harmed. Substance abuse may occur in a misguided attempt to self-treat social phobia.

Prognosis

Mild social phobias seldom interfere with functioning but may consign sufferers to repeated dis-

Table 21–4. *DSM-IV* diagnostic criteria for social phobia.

A. A marked and persistent fear of one or more social or performance situations in which the person is exposed to unfamiliar people or to possible scrutiny by others. The individual fears that he or she will act in a way (or show anxiety symptoms) that will be humiliating or embarrassing. **Note:** In children, there must be evidence of the capacity for age-appropriate social relationships with familiar people and the anxiety must occur in peer settings, not just in interactions with adults.

B. Exposure to the feared social situation almost invariably provokes anxiety, which may take the form of a situationally bound or situationally predisposed panic attack. **Note:** In children, the anxiety may be expressed by crying, tantrums, freezing, or shrinking from social situations with unfamiliar people.

C. The person recognizes that the fear is excessive or unreasonable. **Note:** In children, this feature may be absent.

D. The feared social or performance situations are avoided or else are endured with intense anxiety or distress.

E. The avoidance, anxious anticipation, or distress in the feared social or performance situation(s) interferes significantly with the person's normal routine, occupational (academic) functioning, or social activities or relationships, or there is marked distress about having the phobia.

F. In individuals under age 18 years, the duration is at least 6 months.

G. The fear or avoidance is not due to the direct physiological effects of a substance (eg, a drug of abuse, a medication) or a general medical condition and is not better accounted for by another mental disorder (eg, panic disorder with or without agoraphobia, separation anxiety disorder, body dysmorphic disorder, a pervasive developmental disorder, or schizoid personality disorder).

H. If a general medical condition or another mental disorder is present, the fear in Criterion A is unrelated to it, eg, the fear is not of stuttering, trembling in Parkinson's disease, or exhibiting abnormal eating behavior in anorexia nervosa or bulimia nervosa.

Specify if:
   Generalized: If the fears include most social situations, also consider the additional diagnosis of avoidant personality disorder.

comfort when in their phobic situations. More severe social phobia frequently interferes with functioning substantially and causes great suffering. Individuals with social phobia sometimes change professions to avoid situations that give rise to performance anxiety. The model wages of a person with generalized social phobia are 14% lower than those without the disorder.

Illustrative Case

A medical student ranking in the top 10% of his class sought treatment before making a decision to drop out of medical school during the first clinical rotation in his third year. He had always experienced extreme anxiety whenever called on to speak in class and had successfully avoided such presentations through high school, college, and the first 2 years of medical school. He had taken pains to select a medical school in which he thought formal oral presentations were not required. At the beginning of his junior year, he was informed that he would have to make a "medical advances" presentation 4 months later. Although he quickly developed the topic and was confident of his material, he felt that he could not face the ordeal of making the presentation. Anticipatory anxiety had already begun to mount to a level that interfered with his sleep and performance on the wards.

The student reported that his father had similar anxiety and had given up a career in law for work as an accountant because of his anxiety in moot court during law school.

Treatment was begun with a combination of exposure therapy (with videotape feedback) and drug therapy (a β-blocker). Within 2 weeks (four exposure sessions), the student's anticipatory anxiety abated substantially, and he reported enjoyment of his new-found confidence and improved performance in public speaking. His presentation was a success, and he continued to feel and function well through the rest of medical school.

Epidemiology

Many individuals with social phobia were shy as children; however, most shy children do not develop social phobia. Age at onset is usually around puberty, with peak presentation for treatment in the 20s and few new cases emerging after age 30. Males are almost as likely as females to experience social phobia (the National Comorbidity Survey study 12-month prevalence is 6.6% for males and 9.1% for females). Males predominate among the most severe cases.

Etiology & Pathogenesis

The specific cause of social phobia is unknown. A family history is often discovered, although the relative contributions of heredity and environment have not been determined. As with other phobias, avoidance in a misguided attempt at self-treatment probably increases severity of symptoms and perpetuates dysfunction (Greist et al, 1980).

Treatment

A. Psychotherapy: Many individuals suffering from social and other phobias continue to receive analytic and other dynamic psychotherapies with the ambitious goal of uncovering and working through unconscious psychological causes of the anxiety disorder. Research does not support the effectiveness of these approaches for phobic disorders. Their continued use in the face of evidence supporting more effective treatments indicates that many clinicians find it difficult to abandon models learned while in training.

B. Behavioral Therapy: Exposure therapy in vivo with videotape feedback and in fantasy (for situations that are difficult to produce in real life) is helpful to many individuals with fear of public speaking and other forms of social phobia. At times, paradoxical exaggeration of the feared performance will **decrease** anxiety (eg, asking a patient with fear of writing illegibly to write more illegibly). Although many individuals with social phobias have become convinced that they cannot face their feared situation, a few exposure treatments usually reverse this misapprehension.

C. Drug Treatment: β-Adrenergic blocking drugs are often helpful in decreasing peripheral symptoms of anxiety such as tremor, tachycardia, and sweating. They may be used in a single dose 1 hour or more before entering phobic situations likely to evoke these symptoms. Benzodiazepine antianxiety drugs are sometimes used in combination with β-blockers as well as alone. Gabapentin has also been found effective in treating generalized social phobia and does not cause physical dependency as benzodiazepines do (Pande et al, 1999). Monoamine oxidase inhibitor (MAOI) antidepressants (usually phenelzine) have been shown to be effective in controlled trials for social phobia, although they must be used regularly and require a diet low in tyramine. Controlled trials of selective serotonin reuptake inhibitors (SSRIs) have also been positive (Stein et al, 1998), and they have become first-line treatment for social phobia, now that paroxetine has received FDA approval for an indication in social anxiety disorder.

Frequently, a combination of exposure therapy and β-blocking drugs works well for specific social phobia, and patients who have experienced years of disability achieve substantially higher levels of functioning in a few weeks. For generalized social phobia, SSRIs, MAOIs, and benzodiazepines are pharmacological treatments of choice.

SPECIFIC PHOBIA

Symptoms & Signs, Differential Diagnosis, & Prognosis

Although less incapacitating than agoraphobia or social phobia, specific phobias can have major effects on sufferers' lives.

The most common phobic objects or situations that invoke specific phobias are snakes, spiders, heights, elevators and other small closed spaces, and flying. Fewer individuals seek treatment for specific phobias than for agoraphobia and social phobia, both because many specific phobias remit spontaneously and because it is easier to avoid a specific phobic situation than the multiple situations often associated with agoraphobia and social phobia.

Flying phobia can cause significant problems for those who need to travel because of their work and substantial inconvenience for those who must use surface transportation to cover long distances. Occa-

sionally, insect phobias reach such proportions that individuals remain indoors during the season when the feared insect is active (as with bees). Blood-injury phobia, although less common than some other specific phobias, is of particular interest because it commonly causes fainting. Whereas agoraphobic individuals often fear fainting but seldom if ever faint, individuals with blood-injury phobia actually faint as a result of vasovagal syncope when exposed to their phobic stimulus. Brought on by sight, experience, or discussion of blood, operations, injuries, or even minor pain, blood-injury phobia can lead to long-term avoidance of visits to physicians and dentists as well as other situations that have induced fainting. The *DSM-IV* diagnostic criteria for specific phobia are listed in Table 21–5.

Since individuals with specific phobia can usually successfully avoid their feared object or situation ("I

Table 21–5. *DSM-IV* diagnostic criteria for specific phobia.

A. Marked and persistent fear that is excessive or unreasonable, cued by the presence or anticipation of a specific object or situation (eg, flying, heights, animals, receiving an injection, seeing blood).

B. Exposure to the phobic stimulus almost invariably provokes an immediate anxiety response, which may take the form of a situationally bound or situationally predisposed panic attack. **Note:** In children, the anxiety may be expressed by crying, tantrums, freezing, or clinging.

C. The person recognizes that the fear is excessive or unreasonable. **Note:** In children, this feature may be absent.

D. The phobic situation(s) is avoided or else is endured with intense anxiety or distress.

E. The avoidance, anxious anticipation, or distress in the feared situation(s) interferes significantly with the person's normal routine, occupational (or academic) functioning, or social activities or relationships, or there is marked distress about having the phobia.

F. In individuals under age 18 years, the duration is at least 6 months.

G. The anxiety, panic attacks, or phobic avoidance associated with the specific object or situation is not better accounted for by another mental disorder, such as obsessive-compulsive disorder (eg, fear of dirt in someone with an obsession about contamination), posttraumatic stress disorder (eg, avoidance of stimuli associated with a severe stressor), separation anxiety disorder (eg, avoidance of school), social phobia (eg, avoidance of social situations because of fear of embarrassment), panic disorder with agoraphobia, or agoraphobia without history of panic disorder.

Specify type:
   Animal type
   Natural Environment type (eg, heights, storms, water)
   Blood-Injection-Injury type
   Situational type (eg, airplanes, elevators, enclosed places)
   Other type (eg, phobic avoidance of situations that may lead to choking, vomiting, or contracting an illness; in children, avoidance of loud sounds or costumed characters)

know where spiders hang out, so I stay away from those places"), few experience pervasive anxiety. When such individuals know they must face the source of their phobia, they develop anticipatory anxiety, and when they encounter that source, either intentionally or inadvertently, a situational panic indistinguishable from spontaneous panic may occur.

Differential diagnosis is seldom a problem because of the specific nature of the phobia. Some flying phobia is actually agoraphobia in which the individual fears confinement in the plane's cabin without means of ready egress.

Illustrative Case

A 32-year-old man presented for treatment because he had fainted every time he had had blood drawn since age 12. This experience led to fearful avoidance of doctors and venipuncture in this otherwise healthy and physically fit individual. He sought treatment because he avoided routine health monitoring and might find it difficult to seek care for acute medical problems. He also reported embarrassment about his inability to have blood drawn without fainting unless recumbent. His mother and maternal grandfather also experienced fainting with minor pain.

Epidemiology, Etiology, Pathogenesis, & Treatment

Specific phobias are the most common anxiety disorders. Peak onset is in childhood (fears of strangers, large animals, snakes, the dark, and injury are very common), and a rapid and spontaneous resolution of most of these phobias is the rule, probably because of developmental maturation and natural exposure. In the past, many of these fears had actual survival value for comparatively defenseless small children and would not have been diagnosed as phobias. Their atavistic persistence leads to their definition as phobias. The vast majority of such fears abate without formal treatment. The NIMH-ECA study found that 7% of females and 4.3% of males met *DSM-III* diagnostic criteria for specific phobia. The National Comorbidity Survey using *DSM-III-R* criteria found 12-month prevalence of specific phobias of 13.2% for females and 4.4% for males. That learning plays a part in some specific phobias is most dramatically illustrated by epidemic anxiety (or mass hysteria), such as widespread fainting in schoolgirls after one girl has fainted.

Treatment of specific phobia with exposure therapy is highly successful. Spider phobia, for example, can often be alleviated in a single 2-hour session. One or two "booster" sessions are a prudent follow-up procedure. Patients with flying phobia can be successfully treated with one or two flights in a small plane in which an experienced pilot repeatedly exposes patients to specific phobic stimuli (eg, takeoffs and landings, particular maneuvers, turbulence) until anxiety diminishes to comfortable levels. Blood-

injury phobia should first be treated with the patient recumbent; patients seldom faint when recumbent even if bradycardia occurs. Gradual exposure to the evoking stimulus (eg, a needle) at a rate that does not produce bradycardia is the preferred treatment technique for blood-injury phobia. Most venipuncture phobias can be treated successfully in one or two sessions in a blood-drawing facility.

OBSESSIVE-COMPULSIVE DISORDER

Symptoms & Signs

Obsessions are repetitive, intrusive ideas, images, or impulses. Obsessions commonly focus on harming others, acquiring or spreading contamination, losing things, doubt about having performed routine tasks properly, and transgressing social norms (eg, making unacceptable sexual overtures).

Compulsive rituals are repetitive thoughts or acts usually performed to decrease anxiety or other discomfort associated with obsessions. The acts may be sensible in the abstract, but the frequency and duration of their repetition make them repugnant and inconvenient, even incapacitating. Attempts are usually made to resist rituals, although children and those who have been performing rituals for years may not resist. If prevented from carrying out a ritual, obsessive-compulsive individuals frequently become anxious. Rituals are usually preceded by obsessions, but obsessions do not always lead to rituals. Rituals of cleaning, repeating, checking, tidying, hoarding, and avoiding may consume almost every waking hour. See Table 21–6 for the *DSM-IV* diagnostic criteria for obsessive-compulsive disorder (OCD).

Differential Diagnosis

A classical picture of OCD can emerge as a secondary complication of major depression. Obsessions alone may appear in the context of either depression or schizophrenia, and the distinction between obsessions and delusions can be difficult. There is a tendency to overdiagnose delusions and underdiagnose obsessions. Other attributes of schizophrenia are usually absent in patients with OCD, although some of these patients also suffer from schizotypal personality disorder, which worsens the prognosis.

OCD can usually be differentiated from phobias in the following ways:

1. Phobics are more fearful about confronting the feared object than are obsessive-compulsives, who are usually more concerned about the rituals they will face because of contact with the feared object.
2. The fears of phobics are usually less complex than those of obsessive-compulsives. Phobic fears are more typically focal (eg, fear of fainting while having blood drawn) than the fears of

Table 21–6. *DSM-IV* diagnostic criteria
for obsessive-compulsive disorder.

A. Either obsessions or compulsions:
  Obsessions as defined by (1), (2), (3), and (4):
    (1) Recurrent and persistent thoughts, impulses, or
    images that are experienced, at some time during the
    disturbance, as intrusive and inappropriate and that
    cause marked anxiety or distress. (2) The thoughts,
    impulses, or images are not simply excessive worries
    about real-life problems. (3) The person attempts
    to ignore or suppress such thoughts, impulses, or
    images, or to neutralize them with some other
    thought or action. (4) The person recognizes that
    the obsessional thoughts, impulses, or images are
    a product of his or her own mind (not imposed from
    without as in thought insertion).
  Compulsions as defined by (1) and (2):
    (1) Repetitive behaviors (eg, hand washing, ordering,
    checking) or mental acts (eg, praying, counting, re-
    peating words silently) that the person feels driven to
    perform in response to an obsession, or according to
    rules that must be applied rigidly. (2) The behaviors or
    mental acts are aimed at preventing or reducing dis-
    tress or preventing some dreaded event or situation;
    however, these behaviors or mental acts either are
    not connected in a realistic way with what they are
    designed to neutralize or prevent or are clearly exces-
    sive.

B. At some point during the course of the disorder, the person has recognized that the obsessions or compulsions
  are excessive or unreasonable. **Note:** This does not
  apply to children.

C. The obsessions or compulsions cause marked distress,
  are time consuming (take more than 1 hour a day), or
  significantly interfere with the person's normal routine,
  occupational (or academic) functioning, or usual social
  activities or relationships.

D. If another Axis I disorder is present, the content of the
  obsessions or compulsions is not restricted to it (eg,
  preoccupation with food in the presence of an eating
  disorder; hair pulling in the presence of trichotillomania;
  concern with appearance in the presence of body
  dysmorphic disorder; preoccupation with drugs in the
  presence of a substance use disorder; preoccupation
  with having a serious illness in the presence of
  hypochondriasis; preoccupation with sexual urges or fantasies in the presence of paraphillia; or guilty ruminations
  in the presence of major depressive disorder).

E. The disturbance is not due to the direct physiological effects of a substance (eg, a drug of abuse, a medication)
  or a general medical condition.

Specify if:
  With Poor Insight: If, for most of the time during the
  current episode, the person does not recognize that
  the obsessions and compulsions are excessive or
  unreasonable.

sive checking with doctors are not considered OCD if
the content of obsessions or compulsions is restricted
to that disorder (eg, preoccupation with food in the
presence of an eating disorder, hair pulling in the
presence of trichotillomania, concern with appearance in the presence of body dysmorphic disorder, or
preoccupation with drugs in the presence of substance use disorder, or preoccupation with having a
serious illness in the presence of hypochondriasis).
Nevertheless, these and other obsessive-compulsive
spectrum disorders share some phenomenologic
characteristics with OCD, and some sufferers respond to the same treatments effective in OCD.

Prognosis

Dysfunction is defined in terms of the amount of
time consumed by obsessions and rituals, interference with functioning, control over obsessions and
rituals, and the amount of suffering endured. The disorder usually lasts for decades once it has begun and
runs an undulating course, worsening if the individual becomes depressed and temporarily improving if
the individual can successfully avoid obsessions that
provoke rituals. However, such relief is usually short-
lived, as new obsessions and corresponding rituals
replace those that have disappeared. At its worst, obsessive-compulsive disorder can consume the individual and interfere substantially with family functioning.

Illustrative Case

Ten years before she sought treatment, a 31-year-
old registered nurse noted gradual onset of fears that
she would contaminate needles or intravenous apparatus. Nine years before treatment, she changed from
inpatient to outpatient nursing because of constant
doubt about her skill in safely performing common
nursing tasks. For intramuscular injections, she would
aspirate the syringe two or three times before injecting medication to ensure that the needle was not in a
blood vessel. Cleaning instruments was an ordeal because she often repeated the procedure to ensure
sterility and still felt anxious about the possibility of
contamination. She repeatedly asked for reassurance
from physicians regarding the safety of air bubbles in
syringes. At this point, her worries were confined to
work. As her anxiety and uncertainty in outpatient
work increased, she left clinical medicine and became
a claims adjuster in an insurance company. Her quest
for accuracy led to checking and rechecking of coding, which interfered substantially with the quantity
of work performed and produced feelings of guilt
about not working to her full potential.

As years passed, her concerns spread to the home
setting and her person. She worried that she had become soiled by urine and feces, and this led to rituals
of repeatedly washing her body and clothing. The latter then became impossible because she felt that she
might have put feces, instead of soap, into the wash-

obsessive-compulsives (there are myriad ways
one can become contaminated).

3. Anxiety of phobics is usually greater than that
  exhibited by obsessive-compulsives when both
  confront the things they fear.

So-called compulsive behaviors such as eating, hair
pulling, dysmorphophobia, drug taking, and exces-

ing machine. This "grotesque" thought continued until she was treated with a combination of exposure therapy (she no longer permitted herself to wear gloves or use tissues when touching the telephone, doorknobs, etc) and response prevention, in which she was asked to delay her washing and checking rituals for 3 hours after exposure sessions. With these behavioral treatments, her symptoms diminished rapidly and dramatically, so that she eventually experienced little interference with everyday activities. Common tricyclic antidepressants had not modified her anxiety or rituals at all, but clomipramine, administered after improvement following behavior therapy had stabilized, yielded further worthwhile gains.

Epidemiology

In one-third of obsessive-compulsive individuals, onset of the disorder occurs by the age of 15. A second peak of incidence occurs during the third decade of life. Once established, OCD is likely to persist throughout life with varying degrees of severity. Men are only slightly less likely to suffer this disorder than women. In the NIMH-ECA study 6-month prevalence of OCD was approximately 1.5% and lifetime prevalence was 2.5%. There has been concern about the accuracy of the ECA OCD diagnoses, because only 19.2% of those receiving a lifetime diagnosis continued to meet criteria for the diagnosis 1 year later (Nelson and Rice, 1997).

Etiology & Pathogenesis

OCD clusters in families and appears to have a partly hereditary basis. In individuals with the disorder, once an obsessive thought intrudes, the forces maintaining its recurrence are uncertain. Efforts to demonstrate meaningful linkages between obsessions and unconscious conflict have failed to yield useful treatment techniques or to persuade many psychiatrists that such hypotheses have anything to do with the cause or pathogenesis of the disorder. A more credible behavioral explanation is that once the anxiety or discomfort associated with obsessive thought begins, sufferers gain at least temporary partial relief by performing rituals that are tied in a quasilogical way to their obsessions. However, in time, most rituals must be performed to great excess.

The biochemical and anatomic bases of OCD have not been fully defined, but present research suggests that among any probable contributory factors, dysfunction of serotonin neurotransmission in a circuit involving the orbital cortex, caudate, globus pallidus, and thalamus may play a prominent part.

Treatment

A. Behavioral Therapy: Behavioral therapy employing exposure and prevention of ritualistic responses yields a 60–80% reduction in symptoms for the three-fourths of patients who are able to comply with treatment instructions. Family members are often included as co-therapists. They are instructed to praise the patient when appropriate and to refrain from giving the patient counterproductive reassurance. Many obsessive-compulsives become "reassurance junkies" in their quest for certainty; reassurance can be viewed as a ritual avoidance of the anxiety associated with uncertainty. Behavioral therapy for these patients essentially involves asking them to run the same risks of contamination, uncertainty, and doubt that confront everyone and to stop performing rituals as an excessively costly and ineffective method of gaining transient and illusory certainty of safety.

B. Drug Therapy:

1. Antidepressants—Most antidepressants do not appear to have specific anti–obsessive-compulsive properties, but clomipramine and other potent serotonin reuptake inhibitors (SRIs) (fluoxetine, fluvoxamine, paroxetine, and sertraline proven; citalopram probable) do have anti–obsessive-compulsive effects independent of their antidepressant properties.

2. Anxiolytics—Antianxiety medications have a limited role in the long-term treatment of OCD but are sometimes helpful in the management of acute anxiety.

3. Antipsychotic drugs—Standard antipsychotic medications added to potent SRIs have been shown to be beneficial for patients with concurrent tics. Atypical antipsychotics offer some benefit as augmentation for patients without comorbidities who are unresponsive to SRIs alone.

C. Other Treatment:

1. Electroconvulsive therapy—Electroconvulsive therapy is sometimes helpful in individuals with severe primary depression and secondary obsessions and rituals, but has not been shown to be beneficial for OCD alone.

2. Psychotherapy—Some obsessive-compulsive patients are still treated with dynamic psychotherapy, often for many years, without manifest relief or improvement in functioning. Psychotherapists often point to "intrapsychic" benefits in patients who remain as troubled with obsessions and rituals as when therapy began. Although unfortunate, this example of difficulty in changing treatment methods in the face of strong evidence supporting an effective alternative approach has long been recognized (Kuhn, 1962).

3. Neurosurgery—Anterior cingulotomy, stereotactic limbic leukotomy (combining anterior cingulotomy and subcaudate tractotomy), and anterior capsulotomy (Mindus, 1992) have been shown to help some severely ill obsessive-compulsive patients who have failed to benefit from other treatments.

POSTTRAUMATIC STRESS DISORDER

Symptoms & Signs

The *DSM-IV* diagnostic criteria for posttraumatic stress disorder (PTSD) are presented in Table 21–7.

Table 21–7. *DSM-IV* diagnostic criteria for posttraumatic stress disorder.

A. The person has been exposed to a traumatic event in which both of the following were present:
(1) The person experienced, witnessed, or was confronted with an event or events that involved actual or threatened death or serious injury, or a threat to the physical integrity of self or others. (2) The person's response involved intense fear, helplessness, or horror. **Note:** In children, this may be expressed instead by disorganized or agitated behavior.

B. The traumatic event is persistently reexperienced in one (or more) of the following ways:
(1) Recurrent and intrusive distressing recollections of the event, including images, thoughts, or perceptions. **Note:** In young children, repetitive play may occur in which themes or aspects of the trauma are expressed. (2) recurrent distressing dreams of the event. **Note:** In children, there may be frightening dreams without recognizable content. (3) acting or feeling as if the traumatic event were recurring (includes a sense of reliving the experience, illusions, hallucinations, and dissociative flashback episodes, including those that occur on awakening or when intoxicated). **Note:** In young children, trauma-specific reenactment may occur. (4) intense psychological distress at exposure to internal or external cues that symbolize or resemble an aspect of the traumatic event, (5) physiological reactivity on exposure to internal or external cues that symbolize or resemble an aspect of the traumatic event.

C. Persistent avoidance of stimuli associated with the trauma and numbing of general responsiveness (not present before the trauma), as indicated by three (or more) of the following:
(1) Efforts to avoid thoughts, feelings, or conversations associated with the trauma, (2) efforts to avoid activities, places, or people that arouse recollections of the trauma, (3) inability to recall an important aspect of the trauma, (4) markedly diminished interest or participation in significant activities, (5) feeling of detachment or estrangement from others, (6) restricted range of affect (eg, unable to have loving feelings), (7) sense of a foreshortened future (eg, does not expect to have a career, marriage, children, or a normal life span).

D. Persistent symptoms of increased arousal (not present before the trauma), as indicated by two (or more) of the following:
(1) Difficulty falling or staying asleep, (2) irritability or outbursts of anger, (3) difficulty concentrating, (4) hypervigilance, (5) exaggerated startle response.

E. Duration of the disturbance (symptoms in Criteria B, C, and D) is more than 1 month.

F. The disturbance causes clinically significant distress or impairment in social, occupational, or other important areas of functioning.

Specify if:
Acute: If duration of symptoms is less than 3 months.
Chronic: If duration of symptoms is 3 months or more.

Specify if:
With Delayed Onset: If onset of symptoms is at least 6 months after the stressor.

Many people experience a psychological traumatic stressor "outside the range of usual human experience," but few develop PTSD. Many of those subjected to psychologically traumatic stressors reexperience them in dreams or memory with associated unpleasant feelings; changes in affect and reexperiencing of trauma usually diminish in frequency and intensity (just as recall of pleasant events does) and are not in themselves signs of PTSD.

A diagnosis of PTSD requires the presence of substantial disruption in functioning or suffering associated with reexperiencing the trauma, persistent symptoms of arousal, and signs of numbing or avoidance.

A diagnosis of PTSD cannot be made unless symptoms persist for at least 1 month. PTSD is diagnosed as acute if symptoms last less than 3 months and as chronic if symptoms last 3 months or more; delayed onset should be specified if symptoms became apparent more than 6 months after the trauma.

Differential Diagnosis

Most of the time, the human capacity for recall and associated affect does not provoke substantial dysfunction or suffering and should not be diagnosed as PTSD.

Adjustment disorders involve "a maladaptive reaction to an identifiable psychosocial stressor" but a broader range of less extreme human experiences (eg, the nonviolent death of a relative) and may result in a few of the symptoms found in PTSD (eg, symptoms of arousal, numbing, or avoidance). Intense reexperiencing is less common with adjustment disorders.

Prognosis

Acute PTSD usually responds well to simple measures of support, emotional catharsis, and return to activity if they are promptly applied. Full recovery is the rule rather than the exception. Chronic PTSD, however, is more difficult to treat and may last for decades while causing varying degrees of disability.

Illustrative Case

Four years before seeking treatment, a highly successful truck driver with a 21-year history of accident-free driving had been involved in a two-truck accident in which the other driver was trapped and burned to death despite the patient's effort to free him. In addition to burns received in the rescue attempt, he also suffered a concussion, bruises, and a scalp laceration. While still in the hospital immediately after the accident, the man had nightmares involving repetition of the incident. He became wary about falling asleep, was reluctant to discuss the accident with his family or authorities, and claimed he could not remember much of what happened. The patient seemed markedly distant to close family members and expressed the worry that not much could be counted on in life. Irritability was noted by all, and he appeared to have difficulty concentrating.

Because of the circumstances of the accident, he was not permitted to resume work as a truck driver for more than 9 months until administrative hearings concluded that he had not been at fault. During that interval, his condition remained largely as described, although his nightmares became less frequent and the quality of his relationship with his family improved. When he was allowed to resume work, he felt extreme apprehension and could not bring himself to drive again because of fear that another accident would result. He was also fearful about driving or riding in a car, and he specifically stated that he had "seen what trucks can do." Tricyclic antidepressant medication decreased the frequency of nightmares and improved sleep but had little effect on his anxiety and avoidance. Previous psychotherapy had not been helpful, and exposure therapy did little to ease his distress.

Epidemiology

Since a psychologically traumatic experience is a prerequisite for PTSD, incidence and prevalence figures would ideally be related to several different types of trauma. However, no uniform classification of trauma has been accepted. The potential for high prevalence of PTSD-like phenomena is demonstrated by an 80% incidence of acute posttraumatic syndrome in survivors of the Buffalo Creek flood disaster and a 57% prevalence after 1 year in survivors of the Cocoanut Grove fire; it should be remembered that diagnostic criteria have changed and that some diagnoses were based on unstructured interviews.

A survey of 2500 citizens of St. Louis conducted as part of the NIMH-ECA study found a lifetime prevalence of 1% in both sexes. Fifteen percent of subjects in the study had at least one symptom of PTSD. Of those exposed to psychological trauma "outside the range of usual human experience," 4% satisfied *DSM-III* criteria for the disorder and 20% experienced some symptoms of the disorder. In a group of 15 Vietnam combat veterans who were wounded, 20% fully satisfied *DSM-III* criteria for PTSD and 60% had one or more combat-related symptoms (Helzer, 1987).

Etiology & Pathogenesis

Since different individuals experiencing the same trauma respond differently, the cause and pathogenesis of PTSD involve many factors. The relative contributions of genetic endowment, physical development, psychological maturity, social support, cultural expectations, past experience with trauma, and the nature of the trauma itself are unclear. Psychologically, failure to integrate a traumatic experience into a person's life experiences may lead to an alternating pattern of reexperiencing the traumatic event and defensive numbing when the reexperiencing itself proves traumatic (Horowitz, 1976).

Treatment

A. Acute Posttraumatic Stress Disorder: Excellent evidence gathered in military conflicts from World War II onward indicates that individuals suffering from incapacitating acute PTSD are highly likely to recover fully if they are treated as follows: As symptoms and signs of PTSD emerge in combat and are recognized by fellow soldiers, the affected individuals are removed from the front line and sent to the nearest aid station. There, they are kept in uniform, given food, encouraged to talk about their experiences, and told that their reaction is normal for the trauma they have experienced. They are expected to perform duties within their capabilities, are not permitted to assume the role of patients, and are returned to the front line within 24–72 hours. Sedation is unnecessary and may be counterproductive because of the suggestion of a "sick role" and possible induction of state-dependent learning. The Israeli experience in the 1973 Yom Kippur War found these techniques effective in restoring soldiers to combat fitness and in preventing development of chronic PTSD. This approach appears to include important elements of graduated exposure.

The implications of war experience for acute posttraumatic stress syndromes in civilians are obvious and confirm the old aphorism: "You must climb right back on the horse that throws you."

B. Chronic or Delayed Posttraumatic Stress Disorder: Effective treatments for chronic PTSD are available. Exposure in fantasy or, when it may be done with safety, in real life (eg, asking a woman who has been raped to revisit the site of the rape) has been shown to be helpful to some, but not all, patients. For others, exposure seems a form of reexperiencing that they (and some therapists) view as too distressing and possibly sensitizing. Other behavioral therapists experienced in working with patients suffering from PTSD maintain that exposure is effective for most patients unless they are markedly depressed. Exposure is most helpful for the phobic avoidance and anxiety symptoms associated with this disorder.

Medications are often helpful in relieving dysphoric and depressive symptoms associated with chronic PTSD. In particular, sleep disturbance and nightmares are often alleviated with a variety of antidepressant medications. Antianxiety medications may be of benefit as well, although the risk of dependence must be kept in mind. β-Blocking agents may be helpful if tremor is a major problem. Recently, SSRIs have demonstrated substantial benefit for reexperiencing, arousal, and avoidance/numbing aspects of PTSD (Davidson, 1997). In late 1999, sertraline became the first FDA-approved drug for the treatment of PTSD.

Psychotherapy aimed at integrating the traumatic experience into the patient's sense of self may be helpful. Such therapy should first employ techniques of catharsis and abreaction, which may properly be viewed as a form of exposure in fantasy. If these brief psychotherapeutic approaches prove ineffective, more extensive exploration of the meanings of the trauma may be undertaken, although evidence for the effectiveness of long-term psychotherapy is scant.

GENERALIZED ANXIETY DISORDER

Symptoms & Signs

The *DSM-IV* diagnostic criteria for generalized anxiety disorder are listed in Table 21–8. This diagnosis has been made less frequently in the United States since panic disorder was introduced in *DSM-III* in 1980. In Great Britain and Europe, where panic is usually viewed as extreme anxiety and not as a categorically discrete disorder, a diagnosis of generalized anxiety disorder is more common.

Differential Diagnosis

Several of the symptoms of generalized anxiety disorder are commonly present in mild depression (sometimes called dysphoria or dysthymia). Generalized anxiety disorder usually causes less dysfunction than other anxiety disorders (except specific phobia). Caffeine intoxication and withdrawal from central nervous system depressant substances can mimic generalized anxiety disorder. Because of the substantial overlap in motor tension and autonomic hyperactivity symptoms with those of panic disorder, careful attention to the possibility of panic is essential in distinguishing between generalized anxiety disorder and panic disorder.

Table 21–8. *DSM-IV* diagnostic criteria for generalized anxiety disorder.

A. Excessive anxiety and worry (apprehensive expectation), occurring more days than not for at least 6 months, about a number of events or activities (such as work or school performance).

B. The person finds it difficult to control the worry.

C. The anxiety and worry are associated with three (or more) of the following six symptoms (with at least some symptoms present for more days than not for the past 6 months). **Note:** Only one item is required in children. (1) Restlessness or feeling keyed up or on edge, (2) being easily fatigued, (3) difficulty concentrating or mind going blank, (4) irritability, (5) muscle tension, (6) sleep disturbance (difficulty falling or staying asleep, or restless unsatisfying sleep).

D. The focus of the anxiety and worry is not confined to features of an Axis I disorder, eg, the anxiety or worry is not about having a panic attack (as in panic disorder), being embarrassed in public (as in social phobia), being contaminated (as in obsessive-compulsive disorder), being away from home or close relatives (as in separation anxiety disorder), gaining weight (as in anorexia nervosa), having multiple physical complaints (as in somatization disorder), or having a serious illness (as in hypochondriasis), and the anxiety and worry do not occur exclusively during posttraumatic stress disorder.

E. The anxiety, worry, or physical symptoms cause clinically significant distress or impairment in social, occupational, or other important areas of functioning.

F. The disturbance is not due to the direct physiological effects of a substance (eg, a drug of abuse, a medication) or a general medical condition (eg, hyperthyroidism) and does not occur exclusively during a mood disorder, a psychotic disorder, or a pervasive developmental disorder.

Epidemiology

The National Comorbidity Survey found the 12-month prevalence of generalized anxiety disorder to be 2.0% in males and 4.3% in females.

Etiology & Pathogenesis

As with all of the anxiety disorders, many factors are probably involved in the etiology and pathogenesis of generalized anxiety disorder.

A. Biochemical Theories: The up- and down-regulation of noradrenergic function mediated largely through the locus ceruleus (Redmond, 1977) and demonstration of brain benzodiazepine receptors (Squires and Braestrup, 1977) and their interaction with γ-aminobutyric acid (GABA) (Paul et al, 1980) have stimulated research on the role played by the GABA-benzodiazepine and noradrenergic-locus ceruleus systems. The GABA-benzodiazepine system may be more active in generalized anxiety disorder, whereas the noradrenergic-locus ceruleus system is more often implicated in the etiology of panic.

B. Behavioral Theories: Successful avoidance of noxious stimuli (unconditioned stimulus), which reduces discomfort or trauma (unconditioned response), is usually reinforced in both humans and other species (Kandel, 1983). When avoidance in humans produces unpredictable results, avoidance becomes unreliable, and generalized anxiety is thought to develop.

C. Psychological Theories: A state of generalized anxiety is thought by many dynamic psychotherapists to reflect an unconscious conflict about dangerous emotions, behaviors, or states (eg, anger, depression, injury or death, sexual arousal, hunger, and anxiety itself). Another theory postulates that some individuals with generalized anxiety disorder may seek anxiety-provoking stimuli and maintain themselves in situations likely to evoke high anxiety in order to achieve mastery over anxiety, gain relief through the eventual cessation of such anxiety states, or avoid an even less enjoyable affective state such as anger or boredom.

Prognosis

Generalized anxiety disorder persists for at least 6 months and, commonly, for many years. Untreated, it usually waxes and wanes in response to common stressors and unspecified factors. With treatment (eg, antianxiety medication), symptoms are reduced but usually reemerge when treatment is stopped.

Illustrative Case

For as long as he could remember, a 53-year-old man had "worried" about things that never came to pass; their possible occurrence had little foundation in reality, and if they did occur, they were unlikely to be of serious consequence. He described himself as always feeling tense and restless, sometimes trembling or being on edge, and feeling irritable and easily fatigued. He had trouble falling and staying asleep because of "worries." At times of peak worry, he described symptoms of autonomic distress, including dry mouth, sweating, tachycardia, urinary frequency, and diarrhea. These symptoms were present most days to a greater or lesser degree and never worsened suddenly.

He had engaged in two courses of psychotherapy, each lasting more than 1 year, as well as "relaxation training" and biofeedback. None of these treatments had led to meaningful reduction in symptoms. When benzodiazepines became available, his family physician began treatment with diazepam, which proved remarkably effective over the following 20 years at a dose of 15 mg/d. The patient never increased the dosage, and on repeated occasions, when he or his doctor had attempted to withdraw the medication, symptoms returned.

Treatment

A. Drug Treatment: Benzodiazepine antianxiety drugs are effective in reducing or alleviating symptoms of generalized anxiety in many patients. Return of symptoms is common when benzodiazepines are discontinued. Sedation is the major side effect, and physiological dependence will occur in most patients taking benzodiazepines steadily over several months. Despite this potential, the incidence of benzodiazepine abuse is quite low except in those who abuse other substances, and many patients find these agents effective for generalized anxiety disorder and do not take more than the prescribed dosage.

Buspirone, an azapirone, is also useful in treating generalized anxiety disorder. It does not have sedative effects, does not interact with alcohol, and does not lead to dependence.

Tricyclic antidepressants and venlafaxine have been shown to be effective treatments for generalized anxiety disorder, the latter having recently been approved for this condition by the FDA. They avoid risks of physical dependency associated with benzodiazepine treatment but usually cause more side effects. β-Adrenergic blocking agents and antihistamines have limited roles in the treatment of symptoms associated with generalized anxiety. Barbiturates and meprobamate have been superseded by benzodiazepines, buspirone, and, to a lesser degree, nefazodone, mirtazapine, and SSRIs.

B. Behavioral Therapy: Behavioral therapy has not been of particular benefit in the treatment of generalized anxiety disorder because it is difficult to specify situations or stimuli to which the individual should be exposed. Relaxation and biofeedback are commonly advocated, but their efficacy has not been validated in controlled studies of clinically significant generalized anxiety disorder.

C. Psychotherapy: For decades, dynamic psychotherapy was the treatment of choice for general-

ized anxiety. Unfortunately, evidence from controlled studies supporting the efficacy of this approach is limited at best. Cognitive therapy is being evaluated and has shown some promise (Woodward et al, 1980).

OTHER ANXIETY DISORDERS

DSM-IV formalizes the long-standing recognition that somatic conditions can cause and substances can induce anxiety disorders. Presentations may be typical for the several anxiety disorders alone or may include manifestations associated with the medical condition or substance use/withdrawal. Obviously, management of these secondary anxiety disorders should be directed at identifying and removing or ameliorating the primary causative conditions. Often the anxiety disorders engendered by the medical conditions or substances will then abate without specific treatment, and if treatment is required, it is likely to be more successful. When treatments for what appear to be primary anxiety disorders fail to work as expected, careful rediagnosis may identify comorbid medical conditions or substances that complicate or cause the anxiety disorder.

Anxiety disorder not otherwise specified (*DSM-IV* 300.00) is intended for disorders with prominent anxiety, phobic avoidance, or obsessions and rituals that fail to meet criteria for a specific anxiety disorder, adjustment disorder with anxiety, or adjustment disorder with mixed anxiety and depressed mood. Examples include the following:

1. Fear that one's physical appearance or body odor is offensive, leading to social avoidance
2. Significant symptoms of social phobia related to the social impact of a general medical condition or mental disorder such as Parkinson's disease, dermatological conditions, stuttering, or anorexia nervosa
3. Ambiguous situations in which an anxiety disorder appears present but cannot be identified as primary or secondary
4. Finally, the category of mixed anxiety-depressive disorder has been incorporated into the *International Classification of Disease,* 10th edition (*ICD-10*). These individuals suffer clinically significant symptoms of both anxiety and depression, but fail to meet criteria for either a specific mood or anxiety disorder. There are comparatively few studies of treatments for mixed anxiety-depressive disorder, but clinicians often employ antidepressant medications, which also exert antianxiety effects, and cognitive-behavioral psychotherapies, which are helpful for both anxiety and depressive disorders.

SUMMARY

Anxiety is a common emotion with adaptive value for most individuals most of the time. For some, anxiety is so intense or lasts so long that it becomes maladaptive and is properly diagnosed as a disorder. Treatment of anxiety disorders has improved substantially over the past two decades, with behavioral and drug therapies forming the foundations of effective treatment. Table 21–9 illustrates a synopsis of current treatments for anxiety disorders. Classification is becoming more refined, and understanding of the epidemiological, genetic, developmental, psychological, behavioral, biochemical, and environmental aspects of anxiety is growing steadily (Marks, 1987).

Table 21–9. Clinical approach to anxiety.

Disorder	Treatment[a]
Medical	Treat underlying disorder
Primary depression	Treat depression
Spontaneous panic	TCA, MAOI, BZ, SSRI, CBT
Phobic avoidance	BT
Obsessive-compulsive	BT, CMI, SSRI
Social phobia	MAOI, BZ, GP, SSRI, β-blockers
Generalized anxiety	BZ, Busp, VEN
Posttraumatic stress	BT, SSRI, TCA, MAOI

[a] Abbreviations: BT, behavior therapy; Busp, buspirone; BZ, benzodiazepine; CBT, cognitive-behavioral therapy; CMI, clomipramine; GP, gabapentin; MAOI, monoamine oxidase inhibitor; SSRI, selective serotonin reuptake inhibitor; TCA, tricyclic antidepressant; VEN, venlafaxine.

REFERENCES & SUGGESTED READINGS

Barlow DH: *Anxiety and Its Disorders: The Nature and Treatment of Anxiety and Panic.* Guilford, 1998.

Baxter LR et al: Local cerebral glucose metabolic rates in OCD. Arch Gen Psychiatry 1987;44:211.

Davidson JRT: Posttraumatic stress disorder in primary care: Diagnosis and pharmacologic treatment. Primary Psychiatry 1997;4(2):23.

Greist JH et al: Avoidance versus confrontation of fear. Behav Res Ther 1980;11:1.

Greist JH, Jefferson JW, Marks IM: *Anxiety and Its Treatment: Help Is Available.* American Psychiatric Press, 1986. [Also available as a Warner paperback, 1986.]

Helzer JE, Robins LN, McEvoy LT: Post-traumatic stress disorder in the general population: Findings of the Epidemiologic Catchment Area Survey. N Engl J Med 1987;317:1630.

Horowitz MJ: *Stress Response Syndromes.* Jason Aronson, 1976.

Jenike MA, Baer L, Minichiello WE (editors): *Obsessive-Compulsive Disorders: Theory and Management,* 2nd ed. PSG, 1990.

Kandel ER: From metapsychology to molecular biology: Explorations into the nature of anxiety. Am J Psychiatry 1983;140:1277.

Kessler RC et al: Lifetime and 12-month prevalence of *DSM-III-R* psychiatric disorders in the United States. Arch Gen Psychiatry 1994;51:8.

Kuhn TS: *The Structure of Scientific Revolutions.* University of Chicago Press, 1962.

Marks IM: Genetics of fear and anxiety disorders. Br J Psychiatry 1986;149:406.

Marks IM: *Fears, Phobias and Rituals: The Nature of Anxiety and Panic Disorder.* Oxford University Press, 1987.

Mindus P: Neurosurgical treatment of malignant obsessive compulsive disorder. Psychiatr Clin North Am 1992; 15(4):921.

Myers JK et al: Six-month prevalence of psychiatric disorders in three communities, 1980–1982. Arch Gen Psychiatry 1984;41:959.

Nelson E, Rice J: Stability of diagnosis of obsessive-compulsive disorder in the Epidemiologic Catchment Area study. Am J Psychiatry 1997;154(6):826.

Nutt D, Lawson C: Panic attacks: A neurochemical overview of models and mechanisms. Br J Psychiatry 1992;160:165.

Pande AC et al: Treatment of social phobia with gabapentin: A placebo-controlled trial. J Clin Psychopharmacol 1999;19:341.

Paul SM, Skolnich P, Gallager DW: Receptors for the age of anxiety: Pharmacology of the benzodiazepines. Science 1980;207:274.

Redmond DE Jr: Alterations in the function of the nucleus locus coeruleus: Possible model for studies of anxiety. In: *Animal Models in Psychiatry and Neurology.* Usdin E, Hanin I (editors). Pergamon, 1977.

Squires RF, Braestrup C: Benzodiazepine receptors in rat brain. Nature 1977;266:732.

Stein MB et al: Paroxetine treatment of generalized social phobia (social anxiety disorder): A randomized controlled trial. JAMA 1998;280:708.

Swinson RP et al: Brief treatment of emergency room patients with panic attacks. Am J Psychiatry 1992; 149(7):944.

Somatoform & Dissociative Disorders

22

Richard J. Loewenstein, MD, Shane MacKay, MD, & Stephen D. Purcell, MD

Historically, the somatoform and dissociative disorders have been linked together and viewed as different manifestations of similar psychological processes. Although the phenomena that define these two diagnostic categories are quite different, and the *Diagnostic and Statistical Manual of Mental Disorders (DSM)* has empirically chosen to separate them, psychological factors are believed to have essential etiological significance in most of these disorders.

Recent research has found that it is common for dissociative and somatoform symptoms to coexist in the same individual, either sequentially or simultaneously; that a history of traumatic experiences, particularly subjection to intrafamilial violence in childhood and/or adulthood, reliably predicts numbers of somatoform symptoms markedly higher than found in nonabused controls (McCauley et al, 1995, 1997); and that a history of significant childhood and/or adult trauma or abuse is significantly associated with development of most of the dissociative disorders.

Further, a series of systematic studies from researchers in psychiatry, internal medicine, gastroenterology, neurology, orthopedics, and gynecology have demonstrated higher rates of childhood and adult sexual trauma and abuse compared with controls in patients with unexplained chronic pelvic pain, irritable bowel syndrome (IBS), gastroesophageal reflux disorder (GERD), pseudoseizures, fibromyalgia, late luteal phase dysphoric disorder (LLPDD), morbid obesity, chronic low back pain, and migraine headaches. Studies also have shown that adverse life experiences such as maltreatment and abuse are significantly related to poorer general health status and a variety of poorer outcomes for many medical illnesses (Felitti et al, 1998).

Because interpersonal violence and traumatic experiences are so common in our society, somatoform and dissociative disorders are far more common than had been previously thought. However, only limited epidemiological data exist to document the actual prevalence of these disorders.

SOMATOFORM DISORDERS

As the name implies, the essential feature of the somatoform disorders is the presence of symptoms that suggest somatic (or bodily) disorder. To establish a diagnosis of any one of the somatoform disorders, however, the physical findings and laboratory studies cannot account for the symptoms, and there must be positive evidence—or a strong presumption—that the symptoms have a psychological origin.

Surveys report that during any week, 60–80% of the general population will suffer a somatic symptom. Other studies have shown that 60% percent of visits to a physician in a large HMO studied over many years were for complaints for which no physical or biological difficulties could be discovered. In these studies, another 20–30% of patients were seeking help for disorders with a significant psychological aspect, such as IBS. Somatization is a potentially vast and costly problem in primary care practice. It is particularly important, then, that physicians who are not psychiatrists be familiar with these disorders so that they can recognize and treat them appropriately.

To be sure, apparent somatization is a complex problem with many determinants. These can include undiagnosed or misdiagnosed medical disorders, somatic symptoms due to *DSM-IV* disorders such as anxiety, affective, psychotic, and posttraumatic stress disorders, as well as malingering and factitious disorders. Further, these conditions are not mutually exclusive and more than one can coexist in an individual patient.

There are five subtypes of somatoform disorders: body dysmorphic disorder, somatization disorder, conversion disorder, somatoform pain disorder, and hypochondriasis. In each type, although the symptoms are physical, the specific pathophysiological processes involved are not demonstrable or explicable on the basis of laboratory or other physical diagnostic procedures. A decision tree for the diagnosis of the somatoform disorders is shown in Figure 22–1.

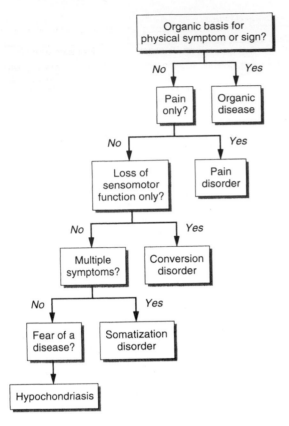

Figure 22–1. Decision tree for diagnosis of the somatoform disorders.

BODY DYSMORPHIC DISORDER

Body dysmorphic disorder (BDD) is covered here only briefly. BDD involves concerns about the body. However, recent research has led to the view that this condition is better conceptualized as part of the obsessive-compulsive disorder (OCD) spectrum, not as one of the somatoform disorders. Recent research suggests that almost 2% of the general population may suffer from this disorder.

This disorder involves the preoccupation with an imagined defect in appearance in a person whose actual appearance is unremarkable. If a slight abnormality is present, the individual's concern is out of proportion to the defect. These patients typically focus on skin wrinkles and blemishes, facial hair, or the shape of the nose, mouth, or jaw. Some patients with this disorder are aware that their concerns are exaggerated. In others, the disorder manifests itself with delusional intensity. These patients typically seek reassurance about their condition, but rarely are relieved by its provision. Many of these patients are severely impaired and unable to function. High rates of psychiatric hospitalization and suicide attempts have been noted among BDD patients.

A majority of BDD patients are thought to seek treatment or referral from dermatologists and/or reconstructive or plastic surgeons for surgical correction of the perceived anomaly. Seven to 15% of patients seeking cosmetic surgery may suffer from this condition (Phillips et al, 1999). Medical interventions and/or reconstructive or plastic surgery almost never resolve these patients' preoccupations, and additional pursuit of medical and/or surgical interventions usually follow. Violence toward physicians by disgruntled BDD patients has occurred. Other BDD patients may attempt suicide when their perceived deformity persists despite surgical interventions.

Physicians should be aware of these patients' insistence on unnecessary surgery or reconstructive procedures and resist pressure for these. BDD patients should be referred for psychiatric consultation despite their reluctance to view their difficulties as mental. Recent studies suggest that these patients, even those with delusional preoccupations, respond preferentially to antidepressants with antiobsessive efficacy, particularly clomipramine and fluvoxamine (Hollander et al, 1999).

SOMATIZATION DISORDER

Historically, somatization disorder has been known as both hysteria and Briquet's syndrome. The diagnosis and treatment of somatization disorder are summarized in Table 22–1.

Symptoms & Signs

According to *DSM-IV*, somatization disorder is characterized by multiple physical symptoms that recur over a period of several years and are either unrelated to an identifiable physical disorder or grossly in excess of physical findings. A diagnosis of somatization disorder cannot be made unless symptoms occur in contexts other than panic attacks and unless symptoms have been severe enough to drive the patient to attempt self-medication with drugs other than aspirin, to seek medical attention, or to make life-style changes. The symptoms are often part of a complicated medical history and may be vaguely defined or presented in a dramatic or exaggerated manner. People with this disorder have usually seen many physicians, sometimes simultaneously. Anxiety and depressed mood are common associated symptoms. When mental health care is sought by people with these disorders, it is usually because of these psychiatric symptoms and not because the physical symptoms are believed to have a psychological basis.

Dissociative disorders and posttraumatic stress disorder (PTSD) commonly coexist with somatization disorder. In one study, patients with PTSD were 90 times more likely to have associated somatization than patients with other psychiatric disorders. Histrionic personality disorder, mixed personality disorder

Table 22–1. Somatoform disorders.

	Somatization Disorder	Conversion Disorder	Somatoform Pain Disorder	Hypochondriasis
Key features	Multiple somatic symptoms without organic basis	Loss or change in physical function due to psychological conflict; usually pseudoneurological symptoms predominate	Preoccupation with pain in the absence of, or in excess of, objective findings	Fear of having, or belief that one has, a serious physical disease
Epidemiology (1.5–3.5% of primary care patients)	0.2–2% of general population	Relatively uncommon	Relatively more common	4–9% in general medical practice
Differential diagnosis	Medical disorders such as systemic lupus erythematosus, multiple sclerosis, porphyria, thyroid disease; psychiatric disorders such as schizophrenia, depression, posttraumatic stress disorder	Medical disorders such as multiple sclerosis, myasthenia gravis, polymyositis, brain tumor, stroke; psychiatric disorders such as dissociative identity disorder, schizophrenia, depression, somatization disorder, factitious disorder, malingering	Coronary artery disease, lumbar disc disease, endometriosis, and reflex sympathetic dystrophy; psychiatric disorders such as dissociative identity disorder, schizophrenia, posttraumatic stress disorder, mood disorders	Medical illness; psychiatric disorders such as mood disorders, anxiety disorders, somatization disorder, schizophrenia
Treatment	Consolidation of care with one primary care physician; group or individual psychotherapy	Psychotherapy, hypnotherapy, drug-facilitated interviews	Specialized multidisciplinary team; consolidation of care; cognitive-behavioral psychotherapy; antidepressant medication	Consolidation of medical care; supportive relationship with primary care doctor; psychotherapy in rare cases

(personality disorder not otherwise specified [NOS]), and, less frequently, antisocial personality disorder are also sometimes present. Concurrent occupational, interpersonal, and marital difficulties are common. The most frequent complaints are of being "sickly," with pain, psychosexual symptoms, and symptoms associated with the neurological, gastrointestinal, and reproductive systems (Table 22–2).

Natural History

The pattern of multiple, recurrent physical symptoms begins most often during the teen years but (by definition) always before age 30. In women, menstrual problems may signal the onset of this disorder, but a wide variety of symptoms may be observed in both sexes. Somatization disorder is a chronic disorder, and spontaneous remission occurs rarely; fluctuations in the number and severity of symptoms do occur, but it is unusual for a year to pass without medical attention being sought.

The impact on the lives of people who have this disorder should not be underestimated. Symptoms may be quite severe and persistent to the point of being incapacitating or disruptive to occupational and interpersonal relationships. Because of the continuing search for medical care from different physicians, there is a risk of substantial iatrogenic complications. Physicians who fail to perceive the psychological basis of the patient's physical complaints may perform unnecessary surgical procedures or prescribe medications aimed at treating physiological abnormalities. Each procedure or treatment may have its own set of adverse reactions or complications, requiring more tests and treatments. There is also a risk of substance use disorder from prescribed analgesics or antianxiety agents. Because of associated depressive thoughts or moods, suicidal threats and attempts occur; when suicide results, it is frequently in association with substance abuse.

Somatization disorder is also exceptionally costly in terms of expenditure of unnecessary health care dollars for hospitalizations, surgery, tests and procedures, and medications. One study found dramatic savings in the cost of medical care when primary care physicians were educated about somatization disorder, recognized patients in their practices with this condition, and made efforts to control unneeded interventions for these patients (Smith et al, 1986).

Table 22–2. *DSM-IV* diagnostic criteria for somatization disorder.

A. A history of many physical complaints beginning before age 30 years that occur over a period of several years and result in treatment being sought or significant impairment in social, occupational, or other important areas of functioning.

B. Each of the following criteria must have been met, with individual symptoms occurring at any time during the course of the disturbance:
   (1) *four pain symptoms:* a history of pain related to at least four different sites or functions (eg, head, abdomen, back, joints, extremities, chest, rectum, during menstruation, during sexual intercourse, or during urination), (2) *two gastrointestinal symptoms:* a history of at least two gastrointestinal symptoms other than pain (eg, nausea, bloating, vomiting other than during pregnancy, diarrhea, or intolerance of several different foods), (3) *one sexual symptom:* a history of at least one sexual or reproductive symptom other than pain (eg, sexual indifference, erectile or ejaculatory dysfunction, irregular menses, excessive menstrual bleeding, vomiting throughout pregnancy), (4) *one pseudoneurological symptom:* a history of at least one symptom or deficit suggesting a neurological condition not limited to pain (conversion symptoms such as impaired coordination or balance, paralysis or localized weakness, difficulty swallowing or lump in throat, aphonia, urinary retention, hallucinations, loss of touch or pain sensation, double vision, blindness, deafness, seizures; dissociative symptoms such as amnesia; or loss of consciousness other than fainting).

C. Either (1) or (2):
   (1) after appropriate investigation, each of the symptoms in Criterion B cannot be fully explained by a known general medical condition or the direct effects of a substance (eg, the effects of injury, medication, drugs, or alcohol), (2) when there is a related general medical condition, the physical complaints or resulting social or occupational impairment is in excess of what would be expected from the history, physical examination, or laboratory findings.

D. The symptoms are not intentionally feigned or produced (as in factitious disorder or malingering).

Differential Diagnosis

The differential diagnosis of somatization disorder obviously includes somatic disorders that present with vague or multiple somatic symptoms. These include multiple sclerosis, systemic lupus erythematosus, hyperparathyroidism, and porphyria. It is important to remember that somatization disorder begins before age 30 and, conversely, that the onset of multiple somatic symptoms later in life usually represents somatic disease. Schizophrenia with multiple somatic delusions and major depression with somatic symptoms may occasionally require differentiation from somatization disorder. In panic disorder, physical symptoms may occur, but only in association with panic attacks. PTSD may coexist with somatization disorder and the intrusive recollections of physical and/or sexual trauma may account for some of the somatoform symptoms, although active history taking must usually be done to elicit this association. Conversion disorder involves certain physical symptoms that occur in the absence of the full clinical picture of somatization disorder. Factitious disorder with physical symptoms is distinguished by the presence of conscious deception to produce symptoms. Dissociative disorders are often accompanied by somatoform symptoms and will be discussed later in this chapter.

Somatization disorder, which does not involve any definitive physiological abnormality, should not be confused with the *DSM-IV* disorder Psychological Factors Affecting Physical Condition by contributing either to the onset or exacerbation of a physical disorder or to the perception that an existing physical disorder has worsened.

Prognosis

Without treatment, the prognosis is poor. Spontaneous remission is rare, and a lifelong pattern of seeking medical attention develops with its attendant interference with other aspects of the patient's life and with iatrogenic complications.

Illustrative Case

A 36-year-old twice divorced woman who worked as a salesclerk entered the hospital emergency room at 2:00 AM complaining loudly that something was wrong with her stomach. She was tearful and agitated, with arms held tightly across her abdomen. She stated that shortly after her evening meal she began to feel nauseated and "bloated" and that she vomited some undigested food. Within minutes of vomiting she began to feel a dull pain in her periumbilical area that gradually became sharper and spread throughout her entire abdomen; when the pain became "unbearable," she decided to come to the emergency room.

As the patient calmed down and became more comfortable, she stated that she had had many similar episodes of abdominal discomfort over the past 15 years but that no doctor had been able to determine the cause. At the age of 18 she had had severe salpingitis requiring removal of the left oviduct, and 2 years later, because of persistent abdominal pain, the right ovary was removed. When she was 22, she underwent cholecystectomy, and over the next 10 years she had three abdominal surgical procedures to correct "adhesions" causing abdominal pain. At various times, she said, physicians had told her that she had "an ulcer" or "colitis," but despite a variety of medical treatments her symptoms had persisted. On further questioning, she also admitted to sporadic episodes of dizziness, chest pain that awakened her from sleep, chronic dysuria, occasional urinary retention requiring catheterization, and chronic low back pain. As she finished relating her history, she commented that "only someone with a poor constitution could be sick for this long." She admitted taking diazepam (10 mg) four times a day for "nerves," phenobarbital (30 mg) four times a day for her gastric symptoms, and "some pain pills whenever I need them"—each medication prescribed by a different physician.

She had been hospitalized for psychiatric treatment several times for overdoses and self-injury but had never continued recommended outpatient psychiatric treatment for long.

Family history was significant for alcoholism in both parents, drug abuse and criminal behavior in male siblings, and depression, attempts at suicide, somatization, and abuse of prescription drugs in female siblings. The patient and her sisters had been removed from the family home when she was 16 because of documented physical and sexual abuse by the patient's father and older brothers. She was placed in several foster homes in which she reportedly was also abused. She had been married twice, both times to abusive alcoholics. Protective services had been involved because of her husbands' abusiveness to her children. Her only "happy time" in childhood was when she was hospitalized for repeated episodes of pyelonephritis.

Except for voluntary guarding on palpation of the abdomen and the old abdominal surgical scars, physical examination was normal.

Epidemiology

The lifetime prevalence rate for somatization disorder in primary care settings may range from 1.5% to 3.5% depending on the sample (Simon and Gureje, 1999). The majority of these individuals will seek medical care within a given year. Families of individuals with somatization disorder may also have higher rates of alcohol abuse, antisocial personality disorder, and attention deficit/hyperactivity disorder. High rates of childhood maltreatment, particularly childhood sexual abuse, have been reported in patients with somatization disorder (Pribor et al, 1993).

Etiology & Pathogenesis

Although the increased incidence among family members suggests a genetic basis for somatization disorder, there is no conclusive evidence of that, and no biochemical theories have been adduced to explain the disorder. The relationship between traumatic experiences and somatization disorder has been studied in several recent reports. A strong relationship between traumatic experiences, somatization, dissociation, and affect dysregulation has been found (van der Kolk et al, 1996).

Traumatic experiences may be physically "remembered" as somatoform symptoms. In addition, individuals with histories of abuse may be more likely to perceive normal body sensations as noxious or painful. Interactions with the medical care system may represent ways to seek repair of a subjectively experienced "bad" body related to having been abused. Receiving medical care may have been among the few benign interpersonal experiences for these patients in childhood. Unfortunately, many of these patients have only disappointing experiences with the medical care system along with additional "damage" to their body due to iatrogenic complications (Scarcini et al, 1994).

Other psychological factors leading to a predominance of somatoform symptoms may include pathological identification with a medically ill parent, immature efforts to deal with dependency needs, and maladaptive resolution of intrapsychic conflicts over anger or sexuality.

Treatment

Chronic somatizers often resist psychiatric referral for their disorder because they regard themselves as physically rather than mentally ill. Thus, physicians who are not psychiatrists often have the only opportunity to help these patients. Specific skills and strategies are required with the overall goals of limiting unnecessary medical consultations, tests, and procedures and facilitating the patient's acceptance of psychiatric treatment. Although these patients may be demanding and time consuming, it is important that the primary care provider not fall into the trap of believing that "nothing is wrong" with these patients. They are psychiatrically ill and create tremendous burdens on the medical care system.

Consolidating the patient's care under a single physician helps to limit unnecessary consultations and tests. In teaching hospitals with frequently rotating house staff, a staff physician may be the most appropriate person to see these patients or to be a consistent supervisor for the house staff. Referral to a behavioral medicine clinic, where medical and psychiatric staff work jointly with patients, may be appropriate. In cases in which patients show a capacity for psychological thinking (insight) or motivation to change, referral to a psychiatrist may be indicated. This should be done openly and with full knowledge of the patient.

In working with these patients, the physician must be willing to tolerate the ambiguity that these patients' symptoms present. It is often not possible to completely reassure these patients (or oneself) with negative results, since there are always more tests that can be performed. Instead, physicians should seek to reassure themselves that acute conditions with significant morbidity and mortality have been ruled out and that coexisting medical disorders (if present) are more or less at baseline. The physician should provide unambiguous feedback to the patient about the lack of physical findings, but in a positive way: "I'm happy to tell you that the findings are normal. I can reassure you that no life-threatening condition is present. That means we can proceed carefully and slowly to work with you on your difficulties. I'm sure you don't want all kinds of unnecessary tests or procedures with all those potential side effects and complications."

Patients should not be placated with unwarranted diagnoses or treated for illnesses they do not have.

The physician should listen carefully and/or inquire gently about psychosocial issues from the patient, such as stressful life events or interpersonal conflicts. When organic factors have been ruled out, the physician should attempt to provide the patient with an explanatory model of how physical symptoms can arise in response to psychosocial stressors.

Psychiatric treatment for this disorder may include behavioral, cognitive-behavioral, psychotherapeutic, and pharmacological approaches. Group therapy has been found helpful in some clinic settings. Substantial improvement may be possible in some cases, but many patients will remain chronically debilitated. In any event, significant reduction in medical care costs can be achieved with better primary care management. Younger age, continued employment and work satisfaction, a significant life event preceding the onset of symptoms, absence of a symptom-contingent compensation payment, and the ability to accept the contribution of psychosocial factors to symptoms are associated with a better response to treatment.

CONVERSION DISORDER

Historically, conversion disorder also has been known as hysterical neurosis, conversion type. The diagnosis and treatment of conversion disorder are summarized in Table 22–1.

Symptoms & Signs

Conversion disorder is characterized primarily by loss or alteration of physical functioning that suggests physical disorder but instead is apparently an expression of psychological conflict or need. The symptom is not under voluntary control and cannot be explained by any physical disorder or known pathophysiological mechanism.

Conversion symptoms suggesting neurological disease of the sensory or motor systems are most common: paresis, paralysis, aphonia, seizures, blindness, anesthesia. Occasionally, the autonomic nervous system or the endocrine system may be involved, as with vomiting or pseudocyesis.

By definition, the diagnosis of conversion disorder is not made when the physical alteration is limited to pain or to a disturbance in sexual functioning—in which case the diagnosis of somatoform pain disorder or sexual dysfunction, respectively, is made. This diagnosis is also precluded when the conversion symptom occurs as one component of somatization disorder (Table 22–3).

Natural History

Conversion disorder may begin at any age, but is most likely to make its first appearance in adolescence or early adulthood. There may be only one episode, or episodes may recur over a lifetime. The natural history of the disorder cannot be described with certainty at

Table 22–3. *DSM-IV* diagnostic criteria for conversion disorder.

A. One or more symptoms or deficits affecting voluntary motor or sensory function that suggest a neurological or other general medical condition.

B. Psychological factors are judged to be associated with the symptom or deficit because the initiation or exacerbation of the symptom or deficit is preceded by conflicts or other stressors.

C. The symptom or deficit is not intentionally produced or feigned (as in factitious disorder or malingering).

D. The symptom or deficit cannot, after appropriate investigation, be fully explained by a general medical condition, or by the direct effects of a substance, or as a culturally sanctioned behavior or experience.

E. The symptom or deficit causes clinically significant distress or impairment in social, occupational, or other important areas of functioning or warrants medical evaluation.

F. The symptom or deficit is not limited to pain or sexual dysfunction, does not occur exclusively during the course of somatization disorder, and is not better accounted for by another mental disorder.

Specify type of symptom or deficit:
  With Motor Symptom or Deficit
  With Sensory Symptom or Deficit
  With Seizures or Convulsions
  With Mixed Presentation

present, but the onset seems most often to be abrupt and in the context of psychosocial stress; though variable, the duration is probably most often short, and resolution is rapid. However, some patients may develop chronic conversion disorders with loss of function persisting for years. In one study, the majority of patients with apparent conversion symptoms were found on follow-up to have clear-cut medical illnesses that must have caused the supposed conversion symptoms or significant psychiatric pathology such as depression or psychosis. Occasionally, a patient with a chronic neurological disorder (eg, epilepsy) may develop symptoms (eg, pseudoepileptic fits) without physical evidence of active disease. It is as if the patient "learned" the conversion symptom from previous experience with neurological illness.

As with the physical symptoms occurring in somatization disorder, the symptoms of conversion disorder can be extremely disruptive and can place the individual at risk for the costs and complications of unnecessary medical or surgical treatment. Actual physical problems may result from the conversion symptoms, eg, contractures or disuse atrophy associated with conversion paralysis. A number of factors have been noted to predispose to the development of conversion disorder, including an antecedent somatic disorder, exposure to others with physical symptoms, severe psychosocial stress, and histrionic and dependent personality disorders. Antecedent histories of trauma, abuse, and dissociation have been strongly associated with conversion symptoms, particularly pseudoseizures.

Differential Diagnosis

The differential diagnosis includes somatic disease and is particularly difficult when the underlying disease characteristically presents with vague neurological symptoms, such as multiple sclerosis. A diagnosis of conversion disorder is suggested when the somatic symptom does not conform to an actual known somatic disorder or does not correspond to the anatomy of the nervous system. Examples would be normal pupillary and electroencephalographic responses to light in someone with "blindness" or "stocking-glove anesthesia," in which numbness in a foot or hand is complete and sharply delimited at the wrist or ankle rather than conforming to the distribution of sensory nerves.

Even when a somatic disorder cannot be identified, the diagnosis of conversion disorder should not be made unless there is also clear-cut evidence that the symptom serves a psychological function. Conversion symptoms may occur as one component of somatization disorder. When this occurs, the diagnosis of conversion disorder is not made. Conversion disorder is common in patients with dissociative identity disorder (see below) and occasionally occurs in patients with schizophrenia. Hypochondriasis involves physical symptoms but without any loss or distortion of bodily function. In both factitious disorder and malingering, physical symptoms are consciously feigned, whereas in conversion disorder they are not.

Prognosis

There are no good data on the natural history of conversion disorder, nor have there been large-scale systematic studies characterizing response to treatment. It is believed that many conversion symptoms may resolve over a period of days to months without treatment; conversely, some conversion symptoms may persist for years in spite of intense efforts at treatment. The prognosis seems to be highly variable, probably has little to do with the specific symptom involved, and is seemingly dependent on the interplay of the individual's psychological makeup, the social environment, and the response to the symptom by people who are important to the patient.

Illustrative Case

A 47-year-old, married, white, right-handed female was seen in psychiatric consultation on the medical unit in which she had been admitted for a presumptive cerebrovascular accident. She had collapsed at her family home and was brought for treatment with apparent paralysis of her right side. On examination, however, weakness was limited to the right arm and right leg with normal reflexes and loss of sensation in the right extremities beginning at the periphery and ending suddenly at the trunk. A staggering and falling gait was noted with a dramatic collapse and fall. All other aspects of the neurological exam were normal. The patient seemed relatively unconcerned

about her difficulties, chatting calmly with fellow patients and staff. Laboratory studies, brain computed tomographic (CT) scan and magnetic resonance imaging (MRI) were all within normal limits.

Review of the psychosocial context of the symptoms indicated that they began during a series of brutal arguments between the patient's husband and her favorite son. The patient's other two sons, as they got older, had been "thrown out" of the family home by their father after repeated physical conflicts over their hours and behavior. The same pattern was being repeated with the youngest son. Although she described herself as "someone who never gets angry," the patient vowed she would "never let him [her husband] do the same thing" to her last son. A series of conflicts had occurred, with the husband threatening to physically attack the son. On the night of the collapse, the patient had found her son and husband beginning a physical altercation. The patient, furious and terrified for her son's safety, had the thought: "I hate these two jerks. If they weren't so big, I'd knock them both out." At that point she experienced a feeling of weakness in her right arm and collapsed on the floor. The men forgot their argument and rushed her to the hospital; they dutifully visited her every day. She had a prior history of two episodes of conversion symptoms in the context of similar family conflicts. She described a childhood history of physical abuse, witness to family violence, and neglect.

Epidemiology

Conversion disorder was described more commonly in the nineteenth century than it is now and was seen predominantly in women. In the twentieth century, conversion symptoms have been reported frequently in male psychiatric battlefield casualties of every war since World War I. Today conversion disorder usually appears in patients seen in nonpsychiatric settings, such as neurology and medical wards and emergency rooms, and among military personnel. *DSM-IV* reports rates of conversion disorder from 10/100,000 to 300/100,000 in general population samples and states that conversion symptoms have been reported as a focus of treatment in 1–3% of outpatient referrals to mental health clinics.

Etiology & Pathogenesis

Conversion disorder is unusual in the *DSM-IV* classification, because a presumed cause (relationship to psychological conflicts or needs) is incorporated into the definition. Classic psychoanalytic notions of conversion propose the following. An unacceptable sexual or aggressive urge is denied conscious awareness and through "repression" becomes unconscious. The mental energy associated with the urge or wish, which would normally push it into conscious experience, is converted into a somatic symptom. This allows the individual to remain unaware of the unacceptable idea and at the same time permits symbolic expression of it. Protection from experiencing the unacceptable idea consciously is considered the "primary gain." The symptom itself elicits from others responses that gratify needs that were not involved in the original symptom production—eg, sympathy and attention, which may gratify dependency or other related needs. This gratification is referred to as a "secondary gain." The source of the symptom, in other words, is primary gain; once established, both primary gain and secondary gain serve to maintain the symptom.

A simpler formulation substitutes the terms "initiating and perpetuating factors" of the conversion symptom for primary and secondary gain. In the illustrative case, the patient's fear and anger, and conflicts over the expression of anger, were the initiating factors. The cessation of fighting and dutiful support of the family members were the perpetuating factors.

Historical Note

The story of the discovery of the psychological mechanisms responsible for conversion symptoms is worthy of a brief digression.

What are now called conversion symptoms were recognized in women by the ancient Greeks and Romans, who believed they resulted from a wandering of the uterus from its normal anatomical position into various other parts of the body, which were adversely affected. The term "hysteria," which in the past was used synonymously with conversion disorder, is derived from the Greek word for uterus. In the Middle Ages, conversion phenomena were given various supernatural and religious interpretations. This is also true today in many ecstatic religious groups and in non-Western cultures.

By the late nineteenth century, conversion symptoms (called hysteria then) had become a legitimate focus of medical and scientific investigation. Prominent researchers included Briquet, Charcot, Janet, and Freud. Classic descriptions of hysteria, dissociation, and hypnotic phenomena were compiled by these clinicians, and a variety of theories were posited to explain them. Paul Briquet suggested that "woes and losses" and other traumatic events and Jean-Martin Charcot and his followers suggested that a degeneration of the nervous system were the underlying causes of hysteria.

Pierre Janet made significant contributions to understanding the psychology of conversion symptoms. Specifically, Janet proposed the psychological mechanism of dissociation, by which selected mental contents could be removed from consciousness (dissociated from experience) but could continue to produce motor and sensory effects. This mechanism was thought to be illustrated by posthypnotic suggestion, in which a directive given to a subject in a hypnotic trance would be carried out after return to the normal waking state of consciousness without any memory by the subject of having received the directive. Janet proposed that traumatic experiences were etiological in the development of dissociative and hysterical phenomena.

Sigmund Freud, at that time a neurologist interested in hysteria, studied with Charcot and Hyppolyte Bernheim, a pioneering French hypnotist. Freud observed the use of hypnosis in treating conversion symptoms and returned to his own practice of neurology to use the new technique in treating his patients. Freud was particularly interested in the psychological theories of hysteria, and his theorizing was given an important boost by an accidental discovery made by a colleague, Josef Breuer. Breuer was treating a woman with hysteria ("Anna O") who in a hypnotic trance produced memories of previously unconscious traumatic events that appeared to be directly and causally related to the hysterical symptoms. Furthermore, the expression of these memories and the associated emotions caused the symptoms to disappear.

Drawing on the concept of the psychological mechanism of dissociation and on these new observations, Freud proposed that emotions associated with the traumatic event were morally unacceptable to the woman, and, because of this, the emotions were forced (repressed) into her unconscious. The mental energy associated with these emotions and expended in denying their expression was then "converted" into a somatic symptom that symbolically represented the traumatic event. Later, Freud abandoned his traumatic theory of conversion, emphasizing conflicts over sexual or aggressive wishes as etiological in the development of conversion symptoms.

At the end of the nineteenth century, J.F.F. Babinski, a student of Charcot, rejected the views of Charcot, Janet, and Freud. He proposed that all hysteria and dissociation were caused by "suggestion" and were not authentic phenomena. This idea had a substantial following until World War I when soldiers with "shell-shock," now conceptualized as posttraumatic stress disorder (PTSD), were shown to develop profound hysterical and dissociative symptoms after experiencing combat trauma.

The controversy about the etiology of hysteria and dissociation continues to this day. Different schools of thought ascribe these phenomena primarily to psychological trauma, intrapsychic conflict, neurobiological abnormalities, and suggestion. However, there is a broad spectrum of somatizing and dissociative individuals. Some or all of these factors may shape the clinical presentation of a given patient.

Treatment

Freud and Janet developed psychological treatment paradigms for patients with conversion disorders. They emphasized the verbalization of traumatic experiences and/or psychological conflicts that underlie the somatoform symptoms. Expression of suppressed emotions related to traumas and conflicts was central to these theories. Also, Janet emphasized transformation of the meaning of the symptoms to help the patient master the traumatic events that were etiological in the development of hysteria.

World War I produced high rates of psychiatric battlefield casualties suffering from shell-shock. Some clinicians emphasized psychological therapies for these conditions. Others proposed interventions such as electrical stimulation and moral exhortation.

Attempts were made during World War II to actively treat soldiers with "traumatic war neurosis" and to reduce battlefield psychiatric morbidity. Pharmacologically facilitated interviews, primarily with amobarbital (Amytal), were common in the treatment of soldiers who developed conversion symptoms as a result of traumatic combat experiences. Sometimes called narcosynthesis or Amytal interview, the intravenous use of a barbiturate to place the patient in a trancelike, relaxed state was combined with psychotherapeutic efforts to encourage the patient to remember traumatic events and emotions associated with the onset of the conversion and/or dissociative symptoms. An emotionally intense reliving of the traumatic experience often occurred, which, when accepted and remembered by the patient, caused the symptoms to disappear. Psychotherapy and hypnotherapy were also employed to treat these symptoms. In World War II these treatments were thought to have reduced substantially the rates of chronic trauma-related conversion and dissociative disorders in combatants as compared with the rates found in combatants in World War I.

In general hospital settings, acute conversion disorders are often treated with some combination of psychotherapy, hypnotherapy, and/or narcosynthesis. These allow alleviation of the acute conversion symptoms in most cases. However, longer-term psychotherapy and/or psychopharmacological interventions are often indicated to treat other psychiatric disorders such as PTSD and mood disorders that are comorbid with the conversion disorder. Family and/or marital therapy may be indicated to intervene in the factors that tend to perpetuate conversion symptoms.

Conversion symptoms that do not respond to acute interventions are treated with long-term psychotherapy, usually combining elements of cognitive, behavioral, supportive, and psychodynamic therapies. Hypnotherapy may be used adjunctively as well. Patients with long-standing conversion symptoms often have a poor prognosis and/or require prolonged courses of psychotherapy to permit improvement. There is no evidence for the effectiveness of any somatic therapy in the treatment of conversion disorder.

SOMATOFORM PAIN DISORDER

The diagnosis and treatment of somatoform pain disorder are summarized in Table 22–1.

Symptoms & Signs

Somatoform pain disorder is diagnosed when the major complaint is preoccupation with pain of at least 6 months' duration in the absence of, or grossly in excess of, explanatory physical findings (Table 22–4). In contrast to conversion disorder, evidence of a psychological factor that might be causing the pain is not necessary for diagnosis of somatoform pain

---

Table 22–4. *DSM-IV* diagnostic criteria for somatoform pain disorder.

A. Pain in one or more anatomical sites is the predominant focus of the clinical presentation and is of sufficient severity to warrant clinical attention.

B. The pain causes clinically significant distress or impairment in social, occupational, or other important areas of functioning.

C. Psychological factors are judged to have an important role in the onset, severity, exacerbation, or maintenance of the pain.

D. The symptom or deficit is not intentionally produced or feigned (as in factitious disorder or malingering).

E. The pain is not better accounted for by a mood, anxiety, or psychotic disorder and does not meet criteria for dyspareunia.

Code as follows:

Pain disorder associated with psychological factors: psychological factors are judged to have the major role in the onset, severity, exacerbation, or maintenance of the pain. (If a general medical condition is present, it does not have a major role in the onset, severity, exacerbation, or maintenance of the pain.) This type of pain disorder is not diagnosed if criteria are also met for somatization disorder.

Specify if:
Acute: duration of less than 6 months
Chronic: duration of 6 months or longer

Pain disorder associated with both psychological factors and a general medical condition: both psychological factors and a general medical condition are judged to have important roles in the onset, severity, exacerbation, or maintenance of the pain. The associated general medical condition or anatomical site of the pain (see below) is coded on Axis III.

Specify if:
Acute: duration of less than 6 months
Chronic: duration of 6 months or longer

Note: The following is not considered to be a mental disorder and is included here to facilitate differential diagnosis.

Pain disorder associated with a general medical condition: a general medical condition has a major role in the onset, severity, exacerbation, or maintenance of the pain. (If psychological factors are present, they are not judged to have a major role in the onset, severity, exacerbation, or maintenance of the pain.) The diagnostic code for the pain is selected based on the associated general medical condition if one has been established or on the anatomical location of the pain if the underlying general medical condition is not yet clearly established— for example, low back, sciatic, pelvic, headache, facial, chest, joint, bone, abdominal, breast, renal, ear, eye, throat, tooth, and urinary.

disorder. Because of the relative frequency of this symptom and the special clinical problems associated with the management of pain, separate diagnostic categories are indicated.

Natural History

Patients with somatoform pain disorder typically make repeated visits to doctors for diagnosis or relief of pain. Many physicians may be consulted successively or simultaneously, and there is an obvious risk of substance use disorder involving prescribed analgesics. Complaints of anxiety or depression are common but are not the predominant symptom, and there is an increased incidence of conversion symptoms. Histrionic personality disorder is an uncommon associated disorder.

This disorder may begin at any age but usually starts in adolescence and young adulthood. It seems to begin suddenly and increases in severity over days to weeks. It may resolve spontaneously or with treatment or may become chronic despite treatment. Severe symptoms may seriously disrupt overall function and expose the individual to iatrogenic complications of medical or surgical treatment.

Differential Diagnosis

Differential diagnosis includes painful physical disorders, such as atherosclerotic coronary artery disease and lumbar disk disease. The dramatic presentation of physical pain out of proportion to physical findings is not sufficient for the diagnosis, since the manner of expressing pain may reflect individual personality traits or cultural factors. Furthermore, pain that shows temporary improvement with placebo medications or suggestion should not be judged to be of psychological origin, since these phenomena also occur with pain caused by somatic disease.

Complaints of pain in somatization disorder, conversion disorder, major depression, and schizophrenia rarely dominate the clinical picture, and the diagnosis of somatoform pain disorder is not made if the pain is judged to be related to any other mental disorder. In somatization disorder, multiple symptoms, in addition to pain, are present. In malingering and factitious disorders, pain is under conscious control, which is not the case in somatoform pain disorder.

Prognosis

There are no good data on the prognosis of somatoform pain disorder. Clinical experience suggests a variable course with chronicity as a frequent characteristic. Better prognosis is found in individuals who continue to participate in regularly scheduled activities, such as work, and who do not allow the pain to become the dominant aspect of their lives.

Illustrative Case

A 32-year-old unemployed college graduate arrived at the emergency room frightened and breathless, complaining of severe substernal chest pain that he characterized as an unbearable "tightness." Except for slight tachycardia, his vital signs and electrocardiogram were normal. Despite reassurance from the physician, he continued to complain of severe pain and demanded "a shot of Demerol." After a time the physician ordered 75 mg of meperidine intramuscularly, after which the patient felt "a little better."

A telephone call to the family physician elicited the following information: There was a strong family history of heart disease, and the patient's father had died suddenly of acute myocardial infarction in his son's presence 4 years earlier. The patient's first episode of chest pain occurred 1 year later, when he was awakened from sleep the night before he was due to appear in court to testify in a legal proceeding contesting his father's will. Since that time he had had bouts of chest pain, usually requiring narcotic analgesia for relief, about twice a month and occasionally as often as three to four times a week. Thorough physical evaluation, including coronary angiography, revealed no organic disease.

Epidemiology

The prevalence of somatoform pain disorder is not known, but the disorder seems to be common in general medical practice. It is more common in women than in men. Familial distribution has not been reported. However, there is an increased familial incidence of painful injuries and illnesses, suggesting that some symptomatology may be learned or may result from identification with an ill family member. Depression and alcohol abuse may be common in families of these patients. As noted above, a history of childhood sexual abuse has been found to be more common in patients with chronic pelvic pain, fibromyalgia, refractory headaches, and chronic back pain, as compared with controls.

Etiology & Pathogenesis

The pain is thought to be of psychological origin. The specific psychological mechanisms involved in pain production are unknown and are probably multiple and variable. It has been proposed that the pain of somatoform pain disorder is a conversion symptom produced by the same mechanisms responsible for the symptoms of conversion disorder. A psychological cause is indicated by the following: (1) a temporal relationship exists between a presumed environmental stimulus (stressor) and pain; (2) the pain enables the person to avoid a noxious activity; or (3) the pain enables the person to obtain added support from the environment. It has also been observed that in certain cases the psychological mechanism appears to be identification, with the individual taking on the attributes (symptoms) of an emotionally significant other person, such as a parent. People with somatoform pain disorder may be less able to experience and verbalize emotions directly; the implication is that emotions are more or less directly translated into physical pain (by unknown mechanisms) rather than being expressed in other ways. Pain may also be a way of physically remembering trauma and abuse ("somatic memory"), eg, genital, rectal, chest, back, face, and/or extremity pain related to injuries incurred while being assaulted. None of these proposed mechanisms are mutually exclusive.

Treatment

In recent years, there has been considerable interest and progress in the treatment of chronic pain. Studies have shown that a multidisciplinary approach (involving neurologists, internists, and anesthesiologists in addition to psychiatrists) to management of pain in an inpatient setting, which includes treatment with psychotropic medications such as antidepressants, can be effective in achieving relief from pain and improving depressive symptoms. The relationship between chronic pain and depression is unclear. In some cases the pain is the most prominent manifestation of the depressive disorder; in other cases the relationship is far more complex. It may be problematic to generalize outcome studies done on patients with chronic pain, not necessarily suffering from somatoform pain disorder, to this psychiatric population. However, since many of these patients have complex psychosocial and medical situations, a multidisciplinary approach is often most helpful in assessing and treating these patients.

There are increasing numbers of multidisciplinary treatment centers for patients with chronic pain, and referral to one of these centers may be appropriate when possible. Specialized treatment methods often include group, milieu, and behavioral approaches to the problem and are aimed at reducing pain-related behavior and increasing normal functioning rather than alleviating pain.

When specialized treatment resources are not available, the physician should attempt to establish a supportive relationship with the patient that helps to prevent unnecessary medical and surgical procedures and treatments. When drugs are involved in treatment, use of sedative and antianxiety agents should be minimized, if possible. The use of opiates should be limited in this patient population since definition of an end point in their use is difficult. Chronic misuse of these substances by patients is common. In some cases it may be possible to achieve control of the patient's use of these drugs only through provision by a single physician in carefully defined amounts.

Most patients should be given a trial of antidepressant medication in the dosages used to treat a major depressive episode. Cognitive and behavioral psychotherapy with adjunctive hypnotherapy may also be helpful. As with treatment of conversion disorder, marital and family therapy is important since the patient's pain syndrome frequently dominates family relationships and maladaptive family patterns may lead to poorer outcome. Intercurrent substance and/or alcohol dependence may require specialized referrals.

HYPOCHONDRIASIS

Hypochondriasis was formerly called hypochondriacal neurosis. A "hypochondriac" is a person who complains about minor physical problems, worries unrealistically about serious illness, persistently seeks professional care, and consumes multiple over-the-counter remedies. The term hypochondriac includes elements of somatization disorder and hypochondriasis. The diagnosis and treatment of hypochondriasis are summarized in Table 22–1.

Symptoms & Signs

The chief manifestation of hypochondriasis is the fear of having (or the belief that one has) a serious physical disease. This fear is based on actual benign symptoms or signs or normal physiological sensations, and it exists despite the absence of evidence of physical disorder to account for the belief—although there may in fact be a coexistent somatic disorder. The misinterpretation of symptoms is quite natural. In hypochondriasis, however, the fear of having a serious disease persists despite medical reassurance, and it interferes with social or occupational functioning.

A person with hypochondriasis may interpret normal functions (heartbeat, peristalsis) or minor abnormalities (tension headache, viral respiratory infection) as evidence of serious disease. The fear of serious disease usually involves multiple organ systems simultaneously or in succession, although in some individuals the fear will center on a single organ system, such as in "cardiac neurosis," in which the unrealistic fear is of heart disease (Table 22–5).

Natural History

Anxiety, depression, and compulsive personality traits are commonly associated with hypochondriasis. When asked about their state of health, hypochondriacal patients usually respond at great length, often expressing frustration with physicians and the inadequate medical care they have received.

This disorder usually begins in adolescence, but may not begin until the fourth decade in men and the fifth decade in women. It is usually chronic, although marked by fluctuations in the intensity with which the belief is held and in the degree of disruption of social and occupational functioning. As with the other somatoform disorders, disruption of the patient's life may be marked (eg, the patient may take to bed and adopt an invalid life-style). The tendency to seek treatment from different physicians increases the risk of unnecessary medical or surgical treatments with their associated costs and complications.

Table 22–5. *DSM-IV* diagnostic criteria for hypochondriasis.

A. Preoccupation with fears of having, or the idea that one has, a serious disease based on the person's misinterpretation of bodily symptoms.

B. The preoccupation persists despite appropriate medical evaluation and reassurance.

C. The belief in Criterion A is not of delusional intensity (as in delusional disorder, somatic type) and is not restricted to a circumscribed concern about appearance (as in body dysmorphic disorder).

D. The preoccupation causes clinically significant distress or impairment in social, occupational, or other important areas of functioning.

E. The duration of the disturbance is at least 6 months.

F. The preoccupation is not better accounted for by generalized anxiety disorder, obsessive-compulsive disorder, panic disorder, a major depressive episode, separation anxiety, or another somatoform disorder.

Specify if:

With Poor Insight: if, for most of the time during the current episode, the person does not recognize that the concern about having a serious illness is excessive or unreasonable.

Differential Diagnosis

The differential diagnosis includes actual serious somatic disease. Occasionally, hypochondriasis will require differentiation from schizophrenia or major depression with somatic delusions. Although the final diagnosis will be based on specific diagnostic criteria, in the person with hypochondriasis the belief that somatic disease exists does not have the rigidly fixed quality of a true delusion, and the possibility that the feared disease does not exist will often be entertained. Differentiation from somatization disorder is usually based on multiple physical symptoms rather than on the fear of having a specific disease.

Prognosis

Most psychiatrists consider hypochondriasis to be a chronic disorder with a very poor prognosis.

Illustrative Case

A 28-year-old salesman sought a medical appointment for "a complete physical examination." He stated that several months ago he had consulted another physician but now was looking for a doctor who could "get to the bottom" of his problems. He expressed some anger because the other physician had refused to perform tests the patient thought were indicated, and he hoped the new doctor would be more helpful.

When asked what was troubling him, the patient said he was sure he had cancer—probably cancer of the stomach. He reported that 4 or 5 years ago he began to have occasional burning sensations in his upper abdomen after meals. He saw several doctors then, all of whom performed multiple diagnostic procedures and pronounced him healthy except for mild indigestion. He began to scrupulously monitor his diet, keeping records of the frequency and intensity of his gastric symptoms. Gradually he began to "suspect the worst" (cancer) and again saw several different physicians, hoping that his cancer could be diagnosed and treated. He began to feel tired at the end of the workday and occasionally thought he felt "swollen glands" in his neck, which suggested that his cancer might be spreading. He cut back on the amount of work he was doing ("to rest more") and broke off a relationship with a woman.

Recently the patient became angry when his last physician refused to repeat diagnostic procedures already done and instead requested records from other physicians. He then made the startling admission that unless the cancer could be diagnosed this time, "I guess I'll have to give up the idea that I have it. But I feel like I do."

Epidemiology

Hypochondriasis is common in general medical practice and seems to occur with equal frequency in men and women. It is not known if there is an increased incidence among family members.

Etiology & Pathogenesis

Hypochondriasis is believed to have its origin in maladaptive attempts to cope with unmet psychological needs or unconscious psychological conflicts, but there is no agreement about the specific psychological mechanisms involved. Some feel the hypochondriacal patient merely shows an excessive self-concern; others suggest that hypochondriasis represents a physical expression of low self-esteem (sick, weak, defective) or protects the individual from awareness of destructive impulses toward others (seeing oneself as being damaged rather than seeing oneself as wishing to damage others). It has recently been proposed that these symptoms result from serious deficits in the ability of a patient to maintain a "sense of the self" (as well integrated or "put together") and that hypochondriacal symptoms must be viewed as one manifestation of this underlying problem. Hypochondriacal patients may have profound difficulty naming or expressing emotions. It is thought that the preoccupation with physical symptoms is related to this inability. Some studies have found increased rates of childhood abuse and neglect in the histories of hypochondriacal patients as compared with other patient groups.

Treatment

Psychotherapy appears to be useful for only a few hypochondriacal patients. Most are resistant to the idea of psychiatric treatment, and it should probably be offered only to highly motivated, insightful patients who will readily accept the recommendation. There is no evidence that somatic treatments are effective.

Because people with hypochondriasis usually present to physicians who are not psychiatrists and are opposed to psychiatric treatment, the general medical practitioner has the best opportunity to be of help. To benefit a hypochondriacal patient, the physician must give up the idea of cure in the usual sense of relieving symptoms. The physician must be able to accept the patient's fears and complaints and recognize that they are manifestations of a chronic psychiatric disorder, that they serve an important (if poorly understood) psychological function, and that they will continue indefinitely. With this approach, the physician may be able to avoid becoming frustrated, angry, or hopeless and will maintain a sensitivity to the patient's social and psychological needs and problems. The possibility exists that a consequence of this supportive doctor-patient relationship will be a reduction in the patient's anxiety, which may result in decreased fears of disease and improved social and occupational functioning. The physician should have fixed, regular appointments of unvarying duration with the hypochondriacal patient and should continue to respond in appropriate ways to physical complaints or true disease while avoiding unnecessary diagnostic or therapeutic procedures. This approach at least prevents "doctor shopping" by the patient and reduces the risk of iatrogenic complications.

SUMMARY

The somatoform disorders are a group of psychiatric syndromes characterized by physical symptoms that suggest the presence of a physical disorder. Physical or laboratory findings must not fully account for the symptoms, and there must be direct or strong presumptive evidence of a psychological origin. People with these disorders usually do not perceive themselves as psychiatrically disturbed and therefore frequently present to nonpsychiatric medical practitioners for treatment. It is important that physicians be knowledgeable about these syndromes in order to avoid unnecessary and potentially harmful diagnostic and therapeutic interventions and to minimize secondary gain in the context of the medical treatment or in the patient's other relationships. More effective management of many of these patients in primary care can help improve their well-being and reduce expenditures for unneeded medical tests and treatments.

DISSOCIATIVE DISORDERS

The dissociative disorders are a group of psychiatric syndromes characterized by disruptions of some aspect of consciousness, identity, memory, motor behav-

ior, or awareness of the environment. The dissociative disorders are dissociative amnesia, dissociative identity disorder or multiple personality disorder, dissociative fugue, depersonalization disorder, and dissociative disorder NOS, a residual category for atypical dissociative disorders.

Additionally, recent studies of individuals acutely traumatized in natural disasters and war have led to the description of "peritraumatic dissociation." The symptoms of this condition include disorientation, amnesia, depersonalization, confusion, and time distortion. In a number of studies, the extent of peritraumatic dissociation was the best predictor of subsequent PTSD and psychopathology in the populations studied. The extent of trauma and capacity to dissociate were also important variables, however. A decision tree for the diagnosis of the dissociative disorders is shown in Figure 22–2.

DISSOCIATIVE AMNESIA

The diagnosis and treatment of dissociative amnesia are summarized in Table 22–6.

Symptoms & Signs

The essential feature of dissociative amnesia (DA) is an inability to recall important personal information, usually of a traumatic or stressful nature, that is more extensive than can be explained by normal forgetfulness (Table 22–7). The memory disturbance is not related to organic mental disorder (see Chapters 5, 16, and 17). There are two basic presentations of DA. The first is a dramatic, sudden disturbance in which extensive aspects of memory for personal information are not available to conscious verbal recall. These patients are often seen in emergency rooms or general medical or neurological services since the sudden development of memory loss requires medical assessment. In addition, during an amnestic episode, some individuals may demonstrate disorientation, perplexity, and purposeless wandering.

Despite its rarity, this type of DA is featured in the media and in most textbooks as representative of the condition. However, a far more prevalent form of DA is a deletion from conscious memory of large aspects of the personal history. Ordinarily, patients do not complain of this difficulty and it is usually discovered only in taking a careful life history. DA typically has a clear-cut onset and offset, so that the person is subjectively aware of a deletion in continuous memory rather than the gradual wearing away characteristic of normal remote memory. A patient may complain that she does not "remember being in third grade," although there is clear memory for other school years. Usually such symptoms are associated with traumatic circumstances, eg, third grade was the year the patient was kidnapped by her estranged father in a custody dispute and reportedly was sexually

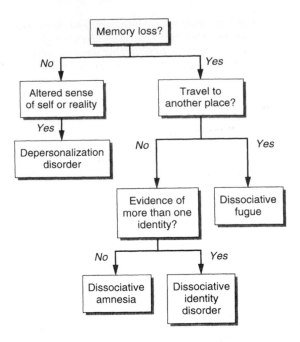

Figure 22–2. Decision tree for diagnosis of the dissociative disorders.

abused by him during that time. In extreme cases, patients may deny recall for their entire childhood or other major life epochs.

Several different types of memory disturbance have been identified in DA. The most common type is "localized" amnesia, the inability to recall events occurring within a circumscribed period (eg, the patient's experiences in combat during a series of battles). Localized amnesia may be "selective"—ie, the memory loss may exist for some events but not for all. "Generalized" amnesia is the inability to recall everything that has happened during the individual's lifetime, including personal identity. "Continuous" amnesia is an unusual memory disturbance in which all events subsequent to a specific time (up to and including the present) are forgotten, so that the individual appears unable to form new memories even though apparently alert and aware. "Systematized" amnesia defines loss of memory for certain categories of information, such as all memories relating to one's family or to a particular person.

Natural History

An acute episode of DA typically begins following a life event that causes severe psychological stress in the affected individual. The precipitating event is often something that threatens the patient's physical or emotional well-being, such as being the victim of a brutal rape or witnessing the injury or death of others. At other times, the precipitating event, although only moderately stressful, may be experienced as ex-

Table 22–6. Dissociative disorders.

	Dissociative Amnesia	Dissociative Identity Disorder	Dissociative Fugue	Depersonalization Disorder
Key features	Memory loss following stressful/traumatic life experiences	Two or more alter identities; switching, transfer of control; amnesia	Travel to a new location; amnesia and/or assumption of new identity	Feeling detached from, or observing, one's mental processes or body
Epidemiology	2–7% of general population using DES and DDIS[a]	May be as high as 1–3% of general population using DES and DDIS[a]; runs in families; related to severe early trauma	More common during war or social dislocation; possibly 0.2% of general population using DES and DDIS[a]	Possibly 2.4% of general population using DES and DDIS[a]
Differential diagnosis	Organic mental disorders: dementia, delirium, transient global amnesia, Korsakoff's disease, and postconcussion amnesia; substance abuse, other dissociative and trauma disorders; malingering, factitious disorder	Dissociative disorders, mood disorders, personality disorders, schizophrenia, seizures, eating disorders, substance abuse disorders, malingering, factitious disorders	Other dissociative disorders; seizure disorder; amnestic disorders, schizophrenia, mania, malingering, factitious disorders	A comorbid symptom of mood, anxiety, psychotic, personality disorder; normal adolescence; epilepsy, brain tumor; substance abuse
Treatment	Psychotherapy, hypnotherapy, drug-facilitated interviews	Long-term, phasic, multimodal psychotherapy; adjunctive hypnotherapy, pharmacotherapy	Psychotherapy, hypnotherapy, drug-facilitated interviews	No effective treatments found; supportive psychotherapy, antidepressants, and antianxiety agents

[a] DES, Dissociative Experiences Scale; DDIS, Dissociative Disorders Interview Schedule.

Table 22–7. *DSM-IV* diagnostic criteria
for dissociative amnesia.

A. The predominant disturbance is one or more episodes of inability to recall important personal information, usually of a traumatic or stressful nature, that is too extensive to be explained by ordinary forgetfulness.

B. The disturbance does not occur exclusively during the course of dissociative identity disorder, dissociative fugue, posttraumatic stress disorder, acute stress disorder, or somatization disorder and is not due to the direct physiological effects of a substance (eg, a drug of abuse, a medication) or a neurological or other general medical condition (eg, amnestic disorder due to head trauma).

C. The symptoms cause clinically significant distress or impairment in social, occupational, or other important areas of functioning.

tremely threatening because of powerful psychological conflicts, eg, participation in an extramarital affair in spite of strong moral disapproval of such behavior. However, patients with this latter configuration of circumstances frequently have had a traumatic history prior to this event, which may predispose them to the development of amnesia. The onset and termination of the episodes are usually sudden. Recovery of memory after an acute amnesia appears to be common if the patient receives appropriate treatment. However, some patients develop a chronic course. Recurrences occur in a subset of patients and single episodes predispose to subsequent ones. DA may be an alternative to a suicide attempt in some patients. Successful suicide has been reported in DA patients in whom the amnesia has been lifted precipitously without adequate psychotherapeutic preparation.

Differential Diagnosis

Memory return following loss of memory as a result of an organic mental disorder is gradual and usually incomplete if it occurs at all. It may be difficult to differentiate between a substance-induced blackout and DA since substance abusers may minimize their substance use. Conversely, DA patients may misattribute their amnesia to alcohol or drugs, since they are frequently more frightened of dissociation than they are of being labeled a substance abuser. However, a careful history, using collateral informants if necessary, may be of assistance in clarifying the situation. Unlike the memory loss in DA, substance-related memory deficits are usually not reversible.

Alcohol amnestic disorder, also called Korsakoff's disease, may be confused with the continuous form of DA. Alcohol amnestic disorder occurs in the context of heavy and prolonged alcohol abuse, often follows an episode of Wernicke's encephalopathy, and is not associated with psychological stress. Unlike the patient with DA, the patient with Korsakoff's disease

is not able to learn new information and shows considerable deterioration in personal functioning.

In amnesia due to brain injury there is usually a history of a clear-cut physical trauma, a period of unconsciousness, and/or clinical evidence of brain injury. The disturbance of recall, although circumscribed, is usually retrograde and encompasses a period of time before the head trauma. In contrast, in DA, the disturbance of recall is almost always anterograde (ie, memory loss is restricted to the period *after* the trauma). The patient with DA is usually highly hypnotizable, which brain-injured patients tend not to be. Hypnosis and/or drug-facilitated interviews may clarify the differential diagnosis. With these specialized techniques, patients with DA commonly recall information for which they had been amnestic. Brain-injured patients will become more confused and show greater memory deficits with sedative drug infusion.

Dissociative fugue may include amnesia but is distinguished from DA by the additional features of travel to a new locale and/or assumption of a new identity. Patients with dissociative identity disorder usually show highly complex forms of chronic DA as well as demonstrating multiple alternate identities. Malingering involving feigned amnesia may be difficult to distinguish from DA. This usually presents with the acute form of amnesia. The motivation for the malingering is usually obvious and may involve wishes to avoid incarceration, military service, etc. However, bona fide patients with DA may also show a secondary gain component in which the DA facilitates avoidance of painful circumstances or unwanted duties. Some individuals who commit violent crimes in states of intense emotion or rage may have genuine amnesia for these events.

Illustrative Case

A 45-year-old divorced left-handed male bus dispatcher was seen in psychiatric consultation on a medical unit. He had a history of hypertension and in the past year had been admitted for chest pain that was thought to be due to ischemia, although he did not suffer a myocardial infarction. He had been followed carefully after that and exhibited no change in his cardiac function or electrocardiogram. Two nights before he had been admitted with an episode of chest discomfort, "light headedness," and weakness in his left arm. Psychiatric consultation was requested as the patient complained of having no memory of any event that occurred in the previous 12 years. Physical and laboratory findings were unchanged from the patient's usual baseline and brain computerized axial tomography scan was normal.

On mental status examination, the patient displayed intact intellectual function but insisted the date was 12 years earlier, denying recall of his entire subsequent personal history and of current events for the past 12 years. He did not recognize his 8-year-old son, insisted that he was unmarried, denied awareness of his current address, life circumstances, and job, and denied recollection of recent political events, such as the current president. He was perplexed by the contradiction between his memory and current circumstances. The patient described a family history of brutal beatings and physical discipline. He was a decorated combat veteran, although he described amnestic episodes for some of his combat experiences. He had been a golden gloves champion boxer noted for his powerful left hand.

He was provided with information about his disorder and given the suggestion that his memory could return as he could tolerate it, perhaps overnight during sleep, or perhaps over a longer time. If this strategy was unsuccessful, hypnosis or Amytal interview was proposed.

On subsequent examination, the patient reported that his memory had returned. Prior to the amnestic episode, he described an escalating series of conflicts at work, in his marriage, and with his son. His wife was discussing a separation and had asked him to discuss this with his son. He felt completely responsible for his coworkers and for the care of his relatives. He had felt panicked, overwhelmed, and enraged. He had felt violently angry at his wife, but had said he would "beat to death anybody who tried to hurt her." He stated he would have attempted suicide, but he "couldn't" because he had too many people relying on him. The amnesia developed after he felt a kind of "paralysis" in his left arm. His wife had rushed him to the hospital and was extremely concerned about his well-being.

He was aware that none of these problems existed 12 years before and that he had unconsciously returned to a happy, less stressful time by losing his memory. The patient was treated with supportive psychotherapy in the hospital and coordination of care was arranged with his cardiologist. The patient responded well to marital and individual psychotherapy and to antidepressant medication.

Epidemiology

There is controversy about the prevalence of DA. General population studies have found as many as 2–7% of the population may have DA (Ferdinand et al, 1995). At the other extreme, others have questioned whether this condition exists at all. However, DA has been described in many populations in both prospective and retrospective studies: combat veterans in all wars since World War I, survivors of childhood sexual and/or physical abuse, concentration camp survivors, victims of torture, survivors of natural disasters, and survivors of genocidal violence in Cambodia and the Balkans, among others (Brown et al, 1998). Systematic studies have shown high correlations between the extent of traumatization and the development of amnesia and have documented events for which the individual reports amnesia. Amnesia

seems less likely to occur with natural disasters than with assaults by human beings, particularly those with greater degrees of threat and violence.

There is also controversy about the accuracy of recall of individuals with amnesia, particularly for childhood sexual abuse. As with most autobiographical accounts, only reliable, independent corroboration can verify a specific recollection. However, studies have shown that there are a number of independently documented cases of accurate recall for childhood sexual and physical abuse after DA abates (Brown et al, 1998). Objective data about memories of childhood abuse may be difficult to acquire, however. Expert consultation may be needed if this becomes a contentious issue in a specific case.

Etiology & Pathogenesis

Animal research on stress and studies of combat veterans, former prisoners of war, and survivors of childhood sexual abuse suggest that DA due to trauma may have a distinct psychobiology involving alterations in the neuronal structure of the hippocampus, possibly due to excess production of glucocorticoid. Decreased hippocampal volume has been found in patients with PTSD as compared to controls and correlates with increased dissociation.

Alterations in the amygdala and other neuronal systems such as the benzodiazepine–γ-aminobutyric acid system, the opiate system, the norepinephrine system, and the corticotropin-releasing factor–hypothalamic-pituitary-adrenal axis system due to extreme stress may all contribute to the manifold memory disturbances caused by trauma. In addition to DA, these include depersonalization, and the various forms of posttraumatic hypermnesia including reexperiencing (flashback) episodes, intrusive posttraumatic imagery, and eidetic engraving of the traumatic experience in memory (Bremner et al, 1993).

From a psychological perspective, dissociation is conceptualized here as a basic part of the psychobiology of the human response to trauma: a protective activation of altered states of consciousness in reaction to overwhelming psychological trauma. Memories and affects relating to the trauma are encoded during these altered states. When the person returns to the baseline state, there is relatively less access to the dissociated information, leading, in many cases, to DA for at least some part of the traumatic events. However, the dissociated memories and affects can manifest themselves in nonverbal forms: posttraumatic nightmares, reenactments, intrusive imagery, and somatoform symptoms. In addition to amnesia for the trauma, the person frequently has dissociated basic assumptions about the self, relationships, other people, and the nature of the world (Loewenstein, 1994).

The concepts of primary and secondary gain, discussed in the section on the etiology of conversion disorder, may also contribute to our understanding of

DA. The primary gain is protection from overwhelming traumatic or stressful experiences. Responses of others may provide gratification of other psychological needs (secondary gain) and thus serve to maintain the amnesia after it is established.

In individuals who develop DA without a specific acute traumatic experience, a preexisting history of trauma usually represents a diathesis for development of amnesia under more ordinary, albeit stressful, circumstances.

Treatment & Prognosis

Many cases of DA resolve spontaneously when the individual is removed from the stressful situation. In general, psychotherapy, frequently augmented by hypnosis or drug-facilitated interviewing, is the treatment of choice. Other than drug-facilitated interviews, there are no known somatic treatments that target DA itself. Psychotherapy must be carefully structured to not overwhelm the amnestic patient when memory is recalled.

Patients with amnesia frequently also have mood and anxiety disorders, as well as PTSD. Pharmacological treatments for these comorbid conditions are usually helpful.

DISSOCIATIVE IDENTITY DISORDER

The diagnosis and treatment of dissociative identity disorder are summarized in Table 22–6.

Symptoms & Signs

Dissociative identity disorder or DID (previously known as multiple personality disorder or MPD) is characterized by the existence of two or more identities or personality states (also called alters, parts, alter identities, etc) within a single individual (Table 22–8). Alter identities are defined as mental constructs, each with its own relatively enduring pattern of thoughts, memories, emotions, perceptions, and subjective experience. Individuals with this disorder demonstrate transfer of behavioral control among alter identities either by state transitions (switching) or interference and overlap of alters who manifest themselves simultaneously. DA is also present in almost all patients with DID.

The florid, dramatic patient with DID depicted in the media and old psychiatric textbooks probably represents fewer than 5% of patients with this disorder. In most patients with DID, the dissociative disorder presents in a covert and subtle fashion. The most typical clinical presentation is one of a refractory psychiatric disorder, usually a mood disorder, or, of particular relevance to primary care, multiple somatic symptoms. Many patients with DID meet diagnostic criteria for somatization disorder and/or other somatoform disorders. Overuse of medical resources is typical of a significant subgroup of these patients.

Table 22–8. *DSM-IV* diagnostic criteria for dissociative identity disorder.

A. The presence of two or more distinct identities or personality states (each with its own relatively enduring pattern of perceiving, relating to, and thinking about the environment and self).

B. At least two of these identities or personality states recurrently take control of the person's behavior.

C. Inability to recall important personal information that is too extensive to be explained by ordinary forgetfulness.

D. The disturbance is not due to the direct physiological effects of a substance (eg, blackouts or chaotic behavior during alcohol intoxication) or a general medical condition (eg, complex partial seizures). **Note:** In children, the symptoms are not attributable to imaginary playmates or other fantasy play.

Alter identities vary in complexity and psychological structure. In some cases, highly developed alter identities are present with marked presentational differences in posture, voice tone, manifest mood, energy, interests, talents, capacities, manifest age, gender, etc. In the majority of cases, however, the alters are relatively limited in their psychological depth and do not manifest with dramatic differences on switching. Alter identities may develop with polarized perceptions and viewpoints: eg, a male multiple with an actively homosexual alter and a hypermasculine homophobic alter. Others seem to sequester neutral information, talents, capacities, and historical information. Alter identities are *not* separate people, although they may perceive themselves as separate persons inhabiting different bodies, unaffected by what happens to one another. All the alters together make up the personality of a single human being. In general, all alters should be held responsible for the behavior of any other alter, despite subjective amnesia or disavowal of behavior.

Developmental, cultural, and social factors, as well as more extensive traumatization, may influence the structuring, complexity, and elaboration of the alter identity "system." For example, some patients with DID with substantial creativity and intelligence may develop far more elaborate alter systems. This secondary structuring is *not* the sine qua non of this disorder. The essential features are the development of the subjectively experienced alter identity states accompanied by state transitions and amnesia.

Natural History

DID is thought to begin in childhood in response to repeated traumatic and/or overwhelming life experiences. In Western cultures these incidents of childhood maltreatment most commonly involve physical and/or sexual abuse, although some patients have reported subjection to long painful childhood medical experiences, wartime dislocation, etc. Studies in the United States, Canada, Europe, Asia, and Latin America have indicated strikingly similar clinical presentations and life history in patients with DID. Across studies, these patients report very high rates of severe, repeated childhood trauma and/or maltreatment, with rates of childhood sexual abuse ranging from about 70% to over 95%. Accordingly, over 80% of patients with DID will meet the diagnostic criteria for PTSD.

In some recent studies, researchers have confirmed patients' reports of childhood trauma by extensive review of childhood medical, social service, and psychiatric records, as well as by corroboration by family members and significant others (Lewis et al, 1997). However, controversy exists about the accuracy of recollection in these patients and some patients with DID will substantially revise their views of their life history as treatment progresses.

Most patients with DID demonstrate marked, repeated episodes of dissociative amnesia. They may have "blackouts," episodes of fugue, bewildering life predicaments, lack of memory for important life events, marked fluctuations in talents and abilities, and acquisition of unexplained possessions. With switching some patients with DID may actually show variable blood pressure and glucose readings, objective changes in visual acuity, and differential responses to drugs, alcohol, and prescription medications. Some primary care physicians have found medical management problematic in these patients due to their marked variability in symptoms.

Most patients with DID are diagnosed in adulthood. With more vigorous case finding and awareness of the sequela of abuse and maltreatment, an increasing group of cases involving children and adolescents has been recognized. Many patients with DID have long, complex, often refractory psychiatric histories, acquiring multiple diagnoses over the years. In addition, a significant subgroup of these patients has substantial difficulties with substance abuse. Some of these patients require social service interventions due to abuse and/or neglect of their own children.

Differential Diagnosis

DID can be mistaken for most other psychiatric disorders. Comorbid mood, anxiety, somatoform, personality, and posttraumatic disorders are common, as are eating disorders and substance abuse. Patients with DID may be mistakenly considered psychotic because they hear the voices of their alter identities and/or experience other bizarre hallucinatory phenomena. However, the dissociative patient commonly experiences "hearing voices" within the mind, not outside it as with true hallucinations. Patients with DID are often frightened of being labeled "crazy" for having pseudopsychotic experiences. True paranoid delusions are uncommon in patients with DID, although mistrust and suspicion of the intentions of others are common, usually secondary to abuse and maltreatment.

Mood swings are common in patients with DID, but often occur over minutes to hours, not days or weeks as in bipolar patients. These very rapid mood changes usually do not respond to mood stabilizers, such as lithium. Chronic depression, anxiety, and dysphoria are common in these patients. They are only partially responsive to psychiatric medications. Severe sleep problems are also present in most cases.

A subgroup of patients with DID may have a somatoform presentation with refractory pain, apparent paralysis, pseudoseizures, multiple sclerosis-like symptoms, etc. A complex subgroup of these patients suffers from bona fide chronic medical disorders such as systemic lupus erythematosus or myasthenia gravis. Their psychiatric pathology complicates their medical management and vice versa. Joint medical and psychiatric management is frequently essential in these cases.

Careful history taking to help recognize chronic amnesia, symptoms of PTSD, a history of early maltreatment, and the presence of alter identities may allow diagnosis of DID, even in cases in which other symptom clusters appear to predominate.

Illustrative Case

A 38-year-old separated white female was seen in urgent psychiatric consultation on a cardiology unit. She had been referred for arrhythmias producing apparent syncopal episodes. These episodes occurred in the hospital but were not associated with significant changes in vital signs or alterations in cardiac function. Mitral valve prolapse was present, however. Neurology consultation was obtained since the patient reported memory difficulties, and members of the staff noted that the patient frequently did not seem to recall what had happened to her from day to day or even hour to hour. An extensive evaluation of electroencephalograms (EEGs), including 24-hour monitoring, was also essentially normal, and alterations in consciousness were not associated with changes in EEG. Physical, neurological, and laboratory examinations, including MRI of the brain, were normal.

Psychosocial history revealed a series of significant recent losses. The patient also described a long history of psychiatric treatment for depression and anxiety with little response to numerous trials of antidepressant medications. She reported no memory for her life before the seventh grade. Psychiatric consultation was called because the patient left her bed one afternoon, dressed herself, and went to the pediatric ward, claiming to be a special education teacher. She used a variant of her name and was about to sing to a group of children when staff intervened. On return to the cardiology unit, she appeared genuinely confused and perplexed, seemed not to recall what had occurred, and was distressed that security and staff were now involved.

On examination, she described a long history of

perplexing memory lapses, such as being told of behavior she could not recall and being called different names by people she did not know (who insisted they knew her), as well as fluctuations in abilities, acquisition of possessions for which she could not account, out of body experiences, and hearing conversations and voices in her head. She denied recall of her early life, feeling as if her "life began when she was 13" after being removed from her abusive family and placed in foster care. Her father reportedly had been incarcerated for physically and sexually abusing his children. Childhood medical records confirmed this information.

She appeared to be shifting states subtly during the interview. When asked if her experience was of having more than one independent part of her mind take control of her behavior, she spontaneously dissociated into a series of alter identities. These alters reported different ages, names, genders, and memories. One took responsibility for the activities on the pediatric unit. Others described symptoms that accounted for the syncopal and seizure-like episodes. Another reported on events in the patient's earlier life. These entities referred to themselves in the first person plural and third person singular and claimed responsibility for the voices heard by the patient.

The patient was transferred to the psychiatric unit. On 1-year follow-up, with appropriate treatment, there had been a significant decrease in somatoform symptoms and medical utilization, as well as improvement in mood and overall adaptation.

Epidemiology

A recent general population study found that 1–3% of the population met diagnostic criteria for DID. This study has been criticized; some have suggested that this figure is too high, considering a more realistic prevalence to be about 0.5% of the population. Still others have suggested that this figure is too low, citing the high rates of childhood maltreatment in the general population. Several studies have shown that DID and other dissociative disorders occur frequently in the family members of patients with DID. Multigenerational families with DID have been described (Braun, 1985).

Etiology & Pathogenesis

The current view is that DID is a developmentally based posttraumatic disorder usually beginning before the age of 6. In DID, overwhelming and/or traumatizing circumstances, accompanied by disturbed caretaker-child attachment and parenting, lead to extreme states of consciousness in the child. These disrupt the normal consolidation of personal identity across shifts in state, mood, and personal and social context. In addition, trauma causes encapsulation of intolerable memories and affects in "dissociative" behavioral states. These dissociative responses may preserve relationships with caretakers, even abusive ones, and allow segregation of traumatic experiences to permit development in other life areas such as academics and social life. Once formed, these entities may show some degree of development relatively independent of other identities in the person. In addition, dissociation and alter identity creation may be used subsequently to cope with more routine, nontraumatic life circumstances. The outcome is a person embodying a number of relatively concretized, more-or-less independent self-states, often in significant conflict with each other.

Recent media-based depictions of DID have posited that the condition is the product of suggestion by clinicians to highly influenceable patients. There are no research studies in clinical populations that have supported this opinion. Conversely, a wealth of studies support the notion of the posttraumatic origin of DID (Gleaves, 1996).

Treatment & Prognosis

Patients with DID range from severely chronically psychiatrically ill individuals with poor psychosocial function to very high functioning people who may be successful professionally and socially. In general, DID is treated as a complex, chronic, trauma-based disorder. Accordingly, a three-stage model is used. In the first, patients are taught techniques to manage symptoms and stabilize their dysfunctional lives. A broad range of psychotherapies may be employed, including cognitive-behavioral, psychodynamic, supportive, and hypnotherapy, to assist the patient with these tasks. Psychopharmacological interventions may be helpful to treat comorbid affective, anxiety, and PTSD conditions. Family, marital, social, and educational interventions may be needed. Homogeneous group therapy for patients with DID may be effective, if carefully structured to focus on current life adaptation, not past traumas. Expressive therapies, such as art and dance therapy, may be helpful for many patients with DID.

After stabilization, some patients may elect to intensively process traumatic memories per se. Premature intensive focus on trauma material, before symptom stabilization is accomplished, usually leads to regression and decompensation in most patients with DID. Finally, once trauma issues are fully resolved, the patient may focus primarily on successful living without domination by posttraumatic symptoms and beliefs. A subgroup of patients with DID may achieve "fusion" in which all identities consolidate into one. The person experiences himself or herself as unified.

On the other hand, another group of patients with DID will never move beyond work on basic symptom and life stabilization. They are seriously and persistently psychiatrically ill and may require repeated psychiatric hospitalizations and partial hospital treatment.

Studies of outcome and cost efficacy in the United States and Canada suggest that proper treatment for patients with DID results in improvement for many of them, as well as reduction in costs for psychiatric and medical care, even for the most severely ill group. Treatment may take years, however, particularly in the more severely ill patients.

DISSOCIATIVE FUGUE

The diagnosis and treatment of dissociative fugue are summarized in Table 22–6.

Symptoms & Signs

The word fugue is derived from the Latin verb *fugere,* which means "to flee." Dissociative fugue is characterized by sudden, unexpected "flights" from home or workplace with an inability to recall some or all of one's past. Some individuals assume a new identity or become confused about their identity (Table 22–9). It is as if the patient is running away from something but is unaware of fleeing. When the episode resolves, many individuals are unable to remember events of the fugue state. Although apparent disorientation and perplexity may occur, this disorder cannot be diagnosed in the presence of organic mental disorder.

The moving about that is part of dissociative fugue is purposeful, in contrast to the confused, dazed activity that may be seen in acute DA. In a typical case, the fugue consists of brief, purposeful journeying during which contacts with other people are minimal. The individual in a fugue usually does not attract attention. The new identity that is produced is frequently quite limited in its development. In rare cases, the assumed identity is quite elaborate, and the individual may take a new name and residence and engage in complex interpersonal relations or occupational activities so that the presence of a mental disorder is not suspected. When a new, complex identity is established, it is often characterized by more gregarious and uninhibited social behavior than was the patient's previous style.

Table 22–9. *DSM-IV* diagnostic criteria for dissociative fugue.

A. The predominant disturbance is sudden, unexpected travel away from home or one's customary place of work, with inability to recall one's past.

B. Confusion about personal identity or assumption of a new identity (partial or complete).

C. The disturbance does not occur exclusively during the course of dissociative identity disorder and is not due to the direct physiological effects of a substance (eg, a drug of abuse, a medication) or a general medical condition (eg, temporal lobe epilepsy).

D. The symptoms cause clinically significant distress or impairment in social, occupational, or other important areas of functioning.

Natural History

The course of this disorder is similar to that described for DA: an episode most often begins in the context of severe psychosocial stress and typically is of a brief duration (hours to days). Fugue may be more common during wartime and during periods of major social dislocation. Occasionally, an episode may last for months and involve complex social activity. Very little is known about the natural history of fugue. Some individuals have recurrent fugue episodes. Some have full recovery of memory for the fugue episode and others do not.

Fugue frequently occurs in the context of severe stress. Depression, suicidal ideation, grief, shame, guilt, and violent impulses may emerge once a fugue is resolved.

Differential Diagnosis

The differential diagnosis includes dementia and organic amnesic disorder, although the distinction is not usually difficult. Unexpected wandering from home can occur in organic mental disorder, but the individual usually does not engage in organized, purposeful behavior (eg, buying airline tickets). The memory disturbance of dissociative fugue may be similar to that in DA, but the latter does not involve purposeful travel or the assumption of a new personal identity.

Complex partial seizures may be associated with a brief journey, but there is no assumption of a new identity and usually no psychosocial precipitating episode. Seizure patients are in an altered state of consciousness, may show repetitive and/or perseverative speech and behaviors, and demonstrate a postictal state. Abnormal electroencephalograms are not associated with dissociative fugue.

Patients with bipolar illness in the manic phase and schizophrenic patients may wander across the country. However, the patient with dissociative fugue displays neither manic nor psychotic symptoms. Some patients with fugue actually have DID. As a result of severe stress, the patient with DID may create a new, amnestic alter that travels away from home. The underlying DID may become apparent only with long-term evaluation of the fugue patient, however.

Malingering may be difficult to distinguish from dissociative fugue, particularly because genuine fugue patients may be escaping some unwanted duty or consequence of misbehavior. Hypnosis and Amytal interviews may not be able to separate malingerers from true dissociative patients. Bona fide dissociative patients, as compared with malingerers, often are enmeshed in bizarre, complex situations in which the actual gain is unclear or minimal.

Illustrative Case

A 32-year-old married schoolteacher and minor town official, after learning of his wife's sexual involvement with another man, left home for work and just disappeared. Two months later, an acquaintance stopped for a meal in a small restaurant in the next state and saw him washing dishes behind the counter. The patient claimed not to know the friend and did not respond to his own name. The friend informed the local police, who found that the patient was unable to remember anything about his life prior to the preceding 2 months. He claimed he had found himself in the town 2 months ago not knowing who he was or how he had gotten there and that he invented a name for himself, moved into a rooming house, and took a job as a dishwasher, hoping he would remember who he was. His employer described him as a quiet and secretive man who nonetheless had been a reliable worker.

Epidemiology

A recent general population study found a prevalence of 0.2% for dissociative fugue. This disorder occurs primarily under conditions of war, natural disaster, or intense personal crisis. Fugue may be more common in males. There are no data on familial patterns of occurrence.

Etiology & Pathogenesis

Little is known about the etiology of dissociative fugue. Most fugues occur in the context of overwhelming life events or in individuals with prior histories of abuse or trauma. The latter amounts to a dissociative diathesis. Psychodynamic theories emphasize the person's conflict over wishing to escape from some circumstance (eg, a terrifying battle in wartime) and moral prohibitions against flight (a fervent belief that wartime cowards should be shot). The amnesia and loss of identity satisfy the wish to flee as well as the prohibition against it.

Treatment & Prognosis

Most fugue patients receive acute treatment in general hospitals and psychiatric facilities. Some fugues resolve completely, although there is frequently some residual amnesia for all or part of the fugue. Psychotherapy with adjunctive hypnotherapy and/or pharmacologically facilitated interviews may help overcome the DA associated with the termination of a fugue. Some patients show persistent amnesia and will undergo a prolonged psychotherapy with adjunctive psychopharmacological and hypnotherapeutic interventions.

DEPERSONALIZATION DISORDER

The diagnosis and treatment of depersonalization disorders are summarized in Table 22–6.

Symptoms & Signs

Historically, the symptoms of depersonalization and derealization have been recognized as part of the clinical picture of a wide variety of mental disorders. Common to both of these symptoms is a temporary disturbance in the subjective experience of reality, so that the usual quality of familiarity associated with perception is replaced by a sense of estrangement or unreality. In depersonalization, the disturbance is in the perception of oneself; in derealization, the alteration is in the perception of the external environment. In depersonalization disorder, the major symptom is that of depersonalization, but as presently defined, the disorder may include the symptom of derealization as well.

Depersonalization disorder is defined in *DSM-IV* as the occurrence of persistent or recurrent episodes of depersonalization, not related to any other mental disorder, that cause marked distress (Table 22–10). The major feature is sudden temporary loss of the sense of one's own reality, manifested as an experience of being detached from or a feeling of being an outside observer of one's body or mental processes. Patients may also describe feeling as though they were mechanical or as though they were in a dream. Reality testing remains intact, but various feelings of self-estrangement or beliefs that the body's physical characteristics have changed may accompany the episode. Various types of automatism or sensory anesthesias may also occur.

Derealization typically involves the perception that objects in the external world have changed in size or shape, or the subjective feeling that other people are automated, mechanical, somehow inhuman, or dead.

All of these distorted perceptions are experienced as being unpleasant and undesired and may be accompanied by anxiety, dizziness, a fear of becoming insane, feelings of depression, obsessive thoughts, or disturbances in the subjective experience of time.

Natural History

Little is known about the natural history of depersonalization disorder. In one recent study, 70% of pa-

---

Table 22–10. *DSM-IV* diagnostic criteria for depersonalization disorder.

A. Persistent or recurrent experiences of feeling detached from, and as if one is an outside observer of, one's mental processes or body (eg, feeling like one is in a dream).

B. During the depersonalization experience, reality testing remains intact.

C. The depersonalization causes clinically significant distress or impairment in social, occupational, or other important areas of functioning.

D. The depersonalization experience does not occur exclusively during the course of another mental disorder, such as schizophrenia, panic disorder, acute stress disorder, or another dissociative disorder, and is not due to the direct physiological effects of a substance (eg, a drug of abuse, a medication) or a general medical condition (eg, temporal lobe epilepsy).

tients with this disorder reported continuous symptoms (Simeon et al, 1997). This disorder often begins in adolescence. Onset may be sudden or gradual. Some individuals report that their symptoms followed an episode of psychoactive substance abuse such as use of cocaine or marijuana.

Differential Diagnosis

Depersonalization is a very common psychiatric symptom and may be associated with depression, anxiety and panic disorders, psychosis, trauma disorders, personality disorders, delirium, and seizure disorders; it is common in normal adolescents. Patients with other dissociative disorders may also have episodic depersonalization symptoms. The diagnosis of depersonalization disorder is made only if the depersonalization symptoms are independent of symptoms of the other mental disorders. Depression may be a result of chronic depersonalization, however. Careful history taking can differentiate the sequence of symptoms in most cases.

Illustrative Case

A 35-year-old lawyer telephoned a psychiatrist and asked for an appointment, saying, "I don't know what's the matter with me, but I'm afraid I'm going crazy." At the first appointment, he explained that for several years he had been having strange "attacks" about once a month. The "attacks" generally occurred during the course of his work, and on two recent occasions he had to leave the courtroom in the midst of a legal proceeding "to get control" of himself. He explained that an "attack" usually was heralded by a sudden feeling of nervousness and awareness that his heart was pounding. This was followed by the experience that all objects in his visual field had diminished to about half their normal size and by the perception that people's actions (his own and others) had lost their usual fluid quality and took on a mechanical, jerky character, "as in silent movies." These symptoms occasionally would be accompanied by the experience that he had become someone else ("I don't know who, but not myself"). On the day he telephoned the psychiatrist, an "attack" had begun while he was driving his car, and the usual symptoms were accompanied by the perception that his arms had become detached from his body and continued to steer the car "on their own."

Epidemiology

A recent study found that 2.4% of the general population met the diagnostic criteria for depersonalization disorder, although some believe that the prevalence is lower (Ross, 1991). In one study, almost two-thirds of individuals exposed to life-threatening accidents reported an episode of depersonalization (Noyes and Kletti, 1977).

Etiology & Pathogenesis

Patients with brain tumors and epilepsy have reported depersonalization. Electrical stimulation of the temporal lobe cortex has been reported to produce depersonalization phenomena, and some psychotomimetic drugs (eg, LSD) produce various distortions of reality (including the sense of reality in the perception of the self) in some individuals. These findings have led to speculations concerning the neurobiological basis of depersonalization phenomena.

In one study about 43% of patients with depersonalization disorder reported a history of childhood trauma such as sexual abuse or witnessing violence. Levels of trauma were less severe than that reported for patients with other dissociative disorders, however.

Treatment & Prognosis

Little is known about effective treatments for patients with this poorly studied disorder. Existing studies suggest that the majority of patients do not respond well to most forms of psychotherapy and psychiatric medications. Some patients may show mild to moderate response to selective serotonin reuptake inhibitor antidepressants and/or benzodiazepines. Many patients therefore are seen in long-term supportive psychotherapies with adjunctive pharmacotherapy.

SUMMARY

In the past decade there has been an explosion in data on dissociative disorders. Most studies have found a significant link between dissociation and the experience of psychological trauma. This association is so strong that some authorities have suggested creating a new category called the trauma disorders that would encompass the dissociative disorders, posttraumatic stress disorder, acute stress disorder, and some of the somatoform disorders, among others. Since, unfortunately, the prevalence of violence and trauma in our society is so great, this idea has the merit of better organizing data about some of these common mental disorders.

REFERENCES & SUGGESTED READINGS

Braun BG: The transgenerational incidence of dissociation and multiple personality disorder: A preliminary report. In: *Childhood Antecedents of Multiple Personality.* Kluft RP (editor). American Psychiatric Press, 1985.

Bremner JD, Marmar CR: *Trauma, Memory, and Dissociation.* Vol 54. American Psychiatric Press, 1998.

Bremner JD et al: Neurobiology of posttraumatic stress disorder. In: *American Psychiatric Association Annual Review of Psychiatry.* Vol 12, pp. 157–179. Oldham JM, Riba MB, Tasman A (editors). American Psychiatric Press, 1993.

Breuer J, Freud S: Studies on hysteria. In: *Standard Edition of the Complete Psychological Works of Sigmund Freud.* Vol 2. Hogarth Press, 1955.

Briquet P. *Traite de l'Hysterie.* Paris, J. Balliere, 1859.

Brown D, Scheflin AW, Hammond DC: *Memory, Trauma, Treatment, and the Law.* Norton, 1998.

Ellenberger HF: *The Discovery of the Unconscious.* Basic Books, 1970.

Felitti VJ et al: Relationship of childhood abuse and household dysfunction to many of the leading causes of death in adults. The adverse childhood experiences (ACE) study. Am J Prevent Med 1998;14(4):245.

Ferdinand RF et al: Assessment of the prevalence of psychiatric disorders in young adults. Br J Psychiatry 1995;166:480.

Fisher C: Amnesic states in war neurosis: The psychogenesis of fugue. Psychoanalyt Quart 1945;14:437.

Ford CV: *The Somatizing Disorders: Illness as a Way of Life.* Elsevier Biomedical, 1983.

Gleaves DH: The sociocognitive model of dissociative identity disorder: A reexamination of the evidence. Psychol Bull 1996;120:42.

Grinker RR, Spiegel JP: *Men Under Stress.* Blakiston, 1945.

Guze SB: Genetics of Briquet's syndrome and somatization disorder. Ann Clin Psychiatry 1993;5:225.

Herman JL: *Trauma and Recovery.* Basic Books, 1992.

Hollander E et al: Clomipramine vs desipramine crossover trial in body dysmorphic disorder. Arch Gen Psychiatry 1999;56:1033.

Janet P: *The Major Symptoms of Hysteria.* Macmillan, 1907.

Kardiner A, Spiegel H: *War, Stress, and Neurotic Illness.* Hoeber, 1947.

Kellner R: Diagnosis and treatments of hypochondriacal syndromes. Psychosomatics 1992;33(3):278.

Kent DA et al: Course and outcome of conversion and somatization disorders. Psychosomatics 1995;36:138.

Lazare A: Conversion symptoms. N Engl J Med 1981; 305:745.

Lewis DO et al: Objective documentation of child abuse and dissociation in 12 murderers with dissociative identity disorder. Am J Psychiatry 1997;154:1703.

Loewenstein RJ: Somatoform disorders in victims of incest and child abuse. In: *Incest-Related Disorders of Adult Psychopathology,* pp. 75–113. Kluft RP (editor). American Psychiatric Press, 1990.

Loewenstein RJ: Diagnosis, epidemiology, clinical course, treatment, and cost effectiveness of treatment for dissociative disorders and multiple personality disorder: Report submitted to the Clinton administration task force on health care financing reform. Dissociation 1994;7(1):3.

Loewenstein RJ: Dissociative amnesia and dissociative fugue. In: *Treatment of Psychiatric Disorders,* 2nd ed. Vol 2, pp. 1570–1597. Gabbard GO (editor). American Psychiatric Press, 1995.

McCauley J et al: The battering syndrome: Prevalence and clinical characteristics of domestic violence in primary care internal medicine practice. Ann Intern Med 1995; 123(17):737.

McCauley J et al: Clinical characteristics of women with a history of childhood abuse: Unhealed wounds. J Am Med Assoc 1997;277(17):1362.

Noyes RJ, Kletti R: Depersonalization in response to life threatening danger. Comprehensive Psychiatry 1977; 18:375.

Phillips KA, Rassmussen SA, Price LH: Treating imagined ugliness. Arch Gen Psychiatry 1999;56:1041.

Pribor EF, Yutzy SH, Dean T, Wetzel RD: Briquet's syndrome, dissociation, and abuse. Am J Psychiatry 1993;150:1507.

Putnam FW: *Diagnosis and Treatment of Multiple Personality Disorder.* Guilford, 1989.

Putnam FW: *Dissociation in Children and Adolescents: A Developmental Perspective.* Guilford, 1998.

Ross C: The epidemiology of multiple personality disorder and dissociation. Psychiatr Clin North Am 1991;14:503.

Ross CA, Joshi S, Currie R: Dissociative experiences in the general population. Am J Psychiatry 1990;147:1547.

Ross CA et al: Structured interview data on 102 cases of multiple personality disorder. Am J Psychiatry 1990;147:596.

Scarini IC et al: Altered pain perception and psychophysical features among women with gastrointestinal disorders and history of abuse: A preliminary model. Am J Med 1994;97:108.

Simeon D et al: Feeling unreal: 30 cases of *DSM-III-R* depersonalization disorder. Am J Psychiatry 1997;154: 1107.

Simon GE, Gureje O: Stability of somatization disorder and somatization symptoms among primary care patients. Arch Gen Psychiatry 1999;56:90.

Smith GR, Monson RA, Ray DC: Psychiatric consultation in somatization disorder. New Engl J Med 1986;314: 1407.

Spiegel DE: The dissociative disorders. In: *American Psychiatric Press Annual Review of Psychiatry.* Vol 10. Tasman A, Goldfinger S (editors). American Psychiatric Press, 1991.

Steinberg M: *Handbook for the Assessment of Dissociation: A Clinical Guide.* American Psychiatric Press, 1995.

van der Kolk B et al: Dissociation, somatization, and affect dysregulation: The complexity of adaptation to trauma. Am J Psychiatry 1996;153(Suppl):83.

Walker EA et al: Relationship of chronic pelvic pain to psychiatric diagnoses and childhood sexual abuse. Am J Psychiatry 1998;145:75.

Walker EA et al: Histories of sexual victimization in patients with irritable bowel syndrome or inflammatory bowel disease. Am J Psychiatry 1993;150:1502.

23

Adjustment Disorder

Daniel S. Weiss, PhD, & Kathryn N. DeWitt, PhD

Other chapters in this text describe psychiatric disorders that are characterized by identifiable symptom patterns. Although these disorders are important subjects of psychiatric research and teaching, they do not account for the emotional problems of a great many individuals who seek help. The patients whose problems comprise the subject matter of this chapter lack some or all of the specific symptoms that would qualify them for the disorders discussed in other chapters. Adjustment disorders are generally associated with difficult life experiences, but the suffering or dysfunction that results is out of proportion to the degree of stress.

The diagnosis of adjustment disorder serves three important functions: (1) it draws attention to people who need professional help, (2) it provides a way of collecting data to devise new subcategories of illness, and (3) it describes specific procedures for distinguishing patients with adjustment disorder from patients with other mental disorders or with normal responses to the problems of life. Patients with "problems in living" but no mental disorder are classified by use of "V" codes (see below).

ADJUSTMENT DISORDER

Establishing a Diagnosis

The *Diagnostic and Statistical Manual of Mental Disorders,* 4th edition (*DSM-IV*) characterizes adjustment disorder as "the development of emotional or behavioral symptoms in response to an identifiable stressor(s) occurring within three months of the onset of the stressor." The reaction may take the form of either "marked distress in excess of what would be expected" or "significant impairment in social or occupational functioning." The disturbance may not have persisted for longer than 6 months after the termination of the stressor. The diagnosis of adjustment disorder is not used when symptoms conform to the specific criteria for another mental disorder (excluding personality disorder or developmental disorder); nor is it used when current distress represents but one instance of a general pattern of overreaction to stressors. For this reason, adjustment disorder is a diagnosis of exclusion.

Four major decisions are involved in the diagnosis of adjustment disorder: (1) establishing a relationship to a psychosocial stressor, (2) evaluating the level and duration of disturbance, (3) ruling out other mental disorders, and (4) evaluating the context of the patient's total personality.

A. Establishing a Relationship to a Psychosocial Stressor:

A 64-year-old retired teacher came to an internist seeking help for a feeling of constant exhaustion. She said that her troubles began months earlier with the death of her husband from kidney disease. She had thought that her problems were due to sadness at her loss, but now that they had lasted unchanged for nearly 6 months, she wondered whether she had "high blood pressure or low blood sugar or some such." She reported that her sleeping patterns had not changed and she had continued her regular pattern of daily walks. The patient and her husband were both accomplished bridge players, and she was an excellent cook; yet neither playing cards nor cooking was pleasurable any more. She still had a good appetite and attended her bridge club regularly, but her lack of enthusiasm was commented on by club members. The patient admitted that she felt she would be better off if she had died too, though she would not do anything to hurt herself. She was able to get around and take care of herself, but life did not seem to have any meaning.

Physical examination and laboratory tests failed to show evidence of any physical disorder. The physician concluded that the symptoms were of psychological origin.

Before a diagnosis of adjustment disorder can be made, the clinician must determine whether the patient's current problem is causally related to a psychosocial stressor. In many cases, a patient or someone who knows the patient may make a causal connection between the stressor and the disturbance. If the current disturbance represents a change in functioning that coincided with the occurrence of the stressor, there is a good cause for suspecting a connection. Symptoms may have appeared within minutes after the onset of stress or may have been long delayed. The *DSM-IV* diagnostic criteria require that the dysfunction be evident within 3 months after the onset of the stressor and persist for no longer than 6 months after the termination of the stressor.

Sometimes there is a logical connection between the kind of stressor and the content of the patient's disturbance, or the patient may report being consciously preoccupied with the stressor, as was the widow (see above). In other cases, patients may be unaware of a connection or even deny it if asked. In more ambiguous circumstances, discerning a connection may depend on the creativity and clinical experience of the clinician. A diagnosis of adjustment disorder is applicable only to patients whose current disturbance is clearly linked to a specific event, as would appear to be the case with the widow, since her exhaustion, suicidal thoughts, and lack of interest in life activities began soon after her husband's death and were not characteristic of her functioning before the event.

B. Evaluating the Level and Duration of Disturbance: The second decision-making process in the diagnosis of adjustment disorder is evaluation of the patient's specific signs and symptoms. A diagnosis of adjustment disorder may be warranted if the following circumstances apply: (1) the patient's symptoms are more severe than would be expected in the absence of some mental disorder, (2) the disturbance leads to significant impairment in social or occupational functioning, (3) the symptoms do not meet the criteria established for other mental disorders, and (4) the duration of symptoms does not exceed 6 months.

A diagnosis of adjustment disorder is used for patients whose response to a stressor is more severe or lasts longer than normally expected but somehow is nonspecific or incomplete. Patients whose reactions exceed expectable limits often are an object of concern to those around them, so that they may come to the physician's office accompanied by a friend or relative, or they may come alone but make a point of having done so at another's urging.

The reactions of others may help the clinician determine whether the patient's response to stress should be diagnosed as adjustment disorder. Responses not indicative of mental disorder may be assigned a V code (see below) to identify the condition that was the focus of medical attention. Responses indicative of some mental disorder by virtue of inappropriate severity or duration are examined more closely so that a specific diagnosis may be assigned. In the illustrative case discussed above, the unchanged nature of the widow's disturbance exceeds the expectable reaction following death of a spouse. Her symptoms are interfering with her social functioning and have been commented on by those around her.

C. Ruling Out Other Mental Disorders (Excluding Personality and Developmental Disorders): Patients are not given a diagnosis of adjustment disorder if their stress response meets the criteria for some other mental disorder. Patients for whom a diagnosis of adjustment disorder is inappropriate include those whose disturbances are organically caused, psychotic in nature, or limited to psychosexual problems, amnesia, loss of integration of

consciousness, or loss of identity. Also eliminated are those whose current disturbances are a single instance of a continuing psychosexual, substance abuse, or impulse control problem; similarly excluded are manic episodes, panic attacks, or phobic avoidance. Many excluded diagnostic categories are defined in part as an untoward reaction to a psychosocial stressor; examples include brief reactive psychosis, somatoform pain disorder, conversion disorders, psychogenic amnesia, psychogenic fugue, depersonalization disorder, and separation anxiety. Each of these diagnoses has additional specific distinguishing features that differentiate it from the nonspecific category of adjustment disorder.

Patients with adjustment disorder show disturbances of mood (either anxiety or depression) and impaired social and occupational functioning (withdrawal, misconduct, inhibition). They usually satisfy some but not all of the criteria for one or more of the following disorders: generalized anxiety disorder, posttraumatic stress disorder, major depressive disorder, dysthymia, cyclothymia, conduct disorder, or avoidant disorder.

In the case of the widow, the symptoms of fatigue, loss of pleasure in formerly satisfying activities, and passive death wishes place her within the spectrum of depressive disorders as set forth in Table 23–1; the depressive disorders include uncomplicated bereavement, adjustment disorder, major depressive disorder, dysthymia, and posttraumatic stress disorder. The patient's symptoms exceed the normal reaction to the death of a spouse. They began soon after her husband's death and continued unchanged for 6 months; they caused concern to her and those around her. Therefore, "uncomplicated bereavement" would be eliminated as a diagnostic consideration, and, by extension, the presence of a mental disorder would be confirmed. The duration of symptoms is insufficient for a diagnosis of dysthymia, which requires that symptoms be continually present for at least 2 years. The death of the patient's husband from kidney disease does not meet the criteria for posttraumatic stress disorder, since the principal stress is not beyond the range of common human experience. A diagnosis of major depressive disorder is inappropriate because the patient demonstrates only three of the eight major symptoms. The diagnosis of adjustment disorder is thus reached by a process of exclusion.

D. Evaluating the Context of the Patient's Total Personality:

A 56-year-old steelworker was brought to a family practitioner by his daughter. The daughter explained that her father had always been considered "difficult" but that lately he had become "nearly impossible," and she was concerned about his health. She reported that her father was known for sayings such as, "I wouldn't trust him as far as I could throw him." He usually kept to himself and was touchy about being taken advantage

Table 23–1. Differential diagnosis of depressed mood in bereavement.

	Type of Death	Duration of Symptoms	Type of Symptoms
Uncomplicated bereavement	Any type	2–3 months; longer by social custom or relationship to deceased	Limited to those normally expected
Adjustment disorder	Any type	Begin within 3 months; may be longer than normally expected; may not persist beyond 6 months	Either impaired social or occupational functioning or symptoms in excess of those normally expected
Major depressive disorder	Any type	Every day for at least 2 weeks	Dysphoric mood plus 4 out of 9 major symptoms (see Table 20–1)
Dysthymia	Any type	Continually present for 2 years, with remissions of 2 months or less	Depressive mood, but symptoms not severe enough for major depression; 3 out of 13 key symptoms present (see Table 20–1)
Posttraumatic stress disorder	Outside the range of usual experience	Immediate or delayed; duration not specified	Reexperiencing of trauma; numbing of responsiveness plus 2 out of 6 additional symptoms (see Table 21–7)

of. For the past 4 months, his suspicions had become frantic—he spent every waking moment worrying about some possible harm that might be done to him until he collapsed exhausted.

The patient seemed haggard and exhausted, though hyperalert during the interview. He nervously scanned the room as he talked and nearly jumped off the examining table when the nurse entered the room. When asked to explain his troubles, he replied that he had come "to get my daughter off my back." He said that although he was very tired, he could not let up, because he knew that "guys from work have it in for me." He had been out of work for 4 months since the local plant had closed. Previously he could "keep those bums in their place" because of his seniority, but now he was less able to defend himself and had to be constantly on the alert.

The patient was in touch with reality. His fears about his coworkers had the flavor of self-fulfilling prophecy and were not out of the realm of possibility, given his customary behavior in social situations. He showed no signs of abnormal thought patterns and was oriented as to time and place. He refused physical examinations and tests. In the absence of additional clinical information, the physician concluded that the patient's symptoms were probably due to psychological causes.

The clinician must assess the patient's personality style to determine whether the current maladaptive response is a unique and striking episode or is simply one aspect of a consistently maladaptive pattern of relating to the environment and oneself, as occurs in personality disorder. In general, a diagnosis of adjustment disorder is made if no diagnosis of personality disorder or developmental disorder alone can account for all of the symptoms and signs or if symptoms of the current stress response are atypical for a preexisting personality disorder.

The functioning of the widow did not meet the criteria for any of the personality disorders. She was capable of warm personal relationships and had a well-developed sense of self. In contrast, the steelworker's

usual manner of relating was compatible with a diagnosis of paranoid personality disorder. His current symptoms of exhaustion, suspiciousness, and hypervigilance were judged to be a stress-related exacerbation of a long-standing and stable dysfunctional personality style. Since the patient did not have symptoms that would lead to a diagnosis of organic delusional syndrome, paranoia, or paranoid schizophrenia, diagnoses of adjustment disorder and paranoid personality disorder were made.

Types

DSM-IV describes six main symptom patterns in adjustment disorder and assigns a code to each. The codes and their corresponding symptoms are set forth in Table 23–2.

The diagnosis of the widow would be classified as adjustment disorder with depressed mood, since all of her symptoms (exhaustion, loss of pleasure, death wishes) lie within the spectrum of depression. The steelworker's predominant symptoms of excessive vigilance against possible attack justify a diagnosis of adjustment disorder with anxious mood.

V Codes for Conditions Not Attributable to Mental Disorder

DSM-IV includes 21 V codes for "conditions that are a focus of attention or treatment but are not attributable to any of the mental disorders noted previously." These codes were adapted from a longer listing of similar conditions in ICD-9-CM (*World*

Table 23–2. Types of adjustment disorder.

Code	Description
309.24	With anxiety
309.0	With depressed mood
309.3	With disturbance of conduct
309.4	With mixed disturbance of emotions and conduct
309.28	With mixed anxiety and depressed mood
309.9	Unspecified

Health Organization's International Classification of Diseases, Injuries, and Causes of Death, 9th edition, with clinical modification codes [CM]) and include categories such as malingering, adult antisocial behavior, noncompliance with treatment for a mental disorder, partner relational problem, and sexual abuse of a child. The reactions of some patients in whom a diagnosis of adjustment disorder is being considered may fall within the limits of a normal and expectable response to a stressful life event; these patients would be assigned an appropriate V code to show the reason for their contact with a health facility. A V code may also be used when information is insufficient to determine whether a mental disorder is present or when the focus of treatment is not related to a coexisting mental disorder, eg, treatment of an uncomplicated marital problem in a person with simple phobia.

Natural History

A. Course and Outcome: The course and outcome of adjustment disorder are less severe and disabling than those of other major psychiatric disorders. A large study by Looney and Gunderson (1978) showed that the problems of persons with this diagnosis tended to be less severe with regard to chronicity, length of treatment, and disposition than those of other major psychiatric disorders.

B. Differential Course and Outcome in Adolescents and Adults: Studies by Andreasen and Hoenk (1982) found important differences in the expression of adjustment disorder in adolescents and in adults. Adolescents with adjustment disorders showed more serious disturbance than did adults with regard to symptoms, required length of treatment, and duration of symptoms before diagnosis. Adolescents also differed from adults with regard to their main presenting symptoms; adolescents were more likely to report disturbance of conduct, whereas adults were more likely to report depressive symptoms. The patient's age was found to be one of the most significant predictors of the outcome of adjustment disorder. About twice as many adolescents as adults experienced an episode of some other psychiatric disorder during a 5-year follow-up period.

In summary, available empirical evidence does indicate that adjustment disorder is less severe than other disorders with regard to both course and outcome. However, for some patients—particularly adolescents—an episode of adjustment disorder may be characterized by distress that is not self-limited and may be recurrent.

Epidemiology

A. General Prevalence: The limited data available on the prevalence of adjustment disorder support the view that the diagnosis is common in the psychiatric population, particularly among adolescents. Fabrega and Mezzich (1987) found that of 6800 psychiatric outpatients, close to 10% met the criteria for adjustment disorder as defined by *DSM-III*. Because the duration of *DSM-III* was only 1 month, the *DSM-III-R* and *DSM-IV* criteria would likely increase the prevalence, at least in the anxiety subtype (Schatzberg, 1990).

B. Differential Prevalence in Adolescents and Adults: The diagnosis of adjustment disorder is frequently made in adolescents. It is not clear whether the disorder is actually more common during adolescence or whether there are other reasons that the diagnosis is more commonly used for patients in that age group.

In spite of arguments and evidence to the contrary, many clinicians believe that significant distress is a common response to physiological and cultural events that normally occur during adolescence. They may therefore automatically classify cases of adolescent psychological disturbance as examples of adjustment disorder.

Frequent use of the diagnosis of adjustment disorder for adolescents may reflect its function as a provisional diagnosis. A crucial requirement of many alternative diagnoses is that the observed disturbance be long-standing and persistent; however, many psychiatric problems first appear during adolescence and persist from then on. The ambiguous picture may force the use of adjustment disorder as a nonspecific diagnosis until the long-range picture is clear.

Finally, researchers have found that some clinicians overuse the category because they are concerned about the adverse effects of applying psychiatric labels such as alcoholism or antisocial personality disorder to young people. The diagnosis of adjustment disorder is seen as less harmful than lifelong stigmatization by other diagnoses.

Careful epidemiological studies should eliminate such diagnostic inaccuracies, so that a more valid estimate of the prevalence of adjustment disorder can be made. In spite of this need, research on adjustment disorder is a relatively neglected area. Meanwhile, the diagnosis should be used with discretion. In an adolescent, there should be strong evidence that current problems are related to some specific event or to some identifiable aspect of the adolescent experience. When the diagnosis is unclear after careful assessment, a diagnosis of atypical psychosis or unspecified mental disorder (nonpsychotic) should be used instead.

Etiology & Pathogenesis

A. Presumed Causal Mechanism: Stress-related disorders are a disruption of the normal process of adaptation to stressful life events. Models of normal adaptation have been developed by Lindemann (1944) and Horowitz (1997), among others. In the Horowitz model, the person experiencing stress passes through regular stages of response, including outcry, in which the person protests that what has happened cannot be true; intrusion and denial, during which the person is either painfully aware of or oblivious to the new reality; working through, when the person becomes better able to integrate the event; and completion, which is marked by function at or above the prestress level.

In adjustment disorder, this process of adaptation does not proceed to completion. The presumed cause is psychic overload, ie, a level of intrapsychic strain that exceeds the individual's ability to cope.

The pattern of disruption may take many forms. Some persons become caught in a seemingly endless stage of denial; they act as if the stressful event had never occurred, avoid all reminders of the stress, and remain emotionally numb or isolated. In others, intrusive symptoms predominate; individuals become so painfully aware of the stressor that they are unable to sleep or control the flood of incoming emotions and images associated with the event. Still others oscillate between symptoms of intrusion and denial, with no overall change in psychological assimilation of the stressor. Any of these patterns may be accompanied by difficulties in interpersonal relationships.

B. Contributing Factors: Several models have been developed to explain why some people can handle stress and even grow as a result, whereas others develop distress of psychopathological proportions. Most models take into account the interaction of the stressor, the situation, and the person.

1. Stressors—Stressors are of two general types: shock-type stressors are time-limited events; continuous stressors are ongoing situations. Most descriptions of adaptation to stress concentrate on shock-type stressors. However, research shows that continuous stressors were more commonly cited as precipitating causes of psychiatric disorders. Adults usually developed adjustment disorder in response to ongoing problems in marriage, finances, work, or school. In adolescents, common stressors were problems with school, parental rejection, or parents' marital problems. Shock-type stressors were less commonly cited precipitating factors.

Research shows that the degree of undesirable change a stressor causes is the most significant aspect of its ability to cause strain. Other characteristics that influence the amount of strain produced by a stressor include whether the event was sudden or anticipated, central or peripheral to the life of the individual, and culturally shared or experienced in social isolation.

2. Situational context—The presence of material and social supports or handicaps can mitigate or exacerbate the strains of adaptation to stress. Pertinent factors in the material environment include economic conditions, occupational and recreational opportunities, and weather conditions. Factors in the social environment include family, friends, neighbors, and cultural or religious support groups. These elements create a supportive or nonsupportive climate for adaptation.

3. Intrapersonal factors—Intrapersonal factors are considered the most crucial in determining whether the response to stress will be normal or dysfunctional. Not all persons with roughly similar stressors and environmental circumstances have similar responses to stress. Some are vulnerable to even minor stressful events, whereas others show an amazing resilience in the face of the most traumatic experiences.

Intrapersonal vulnerability to stressful life experiences may be general or specific. General factors include limitations in social skills or in intelligence, flexibility, and range of coping strategies. The presence of chronic disorders such as organic mental disorder, mental retardation, psychotic disorder, or personality disorder limits the general adaptive capacity of an individual.

Vulnerability to specific types of stressful events or circumstances may arise from relevant life traumas, unresolved conflicts, or developmental issues. Women who lost their mothers in infancy are more likely to develop serious depressive episodes following adult losses. People who have conflicts about aggression may respond to assault by alternately avoiding and provoking fights with others. Individuals who have difficulty making choices respond to the absence of structure in retirement by feeling helplessly directionless. Each of these intrapersonal factors combines with extrapersonal factors and characteristics of the stressor to produce the individual's stress response.

Treatment

A. Controversy About Treatment: The *DSM-III-R* definition of adjustment disorder and its continuation in *DSM-IV* has engendered controversy about treatment. On the one hand, the disorder is expected to eventually remit after the stressor ceases or, if the stressor persists, when a new level of adaptation is achieved. This expectation has led some to argue that treatment is unnecessary and wasteful. Some suggest that treatment may actually interfere with normal coping and result in worsening symptoms and delayed resolution.

On the other hand, adjustment disorder is also defined as being associated with exaggerated symptoms and social or occupational impairment. Clinicians who favor treatment suggest that symptoms must be brought within manageable limits before the patient can begin to cope with the stress. They also point out that in adjustment disorder, duration of symptoms may have exceeded the point of spontaneous remission. Such disturbances become self-sustaining and require some means of interrupting the downward spiral if serious effects on work and social relationships are to be avoided. Proponents of crisis intervention theory maintain that a crisis offers an ideal opportunity for treatment that will act as a catalyst for positive change in coping strategies.

B. General Recommendations: The general recommendation for treatment of adjustment disorder is for brief treatment with periodic reassessments. The primary goals of treatment are to relieve symptoms and assist patients in achieving a level of adaptation that at least equals their functioning before the stressful event. A secondary goal is to foster positive change whenever possible—particularly in areas still vulnerable to recurrent stress-related disorders.

C. Psychosocial Treatment Methods: Mental health professionals most commonly recommend some form of psychosocial treatment for patients with adjustment disorder. Since adjustment disorder is generally thought to arise from vulnerabilities in the patient's psychosocial functioning, treatment measures are designed to have an impact on whatever habits, conflicts, developmental inadequacies, or disturbing social symptoms are thought to be the source of the patient's problem. Such treatments hold the greatest promise for preventing recurrent disorders.

1. Individual psychotherapy is the most common psychosocial treatment for adjustment disorder. The brief psychodynamic psychotherapy described by Horowitz (1989) is a good example. In this approach, the patient's problems are thought to result from the meanings assigned by the individual to the stressful event in relation to unresolved conflicts, previously latent negative self-images, earlier traumatic experiences, and developmental inadequacies. Common psychodynamic techniques of supportive and expressive psychotherapy are used to discover and resolve these meanings.

   Individual behavior therapy differs significantly in theory and technique from individual psychodynamic psychotherapy. In behavior therapy, the patient's problems are seen to be the result of habitually dysfunctional patterns of responding to situations. The goal of treatment is to replace ineffective adaptive response patterns with successful ones. Modeling, coaching, didactic presentations, and carefully designed reinforcement schedules are common techniques. Behavior therapy has usually been considered most appropriate for problems of impulse control, which may occur in adjustment disorder with disturbance of conduct.

2. Family therapy is the second most common treatment for adjustment disorder. In this approach, the focus of diagnosis and treatment is shifted from the individual to the system of relationships in which the individual is involved.

Treatment is designed to alter the functioning of the social network, and, when possible, all relevant family members are included in treatment sessions. Family therapy should be seriously considered in adjustment disorder associated with developmental milestones such as birth of a child, mid-life transition, or retirement. It is also helpful in situations such as family bereavements and marital problems.

3. Self-help groups, in which people who have experienced similar stressful life events come together without a professional facilitator, are increasing in popularity. Group members often gain reassurance from discovering that many of their frightening emotional experiences are common and therefore not "crazy," as they had feared. Members also benefit from having an arena in which they can talk about painful topics without feeling like a burden to family and friends. Group members exchange advice, share coping strategies, and provide support and encouragement. They may also develop new social networks to replace those lost through events such as death or divorce. Community service agencies can be a good source of information on self-help groups.

D. Biomedical Treatment Methods: Medication may be the most commonly used treatment for adjustment disorder, since self-medication with alcohol, caffeine, over-the-counter medications, and street drugs is undoubtedly widespread. Treatment of symptoms of depression and anxiety with prescribed medications is also common. Prescription drugs have the potential advantage of being carefully chosen and continually monitored.

Mental health professionals usually do not treat adjustment disorder with medication. Reasons for this include concerns that the effect of medication is temporary; that alleviating symptoms masks the real problem or interferes with the motivation to find a real, lasting solution; and that patients may develop either psychological or physiological dependence.

Although depressive symptoms are common in adjustment disorder, concerns about side effects of antidepressant medications and the length of time required to achieve effective results persuade most clinicians that their use should be limited to major depressive disorder.

When used, medications are generally considered adjuncts to treatment or as backup treatment when psychological treatments are unavailable or unacceptable to the patient. Medications may be used to bring distress within tolerable limits, so that the patient's coping strategies may be effectively mobilized. When they are used, clinicians should prescribe the lowest effective dosage for the shortest possible duration, together with frequent monitoring of efficacy and side effects.

SUMMARY

Adjustment disorder is one of the more common psychological disorders for which patients seek professional help, particularly from general practitioners. For this reason, all clinicians should have a good working knowledge of the four decision-making procedures used to diagnose adjustment disorder: (1) establishing a relationship to a psychosocial stressor, (2) evaluating the level and duration of disturbance, (3) ruling out other mental disorders (excluding personality or developmental disorder), and (4) evaluating the patient's total personality. Patients with adjustment disorder demonstrate inadequate or incomplete adaptation to life stresses. The treatment of choice is brief psychosocial intervention designed to enhance the patient's ability to cope with the stressful event. When patients feel out of control, appropriate medications may be used to alleviate symptoms to the point that the patient can begin to cope with the stressful situation.

REFERENCES & SUGGESTED READINGS

Andreasen NC, Hoenk PR: The predictive value of adjustment disorders: A follow-up study. Am J Psychiatry 1982;139:584.

Andreasen NC, Wasek P: Adjustment disorders in adolescents and adults. Arch Gen Psychiatry 1980;37:1166.

Fabrega H Jr, Mezzich J: Adjustment disorder and psychiatric practice: Cultural and historical aspects. Psychiatry 1987;50:31.

Horowitz MJ: *Stress Response Syndromes,* 3rd ed. Jason Aronson, 1997.

Horowitz MJ: Brief dynamic psychotherapy. In: *Treatments of Psychiatric Disorders: A Task Force Report of the American Psychiatric Association.* American Psychiatric Association, 1989.

Lindemann E: Symptomatology and management of acute grief. Am J Psychiatry 1944;101:141.

Looney JG, Gunderson EK: Transient situational disturbances: Course and outcome. Am J Psychiatry 1978; 135:660.

Schatzberg AF: Anxiety and adjustment disorder: A treatment approach. J Clin Psychiatry 1990;51:11 (Supplement).

Personality Disorders

24

Charles R. Marmar, MD

Patients with personality disorder are common both in medical and in psychiatric practice. Such people frequently make pressing demands for treatment of their numerous complaints while at the same time resisting appropriate treatment recommendations. Their lack of cooperation may cause resentment and possibly even alienation and burnout in the health care professionals who treat them. The frequently overriding needs of such individuals for self-aggrandizement, their diminished capacity for understanding and respecting the needs of others, and their mistrust and emotional instability lead to maladaptive behavior, including manipulation and exploitation of others. Such individuals are limited in their capacity to participate in mutual give and take with another person.

In this chapter, each major personality disorder is discussed from two perspectives, that of formal psychiatric nosology and that of management of the medically or surgically ill patient with an impaired personality.

Medical illness may have a recurrent, predictable psychological meaning for patients with specific personality disorders. Hidden motives (covert agendas) in the patient's relationship with the physician may lead to problems of overutilization or underutilization of the health care system, substance abuse, and potential negative reactions in the physician. This chapter presents coping strategies for the physician that may increase the chances of patient compliance with medical or surgical treatment and minimize medical complications and interpersonal problems in the care of such patients.

CHARACTERISTICS OF PERSONALITY DISORDERS

The *Diagnostic and Statistical Manual of Mental Disorders,* 4th edition (*DSM-IV*) defines **personality traits** as "enduring patterns of perceiving, relating to, and thinking about the environment and oneself . . . exhibited in a wide range of important social and personal contexts." When these patterns are "inflexible and maladaptive and cause either significant impairment in social or occupational functioning or subjective distress," they constitute **personality disorders.** Such personality disturbances can be recognized

by adolescence or earlier and commonly continue through adulthood; the pathological characteristics have their precursors in early developmental disturbances and remain as enduring qualities of a person. A diagnosis of personality disorder is not appropriate if the disturbance in functioning is episodic, since the symptoms of personality disorder should represent the person's *stable* characteristics and social functioning.

Because elements of character disorders appear early in life, childhood and adolescent disorders correlate strongly with adult personality disorders. For example, a child with conduct disorder frequently presents as an adult with antisocial personality disorder. Similarly, schizoid disorder of childhood or adolescence is linked to schizoid personality disorder of adulthood; avoidant disorder of childhood or adolescence may become avoidant personality disorder of adulthood; oppositional disorder of childhood may become passive-aggressive personality disorder of adulthood; and identity disorder of childhood may become borderline personality disorder in adulthood.

Because individuals with personality disorders exhibit recurrent maladaptive strategies in their interpersonal relationships, they may be markedly dissatisfied with the impact of their behavior on others and with their inability to function effectively. The resulting distress is prevalent in personality disorders; this is contrary to earlier concepts, which asserted that these patients were free from distress. Anxiety and depression are particularly common and may be the primary complaint.

Substantial evidence suggests that individuals with personality disorders—which by definition are long-standing and at times lifelong disturbances in functioning—are at greater risk for various **Axis I** psychiatric disorders, with symptomatic flare-ups occurring during occupational or personal stresses or developmental milestones (adolescence, midlife crisis, aging, etc).

Ucok et al (1998) studied 90 outpatients with bipolar I disorder and 58 controls, and reported that *DSM-III-R* comorbid personality disorders were three times more likely in the bipolar patients. Morgenstern et al (1997) assessed the comorbidity of alcoholism and personality disorder and reported high prevalence rates of alcoholism in both antisocial and borderline personality disorder.

GENERAL DIAGNOSTIC CRITERIA FOR PERSONALITY DISORDERS

The general criteria diagnostic of all personality disorders as specified in *DSM-IV* are given in Table 24–1.

DIFFERENTIATION BETWEEN PERSONALITY DISORDERS & OTHER PSYCHIATRIC DISORDERS

Differentiation from Neurotic Disorders

Because anxiety and depression are common both in personality disorders and in neurotic disorders, these symptoms cannot be used as criteria in making a differential diagnosis; however, in making a differential diagnosis other factors are useful. Individuals with personality disorders have **alloplastic** defenses and react to stress by attempting to change the *external* environment. For example, such patients often deal with a potential disappointment by threatening to retaliate and in that way manipulate another person to gratify rather than disappoint them (Berman and McCann, 1995). In contrast, patients with neurotic disorders have **autoplastic** defenses and react to stress by changing their *internal* psychological processes. For example, neurotic patients might rationalize that a disappointment is of no great importance.

Another distinguishing factor is the difference in self-awareness manifested in patients with the two types of disorders. Patients with personality disorders

Table 24–1. *DSM-IV* general diagnostic criteria for personality disorders.

A. An enduring pattern of inner experience and behavior that deviates markedly from the expectations of the individual's culture. This pattern is manifested in two (or more) of the following areas:
(1) cognition (ie, ways of perceiving and interpreting self, other people, and events), (2) affectivity (ie, the range, intensity, lability, and appropriateness of emotional response), (3) interpersonal functioning, (4) impulse control.

B. The enduring pattern is inflexible and pervasive across a broad range of personal and social situations.

C. The enduring pattern leads to clinically significant distress or impairment in social, occupational, or other important areas of functioning.

D. The pattern is stable and of long duration, and its onset can be traced back at least to adolescence or early adulthood.

E. The enduring pattern is not better accounted for as a manifestation or consequence of another mental disorder.

F. The enduring pattern is not due to the direct physiological effects of a substance (eg, a drug of abuse, a medication) or a general medical condition (eg, head trauma).

frequently perceive character deficits as **egosyntonic,** ie, acceptable, unobjectionable, and part of the self. For example, patients with such a disorder disavow personal responsibility for hurting another person, have difficulty in appreciating the pain they have inflicted on another, and attribute blame to another person. In contrast, individuals with neurotic disorders perceive personal shortcomings as **egodystonic,** ie, unacceptable, objectionable, and alien to the self. Patients with neurotic disorders blame and chastise themselves for disappointing or hurting a valued person through their shortcomings.

Differentiation from Psychotic Disorders

Although there may be severe disturbances in social and occupational functioning in individuals with personality disorders, persistent psychotic features such as formal thought disorder (as manifested by loosening of associations), delusions, and hallucinations are absent. Transient psychotic states, or "micropsychotic episodes," in people with severe borderline personality disorders are important exceptions (see below). The quality of the psychotic disturbance in borderline personality disorder is different from that in schizophreniform psychoses; episodes are short-lived, directly related to a given situation, and usually self-limited, and they normally do not require hospitalization or medication. (See Chapter 19 for a discussion of brief reactive psychoses.)

Differentiation from Organic Mental Disorders

Individuals with uncomplicated personality disorders have a clear sensorium; are oriented as to time, place, and person; and show normal intellectual functioning, so that memory for recent or remote events, fund of general knowledge, ability to perform calculations, and so on are within normal limits. Individuals with personality disorders may of course develop dementia or delirium later in life and in certain cases may be at greater risk for such disorders (eg, through sustained alcohol or substance abuse). Multiple diagnoses are warranted in such patients.

PARANOID PERSONALITY DISORDER

Symptoms & Signs

The diagnostic criteria for paranoid personality disorder are summarized in Table 24–2.

According to *DSM-IV,* the essential feature of paranoid personality disorder is "a pattern of pervasive distrust and suspiciousness of others such that their motives are interpreted as malevolent." These symptoms and signs are characteristic of the patient's long-term functioning and are not episodic in character or limited to particular episodes of illness. They are also associated with significant impairment in

Table 24–2. *DSM-IV* diagnostic criteria for paranoid personality disorder.

A. A pervasive distrust and suspiciousness of others such that their motives are interpreted as malevolent, beginning by early adulthood and present in a variety of contexts, as indicated by four (or more) of the following: (1) suspects without sufficient basis that others are exploiting, harming, or deceiving him or her, (2) is preoccupied with unjustified doubts about the loyalty or trustworthiness of friends or associates, (3) is reluctant to confide in others because of unwarranted fear that the information will be used maliciously against him or her, (4) reads hidden demeaning or threatening meanings into benign remarks or events, (5) persistently bears grudges, ie, is unforgiving of insults, injuries, or slights, (6) perceives attacks on his or her character or reputation that are not apparent to others and is quick to react angrily or to counterattack, (7) has recurrent suspicions, without justification, regarding fidelity of spouse or sexual partner.

B. Does not occur exclusively during the course of schizophrenia, a mood disorder with psychotic features, or another psychotic disorder and is not due to the direct physiological effects of a general medical condition.

Note: If criteria are met prior to the onset of schizophrenia, add "premorbid," eg, "paranoid personality disorder (premorbid)."

work and personal relationships. Patients are hostile, stubborn, and defensive, and they avoid intimacy. They are rigid and uncompromising, interested primarily in inanimate objects rather than human relations, extremely sensitive to rank, and disinterested in the arts and esthetics.

Natural History & Prognosis

Systematic data are not available.

Differential Diagnosis

In paranoid schizophrenia and paranoid disorders, there are persistent psychotic symptoms, including delusions and hallucinations, that are not features of paranoid personality disorder. Individuals with paranoid personality disorder may develop paranoid psychoses, however, at which time an additional diagnosis is justified.

Illustrative Case

A 52-year-old man was referred for psychiatric evaluation after a medical workup revealed no basis for his persistent headaches. The headaches had begun 6 months earlier, at about the same time that he became preoccupied with the possibility that his supervisor wanted to fire him. They had an argument about the vacation schedule, and he felt that he was being taken advantage of unfairly, since coworkers with less seniority had more favorable schedules. After the argument, he had seen his supervisor joking with one of the other mechanics and had assumed that he was the object of their derision.

Although emotionally distant, the patient had been

a loyal, serious, hardworking, and productive employee and had stayed at the same company for the past 18 years. He could always be counted on to do a good job, but he tended to be excluded by other workers, who found him unable to relax and make jokes. He had been married for 25 years to a school librarian and described his marriage as satisfactory: "She's always there, but she doesn't make a lot of demands on me." They had decided not to have children, because "they're disruptive, unpredictable, demanding, take whatever they can get out of you, and then go off on their own."

In the interview, the patient appeared tense and vigilant, and seemed to search for verbal or nonverbal clues indicating that the interviewer did not have his best interests at heart. When the interviewer suggested that he might have provoked his supervisor, he snapped back irritably that the interviewer, like most people, misunderstood him. The patient was understandable and goal-directed in his thinking, and there was no evidence of well-formed delusions or hallucinatory experiences. He admitted that he might be overreacting to the altercation with his supervisor. He noted that this had happened several times before and that in each instance he had later been reassured that he was a valued employee.

Epidemiology

The prevalence has been reported to be 0.5–2.5% in the general population, 2–10% in psychiatric outpatients, and 10–30% among psychiatric inpatients.

Paranoid personality disorder is more commonly diagnosed in men than in women. A familial pattern has been suggested with increased prevalence among first-degree relatives of probands with chronic schizophrenia as well as those with delusional disorders, persecutory type. The relationship of paranoid personality disorder to paranoid schizophrenia and paranoid disorder is uncertain.

Etiology & Pathogenesis

The specific causes of paranoid personality disorder are not known. However, genetic predisposition may play a role, and it is likely that someone in the patient's family has a paranoid disorder. Early childhood deprivation or child abuse alone or in concert with genetic susceptibility may lead to a paranoid sense of mistrust.

Treatment

An honest, respectful attitude is important in psychotherapeutic treatment of patients with paranoid personality disorder. The therapist must pay attention to the degree of closeness shown toward the patient, since too much intimacy, warmth, and empathy may be seen as an intrusive attempt at control. Deep psychological interpretations tend to increase feelings of suspicion rather than clarify conflicts about warded-off feelings or intentions. The therapist can reduce the chances of being perceived as yet another enemy by insisting on prompt and repeated examination of the patient's distorted image of the therapist (reality testing) in a firm but noncritical way.

The therapist should readily acknowledge and confirm any errors, feelings of irritation, or lapses in consideration, because patients with paranoid personality disorder will interpret denials of such behavior as proof of covert persecutory intentions. A tactful and polite but not overly elaborate apology by the therapist can do much to restore the patient's trust.

Paranoid Personality Disorder in Medical Practice

The paranoid patient's underlying mistrust, hypersensitivity to slights, fear of dependency, and underlying sense of shame and vulnerability are heightened during illness or even with the threat of illness. A trusting relationship between the physician and the patient is essential to ensure compliance with surgical or pharmacological treatments. A low-key and friendly but not overly intimate attitude on the part of the physician effectively counters the paranoid patient's dual expectations of being disregarded as worthless on the one hand and being intruded upon on the other. In the first few visits, the therapist can ask the patient about previous doctor-patient relationships, particularly about both the helpful and the irritating elements. Inquiring whether the patient has ever abruptly terminated treatment with another physician because of actual or fantasied injury or betrayal is valuable with any patient, but may be particularly informative with a paranoid patient, since the physician can establish an effective working relationship and avoid the pitfalls encountered in the patient's previous relationships with health care professionals.

A physician who is being berated by a paranoid patient and who can acknowledge—without being defensive or attacking or encouraging the patient's distorted view—that the patient's pain and fear aroused by aspects of the physician-patient relationship are real is creating an invaluable opportunity to provide an atmosphere in which the patient can feel safe in working toward clarification of past difficulties. For paranoid patients, the primary problem in the doctor-patient relationship is frequently not any actual failure in treatment but rather the patient's subjectively distorted image of the physician as an individual with malevolent intentions, a fear that proves "justified" when difficulties occur in diagnosis or treatment.

In a discussion of the hostile, suspicious, and recalcitrant patient in medical practice, Dennis Farrell offers the following case (personal communication) as an example of the need by the medical staff to provide clear explanations of all procedures undertaken in treating such patients.

Illustrative Case

A 42-year-old man with paranoid personality disorder who had presented at a medical clinic for treatment had a history of changing doctors and of not complying with prescribed medical regimens. The patient scowled when he was handed a prescription for medication, and the medical student assigned to work with the patient noted the patient's reaction aloud. The patient muttered a comment about "cheap medication," and the student asked him to explain the remark. It appeared that when the dosage of the patient's medication had recently been changed, the patient had not received an adequate explanation and had merely been told that he was receiving the same medication. The patient concluded that the doctors had decided to give him some cheap, second-rate medicine because he was a clinic patient. The patient thought that there was no good reason why the same medication should look different unless it was in some way inferior. When the medical student expressed genuine interest in the patient and offered a clear explanation of why the dosage had been changed, the patient felt comfortable in taking the medication as prescribed.

SCHIZOID PERSONALITY DISORDER

Symptoms & Signs

The diagnostic criteria for schizoid personality disorder are presented in Table 24–3. According to *DSM-IV,* the disorder is characterized by "a pervasive pattern of detachment from social relationships and a restricted range of expressions of emotions in interpersonal settings." Patients have difficulty in expressing hostility. They are excessively self-absorbed and

Table 24–3. *DSM-IV* diagnostic criteria for schizoid personality disorder.

A. A pervasive pattern of detachment from social relationships and a restricted range of expression of emotions in interpersonal settings, beginning by early adulthood and present in a variety of contexts, as indicated by four (or more) of the following:
(1) neither desires nor enjoys close relationships, including being part of a family, (2) almost always chooses solitary activities, (3) has little, if any, interest in having sexual experiences with another person, (4) takes pleasure in few, if any, activities, (5) lacks close friends or confidants other than first-degree relatives, (6) appears indifferent to the praise or criticism of others, (7) shows emotional coldness, detachment, or flattened affectivity.

B. Does not occur exclusively during the course of schizophrenia, a mood disorder with psychotic features, another psychotic disorder, or a pervasive developmental disorder and is not due to the direct physiological effects of a general medical condition.

Note: If criteria are met prior to the onset of schizophrenia, add "premorbid," eg, "schizoid personality disorder (premorbid)."

detached, and they engage in daydreaming. Their work performance is generally better than their ability to participate in interpersonal relationships. They appear to derive little pleasure from intimacy and live for the most part as isolated loners.

Natural History & Prognosis

Onset is in early childhood. Prospective studies indicate that the majority of shy children do not go on to develop schizoid personality disorder. However, once the pattern is established, it tends to be stable during adolescence and throughout adulthood.

Differential Diagnosis

Schizoid personality disorder must be differentiated from schizotypal personality disorder, in which there are eccentricities of communication and behavior and in which a positive family history of schizophrenia occurs more frequently. Schizoid personality disorder must also be differentiated from avoidant personality disorder, in which there is social withdrawal despite a desire for acceptance; this withdrawal in the avoidant personality results from an exquisite sensitivity to rejection. People with schizoid personality disorder do not directly experience or acknowledge a wish for closeness.

Illustrative Case

A 32-year-old assistant professor of philosophy presented for psychiatric evaluation, primarily to satisfy a request from his aging parents. They were worried about their son's impoverished social life and wanted to see him happily married so they could die in peace, knowing that their son would not be alone in the world. He was not overtly dissatisfied with his life and found gratification in his theoretical writings and occasional intellectual debates with colleagues. He did not seem to feel the loneliness that troubled his parents. He said that it was not a matter of wishing to be included in the company of others or feeling shy about forming an attachment but that he simply had no wish to be close to others.

When the patient was not working, he spent his evenings and weekends refining a mathematically elaborate system for winning at blackjack. In testing this theory, he always visited the casinos alone. He said that as a child he had preferred to read about politics and religion rather than participate in sports or associate with other children, and he felt that he had been a loner all his life.

In the interview, the patient appeared timid. He was unable to sustain eye contact, and he provided circumscribed, emotionally barren responses to questions. He fidgeted and appeared to be counting the minutes until he could leave the room. When asked if he resented being asked to come to the interview to relieve his parents' anxieties, he answered in the affirmative, but without any apparent feeling. The in-terviewer found it difficult to empathize with the patient, since he seemed so remote and uninvolved in the discussion.

Epidemiology

There is little evidence linking schizoid personality disorder to schizophrenia, in contrast to schizotypal personality disorder, which is considered part of the spectrum of schizophrenic disorders. The prevalence of schizoid personality disorder has not been established.

Etiology & Pathogenesis

It is not clear whether there is a genetic predisposition to development of schizoid personality disorder. Important psychological factors include a cold, unempathic, emotionally impoverished childhood as shown by retrospective (not prospective) studies.

Treatment

Long-term psychotherapy has been useful in selected cases. The course of therapy involves gradual development of trust. If this can be achieved, the patient may share long-standing fantasies of imaginary friendships and may reveal fears of depending on others. Patients are encouraged to examine the unrealistic nature of their fears and fantasies and to form actual relationships. Successful psychotherapy will produce gradual change.

Group psychotherapy may be helpful. A prolonged period of silent withdrawal may often be followed by gradual involvement in the group process. It is important for the group leader to protect the schizoid patient from criticism by other members for not participating verbally in the early, affiliative phase of the group.

Schizoid Personality Disorder in Medical Practice

The person with schizoid personality disorder sustains a fragile emotional equilibrium by avoiding intimate personal contact and thereby minimizing conflict that is poorly tolerated. Illness is not only a threat to personal integrity but also necessitates seeking treatment from a health care team that may seem to impose a demand for dependent involvement that is hard for this type of patient to accept. For this reason, the patient may delay seeking help until symptoms become severe. Once treatment has started, the patient frequently appears detached, as though unappreciative of the help being offered. Such individuals may dissociate the tolerable, technical aspects of treatment from its frightening interpersonal context.

The physician should appreciate the need for privacy in a person with schizoid personality disorder and should maintain a low-key approach that focuses on the technical elements of treatment. Such a focus will demonstrate caring and let the patient know that caretakers will not press beyond comfortable limits. The patient should be encouraged to maintain daily routines so that a sense of "life as usual" can counteract the worry that illness will shatter the patient's efforts to remain detached and uninvolved. Knowledge of the patient's usual pattern of functioning will counteract any tendency on the part of the health care team to become personally overinvolved or to be too zealously concerned with providing social supports for the patient.

SCHIZOTYPAL PERSONALITY DISORDER

Symptoms & Signs

The diagnostic criteria for schizotypal personality disorder are presented in Table 24–4. According to *DSM-IV*, the disorder is characterized by "a pervasive pattern of social and interpersonal deficits marked by acute discomfort with and reduced capacity for close relationships as well as by cognitive or perceptual distortions and eccentricities of behavior." The patient suffers from anxiety, depression, and other dysphoric mood states. If features of borderline personality disorder are present, both diagnoses may be assigned. Reactive psychoses and eccentric convictions occur. The patient also demonstrates magical thinking, as illustrated by superstition and by a belief in clairvoyance and telepathy. Speech is character-

Table 24–4. *DSM-IV* diagnostic criteria for schizotypal personality disorder.

A. A pervasive pattern of social and interpersonal deficits marked by acute discomfort with, and reduced capacity for, close relationships as well as by cognitive or perceptual distortions and eccentricities of behavior, beginning by early adulthood and present in a variety of contexts, as indicated by five (or more) of the following: (1) ideas of reference (excluding delusions of reference), (2) odd beliefs or magical thinking that influences behavior and is inconsistent with subcultural norms (eg, superstitiousness, belief in clairvoyance, telepathy, or "sixth sense"; in children and adolescents, bizarre fantasies or preoccupations), (3) unusual perceptual experiences, including bodily illusions, (4) odd thinking and speech (eg, vague, circumstantial, metaphorical, overelaborate, or stereotyped), (5) suspiciousness or paranoid ideation, (6) inappropriate or constricted affect, (7) behavior or appearance that is odd, eccentric, or peculiar, (8) lack of close friends or confidants other than first-degree relatives, (9) excessive social anxiety that does not diminish with familiarity and tends to be associated with paranoid fears rather than negative judgments about self.

B. Does not occur exclusively during the course of schizophrenia, a mood disorder with psychotic features, another psychotic disorder, or a pervasive developmental disorder.

Note: If criteria are met prior to the onset of schizophrenia, add "premorbid," eg, "schizotypal personality disorder (premorbid)."

ized by idiosyncratic construction and phrasing, leading to a peculiar, stilted quality to communication.

Natural History & Prognosis

The prevalence in the community has been estimated at 3%.

Differential Diagnosis

The differential diagnosis should include schizoid personality disorder, in which behavioral and communicative oddities do not occur, and schizophrenia, in which formal thought disorder occurs.

Illustrative Case

A 34-year-old single woman presented at a community mental health center complaining of feelings of detachment and unreality. She said she felt cut off from her environment, as though she were looking out at the world through "semitransparent gauze." She also complained that when she was walking in the evening, moving shadows cast by the wind blowing through the trees created the frightening illusion of a potential assailant. She momentarily visualized a menacing figure, only to realize it was merely an illusion. This experience occurred repeatedly.

The patient had supported herself over the past few years by tea leaf and palm reading and other forms of fortune-telling. She said that this choice of occupation followed from her long-standing belief that she possessed special powers. During adolescence, she had claimed to be clairvoyant. She was regarded as either odd or fascinating by her acquaintances. She was deeply superstitious and preoccupied with numbers, colors, and dates. For example, she traveled on airplanes only when the day of the month, the flight number, and the scheduled arrival time were even numbers.

The patient's relationships usually involved superficial acquaintances, primarily people who shared her superstitious belief systems. She spent long periods daydreaming and fantasizing that she was a beautiful woman who would achieve great prominence by foretelling important world events. Such daydreams usually occurred after she experienced insults or slights.

At the interview, the patient was colorfully dressed in a juxtaposition of clashing, gypsy-like styles that gave her a patchwork, disheveled appearance. Although she showed no frank disorder of speech such as incoherence or gross loosening of associations, her language was stilted, and she used inappropriately formal and technical terms in a disjunctive fashion that made her speech difficult to follow. There was no evidence of delusions or hallucinations. When she was asked about a family history of mental disorder, she replied that an older sister had undergone several psychiatric hospitalizations and was currently receiving antipsychotic drugs.

Epidemiology

The incidence of schizophrenia is increased in first-degree relatives of individuals with schizotypal personality disorder.

Etiology & Pathogenesis

Schizotypal personality disorder shares a genetic relationship with schizophrenia, as shown by family, twin, and adoption studies, which have demonstrated that these disorders occur more often in genetically related family members than in unrelated individuals.

Treatment

The physician must exercise tact when exploring idiosyncratic belief systems during psychotherapy. Antipsychotic medication is useful in patients with pronounced psychotic manifestations, particularly during stress.

Schizotypal Personality Disorder in Medical Practice

The problems encountered in the management of schizotypal patients and the management approaches used are similar to those for schizoid patients, as described above. The physician must also be able to help the patient with reality testing and differentiating fantasy from fact. In this respect, management techniques are similar to those used for patients with paranoid and borderline personality disorders and patients with psychotic disorders. Occasionally, the physician may consider the use of antipsychotic medications if the patient becomes frankly psychotic. If psychosis persists, the possibility of a coexisting mental disorder must be considered, and psychiatric consultation is indicated.

HISTRIONIC PERSONALITY DISORDER

Symptoms & Signs

The diagnostic criteria for histrionic personality disorder are summarized in Table 24–5. *DSM-IV* states that the essential feature of this disorder is "pervasive and excessive emotionality and attention-seeking behavior."

Patients with histrionic personality disorder experience reactive dysphoria in the face of loss or rejection as well as difficulty with linear, analytic thought, although they are often creative and imaginative. Patients are impressionable, suggestible, and intuitive, ie, they "play hunches" instead of thinking decisions through methodically. They draw attention to themselves by their dramatic, lively, and at times seductive social behavior. There is a tendency toward somatization, with dramatic and shifting presentations of physical symptoms.

Natural History & Prognosis

Systematic data are not available.

Table 24–5. *DSM-IV* diagnostic criteria for histrionic personality disorder.

A pervasive pattern of excessive emotionality and attention seeking, beginning by early adulthood and present in a variety of contexts, as indicated by five (or more) of the following: (1) is uncomfortable in situations in which he or she is not the center of attention, (2) interaction with others is often characterized by inappropriate sexually seductive or provocative behavior, (3) displays rapidly shifting and shallow expression of emotions, (4) consistently uses physical appearance to draw attention to self, (5) has a style of speech that is excessively impressionistic and lacking in detail, (6) shows self-dramatization, theatricality, and exaggerated expression of emotion, (7) is suggestible, ie, easily influenced by others or circumstances, (8) considers relationships to be more intimate than they actually are.

Differential Diagnosis

Histrionic personality disorder must be differentiated from somatization disorder, borderline personality disorder, and narcissistic personality disorder. These three disorders may coexist in some combination with histrionic personality disorder, in which case all relevant diagnoses may be assigned.

Illustrative Case

A 32-year-old single professional photographer sought psychiatric treatment because of repetitive disappointments in her love relationships. She had achieved considerable success in her career over the past few years but was unmotivated to work after the recent breakup of an affair with an older man, one of the teachers at an art institute she had attended. The affair had begun when he was unhappily married, and during the course of the relationship, he had left his wife. After the separation, the patient grew disenchanted as she began to note his unattractive character traits. Instead of becoming more available to her emotionally, he became preoccupied with work, and she felt left out. In her own words, "His work became his mistress, and I felt like the other woman, abandoned, except for diversionary relief when he needed some entertainment."

The patient went on to describe several other disappointing love relationships that had occurred over the past few years and seemed unaware that she repeatedly chose powerful and attractive but self-absorbed men. She was the youngest of three daughters. Her father was an architect and her mother an interior decorator. Her older sister had a congenital heart defect; in the patient's view, "She got all the attention. My achievements were taken for granted, but a big deal was made out of everything she could do."

At the interview, the patient appeared attractive and chic. Her manner of relating to the interviewer was dramatically intense as she gestured widely and maintained unwavering eye contact. She showed labile emotional shifts from sadness to shame to anger as she reviewed aspects of her love relationship. Her thinking was organized and coherent but vague and highly emotional, with sparse detail in her descriptions of the difficulties in her relationships.

Epidemiology

The prevalence has been estimated to be 10–15% of psychiatric outpatient and inpatient populations.

Etiology & Pathogenesis

The causes of histrionic personality disorder are mainly psychological; in better-functioning patients, these are typically unresolved oedipal problems. The more immature, dependent (so-called oral) hysteric has a history of disturbance early in life in attachments and separation.

Treatment

Long-term psychoanalytic psychotherapy is the treatment of choice and should focus on developing the patient's insight into the reasons for repetitive difficulties in sustaining love relationships and on promoting autonomous self-expression. The therapist should also help the patient think more clearly and systematically, so that information processing and decision making are not distorted by vagueness or failure to attend to relevant details.

Histrionic Personality Disorder in Medical Practice

For people with histrionic personalities, self-esteem is heavily centered in perception of their body image, with physical prowess and attractiveness being prized attributes. Men with histrionic personality disorder may, when physically ill, display hypermasculine ("macho") behavior to counteract their perception of themselves as weak. Such counterphobic behavior may worsen the course of illness. Such men may act in an overtly seductive fashion toward female physicians and other members of the health care team. Women with histrionic personality disorder may attempt to reaffirm their sense of self-worth by exhibiting dependent and coquettish behavior in an attempt to evoke reassuring admiration from their male physicians. Patients of both sexes may attempt to draw the physician into a rescuing, admiring role in order to ward off anxiety associated with the threat to self-esteem that is posed by the illness.

The physician must be able to provide maximal emotional support and interest in order to lessen the patient's anxiety but at the same time must avoid entering into a close personal relationship that might be misinterpreted as sexual. The physician must also avoid fostering magical expectations of cure. The physician should adopt a kindly but objective stance and should periodically provide a clear explanation of the disorder and plans for treatment so as to foster trust and firmly counteract the patient's denial of illness. Such patients tend to fluctuate between a state of overwhelming anxiety about the potential loss of capacities (intrusions or flooding of affect) and a state of numbing and apparent disregard (*la belle indifférence*). A flexible approach combining support or tactful confrontation as appropriate will help the patient gain a realistic understanding of the disorder and cooperate with treatment. The patient's capacity for overly dramatic expression and the shifting focus of somatic distress raise the risk that the physician will dismiss the complaints as those of a hypochondriac or even as the conscious manipulations of a malingerer. The histrionic patient will challenge the physician's diagnostic acumen, since serious illness, conversion symptoms, and dramatization of minor somatic disturbances may coexist or evolve sequentially within the same individual.

Leigh and Reiser (1980) illustrate the difficulty that a patient with histrionic personality disorder has in coping with physical illness.

Illustrative Case

A 59-year-old married businessman had severe chest pain and was admitted to the intensive care unit after an electrocardiogram and serum enzyme determinations confirmed that he had suffered a massive myocardial infarction. Absolute bed rest was prescribed in order to minimize the threat of further myocardial damage. The patient prided himself on his physical prowess, and when his physician empathically commented on how frightening the attack must have been for him, the patient replied, "No. I didn't get frightened at nothing—nothing scares me. All I did was holler up to my wife. I've got a bull voice—you know what I mean: I can't help myself. You understand. I got a powerful chest, so it comes out strong."

The patient presented a problem in management because, in an effort to ward off the anxiety associated with his illness, he persuaded himself that a daily exercise program would hasten his rehabilitation, and despite the admonitions of the intensive care unit staff, he began repeatedly lifting up his bed in order to improve his circulation. He told one of the nurses, "My doctor thinks I had a heart attack. All I need is to get my strength back, which I lost from being in here too long." His denial and counterphobic behavior precipitated a burst of cardiac arrhythmias that required urgent medical treatment and subsequent psychiatric consultation.

Appropriate psychological management of this patient would include a review of the events leading up to his admission to the hospital, tactful confrontation of his defensive need to appear invincible, and step-by-step efforts to help him gradually accept his real vulnerabilities while countering his fear of being a "cardiac cripple." The physician's admiration of the patient's efforts to cope more adaptively would help restore the patient's sense of self-esteem and safety.

NARCISSISTIC PERSONALITY DISORDER

Symptoms & Signs

The diagnostic criteria for narcissistic personality disorder are listed in Table 24–6. The disorder is characterized by *DSM-IV* as "a pervasive pattern of grandiosity, need for admiration, and lack of empathy." An exaggerated sense of self-importance is manifest in a pretentious, boastful overestimation of abilities and accomplishments, fantasies of beauty, brilliance, and unlimited success, and preoccupation with restitution for not having been recognized for their "true" talents. They believe that they are exempt from the duties and responsibilities of everyday people who are beneath them. They crave excitement to ward off boredom and emptiness.

Brief reactive psychoses may occur; in psychodynamic theory, these represent fragmentation of a coherent sense of self under psychosocial stress. This fragmentation is experienced as a loss of the sense of continuity of oneself as worthwhile and lovable in the face of a current disappointment, criticism, or rejection. Depression is common, as is chronic intense envy. Defensive self-delusion or lying to oneself by distorting the facts so that a feeling of self-importance is preserved ("sliding of meanings") is also seen. The patient may pretend to have certain feelings in order to impress others.

Natural History & Prognosis System

Systematic data are not available.

Differential Diagnosis

Individuals with narcissistic personality disorder lack the impulsivity, self-destructiveness, and instability of those with borderline personality disorder,

---

Table 24–6. *DSM-IV* diagnostic criteria for narcissistic personality disorder.

A pervasive pattern of grandiosity (in fantasy or behavior), need for admiration, and lack of empathy, beginning by early adulthood and present in a variety of contexts, as indicated by five (or more) of the following:
(1) has a grandiose sense of self-importance (eg, exaggerates achievements and talents, expects to be recognized as superior without commensurate achievements), (2) is preoccupied with fantasies of unlimited success, power, brilliance, beauty, or ideal love, (3) believes that he or she is "special" and unique and can only be understood by, or should associate with, other special or high-status people (or institutions), (4) requires excessive admiration, (5) has a sense of entitlement, ie, unreasonable expectations of especially favorable treatment or automatic compliance with his or her expectations, (6) is interpersonally exploitative, ie, takes advantage of others to achieve his or her own ends, (7) lacks empathy, is unwilling to recognize or identify with the feelings and needs of others, (8) is often envious of others or believes that others are envious of him or her, (9) shows arrogant, haughty behaviors or attitudes.

---

are less impulsively aggressive than those with antisocial personality disorders, and have far greater contempt for the sensitivities of others than those with histrionic personality disorders. The grandiosity of narcissistic personality disorder is stable across time and not mood driven, as seen in hypomanic behavior or stimulant abuse.

Illustrative Case

A 38-year-old recently divorced and infrequently employed actor, the father of an 8-month-old son, sought help because of depression. He had left his wife and son 6 weeks earlier because he could no longer tolerate his wife's "slavish devotion to our baby boy; I may as well not exist as far as she's concerned." He complained that since his wife had become pregnant she was disinclined to admire his acting abilities and less interested than before in sympathizing with his envy of actors who obtained better and more frequent employment.

The patient was the eldest child and only son of a materially successful but emotionally withholding, punitive, and sniping father who, in the patient's view, magnified his son's slightest imperfections. The patient described his mother as an indulgent and admiring woman who frequently made excuses for him. His two younger sisters were competent in their professions, and their success was a source of shame and guilt for him.

The patient had experienced a rapid turnover in friendships, since he initially idealized people and then impulsively trashed the relationships when he was frustrated or disappointed. Before his marriage he had fancied himself as a Don Juan, saying, "I had women on a string, but after a while I couldn't stand their vanity and pettiness."

In the interview, the patient presented as an expensively dressed, well-groomed, and handsome man who tried to project a smooth, self-assured facade. There was, however, a palpable undercurrent of insecurity, loneliness, and depression. His distraught feelings had a quality of caricature to them that was evident to the interviewer. He presented himself as a colleague rather than a patient, and provided his own formulations for his psychological difficulties in an effort to save face. Although there were no gross abnormalities of thinking or perception, he presented an apparently distorted account of his role in his marital and occupational difficulties and cast himself in a better light than was warranted. He blamed an external power, which lent a quality of self-delusion to his version of his interpersonal difficulties.

Epidemiology

Prevalence estimates for narcissistic personality disorder are 1% in the general population and 2–16% in psychiatric outpatient and inpatient samples.

Etiology & Pathogenesis

In normal psychological development, all very young children have an exaggerated sense of their own importance as well as an idealized view of parental figures as protective, powerful, and immortal. These immature, idealized views of the self and others are modified as children learn to face gradual, tolerable disappointments with the empathic support of their caretakers. The result of this process is that healthy adults can accept their own realistic limitations, tolerate criticism and setbacks, and still maintain an overall positive self-regard. In contrast, the early life experiences of individuals with narcissistic personality disorder were described by Kohut (1971) as marked by premature, repeated, and intense injuries to self-esteem as well as by radical disillusionment in parental figures rather than by gradual and tolerable disappointments in themselves and important caretakers. The long-term sequelae in adulthood are characteristic disturbances in self-esteem, with alternating idealization and devaluation of others that is accompanied by alternating grandiose and inferior images of the self.

Treatment

Long-term psychoanalytic psychotherapy and psychoanalysis have been attempted with these patients, although their use has been controversial. The goal is to increase the patient's capacity to tolerate disappointments, to appreciate the needs of others, and to develop healthy self-esteem.

Narcissistic Personality Disorder in Medical Practice

Narcissistic patients try to sustain an image of perfection and personal invincibility for themselves and attempt to project that impression to others as well. Physical illness may shatter this illusion, and a patient may lose the feeling of safety inherent in a cohesive sense of self. This loss precipitates a panicky sensation of insecurity, and the patient feels a sense of personal fragmentation. The narcissistic individual shares with the histrionic personality a concern about loss of admiration and approval, but the person with narcissistic personality disorder shows a more disturbed response to illness. The histrionic patient's idealization of the physician stands in contrast to the narcissistic patient's frequent contemptuous disregard for the physician, who is denigrated in a defensive effort to maintain a sense of superiority and mastery over illness.

Health care professionals must convey a feeling of respect and acknowledge the patient's sense of self-importance so that the patient can reestablish a coherent sense of self, but at the same time they must avoid reinforcing either pathological grandiosity (which may contribute to denial of illness) or weakness (which frightens the patient). An initial approach of support followed by step-by-step confrontation of the patient's vulnerabilities may enable the patient to deal with the implications of illness with feelings of greater subjective strength. The increased self-confidence may reduce the patient's need to attack the health care team in a misguided effort at psychological self-preservation and ease the pressure to provide perfect care, since the patient's antagonistic feeling of entitlement (defined by *DSM-IV* as an "unreasonable expectation of particularly favorable treatment") is reduced.

The following case shows the difficulty encountered in medical management of the narcissistic personality.

Illustrative Case

A partner in a prestigious law firm was admitted to the specialized endocrine service of a teaching hospital for investigation of inflammation of the thyroid gland. The patient had sought consultation with the chief of the endocrine service after seeing the endocrinologist's recent research findings reported on network television and characterized as a glamorous, high-technology innovation. The patient recalled thinking at the time, "Finally, here is a doctor who can understand the complexities of my illness!"

When the patient arrived at the endocrine service, he was greeted by the junior resident, who introduced himself and explained that he would be responsible for the patient's day-to-day care, while the chief of the service would consult on major diagnostic and treatment issues. The lawyer flew into a rage and shouted, "No damn wet-behind-the-ears student doctor is going to lay a hand on me!"

The resident attempted to calm the patient and agreed to ask the chief of the service to mediate the dispute. When the chief arrived and was informed of the situation, his previous experience in dealing with influential patients enabled him to grasp the nature of the lawyer's narcissistic rage, the underlying sense of entitlement and fear that motivated it, and the embarrassment of the resident who was the unwitting target of the tirade. He welcomed the patient and apologized for not being able to meet him at the time of admission. He introduced the resident as "one of our brightest young colleagues—we are expecting great things from him" and continued, "He and I will work closely together to get to the bottom of your problems."

The lawyer was reassured by this respectful apology and the statement of confidence in the junior resident. The chief of the service had in effect transferred his reputation for excellence to his younger colleague ("passed the baton") and had thereby imbued the resident with the charismatic healing qualities the narcissistic patient needed in order to feel the trust necessary for a successful therapeutic relationship with the health care team.

ANTISOCIAL PERSONALITY DISORDER

Symptoms & Signs

The diagnostic criteria for antisocial personality disorder are set forth in Table 24–7. *DSM-IV* states that this disorder is characterized by "a pervasive pattern of disregard for and violation of the rights of others that begins in childhood or early adolescence and continues into adulthood." The antisocial features are reflected in poor job performance, academic failure, participation in a wide variety of illegal activities, recklessness, and impulsive behavior.

The patient with antisocial personality disorder also experiences a feeling of subjective dysphoria, characterized by tension, depression, inability to tolerate boredom, and a feeling of being victimized. There is also a diminished capacity for intimacy.

Natural History & Prognosis

Antisocial personality disorder tends to remit with time. After 21 years of age, the remission rate is about 2% of all patients each year. As destructive social behavior diminishes, patients tend to develop hypochondriacal and depressive disorders.

Differential Diagnosis

If characteristic features of antisocial personality disorder are present but the person is younger than 18 years of age, a diagnosis of conduct disorder is appropriate. When criminal behavior is present without other features of antisocial personality disorder, the appropriate diagnosis is adult antisocial behavior, usually without the precursory signs seen in adolescents with conduct disorders.

Table 24–7. *DSM-IV* diagnostic criteria for antisocial personality disorder.

A. There is a pervasive pattern of disregard for and violation of the rights of others occurring since age 15 years as indicated by three (or more) of the following:
(1) failure to conform to social norms with respect to lawful behaviors as indicated by repeatedly performing acts that are grounds for arrest, (2) deceitfulness, as indicated by repeated lying, use of aliases, or conning others for personal profit or pleasure, (3) impulsivity or failure to plan ahead, (4) irritability and aggressiveness, as indicated by repeated physical fights or assaults, (5) reckless disregard for safety of self or others, (6) consistent irresponsibility, as indicated by repeated failure to sustain consistent work behavior or honor financial obligations, (7) lack of remorse, as indicated by being indifferent to or rationalizing having hurt, mistreated, or stolen from another.

B. The individual is at least age 18 years.

C. There is evidence of conduct disorder with onset before age 15 years.

D. The occurrence of antisocial behavior is not exclusively during the course of schizophrenia or a manic episode.

Illustrative Case

A 21-year-old divorced independent trucker was referred for pretrial psychiatric evaluation after being charged with interstate transportation of stolen property. He had a history of repeated criminal offenses, prison terms, and psychiatric disturbance during childhood and adolescence. He had been apprehended 4 weeks earlier when a random road inspection revealed stolen automobile parts hidden among cartons of groceries.

About 8 months before his latest arrest, the patient had suddenly abandoned his wife when he learned from an acquaintance that she sometimes flirted with customers at the sandwich shop where she worked.

The patient was the second in a family of four boys. His alcoholic father was episodically violent toward him when drunk, and his mother was absent long hours while she worked to support the family.

During childhood, the patient had been evaluated and briefly treated in a community mental health center after he had been caught setting fire to an abandoned warehouse. During adolescence, he had received counseling from a school psychologist because of a consistent pattern of antisocial behavior, including car theft, joyriding, drunk driving, driving with a suspended license, truancy, and stealing money from his mother. While he was growing up, he had no close friendships, although he was a peripheral member of a hot-rod gang. Though sexually active from a young age and proud of his sexual prowess, he was mistrustful of women and became easily bored with the same partner.

In the interview, the patient appeared nonchalant and composed, with an apparent equanimity that was incongruent with the seriousness of his situation. He made eye contact with the interviewer but appeared to be looking through the interviewer rather than at him. There was an unspoken but clearly communicated disregard for the interviewer's authority. There were no major disturbances in thought, perception, or mood, with the exception of a lack of remorse or anxiety when he was confronted with his lifelong pattern of destructive behavior and the seriousness of the charges presently lodged against him.

Epidemiology

Onset of antisocial personality disorder is before age 15, frequently around puberty in girls and quite early in childhood for boys. The disorder is more prevalent in men, with incidence being about 3% for men and 1% for women. Prevalence is increased in lower socioeconomic groups. Family histories are often positive for antisocial personality disorder, with increased incidence in the fathers of both male and female patients with this disorder. Evidence suggests that this familial occurrence results from both genetic and environmental causes; the relative contribution of each factor is unknown. Antisocial personality disorder may be diagnosed in as many as 75% of prison inmates.

Etiology & Pathogenesis

A. Genetic and Biological Factors: Robins (1966) found an increased incidence of sociopathic characteristics and alcoholism in the fathers of individuals with antisocial personality disorder. Within the families of these individuals, male relatives have increased rates of antisocial personality disorder and substance abuse disorders, whereas female relatives have increased rates of somatization disorder. Adoption studies support the role of both genetic and environmental contributions to the development of the disorder. In a retrospective study of this disorder, Raine et al (1990) reported that indices of psychophysiological underarousal at age 15 were predictive of criminality at age 24 years. Criminals had significantly lower heart rates and skin conductance activity and more slow-frequency electroencephalographic activity than noncriminals.

B. Psychological Factors: Bowlby (1944) correlated antisocial personality disorder with maternal deprivation in the child's first 5 years of life. Glueck and Glueck (1968) reported that the mothers of children who developed this personality disorder show a lack of consistent discipline, a lack of affection, and an increased incidence of alcoholism and impulsiveness. These qualities contribute to failure to create a cohesive home environment with consistent structure and behavioral boundaries. In the prospective study, children found to be at risk by age 6 frequently showed features of antisocial personality at 18 years.

Treatment

In a review of the effectiveness of treatments for antisocial personality disorder Garrido et al (1995) concluded that treatment is more effective with those subjects who are not currently abusing drugs, who have less serious histories of criminality, and who are treated in an institutional setting such as an inpatient unit or a prison rather than in an outpatient setting. As an example Dolan (1998) describes a therapeutic community program for antisocial patients and those with other violent personality disorders that is successful in reducing not only impulsive behaviors but also physical health problems, rates of incarceration for criminal offenses, and core features of personality disorder.

Antisocial Personality Disorder in Medical Practice

The relationship between a physician and a patient with antisocial personality disorder is characterized by mutual feelings of suspicion and, at times, hostility. The antisocial person's mistrust of the physician stems from unwarranted generalizations about physicians that are based in part on early abusive experiences at the hands of parental caretakers, particularly during the formative periods of childhood and adolescence. The physician's mistrust of the antisocial patient may well be grounded in unpleasant personal experience. Persons with antisocial personality disorder may feign physical symptoms to obtain narcotic analgesics for substance abuse, may attempt to defraud third-party health care payment sources by seeking reimbursement for services not rendered, or may be delinquent in payment for services they have actually received. Unfortunately, individuals with antisocial personalities are at least as vulnerable to physical illness as any other type of patient and are in fact at higher risk for illnesses associated with substance abuse and stress because of their chronic unstable interpersonal and occupational adjustments. The physician is therefore challenged to find a way to create an effective therapeutic alliance. A firm, nononsense approach that is not punitive but conveys a streetwise awareness of the patient's potential for manipulation will encourage respect without aggravating the patient's hostility against authority.

Illustrative Case

A 25-year-old man presented for an initial visit to a local general practitioner and complained of recurrent backache. He said that he had tried many analgesics in the past and found that they either were ineffective or caused intolerable side effects, with the exception of high doses of codeine. Physical examination revealed significant disease of the lumbosacral spine secondary to a congenital defect in the alignment of the vertebrae.

Alerted by the patient's specific request for a potentially addictive narcotic that also had high resale value in the illicit drug market, the physician inquired further into the patient's work and occupational history. A typical unstable pattern of impulsive and manipulative interpersonal relations was identified, including an irregular work history and other features characteristic of antisocial personality disorder. A respectful but appropriately tough tone of inquiry into the patient's previous use of analgesics revealed a history of morphine addiction following lower back surgery. Denial of the patient's request for codeine led to an angry outburst, with the patient declining alternative treatment. Several months later, however, the patient reappeared with legitimate complaints of upper respiratory tract infection. He told the physician, "I came back to see you again because I figure you're nobody's fool, but you're not going to lecture me about how I should live my life either."

BORDERLINE PERSONALITY DISORDER

Symptoms & Signs

The diagnostic criteria for borderline personality disorder are set forth in Table 24–8. As described by

Table 24–8. *DSM-IV* diagnostic criteria for borderline personality disorder.

A pervasive pattern of instability of interpersonal relationships, self-image, and affects, and marked impulsivity beginning by early adulthood and present in a variety of contexts, as indicated by five (or more) of the following:
(1) frantic efforts to avoid real or imagined abandonment. **Note:** Do not include suicidal or self-mutilating behavior covered in Criterion 5. (2) a pattern of unstable and intense interpersonal relationships characterized by alternating between extremes of idealization and devaluation, (3) identity disturbance: markedly and persistently unstable self-image or sense of self, (4) impulsivity in at least two areas that are potentially self-damaging (eg, spending, sex, substance abuse, reckless driving, binge eating). **Note:** Do not include suicidal or self-mutilating behavior covered in Criterion 5. (5) recurrent suicidal behavior, gestures, or threats, or self-mutilating behavior, (6) affective instability due to a marked reactivity of mood (eg, intense episodic dysphoria, irritability, or anxiety usually lasting a few hours and only rarely more than a few days), (7) chronic feelings of emptiness, (8) inappropriate, intense anger or difficulty controlling anger (eg, frequent displays of temper, constant anger, recurrent physical fights), (9) transient stress-related paranoid ideation or severe dissociative symptoms.

DSM-IV, borderline personality disorder is characterized by "a pervasive pattern of instability of interpersonal relationships, self-image, and affects and marked impulsivity that begins by early adulthood and is present in a variety of contexts."

Individuals with borderline personality disorder are preoccupied with threats of real or imagined abandonment. At the same time, intimacy often leads to fears of merger with subjugation of identity to the other person. The patient alternates between the wish for closeness and the need for distance. There are also sudden identity shifts with rapid change in values, goals, and career choices. Impulsivity is reflected in behaviors such as substance abuse, overeating, gambling addictions, unsafe sex, promiscuity, excessive spending, or reckless driving.

The patient with borderline personality disorder is vulnerable to development of transient reactive psychoses (micropsychotic episodes) and may be chronically depressed. Borderline personality disorder may coexist with schizotypal, histrionic, narcissistic, or antisocial personality disorder.

Natural History & Prognosis

Follow-up studies by Werble (1970) and by Carpenter et al (1977) suggest that the clinical picture in patients with borderline personality disorder is chronically unstable but that the disorder does not deteriorate into schizophrenia. In both studies, symptoms were present over long periods, and patients experienced major disturbances in social functioning and enjoyed little satisfaction from their low quality of life. These individuals were unlikely to marry. The patients in the two studies were suffering from a se-

vere form of borderline personality disorder; the prognosis is better for individuals with higher levels of functioning. For example, 57 former inpatients with borderline personality disorder were studied by Links et al (1998) at baseline and 7 years later. At follow-up approximately 50% had remitted. Those who met criteria at 7-year follow-up had more severe borderline features and greater comorbid personality disorder diagnoses at baseline.

Epidemiology

Estimates of the prevalence of borderline personality disorder vary from 2% of the general population to 10% of individuals in outpatient and 20% of individuals in inpatient psychiatric clinics.

Differential Diagnosis

If an individual with characteristics of borderline personality disorder is under 18 years of age, the appropriate diagnosis is identity disorder.

Borderline personality disorder must be differentiated from cyclothymic disorder, in which there are hypomanic periods.

Illustrative Case

A 25-year-old single graduate student was brought to a crisis clinic by her girlfriend, who had become worried after the patient expressed a wish to commit suicide. Two weeks earlier, the patient's boyfriend had left for a summer vacation trip to Europe. The vacation had initially been planned as a joint trip, but the patient had persuaded her boyfriend to go alone so they could have a period of independence from each other. She was worried that they were becoming psychologically enmeshed and "like Siamese twins," a view that threatened her chronically fragile sense of separateness and autonomy. In the 2 weeks since his departure, she had grown progressively more distraught and had felt a panicky sense of abandonment, emptiness, and loss of all positive feelings and memories of her relationship with her boyfriend, all of which contributed to a sense of unreality about her life. She considered taking an overdose of drugs, because "nothing else would numb the pain I feel." She had also harbored an increasing sense of rage at being left behind, because "he didn't understand that I was only testing his loyalty when I told him to go alone."

The patient's current relationship, like her previous love relationships, had been characterized by periods of intense intimate contact alternating with flights into independence. She felt she could not achieve a comfortable compromise that would enable her to feel close to another person yet preserve a sense of her own separateness. Although she was a gifted student, she had enrolled in three widely different graduate programs after having made abrupt shifts in her career training just when she was nearing completion of any one program. Her academic interests were scattered over the fine arts, social sciences, and business. She was by her own description a "chameleon" who had no strong preferences of her own. She was powerfully influenced by charismatic teachers whose value systems and career goals she would make her own in an effort to counter her inner sense of emptiness and lack of direction.

The patient was an only child whose mother became bedridden with rheumatoid arthritis when the patient was between 18 and 30 months of age. Her mother made a partial recovery but struggled with physical pain and depression during subsequent relapses. Her parents were divorced when the patient was 9 years of age, and her father subsequently maintained only a distant relationship with the family. After her parents' divorce, the patient felt even more responsible for the health and happiness of her mother than she had before. She was made to feel guilty for placing her own social and intellectual needs ahead of those of her mother. In her view, "Every step I took toward becoming my own person was a step closer to destroying my mother."

In the interview, she presented as an appealing young woman who seemed distraught, somewhat disheveled, and physically exhausted. In describing her separation from her boyfriend, she oscillated between uncontrollable sobbing and furious rage, but was able to regain her composure in responding to the structuring and supportive remarks of the interviewer. There was no evidence of delusions or hallucinations. Her sensorium was clear, although she reported a subjective sense of disorientation and unreality that she attributed to the change in her world as a result of her boyfriend's absence.

Etiology & Pathogenesis

A. Genetic and Biological Factors: Kemberg (1975) and Klein (1977) have suggested that patients with borderline personality disorder have a "constitutionally based" inability to regulate affects, particularly anger. There may be a relationship between borderline personality and depressive illness, which is prevalent in first-degree relatives of patients with borderline personality disorder.

B. Psychological Factors: Kemberg hypothesized an arrest in normal psychological development, with failure to integrate ambivalent feelings originally aroused against the primary caretaker but later occurring in other close relationships as well. The primitive defenses ordinarily relinquished in early childhood are prolonged into adulthood, and patients tend to have distorted appraisals of others, who are perceived as virtual caricatures that are either all good or all bad. This all-or-nothing thinking extends to an exaggerated view of physical symptoms as well, so that the patient tends to feel that he or she is either completely well or deathly ill. The threat of physical illness is exaggerated to terrifying proportions.

Mahler (1971) and Masterson (1972) have hypothesized that borderline personality disorder results after a disturbance occurring in children between 16 and 25 months of age during the rapprochement subphase of separation-individuation. In this phase, the child practices independent behavior and returns to the primary caretaker for approval, admiration, and emotional "refueling." The critical, rejecting parent or the suffocating, smothering parent interferes with optimal progression of attachment-separation sequences.

Treatment

A. Psychological Treatment Measures: Controversy exists about which of the two dominant psychological approaches is more effective in the treatment of borderline personality disorder. Long-term psychoanalytic psychotherapy with some supportive modifications tries to develop trust early in treatment and progresses to deeper exploration with time. The other approach is long-term, more reality-oriented supportive psychotherapy that does not focus on unconscious fantasies and attempts instead to provide structure and prevent the deterioration or overstimulation sometimes seen in more insight-oriented approaches. Behavioral contracting is useful for setting limits with borderline patients (Selzer et al, 1987). Linehan (1987) has developed an approach designated dialectical behavior that combines behavioral interventions in a supportive framework. Beck and Fernandez (1998) reported on 50 studies of cognitive-behavioral treatment for anger management with applicability to borderline personality disorder and found large treatment effect for this approach.

B. Drug Treatment Measures: Klein (1977) advocates the use of monoamine oxidase inhibitors for patients with borderline personality disorder who are sensitive to rejection. These patients experience intensely unpleasant affects, particularly anxiety and depression, when they feel rejected. The use of other antidepressant and antianxiety agents may become necessary at certain times. During brief reactive psychoses, low doses of antipsychotic drugs may be useful, but they are usually not essential adjuncts to the treatment regimen, because such episodes are most often self-limiting and of short duration. Selective serotonin reuptake inhibitors are useful for mood regulation and impulse control. Mood-stabilizing agents including lithium and carbamazepine may be useful when impulse dyscontrol is a prominent feature (Eichelman, 1988; Coccaro, 1998).

Borderline Personality Disorder in Medical Practice

Persons with borderline personality disorder have marked difficulty in differentiating reality from fantasy, so that a minor health problem may be perceived as a life-threatening event. Loss of perspective and miscommunication with the physician may occur as a result. Such patients frequently delay in presenting for medical treatment. They fear the worst with regard to the diagnosis, and they mistrust physicians because of their previous experiences with unreliable caretakers. Some patients may have a subconscious need to suffer in order to expiate guilty feelings. Once they have delivered themselves to the health care team, these patients ward off their catastrophic fear of being damaged by imperfect caretakers by imagining them as all-good. If any problems occur, patients switch abruptly to an all-bad image of medical personnel; the omnipotent rescuer becomes the persecutory invader. The patient may bolt from treatment and attempt to resurrect an idealized relationship with a new doctor, only to be painfully disillusioned later. Patients with borderline personality disorder may interpret any "intellectual" errors in diagnosis or treatment on the part of the health care team on an emotional level. They see themselves as having been rejected, callously disregarded, and abandoned to struggle with their illnesses alone because they are unworthy of the time and interest of their physicians.

The physician should provide clear, nontechnical answers to questions to counter any elaborate fantasies about the dangers of the illness or its treatment. Honest but not overly dramatic information should be provided about the course of the illness and potential side effects of treatment. The physician should be careful to avoid encouraging the patient to idealize the physician and should not be drawn into the patient's denigration of other physicians. More frequent periodic checkups may reassure the patient of the physician's empathy and interest and may provide closer monitoring of illness; they also reduce the chances that the patient will create a frightening mental scenario out of proportion to any genuine threat. Although the physician should offer reassurance, this should not be premature, since it may deprive the patient of an opportunity to spell out these fearful expectations about the illness and may deny the physician a chance to clarify the often idiosyncratic and unexpected nuances of the patient's beliefs about the illness. The physician's tolerance of the patient's episodic angry outbursts demonstrates to the patient that the physician cannot be destroyed by the patient's strong negative feelings and that the physician will not retaliate by leaving the patient to a self-fulfilling prophecy of abandonment.

Illustrative Case

A 29-year-old man was admitted to the chest service of a community hospital for investigation of an undiagnosed lesion found during a routine annual physical examination. The night before a scheduled biopsy, the patient had a nightmare in which he was lying on the operating table surrounded by medical personnel. The two surgeons who were attending him appeared kindly at first, but as the dream progressed, their expressions grew more threatening. He finally awoke when the surgeons were transformed into vampire-like creatures. When the nursing staff arrived at the patient's bedside after the nightmare, he was extremely agitated. He was hyperventilating, complained of a pounding headache, and shouted that he was going to die. After the nurses encouraged him to talk about his fears, he said that he was convinced he had lung cancer that had spread to his brain, and he felt that his severe headache supported this self-diagnosis. The nurses explained that he probably had a tension headache because of anxiety about the biopsy, and they showed him a relaxation exercise that relieved his headache and enabled him to gain a more realistic perspective on his situation. The biopsy revealed a benign fibrous cyst that was treated without complication.

AVOIDANT PERSONALITY DISORDER

Symptoms & Signs

The diagnostic criteria for avoidant personality disorder are summarized in Table 24–9. Features of the disorder, as outlined by *DSM-IV,* include social discomfort, hypersensitivity to criticism and rejection, and timidity. The patient with avoidant personality disorder also experiences depression, anxiety, and anger for failing to develop social relations.

Natural History & Prognosis

Avoidant traits are usually first manifest in early childhood as shyness, which may intensify during adolescence and young adulthood. Early adulthood developmental demands for intimacy may exacerbate the condition. There is frequently a reduction in the intensity of the features during middle age.

Differential Diagnosis

Avoidant personality disorder must be differentiated from schizoid personality disorder, social pho-

Table 24–9. *DSM-IV* diagnostic criteria for avoidant personality disorder.

A pervasive pattern of social inhibition, feelings of inadequacy, and hypersensitivity to negative evaluation beginning by early adulthood and present in a variety of contexts, as indicated by four (or more) of the following:
    (1) avoids occupational activities that involve significant interpersonal contact because of fears of criticism, disapproval, or rejection, (2) is unwilling to get involved with people unless certain of being liked, (3) shows restraint within intimate relationships because of the fear of being shamed or ridiculed, (4) is preoccupied with being criticized or rejected in social situations, (5) is inhibited in new interpersonal situations because of feelings of inadequacy, (6) views self as socially inept, personally unappealing, or inferior to others, (7) is unusually reluctant to take personal risks or to engage in any new activities because they may prove embarrassing.

bia, and avoidant disorder of childhood or adolescence (when the disorder occurs before age 18).

Illustrative Case

A 34-year-old single professional musician sought psychiatric treatment to deal with chronic feelings of insecurity, inferiority, and shyness. Although she was a gifted and sensitive musician, success in her career had not been matched by parallel gratifications in her social life. She came for treatment several weeks after a man in her orchestral group had moved to a different city. She was particularly fond of this man although reticent about approaching him on other than a superficial, chatty basis. She had fantasized their falling in love and was disheartened when he moved away before a deeper relationship could develop.

The disappointment she experienced in this potential relationship was a recurring pattern for the patient. She very much wanted to fall in love and be married but felt that any attractive, intelligent, and caring man would reject her. She was an esteemed member of her musical group but was perceived as someone who kept to herself and lived on the periphery of the group; she gave the impression of being a loner—all despite her wish to be one of the "in" group.

The patient described herself as having been a shy, insecure child and adolescent. Her role among her peers at school had closely paralleled her present position in the social structure of the orchestra. She had always felt that she was on the outside looking in, wanting to become involved but frightened that she would not be accepted. She had often daydreamed about artistic and social successes.

In the interview, the patient appeared to be a soft-spoken, articulate woman who seemed embarrassed by her situation and gave a low-key presentation of herself. She displayed no oddities of speech or behavior. Her mood was sad when she talked about her disappointment in the fantasied love relationship, but signs of a major depressive disorder were absent.

Epidemiology

The prevalence of avoidant personality disorder in the general population is estimated to be 0.5–1.0%, with rates of 10% reported in outpatient psychiatric settings. Avoidant personality disorder is equally frequent in women and men.

Etiology & Pathogenesis

A complex interaction of early childhood environmental experiences and innate temperament plays a role in the occurrence of avoidant personality disorder, but definitive studies concerning the cause have not yet been conducted. Avoidant disorder of childhood and adolescence is said to predict avoidant personality disorder of adulthood.

Treatment

Psychoanalytic psychotherapy is useful in selected patients with avoidant personality disorder. The therapist must expend considerable effort in establishing an effective therapeutic alliance, because their exquisite sensitivity to rejection often causes these patients to abandon treatment abruptly. Assertiveness training and training in general social skills may also be helpful. Group therapy may desensitize the patient to the exaggerated threat of rejection.

Avoidant Personality Disorder in Medical Practice

When a person with avoidant personality disorder falls ill, preexisting shyness and insecurity may intensify. Because the person is already sensitive to social rejection, he or she may feel further stigmatized by the illness and uncomfortable about asking for help and attention from the physician. Embarrassment about being scrutinized during physical examination may also contribute to downplay of symptoms and delay in seeking help.

Tact and timing—particularly in history taking and physical examination—are of the utmost importance in establishing the gradual deepening of trust and rapport required to form a satisfactory working relationship with these patients. This approach encourages the patient with avoidant personality disorder to disclose physical symptoms frankly and without undue embarrassment. The physician needs to steer a middle course between inadvertently cooperating with the patient to minimize complaints and possibly missing the diagnosis on the one hand and adopting an overly intrusive approach that may threaten the patient's sense of privacy and modesty and perhaps contribute to noncompliance on the other. A low-key approach that emphasizes the physician's friendliness and availability and includes prompt return of phone calls, respect for punctuality at appointments, and periodic reassurance of the physician's personal interest and commitment will counter the patient's normal inclination to see himself or herself as unimportant or undeserving of the physician's attention.

Illustrative Case

A 23-year-old woman sought consultation with a dermatologist because of an extensive reaction following exposure to poison oak. The patient had delayed seeking help by persuading herself that she was overreacting and using a variety of home remedies that failed to stop the spread of the rash. When she finally requested an appointment, the receptionist inquired about the urgency of the problem in order to appropriately schedule the appointment. The patient replied, "Well, uh, it's not that bad, but it's sort of uncomfortable; I also have a mild fever."

The alert receptionist recognized the tentative quality of this response and brought the physician to the telephone. After more detailed inquiry into the severity of symptoms, an immediate appointment was arranged, and examination revealed a moderately severe allergic reaction with superimposed bacterial infection. The dermatologist took the time to explore the patient's ambivalence about seeking consultation without at the same time making her feel that she was being criticized. He explained the necessity for close follow-up examination in a low-key, friendly manner devoid of arrogance or pretense. He appeared genuinely unhurried and not overly burdened by the pressures of his practice, and he gave an impression of accessibility that was conveyed more through nonverbal communication than by anything he said. His manner of relating to the patient contradicted her stereotype of the doctor as one of the busy professionals who have better things to do with their time than "pander to my self-indulgent concerns." This new view of physicians made it more comfortable for her to comply with the recommendations for follow-up visits and easier for her to think about seeking consultation for future problems.

DEPENDENT PERSONALITY DISORDER

Symptoms & Signs

The diagnostic criteria for dependent personality disorder are listed in Table 24–10. According to *DSM-IV,* the disorder is characterized by "a pervasive and excessive need to be taken care of that leads to submissive and clinging behavior and fears of separation."

The person with dependent personality disorder may be anxious and depressed and may experience

---

Table 24–10. *DSM-IV* diagnostic criteria for dependent personality disorder.

A pervasive and excessive need to be taken care of that leads to submissive and clinging behavior and fears of separation, beginning by early adulthood and present in a variety of contexts, as indicated by five (or more) of the following:

(1) has difficulty making everyday decisions without an excessive amount of advice and reassurance from others, (2) needs others to assume responsibility for most major areas of his or her life, (3) has difficulty expressing disagreement with others because of fear of loss of support or approval. **Note:** Do not include realistic fears of retribution. (4) has difficulty initiating projects or doing things on his or her own (because of a lack of self-confidence in judgment or abilities rather than a lack of motivation or energy), (5) goes to excessive lengths to obtain nurturance and support from others to the point of volunteering to do things that are unpleasant, (6) feels uncomfortable or helpless when alone because of exaggerated fears of being unable to care for himself or herself, (7) urgently seeks another relationship as a source of care and support when a close relationship ends, (8) is unrealistically preoccupied with fears of being left to take care of himself or herself.

---

intense discomfort when alone for more than a short time. The patient is often intensely preoccupied with the possibility of abandonment. Dependent personality disorder may coexist with another personality disorder such as schizotypal, histrionic, narcissistic, or avoidant personality disorder.

Natural History & Prognosis

The prognosis is unknown.

Differential Diagnosis

Dependent personality disorder must be differentiated from histrionic and avoidant personality disorder as well as the more severe personality disorders, including narcissistic, borderline, and schizotypal personality disorder.

Illustrative Case

A 32-year-old married postal worker presented for psychiatric evaluation because she was considerably upset after receiving a job promotion. She had earlier refused several promotions because she had not wanted to assume the responsibility for supervising others. She was now being forced either to accept a promotion or to leave her position. She desperately wished to maintain her present rank despite the fact that she had an excellent work record and was regarded by management as a good candidate for the supervisory position.

The patient's husband was an ambitious and domineering man who "ruled the roost" in the family, just as her father had done when she was growing up. She was aware that she suppressed her own needs in favor of meeting those of her husband, and although she was occasionally frustrated because of this, she admired his strength of character and felt relieved to know that someone was in control.

The patient was the youngest child in her family and had two older brothers who had enjoyed fussing over their baby sister and of whom she said, "To them I was a real live doll to play with." When she was growing up, she had been hesitant to compete academically and had felt socially stigmatized as the "square" in her peer group.

During the interview, the patient seemed to be quiet, passive, and deferential and appeared younger than her stated age. She cooperated enthusiastically during the interview and in fact seemed eager to anticipate the interviewer's questions in an effort to appear likable. There were no abnormalities of thought, perception, or sensorial functioning. Although she seemed mildly anxious, her symptoms did not meet the diagnostic criteria for anxiety disorder.

Epidemiology

In the Midtown Manhattan Study, Langner and Michael (1963) found that 2.5% of the patients in their sample had passive-dependent traits such as those seen in dependent personality disorder. The diagnosis of passive-dependent personality disorder is made more frequently in women than in men, and it is more common in the youngest child of a family. Dependent personality disorder is the most prevalent personality disorder in psychiatric settings.

Etiology & Pathogenesis

A. Genetic Factors: Gottesman (1963) found that the presence of submissiveness or dominance was more highly correlated in identical twins than in fraternal twins, which supports the hypothesis that dependent personality disorder has a genetic component.

B. Psychological Factors: A disturbance at the oral stage of psychosexual development is believed to occur in patients who later develop dependent personality disorder; it takes the form of maternal deprivation rather than overgratification during early attachment (see Chapter 4).

Treatment

Long-term psychoanalytic psychotherapy is the treatment of choice and should focus on the patient's exaggerated fears of damaging others or himself or herself by pursuing autonomy and becoming his or her own person. Assertiveness and social skills training and cognitive-behavioral treatments aimed at increasing autonomy may also be useful.

Dependent Personality Disorder in Medical Practice

Patients with dependent personality disorder may make a dramatic appeal for caretaking, with urgent and inappropriate demands for immediate attention to their medical complaints, which have an exaggerated quality. If they fail to receive a prompt response, they may erupt in angry outbursts that threaten important emotional ties, including those with the physician. Since illness provides secondary gains in the form of caretaking and attention, such patients tend to be passive participants in the healing partnership rather than seeking active solutions. The well-known oral characteristics of dependent persons may be expressed in food, alcohol, and drug problems. The physician must be particularly alert to the possibility of abuse of sedatives, hypnotics, tranquilizers, and analgesics. Patients with dependent personality disorder are overly compliant in their acceptance of medical treatment and may search for gratification of their unmet needs for dependence by seeking unnecessary procedures while minimizing the associated hazards.

The physician should provide reassurance and convey an impression of being available and accessible to the patient but should be careful to explain clearly and firmly the realistic limits of such availability. The physician can provide help in other ways, eg, coordinating support services and instituting flexible appointment scheduling, in which the patient assumes some responsibility for establishing the timing of appointments. Physicians treating these patients must guard against "burnout" and the hostile rejection that may be aroused by these patients' strong needs for dependence. The patient's exaggerated compliance with the treatment regimen may lead to overutilization of medical care systems, which health care professionals need to be aware of. Other members of the health care team, including nurses and physical therapists, may play an important role in communicating the physician's interest and concern and in alleviating physical discomfort, so that the burden of meeting needs for dependence is distributed throughout the team rather than being focused exclusively on any one member.

Illustrative Case

A 45-year-old man was admitted to the hospital for surgical repair of damaged cartilage in his left knee. On the evening of admission, the resident on the surgical service completed the preoperative physical examination and noted the following in the chart: "Except for the damaged medial meniscus in the left knee, the patient is in remarkably good health. He does, however, present a psychological management problem. He has made frequent requests for analgesics and bristled with irritation when I was called away to the emergency room before I could complete the physical examination. When I returned, the nurse assigned to his care remarked that the patient acted as though this were a Hilton hotel and that he regarded his pain and anxiety as the only concerns of the hospital staff."

The resident held a meeting with the nurse, the physical therapist, and other members of the health care team in order to prevent further development of hostile reactions on the part of the staff toward this patient and to develop a management strategy. They agreed to meet the patient's requests for attention within realistic limits but decided that the burden of care would be distributed across the entire team. They also decided that a premedical student summer volunteer should be assigned to the patient. This decision proved mutually rewarding, since it alleviated the patient's anxiety about being alone at a time when he felt vulnerable and provided the student volunteer with a glimpse of the way patients may react to illness.

COMPULSIVE PERSONALITY DISORDER

Symptoms & Signs

The diagnostic criteria for compulsive personality disorder are listed in Table 24–11. According to *DSM-IV*, the essential feature is "a preoccupation with orderliness, perfectionism, and mental and interpersonal control at the expense of flexibility, openness, and efficiency."

Table 24–11. *DSM-IV* diagnostic criteria for obsessive-compulsive personality disorder.

A pervasive pattern of preoccupation with orderliness, perfectionism, and mental and interpersonal control, at the expense of flexibility, openness, and efficiency, beginning by early adulthood and present in a variety of contexts, as indicated by four (or more) of the following:

(1) is preoccupied with details, rules, lists, order, organization, or schedules to the extent that the major point of the activity is lost, (2) shows perfectionism that interferes with task completion (eg, is unable to complete a project because his or her own overly strict standards are not met), (3) is excessively devoted to work and productivity to the exclusion of leisure activities and friendships (not accounted for by obvious economic necessity), (4) is overconscientious, scrupulous, and inflexible about matters or morality, ethics, or values (not accounted for by cultural or religious identification), (5) is unable to discard worn-out or worthless objects even when they have no sentimental value, (6) is reluctant to delegate tasks or to work with others unless they submit to exactly his or her way of doing things, (7) adopts a miserly spending style toward both self and others; money is viewed as something to be hoarded for future catastrophes, (8) shows rigidity and stubbornness.

Patients with compulsive personality disorder experience distress associated with indecisiveness and difficulty in expressing tender feelings. They are generally depressed and feel suppressed anger about feeling controlled by others, and they demonstrate extreme sensitivity to social criticism and excessively conscientious, moralistic, scrupulous, and judgmental behavior. Painstaking attention to details or the need for a perfect product interfere with creativity and generativity. Work may be pursued to the exclusion of leisure. Miserly attitudes and "packrat" behavior interfere with generosity and adaptability to change.

Natural History & Prognosis

Full-blown Axis I obsessive-compulsive disturbances may break out periodically and remit. Kringlen (1965) noted the presence of characteristics of compulsive personality disorder in 72% of individuals who developed symptoms of obsessive-compulsive disorder. Despite the compulsive individual's worry about the loss of impulse control, the incidence of sexual or aggressive behavior that is out of control is not higher in individuals with compulsive personality disorder than it is in the general population. The risk of major depressive episodes appears to be increased during midlife crisis.

Differential Diagnosis

Compulsive personality disorder must be distinguished from obsessive-compulsive disorder, in which the patient experiences obsessive thoughts (eg, intrusive, unwanted impulses to shout obscenities or handle feces in an ordinarily controlled, moralistic, and meticulous person) or compulsive behavior (eg, repeated checking and rechecking of door locks) (see

Chapter 21). The two disorders may coexist, in which case both diagnoses are warranted. Compulsive personality disorder must also be differentiated from schizoid and paranoid personality disorders. Obsessive traits (often seen in persons successfully engaged in professional careers) must be distinguished from full-blown compulsive personality disorder (which is maladaptive and interferes with normal functioning).

Illustrative Case

A 43-year-old senior vice president in an accounting firm sought psychiatric treatment because of a chronic sense of personal dissatisfaction. He had risen rapidly to the highest management level in his firm, but he derived no internal sense of pride and satisfaction. Reporting on this chronic feeling of dissatisfaction, he said, "When I successfully complete a project, it is a reprieve from my fearful expectations; when I experience a setback, it confirms my worst fears."

The patient's wife was a caring and competent woman who was a special education teacher. They had two children. The wife was a lively, articulate, and emotionally spontaneous person who had complained in the past about her husband's emotional remoteness and lack of adventuresome spirit. He felt great affection for his wife and children but was afraid to commit himself emotionally to these relationships, saying, "What if I allow myself to give and receive the love that I crave, and then something happens to them? I would be devastated." The patient was the eldest son of two professional parents. While growing up, he had been extremely well provided for materially but had felt a lack of warmth and intimacy at home. His primary involvement with his family had centered around performance, and he felt pressured to succeed in school and sports. He felt that the family had placed little value on the quiet unstructured times of just enjoying one another's company. He had excelled in school but felt driven, and he had feared that his competitive strivings alienated him from his peers. In addition, he had felt stigmatized when he was left out of social activities during adolescence.

At the interview, the patient was dressed conservatively in somber tones and was meticulously groomed. He was reserved, emotionally distant from the interviewer, and provided a carefully detailed account of his unhappiness. His manner was that of a colleague consulting with another professional about a third person's difficulties rather than that of a patient visiting a doctor. There was no evidence of delusions, hallucinations, or disturbance in consciousness. His thinking was characterized by marked intellectualization and rationalization, a tendency to veer away from emotion-laden topics, and preoccupation with details to the exclusion of understanding the overall issues. Although he said that he felt a chronic sense of unhappiness in his life, he denied the presence of vegetative or other specific symptoms of depression.

Epidemiology

Compulsive personality disorder is frequently diagnosed in men and is believed to be common, particularly in the oldest children of a family. Prevalence is estimated to be 1% in community samples and 5–10% in psychiatric settings.

Etiology & Pathogenesis

A. Genetic Factors: Twin and adoption studies have demonstrated that there is a genetic contribution to compulsive personality disorder.

B. Psychological Factors: According to Freud, compulsive personality disorder is caused by arrest at the anal level of psychosexual development that results in repetitive power struggles with authority figures, dominance-submission conflicts, and emotional withholding. According to Erikson, disturbance in the stage of development characterized by the issue of autonomy versus shame and self-doubt predisposes to development of compulsive personality disorder (see Chapter 4). Family life is characterized by constrained emotions, and members are often criticized and socially ostracized if they express anger.

Treatment

Insight-oriented psychoanalytic psychotherapy is the treatment of choice. The focus must be on feelings rather than thoughts and would emphasize the clarification of the defenses of isolation of affect (intellectualized distancing from emotions) and displacement of hostility.

Group and behavioral therapy may be helpful in developing skills in achieving intimacy.

Compulsive Personality Disorder in Medical Practice

When they are confronted with physical illness, individuals with compulsive personality disorder are particularly troubled by the sense of loss of control over bodily functions. Feelings of shame and vulnerability for being in a weakened condition are typical. The patient also feels angry about the disruption of routines and is fearful of relinquishing control to the health care team. There may be exaggerated worries about submitting to authority figures. Under pressure from the many emotional aspects of the illness, the patient may be apprehensive about the possibility of giving way to emotional outbursts. The patient will attempt to ward off these anxieties by redoubling efforts at composure and presenting a precisely detailed, orderly account of progression of symptoms in an emotionally detached manner.

A scientific approach on the part of the physician—as conveyed in thorough history taking and careful diagnostic workups—is reassuring and fosters the trust necessary for an effective therapeutic alliance. A well-articulated account of the disease process and treatment alternatives reassures the patient that someone is in control and that the doctor respects the patient's capacities to participate as an informed partner in the healing process. The reassurance provides a foundation on which the patient can begin to reconstruct a sense of order in everyday life.

Patients with compulsive personality disorder are not reassured by vague impressionistic overviews of their prognosis. Patients feel most comfortable when the doctor provides documentary evidence in the form of specific laboratory test results, eg, electrocardiograms or x-rays, or cites actual reports from the literature when presenting statistics about risk factors.

The healing process may be promoted by harnessing the innate thoroughness of the patient through encouraging self-monitoring activities such as measurement of fluid intake and output and weight fluctuations and control of graduated exercise programs. When feasible, patients can take over management of more routine procedures, such as changing their surgical dressings. Meticulous adherence to treatment protocols will restore morale as patients regain a sense of mastery and dignity in taking charge of their lives. The physician must remain alert to the possibility that compulsive patients may wish to carry this self-healing process too far and cross the boundaries of their competence while stubbornly resisting the expertise offered by the health care team.

Illustrative Case

A 47-year-old woman who was an executive in a large accounting firm developed symptoms of unexpected weight loss and dizziness. Measurement of fasting blood glucose levels and urinalysis confirmed the diagnosis of adult-onset diabetes. The patient reacted to this news by conducting an extensive search of the literature on diabetes and by requesting that her internist refer her to an endocrinologist for further evaluation. The internist, who had known the patient for a long time, was empathically aware of how emotionally out of control the patient felt and promptly referred the patient to an endocrinologist, who confirmed the diagnosis and provided a detailed description of the nature and expected course of the illness and alternative treatment strategies. The patient was reassured by the consensus of opinion shown by the two trusted experts and agreed to work with her internist in developing a treatment plan.

Although the patient was initially jolted into a state of panicky confusion by what she termed the "internal rebellion of my body," she regained a sense of order and predictability as she became an active partner in the healing process. Through a program of strict dietary control, weight loss, and exercise (which the patient meticulously pursued), she was able to bring her metabolic status within normal limits and thus avoided the need for exogenous insulin. In a 1-year follow-up appointment with the endocrinologist, the patient was complimented on her courageously disciplined response to the illness. When she was asked what had been most helpful in assisting her to cope with the problem, she replied, "Both you and my regular doctor had faith in my capacity to understand the illness and make informed choices about treatment, and you both supported my resolve to fight back. When I first became ill, I felt like a rudderless ship tossed about in dangerous waters. You were like a safe harbor, but even more important, you helped me regain the confidence that I could sail again on my own power."

PERSONALITY DISORDER NOT OTHERWISE SPECIFIED

This category is useful for individuals with passive-aggressive features, self-defeating patterns, or features of several personality disorders that do not meet the full diagnostic criteria for any specific personality disorder. The following two clinical case examples illustrate personality disorder with passive-aggressive features and personality disorder with self-defeating patterns.

Illustrative Case (Personality Disorder with Passive-Aggressive Features)

A 47-year-old man reluctantly sought psychiatric treatment when progressive financial and marital difficulties led to insomnia. Despite his reputation as a capable housing contractor, he had repeatedly been unable to meet his deadlines with both homeowners and subcontractors. He would often forget important appointments, drag his heels on commitments, and make excuses for being behind schedule, while inwardly feeling, "I'll do it in my own sweet time." His wife was threatening to leave him because she was unable to obtain his help around the house; she felt that she had to ask him 10 times to do anything, and even when he complied, he made only a half-hearted effort.

The patient was the youngest son in his family and had two older brothers who, he recalled with some bitterness, had teased and bullied him. He described his father as "the head honcho of the house," who had been more interested in maintaining peace and quiet than in being emotionally close to his sons. He felt his mother had been more caring but overinvolved in his life: "She had to know about every nook and cranny of my life and couldn't tolerate my keeping any secrets from her." As an adolescent he had enjoyed sports but had been prone to outbursts of righteous indignation when he felt he was being

treated unfairly. He had been a good student but had been episodically disruptive in the classroom, particularly with strict male teachers. As an adult he had several close friends, but these relationships were strained because of his stubborn refusal to compromise on social plans and his chronic tardiness.

The patient arrived 20 minutes late for the interview and said that traffic had been heavy across town, when in actuality he was familiar with the traffic patterns and simply had not allowed enough time to ensure his prompt arrival. He indicated that he made the appointment reluctantly and only because of his wife's nagging complaints about his uncooperativeness at home. He provided little spontaneous information during the interview, so that the psychiatrist had great difficult in obtaining useful data. The patient denied that he was in any way "testing" the psychiatrist when the latter tactfully confronted him about his provocative, obstructionist style. Mental status examination revealed no disorder of sensorium, thought organization, or perception, and although the patient's mood was irritable, he did not demonstrate any features of a major mood disorder.

Passive-Aggressive Personality in Medical Practice

Individuals with passive-aggressive personality features may be a source of considerable irritation to physicians, since they tend to make a dramatic display of their suffering while at the same time only minimally acknowledging the actual help they are receiving and exaggerating their continuing discomfort. Such patients derive secondary gains from remaining ill; eg, they have a means of punishing the envied and resented authority figures in their life, including physicians. They may attempt to place the responsibility for getting well on the physician's shoulders while they themselves subtly fail to cooperate with the treatment procedures. Such patients tend to forget appointments and be late in paying their accounts, and the physician finds little reward in treating them. The physician may then feel a sense of resentfulness and guilty responsibility, since the patient seems neither to improve nor to cooperate with the help offered but still seems to require the physician's attention.

The physician should take the time to acknowledge and empathize with the suffering of these patients before steering the conversation toward specific treatment recommendations. Such patients will then feel understood rather than forced into giving up their suffering before they are prepared to do so. Information is often presented to the patient more effectively in the form of questions rather than statements, such as "What will happen to you if you don't take your medication?" or "What do you think would be a fair fee for this treatment?" This approach encourages the patient's cooperation rather than inviting rebelliousness. If physicians understand that these patients have an investment in illness as a means of passively gaining control, they in turn need not feel weak or guilty because patients do not seem to improve.

Physicians should be alert to subtle forms of noncompliance; eg, patients may deliberately ask for information about treatment procedures so that they may later blame the physician for difficulties in treatment. A nonpunitive but frank discussion about the ways in which patients subtly undermine their own well-being may prevent such passive-aggressive patterns.

Illustrative Case (Personality Disorder with Self-Defeating Patterns)

A 38-year-old man sought psychiatric treatment because of depression and loneliness following the breakup of a love relationship. He had been involved for 8 months with an attractive, intelligent, and caring woman. The breakdown of this relationship was particularly painful to him because the woman, unlike most women with whom he had been involved, had been genuinely committed to deepening the relationship. His earlier pattern had been to involve himself with self-absorbed, emotionally aloof partners who "trashed him in favor of someone more interesting."

He initially portrayed his current disappointment as yet another confirmation of his view that the world would victimize him and was not aware of having provoked the separation by repeatedly frustrating his lover's efforts to show him affection.

In the interview, he presented himself as a downtrodden victim who seemed impervious to help and who seemed convinced in advance that treatment would be of no value. The mental status examination revealed no disorder of sensorium, thought organization, or perception. Although his mood was both sad and irritable, he did not demonstrate the prototypical features of major depressive episode.

Self-Defeating Personality in Medical Practice

Patients with personality disorder with self-defeating patterns present a special treatment challenge for the physician. Such patients frequently have an unconscious need to defeat the physician's efforts to effect a cure. Often, they overreact to minor side effects of treatment, discontinue treatment against medical advice, or develop symptom substitution. It is difficult to recruit the patient's active cooperation. When treatment is successful, such individuals frequently place themselves at risk for relapse by neglecting nutritional and exercise needs, abusing alcohol and drugs, or not complying with rehabilitation programs.

When treating self-defeating patients, it is useful for the physician to maintain the perspective that the course will be long-term and often complicated. The physician should resist the patient's witting or unwitting invitation to perform miracles only to be defeated by the patient's compulsive need to undermine help when it is offered. The physician should also anticipate the patient's difficulty in cooperating with treatment. Referral for psychiatric treatment, although initially met with reluctance, may later be accepted as patients gradually gain insight into their own role in self-defeating patterns.

PATIENTS WITH MIXED PERSONALITY DISORDERS

The descriptions provided above present the personality disorders as discrete diagnostic entities to point out the distinctive characteristics of each disorder and thereby provide some framework around which to organize clinical observations. As is also sometimes the case in medical patients, psychiatric patients may show features of more than one disorder simultaneously, so that careful management using a skillful synthesis of the approaches described for each separate disorder is imperative, eg, for a patient with mixed compulsive and narcissistic personality disorder or one with mixed histrionic and borderline personality disorder. The problem is analogous to that encountered in medical management of multisystem disease, eg, coexisting diabetes and hepatitis. In the case of combined personality disorders, the physician must avoid minimizing or overemphasizing any one element at the expense of a balanced "systems" approach.

MANAGEMENT OF THE "HATEFUL" PATIENT

A common theme in this chapter is the resentment that may be aroused in physicians and other caretakers by certain patients with personality disorder. Groves (1978) describes the four types of patients with personality disorder who are most likely to evoke an attitude of dislike or even hatred in their physicians: dependent clingers, entitled demanders, manipulative help rejectors, and self-destructive deniers. The similarity of these four diagnostic categories to specific personality disorders described in *DSM-IV* is readily apparent. The dependent clinger corresponds to dependent personality disorder, the entitled demander to narcissistic personality disorder, the manipulative help rejector to passive-aggressive or borderline personality disorder, and the self-destructive denier to histrionic or borderline personality disorder.

Groves frankly acknowledges the dislike that physicians often feel for certain patients. Although conscious recognition and acceptance of negative feelings toward a patient run counter to the idea of the physician as an unfailingly kind and generous healer of the sick, the denial of such feelings when they really exist can lead to only further disturbances in management of the patient. Recognizing feelings of resentment is an important cornerstone in develop- ing an appropriate management strategy that will create a strong working alliance between the physician and the patient in order to facilitate healing.

REFERENCES & SUGGESTED READINGS

Beck R, Fernandez E: Cognitive-behavioral therapy in the treatment of anger: A meta-analysis. Cog Ther Res 1998; 22:63.

Berman SM, McCann JT: Defense mechanisms and personality disorders: An empirical test of Millon's theory. J Personality Assess 1995;64:132.

Bowlby J: Forty-four juvenile thieves. Int J Psychoanal 1944;25:19.

Carpenter WT, Gunderson JG, Strauss JS: Considerations of the borderline syndrome: A longitudinal comparative study of borderline and schizophrenic patients. In: *Borderline Personality Disorders: The Concept, the Syndrome, the Patient.* Hartocollis P (editor). International Universities Press, 1977.

Coccaro EF: Clinical outcome of psychopharmacologic treatment of borderline and schizotypal personality disordered subjects. J Clin Psychiatry 1998;59:30.

Dolan B: Therapeutic community treatment for severe personality disorders. In: *Antisocial, Criminal and Violent Behavior.* Millon T, Simonsen E (editors). Guilford Press, 1998.

Eichelman B: Toward a rational pharmacotherapy for aggressive and violent behavior. Hosp Commun Psychiatry 1988;39:31.

Freud S: Three essays on the theory of sexuality (1905). In: *Standard Edition of the Complete Psychological Works of Sigmund Freud.* Vol 7. Hogarth Press, 1964.

Garrido V, Esteban C, Molero C: The effectiveness in treatment of psychopathy: A meta-analysis. Issues Criminol Legal Psychol 1995;24:57.

Glueck S, Glueck E: *Delinquents and Nondelinquents in Perspective.* Harvard University Press, 1968.

Gottesman II: Heritability of personality: A demonstration. Psychol Monogr 1963;77:1.

Groves JE: Taking care of the hateful patient. N Engl J Med 1978;298:883.

Horowitz MJ: Sliding meanings: A defense against threat in narcissistic personalities. Int J Psychoanal Psychother 1975;4:167.

Kahana R, Bibring G: Personality types in medical management. In: *Psychiatry and Medical Practice in the General Hospital.* Zinberg N (editor). International Universities Press, 1964.

Kemberg O: *Borderline Conditions and Pathological Narcissism.* Jason Aronson, 1975.

Klein D: Psychopharmacological treatment and delineation of borderline disorders. In: *Borderline Personality Disorders: The Concept, the Syndrome, the Patient.* Hartocollis P (editor). International Universities Press, 1977.

Kohut M: *The Analysis of the Self.* International Universities Press, 1971.

Kringlen E: Obsessional neurotics. Br J Psychiatry 1965; 111:709.

Langner TS, Michael ST: *Life Stress and Mental Health.* Free Press, 1963.

Leigh H, Reiser MF: *The Patient: Biological, Psychological, and Social Dimensions of Medical Practice.* Plenum Press, 1980.

Linehan M: Dialectical behavior therapy for borderline personality disorder. Bull Menninger Clin 1987;51:261.

Links PS, Heslegrave R, vanReekum R: Prospective follow-up study of borderline personality disorder: Prognosis, prediction of outcome, and Axis II comorbidity. Can J Psychiatry 1998;43:265.

Mahler MS: A study of the separation-individuation process and its possible application to borderline phenomena in the psychoanalytic situation. Psychoanal Study Child 1971;26:403.

Masterson JF: *Treatment of the Borderline Adolescent: A Developmental Approach.* Wiley, 1972.

Morgenstern J, Langenbucher J, Labouvie E, Miller KJ: The comorbidity of alcoholism and personality disorders in a clinical population: Prevalence rates in relation to alcohol typology variables. J Abnorm Psychol 1997;106:74.

Raine A, Venables PH, Williams M: Relationships between central and autonomic measures of arousal at age 15 years and criminality at age 24 years. Arch Gen Psychiatry 1990;47:1003.

Robins: In: *Deviant Children Grown Up: A Sociological and Psychiatric Study of Sociopathic Personality.* Williams & Wilkins, 1966.

Schulsinger F: Psychopathy, heredity, and environment. Int J Ment Health 1972;1:190.

Selzer M, Koeningsberg H, Kernberg O: The initial treatment contract in the treatment of borderline patients. Am J Psychiatry 1987;144:927.

Ucok A, Karaveli D, Kundacki T, Yaziki O: Comorbidity of personality disorders with bipolar mood disorders. Comp Psychiatry 1998;72.

Werble B: Second follow-up study of borderline patients. Arch Gen Psychiatry 1970;23:307.

25 Sexual Dysfunction, Gender Identity Disorders, & Paraphilias*

S. Michael Plaut, PhD, & Gregory K. Lehne, PhD

The *Diagnostic and Statistical Manual of Mental Disorders,* 4th edition (*DSM-IV*) (American Psychiatric Association, 1994) classifies sexual disorders in three categories—sexual dysfunctions, gender identity disorders, and paraphilias. They will be discussed in turn, highlighting etiological factors, treatment modalities, and ways in which the physician who is not a specialist in the treatment of sexual dysfunction can assist patients who present with sexual concerns.

SEXUAL DYSFUNCTIONS

There are three general subtypes of sexual dysfunctions, as currently classified. The first, consisting of six specific diagnostic categories, involves dysfunctions of the three phases of the sexual response cycle—desire, arousal (or excitement), and orgasm. Desire disorders include hypoactive sexual desire (formerly inhibited sexual desire) and sexual aversion disorder. Arousal disorders include female sexual arousal disorder and male erectile disorder. Orgasm disorders include inhibited orgasm in women and men and premature ejaculation in men. A second type of dysfunction is the sexual pain disorders, dyspareunia and vaginismus. A newly added third classification denotes sexual dysfunctions as outlined above that are related either to medical conditions or to substance use.

Only a few years ago, the dysfunctions of the sexual response cycle were generally described as either impotence in the case of men or frigidity in the case of women. The recent diagnostic distinctions among the various subtypes of sexual dysfunction reflect the increased knowledge about the basis for these dysfunctions and the development of specific treatment procedures for each.

Despite recent advances, the treatment of sexual dysfunction remains complex for a number of reasons. First, there is still much to learn about the sexual response cycle and its physiological foundations. Second, the causes of sexual dysfunction are varied, and treatment procedures must be both flexible and customized to the needs of the patient. Third, and perhaps most important, sexuality is still a very difficult topic for most people in our culture to discuss openly, either with their intimate partners or with the health professionals to whom they may wish to bring a concern. Health professionals are likely to suffer from the same culturally based inhibitions; although they may have been given some factual knowledge about sexuality as part of their training, they may be no more comfortable discussing these issues with a patient than a patient is with them.

Sexuality is a vital part of everyone's life, and there are many reasons why a patient may need to discuss sexual issues with a professional. They may have simple questions or developmental concerns (eg, appropriateness of masturbation in children, normality of penis size, changes in sexual function with age). A person's sexual function may have been affected by a medication, illness, surgery, or sexual trauma, or by more subtle factors such as fear of intimacy or performance anxiety. For these reasons, any health professional should be comfortable exploring the possibility of sexual concerns, realizing that many patients, because of their discomfort with the topic, are not likely to volunteer these concerns spontaneously, however serious. A health professional should also know how and to whom a patient may be referred for more specialized evaluation and treatment. This discussion will focus primarily on the psychosocial aspects of the evaluation and treatment of sexual dysfunctions, based on knowledge and techniques developed over the past two decades.

For the sake of simplicity, couples will be assumed to be heterosexual throughout this discussion. However, gay and lesbian couples may present with similar concerns, and most of the issues and techniques described here will apply. When working with homosexual couples, however, it is particularly important that the clinician neither stereotype the sexual behavior of homosexual individuals nor apply heterosexual

---

* Portions of this chapter were originally published in Spanish as Plaut SM: Evaluacion y tratamiento de las disfunciones sexuales [Evaluation and treatment of sexual dysfunctions]. In: *Integración en Psicológio.* Opazo R (editor). Santiago, Chile: Centro Cientáifico de Desarrollo Psicológico, 1992:210–225.

stereotypes to their behavior. Rather, he or she should be aware of issues pertinent to homosexual men and women (Nichols, 1989).

SEXUAL RESPONSE CYCLE

The sexual response cycle has been described by Masters and Johnson and modified for diagnostic purposes by Kaplan. Four basic phases are generally recognized:

A. Appetitive or Desire Phase: In this phase, one or more stimuli (eg, visual, olfactory, tactile, fantasies) engender a desire to engage in sexual activity.

B. Excitement or Arousal Phase: This phase includes the individual's feelings of sexual pleasure and accompanying physiological changes. The major change in both men and women is pelvic vasocongestion with accompanying myotonia. In men, this results in penile tumescence, stimulation of Cowper's gland, drawing of the scrotum and testicles closer to the body, and penile erection. In women, pelvic congestion and myotonia result in engorgement of the vessels of the external genitalia and the vaginal lining, sweating (transudate production) of the vagina, which produces lubrication, increased tension of the pubococcygeal muscle surrounding the vaginal orifice, development of the orgasmic platform, increased sensitivity and enlargement of the clitoris, and "ballooning" of the inner two-thirds of the vagina. Breast tissue frequently engorges, with accompanying nipple erection and sensitivity. The period of time during which a level of sexual arousal is maintained is referred to as the plateau phase.

C. Orgasmic Phase: In both men and women, generalized muscle tension is followed by muscle contractions, resulting in involuntary pelvic thrusting and heightened sexual sensations. With the release of muscle tension, there are rhythmic contractions of the pelvic and perineal muscles. In women, contractions occur in the lower third of the vagina and in the uterus, which has been elevated in relation to the other pelvic structures (orgasmic platform). In men, contractions of the prostate, seminal vesicles, and urethra propel seminal and prostatic fluids to the exterior while the bladder sphincter closes.

D. Resolution Phase: In both sexes, vasocongestion and myotonia become less intense, and there is general body relaxation. Men experience a physiological refractory period before erection and orgasm can occur again. Vasocongestion and myotonia subside less quickly in women, and the clitoral and perineal tissues are sensitive enough to respond almost immediately to continued stimulation.

Most sexual dysfunctions are related to disturbances in one or more phases of the sexual response cycle. The disturbance may be physiological, psychological, or both. For example, a man who feels strong desire for a partner (psychological) may find that he is not being aroused, as evidenced by an absent or partial erection (physiological). Similarly, a woman who is sexually aroused by her partner and responding physiologically may be unable to reach orgasm as she begins to worry about losing control. Specific sexual dysfunctions will be described later in this discussion.

INTERVENTIONS

Levels of Intervention—The PLISSIT Model

The PLISSIT model has been proposed to characterize the stepwise approach to counseling a person with a sexual problem. The first level of intervention is the giving of *permission*—for example, to discuss sex openly, to use the language of sex without guilt, or to engage in certain sexual behaviors that are generally considered normal. In providing such permission, the clinician must take care not to insist that the patient violate any strongly held values. The clinician may also provide *limited information* about sexual development, male-female differences, genital anatomy, etc. *Specific suggestions* may be provided that will enhance sexual pleasure or function, such as varying time or location of sexual activity, using certain sexual techniques, approaching a partner more effectively, or rejecting a partner in a supportive way. It may be important to ask the patient specifically about the use of safe sex procedures, to explain such procedures to them, and to recommend HIV testing, particularly if he or she is in a new relationship or is involved with multiple partners.

In many cases, suggestions may take the form of videotapes or assigned reading, which some therapists call "bibliotherapy." A few books often found useful for this purpose include those by Barbach (1976, 1984, 1985), Friday (1973, 1980), Heiman and LoPiccolo (1988), Penner and Penner (1981), and Zilbergeld (1999). Increasingly, the Internet is providing a source of self-help for people with sexual questions and concerns. For example, Gotlib and Fagan (1997) have assembled a Web site that refers to a number of other useful sex-related sites.

Many times, a sexual concern can be dealt with by utilizing only the first three levels of counseling. However, if a dysfunction is clearly present, *intensive therapy* should be undertaken by someone who is skilled in the techniques of sex therapy, in which cases all four levels of intervention are usually involved. In cases in which a dysfunction is shown to have a medical basis, appropriate medical treatment may be provided as well.

Basic Considerations in Sex Therapy

Modern sex therapy was developed in the late 1960s with the pioneering work of Masters and Johnson, who demonstrated the value of behavioral therapy techniques in alleviating sexual symptoms.

Treatment was done in an intense, 2-week format, using male and female cotherapists. Later, Kaplan showed that the same techniques could be effective in the more traditional 1-hour-per-week therapy format, using a single therapist. Whereas the treatment format of Masters and Johnson has the advantage of focusing on the sexual problem in a protected environment, the more spaced format has the advantage of flexibility for both patient and therapist while also integrating the ongoing treatment into the patient's normal life-style.

Basic Premises of Sex Therapy

A central precept of the Masters and Johnson technique is that the sexual response is a *natural function*—that is, barring any medical disturbance to the normal cycle, sexual responses will occur under appropriate psychosocial or tactile stimulation, unless something else in the intrapsychic or interpersonal environment blocks these responses. Kaplan referred to these factors as the **immediate causes** of sexual dysfunction. These may include things such as performance anxiety, absence of fantasy, inability to immerse oneself in a sexual situation (or "spectatoring"), or difficulties in seducing or arousing one's partner.

Deeper causes, such as psychodynamic issues, relationship problems, or early conditioning, may also be involved in the etiology of sexual dysfunctions. However, a short-term behavioral approach focused on the immediate causes of the dysfunction is often more successful and more economical than longer-term insight-oriented therapy. In most cases, the therapist must approach the presenting problem at more than one level of intervention. For example, concomitant problems in the couple's relationship often demand the simultaneous attention to communication and control issues or the need to deal with a partner's fear of intimacy or fear of separation.

Table 25–1 outlines examples of both immediate and deeper causes of sexual dysfunction, many of which will be described more fully throughout the chapter.

There may be no direct correspondence between specific deeper causes and specific dysfunctions, which become the final common pathway for a number of possible precipitating factors. For example, a woman's history of incest may be reflected sexually in hypoactive desire (or sexual aversion), anorgasmia, vaginismus, or a combination of these, or she may show no sexual pathology at all.

A. The Couple as the Patient: Another central premise on which the Masters and Johnson techniques were developed is the conviction that *the couple is the patient.* Thus, although one person may present with a sexual symptom, it is usually important that within treatment one partner is not blamed for the problem. Treatment should elicit the cooperation and support of the other partner, and the sexual

Table 25–1. Etiology of sexual dysfunctions.

I. Immediate causes
  A. Performance anxiety—fear of inadequate performance
  B. Spectatoring—critically monitoring one's own sexual performance
  C. Inadequate communication with partner regarding sex
  D. Fantasy
    1. Absence of fantasy
    2. Distracting thoughts
    3. Antifantasy—fantasies incompatible with sexual arousal

II. Deeper causes
  A. Intrapsychic issues
    1. Early conditioning
    2. Sexual trauma
    3. Depression
    4. Anxiety
    5. Guilt
    6. Fear of intimacy or separation
  B. Relationship issues
    1. Lack of trust
    2. Power and control issues
    3. Anger at partner
  C. Sociocultural factors
    1. Attitudes and values
    2. Religious beliefs
  D. Educational and cognitive factors
    1. Sexual myths (gender roles, age and appearance, proper sexual activity, performance expectations)
    2. Sexual ignorance

problem should be evaluated and treated as a relationship issue. Indeed, the other partner may display sexual symptoms (eg, absence of desire) in the course of treating the presenting problem, particularly if the original symptom was in some way functional for the partner.

Of course, there may be times when the person who presents with a sexual symptom has no partner, or the partner may refuse to participate in treatment. In such instances it is usually best to do what one can with the individual patient while explaining clearly the therapist's conviction that treatment done in the context of the relationship is more likely to be effective. Some sexual dysfunctions, such as a global anorgasmia, premature ejaculation, or vaginismus, can at least initially be treated through the use of individual therapy and/or masturbation exercises.

B. Education and Reassurance—Reframing One's Concept of Sexuality: Another extremely important aspect of sex therapy is the need to educate patients about various aspects of sexuality or to help restructure or *reframe* their conception of what sexuality is, or what it can be. This does not mean that a therapist imposes his or her ideas of what sex should be on the patient. If both members of a couple are satisfied with their level of activity or with their sexual repertoire, the therapist should not advocate personal beliefs concerning enhanced sexual practices. However, when two partners are incompatible in their approach to sex, or if advancing age, disability, or illness affects certain aspects of sexual activity, a broader approach to sex can have a freeing effect, thus allowing the couple to relate to each other in a more satisfying way. For example, if sex is seen primarily as a reproductive act that focuses on vaginal intercourse, the therapist can help the patient to understand that sex can also serve other functions. It can be seen as a recreational activity—as fun! It can be seen as the expression of caring and affection. It can be seen simply as a release of sexual energy. It can be any combination of these four things at different times for the same couple.

The reproductive focus of sexuality in our culture also often leads to an excessive focus on genitals, genital contact, and orgasm as goals of a fulfilling sexual response. Men and women often differ in this regard, as women more typically prefer a slower, whole-body approach to a sexual encounter than do men. Excessive focus on genitals, intercourse, orgasm, and performance only tends to heighten the level of anxiety in the man who experiences erectile problems or the woman who suffers from vaginismus or hypoactive desire. One of the major accomplishments of sex therapy can be a broadening of the couple's approach, so that sexual practices become more varied and creative, anxiety about specific practices diminishes, and the needs of both members of the couple are met.

A third aspect of reframing may be helping the couple to become more immersed in a sexual experience—leaving their daily cares outside the bedroom, being comfortable with a variety of sexual fantasies, and being involved in *experiencing* sex, rather than watching themselves perform, or what Masters and Johnson called "spectatoring." Fantasy is difficult or uncomfortable for some people to experience, as they may have paraphilic fantasies or fantasies about partners other than the one to whom they are making love at the moment, or they may feel pressure from their partner to disclose their fantasies. People often need to be assured that in most cases, sexual fantasies—even unusual ones—are natural and that they can be kept private.

George was a 46-year-old male who had never experienced a sexual relationship with a woman but now had a steady female partner, a divorcee who was frustrated by his inability to maintain an erection when attempting intercourse, particularly since he was able to masturbate privately with a full erection. In a private session, he disclosed that he could masturbate only by fantasizing about a large woman spanking him and then having intercourse with him in the female superior position. Not only was his real partner a slightly built woman who did not fit his fantasy, but he felt guilty about utilizing his functional fantasy when he was with her. The therapist helped him to feel comfortable using the fantasy while with his partner but not disclosing the fantasy to her. As his erectile capacity improved with the aid of sensate focus exercises, he began to become aroused by

fantasies of his actual partner. The therapist encouraged him to "replay" the new fantasy "tapes" he was accumulating, and the paraphilic fantasy gradually faded away.

C. Respecting the Patient's Values: One of the most important qualities of a sex therapist is his or her ability to deal with sexual values and attitudes—both the therapist's and the patient's. Many programs for health professionals in sexuality education require trainees to participate in a values clarification or Sexual Attitude Reassessment (SAR) workshop, which may also be required for certification. By taking a few days to openly and confidentially discuss their sexual attitudes and experiences with a group of peers, clinicians can clarify their own sexual values while developing an understanding of and a respect for the values and attitudes of others. By gaining an appreciation of the range of sexual values, they are less likely to impose their own values on the patient while finding it easier to work within the patient's own value system. The SAR experience can also increase the ability of the clinician to communicate more easily about sexual matters and to use the language of sexuality with less apprehension or anxiety.

The patient's experiences and values may differ sharply from those of the clinician, and it is important that the clinician work effectively within the patient's framework. Couples who are not married will appear for treatment of a sexual dysfunction. An orgasmic woman or a male experiencing premature ejaculation may be unwilling to masturbate, when masturbatory exercises would appear to be an important component of the treatment of choice. The sexual fulfillment of a lesbian couple may involve the kind of manual stimulation of the genitals that many heterosexual individuals consider foreplay. In these and other instances, the clinician must be open, understanding, and flexible if the needs of the patient are to be met.

As mentioned earlier, the clinician should also take care to let the patient ultimately set the therapeutic agenda, as illustrated in the following case example:

Dorothy and Bob, a newly married couple, presented with unconsummated marriage, expressed as the husband's inability to ejaculate intravaginally. Because of the highly religious background of the couple and their general discomfort with sexuality, a regimen of sensate focus exercises was begun and readings were recommended. The couple was aggressive and anxious for a cure, which they defined as a successful pregnancy, and they "cheated" in the second week of treatment by having successful intercourse, even though (or perhaps because!) they had been instructed not to engage in any genital contact. On the fifth week, they announced that Dorothy was pregnant and terminated therapy despite the therapist's expressed feeling that there were additional relationship issues underlying the sexual problem that might be addressed in continued therapy. However, the couple had gotten what they came for—basically, permission to express themselves to each other in a sexual way, resulting in their desired goal of pregnancy. Nine months later, the therapist received a baby announcement in the mail!

Whatever techniques may be used in treating these dysfunctions, there can be no substitute for the therapists' comfort level, skill, creativity, flexibility, humor, sensitivity, patience, and warmth in making this process work. The couple presenting with a sexual problem should be able to leave therapy feeling good about sex, however they may define it, and they need to feel good about themselves as sexual people. In this frequently uncomfortable area, the sensitive, prepared professional can both provide relief and facilitate growth, often with relatively little of the right kind of help and support.

D. Qualifications of a Sex Therapist: There are two or three professional organizations that certify individuals in sex therapy. These organizations have developed standards of training and practice that health professionals are expected to meet if they are to be certified. Since certification as a sex therapist is typically not a legal requirement for the practice of sex therapy, many well-trained sex therapists are not certified as such. However, a referring clinician should be aware of the qualifications normally expected of a competent sex therapist.

A sex therapist should first be qualified in a recognized health care field, such as medicine, psychology, social work, or psychiatric nursing. It is helpful if the therapist already possesses good skills as an individual or couples therapist, as these skills are important to the effective treatment of sexual dysfunction.

The therapist should have a thorough knowledge of the sexual response cycle, the effects of illness, medication, and substances such as alcohol on sexual function, and the effects of intrapsychic and cultural factors on sexual attitudes and function. The therapist's approach to the multidimensional nature of the sexual response must be balanced so that an awareness of all possible causes of a dysfunction is maintained. This awareness should be evident in the comprehensive approach to evaluation and in the therapist's willingness to consult with and refer to professionals in other relevant specialties, as may be necessary. For example, an erectile dysfunction can result from a combination of any number of neurological, endocrinological, circulatory, or behavioral factors. It may often be necessary to refer a patient for a medical workup, treatment of a substance abuse problem, or individual therapy before an appropriate treatment plan can be developed for the presenting sexual problem.

The behavioral and cognitive techniques that are the hallmark of modern sex therapy also require special skill. These techniques and their applications will be discussed in some detail later.

EVALUATION OF SEXUAL PROBLEMS

The evaluation of a presenting sexual problem involves identifying both the immediate and deeper causes of the problem and developing an initial treatment plan. In keeping with the central idea that "the couple is the patient," equivalent histories are taken from both members of the couple. Detailed descriptions of evaluation procedures are beyond the scope of this discussion. However, it may be of value to highlight some of the key issues that should be addressed in conducting the initial interviews.

Some therapists obtain background information from the patient in the form of pencil-and-paper tests or questionnaires. Formal testing may include general assessments (eg, MMPI-2, SCL-90), assessments of sexual function (eg, LoPiccolo's Sexual Interaction Inventory, Derogatis Sexual Function Inventory), or inventories of relationship status (eg, Dyadic Adjustment Inventory). Questionnaires may gather pertinent data such as ages and number of children, household occupants, religious background, names of physicians and time of last physical examination, illnesses, surgeries, and present medications, a brief description of the presenting problem, and the patient's expectations for therapy.

The first two parts of the psychosexual evaluation are the *description of the chief complaint* and what Kaplan calls the *sexual status examination*. These are important, as they help determine the relative contributions of medical and psychosocial factors and enable the therapist to identify the immediate causes of the sexual problem.

Description of the Chief Complaint

This phase of the evaluation should include a description of the problem, its history, and why the patient sought help at the present time. It is here that clear communication and definition of terms need to be established. What does the patient mean by "having sex" or "making love" or "partial erection" or "pain during intercourse?" Does "having sex" mean (only) vaginal intercourse? Is the "partial erection" sufficient for penetration? Is the pain experienced during intercourse deep in the vagina or at the entrance? And so on. A reluctance to communicate in detail may prevent an adequate definition of the problem. The clinician should take care not to assume that the patient means one thing when something quite different might be meant.

A critical aspect of the description of the chief complaint is the determination of whether the symptoms are global or situational—that is, under what conditions the symptoms occur. This will help the clinician to determine (1) whether a medical examination might aid in a complete diagnosis and (2) the extent to which the symptoms are relationship related. For example, if a patient presents with an erectile problem, the clinician should attempt to determine whether the patient experiences erections in masturbation or on awakening, and whether the onset of symptoms was sudden or gradual. The more global the symptoms and the more gradual the onset, the more likely it is that the problem has a medical etiology. If the erectile problem occurs primarily in the context of the patient's current relationship, it is important to know whether the problem began at the beginning of the relationship or whether it was related to a specific event or situation that occurred since the relationship began (eg, moving in together, marriage). Does the problem occur with all partners, or perhaps with certain kinds of partners, such as those for whom the patient has strong feelings?

Sexual Status Examination

The sexual status examination is the patient's account of a recent or typical sexual encounter. The clinician can play an important role in helping patients feel more comfortable discussing their sexual activity in detail, pointing out its importance to the clinician's understanding of the problem. This is the clinician's way of determining the often subtle immediate causes of symptoms, and it should be done during each session in order to elucidate both progress and problems. The sexual status examination should assess all three phases of the sexual response cycle—desire, arousal, and orgasm. The clinician should determine the conditions under which the sexual encounter took place (eg, time of day, location, ambiance), who initiated it, what took place, what problems occurred, if any, how each partner responded to problems, and how the encounter ended. The clinician should also attempt to determine what thoughts or feelings accompanied any problems experienced during the encounter, which may be reassessed during individual interviews, as necessary.

> Barbara was referred by her gynecologist with a diagnosis of intermittent vaginismus that had no apparent medical basis. She was in a good marital relationship and had enjoyed successful intercourse until shortly after the birth of her first child. She displayed a relatively low threshold for anxiety in many areas. She was assigned dilator exercises and, with her husband, sensate focus exercises. Sexual status examinations over the first 3 weeks of treatment revealed a pattern of anxiety at times when she had reason to fear that their young son would either hear the couple making love or enter the room. Once this pattern was revealed to both the therapist and the couple, and measures were taken to minimize the possibility of the child witnessing their sexual encounters, the symptoms quickly abated, and the therapy ended after the seventh week.

It is often useful to know the conditions under which the woman is orgasmic. Many women do not experience orgasm during intercourse without specific clitoral stimulation. This knowledge may have implications for the therapy if, for example, either partner is uncomfortable with oral or manual stimulation of the genitals or if a complaint of premature ejaculation is based solely on the relative occurrence of male and female orgasm.

When appropriate, it may be useful to do a detailed account of masturbatory practices, dreams, or fantasies, as these may provide keys to the immediate causes of sexual symptoms while also aiding in the development of suitable behavioral assignments. The case of George, presented earlier, illustrates the value of doing a sexual status examination on a reported fantasy. In the following case, knowledge about a patient's masturbatory practices was helpful in developing suitable initial assignments.

> Herb presented with a complaint of premature ejaculation, the treatment of which typically begins with masturbation exercises done in a situation that approaches the environment in which the patient might have a sexual encounter with a partner. During the evaluation, it was determined that the patient had always masturbated in the shower, and never in bed. Without that information, a simple prescription of masturbation exercises would not have served the intended purpose. The therapist was able to help the patient feel comfortable learning to masturbate in bed before stop-start exercises (to be described later) were begun.

Medical & Psychiatric Histories

The medical history should concentrate on illnesses, surgeries, and medications that are likely to cause or exacerbate sexual dysfunction, such as diabetes, vaginal infections, or circulatory problems. Assessment of drug use should include smoking, alcohol, illicit drugs, and both prescription and over-the-counter medications. For example, over-the-counter antihistamines may inhibit vaginal lubrication. If appropriate, the couple should be asked about menstrual cycling, the couple's sexual practices during menstruation, contraceptive use, and plans for having children. At times, a couple will have stopped using contraception because "we're not having sex anyway." Unless they are trying to get pregnant, the clinician should encourage the couple to begin or resume whatever contraceptive practices they may wish to use. This will minimize another possible source of anxiety regarding sexual success while helping the couple learn to integrate contraceptive use comfortably into their sexual encounters.

The psychiatric history focuses on previous or existing emotional problems and treatment, as well as a brief family history of psychiatric problems. In most cases, existing psychiatric problems, such as substance abuse or psychosis, should be stabilized before sex therapy is attempted. If a patient is in ongoing individual therapy, the sex therapist should establish consent and communication with the other therapist. Financial considerations may necessitate suspension of individual therapy while sex therapy is in progress.

Family & Sexual Histories

The family history concentrates on relationships in the home during childhood and adolescence, with special attention to the patient's perception of the intimate relationships of parents or other caregivers. This is followed by the sexual history, which includes a description of sexual learning and modeling as well as accounts of sexual experiences, both with and without partners. Patients should specifically be asked about any unwanted sexual experiences including, but not limited to, rape, incest, or other traumatic sexual encounters. The response of both the patient and the family to these experiences should be assessed, as well as any treatment related to these events and the patient's current feelings about them. These questions should be asked of men as well as women, as it is not unusual for men to have experienced an event that they may not have previously identified as a sexual trauma. Such incidents may include incest, sexual contact with older individuals, overexposure to nudity or sexuality in the home, and threats of castration.

Relationship History & Status

Relationship history and status are usually assessed gradually throughout the evaluation, although specific questions may remain at the end. Depending on the nature and age of the relationship, the clinician should determine how the relationship began, how the partners feel about each other (both positive and negative feelings are important), how the relationship may be different from previous relationships, whether there are any problems with intimacy, whether communication and control issues exist, and whether there are plans for cohabitation, children, marriage, etc.

Individual Sessions

Each member of the couple should be seen alone for at least part of a session, with an invitation for further individual sessions as needed and the agreement that any information presented as confidential will be maintained as such. The clinician may introduce these sessions with the assurance that any well-functioning couple has "secrets" that they may not feel comfortable sharing with their partner, but that such information may be useful to the therapist. Both partners are asked whether there is anything about the relationship or about their own development that they are not comfortable disclosing in the partner's presence, but that may be important for the clinician to know. The clinician may also ask about the nature of the person's fantasies and how comfortable he or she is with fantasy. At this session it is also important to ask about any other ongoing sexual relationships. The clinician may point out that such relationships, although the patient's business, may impede the therapeutic process, and that for the duration of therapy it is best that they be discontinued. It is in response to

this question that a patient experiencing erectile problems or problems with lack of desire may admit good performance with another partner, signifying problems in the primary relationship that need to be addressed in therapy. At times, the sudden abandonment of a sexual affair will lead to an almost instantaneous "cure" by encouraging a focus on the primary partner.

Considerations in Overall Assessment

In evaluating the presenting problem, it often becomes clear that the presenting symptom is secondary to a more primary sexual problem, and the therapy must take both into account. For example, lack of desire in a male may be secondary to an erectile problem. Vaginismus is frequently secondary to an underlying hypoactive desire or sexual aversion. A good understanding of the conditions under which symptoms present themselves as well as the history of the presenting problem will clarify the real nature of the problem and enable the clinician to develop an appropriate treatment plan. The case of Kathy and Don, presented later, illustrates this point.

When it appears that there may be a medical etiology to a sexual dysfunction, the patient should be referred to a physician who is knowledgeable about current diagnostic and treatment techniques, respectful of the psychosocial aspects of sexual dysfunction, and comfortable dealing with sexual issues. It is of utmost importance that the various professionals involved in a case communicate clearly about the patient's status (Maurice, 1999).

TREATMENT TECHNIQUES

As indicated earlier, modern sex therapy often involves the combined use of a number of therapeutic techniques, customized to the needs of particular patients. These may include behavioral, cognitive, individual, couples, or medical approaches, as appropriate. Since it is the behavioral and cognitive techniques that are most characteristic of sex therapy, this discussion will focus on these techniques in some detail. Even though the importance of these techniques has sometimes been downplayed in recent years, they still often represent the most effective and most conservative approach to the treatment of sexual dysfunctions. In addition, because of their apparent simplicity, the classic behavioral techniques may be used in a somewhat rigid textbook style by therapists who are not well skilled in their proper use, although this often results in unsatisfactory outcomes that either remain uncorrected or result in searches for more effective therapy. The subtleties emphasized earlier as important to the determination of sexual status are equally important in the prescription and follow-up of behavioral assignments.

The cornerstone of behavioral sex therapy is the

sensate focus technique developed by Masters and Johnson. It is often applied, with appropriate variations, in the treatment of all sexual dysfunctions because of its ability to help the couple broaden their approach to sexuality while reducing the frequently threatening focus on mutuality, performance, genital stimulation, and orgasm. This technique will be described in some detail. Treatment methods that are more germane to specific sexual dysfunctions will then be discussed.

Sensate Focus

The typical first stage of sensate focus involves two 1-hour sessions per week in which the partners stimulate each other in turn, one being the active and the other the passive partner. Depending on the nature of the presenting problem, one or both partners may be instructed to take the initiative in planning the sessions. At this stage, genitals and breasts are off limits to both partners. This is generally the case not only during the exercises but at all other times prior to the next therapy session. Individuals are asked to touch their partner, not specifically to give pleasure to their partner but *for their own interest.* They are also asked to be prepared to provide the therapist with a complete account of their experience at the following session (sexual status examination).

At the next session, the therapist will assess the experiences and perceptions of the two partners, with particular emphasis on what each learned about himself or herself and about their partner, and how they communicated about the exercises. Couples will sometimes complain about the contrived nature of the exercises and the lack of spontaneity. The therapist may help the couple realize that such concerns often reflect a reluctance to take verbal initiative for a sexual encounter by expressing personal desires out of either a sense of discomfort with the language of sexuality or a fear of rejection.

Resistance to exercises may also take the form of noncompliance, either by avoiding them altogether or "cheating" by engaging in genital play or even intercourse. In the former case, it is usually best for the therapist not to confront the patient immediately but to bypass the resistance by accepting the patients' explanations for their avoidance (which may often be quite valid, such as a family crisis, unexpected guests, etc) and simply repeating the assignment for the following week. If the avoidance persists, the therapist can point out patterns in the couple's behavior and either confront or interpret the resistance, as appropriate.

At its best, cheating on assignments by having sexual intercourse may simply be the result of the paradoxical nature of the restrictive assignment and result in an almost instant cure. More often, it represents problems of control and communication within the relationship, and these can then be dealt with as such. These instances of noncompliance will often help

both therapist and couple focus on relationship problems that either underlie or accompany the sexual symptoms.

Even at the first stage of sensate focus, the therapist needs to be flexible in defining the assignment so that it meets the specific needs of the couple. This need may be easily overlooked, since nongenital contact would seem to represent the most elemental form of physical intimacy. However, if one or both members of the couple are uncomfortable with nudity or with the environment that typically represents a sexual encounter (eg, bed and bedroom), it may be necessary to begin the exercises at a less threatening level. For example, taking a shower together is more easily perceived as a functional activity but can also help promote a basic level of physical intimacy. If nudity is a problem, it can be suggested that the couple wear agreed-on articles of clothing during initial exercises, or that lights be dimmed. In setting such boundaries it is important that restrictions apply equally to both members of the couple, regardless of who exhibits the anxiety to a given form of contact.

In some cases, it may be necessary to recommend anatomic restrictions in addition to breasts and genitals, as illustrated in the following case:

Kathy and Don, her husband of 10 years, presented with vaginismus and indicated that they had been to three previous therapists without success. The evaluation disclosed an underlying sexual aversion, which was exacerbated by Don's tendency to focus on intercourse when initiating a sexual encounter. Kathy would either reject his advances or would reluctantly allow him to have an orgasm intrathecally in order to provide him with minimal satisfaction. She could masturbate easily but was frightened by the prospect of sex with her husband, as any approach represented the prospect of intercourse and pain. Although the vaginismus itself was partially related to complications of minor surgery for a labial abnormality, the history revealed suggestions of early sexual trauma, although memories of this were unclear. Initial exercises were done with light clothing, as Kathy was uncomfortable with frontal breast exposure. She would also become very tense whenever Don touched her stomach or inner thighs. As a result, the therapist recommended that those areas as well as the area between the breasts be off limits to touch. With the consequent reduction in anxiety, Kathy was able to enjoy the stimulation of other areas of her body, and with less preoccupation with her anticipated experience as the passive partner, was also able to stimulate her husband. In addition, the couple learned to communicate more effectively about their desires and feelings. Kathy was invited to participate in setting restrictions in subsequent assignments, and both clothing and anatomic restrictions were very gradually and successfully reduced.

The second stage of sensate focus typically involves the lifting of restrictions on breast and genital contact. The couple is encouraged to continue the whole-body stimulation, as before, touching breasts and genitals *in that context,* rather than *instead of* other areas of the body. It is also suggested that the body not be touched so that touch appears to *lead to* genital contact. In fact, this phase of the exercises encourages the couple to reconsider the typical characterization of intimate touch as foreplay and to see it as a pleasurable and fulfilling act in itself. It is suggested that genitals be touched, not in a manner that might *deliberately* induce an orgasm, but with the same sense of detailed interest with which other areas of the body were touched during the previous phase of the exercises. In some cases, anatomic models, photos, art, or even videos may be used to prepare the couple for these exercises. The couple is encouraged to notice what *specific* areas of the body, including breasts and genitals, may be arousing or unpleasant so that each will be more aware of these sensations.

The third stage of sensate focus varies widely, as the assignments depend more than before on the symptoms being treated. If an erectile dysfunction is being treated, for example, the couple may be asked to manually stimulate each other to orgasm. Assuming the male partner is having firm erections by this time, he may then be asked to stimulate himself to orgasm against the outer genitalia of his partner. Eventually, intercourse without thrusting (sometimes called "quiet vagina") will be recommended, followed by active intercourse.

Treatment of patients presenting with vaginismus or premature ejaculation may involve individual exercises (eg, use of dilators or masturbation with stop-start exercises) as well as sensate focus exercises, often assigned simultaneously, with the third stage of the sensate focus exercises typically involving the partner in the individual exercises. These procedures will be described more fully below.

In some cases, it may be impossible to cure a specific sexual dysfunction because the problem has a medical etiology and is not treatable. For example, a male patient may refuse all forms of medical intervention (see below), or certain behaviors may be compromised as a result of paralysis, surgery, or a chronic disability. In such cases, sensate focus exercises can help the couple discover forms of pleasure and arousal that are either new to them or that they had not previously attempted.

Just as some couples may express concerns about the lack of spontaneity in doing sensate focus exercises, other couples may complain about the lack of spontaneity engendered by the need to put on a condom, insert a diaphragm, or do the procedures necessary to prepare a handicapped person for a sexual encounter (eg, transfer from a wheelchair, emptying colostomy bags, dealing with urinary incontinence). In such cases, the therapist can help the couple make these activities a part of sex play, helping them to realize also that arousal that subsides because of interruptions (eg, loss of erection) will return if the idea of sex as a natural function is preserved.

In summary, the use of behavioral exercises should be creative and flexible, and combined appropriately with other therapeutic modalities, so that the specific needs of the patient are met. The need for patience, support, and attention to detail on the part of the therapist cannot be overemphasized in developing and maintaining an effective treatment plan.

Treatment of Specific Dysfunctions

The rest of this discussion will highlight issues that are often important in the evaluation and treatment of specific sexual dysfunctions. For more information regarding each dysfunction see, eg, Kaplan (1974, 1979, 1987), Masters and Johnson (1970), and Leiblum and Rosen (1989).

A. Desire Disorders:

1. Hypoactive sexual desire—Desire-phase disorders have gained increasing prominence in recent years for a number of reasons. The AIDS crisis has encouraged a greater level of monogamy among both homosexual and heterosexual couples. This tendency may encourage couples to deal directly with issues of intimacy and sexuality, rather than to run from them. Unresolved issues of control and communication may lead to a sexual withdrawal. The increase in the number of dual-career couples raises issues of priority between relationship and career; couples often complain that there just isn't *time* for sex. As couples become bound up in career, children, and other activities, they may gradually lose the seductiveness and romance that initially kindled the relationship. The increasing status of women in many industrialized societies as well as their increased comfort with sexual expression have often led them to be more assertive in sexual relationships. Thus, a woman may be more likely to withdraw from sex when a relationship is dysfunctional or when the partner is insensitive to her sexual needs. Women who have been sexually abused may be more likely to express their anxiety regarding sexual activity than they were before. Men may be more threatened by a woman's assertiveness and feel an increased pressure to perform. As people grow older, they may feel that they have lost their attractiveness, or their youthful image of a sexual person may lead them to consider their partners unattractive. Because of the intrapsychic and relationship issues so often at the heart of hypoactive desire, this dysfunction is generally less responsive to a purely behavioral approach than are most of the others, and treatment more often utilizes individual and/or couples therapy in addition to behavioral sex therapy. As shown in Table 25–2, the primary *DSM-IV* diagnostic criterion for this disorder is the persistent absence or deficiency of sexual fantasies and desire.

The therapist must first determine whether there is a true hypoactive desire, or whether the couple is exhibiting only a sexual incompatibility. For example, if one member of the couple is a morning person and the other is a night person in terms of their circadian

Table 25–2. *DSM-IV* diagnostic criteria for hypoactive sexual desire disorder.

A. Persistently or recurrently deficient (or absent) sexual fantasies and desire for sexual activity. The judgment of deficiency or absence is made by the clinician, taking into account factors that affect sexual functioning, such as age and the context of the person's life.

B. The disturbance causes marked distress or interpersonal difficulty.

C. The sexual dysfunction is not better accounted for by another Axis I disorder (except another Sexual Dysfunction) and is not due exclusively to the direct physiological effects of a substance (eg, a drug of abuse, a medication) or a general medical condition.

rhythms and readiness for sex, they may need sex therapy less than they need to be encouraged to communicate and compromise with regard to sexual— and perhaps other—aspects of their relationship.

During the evaluation special attention should also be given to the extent to which there is sexual desire that is not acted on or that is acted on through masturbation or with other partners. The therapist should also determine the kinds of stimuli that have aroused the patient in the past and how effective the stimuli are at present. It is particularly important to attend to sexual fantasy in patients with hypoactive desire. Patients may say they are unable to fantasize, may experience distracting thoughts during sex, or may exhibit what have been called **antifantasies,** that is, fantasies that are incompatible with sexual arousal.

> Tom and his wife, Karen, came for treatment complaining of hypoactive desire on Tom's part. When the therapist prescribed sensate focus exercises, he also recommended a body lotion, which was creamy white in color. In the following session, Tom described dripping the lotion on Karen's stomach from a height of about two feet, saying that it reminded him of bird droppings. Karen remarked, "You could at least have said that it reminded you of semen!"

As mentioned earlier, a hypoactive desire often reflects intrapsychic or relationship problems that require individual or couples therapy. However, behavioral sex therapy can be useful in helping the couple to focus on the sexual aspects of their relationship. One of the first roles of the therapist is to encourage the couple to define sex as a priority in their life and to make the time for it, dispelling the "myth of spontaneity." It may first be necessary to encourage the couple to spend time together for *any* reason, without television, friends, and other third parties. In addition, busy people sometimes forget how to play! The question of who initiates sex is often raised by the couple. The therapist may need to point out that, as in other roles filled by each member of the couple, it is rarely a 50–50 proposition. It is normal for one partner to initiate sex more frequently. Problems develop when one partner never initiates, always re-

jects, or simply goes along with a request for sex to placate the initiator.

With regard to rejection, the couple may need to be reminded that people sometimes do not initiate sex because of a fear of rejection and that a partner can say "no" in a supportive way. At times, a partner may complain about the way in which he or she is approached. A 17-year-old newlywed said, "I wish he would at least touch my *arm* first!" Men who are genitally oriented may initiate sex less frequently with age, as erectile capacity diminishes, and this is one of the areas in which reframing and sensate focus can be of immense benefit by helping the male partner become aware of a greater potential for sexual arousal and enjoyment. When concerns of relative interest are an issue sensate focus can aid in showing that sex does not always have to be mutual, and no component of sexual activity is an absolute *must* for sex to be an enjoyable experience. Partners can set limits in terms of time or activity, or a single sexual encounter can be totally one sided, as long as there is a balance over the long term.

Treatment of hypoactive desire can also include direct work with fantasy material. To the extent that partners can discuss fantasy with each other, they can act out these fantasies with each other. One partner may be aroused by certain clothing or perfume or by certain seductive behaviors, and this can become part of the ambiance and play of sex. Exercises in guided imagery can sometimes help couples make fantasies more vivid and can help them become more immersed in their sexual experience. Do their fantasies involve various sensory modalities? Do they watch a fantasy scene, as if on television, or are they a participant in the fantasized experience? And so on.

2. Sexual aversion—Working with fantasy is also important in patients with a sexual aversion, which involves not only a lack of interest in sex but an active avoidance of even the *possibility* of a sexual encounter. The *DSM-IV* diagnostic criteria for sexual aversion disorder are listed in Table 25–3. A patient whose image of sex is a negative one can be helped to develop positive fantasy associations by helping him or her to identify and utilize any fantasies that are found to be arousing, as therapy proceeds. Whatever therapeutic procedures are used, the therapist must take care to proceed in small, discreet steps that are

Table 25–3. *DSM-IV* diagnostic criteria for sexual aversion disorder.

A. Persistent or recurrent extreme aversion to, and avoidance of, all (or almost all) genital sexual contact with a sexual partner.

B. The disturbance causes marked distress or interpersonal difficulty.

C. The sexual dysfunction is not better accounted for by another Axis I disorder (except another Sexual Dysfunction).

manageable for the patient, as was described in the case of the couple in the section on sensate focus exercises.

Some patients who are aversive to sex experience panic reactions at the prospect of a sexual encounter. The therapist should determine whether the patient experiences panic attacks under other circumstances and, if so, how those have been dealt with. Some therapists have found brief courses of anxiolytic medication useful in sex therapy with such patients. If such medications are used, it is important to be watchful of relevant side effects, such as insomnia, inhibition of orgasm, or priapism.

B. Sexual Arousal Disorders: The *DSM-IV* diagnostic criteria for sexual arousal disorders are outlined in Table 25–4.

1. Female sexual arousal disorder—Female sexual arousal disorder is diagnosed rarely, if at all. Since insufficient vaginal lubrication is a criterion for diagnosis, dyspareunia or painful intercourse is likely to be a consequence and thus a more likely diagnosis. Dyspareunia will be discussed later in this chapter.

2. Male erectile disorder—The basic behavioral techniques for treating male erectile disorder were described earlier in the discussion of sensate focus exercises. Evaluation by the mental health professional needs to account for the possibility of a medical basis, and any doubt that the symptoms are not purely psychogenic should lead to referral to a urologist who is knowledgeable of and skilled in the appropriate methods of medical evaluation. Any patient whose erectile dysfunction was gradual in onset, whose erection is partial or nonexistent under all conditions, or who discloses a history of illness or medication known to cause erectile failure should certainly be referred to an appropriate physician.

Table 25–4. *DSM-IV* diagnostic for sexual arousal disorder.

Female sexual arousal disorder

A. Persistent or recurrent inability to attain, or to maintain until completion of the sexual activity, an adequate lubrication-swelling response of sexual excitement.

B. The disturbance causes marked distress or interpersonal difficulty.

C. The sexual dysfunction is not better accounted for by another Axis I disorder (except another Sexual Dysfunction) and is not due exclusively to the direct physiological effects of a substance (eg, a drug of abuse, a medication) or a general medical condition.

Male erectile disorder

A. Persistent or recurrent inability to attain, or to maintain until completion of the sexual activity, an adequate erection.

B. The disturbance causes marked distress or interpersonal difficulty.

C. The erectile dysfunction is not better accounted for by another Axis I disorder (other than a Sexual Dysfunction) and is not due exclusively to the direct physiological effects of a substance (eg, a drug of abuse, a medication) or a general medical condition.

A complete description of an appropriate medical workup is beyond the scope of this discussion. Frequently used techniques for the evaluation of erectile dysfunction in addition to a genital and prostate examination may include determination of nocturnal penile tumescence (NPT) and buckling pressure in a sleep laboratory or with the aid of a home monitor, measurement of penile blood flow using Doppler techniques and imaging, glucose tolerance tests, determination of the levels of testosterone, follicle-stimulating hormone (FSH), luteinizing hormone (LH), prolactin, and thyroid hormone, and perhaps electromyography, a corpora cavernosagram, and an arteriogram. Using the right combination of tests, the physician can determine the extent to which the disorder may have a neurological, hormonal, or circulatory basis.

It is always possible that there is a psychogenic component to a medically based erectile dysfunction or vice versa, and it may be important for the urologist and sex therapist to maintain close contact so that the patient is treated appropriately. Even a totally medical intervention, such as a penile implant, may require counseling that involves the partner as well as the symptomatic patient.

Medical interventions are becoming increasingly sophisticated as well. There are different types of penile implants, ranging from inflexible to inflatable, and varying in cost and risk of malfunction. Self-injection of papaverine or prostaglandin E has recently been introduced as a therapeutic technique appropriate for some men, as has the use of a vacuum pump. The latter has a chamber placed over the flaccid penis from which the user pumps air. The penis becomes erect in the rarefied environment of the chamber, and the erection is maintained by a constricting band once the chamber is removed.

The most recent and exciting advance in this field has been the appearance of erection-enhancing medications, such as sildenafil (Viagra), which operate on specific penile enzymes in the presence of sexual stimulation. Choice of these methods depends on a number of factors, including etiology of the dysfunction, cost, and the tendency of the patient to comply with one method or another.

C. Orgasm Disorders:

1. Female and male orgasmic disorders—The number of women presenting with anorgasmia, or preorgasmia as it is sometimes called, seems to have decreased somewhat over the past few years, probably because of the generally reduced sexual inhibition among women and the availability of self-help books and articles (eg, Barbach, 1984; Heiman and LoPiccolo, 1988). Although inhibited male orgasm, or retarded ejaculation, is less frequent in men than erectile dysfunction, it may be more difficult to treat, as it often involves deeper intrapsychic issues that may sometimes require individual insight-oriented therapy as well as behavioral sex therapy. Comments on the evaluation and behavioral treatment of men and women will be combined unless noted. Diagnostic criteria for inhibited female and male orgasm are shown in Tables 25–5 and 25–6, respectively.

Evaluation should investigate the meaning of orgasm for the patient. Is it a symbolic expression of a seemingly irreversible commitment, perhaps related to the never-ending search for the perfect partner? Does it represent a loss of control, which is threatening to the patient in some way? In some cases, orgasmic difficulty may reflect a discomfort with genitalia, poor body image, difficulty with fantasy, or a reluctance to communicate sexual needs to one's partner.

If the anorgasmia or retarded ejaculation is global, the therapist may begin with masturbation exercises, encouraging the use of fantasy. In women, this often includes self-examination in order to increase the patient's level of comfort with her body and to help her become better aware of arousing stimuli. Kegel exercises—the tightening and release of the pubococcygeal muscles at the entrance to the vagina—are often a useful adjunct. The probability of orgasm in both men and woman can sometimes be enhanced by encouraging the patient to fake orgasm, mimicking some of the somatic responses that usually accompany the orgasmic response, such as arching of the back, curling of the toes, increased rate of breathing, and vocalization. This helps reduce the embarrassment often involved in abandoning oneself to the natural orgasmic process.

Work with the couple should emphasize communication and cooperation regarding the arousal process and specific arousing—or nonarousing—stimuli. In the case of men who can ejaculate in masturbation but not intravaginally, a gradual approach is recommended, perhaps beginning by masturbation in the partner's presence but with her facing away from the male, then moving ever closer to intravaginal ejaculation in appropriately discrete steps. Another technique sometimes found useful is to ask the male to masturbate and then to place some of his semen into

Table 25–5. *DSM-IV* diagnostic criteria for female orgasmic disorder (formerly inhibited female orgasm).

A. Persistent or recurrent delay in, or absence of, orgasm following a normal sexual excitement phase. Women exhibit wide variability in the type or sexual intensity of stimulation that triggers orgasm. The diagnosis of Female Orgasmic Disorder should be based on the clinician's judgment that the woman's orgasmic capacity is less than would be reasonable for age, sexual experience, and the adequacy of sexual stimulation she receives.

B. The disturbance causes marked distress or interpersonal difficulty.

C. The orgasmic dysfunction is not better accounted for by another Axis I disorder (except another Sexual Dysfunction) and is not due exclusively to the direct physiological effects of a substance (eg, a drug of abuse, a medication) or a general medical condition.

Table 25–6. *DSM-IV* diagnostic criteria for male orgasmic disorder (formerly inhibited male orgasm).

A. Persistent or recurrent delay in, or absence of, orgasm following a normal sexual excitement phase during sexual activity that the clinician, taking into account the person's age, judges to be adequate in focus.

B. The disturbance causes marked distress or interpersonal difficulty.

C. The orgasmic dysfunction is not better accounted for by another Axis I disorder (except another Sexual Dysfunction) and is not due exclusively to the direct physiological effects of a substance (eg, a drug of abuse, a medication) or a general medical condition.

his partner's vagina. This process may help the patient to overcome a symbolic barrier to fertilization.

2. Premature ejaculation—When a patient presents with a complaint of premature (or as some therapists call it, rapid) ejaculation, the therapist should first ascertain the couple's definition of "premature." Couples in which the woman is orgasmic during intercourse will sometimes define "premature" in terms of the latency to the **woman's** orgasm, which may be unrealistic. Definitions in the literature vary somewhat, but the main issue is typically whether the male has sufficient control over his time of ejaculation (Table 25–7).

A number of possible reasons for premature ejaculation have been proposed. These include early conditioning resulting from rapid masturbation or intercourse during adolescence, a lack of awareness of bodily sensations, or a general "somatic vulnerability," which may be reflected in other behaviors in which the patient engages (eg, sweaty palms when shaking hands). In some cases, a fear of intimacy or fear of separation may be involved in premature ejaculation as it often is in other sexual disorders.

Classic behavioral treatment involves either the squeeze technique, introduced by Masters and Johnson, or the stop-start technique, originally developed by Seman, a urologist. In the squeeze technique, the woman stimulates her partner's penis until just before he reaches the point of ejaculatory inevitability, at which time she squeezes the penis in a certain way, preventing the ejaculation response. This process is

Table 25–7. *DSM-IV* diagnostic criteria for premature ejaculation.

A. Persistent or recurrent ejaculation with minimal sexual stimulation before, on, or shortly after penetration and before the person wishes it. The clinician must take into account factors that affect duration of the excitement phase, such as age, novelty of the sexual partner or situation, and recent frequency of sexual activity.

B. The disturbance causes marked distress or interpersonal difficulty.

C. The premature ejaculation is not due exclusively to direct effects of a substance (eg, withdrawal from opioids).

repeated a number of times before ejaculation is permitted to occur. In the stop-start method, stimulation is simply stopped at the same point, allowing sexual tension to abate while the erection is maintained. Some therapists not only consider this latter method more natural, but believe that it lends itself more readily to masturbatory exercises, which typically precede exercises involving the couple.

During masturbation exercises, the patient is asked to use an environment similar to that used with a partner—typically a bed in a bedroom. He lies on his back to minimize physical distraction and may be asked to masturbate with his nonpreferred hand in order to enhance awareness. He is instructed to utilize normal, arousing fantasies rather than distracting thoughts, as patients often do in an effort to delay ejaculation. He first masturbates to orgasm to become better acquainted with the responses that accompany the approach to orgasm. He then introduces the stop-start method, stopping briefly three times before ejaculating after the fourth stimulation period. In later exercises, a lubricant may be introduced to approximate the more arousing feeling of a lubricated vagina. After he achieves a reasonable level of masturbatory control, the partner is introduced, perhaps initially with nongenital sensate focus exercises, after which *she* provides the penile stimulation. This leads gradually to intravaginal exercises and intercourse as in the treatment of erectile dysfunction, described earlier.

D. Sexual Pain Disorders:

1. Dyspareunia—*DSM-IV* defines functional dyspareunia as coitus associated with recurrent and persistent genital pain in either sex (Table 25–8). Most reports of dyspareunia are from women, but it is also reported by men on occasion. Although the problem is frequently associated with a medical condition such as vaginitis, endometriosis, or complications of a surgical procedure, there are often cases in which no medical basis can be found. In these instances, psychotherapy or sex therapy becomes the treatment of choice. Working closely with a gynecologist who is knowledgeable about sexual dysfunction and dyspareunia can be invaluable in making an appropriate diagnosis and providing appropriate treatment.

In evaluating a report of dyspareunia, it is important to assess the relationship, the patient's comfort

with his or her sexuality, and the patient's comfort with fantasy. Problems in any of these could inhibit the patient's desire or ability to become aroused, resulting in poor lubrication and an absence of the other components of the arousal response that facilitate sexual intercourse. For this reason, the approach to therapy should be flexible and often requires a combination of techniques to address the various levels of etiological factors.

2. Vaginismus—Vaginismus, the involuntary constriction of the muscles at the entrance to the vagina, is usually considered to be the most curable of all sexual dysfunctions (Table 25–9). In its simplest form, it is treated with the aid of dilators, usually made of rubber, plastic, or ceramic material of gradually increasing diameter. These are inserted into the vagina, using an appropriate lubricant, either by the patient herself or by her partner. Done in conjunction with Kegel exercises, this usually permits penile entry after a rather short course of treatment.

In practice, however, vaginismus is often combined with or is symbolic of a hypoactive desire, and thus treatment may involve individual or couples therapy as well as behavioral and cognitive treatment, including sensate focus exercises. If it is related to a vaginal infection or complications of vaginal or labial surgery, close collaboration with the patient's gynecologist may be important to successful treatment.

Evaluation should determine the conditions under which vaginismus occurs (eg, only with a partner or with other attempts at insertion, such as a speculum). The patient should be asked whether she uses tampons and, if appropriate, whether masturbation involves insertion of dildos or vibrators. Medical history should include inquiries regarding vaginal infection or surgery. Other issues often involved in the etiology of vaginismus are situational anxiety (eg, fear of children entering the room), past sexual trauma, family of origin issues (eg, parental attitudes toward sex), problems in the current relationship, or, more specifically, how the partner approaches the woman sexually.

E. Sexual Dysfunctions Related to Medical Conditions:

As shown in Table 25–10, a sexual dysfunction can be diagnosed as being related to a medical condition if warranted by a history, physi-

---

Table 25–8. *DSM-IV* diagnostic criteria for dyspareunia.

A. Recurrent or persistent genital pain associated with sexual intercourse in either a male or a female.

B. The disturbance causes marked distress or interpersonal difficulty.

C. The disturbance is not caused exclusively by Vaginismus or lack of lubrication, is not better accounted for by another Axis I disorder (except another Sexual Dysfunction) and is not due exclusively to the direct physiological effects of a substance (eg, a drug of abuse, a medication) or a general medical condition.

Table 25–9. *DSM-IV* diagnostic criteria for vaginismus.

A. Recurrent or persistent involuntary spasm of the musculature of the outer third of the vagina that interferes with sexual intercourse.

B. The disturbance causes marked distress or interpersonal difficulty.

C. The disturbance is not better accounted for by another Axis I disorder (eg, Somatization Disorder) and is not due exclusively to the direct physiological effects of a general medical condition.

Table 25–10. *DSM-IV* diagnostic criteria for sexual dysfunction caused by a general medical condition.

A. Clinically significant sexual dysfunctions that result in marked distress or interpersonal difficulty predominates in the clinical picture.

B. There is evidence from the history, physical examination, or laboratory findings that the sexual dysfunction is fully explained by the direct physiological effects of a general medical condition.

C. The disturbance is not better accounted for by another mental disorder (eg, Major Depressive Disorder).

cal examination, or laboratory findings. For example, a chronic condition such as diabetes or a spinal cord injury may affect one or more stages of the sexual response cycle (ie, desire, arousal, orgasm) or may cause painful intercourse or orgasm. Subcategories of this diagnosis allow the clinician to distinguish among the various sexual dysfunctions that may be affected by such a condition.

F. Substance-Induced Sexual Dysfunction: A sexual dysfunction may also be related to the use of or withdrawal from a prescribed medication or other substance. The criteria for using this diagnosis are given in Table 25–11. Additional subcategories permit the clinician to indicate the nature of the substance involved (eg, amphetamines, alcohol, cocaine).

GENDER IDENTITY DISORDERS

Gender identity disorders are a relatively new category of psychiatric disturbance that continues to be subject to confusion and controversy. Cross-gender behavior has been described since antiquity and en-

Table 25–11. *DSM-IV* diagnostic criteria for substance-induced sexual dysfunction.

A. Clinically significant sexual dysfunction that results in marked distress or interpersonal difficulty.

B. There is evidence from the history, physical examination, or laboratory findings of substance intoxication, and the symptoms in Criterion A developed during, or within a month of, significant substance intoxication.

C. The disturbance is not better accounted for by a sexual dysfunction that is not substance-induced. Evidence that the symptoms are better accounted for by a sexual dysfunction that is not substance-induced might include: the symptoms precede the onset of the substance abuse or dependence; persist for a substantial period of time (eg, about a month) after the cessation of acute withdrawal or severe intoxication; are substantially in excess of what would be expected given the character, duration, or amount of substance used; or there is other evidence suggesting the existence of an independent non–substance-induced sexual dysfunction (eg, a history of recurrent non–substance-related episodes).

tered the medical literature as a distinct condition in the nineteenth century. However, gender disorders were not added to the *DSM* until the third edition in 1980, first as psychosexual disorders and then, in *DSM-III-R*, as disorders first evident in infancy, childhood, or adolescence. In *DSM-IV*, sexual and gender identity disorders have all been grouped together in the same section. The gender identity disorders are essentially disturbances in an individual's sense of masculinity or femininity, which interact with social conceptualizations of gender and sexual orientation.

DEFINITIONS

Sex is defined on the basis of the physical appearance of the genitals (gonadal sex or sex phenotype) or in some cases on the basis of the chromosomes (genotype). Socially, sex is partitioned into two complementary categories: male or female. Newborns with intersex conditions, such as hermaphroditism, are assigned to one sex for rearing.

Gender refers to the individual's status as male or female (or in some rare cases intersex) including personal experience and social and legal identification. Gender is phenomenologically broader than genital anatomy. **Gender identity** is the private experience of gender role as male or female in self-awareness and behavior. **Gender role** refers to the public manifestation of gender identity, everything a person says or does (including sexual behavior) that indicates a status as either male or female. The definitional content of gender statuses varies among groups. Gender includes components of erotic or sexual orientation. For most individuals, gender identity and role are integrated (as gender identity/role) with a unity and persistence.

Gender identity disorders can occur when a person does not experience a unity and persistence of the personal experience of gender identity and the social expression of gender role. **Gender dysphoria** is the pathological state of dissatisfaction and subjective incongruity between the sex phenotype (genital anatomy and secondary sexual characteristics) and the gender identity and role. Gender dysphoria is expressed as a body image disorder, for which the treatment has been a combination of psychotherapy and the alteration of the body through medical and surgical procedures.

Transsexualism as a diagnostic label was dropped from *DSM-IV* but is still used as a descriptive term in the professional and popular literature. Properly considered, transsexualism refers to a process of sex reassignment. Labeling a person as a transsexual might also reflect the status of having completed sex reassignment, as a resolution of an underlying gender dysphoria or gender identity disorder. However, many individuals with gender identity disorders never seek or complete sex reassignment. So the synonymous use of the term transsexualism for gender identity disorder can be misleading.

Gender identity disorders in children and in adolescents and adults are described together in *DSM-IV,* although the diagnostic criteria and nature of the syndrome vary greatly, and they are assigned different code numbers. For clarity of discussion, these two categories of gender identity disorders are separated in the following sections.

GENDER IDENTITY DISORDERS IN CHILDREN

Symptoms & Signs

Identification with the other gender combined with a discomfort with the child's own sex are the defining characteristics of gender identity disorders. Specific *DSM-IV* criteria are given in Table 25–12.

Boys, much more often than girls, come to the attention of physicians for exhibiting preferences for cross-sex-role activities. Cross-gender behavior in boys includes wearing female attire (or draping scarves and towels as facsimiles) and mimicking stereotypic female gestures and body language. They

Table 25–12. *DSM-IV* diagnostic criteria for gender identity disorders in children.

A. A strong and persistent cross-gender identification (not merely a desire for any perceived cultural advantages of being the other sex), manifested by at least four of the following:

   (1) repeatedly stated desire to be, or insistence that he or she is, the other sex

   (2) in boys, preference for cross-dressing or simulating female attire; in girls, insistence on wearing only stereotypic masculine clothing

   (3) strong and persistent preferences for cross-sex roles in make-believe play or persistent fantasies of being the other sex

   (4) intense desire to participate in the stereotypical games and pastimes of the other sex

   (5) strong preference for playmates of the other sex

B. Persistent discomfort with his or her sex or sense of inappropriateness in the gender role of that sex.

   In boys, assertion that his penis or testes are disgusting or will disappear or assertion that it would be better not to have a penis, **or** aversion toward rough-and-tumble play and rejection of male stereotypical toys, games, and activities.

   In girls, rejection of urinating in a sitting position, assertion that she has or will grow a penis, or assertion that she does not want to grow breasts or menstruate, **or** marked aversion toward normative feminine clothing.

C. The disturbance is not concurrent with a physical intersex condition.

D. The disturbance causes clinically significant distress or impairment in social, occupational, or other important areas of functioning.

may express interest in women's clothing, make-up, jewelry, and hairstyling. Play with dolls (particularly Barbie dolls) and domestic play acting are common. There may be artistic and dramatic interests, including a preference for female roles in play acting. Favorite stories have female heroines. They may choose girls for their friends and prefer to associate with adult women rather than men. They avoid rough and tumble play and team sports with other boys. There may be a general lack of interest in stereotypic boys' toys and play activities. Boys with these characteristics are often labeled as "sissy boys," a derogatory term that is also used in the professional literature as in "the sissy boy syndrome." Discomfort may be associated with rejection and teasing by family or peers. Gender identity disorders are characterized by an extreme rejection of masculinity and embracing of femininity, not just some appearance of effeminacy.

Girls may be identified as tomboys but are rarely brought for professional evaluation of gender identity disorder. Active interest and participation in athletics and sports, which includes playing mostly with male peers, and refusal to wear dresses are the most common signs. However, these signs are frequently present in girls who do not experience any distress and thus would not meet diagnostic criteria for a gender identity disorder.

For both boys and girls, the stated desire to be the other sex is infrequent or episodic and mostly found in younger children. Rejection of their own genital characteristics is rarely evident to adults, although some cases of genital self-mutilation in boys are documented.

Natural History

Overt behaviors may be evident as early as age 2–3, and many characteristics subside by age 8 with or without any treatment. Extreme gender-nonconformist behavior can lead to social ostracization from the peer group and to teasing. Distress associated with social impairment is the most common complaint. This can lead to sequelae of poor self-concept and depression. There may also be problems in interactions within the family.

Gender identity disorders of childhood are infrequently diagnosed or referred for treatment. The actual incidence is unknown and may vary according to social standards of sex role stereotyping. There is no association with any single pattern of child rearing or family dynamics. Family dynamics may influence the severity of the presenting problems, particularly in cases in which there are conflicts between parents, pathological encouragement of gender-atypical behavior, or extreme rejection of it.

Most boys diagnosed with gender identity disorder of childhood are socially extreme examples of "sissy boys." Most clinicians used to believe that these boys would continue to show gender problems as they grew up and that many of them would later seek sex reassignment. However, longitudinal follow-up research shows that at least three-quarters of them grew up to be homosexual or bisexual males without gender identity problems (Green, 1987). Many are not noticeably effeminate as adults. Few develop into adults who seek sex reassignment.

There is greater social acceptance of masculine behavior in girls than of feminine behavior in boys. This is probably a reflection of social sex-role bias: femininity devalues males but masculinity enhances females. Social rejection and teasing and family problems are less severe for tomboyish girls, and their self-concepts are often positive. Some tomboyish girls grow up to be lesbians, but most are probably heterosexual or bisexual. Few seek sex reassignment in adulthood.

Gender nonconformity in both boys and girls is the most evident childhood indicator of adult homosexuality. Gender identity disorders of childhood are rarely indicative of any psychiatric disorder of adulthood. Few children diagnosed with gender identity disorders later meet the criteria for gender identity disorders of adulthood and sex reassignment. There is controversy over whether gender identity disorders of childhood should be considered a psychiatric disorder, since they simply may be the juvenile manifestation of homosexuality, which is not pathological.

Treatment

Cross-gendered interests and behaviors can be troublesome for children and upsetting for parents. Parents worry about what the likely outcomes will be. Boys severely stigmatized by peers may develop poor self-concepts and later act in self-destructive ways that may have serious health consequences (including increased risk of suicide or AIDS). Therefore, psychological intervention is helpful for the children and their families. Treatment is not likely to change the outcome in terms of sexual orientation but may help the adjustment of the individuals in the family system.

Treatment usually involves an evaluation of the child and the family system. The parents are then given assistance in developing positive ways to help the child reduce the expression of the gender-atypical behavior or minimize the negative social consequences of such behavior. Depending on the family issues, the parents may be seen individually, as a couple, or in a support group with other parents of children with gender problems. In some cases, the child might participate in behavioral treatment to help modify problematic gender behavior. Child therapy may also be helpful if there are significant family problems or significant anger or depression. Otherwise, the child may not be seen regularly except for follow-up evaluations.

GENDER IDENTITY DISORDERS IN ADOLESCENTS OR ADULTS

Symptoms & Signs

Adolescents or adults with gender identity disorders usually present with a request for sex reassignment or sometimes with confusion about sexuality and gender status. These individuals frequently are self-diagnosed as **transsexuals** and may have some sophistication about the diagnostic criteria.

DSM-IV criteria include "a strong and persistent cross-gender identification . . . manifested by symptoms such as a stated desire to be of the other sex, frequent passing as the other sex, desire to live or be treated as the other sex, or the conviction that one has the typical feelings and reactions of the other sex." Some individuals may seek sex reassignment because they believe that the other sex has more advantages or opportunities in life. This belief may be present but should not be the basic justification for cross-gender identification. Cross-dressing is usually present but is not diagnostically discriminating unless it has been full time. Males are likely to have cross-dressed. Females may not have cross-dressed to the extent that they passed themselves off as males, although their dress styles may never have been stereotypically feminine.

"Persistent discomfort with his or her sex or sense of inappropriateness in the gender role of that sex" is the other important *DSM-IV* diagnostic criterion. Sometimes this is manifested as a "belief that one was born the wrong sex," or a "preoccupation with getting rid of his or her primary and secondary sex characteristics," according to *DSM-IV.* This is usually expressed by seeking procedures to physically alter the appearance through administration of sex hormones, electrolysis for males, plastic surgery to improve cross-gender appearance, and sex reassignment surgery to remove the reproductive organs and/or reconstruct the genitalia.

The difficulty in using *DSM-IV* diagnostic criteria is that most of the symptoms are verbally expressed by the patient or manifested under the control of the patient. Patients can be deceptive when they are seeking medical or surgical treatment from the physician. Some gender-dysphoric individuals believe they should be able to receive hormonal or surgical treatment on demand, without psychological evaluation or treatment. The patient's physical appearance at the clinician's office is not sufficient evidence for the strength or persistence of the cross-gender identification. Part of the diagnostic process therefore involves evaluating and treating the patient over a period of time (usually 1–2 years), so that the clinician can personally assess the persistence of the gender identity disorder. In *DSM-III-R,* 2 years was the criterion for persistence, but *DSM-IV* does not specify a time criterion. Other sources of information, beyond the patient's self-report, may also cautiously be used to assess the persistence of the gender identity disorder. These include a review of the patient's previous medical records, interviews with other informants, or the presentation of evidence by the patient such as photo IDs or references indicating a history of working in the other gender role.

DSM-IV states that gender identity disorders are "not concurrent with a physical intersex condition" (these would be diagnosed as gender identity disorder not otherwise specified). To be considered a disorder there should also be significant distress or impairment in functioning. Diagnosis of a gender identity disorder is not a recommendation for sex reassignment procedures but is the start of a process that for some patients will culminate in sex reassignment.

For adults, the sexual attraction of the patient may be specified as part of the diagnostic process (sexually attracted to males, females, both, neither). Sexual orientation does not affect the diagnosis.

Differential Diagnosis

The differential diagnoses typically involve transitory or episodic cross-dressing or desire for sex reassignment.

Some gay males, "drag queens," or lesbians may go through periods of time in which they think their lives would be better if they were the other sex. This desire may be more intense in periods of depression or lovesickness, or if they are experiencing social rejection and ridicule. It is rare, however, for homosexuals to express long-term interest in getting rid of their genitalia. Only by following these individuals over time, is it possible to distinguish those individuals who are good candidates for surgical sex reassignment from those who are not. Some individuals may go through hormonal sex reassignment, for example, and be quite comfortable with a status as a "lady with a penis" without seeking social or genital reassignment. Many of the individuals who ultimately complete sex reassignment report that they thought they were homosexual for a period of their history.

Heterosexual males who cross-dress episodically, primarily for sexual excitement but sometimes to calm themselves or to relieve stress, may present with confusion about gender identity. In some cases, these individuals suffer from the paraphilia of transvestic fetishism with gender dysphoria. Some transvestite individuals will later be diagnosed as having a persistent gender identity disorder and may become candidates for sex reassignment. A history of cross-dressing for sexual arousal does not preclude a diagnosis of gender identity disorder. However, a dual diagnosis is never made, and the diagnosis of gender identity disorder takes precedence over transvestism.

Episodic gender identity complaints may occur during psychotic episodes, as in schizophrenia, or as a separate personality in multiple personality disorder.

Etiology & Prognosis

The cause of gender identity disorders in adolescents and adults is not known. Patients typically report the onset of their awareness of gender dysphoria in early childhood. In many cases, however, they did not exhibit cross-gendered behaviors that were noticed by others. Few mature individuals with this disorder have a documented history of gender identity disorder of childhood. In other cases, the onset of the disorder would appear to be in adolescence or adulthood, sometimes after marrying and raising a family.

There are several different patterns for gender identity disorders, which may reflect different etiologies and prognoses. However, research is still preliminary, and there is no consensus about any typology. One group of males reports a period of identification as male homosexuals; some of these were effeminate boys. Another group of males had what appeared to be conventional, even macho, masculine heterosexual histories, although they may have reported underlying gender dysphoria. Still another group of males had a history of heterosexual transvestism that evolved into a gender identity disorder later in adulthood. Females with gender identity disorder often describe tomboyish histories and sexual interests in females, although usually not to the extreme that would bring them to professional attention. Asexual individuals seeking sex reassignment also report childhood histories of gender dysphoria, even though they did not exhibit cross-gendered behaviors that aroused the suspicions of others or resulted in referral for evaluation.

Once diagnosed, gender identity disorders of adolescence and adulthood are usually chronic until the individual is rehabilitated in the desired gender identity and role. However, there may be periods of remission, and rehabilitation may not in all cases extend to surgical sex reassignment. Following reassignment, the frequency of satisfaction is very high with remission of most pathology associated with gender dysphoria.

Treatment

Gender identity disorders are treatable through psychotherapy and sex reassignment rehabilitation. Psychotherapy alone has not been effective in alleviating profound gender dysphoria, nor has it eliminated the preoccupation with altering sexual characteristics that individuals with gender identity disorders report. Psychotherapy as a part of sex reassignment rehabilitation helps ensure that those individuals who undergo sex reassignment will benefit from the procedures and be satisfied with the outcome.

Treatment progresses as follows. There is an initial evaluation, which includes screening for psychopathology. Psychological problems are addressed in therapy, while the patient explores whether a transition to the other gender role will help alleviate symptoms of gender dysphoria. Male patients may commence electrolysis and in some cases speech therapy. Patients develop their style of cross-dressing to fit in with their life-styles and work. The patient begins to live as much as possible in the desired gender role, notifying others and changing jobs as necessary. This is called the *real life experience*. The mental health professional may act as a coach as the individual goes through this transition. The ability to work or support oneself is a necessary part of rehabilitation.

Following a medical evaluation, hormonal reassignment (estrogen or testosterone) is the next stage in treatment. This produces dramatic results for female-to-male transsexuals through growth of facial hair and deepening of the voice. In male-to-female transsexuals, breast growth and redistribution of body fat may reduce the amount of artifice necessary for social presentation. By this time, the patient is living and working in the desired gender role full time, and may have a legally changed name consistent with the new gender role.

Surgical sex reassignment is the final stage of treatment, followed by change of legal sex status, completing the process. Surgery is performed only on adults and only following a minimum of 1 year of real life experience living full time in the new gender role. The results of genital sex reassignment surgery for male-to-female transsexuals are highly passable and functional. Female-to-male transsexuals usually undergo a mastectomy and chest reconstruction, including reconfiguration of the nipple, and oophorohysterectomy. They often defer genital reconstruction or phalloplasty.

Patients may stop their progression in the real life experience at any time, or slow their rate of change according to their circumstances. Some give up the process and revert to living in their birth gender role. Health insurance does not usually pay the cost of surgical sex reassignment procedures.

The Harry Benjamin International Gender Dysphoria Association has established minimal standards of care (Levine, 1999). Medical and psychiatric problems should be assessed and treated before hormonal or surgical sex reassignment procedures are recommended. The treating psychotherapist should document, independently of the patient's self-report, that the gender dysphoria has existed continuously for at least 2 years. The patient should have been in psychotherapeutic treatment or documented living full time in the desired sex role for at least 3 months before recommendation for hormonal reassignment and 12 months before surgical reassignment. Successful participation in the real life experience is highly related to positive outcomes of sex reassignment. Following this type of protocol, 85–97% of transsexuals report satisfaction with their rehabilitation (Green and Fleming, 1990).

GENDER IDENTITY DISORDER NOT OTHERWISE SPECIFIED

This is a residual category for individuals who present with complaints of discomfort with their own sex or identification with the other gender but do not meet the criteria for a gender identity disorder of childhood or of adolescence and adulthood.

Individuals with intersex conditions such as hermaphroditism, androgen insensitivity syndrome, or congenital adrenal hyperplasia who are also experiencing gender confusion or dysphoria would be given this diagnosis.

Transient or stress-related cross-dressing in which the chronicity of the gender complaint cannot be determined might be diagnosed as not otherwise specified while the clinician worked with the patient to see whether the gender identity problem persisted. The most common differential diagnosis is transvestism with gender dysphoria.

Some individuals also present with a preoccupation with reducing or eliminating some of their own sexual characteristics but do not wish to alter their gender to the other sex. These are body image disorders involving the primary or secondary sexual characteristics, without a desire for sex reassignment. In males, this includes desire for castration, removal of the penis, or in some cases reversing the process of puberty such as growth of body hair and voice change.

PARAPHILIAS

Paraphilias are psychosexual disorders characterized by recurrent, intense sexual fantasies, urges, or behaviors involving atypical or unacceptable sexual content. They are the sexual equivalents of obsessions and compulsions, focusing on aspects of human sexuality that do not have the goal of mutual sexual arousal with a partner. The term "paraphilia" comes from the Greek for love (*philia*) that is "aside" (*para*) in the sense of being altered or modified, a deviation in the object of attraction. Paraphilia has replaced the older terms of sexual perversion or deviation.

Symptoms & Signs

The paraphilias all involve "recurrent intense sexually arousing fantasies, sexual urges, or behaviors" that have been present for more than 6 months, according to *DSM-IV* criteria. These urges and fantasies are not the transitory or variant sexual scenarios imagined by the sexually adventurous. They do not change readily, are difficult to keep out of sexual consciousness, and have a power that at times makes it difficult to resist acting them out. Paraphilias are manifested in imagery, which may exist as a sexual fantasy or be associated with erection or orgasm in masturbation or other sexual behavior. The *DSM-IV* diagnostic criteria also state that the "fantasies, sexual urges, or behaviors cause significant distress or impairment." Solo masturbation for some affected individuals is hypersexual, to the extent that it occurs many times per day. Because acting out some paraphilias may involve illegal acts, many individuals with paraphilias are reluctant to acknowledge public acts or acts with a partner.

The paraphilias are named for the sexual content that is the primary focus of the sexual fantasy. There are over 40 named paraphilias (Money, 1999), although only the more common ones for which people seek psychiatric help are listed in *DSM-IV*. This content may be independent of sexual orientation. Although some paraphilias usually occur only in heterosexuals, for most a person may be heterosexual, homosexual, or bisexual. Some paraphilias are distinguished by a preoccupation with objects as essential for maximal sexual arousal, primarily items of clothing or materials, as in **fetishism**, or by wearing the clothing of the other sex, as in **transvestic fetishism.** Other paraphilias derive their excitement from the lack of a mutual relationship with the partner, for example, **exhibitionism, voyeurism,** or **frotteurism** (illicit sexual touching or rubbing). **Sexual masochism** and **sadism** focus on humiliation and suffering. In **pedophilia** the fantasized partners are prepubescent children. These paraphilias are discussed in detail in the following sections.

Some paraphilic fantasies are very elaborate and may involve content from several different general paraphilic themes. Thus, for example, **sadistic pedophilia** involves fantasies of the humiliation and suffering of prepubescent children. Paraphilias may be acted out through masturbation accompanied by the paraphilic fantasy, sometimes incorporating relevant props. Some paraphilias are acted out with partners. The paraphilic ritual provides indications of the underlying sexual fantasy, although the ritual may act out only some select portion of the fantasy. The paraphilia is diagnosed, insofar as possible, based on the elaborated fantasy, not just the behavior. Thus, a man who masturbates his exposed penis while watching unsuspecting children and having fantasies about sadistic acts with the children would be diagnosed with sadistic pedophilia (a sexual disorder not otherwise specified in *DSM-IV*), not with the separate diagnoses of voyeurism, exhibitionism, sadism, and pedophilia, unless these fantasies recurrently occurred independently of each other. Sometimes two or more independent paraphilias may exist in the same individual, with no overlap or shared content. Each of the independent paraphilias must have been independently and recurrently present in fantasies for at least 6 months to meet diagnostic requirements for two or more paraphilic diagnoses.

The content of common paraphilic fantasies may occur occasionally in the sexual imagery of individuals with generally conventional sexualities. Or an individual may engage in occasional behaviors or acts involving atypical sexual content. This behavior may be playful and experimental, particularly with a consenting partner. It may be **regressed** in situations of stress or associated with organic impairment. The criteria of recurrent and intense sexual urges, fantasies, or behaviors over at least 6 months must be met before a paraphilia can be diagnosed. For a patient with a paraphilia, the atypical sexual imagery is often necessary for sexual arousal, sometimes to the extent of being intrusive during conventional sexual activity. In some cases, particularly with aging and experience, the paraphilic fantasies may evoke more of a feeling of relief from tension or produce feelings of calm and comfort rather than sexual arousal.

Paraphilias are diagnosed almost exclusively in males, although they may also occur in females. Usually the onset is reported in the sexual fantasies of adolescence. Critical events or early indicators of paraphilic arousal may be reported as early as age 3–5. In other cases, the recognition of paraphilic interests is delayed into adulthood. Paraphilias may be associated with sexual dysfunction, since the sexual arousal is associated with a fantasy scenario rather than the partner. There is usually impairment in sexual or social relationships. Paraphilic imagery and behavior may seriously distract the individual from work and everyday activities. Paraphilic behavior may also be embarrassing or illegal if acted out with a nonconsenting partner.

Individuals with paraphilias may not report feeling distress and may justify their sexual interests as variant sexualities. Others feel shame or guilt about their sexual interests and can be depressed. Referral for treatment is usually a result of problems with partners or potential for legal charges.

Epidemiology & Etiology

The incidence of paraphilias is not known but is believed to be low. The incidence of specific paraphilias varies in different societies and historical periods. Paraphilias have been identified mostly in men but also exist in women.

The cause of paraphilias is not known, however the content of many paraphilic fantasies seems to be associated with childhood experiences. Although the expression of paraphilic fantasies typically begins in adolescence, the disorder does not seem to be caused by adolescent or adult experiences except perhaps in rare cases of severe trauma.

Treatment

Paraphilias are generally chronic conditions that some individuals can learn to control. The treatment for the different paraphilias is similar, although some adjustments are made in association with the differing contents. Compulsive paraphilic acting out that poses a risk to others or is not well controlled may be treated in inpatient settings. Medications that reduce testosterone may be used to decrease the intensity of the sexual urges and facilitate self-control. Individual psychotherapy and group treatment can examine issues concerning the origin of the paraphilia and its effects on an individual's personality development and life-style. Cognitive and behavioral techniques are favored; psychodynamic approaches are not generally believed to be effective. Techniques for reducing inappropriate sexual arousal and controlling undesirable sexual behavior are developed. Patients attempt to increase socially acceptable heterosexual or homosexual sexual arousal and may participate in training to improve social skills and help develop relationships. Cognitive distortions are challenged, and understanding of societal and victims' points of view is enhanced. The patient must learn to identify and avoid risk situations. Relapse prevention planning is part of the therapeutic process, and patients may need to be maintained in long-term follow-up.

FETISHISM

Fetishism is distinguished by sexual fantasies or arousal that primarily focus on objects. Common fetishes involve items of clothing such as undergarments or leg- and footwear. The tactile or olfactory qualities of the items are usually important, particularly with fetishes involving leather, rubber, or silky material. The items are used in masturbation or worn by the individual or partner during sexual activity. Many of the fetishes have some erotic qualities for individuals with conventional sexual interests. In fetishism, sexual arousal in the absence of the fetish items may be difficult, and the item, rather than the partner, is the focus for arousal. Fetishism is found in both men and women.

Cross-dressing in female clothing for sexual arousal is diagnosed as transvestic fetishism. The use of sex toys such as vibrators or vacuum pumps for genital stimulation is not considered fetishistic, because they are designed to be used for this purpose either individually or with a partner. They function primarily through direct physical stimulation of the genitalia rather than through imagery.

Fetishes may appear to be benign, although they can interfere with sexual relationships if the partner feels neglected in favor of the objects. However, in some noxious sex offenses involving sadism, serial rape, or lust murder, it is common for the perpetrator to have fetishistic interests.

TRANSVESTIC FETISHISM

Transvestic fetishism is diagnosed only in heterosexual males who experience intense sexual urges and sexually arousing fantasies involving cross-dressing. Usually the men report episodes of actual cross-dressing associated with sexual arousal and masturbation. They may dress in women's clothes fully or wear only women's undergarments. Some men involve their female sexual partners with their cross-dressing. Sexual experiences with males when cross-dressed are usually only experimental. Men may report embarrassment, guilt, and shame and at times throw away all female apparel and suppress interests in cross-dressing. If the man reports persistent discomfort with his masculine gender identity or role, "with gender dysphoria" should be noted as part of the diagnosis.

The differential diagnosis with gender identity disorders can be difficult in men who may cross-dress frequently for relief of stress, with infrequently reported sexual arousal or no current sexual relationship. Some men who had previously met the diagnostic criteria for transvestic fetishism go on to seek sex reassignment, although for most men the cross-dressing activities remain similar throughout their lives, with some decrease in frequency with aging. Transvestic fetishism can also be combined with other paraphilias, such as masochism. In some types of sexual masochism, cross-dressing and a variety of other activities are used for humiliation, without arousal associated with the clothing; these cases would not be considered transvestic fetishism. Cross-dressing for entertainment (but not sexual purposes) in homosexuals or female impersonators is not fetishistic.

Childhood episodes of being punished by being cross-dressed are reported by some men with histories of transvestic fetishism. Many transvestites report episodes of cross-dressing as a child and in most cases in adolescence.

EXHIBITIONISM

In exhibitionism, the sexually arousing fantasies involve exposing the genitals to an unsuspecting stranger. Almost always, this involves a heterosexual male exposing his penis to an adolescent or adult woman. However, this disorder may be underreported in women. There is no attempt at further sexual activity with the target female. Erection or masturbation may occur during the act, or the episode may be recalled later for sexual arousal and masturbation. Usually the fantasy focuses on the reaction of the female (surprise, shock, disgust, or interest), but there may be other fantasies of the female becoming sexually aroused or approaching the male for sexual activity.

In some cases there may be rape fantasies, which should be diagnosed as a paraphilia not otherwise specified (**rapism** or **raptophilia**). Exposure to children may be indicative of pedophilia rather than exhibitionism. In both of these examples, the exposure is a prelude in fantasy to other sexual activities, which the individual has not acted out, rather than being the goal and end point of sexual fantasy and activity.

Exhibitionism tends to be highly compulsive in younger men, with frequent episodes starting in the teens, but then decreasing in severity in older men.

VOYEURISM

Voyeurism is the counterpart of exhibitionism, in which the man repeatedly watches unsuspecting persons undressing or engaging in sexual activity. Usually the target is female, and the man masturbates while watching. What distinguishes this as a disorder is the recurrent fantasies and compulsive pattern of behavior lasting at least 6 months. Men with this disorder spend large amounts of time going around or waiting for an opportunity to observe a target woman. Voyeurism may be reported as exhibitionism when the target woman sees the man masturbating and thinks he is exposing himself to her. Voyeuristic acts may also be part of stalking for rape or a sexual obsession with a specific woman; these would be diagnosed as sexual disorders not otherwise specified.

FROTTEURISM

Frotteurism involves unsuspecting or nonconsenting partners; the sexual fantasy or arousal focuses on surreptitious touching or rubbing. Typically, the man may touch or fondle erogenous zones of the target female such as buttocks, breasts, thighs, or genitalia. Other men rub their penis, usually with an erection, against the buttocks or crotch of an unsuspecting woman. Males are rarely targets for men with this disorder.

When children are the targets, the diagnosis is usually pedophilia. It is the furtive nature of the contact that is the stimulus for sexual excitement in frotteurism. Touching as an overture to more involved sexual contact is not frotteurism, nor is touching associated with poor judgment, as in mental retardation, deficient social skills, or problems with impulse control.

PEDOPHILIA

Pedophilia, according to *DSM-IV,* involves "over a period of at least 6 months, recurrent intense sexually arousing fantasies, sexual urges, or behaviors involving sexual activity with a prepubescent child or children (generally age 13 years or younger)." The person must be at least 16 years old and more than 5 years older than the child. Although most pedophiles are males, there is a growing literature regarding sexual behavior between women and children.

The sexual attraction of the pedophile should be specified as to males, females, or both. Attraction to girls is more common than attraction to boys. However, pedophiles who are attracted to boys tend to have had more involvement with different children than those attracted to girls. Pedophiles attracted to both sexes usually prefer younger children. Pedophiles typically have highly specific age ranges and physical characteristics that define the children whom they find arousing. There is great variety in the types of sexualized activities they engage in with children. Some pedophilic relationships involve close emotional bonding.

Pedophilia is also coded as **exclusive type,** for individuals who are attracted only to children, or **nonexclusive.** Most male pedophiles who are attracted to boys are not interested in mature males and thus would not be considered homosexual. Nonexclusive pedophiles are usually heterosexual in terms of their adult sexual interests. Nonexclusive pedophilia may be also coded if **limited to incest.** Nonexclusive pedophilia also might be found in examples of regressed behavior, particularly if the sexual fantasies or behavior are manifested with reference to only one child and situation. Nonexclusive or regressed pedophilic behavior may be more likely to occur during times of stress. However, a diagnosis of pedophilia requires at least 6 months of recurrent sexually arousing fantasies, urges, or behaviors; isolated sexual activity with children is not sufficient evidence for diagnosis.

Some cases of pedophilia are associated with histories of having been sexually abused as a child. Pedophilia can also coexist with sexual sadism or lust murder, although this is rare. In most cases, pedophiles attempt to develop otherwise positive relationships with children.

Although adolescents may be defined as children according to the law, a primary and exclusive sexual attraction to adolescents in an adult would be **ephebophilia,** a paraphilia not otherwise specified.

SEXUAL MASOCHISM

DSM-IV defines sexual masochism as intense sexually arousing fantasies, sexual urges, or behaviors, recurrent over a period of at least 6 months, "involving the act (real, not simulated) of being humiliated, beaten, bound, or otherwise made to suffer." In addition, there should be clinically significant distress or impairment. Most masochism, as found in heterosexual or homosexual sadomasochistic scenes, involves consensual simulated acts and thus would not be considered disordered. Suffering as the unintentional result of sexual activity is also not considered masochistic.

Masochistic fantasies are common but are not often enacted in reality in the repetitive way characteristic of paraphilic masochism. Masochism is one of the more common paraphilias for which women seek treatment. Masochistic sexual practices can be life threatening, including masturbatory activities such as **asphyxiophilia,** which may involve strangulation and self-torture for sexual arousal.

SEXUAL SADISM

Sexual sadism, according to *DSM-IV,* involves "over a period of at least 6 months, recurrent intense sexually arousing fantasies, sexual urges, or behaviors involving acts (real, not simulated) in which the psychological or physical suffering (including humiliation) of the victim is sexually exciting to the person." In addition, there should be clinically significant distress or impairment.

Acting out sexual sadism with consenting partners usually involves only simulated acts. However, the sadist may be distressed and seek treatment because of the concern that he will lose control and actually injure the partner. Although sadism exists as a disorder in women, in heterosexual practices women are more often acting out the fantasies of their masochistic partners rather than expressing their own paraphilic sadistic fantasies. In extreme cases, sexual sadism may be acted out with nonconsensual partners in rape or lust murder.

PARAPHILIA NOT OTHERWISE SPECIFIED

Most other paraphilias are variants or combinations of common paraphilias, with some distinctive characteristics that have led to their being given individual names. Some unnamed paraphilias are very individualistic and involve elaborate rituals combining elements of other more common paraphilias.

For example, **telephone scatophilia** is a variant of exhibitionism/voyeurism in which the telephone is used to act out sexual fantasies and to elicit a reaction to sexual content from the listener or is used to eavesdrop on an individual's private sexual thoughts. Consensual telephone sex, including commercial sex lines, would not be considered paraphilic unless it became a compulsive substitute for other sexual outlets, and significantly distressed the participant or caused impairment. Sexual activity over the Internet may be a technologically updated version of telephone scatophilia.

Partialism is a variant of fetishism, in which the sexual urges and fantasies focus exclusively on a body part instead of an object. Partialism for feet and hair are examples. An interest in sexual body parts, such as breasts or penises, would not be considered partialism unless preoccupation with it was distressing or involved compulsive behavior in which the affected individual did not resist urges to touch those parts and did not attempt to engage in any other type of sexual behavior. **Acrotomophilia,** in which the sexual focus is on partners who are amputees, is a variant of partialism.

Sexual focuses on feces (**coprophilia**) or urine (**urophilia**) infrequently come to the attention of clinicians, as does a sexual preoccupation with enemas (**klismaphilia**). More infamous paraphilias such as **necrophilia** (corpses) and **zoophilia** (animals, as a primary focus of sexual urges and fantasies) are also rare in practice.

SEXUAL DISORDER NOT OTHERWISE SPECIFIED

There are other sexual disturbances that are associated with marked distress or preoccupations. One group of problems involves feelings of inadequacy concerning sexual performance or characteristics of masculinity or femininity. For example, there might be persistent concerns about the size or appearance of personal sexual characteristics in the absence of any physical evidence of inadequacy. Lovesickness can involve patterns of sexual relationships without interpersonal bonding, sex without love or love without sex. **Erotomania** is the delusional belief that there is a mutual love affair with a partner who is uninterested. Other problems include persistent confusion and distress about one's sexual orientation.

The concept of **sexual addiction** is becoming increasingly popular among some mental health professionals. It is used to refer to compulsive sexual behavior that is otherwise conventional in content and does not meet diagnostic criteria for paraphilia. Use of the term sexual addiction implies recommendations for participation in "sexaholic" or "sex addict" 12-step programs and self-help support groups. Some individuals with paraphilias also find these groups helpful. Sexual addiction, however, is not an accepted psychiatric diagnosis.

REFERENCES & SUGGESTED READINGS

American Psychiatric Association: *Diagnostic and Statistical Manual of Mental Disorders,* 4th ed. American Psychiatric Association, 1994.

Barbach L: *For Yourself: The Fulfillment of Female Sexuality.* Doubleday, 1976.

Barbach L: *For Each Other: Sharing Sexual Intimacy.* Signet, 1984.

Barbach L: *Pleasures: Women Write Erotica.* Harper & Row, 1985.

Blanchard R, Steiner BW (editors): *Clinical Management of Gender Identity Disorders in Children and Adults.* American Psychiatric Press, 1990.

Bradford JM, Greenberg DM: Pharmacological treatment of deviant sexual behaviour. Annu Rev Sex Res 1996;7:283.

Bradley SJ, Zucker KJ: Gender identity disorder: A review of the past 10 years. J Am Acad Child Adolesc Psychiatry 1997;36:872.

Bullough B, Bullough VL (editors): *Gender Blending.* Prometheus, 1997.

Butler RN, Lewis MI: *Love and Sex after 60.* GK Hall, 1996

Crenshaw TL, Goldberg JP (editors): *Sexual Pharmacology: Drugs That Affect Sexual Functioning.* Norton, 1996.

Denny D (editor): *Current Concepts in Transgender Identity.* Garland, 1998.

Di Ceglie D (editor): *A Stranger in My Own Body: Atypical Gender Identity Development and Mental Health.* Kamac Books, 1998.

Elliott M (editor): *Female Sexual Abuse of Children.* Longman, 1993.

Friday N: *My Secret Garden: Women's Sexual Fantasies.* Pocket Books, 1973.

Friday N: *Men in Love: Men's Sexual Fantasies.* Delacorte Press, 1980.

Goldstein I et al: Oral sildenafil in the treatment of sexual dysfunction. N Engl J Med 1998;338:1397.

Gotlib DA, Fagan PJ: The meanstreets of cyberspace. J Sex Educ Ther 1997;22.

Green R: *The "Sissy Boy Syndrome" and the Development of Homosexuality.* Yale University Press, 1987.

Green R, Fleming D: Transsexual surgery follow-up: Status in the 1990s. Annu Rev Sex Res 1990;1:163.

Hanson RK, Bussiere MT: Predicting relapse: A meta-analysis of sexual offender recidivism studies. J Consult Clin Psychol 1998;66:348.

Heiman JR, LoPiccolo J: *Becoming Orgasmic: A Sexual and Personal Growth Program for Women.* Prentice Hall, 1988.

Israel G, Traver D: *Transgender Care: Recommended Guidelines, Practical Information & Personal Accounts.* Temple University Press, 1997.

Kaplan HS: *The New Sex Therapy.* Brunner/Mazel, 1974.

Kaplan HS: *Disorders of Sexual Desire.* Brunner/Mazel, 1979.

Kaplan HS: *The Evaluation of Sexual Disorders.* Brunner/Mazel, 1983.

Kaplan HS: *Sexual Aversion, Sexual Phobias, and Panic Disorder.* Brunner/Mazel, 1987.

Kirk S, Rothblatt M: *Medical, Legal & Workplace Issues for the Transsexual.* Together Lifeworks, 1995.

Laws DR, O'Donohue W (editors): *Sexual Deviance: Theory, Assessment, and Treatment.* Guilford, 1997.

Leiblum SR, Rosen RC (editors): *Principles and Practice of Sex Therapy,* 2nd ed. Guilford, 1989.

Levine SB: The newly revised standards of care for gender identity disorders. J Sex Educ Ther 1999;24.

Marshall WL et al: *Sourcebook of Treatment Programs for Sexual Offenders.* Plenum, 1998.

Masters W, Johnson V: *Human Sexual Response.* Little, Brown, 1966.

Masters W, Johnson V: *Human Sexual Inadequacy.* Little, Brown, 1970.

Mathews R et al: Juvenile female sexual offenders. Sexual Abuse 1997;9:187.

Maurice WL: *Sexual Medicine in Primary Care.* Mosby, 1999.

Money J: *The Lovemap Guidebook.* Continuum, 1999.

Nichols M: Sex therapy with lesbians, gay men, and bisexuals. In: *Principles and Practice of Sex Therapy,* 2nd ed. Leiblum SR, Rosen RC (editors). Guilford, 1989.

Penner C, Penner J: *The Gift of Sex: A Christian Guide to Sexual Fulfillment.* Word Publishing, 1981.

Schmidt CW: Sexual psychopathology and *DSM-IV.* Am Psychiatr Press Rev Psychiatry 1995;14:719.

Sipski ML, Alexander CJ: *Sexual Function in People with Disability and Chronic Illness: A Health Professional's Guide.* Aspen, 1997.

Zilbergeld B: *The New Male Sexuality,* rev. ed. Bantam, 1999.

Zucker KJ, Bradley SJ: *Gender Identity Disorder and Psychosexual Problems in Children and Adolescents.* Guilford, 1995.

Eating Disorders

26

Kim Norman, MD

This chapter provides an overview of the major eating disorders: anorexia nervosa, bulimia, and obesity. Binge eating disorder is discussed as a subset of bulimia and of obesity. In reading this review, keep in mind that eating disorders are not illnesses per se but behavioral syndromes that develop in individuals who manifest a broad spectrum of psychological, biological, and sociocultural characteristics. Recognition of the psychophysiological impact of associated medical complications and identification of psychiatric comorbidity are of critical importance in the diagnoses and treatment of these disorders. A thorough history, including eating behavior and body image, a comprehensive psychiatric assessment, and a complete medical evaluation are essential for the successful treatment of eating disorders.

ANOREXIA NERVOSA

Anorexia nervosa is a complex disorder manifested by physiological, behavioral, and psychological changes and characterized by morbid fear of fatness, gross distortion of body image, and unrelenting pursuit of thinness. The name is actually a misnomer, since true anorexia (loss of appetite) does not usually occur until late in its course. Although it typically begins in adolescence, the range of onset is between 10 and 30 years.

Symptoms & Signs

Individuals with anorexia nervosa go to incredible extremes to lose weight. They begin by drastically reducing caloric intake, with virtually complete avoidance of high-carbohydrate and fat-containing foods. They exercise incessantly—walking, running, swimming, cycling, dancing, and performing calisthenics. Hyperactivity is dramatic and persists even when weight loss has resulted in cachexia. Some patients alternate fasting with bulimia—episodes of uncontrolled gorging without awareness of hunger or satiation. Such eating binges are often followed by self-induced vomiting. Huge quantities of laxatives are commonly consumed. Diet pills and diuretics may also be abused in the effort to lose weight. There are two types of anorexia nervosa: Patients who engage in binge eating and purging behavior are diagnosed as having the binge eating/purging type and patients who simply starve themselves are diagnosed as having the restricting type.

The eating behaviors of anorexics are often peculiar and may be bizarre. The diet may be exceedingly monotonous or highly eccentric. Large quantities of food may be hoarded or small amounts of food may be hidden around the house. Although they eat very little, anorexics are obsessively preoccupied with food and cooking. Food portions are carefully measured, and small meals may be eaten over many hours. Food is often stored, prepared, served, eaten, and disposed of in a specific, ritualistic fashion. Patients with anorexia nervosa are usually highly secretive and often lie to protect the privacy of their eating behaviors. Kleptomania and stealing are sometimes associated with this disorder, particularly among individuals who also have episodes of bulimia.

Although these features of anorexia nervosa can occur in individuals with a variety of premorbid personality structures and traits, a fairly consistent profile of emotional and psychological manifestations common to all patients with this disorder has been described. Clinicians generally agree that the unrelenting pursuit of thinness manifests an underlying psychological struggle to maintain a sense of personal autonomy and self-control. On the surface, patients are stubbornly defiant and fiercely independent. They insist they are happy, fully aware of their condition, and completely capable of taking care of themselves. But underneath they are stricken with a paralyzing sense of helplessness and ineffectiveness, with control over eating and body size the only mechanisms through which a sense of autonomy and mastery can be sustained. This important insight into the psychology of anorexia nervosa was discovered in 1962 by Hilde Bruch, who also described two other essential features of this disorder: a characteristic misperception of internal body cues, so that patients are unable to differentiate their own feelings and needs from those of others; and a disturbance of body image, so that patients see themselves as grotesquely fat even when exceedingly thin. These cognitive and perceptual distortions accentuate the sense of personal ineffectiveness and reinforce the need to continue the pursuit of thinness to maintain a sense of control.

The lack of confidence in basic self-control is compounded by feelings of personal mistrust. Patients fear they will give in to overwhelming impulses and, so far as eating is concerned, gorge themselves into obesity. Individuals with anorexia nervosa also tend to view themselves in terms of absolutes and polar opposites. Behavior is either all good or all bad; a decision is either completely right or completely wrong; and a person is either absolutely in control or totally out of control. Thus, the gain of an ounce may produce the same sense of horror as would the gain of 100 pounds. Self-mistrust and the tendency to view the world in absolutes reinforce the exaggerated need to maintain rigid control over what is and is not eaten.

Patients with anorexia nervosa often express fear about becoming adults, since that would mean either tolerating intense loneliness or entering the world of interpersonal and sexual relationships. Although desperate for contact, they are mistrustful of relationships. They are often frightened of sexuality and usually avoid sexual encounters. When they do engage in sexual activity, it is usually without enjoyment.

Low self-esteem is invariably present, with the ability to lose weight being the only thing many patients like about themselves. Patients with anorexia nervosa describe intense feelings of inner shame about their bodies in general, with their fat content a specific object of disgust.

Psychiatric Comorbidity

Two-thirds of patients with anorexia nervosa and three-fourths of patients who meet diagnostic criteria for both anorexia nervosa and bulimia nervosa are also diagnosed with at least one mood disorder on presentation. Of patients with anorexia nervosa, up to 60% are diagnosed with major depression and about 33% with anxiety disorders at intake. Obsessive-compulsive disorder accounts for one-half of the associated anxiety disorders, but generalized anxiety disorder, phobias, and panic disorder are also common. The lifetime risk of affective disorder in patients with anorexia nervosa is reported to range from 84% to a nearly universal 98%.

Personality disorders are diagnosed in at least 20% and as many as 80% of patients with anorexia nervosa. Patients with the restricting type of anorexia nervosa tend to exhibit Cluster C (anxious) personality disorders, such as avoidant, dependent, and compulsive, with Cluster A (odd) disorders, such as paranoid and schizoid, sometimes present. The Cluster B (dramatic) personality disorders, such as borderline, histrionic, and narcissistic, tend to be present only in patients with anorexia nervosa binge eating/purging type. Patients with anorexia nervosa also present a lifetime risk of alcohol, amphetamine, and other substance abuse problems, which may be concurrent with the eating disorder.

In addition, starvation is known to produce psychiatric symptoms such as dysphoria, anxiety, obsessiveness, and hyperactivity, which complicate the diagnosis of comorbidity. This phenomenon further underscores the importance of ending starvation and reversing malnutrition as the essential first steps in treating anorexia nervosa.

Medical Complications

A weight loss of at least 15% of the baseline or ideal body weight is necessary to establish the diagnosis of anorexia nervosa. In addition to weight loss, a number of physical signs of anorexia nervosa can be attributed to weight loss, malnutrition, and generalized stress. Amenorrhea or oligomenorrhea, independent of weight loss and often preceding initial weight loss, is always present in women. Anorexia nervosa with premenarcheal onset often results in short stature and delayed breast development. Prolonged amenorrhea in women with anorexia nervosa may lead to the development of osteoporosis. Patients frequently complain of epigastric distress, and gastric emptying time is indeed prolonged. Vomiting, constipation, cold intolerance, headache, polyuria, and sleep disturbances are also commonly reported. In addition to emaciation, physical findings may include edema, lanugo, dehydration, low blood pressure, bradycardia, arrhythmias, diminished cardiac mass, and infantile uterus. Males with anorexia frequently have hemorrhoids and experience loss of libido.

Laboratory findings include abnormalities of vasopressin secretion, prepubertal plasma levels of follicle-stimulating hormone and luteinizing hormone, and a diminished response to gonadotropin-releasing hormone. Estrogen is at postmenopausal levels. Males have low testosterone. There is abolition or reversal of the normal circadian rhythm of plasma cortisol, the metabolic clearance rate of cortisol is reduced, and there is incomplete suppression of adrenocorticotropin and cortisol by dexamethasone. There is diminished growth hormone response to insulin-induced hypoglycemia, arginine stimulation, and levodopa. Glucose tolerance test curves may be flat. Plasma levels of triiodothyronine (T_3) are reduced, and levels of plasma reverse-T_3 may be elevated. Blood urea nitrogen and creatinine may be elevated, renal calculi may form, the glomerular filtration rate may be reduced, and renal failure is possible. Hematological abnormalities may include leukopenia with a relative lymphocytosis, thrombocytopenia, and anemia. Bone marrow aspiration reveals hypocellularity with large amounts of gelatinous acid mucopolysaccharide. The erythrocyte sedimentation rate is low, and plasma fibrinogen levels are reduced. Hypercarotenemia, hypercholesterolemia, and hypomagnesemia are common findings. Hypophosphatemia if present is an ominous sign, associated with rapid decompensation. Self-induced vomiting may produce a metabolic hypokalemic alkalosis. Electroencephalographic patterns may be abnormal, and the electrocardiogram may show flat or inverted T waves, ST depression, and increased intervals.

Refeeding edema frequently complicates the treatment of anorexia nervosa and, when severe, may increase the risk of congestive heart failure. Death, which occurs in 10–22% of patients, is caused by starvation and its complications (including pneumonia and other infections, cardiac arrhythmia, congestive heart failure, and renal failure) or by suicide. Patients who purge by vomiting or by abusing laxatives or diuretics are at risk for sudden death due to fluid and electrolyte imbalance.

Natural History

The onset of anorexia nervosa often follows new life situations in which the patient feels inadequate or unable to cope. Such changes may be biological, such as the onset of puberty; psychological, such as the stages of adolescence; or social, such as entering high school or college. The onset of anorexia nervosa may also follow the breakup of a relationship or the death of a relative or friend.

Typically, anorexia nervosa begins in individuals who are at normal weight or are slightly to moderately overweight. Dieting is initially supported, even actively encouraged, by family and friends as well as, in many cases, by dance teachers and sports coaches. The patient is thus praised for the initial weight loss and takes pleasure in the achievement. Once the original weight reduction goal is attained, however, a new one is immediately set. Ostensibly, this is for "insurance" to offset future weight gains, but weight loss in the pursuit of thinness soon becomes an objective in itself.

Patients usually come to medical attention not because of weight loss but because of complaints such as amenorrhea, edema, constipation, or abdominal pain. They may complain of specific "food allergies" and ask for aids in dieting such as diet pills or diuretics. Patients may also present as medical emergencies, since the complications of dieting or vomiting, such as dehydration and fluid and electrolyte imbalance, may be severe. The patient may be brought in by parents, who become worried when weight loss is extreme or are alarmed by bizarre eating habits and personality changes.

The course of anorexia nervosa is variable. There may be a single episode with complete recovery, or multiple episodes spanning many years. A single episode may also be chronic and unremitting. Complete or partial recovery may occur spontaneously in some cases or may follow treatment. Both single episodes and fluctuating courses may progress to death.

Differential Diagnosis

Anorexia nervosa must be distinguished from weight loss caused by medical illnesses such as neoplasms, tuberculosis, hypothalamic disease, and primary endocrinopathies (anterior pituitary insufficiency, Addison's disease, hyperthyroidism, and diabetes mellitus). These can generally be diagnosed on the basis of thorough histories, physical examinations, and laboratory studies. Patients with these medical illnesses do not present with the dread of fatness, unrelenting pursuit of thinness, and hyperactivity that characterize anorexia nervosa.

Weight loss frequently occurs in patients with depressive disorders or certain schizophrenic disorders characterized by peculiar eating habits prompted by delusions about food. Patients with other disorders also lack preoccupations with caloric intake, obsessions with body shape and size, and hyperactivity. Patients with somatization disorder may manifest weight fluctuations, vomiting, and peculiar food habits, but weight loss is usually not severe, and amenorrhea for longer than 3 months is unusual.

To establish the diagnosis of anorexia nervosa, patients should satisfy the *Diagnostic and Statistical Manual of Mental Disorders,* 4th edition (*DSM-IV*) diagnostic criteria listed in Table 26–1. Subtyping takes into account the findings that patients with a mixture of anorexia nervosa and bulimia nervosa have a higher association of both Axis I and Axis II comorbidity, present greater medical risks as a result of fluid and electrolyte imbalance, and may have a worse prognosis than patients with anorexia nervosa alone.

Prognosis

There is marked variability in the prognosis for patients with anorexia nervosa. About 40% are completely recovered at follow-up and 30% are improved, but 20% remain unimproved or severely

---

Table 26–1. *DSM-IV* diagnostic criteria for anorexia nervosa.

A. Refusal to maintain body weight at or above a minimally normal weight for age and height (eg, weight loss leading to maintenance of body weight less than 85% of that expected; or failure to make expected weight gain during period of growth, leading to body weight less than 85% of expected).

B. Intense fear of gaining weight or becoming fat, even though underweight.

C. Disturbance in the way in which one's body weight or shape is experienced; undue influence of body weight or shape on self-evaluation, or denial of the seriousness of the current low body weight.

D. In postmenarchal females, amenorrhea, ie, the absence of at least three consecutive menstrual cycles. (A woman is considered to have amenorrhea if her periods occur only following hormone, eg, estrogen, administration.)

Specify type:
 Restricting type: During the episode of anorexia nervosa, the person does not regularly engage in binge eating or purging behavior (ie, self-induced vomiting or the misuse of laxatives or diuretics).
 Binge Eating/Purging type: During the episode of anorexia nervosa, the person regularly engages in binge eating or purging behavior (ie, self-induced vomiting or the misuse of laxatives or diuretics).

impaired. The mortality rate for this disorder is as high as 22% in some studies, with suicide reported in 2–5% of chronic cases.

The presence of nonanorexic psychiatric impairments such as depression, anxiety, and agoraphobia is common at follow-up. Indicators of a favorable prognosis include a good premorbid level of psychosocial adjustment, early age at onset, less extreme weight loss, and less denial of illness at presentation. Unfavorable prognostic factors include poor premorbid level of psychosocial adjustment, low socioeconomic status, extreme weight loss, greater denial of illness, and the presence of bulimia, vomiting, and laxative abuse. These indicators are all relative, since no single feature or set of factors can reliably predict the prognosis for any given individual.

Complete recovery in less than 2 years is unusual. The recovery rate is positively correlated with length of time at follow-up, ie, the more time that passes before follow-up, the greater the likelihood of finding recovery. Thus, clinicians will do well to remember the words of William Gull (1874), who described anorexia nervosa: "As regards prognosis, none of these cases, however exhausted, are really hopeless while life exists."

Illustrative Case

A 17-year-old high school senior began dieting to improve her appearance. Although her family initially encouraged her, the parents became alarmed as her weight dropped precipitously and she became cachectic. She was obsessed with food and exercise and avoided friends, and for the first time her school grades dropped from straight As to Cs and Ds. Her parents reported a change in personality from sweet and compliant to argumentative and stubborn. Although everyone told her she was too thin, she saw herself as grotesquely obese. She resented her family's pressure to gain weight and perceived them as being controlling and manipulative. She wanted to continue dieting and reported that her only concerns were that she was cold all the time, had trouble sleeping, could not concentrate well ("I feel in a fog"), and could not keep still.

The patient was hospitalized on a psychiatric unit when persistent bradycardia and hypotension resulted in episodes of fainting. Despite her verbal protests, she appeared relieved by the decision to be admitted. A behavior modification protocol was implemented, and she began to eat normally again. Her baseline personality returned as her weight goal was achieved.

In individual psychotherapy, she revealed that she was terrified about graduating from high school and leaving home to go to college. She felt she lacked the ability to take care of herself and did not have confidence that she could make friends or succeed academically away from home. She also worried that her parents, who seemed to fight all the time, would break up when she left home. She felt powerless and

her life seemed out of control; dieting had become the only thing she felt competent to do.

Although apprehensive at first, the patient seemed most responsive to family therapy. She was pleased by her parents' resolve to work out their marital problems and reported that for the first time in years she could imagine liking herself.

Individual and family therapy continued for 1 year after discharge, during which time the patient was able to maintain a normal weight. She elected to remain in therapy during her freshman year of college and continued to thrive.

Epidemiology

The prevalence of anorexia nervosa among women in the United States and western Europe is between 0.7% and 2.1% of the population. Males constitute 10–15% of patients with anorexia nervosa.

Etiology & Pathogenesis

A. Biological Factors: The number of hormonal changes in anorexia nervosa, as outlined above, suggests a hypothalamic-endocrine origin. However, the changes all appear to be secondary to the effects of starvation, weight loss, malnutrition, and stress, and no evidence of primary hypothalamic dysfunction has been adduced in any of the cases.

There is an increased risk for the disorder in biological siblings of patients with anorexia nervosa, and recent studies have shown a higher concordance rate for monozygotic than for dizygotic twins. However, the fact that anorexia nervosa tends to occur primarily in individuals of the upper and middle socioeconomic classes, and the trend for rates to increase in societies in accordance with exposure to Western culture, argue against an exclusive biological origin. Given that the physiological changes in anorexia nervosa (primary or secondary) definitely contribute to its pathogenesis, the clinical features must be viewed as resulting from interacting biological and psychological factors.

Despite its high association with affective disorders, anorexia nervosa is not viewed as simply a variant of affective illness. This is so because the unrelenting pursuit of thinness and distortion of body image are not typical of affective disorders and because the natural course and outcome of anorexia nervosa differ from those of affective disorders.

B. Psychological Factors: A number of psychological theories have been proposed to account for anorexia nervosa. Classical psychoanalysts have emphasized the avoidance of sexuality. They view self-starvation as a rejection of the wish to be pregnant and refusal of food as a behavioral response to fantasies of oral impregnation. Amenorrhea has been viewed as a symbolic manifestation of the wish to be pregnant. More recently, theorists have stressed impairment in the mother-child relationship as the primary cause. Such theorists view the characteristic struggle for autonomy as a manifestation of the failure to master conflicts associated with the process of separation and individuation. (See Chapter 4 for a discussion of these conflicts.) The cognitive and perceptual deficits associated with anorexia nervosa, such as the distortion of body image, may also arise from impairments in early childhood development. For example, repeated invalidation of a child's perceptions by overly intrusive parents who "know too well" what a child thinks, feels, and needs can result in development of a sense of personal mistrust characteristic of patients with this disorder.

In recent years, family systems theorists have argued that anorexia nervosa is the result of dysfunctional family interactions. The function of the child who develops anorexia nervosa is to maintain the status quo, allowing the family to remain enmeshed, overinvolved, rigid, overprotective, and unable to handle conflicts openly. The child's illness may also provide the vehicle through which parents are able to fulfill their own unresolved dependency needs. (See Chapter 35 for a discussion of family dynamics.)

C. Cultural Factors: Anorexia nervosa occurs predominantly in upper-class families and may represent an exaggeration or caricature of class values that emphasize youth and thinness as virtues. In this regard, it is important to consider a feminist perspective on anorexia nervosa. Feminist writers such as Gloria Steinem and Naomi Wolf argue that a male-dominant culture prevents women from ever being comfortable with their bodies and therefore disempowers them. Models with expressions of angst and emaciated bodies dominate fashion magazines. Men are considered desirable if they attain professional success; women must have cover girl faces and centerfold figures. Thus, Luciano Pavarotti, though large, is an international sex symbol, whereas the equally talented and equally large diva is the proverbial "fat lady who sings." Studies show that women, when asked about the shape and size of their bodies, usually respond disparagingly, eg, "my hips are too big." Men respond in terms of performance, eg, "I can run 10 miles and lift 200 pounds." Women tend to view their bodies as farther from their ideal weight than they actually are; men see themselves as closer. These differences may explain why anorexia and bulimia nervosa occur nine times more often in females than in males.

The abundance of theories reflects the multidimensional nature of this disorder. No single theory offers a satisfactory explanation of the origin of anorexia nervosa, but each has contributed a valuable perspective on treating this puzzling and life-threatening disorder.

Treatment

Treatment approach to anorexia nervosa is summarized in Table 26–2.

The initial goal of treatment is to counteract the ef-

Table 26–2. Treatment approach to anorexia nervosa.

1. *Assess and treat the medical complications of starvation.* Determine whether purging is present, and treat for dehydration and electrolyte imbalance as necessary.

2. *Decide whether hospitalization is necessary.* If dizziness, light-headedness, or fainting from bradycardia or hypotension is reported, if any sign of congestive heart failure is present (including reports of dyspnea on exertion), if fluid and electrolyte balance cannot be maintained, if excessive exercise presents a risk of congestive heart failure and cannot be monitored safely as an outpatient, if cognitive impairment from starvation precludes the utility of outpatient psychotherapy, or if the patient reports mental exhaustion from battling food and eating issues, then hospitalization is essential. Hospitalization is also indicated when reasonable outpatient efforts have failed.

3. *Complete laboratory investigation.* This includes full electrolyte profile including potassium, magnesium, calcium and phosphates, glucose, complete blood count, erythrocyte sedimentation rate, total protein, albumin, liver function tests, renal function tests, thyroid function tests, iron, folate, B_{12}, electrocardiogram, chest x-ray, and bone density studies.

4. *Restore nutritional balance through normal eating and encourage weight gain.* This often involves setting up a behavior modification protocol. Low-dose neuroleptics or benzodiazepine-class anxiolytics may be used if fear of weight gain is excessive. Cyproheptadine may be useful to encourage weight gain in cases where weight loss is extreme.

5. *Diagnose and treat psychiatric comorbidity.* The presence of affective disorder may warrant the use of antidepressant medications. These medications may not be particularly effective when patients are significantly underweight but may be very effective when weight gain has occurred. Issues stemming from personality disorders should be addressed in psychotherapy.

6. *Identify and treat underlying ideas, attitudes, and psychological conflicts.* Treat with cognitive and/or psychodynamically based psychotherapy.

7. *Assess the family.* Utilize family therapy to facilitate support for the patient and to address family dynamics that may be contributing to the patient's development of illness.

8. *Provide ongoing support.* Support healthy diet and exercise habits; constructive approaches to self, family, and interpersonal problems; enhanced self-esteem; and sense of autonomy with ongoing psychotherapy.

fects of starvation by promoting weight gain and restoring normal nutritional balance. In mild cases, this may be accomplished on an outpatient basis; in moderate to severe cases, an initial period of hospitalization is usually required.

Weight gain may be accomplished by hyperalimentation or total parenteral nutrition. However, because of the risks of intravenous feedings, most programs utilize behavior modification protocols based on the principles of operant conditioning. Although behavior modification may be effective in promoting initial weight gain, most outcome studies have concluded that behavior modification alone is not sufficient treatment. Lasting recovery occurs only when such methods are used in conjunction with psychotherapy, which addresses the underlying psychological conflicts. Clinicians should also be advised that too rapid weight gain may cause dangerous gastric dilatation or precipitate congestive heart failure.

Drug therapy may be useful in some cases. Some clinicians have considered the perceptual and body image disturbances characteristic of anorexia nervosa to be manifestations of psychosis, and chlorpromazine and similar drugs have facilitated weight gain in some patients. However, it is not clear whether the benefits of such medications result from their antipsychotic or their sedative effects. Anxiolytics, such as clonazepam, may be helpful in reducing the overwhelming anxiety associated with eating. Recent studies suggest that the serotonin reuptake blockers fluoxetine and clomipramine may help the depression and obsessions associated with anorexia nervosa, however, antidepressants, which have helped some patients, tend to be ineffective until weight loss has been restored. Cyproheptadine, an appetite stimulator and serotonin antagonist, has proved helpful in the treatment of a subgroup of anorexic patients with particularly severe symptoms and a history of birth trauma.

Although psychoanalysis has not been generally effective in the treatment of anorexia nervosa, psychodynamically oriented psychotherapies that provide support to the patient and focus on issues relating to the struggle for autonomy and personal control are often successful. Cognitive behavioral therapy, which challenges irrational beliefs about food, eating, and body size, and teaches patients strategies for reducing anxiety associated with behavioral change, is often effective. Family therapies, which view the symptoms of anorexia nervosa in the context of family structure and dysfunction, are also effective, particularly in the treatment of children, teenagers, and adults still living at home.

To effectively treat anorexia nervosa, biological, psychological, and behavioral changes must all be addressed. Effective treatment programs should not be welded to any single approach. Clinicians should be familiar with various methods of treatment and use them singly or in combination as called for.

BULIMIA NERVOSA

Bulimia nervosa is the episodic, uncontrolled binge eating of large quantities of food over a short period of time. It was originally described in the late 1950s as a pattern of behavior in some obese individuals. In the 1960s and early 1970s, it was recognized as a commonly associated feature of anorexia nervosa. Recently, it has been identified as a distinct disorder that occurs in persons of normal weight who are not obese and do not have anorexia nervosa. To establish the diagnosis of bulimia nervosa, the *DSM-IV* requires some form of compensatory behavior to prevent weight gain, such as purging. A number of normal-weight individuals engage in episodes of binge eating but do not engage in any compensatory behavior. The authors of *DSM-IV* elected not to include a separate diagnosis of binge eating disorder. However, the diagnostic and treatment considerations are the same for these individuals as for those who meet the full diagnostic criteria for bulimia nervosa.

Symptoms & Signs

The essential feature of bulimia nervosa is the episodic, uncontrolled gorging of large quantities of food in short periods of time. Patients are aware of their disordered eating habits and distinguish eating binges from simple overeating. They are usually unaware of hunger during binges and do not stop eating when satiated. They express fear about not being able to stop eating voluntarily and report that binges end only when nausea or abdominal pain becomes severe, when they are interrupted or fall asleep, or when they induce vomiting.

Binges are usually preceded by depressive moods in which the patient feels sad, lonely, empty, and isolated; or by anxiety states with overwhelming tension. These feelings are usually relieved during the binges, but afterward patients typically report a return of depressive mood with disparaging self-criticism and feelings of guilt.

Binges usually occur in secret. They may last from a few minutes to several hours (typically less than 2 hours, with a median reported time of about 1 hour). Most binges are spontaneous, but some may be planned. The frequency of binges ranges from occasional (two or three times a month) to many times a day. The quantity of food consumed varies but is always large. Bulimics report consumption of 3–27 times the recommended daily allowance for calories on binge days, and some claim to spend in excess of $100 a day on binge foods. The food consumed is usually high in carbohydrates and of a texture that is easily swallowed. Patients often report eating the "junk foods" they ordinarily deny themselves but frequently eat whatever is available. Though high-carbohydrate foods are most commonly consumed, the nutritional content of binge foods varies. Although it is uncommon, some bulimics may eat huge quantities of vegetables, such as 7 pounds of carrots, at a single sitting.

Self-induced vomiting is very common but is not essential for the diagnosis. Some patients maintain normal weight by alternating binges with long periods of fasting, and many exercise excessively. (These patients are often referred to as "exercise bulimics.") Those who do vomit may use emetics such as ipecac syrup or induce vomiting by activating the gag reflex. Lesions on the back of the hand may be evidence of this. Many report that they no longer need chemical or mechanical stimulants to induce emesis, as they can simply vomit at will. Laxative abuse is commonly associated with bulimia, the use of diuretics is not unusual, and rumination may occur.

Patients with bulimia are usually self-conscious about their behavior and often go to great lengths to conceal it. They are very concerned about their physical appearance, with self-esteem overly dependent on perception of body size and shape. Sexual adjustment may be disturbed, with behavior ranging from promiscuity to restricted sexual activity. A number of other symptoms related to poor impulse control are commonly associated with bulimia, such as alcoholism, drug abuse, stealing, self-mutilation, and suicidal gestures and attempts.

Most patients experience weight fluctuations, with weight typically ranging from slightly underweight to slightly overweight. Other symptoms associated with bulimia include edema of hands and feet, headache, sore throat, painless or painful swelling of parotid and salivary glands, erosion of tooth enamel and severe caries, feelings of fullness, abdominal pain, and lethargy and fatigue. Light-headedness, dizziness, syncope, and seizures may occur if vomiting is severe. Menstrual irregularities are common, but amenorrhea is usually not sustained.

Bulimia is usually not incapacitating except in extreme cases, where binge/purging is a virtual full-time preoccupation. When vomiting is excessive, dehydration and electrolyte imbalances can occur and may result in medical emergencies. Deaths from gastric dilatation and rupture have been reported.

Psychiatric Comorbidity

There is a high association of affective disorders with bulimia nervosa, with lifetime rates of over 80%. Major depression is most common, occurring in one-third of patients with bulimia nervosa and more than one-half of patients with mixed bulimia nervosa and anorexia nervosa. Depression may precede, follow, or coincide with bulimia. Studies suggest that depression and bulimia operate independently, although both tend to improve with treatment. Anxiety disorders including generalized anxiety disorder, panic disorder, obsessive-compulsive disorder, social phobia, and posttraumatic stress disorder occur in nearly 60% of cases. Patients with bulimia nervosa also have a significant lifetime risk for alcohol and substance abuse, which may be concurrent with their eating disorder.

Personality disorders are commonly associated with bulimia nervosa, with rates ranging from 22% to 77% in published studies. Cluster B (dramatic) personality disorders including borderline personality disorder are most common, but Cluster C (anxious) personality disorders, including avoidant personality disorder, are frequently diagnosed.

Medical Complications

The most serious medical complications of bulimia nervosa are caused by the cardiovascular effects of fluid and electrolyte imbalance. Purging behavior, including vomiting and laxative and diuretic abuse, may cause life-threatening cardiac arrhythmias. Orthostatic hypotension associated with light-headedness and dizziness; headaches, insomnia, and fatigue; dental caries and erosion of tooth enamel; and gastritis and esophagitis are common. Benign enlargement of the parotid and salivary glands occurs in about 25% of patients. The presence of a skin lesion on the back of the hand is a frequent sign of active behavior. In addition to hypokalemia, blood tests may show hypomagnesemia, disturbances in acid-base balance, and elevated serum amylase. Electrocardiogram changes such as ST segment depression and U waves may occur. Cardiomyopathy from emetine poisoning may develop in patients who use ipecac syrup to induce vomiting and may result in death. Patients who use baking soda to induce vomiting are at risk for developing life-threatening acid-base imbalance. Patients with bulimia nervosa are at increased risk for developing seizures. They may have irregular menses or be amenorrheic.

Natural History

Bulimia typically begins in adolescence or young adulthood in individuals consciously trying to stay slim. Some report a history of anorexia nervosa and others report a history of obesity. The onset often follows changes in living situations such as leaving home, starting college, changing jobs, or becoming involved in new relationships.

The course is usually chronic, and patients often engage in such behavior for years before seeking treatment. The chronicity of the illness may be punctuated by brief remissions in which the behavior is absent or the frequency and severity of the symptoms are reduced. Many report experiencing periods of relative improvement and other periods of worsening symptoms.

Differential Diagnosis

The *DSM-IV* diagnostic criteria for bulimia are listed in Table 26–3.

If the patient also satisfies the diagnostic criteria for schizophrenia or anorexia nervosa, that should be the diagnosis. Severe weight loss does not occur in bulimia, and amenorrhea is unusual.

In diagnosing bulimia, it is necessary to rule out neurological disease, such as epileptic-equivalent seizures, central nervous system tumors, Klüver-Bucy–like syndromes, and Kleine-Levin syndrome. Klüver-Bucy syndrome includes visual agnosia, compulsive licking and biting, exploration of objects by mouth, inability to ignore any stimulus, placidity, hypersexuality, and hyperphagia. This syndrome is very rare and unlikely to present a problem in differential diagnosis. Kleine-Levin syndrome occurs chiefly in males and is characterized by hyperphagia and periods of hypersomnia lasting 2–3 weeks.

Table 26–3. *DSM-IV* diagnostic criteria for bulimia nervosa.

A. Recurrent episodes of binge eating. An episode of binge eating is characterized by both of the following:
(1) eating, in a discrete period of time (eg, within any 2-hour period), an amount of food that is definitely larger than most people would eat during a similar period of time under similar circumstances, and (2) a sense of lack of control over eating during the episode (eg, a feeling that one cannot stop eating or control what or how much one is eating).

B. Recurrent inappropriate compensatory behavior to prevent weight gain, such as self-induced vomiting; misuse of laxatives, diuretics, or other medications; fasting; or excessive exercise.

C. The binge eating and inappropriate compensatory behaviors both occur, on average, at least twice a week for 3 months.

Prognosis

Bulimia nervosa is often a chronic illness characterized by multiple periods of relapse and remission. Many patients show significant improvement following brief psychotherapy and/or the administration of medication, and recovery rates (up to 85% in some series) definitely improve over time. Although outcome studies vary in their definition of recovery, and many more studies are needed, both patients and clinicians should be very encouraged by currently available data.

Illustrative Case

A 20-year-old woman sought outpatient treatment for her binge eating and vomiting behavior. Her symptoms began at age 17, when she was a college freshman. Although very bright and attractive, she worried about whether men would like her. Her weight was normal for height and age, but she decided to lose a few pounds in the spring to "be prepared for bathing suit season." She went on a diet together with her roommate, who suggested vomiting after meals.

The patient reported binging three or four times a week, usually in the evening and always when alone. She usually felt depressed and anxious when the urge to binge became overwhelming. She typically binged on breads and sweets. It was not unusual for her to eat a half-gallon of ice cream, a box of cookies, and a loaf of bread during a binge, which typically lasted about 30–45 minutes. She felt relief from her depression and anxiety during binges and reported sensations of warmth, safety, security, and unconditional acceptance. She ended the binges when her stomach ached, at which time she induced vomiting mechanically. After vomiting, she felt guilty and angry at herself for giving in to her impulses and being out of control.

The patient was 5 feet 6 inches tall. Her weight had fluctuated between 110 and 150 pounds since the onset of her bulimia. Although she weighed 122

pounds at the start of treatment, she reported wishing she weighed 15–20 pounds less. She took large doses of laxatives daily and occasionally used diuretics. She had taken amphetamines in the past and was worried about her increasing dependence on alcohol. She complained of spending up to $60 on a single binge and reported stealing food from grocery stores.

She described self-hatred as a result of her behavior and told of superficially cutting her wrists on two occasions, which she characterized as "semisuicide attempts." She had been too embarrassed to discuss her symptoms and felt she might be the only person in the world with such a bizarre disorder. The patient decided to seek treatment after reading an article about the medical dangers of bulimia. She was surprised by the article, which reported that the disorder had a high incidence.

She entered individual psychotherapy and attended a support group for women with bulimia. Her symptoms improved during the first 6 months of treatment, with the frequency of binges dropping to once a week. A trial of fluoxetine was begun and resulted in complete remission of binge eating and purging behavior. She decided to continue in therapy, not only to better understand her eating disorder but also to work on long-standing problems related to low self-esteem and difficulty in social relationships.

Epidemiology

Between 1% and 3% of young adult females in the United States meet the diagnostic criteria for bulimia nervosa. As many as 40% of young adults engage in episodic binge eating but do not meet the diagnostic criteria. Bulimia nervosa occurs in 0.2% of adolescent boys and young adult males and accounts for 10–15% of bulimics identified in community-based studies.

Etiology & Pathogenesis

The cause is not known. The episodic, uncontrolled nature of the eating behaviors has led some investigators to suggest that bulimia may be a variant of complex partial seizure disorder. However, the few electroencephalographic abnormalities reported in patients studied during the testing of this hypothesis did not correlate with treatment response to phenytoin.

The strong association between bulimia nervosa and affective disorders together with the tendency of bulimic behavior to respond to antidepressant medication has led to the hypothesis that the disorder is the result of imbalance in the dopamine, norepinephrine, and serotonin systems in the brain. Some studies have suggested that neuropeptides such as cholecystokinin, which regulate appetite and satiety in the brain, may be abnormal in patients with bulimia nervosa, but the evidence is far from conclusive.

Psychodynamic theories emphasize the symbolic nature of eating binges as representing gratification of sexual and aggressive wishes. Self-deprecation and self-induced vomiting following binges may thus represent guilt-induced self-punishment for fantasized transgressions.

Psychologists have also noted that the binge-vomiting cycle may represent a ritual acceptance and taking in followed by a rejection of symbolic love objects. Bulimia may thus represent an attempt to control the external environment. Patients with bulimia are noted to have low self-esteem, and the vomiting may represent a symbolic purging of bad aspects of the self. Patients with bulimia tend to be overconcerned with body image and often have impaired object relationships that are recapitulated in their eating behaviors.

As with anorexia nervosa, cultural emphasis on a thin, youthful appearance as the singular and overly valued standard of beauty may contribute to the increasing incidence of this disorder.

Sexual abuse may also be a risk factor for the development of bulimia nervosa.

Treatment

Treatment approaches to bulimia nervosa are outlined in Table 26–4.

Multiple studies have been published describing the efficacy of both psychotherapy and psychopharmacology in the treatment of bulimia nervosa.

Table 26–4. Treatment approaches to bulimia nervosa.

1. *Evaluate and treat the medical complications associated with bulimia nervosa.* Replace fluid and electrolytes as necessary. Monitor electrolytes on regular basis. Refer for dental evaluation.

2. *Ascertain the mechanism of purging.* Educate patients regarding the medical dangers of chemical purgatives such as ipecac and baking soda as well as of diuretic and laxative abuse.

3. *Hospitalize when necessary.* If fluid and electrolyte balance cannot be maintained, if episodes of fainting occur, if concentration impairment makes employment or schoolwork impossible to perform, or if binge eating and purging behavior are the dominant activities in one's life, then a brief hospitalization to break the cycle and initiate treatment is necessary.

4. *Diagnose and treat comorbidity.* The presence of an affective disorder is an indication for treatment with an antidepressant medication if such treatment has not already been initiated on the basis of bulimic symptoms alone. Indeed, a trial of antidepressant medication is generally indicated for bulimia nervosa and is often effective even in the absence of concurrent affective disorder. Issues pertaining to personality disorders, when present, should be addressed in psychotherapy.

5. *Identify and address psychological and cognitive underpinnings of bulimic behavior.* Psychodynamically oriented and cognitive-behavioral treatments that address attitudes and feelings related to self and body images are effective treatment modalities. Such treatments may be particularly effective for many patients when combined with antidepressant medications. Support groups are also often helpful in the treatment of bulimia nervosa.

Dynamically based psychotherapies, particularly those that focus on interpersonal conflicts, eg, assertiveness, negotiation of needs, intimacy fears, etc, are effective, but cognitive-behavioral therapies are by far the most studied. Such therapies focus on the thought patterns and feeling states that lead to episodes of binge eating and purging with special emphasis on attitudes pertaining to body weight and shape. Coping strategies for handling the feelings associated with these attitudes, such as maintaining a food journal that includes both "what you are eating, and what's eating you," are suggested to the patient. Patients are expected to eat structured meals and their irrational fears regarding weight gain are addressed. Obsessive preoccupation with body shape and size is challenged, as patients are helped to better tolerate painful affect, and to be more direct in interpersonal problem solving.

Psychoeducational approaches are also helpful. For example, advising patients to not fast during the day, because fasting leads to binge eating (the normal tendency to purchase more groceries, including more "junk foods," if shopping while hungry is an easily recognized example of this phenomenon), usually results in symptom reduction. Patient education and cognitive-behavioral approaches can be easily implemented in primary care settings.

Group therapies, including psychodynamic, cognitive-behavioral, and self-help formats, are usually recommended.

The most dramatic reports of treatment success are of studies using pharmacological therapies, with antidepressant medications being particularly effective. Tricyclic antidepressants, monoamine oxidase inhibitors, and selective serotonin reuptake inhibitors such as fluoxetine, sertraline, and paroxetine have all shown efficacy in the treatment of bulimia nervosa, with responses ranging between reduction of binge eating and/or purging behavior to complete remission of symptoms. The antidepressant venlafaxine and the antiobsessional drug fluvoxamine also have proven efficacy. The antidepressant bupropion is contraindicated in anorexia nervosa and bulimia nervosa because of an increased risk of seizures. Studies show that if one antidepressant is ineffective or poorly tolerated, a trial of an alternative antidepressant may be successful. Mood-stabilizing drugs such as carbamazepine and valproic acid are sometimes helpful (lithium is contraindicated because of the electrolyte imbalance that is commonly present in bulimia nervosa). Anxiolytics may also play a helpful role in some cases, but their potential for abuse necessitates careful monitoring.

PICA & RUMINATON DISORDER OF INFANCY

Pica is the persistent (more than 1 month) ingestion of nonnutritive substances inappropriate for developmental age and unacceptable as cultural practice. Pica encompasses a wide variety of populations including toddlers who eat paint chips, pregnant women who consume starch and clay (the two largest groups), severely retarded children and adults who eat feces, and anxious adults who chew fingernails or pencils. Pica may be caused by poor nutrition, mineral deficiencies, or psychosocial deprivation. The condition is very responsive to nutritional and psychosocial intervention.

Rumination is a rare syndrome of infancy in which swallowed food is repeatedly returned to the mouth, pleasurably sucked on or rechewed, and then swallowed again. Rumination disorder is apparently caused by severe physical and emotional neglect, since it readily responds to substitution of caretakers. The behavior may be the deprived infant's attempt at self-stimulation. Rumination behavior has also been reported in adults, where it is usually associated with stress, such as acute medical illness or surgery, losses, such as a death in the family or being fired from a job, or psychiatric illness, such as depression. Effective treatments include biofeedback and relaxation exercises. Treatment for the associated stress disorders and depression with psychotherapy and/or psychopharmacology is also effective in reducing rumination behavior.

OBESITY

Simple obesity is not included among the eating disorders in *DSM-IV.* However, when there is evidence that psychological factors play a substantial etiological role in a specific case, this may be documented by noting "psychological factors affecting physical condition" in the diagnosis.

Symptoms & Signs

Despite the absence of clear-cut psychological and behavioral profiles associated with the development of obesity, there is a subgroup of obese individuals that manifests emotionally based patterns of overeating. Between 25% and 50% of participants in weight control programs report severe problems with binge eating, with women $1^1/_2$ times more likely to report this pattern than men. The eating binges are related to emotional stresses, and these individuals are more likely than nonbingers to have coexisting psychiatric disorders. *DSM-IV* established research criteria for diagnosing these individuals as having binge-eating disorder. This diagnosis is differentiated from bulimia nervosa only by the absence of compensatory behavior such as purging, fasting, or excessive exercising.

As many as one-third of obese patients have severe disparagement of body image. They feel that their bodies are grotesque and that others view them with hostility and contempt. Such feelings are reinforced by social attitudes, since fat people are often discriminated against and viewed by others as lazy, weak, self-destructive, and responsible for their condition. They also manifest low self-esteem and a negative self-concept.

Although many obese individuals tend to eat in response to emotional cues such as feelings of anxiety, fear, loneliness, boredom, and anger, so do many persons of normal weight. Obese individuals tend to chew less and eat more rapidly than other people, but both groups are strongly influenced by the eating behaviors of those around them.

Obese adults are usually physically less active than others, but this may be a consequence rather than a cause of obesity. Obese children are not less active than their normal-weight peers.

Dieting itself can be a significant biological and psychosocial stress factor. Dieting may cause feelings of frustration, agitation, irritability, and heightened emotional reactivity in otherwise normal persons. Thus, some of the emotional features traditionally attributed to obese persons may be a consequence of attempts to lose weight by dieting rather than a cause of their condition.

Psychiatric Comorbidity

As noted, as many as 50% of obese individuals engage in recurrent binge eating. Approximately one-fourth of obese binge eaters meet the diagnostic criteria for major depression compared with fewer than 5% of nonbingers. Obese binge eaters are twice as likely as nonbingers to have anxiety disorders, four times as likely to suffer from social phobia, and three times as likely to have drug or alcohol problems than nonbingers.

Medical Complications

It is estimated that more than 90% of cases of Type II diabetes, 70% of gallstones, 60–70% of coronary artery disease, 11% of breast cancers, and 10% of colon cancers are attributable to obesity.

Excess weight may cause low back pain, aggravation of osteoarthritis (particularly of the knees and ankles), and huge calluses on the feet and heels. Obesity may be associated with amenorrhea and other menstrual disturbances. The lower ratio of body surface area to body mass leads to impaired heat loss and increased sweating. Intertrigo in tissue folds, itching, and skin disorders are common. There is often mild to moderate swelling of hands and feet.

In massively obese persons, pressure of fatty tissue on the thorax combined with pressure of intra-abdominal fat on the diaphragm may reduce respiratory capacity and produce dyspnea on exertion. This condition may progress to the so-called pickwickian syndrome, characterized by hypoventilation with hypercapnia, hypoxia, and somnolence.

Natural History

Obesity can begin in childhood, adolescence, or adulthood. Amounts of body fat also increase with age even when weight remains constant. Obesity is usually a chronic and progressive condition. It is estimated that 300,000 deaths per year are caused by weight-related conditions, making obesity second only to cigarette smoking as the leading cause of preventable death in the United States.

Differential Diagnosis

Body mass index, or BMI, which is calculated by dividing weight in kilograms by height in meters squared, is the standard for determining obesity. A BMI under 25 is considered normal, with no weight-associated health risk. A BMI of 25–30 is considered overweight, with low to moderate health risk. Obesity is diagnosed by a BMI over 30, with high associated health risk. A BMI over 35 has a very high risk of weight-related health problems, and morbidly obese individuals (a BMI greater than 40) are at extremely high risk, with mortality rates up to 90% greater than those for normal-weight individuals.

In assessing obesity, the clinician must rule out medical illnesses such as hypothyroidism.

Prognosis

Although the prognosis for short-term weight loss has improved with the advent of new dieting and exercise strategies and the development of behavior modification programs, the long-term prognosis for losing excess weight and keeping it off remains poor, with few patients losing more than 40 pounds and most regaining the weight they lose. It is estimated that if an obese child does not achieve nearly normal weight by the end of adolescence, the odds against doing so later are 28:1. Morbidity and mortality rates for obese individuals increase in direct proportion to increases in the BMI.

Epidemiology

It is estimated that 34% of adults in the United States are obese. The prevalence increases with age up to age 50, at which point it falls sharply in accordance with the increased mortality rate. Obesity is more common in women, particularly after age 50, because of the higher mortality rate among obese men after that age. Obesity is also more common among minorities and low-income populations. It has been estimated that about 25% of children and 20% of adolescents are significantly overweight.

Family studies of obesity show that 40% of adolescents studied at age 15 who had one obese parent were obese, whereas 80% of those with two obese parents were obese. This compares to only a 10% incidence of obesity among adolescents whose parents are of normal weight. Studies of monozygotic and dizygotic twins suggest genetic factors, but environmental influences are also present. Adoption studies have shown conflicting evidence for genetic transmission. Evidence for the heritability of somatotypes is stronger than for obesity. This fact may be significant in that even a moderate degree of ectomorphic body habitus may protect against the development of obesity.

Etiology

Although there is great variability in weight among humans, individuals show remarkable consistency over time. Humans who agree to increase or decrease their weights for experimental purposes generally return to their starting weights when allowed to eat freely. Such observations have led to the theory that there is a biological set point for body weight in humans. This is supported by animal studies in which lesions of the ventromedial hypothalamus cause hypo- and hyperphagia, respectively. To the extent that the "set point theory" is applicable to humans, many obese individuals may be dieting in opposition to biological factors that make dieting far more difficult for them than for other people.

Weight gain can occur as a result of an increase in either the number or the size of fat cells. The fat cells of adults with juvenile-onset obesity may be about the same size as those of normal-weight persons, but there may be up to five times as many. Persons with adult-onset obesity may have a normal number of larger-than-normal fat cells. In studies in which fat cell number and size were determined, individuals tended to stop losing weight when fat cell size returned to normal. Since fat cells once formed do not disappear, fat cell number may determine the lower limit of weight for persons who by dieting have worked to reduce cell size to normal. There are two periods of cellular proliferation in normal-weight children: birth to 2 years of age and 10–14 years of age. In obese children, the period may extend well past 2 years of age, with consequent hypercellularity of fat tissue early in life. Although this may be partly under genetic control, the cellular theory of obesity thus has important implications regarding nutritional practices and weight regulation for children.

The gene governing the storage and breakdown of fat, and leptin, the protein it codes for, have been identified. Leptin has been shown to resolve obesity in genetically deficient mice, however, human trials have failed to consistently produce weight loss. There are multiple central nervous system chemical regulators of appetite, including several neuropeptides, the endogenous opiates, serotonin, dopamine, and norepinephrine. Their role in obesity, however, has not been established.

Early psychoanalytic theories of obesity held that obese individuals had unresolved dependency needs and were fixated at the oral level of psychosexual development. The symptoms of obesity were viewed as depressive equivalents, attempts to regain "lost" or frustrated nurturance and care. Recent studies have failed to demonstrate an increased incidence of psychopathological disorders in obese compared to normal-weight individuals. However, a subgroup of juvenile-onset obese subjects has gross disturbances in body image, ie, they view their bodies as hideous and loathsome and feel that others view them with contempt. They have a negative self-concept, are very self-conscious, and have impaired social functioning. Such experiences may contribute to the development and maintenance of obesity. Furthermore, since obese individuals are often discriminated against socially and are perhaps less often the object of sexual desire than normal-weight individuals, the maintenance of obesity may in some cases reflect an unconscious wish to remain isolated to avoid conflicts relating to sexuality or emotional intimacy.

Although there is no specific family constellation that predisposes to obesity, members of families lacking in warmth and love may use food and overeating as a substitute for love. The mothers in such families are often lonely individuals whose own childhoods were marked by social, economic, or emotional deprivation. Such mothers may unconsciously wish to have fat children. Identification with their "well-fed, well-cared-for" children may compensate for earlier deprivation. Such families may also equate physical size and the state of being "well fed" with physical and emotional strength. Obese children in such families may thus actually fear weight loss by concretely interpreting it as a loss of physical strength and emotional well-being.

The higher incidence of obesity among lower socioeconomic classes has been noted. In some societies in which food is scarce, obesity may be valued as a symbol of prosperity. In affluent countries such as the United States, value is instead placed on thinness, perhaps because foods low in calories but of high nutritional value are more expensive and unaffordable to the poor.

The definition of obesity may itself be culturally determined. Since 1943, revisions in standard height and weight charts have steadily lowered the ideal weights for women. The ideal weight for an average 5 foot 4 inch woman in 1943 was approximately 130 pounds; in 1980 it was under 120 pounds. Ideal weights for men have also been lowered, though not as much, and in 1974 the ideal weight for an average 5 foot 10 inch man was actually higher than the corresponding standard in 1943. These revisions have not been based on morbidity or mortality statistics but on measurements of the heights and weights of 25-year-old graduate students. Such standards do not take into account the fact that the percentage of body fat increases with age but instead reflect the fashion trends of the youthful, affluent college populations. For women, the steady decline in ideal weight reflects the upper-class emphasis on fashion model thinness as the standard of beauty. For men, there is

greater acceptance of a wider variety of body types. Attractive men may be thin, eg, long-distance runners and basketball players; or bulky, eg, weight lifters and football players. This broader range of acceptability may account for the less consistent downward trend in ideal weights for men listed in standard charts.

If the 1980 standards for ideal weights are accepted, and if obesity is defined as weight at least 20% above ideal, then the average American woman is by definition obese, and the average American man is on the verge of obesity.

Treatment

Table 26–5 summarizes treatment approaches to obesity.

Surgical procedures, such as intestinal bypass operations and gastric stapling, are effective in producing weight loss and in improving psychosocial functioning. These surgical procedures may also produce biological change, perhaps by lowering the body weight set point. However, risks of surgery and anesthesia, which are greater in obese individuals, plus the possibility of postoperative complications such as

---

Table 26–5. Treatment approaches to obesity.

1. *Assess and treat medical complications of obesity.* Patients must be monitored for hypertension, diabetes mellitus, heart disease, and fluid and electrolyte changes during weight loss.

2. *Assess diet and exercise habits.* Patients with binge-eating behaviors should be identified. A diet and exercise program should be prescribed in conjunction with an internist.

3. *Diagnose and treat psychiatric comorbidity.* Patients with affective disorders and binge-eating behaviors may be considered for treatment with antidepressant medications, particularly selective serotonin reuptake blockers.

4. *Identify psychological and cognitive underpinnings of obesity.* Cognitive-behavioral and dynamically oriented psychotherapies may be particularly helpful for obese individuals with affective disorders or with binge-eating patterns of behavior and for those who manifest extreme disparagement of self and body image. Support groups may also be helpful to these individuals.

5. *Consider antiobesity medications.* Appetite suppressants may be useful for some obese individuals who fail to respond to diet, exercise programs, and supportive psychotherapy. These medications must be reserved for significantly overweight patients (BMI >30), should be used for a short period of time, and should not be combined with serotonin reuptake blockers. Their use must be carefully monitored and they should be given only in conjunction with therapeutic modalities. Lipase inhibitors may also be helpful, but their safety and efficacy are still under investigation.

6. *Consider surgical procedures as last resort.* Surgical procedures such as gastric stapling, intestinal bypass, and intragastric balloons should be considered only for morbidly obese individuals who have failed all other treatment interventions.

malabsorption syndromes following bypass procedures should limit the indications for these interventions to the treatment of massive and morbid obesity that has not responded to conservative management. Wiring the jaws shut to prevent the intake of solid food may help some individuals, particularly when used in preparation for surgery. The use of intragastric balloons, a noninvasive method of gastric restriction, may also be effective. It should be noted that surgical interventions are never curative by themselves, as many patients regain the weight they lose within 2 years of the procedures.

Amphetamines were once widely prescribed as anorexigenic agents in the treatment of obesity. However, their high potential for abuse limits their use as diet aids. Furthermore, tolerance develops easily. Anorexigenic drugs with low abuse potential include sibutramine, diethylpropion, phentermine, and mazindol. Their effectiveness is modest and side effects, primarily anxiety and insomnia, are comparable.

The combination of the serotonin enhancer fenfluramine with the sympathomimetic amine phentermine was widely prescribed in the mid 1990s. The practice of prescribing "fen-phen" was abruptly halted in 1997 with the discovery of heart valve lesions in a large number of these patients. Fenfluramine has since been withdrawn from the market, and although phentermine remains available, it should not be combined with other serotonin-enhancing agents. Given the limited efficacy and significant risks of appetite suppressants, their use should be limited to patients who are significantly overweight (BMI greater than 30) and they should be used only for brief periods of time.

Other selective serotonin reuptake inhibitors may also be useful in the treatment of obesity, particularly with patients who engage in binge eating and who have coexisting affective disorders. Hope for the future may also lie with a new class of drugs called lipase inhibitors, which act directly on the gastrointestinal tract to block the absorption of fat.

Exercise regimens are recommended as part of most treatment plans. Exercise is helpful not only because of the increase in caloric expenditure but because physical activity (in otherwise sedentary individuals) is associated with decreased appetite and increased basal metabolism. This latter effect may offset the estimated 15–30% decrease in basal metabolic rate that occurs with caloric restriction and weight loss from dieting. Exercise also increases the proportion of weight loss from fat as opposed to lean body tissue. Exercise combined with low-calorie diets will result in weight loss; the difficulty, of course, is in motivating patients to comply with a disciplined regimen.

Support groups such as Overeaters Anonymous and Weight Watchers may be helpful in motivating some individuals to lose weight. In recent years, behavior modification programs have been shown to be effective in reducing the high dropout rate associated with most weight reduction programs, particularly when deposits of money are required and sums are refunded with regular attendance or weight loss. Behavioral programs have been shown to be effective in the short run, but weight tends to be regained. Psychoanalysis and psychoanalytically oriented psychotherapy have not traditionally been regarded as being effective in the treatment of obesity. In their classic 1983 study, Rand and Stunkard suggest a more optimistic outlook. Of 84 men and women treated by 72 psychoanalysts, 72 had weight losses comparable to what was achieved by other methods, even though only about 6% of obese persons who entered treatment did so because of their obesity. Analysts also reported dramatic improvements in body image perceptions in their patients. Whereas 40% of obese patients showed marked body image disturbances at the start of treatment, only 14% continued to have such problems at termination. This study suggests that psychoanalytic psychotherapy may be effective in some cases, particularly for patients with disturbances of body image and self-concept.

SUMMARY

Abnormal eating behavior may arise as an attempt to calm and soothe unpleasant emotions, as an effort to resolve intrapsychic conflicts around aggression, sexuality, and interpersonal relationships, or as an attempt to act out issues on behalf of a dysfunctional family. Biological factors may play a role by directly affecting the physiology of fat accumulation or indirectly by predisposing to affective disorders (anxiety and depression) commonly associated with eating disorders. Cultural factors such as society's preoccupation with youth and thinness also play a major role. Eating disorders clearly provide a clinical paradigm for the biopsychosocial model.

REFERENCES & SUGGESTED READINGS

Agras WS: Pharmacotherapy of bulimia nervosa and binge eating disorder: Longer-term outcomes. Psychopharm Bull 1997;33:433.

Bruch H: Perceptual and conceptual disturbances in anorexia nervosa. Psychosom Med 1962;24:187.

Carlat DJ et al: Eating disorders in males: A report of 135 patients. Am J Psychiatry 1997;154:1127.

Fairburn CG, Wilson GT (editors): *Binge Eating: Nature, Assessment and Treatment.* Guilford Press, 1996.

Federman DG, Kirsner RS, Federman GS: Pica: Are you hungry for the facts? Connecticut Med 1997;61:207.

Garner D, Garfinkle P (editors): *Handbook of Treatment for Eating Disorders.* Guilford Press, 1997.

Gull WW: Anorexia nervosa. Trans Clin Soc (Lond) 1874; 7:22.

Herzog DB et al: Comorbidity and outcome in eating disorders. Psychiatr Clin North Am 1996;19:843.

Rand CSW, Stunkard AJ: Obesity and psychoanalysis: Treatment and four-year follow-up. Am J Psychiatry 1983;140:1140.

Soykan I et al: The rumination syndrome: Clinical and manometric profile, therapy, and long-term outcome. Dig Dis Sci 1997;42:1886.

Steinmen G: *Revolution from Within: A Book of Self Esteem.* Little, Brown, 1993.

Thiels C et al: Guided self-change for bulimia nervosa incorporating use of a self-care manual. Am J Psychiatry 1998;155:947.

Walsh TB et al: Medication and psychotherapy in the treatment of bulimia nervosa. Am J Psychiatry 1997;154:523.

Werne J (editor): *Treating Eating Disorders.* Jossey-Bass, 1996.

Wolf N: *The Beauty Myth: How Images of Beauty Are Used Against Women.* Anchor, 1992.

Factitious Disorders

27

Stuart J. Eisendrath, MD, & Gemma G. Guillermo, MD

The term "factitious" means "willfully produced." Factitious disorders are disorders in which the individual produces the signs or symptoms of illness. The illness may be manifested either by physical or psychological symptoms. The patient's primary goal is to receive medical, surgical, or psychiatric care; secondary motivations involve obtaining drugs or financial assistance.

In this century formal attention to these disorders began with Asher, who in 1951 coined the term **Munchausen's syndrome** to denote a disorder observed in certain patients who traveled widely in England, presenting at hospitals and surgeries with plausible but dramatic stories of medical illness that resulted in numerous hospitalizations and operations. The clinical histories of these patients and their diagnoses revealed that their primary purpose was to seek and receive medical care rather than to be cured. Asher noted that the patients told elaborate tales, often in a quite entertaining manner; he therefore named the syndrome after Baron von Münchhausen, an eighteenth-century German soldier and raconteur known for his tall tales.

Patients with Munchausen's syndrome usually have a history of repeated hospitalizations extending over years, have adopted the role of patient as a career, and have notable characteristics of sociopathy, imposture, perigrination, and marked resistance to treatment. However, Reich and coworkers (1983) found that these patients represent a small subset of those with factitious disorder with physical symptoms, the majority of whom do not have Munchausen's syndrome, but instead have intermittent and mild physical illness (eg, factitious dermatitis), do not seek invasive interventions, often have stable family and work roles, and have episodes of illness that usually occur in reaction to a specific stressor.

Other patients with factitious disorders produce psychological symptoms to obtain psychiatric care. Still others display both physical and psychological factitious symptoms, either alternately or concurrently. Finally, some patients act to produce illness in others; usually it involves mothers doing so with their children, but it can also involve caregivers in a healthcare setting who produce illness or even death in their patients. These last individuals are categorized under the heading of factitious disorder by proxy. However, it has been suggested that these individuals are criminals and should be categorized with a V code diagnosis and not a psychiatric disorder. The *DSM-IV* criteria for the factitious disorders are outlined in Table 27–1.

FACTITIOUS DISORDER WITH PHYSICAL SYMPTOMS

Symptoms & Signs

Any organ system will serve as a site of pain or other symptom for a patient with factitious illness, and histories compatible with virtually every known disease have been described by these patients. Laboratory abnormalities have also been produced, including anemia, hypokalemia, hematuria, hypoglycemia, coagulopathies, and hyperamylasuria. The choice of

Table 27–1. *DSM-IV* diagnostic criteria for chronic factitious disorder.

Factitious disorder

A. Intentional production or feigning of physical or psychological signs or symptoms.

B. The motivation for the behavior is to assume the sick role.

C. External incentives for the behavior (such as economic gain, avoiding legal responsibility, or improving physical well-being, as in malingering) are absent.

D. The behavior is not better accounted for by another mental disorder.

Code based on type

300.16 With Predominantly Psychological Signs and Symptoms: If psychological signs predominate in the clinical presentation.

300.17 With Predominantly Physical Signs and Symptoms: If physical signs and symptoms predominate in the clinical presentation.

300.18 With Combined Psychological and Physical Signs and Symptoms: If both psychological and physical signs and symptoms are present but neither predominate in the clinical presentation.

300.19 Factitious Disorder Not Otherwise Specified: This category is for disorders with factitious symptoms that do not meet criteria for a specific factitious disorder. For example, factitious disorder by proxy, ie, the intentional production or feigning of physical signs or symptoms in another person who is under the individual's care for the purpose of indirectly assuming the sick role.

organ system is limited only by the patient's creativity and available resources. The means by which patients produce evidence of illness may be startling to the unsuspecting medical practitioner. One patient produced an elevated rectal temperature by alternately relaxing and contracting the anal sphincter to generate heat. Another patient produced spurious evidence of pancreatitis by spitting saliva into his urine sample so that the salivary amylase would elevate urinary amylase readings. Patients have produced hypoglycemia by injecting insulin, and the spurious source was detected only by peptide studies.

A patient with Munchausen's syndrome may present to the emergency room with a classic history of myocardial infarction, bleeding ulcer, pulmonary embolism, etc. On admission, these patients often loudly demand attention from the medical staff and may request high doses of narcotic analgesics. They are usually familiar with medical terminology and procedures and may even suggest additional diagnostic tests to the attending physician. An important recurring symptom pattern is that these patients frequently request invasive diagnostic or therapeutic procedures. They often ask for surgery, saying, "I know that's the only thing that will help me."

Patients with Munchausen's syndrome, who represent a subset of the broader category of chronic factitious illness, frequently travel from hospital to hospital, often over wide distances. Typical patients with chronic factitious illness do not travel unless forced to do so, usually because of rejection by a local hospital or physician. When traveling, these patients often exhibit certain sociopathic characteristics such as lying without showing any feelings of guilt. They often take on the role of impostor, assuming the identity of a war hero, a lawyer, or even a doctor, and then disclose clues to the imposture, since part of what they are trying to achieve is to reveal their ability to dupe the hospital staff. When the imposture is discovered, they move on to repeat the pattern before a new group in a new hospital or city. Characteristically, these patients abuse narcotic analgesics and are strident in their demands for them. If the staff is reluctant to comply with their requests, they become angry and arrogant. If confronted with damaging documentation of their overuse of drugs or the possibility that their disease is factitious, these patients typically threaten litigation and leave the hospital against medical advice.

Once the suspicion of false illness arises, detection is usually not difficult. A patient with bacterial abscesses has them only in areas accessible to self-inoculation. Unusual bacterial flora are noted on culture of the abscesses and indicate oral or fecal contamination. The major clue to detection lies in examination of the patient's background. In almost all cases, patients with factitious illness have worked in the health care field. When a patient with such a background presents with a chronic medical problem not fully explained by normal pathophysiological mechanisms, the possibility of factitious disease should be considered.

The psychiatric symptoms of these patients are quite varied. Normal individuals, given sufficient emotional distress, might resort to factitious disease as a coping mechanism. Patients with borderline personality who tend to act impulsively and have difficulty tolerating anger or depression may briefly decompensate into psychosis. Borderline patients tend to view everybody, including the staff on the medical-surgical floor, as either "good people" or "bad people" and may struggle to escape from or defeat the "bad ones." There is often controversy among the staff, with some taking the role of advocate for the patient and others acting with retaliatory anger.

Patients with factitious illness can produce illness at three levels. At the first level individuals give a **fictitious history** consistent with a known diagnosis, but with no supporting physical evidence. The second level involves the **simulation of signs of illness;** for example, an individual pricks a finger with a pin and squeezes a few drops of blood into a urine sample to give the appearance of hematuria and support a factitious history of renal stone. The most dangerous level involves patients who actually produce **abnormal pathophysiological states.** Individuals in this category take anticoagulants, thyroid, or insulin or inject themselves with foreign substances.

Natural History

Because only a few patients with chronic factitious illness with physical symptoms have had the benefit of careful psychological study, the natural history of the disorder is unclear. Most patients have a deprived early childhood, and many have had hospitalizations during the first 5 years of life for some medical problem. Children who stay home from school feigning illness are at risk for this disorder. Clinically significant factitious illness usually develops in the teen or early adult years.

Differential Diagnosis

Factitious disorder is an example of an abnormal illness-affirming behavior. Other examples of illness-affirming behaviors include hypochondriasis, somatization disorder, conversion disorders, somatoform pain disorders (psychalgia), and malingering. All of these must be included in the differential diagnosis of factitious disorder. The most important diagnostic problem for the clinician is to differentiate between true medical illness and factitious disorder. Even people with clear histories of factitious disorder develop medical or surgical disorders that must always be suitably investigated. Patients who perform self-destructive acts requiring medical care must also be distinguished. For example, the schizophrenic patient who performs some act of self-mutilation as part of a delusional psychosis certainly has produced the physical illness, but this differs from factitious disorders in that the behavior results from acting in accordance with the delusion (eg, to escape persecutory voices) rather than acting to obtain medical care. Other behavior, such as persistent substance abuse or suicide attempts may also cause the patient to receive medical attention, however, this not the primary goal.

Individuals with illness-affirming behavior originate or amplify the idea that they are ill in order to achieve unconscious goals. As shown in Table 27–2, in patients with hypochondriasis, somatization disorder, conversion disorders, and somatoform pain disorders, the production of illness-affirming symptoms or signs is entirely unconscious. These patients are not aware that they are exaggerating or focusing on normal bodily sensations. They are also unaware of the motivations for this behavior. An observer who is aware of the environmental situation might make psychodynamic inferences about the goal of such behavior, such as hysterical paralysis serving to avoid family conflict.

The distinction between malingering and factitious disorder can be subtle and the terms are often used interchangeably among clinicians, which is incorrect. The malingerer is aware of the conscious production of the signs or symptoms of a disease state as well as the motive for this production. The motive most often involves an external incentive such as avoiding work, evading a distasteful environment (eg, military service or jail), obtaining money (from lawsuits or insurance claims), or appropriating medications (eg, opioids). An outside observer would be able to recognize the malingerer's motivation without having to make a psychological formulation.

Patients with factitious illness are aware that they produce the illness but do not know why. This is analogous to the phobic patient who consciously avoids the feared object but cannot explain why. Motivation for feigning illness is entirely unconscious, and an observer would be unaware of a reason for the behavior without resorting to some psychological inference. An algorithm for differentiating abnormal illness-affirming behaviors is shown in Figure 27–1.

Prognosis

The prognosis for factitious disease with physical symptoms varies considerably. For the majority of

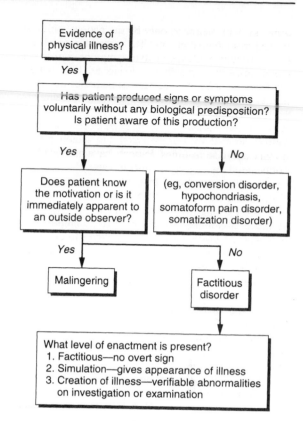

Figure 27–1. Decision tree for the identification of factitious physical disorders. (Reprinted, with permission, from Eisendrath, 1984.)

patients without Munchausen's syndrome (Illustrative Cases 1 and 2), there is good potential for successful psychiatric treatment. For patients with the full syndrome, however, the prognosis is dismal, since they appear to have adopted patienthood as their sole career. Their lack of social supports, wandering, and sociopathy contribute to the refractory nature of their condition. It appears that the intermittency of illness production rather than the level of illness production is the best predictor of response to psychiatric intervention.

Illustrative Case 1

A 30-year-old woman who worked as an x-ray technician was evaluated for skin lesions—superficial excoriations surrounded by normal skin, occurring over the inner thigh and pubic mound. A gynecological assessment for spotty bleeding revealed similar vaginal lesions. Her symptoms had developed a few weeks after she underwent a total abdominal hysterectomy and bilateral salpingo-oophorectomy for a ruptured ectopic pregnancy—her first attempt at childbearing.

The dermatologist used skin patching to determine that the lesions were factitious and referred the pa-

Table 27–2. Differential diagnosis of factitious disorder.

	Illness Production	Motivation
Hypochondriasis, somatization disorder, conversion reaction, pain disorder with psychological factors	Unconscious	Unconscious
Factitious disorder	Conscious	Unconscious
Malingering	Conscious	Conscious

tient for psychiatric consultation. The psychiatrist learned from the patient and her husband that she had suffered significant depressive symptoms since her surgery. She noted that she "no longer felt like a whole woman" and had lost interest in sex. Her lesions were seen as an attempt to solve her problem by believing that "something's wrong down there." The vaginal bleeding was an attempt to produce a semblance of menstruation. She was referred for ongoing psychotherapy to help her deal with her sense of "lost womanhood."

Illustrative Case 2

A 30-year-old divorced registered nurse with a history of abdominal pain, nausea and vomiting, and hematemesis was admitted to a general hospital for evaluation. At the admissions desk she said, "I think I'll need surgery." She reported a 10-year history of peptic ulcer disease, for which she had been treated surgically. She had also had a cholecystectomy and several laparotomies for possible bowel obstruction. She described several episodes of septic shock for which no originating locus of infection had been found. She had several surgery scars on her abdomen and numerous cutdown sites on her arms and legs. There was a tenderness to deep palpation in the epigastric region but no rebound tenderness. Stool was negative for occult blood. Endoscopy revealed modest gastric irritation, presumably secondary to bile reflux. Because one of her physicians felt there was a strong psychosocial component to her pain complaints, psychiatric consultation was obtained. The patient was at first angry about the consultation but agreed to participate. She complained to the psychiatrist that pain precluded intercourse with her boyfriend. In fact, the current pain had begun just when the relationship had become a sexual one.

The family history disclosed that she had been reared by a cold, distant, and competitive mother who frequently criticized and humiliated her. The patient's father had raped her, according to her report, on two occasions when she was 12 and 13 years old. The patient felt guilty for perhaps having "unconsciously encouraged" her father's advances.

The consultant suggested psychotherapy and doubted that surgery would affect her pain complaints, because they seemed to serve an important psychological function in relieving sexual guilt. Surgery was performed, however, and she did well until 6 days postoperatively, when she went into septic shock. One day prior to that event, the patient's boyfriend had brought her a diamond engagement ring. No cause was discovered for the patient's sepsis. Blood cultures yielded multiple organisms. In reviewing her earlier history of septic episodes and in exploring the similarity between the current episode of sepsis and the patient's previously reported episodes, the psychiatrist gently explored the possi-

bility that she had felt guilty about the engagement. After several sessions, she admitted she had injected urine intravenously because she felt guilty about her boyfriend being too nice to her. The patient was then referred for ongoing outpatient psychotherapy.

In psychotherapy, she admitted that many of her symptoms were factitious but she could not fully understand why she had committed the acts. With treatment she was able to understand that the pain of her illnesses and surgery served psychologically to relieve her of guilt through self-punishment.

This patient had not been specifically confronted about her factitious disorder. Establishing rapport and suggesting that her engagement precipitated her septicemia allowed her to admit her actions and enter psychotherapy.

Epidemiology

Only a few studies have investigated the prevalence of factitious disease. Factitious illness may be incorrectly diagnosed or unidentified because of its typical psychopathological features, in particular the use of aliases, hospital wanderings, and abrupt self-discharges from hospitals without medical follow-up. The difficulty in identifying cases of factitious illness is even greater when the patient resorts to factitious symptoms rarely and intermittently. Factitious illness may also occur in patients who have documented organic illness, in which case diagnosis may be even more difficult. On the other hand, some individuals tend to be overreported in the medical literature as they go from hospital to hospital.

The best epidemiologic studies have been described in patients with fever of unknown origin. In a study at the National Institutes of Health, over 9% of such patients were diagnosed as having factitious fevers. A similar study at Stanford indicated factitious fever in 3% of such patients. It appears likely that factitious disorders are more often seen at tertiary care centers where complex diagnostic problems are referred for evaluation.

Some reports indicate that this disorder occurs with increased (3:1) frequency in females, but in individuals with the full Munchausen's syndrome, males appear to outnumber females by a ratio of 2:1. In all studies, the health care field was the usual occupation of patients with factitious illness: nurses, ward clerks, physical therapists, x-ray technicians, and (less often) physicians.

Etiology & Pathogenesis

The psychodynamic origin of adult factitious disorders is believed to lie in early childhood experiences. Emotional and sometimes physical deprivation in childhood is a common feature of the developmental history. Early deprivation leads to a disturbance of self-image in these patients. Many authors have noted that patients with factitious disorders often have borderline personality characteristics. The borderline patient has a developmental difficulty during the separation-individuation (toddler) phase of childhood. When separation is not successfully achieved, the individual enters adult life with a poor self-image, feeling "needy" and dependent on others but expecting that their needs will continue to be frustrated by authority figures.

The history often includes a period of hospitalization during early childhood, when the patient's needs were met by nurses and doctors who provided care and kindly ministrations. In other instances, a childhood hospitalization (and perhaps operation) was extremely frightening to a helpless and vulnerable toddler. Thus, childhood hospitalization may serve as a positive reinforcing experience or a major traumatic event. In still other instances, a patient's sense of vulnerability and helplessness results from the loss of a parent who was hospitalized.

The developmental history may uncover several major themes in a patient with factitious illness. The first involves the patient's sense of needing to be taken care of. The hospital provides a socially sanctioned way to receive bodily ministrations and be an object of concern to symbolic parental figures, mainly doctors and nurses. Because of past experiences, however, the patient's desire to be taken care of is often accompanied by expectations of disappointment. Thus, these patients frequently present with a veneer of eager compliance that covers an underlying attitude of hostility and wariness.

Masochism is the second major theme. Anger over past deprivations often makes these individuals anxious and guilty. Invasive operations and diagnostic procedures serve as "punishment" to relieve feelings of guilt; they also enable to patient to replay early childhood experiences during which the parents provided care as well as pain. Doctors and nurses thus represent parental figures of early childhood. Occasionally, these patients also develop positive feelings, which may have sexual features, toward people in their lives, including their doctors and nurses. This causes just as much discomfort as their anger and hostility. Invasive and painful procedures may then serve to assuage feelings of guilt about positive as well as negative responses. Certain behaviors may then function as punishment for those feelings or as a symbolic representation of the wishes involved with them. For example, a female patient who feels guilty about sexual arousal may invite a male physician to operate on her, an act that has both sexual and punitive symbolism.

A third major theme is mastery of an early trauma. Hospitalized children may feel extremely vulnerable. When repeating the experience as adults, they may hope to control the situation as they could not in childhood. This theme is often observable when patients appear to be unconcerned about their clinical status as physicians feverishly perform diagnostic workups.

The patient with factitious illness may also utilize disease to master a relationship with a parental figure. The feigned illness may provide retaliatory gratification, represented by victory over authority figures who are unable to control the symptoms. In accomplishing this, the patient ignores the fact that the victory is a Pyrrhic one. It is the patient who is disabled and ill.

Patients with factitious illness commonly allow their fabrications and actions to be discovered. They may leave a syringe on the bedside table or let other patients see them performing their deceptive actions. By allowing themselves to be discovered, the patients show their contempt for the staff while at the same time provoking the staff to anger. The staff's first reaction may be a feeling of having been duped and deceived. They may then react angrily by confronting or immediately discharging the patient; this provides justification for the patient's belief in mistreatment by parental figures.

Treatment

There is growing evidence that patients with factitious disorders are responsive to psychiatric interventions. Although patients with Munchausen's syndrome are generally considered untreatable, the vast majority of patients with factitious disorder do not fall in this category.

After the factitious disorder has been identified by the primary physician, treatment should begin with a psychiatric consultation. Since patient treatment is based on an implicit foundation of honesty, the consultant must allow the staff and the physician to ventilate their anger at having been deceived and duped by these patients. The psychiatric consultant can help inform the staff about the psychopathological features of the patient's illness. This is important because it prevents staff members from acting out their anger. Operations and invasive diagnostic procedures should be avoided unless clearly indicated. If the staff does not act out of anger, the first step toward treating the patient has been accomplished—recognizing that the factitious behavior is a psychopathological symptom, not merely a hostile attack on the physician.

Two broad approaches are usually taken by psychiatric consultants in dealing with these patients. A standard approach has been to have the primary physician confront the patient diagnosed with the factitious disorder in a nonpunitive manner: "We know you have been producing this disorder, and we realize that you must be in great distress to have used this way of getting help. We'd like you to have a more appropriate form of help from our psychiatrist." The psychiatrist, who is often present during the confrontation, then tries to assist the patient by acting as an ally rather than as a prosecutor.

Confrontational approaches often produced few results except to humiliate the patient and drive him or her to another hospital; nonconfrontational techniques have recently been used with more success. These techniques involve interpreting the patient's behavior and feelings in terms of how they affect the patient's physical condition, without specifically revealing to the patient that their condition has been diagnosed as factitious (see Illustrative Case 2). This often helps these patients feel better understood and may lead them to enter psychotherapy and eventually admit to the factitious nature of the disorder on their own.

Patients diagnosed with factitious disorder can be referred for ongoing psychiatric management once the medical condition permits discharge. Most choose outpatient rather than inpatient psychiatric treatment. It is often quite helpful to involve the family, since valuable information can sometimes be obtained from them. The family may also be helpful in setting behavioral limits once the patient leaves the hospital. Occasionally, antidepressants and, more rarely, antipsychotics have been utilized with success in patients who show evidence of underlying depression or psychosis.

Management of patients diagnosed with factitious disorder requires a psychotherapist familiar with patients who act out. These patients need substantial assistance in learning to talk about their feelings rather than acting out their distress. Therapy is aimed at increasing the patient's autonomy and self-esteem while diminishing the sense of helplessness, vulnerability, and anger.

Another nonconfrontational approach is to offer the patient a face-saving way to relinquish the factitious symptom. For example, the patient might be told that unless the condition improves with a new medical treatment (eg, a trial of medication, a final surgical procedure, relaxation training, or biofeedback training) the physician's suspicion of factitious disorder will be confirmed. This strategy allows the patient the option of recovering without necessarily admitting that the disorder was factitious.

FACTITIOUS DISORDER WITH PSYCHOLOGICAL SYMPTOMS

Symptoms & Signs

Patients with factitious disorder with psychological symptoms often present with manifestations a lay person would regard as typical of psychiatric illness (Table 27–1). Recently there have been reports of individuals presenting to Veterans Administration hospitals with factitious complaints of posttraumatic stress disorder. On investigation, it was discovered that many of these patients were never in combat, never in Vietnam, and sometimes never even in the military. Rigorous review of medical records often revealed the diagnosis. Group therapy with true Vietnam combat veterans also often led to identification of these factitious patients by the veterans.

Patients with factitious psychiatric disorders may be familiar with psychiatric entities and present to psychiatric hospitals with plausible histories. The motive is the wish to assume the role of a psychiatric patient. The unconscious motivations are similar to those of the patient with chronic factitious disorder with physical symptoms. Popli et al (1992) described several of these cases. One difference between psychological and physical disorders is that verification of the diagnosis of psychological disorder rests with the patient: unless the patient admits falsifying the psychiatric history or there is conclusive psychological diagnostic testing (requiring the patient's cooperation), it may be impossible to prove that the patient does not have a psychiatric disease. With factitious physical disorders, there is usually some objective evidence that does not rely on the patient's cooperation. The patient who feigns psychiatric factitious disorder often has a true psychiatric disorder (eg, borderline personality disorder), but not the one being feigned. It also appears that some patients can present with both factitious psychological and factitious physical disorders at either the same time or in alternating fashion.

Differential Diagnosis

The major differential diagnostic problem is malingering. Malingerers are aware of their motivation, whereas the motivation for illness in patients with factitious disorder is unconscious and can be arrived at only by inference. Other differential diagnoses to be considered include brief reactive psychosis, schizophrenia, and organic psychosis. Occasionally, patients with borderline personality disorder may decompensate into psychosis for brief periods and may be difficult to differentiate from those with factitious disorder. The environmental context as well as an adequate history corroborated by family or friends usually clarifies the diagnosis.

Prognosis, Epidemiology, Etiology, & Treatment

Little is known about the incidence of factitious psychological disorders. In one study (Nicholson and Roberts, 1994), the prevalence of psychological factitious disorders was found to be 0.14% of inpatient psychiatric admissions. The causes, psychodynamics, and treatment are probably similar to those of patients with chronic factitious illnesses of a physical nature. Patients with factitious psychological disorder typically come from emotionally depriving families. They are a bit closer to treatment, since they have presented themselves in a psychiatric setting to begin with. However, the only completed outcome study (Pope et al, 1982) suggests that patients with factitious psychological disorders have a poorer prognosis than if they had a true major mental disorder. As the study concluded, "It appears that acting crazy may bode more ill than being crazy." All of their patients had recurrent hospitalizations and poor social functioning.

Illustrative Case

A 40-year-old man presented to a psychiatric emergency service at a general hospital complaining of severe depression. He described severe early morning awakening, loss of appetite, marked weight loss, and suicidal ideation. He was admitted to the inpatient psychiatric unit, where he told his attending psychiatrist that he had had similar episodes of depression in the past (in a distant state) that had responded to antidepressants and inpatient psychiatric treatment. He claimed he had no living relatives, that his wife had recently died of breast cancer, and that her death had precipitated the current episode of depression.

By chance, a new psychiatrist on the unit recognized the patient from another hospital in a nearby city. The psychiatrist told the staff that the patient was well known for feigning psychiatric illness. When not being observed by psychiatric staff, the patient showed no signs of clinical depression. The patient was known to have several brothers and sisters and had never been married. Confronted with this information, the patient's apparent mood abruptly shifted from depression to defensive anger. He threatened litigation and signed out against medical advice. Since the patient was already receiving a disability pension, no apparent motivation for his behavior was determined during the hospitalization.

FACTITIOUS DISORDER WITH PHYSICAL & PSYCHOLOGICAL SYMPTOMS

Some patients with factitious disorder display both physical and psychological symptoms, either alternately or concurrently. Most commonly, these patients initially feign a physical disorder; when this is discovered, they then feign psychiatric symptoms. For example, a 34-year-old man was admitted to a coronary care unit to rule out myocardial infarction. When it became clear that he had had numerous similarly negative evaluations, he immediately claimed he was depressed because his wife and children had been killed in an automobile accident. Family members revealed that he had never been married. The treatment strategy for these individuals usually consists primarily of psychotherapy.

FACTITIOUS DISORDERS NOT OTHERWISE SPECIFIED

This category is reserved for factitious disorders that do not meet criteria for any other specification in this category. The most commonly recognized disorder in this group is factitious disorder by proxy (FDP), which is defined in the *DSM-IV* as "the deliberate production or feigning of physical or psychological signs or symptoms in another person who is under the individual's care." The perpetrator in FDP may be a parent, babysitter, other relative, or, in an occupational setting, a health caregiver. Most frequently, however, the disorder involves a mother producing signs and symptoms of disease in one or more of her children. Since Meadow (1977) first described this entity, it has become widely recognized in pediatric centers.

In this syndrome, a child (typically an infant) appears to have a disorder often involving induced or simulated bleeding, seizures, apnea, diarrhea, vomiting, fever, electrolyte disturbance, or rash. There is usually a history of multiple visits to physicians and emergency rooms. Often other children in the family may have had similar episodes of illness or unexplained death. Typically the mother appears as highly involved and knowledgeable about her child's disorder. In many instances the mother appears "perfect," and the family physician is usually astounded to learn of the true diagnosis. The illness improves or vanishes if the mother is removed from the child. There are often inconsistencies in the history the mother gives. Another clue to the presence of this disorder is a mother who appears more concerned with the medical care, such as seeking invasive testing, than with her child's emotional state (Rand, 1993). The differential diagnosis for this entity is usually a rare disease that is not easily diagnosed.

This disorder is generally thought to be related to serious emotional disturbance in the mother such as a borderline personality disorder. Psychosis, however, is rarely present in the mothers, who are typically socially adept. In some instances, the mother may be attempting to act out sadistic impulses toward the child as a displacement from herself or others. In other instances, the mother may be seeking to atone for some unconscious guilt. Schreier (1992) believes these mothers may be using the child to actuate a sadomasochistic relationship with the pediatrician, who is seen as a symbolic parental figure. When the disorder arises in the setting of divorce, it may be accompanied by false accusations by the mother of sexual abuse perpetrated on the child by the father (Meadow, 1993).

Once diagnosed, the treatment of this condition begins with notification of child abuse authorities. In many instances criminal charges are appropriate. Usually psychiatric treatment for the mother is indicated, and this is usually long-term psychotherapy under court supervision. In the case of children, the child is often separated from the mother and returned, even for visits, only under carefully monitored situations. In some cases family therapy involving the child and the father may be useful. The child, if old enough, usually needs psychotherapeutic efforts, particularly if he or she had actively colluded with the perpetrator. The management of FDP requires well-coordinated efforts from social, pediatric, and psychiatric services, as well as the courts.

In addition to mothers producing symptoms in children, FDP appears to exist within occupational settings. Media attention and published studies have been focusing on growing evidence of hospital epidemics of FDP, most involving registered nurses being linked to an epidemic of suspicious deaths in hospital intensive care units. In 1988, the first systematic investigation of nurses charged with serial murder

was published by Yorker. Since then, the use of FDP as a paradigm for understanding serial deaths caused by health care professionals has been gaining acceptance. Accurate diagnosis of FDP involves collecting corroborative data from sources other than the individual's caretaker. Family physicians, fathers, siblings, and court videotaping have been extremely helpful in cases involving children. Although a rare phenomenon, improved surveillance and heightened recognition of the phenomenon may uncover cases of FDP in an occupational setting.

REFERENCES & SUGGESTED READINGS

Aduan RP et al: Factitious fever and self-induced infection. Ann Intern Med 1979;90:230.

Asher R: Munchausen's syndrome. Lancet 1951;1:339.

Bursten B: On Munchausen's syndrome. Arch Gen Psychiatry 1965;13:261.

Eisendrath SJ: Factitious illness: A clarification. Psychosomatics 1984;25:119.

Feldman M, Eisendrath SJ: *The Spectrum of Factitious Disorders.* American Psychiatric Press, 1996.

Gavin H: *Feigned and Factitious Diseases.* Churchill, 1843.

Meadow R: Munchausen by proxy. Lancet 1977;2:342.

Meadow R: False allegations of abuse and Munchausen syndrome by proxy. Arch Dis Child 1993;68:444.

Nicholson SD, Roberts GA: Patients who (need to) tell stories. Br J Hosp Med 1994;51:546.

Pankratz L: Continued appearance of factitious posttraumatic stress disorder. (Letter) Am J Psychiatry 1990;137:165.

Pope H, Jonas JM, Jones B: Factitious psychosis: Phenomenology, family history, and long-term outcome of nine patients. Am J Psychiatry 1982;139:1480.

Popli AP, Prakash SM, Dewan MJ: Factitious disorders with psychological symptoms. J Clin Psychiatry 1992;53:315.

Rand DC: Munchausen syndrome by proxy: A complex type of emotional abuse responsible for some false allegations of child abuse in divorce. Issues Child Abuse Accus 1993;5:135.

Reich P, Gottfried LA: Factitious disorders in a teaching hospital. Ann Intern Med 1983;99:240.

Schreier HA: The perversion of mothering: Munchausen syndrome by proxy. Bull Menninger Clin 1992;56:421.

Shafer N, Shafer R: Factitious diseases including Munchausen's syndrome. NY State J Med 1980;80:594.

Yorker BC: Nurses accused of murder. Am J Nurs 1988;88:1327.

Childhood Mental Disorders & Child Psychiatry

28

Roberta Huberman, MD, Linda Cahill, MD, & Mary Witt, MD, MPH

Child psychiatry is a relatively young specialty, with the first Board certification examination conducted in 1959. However, the disorders child psychiatrists treat have been recognized for centuries. In the 1400s there were references to nightmares, bedwetting, and children's good and bad mental habits. A treatise from 1799 contains a description of a 10-year-old boy who was "an unrelenting foe to all china, glass and crockery," and "incapable of forming a friendship and inaccessible to any kindness shown him."

The roots of child psychiatry lie in diverse areas including pediatrics, adult psychiatry, the juvenile justice system, schools, child welfare, psychology, psychometrics, ethnology, the mental hygiene movement, and child guidance clinics.

Child psychiatrists address numerous problems: Why is a child worried, unhappy, or nervous? Why do some infants fail to thrive although otherwise physically well? What is the nature of some children's impaired intellectual functioning, and why do others have problems in school despite adequate intelligence? Why do some children appear odd and socially distinctive from their peers? What is the basis for delay or peculiarity in talking? Why is a child misbehaving or committing criminal acts? What is causing a child to move strangely? Why is a child overactive? Why are some parents negligent or cruel to their children? How are children affected by acute or chronically traumatic situations? And, perhaps most importantly, how can all these children be helped?

Some mental disorders are diagnosed only in children, such as reactive attachment disorder of infancy or early childhood, in which a child manifests either indiscriminate sociability or responds to people in an inhibited or ambivalent way because of grossly negligent emotional or physical caretaking. Other disorders, such as mental retardation, are usually first diagnosed early, but will continue to be present throughout the life span. There are disorders that are usually diagnosed in childhood, such as conduct disorder, that often result in a specific adult diagnosis (antisocial personality disorder). Finally, many disorders of adults may be diagnosed in children, using the same or slightly modified criteria used for adults.

In the *Diagnostic and Statistical Manual of Mental Disorders,* 4th edition (*DSM-IV*) the distinction is retained between disorders usually first diagnosed in infancy, childhood, or adolescence and other disorders. However, where research indicates it is appropriate, there has been a shift toward using the same criteria (applied in an age-appropriate way) to diagnose children as used for adults, eg, for disorders such as anxiety disorders, mood disorders, adjustment disorders, or schizophrenia.

Table 28–1 lists *DSM-IV* disorders first diagnosed in children, and Table 28–2 identifies some other disorders that can be diagnosed in children. Because the number of psychiatric conditions seen in children is so great, this chapter will focus on only a few, chosen to illustrate the range of childhood psychopathology. For information on disorders not described here, a standard child psychiatry text or the suggested readings at the end of this chapter should be consulted.

DIAGNOSTIC ASSESSMENT IN CHILD PSYCHIATRY

The basic principles of comprehensive history taking, careful observation, and skillful eliciting of signs and symptoms apply to the assessment of children, but there are several additional features of child evaluation that require emphasis. An outline for a written child assessment is shown in Table 28–3.

Developmental Approach

Because children are rapidly changing physically, psychologically, cognitively, and emotionally, they need to be evaluated in a developmental context. This means that children are compared to others of the same age. Are they the same height and weight as their agemates? Where do they place on standard growth charts? Is their intellectual developmental on par? How are they doing in school and what does psychometric testing show? Are they where they should be emotionally? Marked anxiety at separation from a parent is usual in a 1-year-old but unusual in a 6-year-old child. Is their behavior similar to that of their peers or are they babyish, aggressive, or withdrawn in comparison? How clumsy are they for their age? Age-comparative evaluation allows the 7-year-

Table 28–1. *DSM-IV* disorders usually first diagnosed in infancy, childhood, or adolescence.

Mental Retardation
Mild Mental Retardation
Moderate Mental Retardation
Severe Mental Retardation
Profound Mental Retardation
Mental Retardation, Severity Unspecified

Learning Disorders
Reading Disorder
Mathematics Disorder
Disorder of Written Expression
Learning Disorder NOS

Motor Skills Disorder
Developmental Coordination Disorder

Communication Disorders
Expressive Language Disorder
Mixed Receptive-Expressive Language Disorder
Phonological Disorder
Stuttering
Communication Disorder NOS

Pervasive Developmental Disorders
Autistic Disorder
Rett's Disorder
Childhood Disintegrative Disorder
Asperger's Disorder
Pervasive Developmental Disorder NOS

Attention-Deficit and Disruptive Behavior Disorders
Attention-Deficit/Hyperactivity Disorder
    Combined Type
    Predominantly Inattentive Type
    Predominantly Hyperactive-Impulsive Type
Attention-Deficit/Hyperactivity Disorder NOS
Conduct Disorder
Specify type: Childhood-Onset Type/Adolescent-Onset Type
Oppositional Defiant Disorder
Disruptive Behavior Disorder NOS

Feeding and Eating Disorders of Infancy or Early Childhood
Pica
Rumination Disorder
Feeding Disorder of Infancy or Early Childhood

Tic Disorders
Tourette's Disorder
Chronic Motor or Vocal Tic Disorder
Transient Tic Disorder
Specify if: Single Episode/Recurrent
Tic Disorder NOS

Elimination Disorders
Encopresis
    With Constipation and Overflow Incontinence
    Without Constipation and Overflow Incontinence
Enuresis (Not a result of a General Medical Condition)
Specify type: Nocturnal Only/Diurnal
Only/Nocturnal and Diurnal

Other Disorders of Infancy, Childhood, or Adolescence
Separation Anxiety Disorder
Specify if: Early Onset
Selective Mutism
Reactive Attachment Disorder of Infancy or Early Childhood
Specify type: Inhibited Type/Disinhibited Type
Stereotypic Movement Disorder
Specify if: With Self-Injurious Behavior
Disorder of Infancy, Childhood, or Adolescence NOS

Table 28–2. Selected additional disorders that may be diagnosed in children.

Delirium
Dementia
Substance-related disorders
Schizophrenia
Depressive Disorders
Bipolar Disorders
Anxiety Disorders
Panic Disorder
    Agoraphobia Without History of Panic Disorder
    Specific Phobia
    Social Phobia
    Obsessive-Compulsive Disorder
    Posttraumatic Stress Disorder
    Acute Distress Disorder
    Generalized Anxiety Disorder
    Anxiety Disorder Due to a General Medical Condition
Somatoform Disorders
Gender Identity Disorders
Eating Disorders
Sleep Disorders
Adjustment Disorders
Other conditions that may be a focus of clinical attention
    Relational Problems (parent-child, sibling)
    Abuse or Neglect

Table 28–3. Outline for written child assessment.

Identifying Information
Age, ethnicity, school grade, living arrangements, known medical conditions, referral source

Chief complaint or presenting problems
May differ for varied informants

History of present illness

Past psychiatric history and treatment

Developmental history
Pregnancy, delivery, early infancy, temperament, motor and language milestones, toileting, significant separations, onset of puberty

School history
Daycare, preschool, academic performance, learning problems, school avoidance, special education, extracurricular interests, school behavior, vocational training, future plans

Personal history
Relationships with others (friends, caretakers, family, teachers), sexual history, gender identification, drug, alcohol, and nicotine use

Medical history
Includes dates of most recent physical exam, vision and hearing tests

Family history
Genogram with relatives' age, health, and occupation, past history of medical problems in family members (psychiatric, behavioral, learning disorders) religious, cultural, and educational attitudes.

Review of systems
Physical and psychiatric

Mental status exam

Case formulation
Summary of case

Diagnosis (Axis I–V)

Differential diagnosis

old child who functions at the appropriate age level in everything except the ability to pay attention to be distinguished from the 7-year-old child who operates at a younger level in all spheres.

In addition to comparing children to their age-mates, each aspect of the child's development from birth to the present should be evaluated. Domains to be assessed include gross and fine motor control, language, and social, emotional, and cognitive development. This kind of longitudinal approach allows the 6-year-old child who never gained bladder and bowel control to be distinguished from the 6-year-old child who had control of elimination at age 4 but lost it later in the context of severe environmental stress, such as the birth or death of a sibling or a contentious parental divorce.

Familiarity with developmental norms is essential to child assessment. Experience with children can help gain this familiarity, but there are also screening tests (eg, Denver Developmental Screening Test) and summaries of comparative development to assist with this (see Chapter 4).

Use of Age-Appropriate Methods in Interviewing the Child

Children are usually brought to an interview by their parents or other adults. Often they have not been told either the reason for the visit or the methods to be used in psychiatric exploration. Therefore, child psychiatrists often set the stage by explaining that they are "talk doctors" or "worry doctors," and they are familiar with children's concerns. Since most children associate doctors with extensive physical examinations and often with injections, psychiatrists explain that they are not "shot" doctors and that the interview will consist of talking, playing, and perhaps some tasks such as drawing, catching a ball, or standing on one foot. The child should be told that the psychiatrist will probably speak with other family members as well.

Since the child's capacity to relate to others is one of the things being evaluated, it is important to put the child at ease. For a very young child this may be accomplished by allowing the parent to remain in the room. For an adolescent, it is usually better to see the patient alone initially and offer realistic explanations about the degree of confidentiality that can be expected.

Language should be geared to the child's level of comprehension, and it is wise to verify that you are being understood. With young children words for emotional states may need to be clarified. "Do you feel bad?" may be heard as "Are you a bad person? Do you misbehave?" With adolescents, it is risky to try to use slang, since this changes so rapidly that what was in style a year ago may be hopelessly old-fashioned today.

In the actual interview, a productive approach is to interweave conversation and questioning with play.

Much of the verbal inquiry will be straightforward: "How long have you been having problems in school?" and "Do your mommy and daddy fight a lot?" are questions many children will answer. You also want to gain information regarding inner conflicts of which the child is either unaware or is not yet ready to share. This can be done by asking questions that approach the topic more tangentially: "I once knew a girl who was sad. Can you think of something that could make a girl sad?" or "If you had three wishes, what would they be?" "If you could take only one person to a desert island with you, who would you take?" "If you could be any animal, what would you be? Why?" The rough, aggressive 8-year-old boy who wants to be a kitten so people would pet and feed him is providing a lot of information, as is the 7-year-old girl, known to have been sexually abused but denying any emotional distress, who says she wants to be an elephant because then she would be so big no one could ever hurt her.

Another good method to learn about a child's inner world is through play. Children can often reveal feelings and concerns through play that they cannot report narratively. With only a doll house, doll figures, crayons, and paper, much information can be obtained, although child psychiatrists usually have additional toys available such as blocks, puppets, Play-Doh, board games, guns, and soldiers. In play, children frequently act out family conflicts, issues of abuse and neglect, specific traumatic events, and concerns about peers, school, and self-image.

Drawings are also very useful, particularly kinetic family drawings in which children are asked to draw a picture of their family doing something. Another standard drawing task is to draw a person, then a person of the gender opposite to the first. Some adolescents who may be difficult to engage in conversation will enthusiastically draw pictures that provide very clear statements about their view of themselves, their families, and the world in which they live.

Family Assessment

At least one caretaking adult usually accompanies a child to the initial evaluation. Most often this is a parent, but sometimes both parents, a guardian, a foster parent, or a social worker will come. The adult can provide much of the background information including medical history, family history, prenatal, neonatal, and developmental history, and an adult's perspective on the presenting problem and history of the present illness. When one or both parents are present, information about family relationships can often be directly assessed by observation. Evaluation of family dynamics as well as of emotional problems of other family members is crucial, since the child's symptoms may be a "cry for help" in an attempt to alleviate or cope with problems of other family members, eg, serious strife between parents, a severely depressed parent, or a disturbed sibling.

Although parents may express certainty in their view of their child's problems, studies have shown that often they are not aware of emotional symptoms in their children such as anxiety, depression, or even suicidality. Reports of behavioral symptoms, particularly substance use or delinquent acts, may also be divergent.

Use of Information from Multiple Sources

In addition to the interview with parents and child, information from schools, social work agencies, baby sitters, daycare providers, pediatricians, court records, child abuse registries, and other family members may also be required. Children behave differently in different settings. A child whose parents cite few attentional problems at home, commenting on the child's ability to stay glued to the TV set when fast-paced cartoons are on, may be the same child whose teacher describes a restless, inattentive student in the classroom. Besides actual differences in behavior, children may be perceived differently by the various adults in their life. A depressed parent may be so self-absorbed that the child's own sadness goes unnoticed at home but is apparent to visiting grandparents. An abusive parent may exaggerate the provocative nature of a child's behavior to justify harsh discipline, whereas the after-school center describes an engaging but needy youngster.

Child Mental Status Examination

As with adults, the mental status examination is not a specific examination conducted sequentially but rather an organized summary of many observations gathered throughout the time spent with the child. Table 28–4 provides a sample outline for a mental status examination of a child. **Appearance** covers such physical characteristics as height and weight for age, attractiveness, dysmorphic features, cutaneous lesions, scars, bruises, excoriations, perceptual or motor disabilities, hygiene, neatness, and appropriateness of clothing for age, size, gender, and weather conditions. **Motor activity** includes qualitative and quantitative assessment, eg, amount relative to age norms, type (coordinated, clumsy), abnormal movements (tics, stereotypies, rocking, twirling, hand flapping, choreoathetosis), and right and left preference (hand, foot, and eye). **Behavior** refers to both overall impression (age appropriate or immature, distractible,

---

Table 28–4. Child mental status examination.

Appearance
Motor activity
Behavior
Speech
Language
Social relatedness
Affect and mood
Cognitive functioning
Thought process and content

---

impulsive, reflecting short attention span, listless, engaged, aggressive, oppositional, provocative, destructive, perseverative) and presence of specific actions (nail biting, thumb sucking, picking at self, masturbation, sexualized posturing, self-injurious acts). Speech and language are frequently confused. **Speech** is the physical production of sound and includes attributes such as articulation, rate, rhythm, stutter, loudness, raspiness, and whininess. **Language** is communication, which is usually through speech but may also be nonverbal (body language, sign language, and mime), and has both expressive and receptive components. Some aspects of language to assess are age appropriateness, vocabulary, use of sentences, mean length of utterance, spontaneous content, pressured speech, neologisms, echolalia, pronoun reversals, communicative intent, and nonverbal communication. **Social relatedness** refers to the child's range of social behaviors and interactions, such as amount of eye contact, physical proximity, ease of separation from caretaker, friendliness or shyness, and whether interested or withdrawn. **Affect and mood** are assessed much as in adults, with special attention to children's less mature ability to clearly describe internal emotional states. **Cognitive functioning** can be difficult to assess because the cognitive norms are so different for various ages. Functions on which to focus include orientation, vocabulary, fund of knowledge, attention, memory, intactness of perceptual senses, visual motor ability to copy designs such as a circle, cross, or diamond, and ability to read or do arithmetic. **Thought process and content** covers spontaneous content of discourse, hallucinations, delusions, loose associations, tangentiality, nightmares, dreams, suicidal or homicidal ideation, projective questions (three wishes, hero, favorite animal, favorite movie or TV show, happiest/saddest memory), and nature and content of play and of drawings. The richness and content of fantasy life should be noted, and the quality of age-appropriate reality testing should be assessed.

Adjuncts to Diagnosis

Contemporary child psychiatrists use the full array of diagnostic tools to supplement their clinical observations. Standard laboratory tests as well as chromosome analysis, electroencephalogram (EEG), drug screens, lead levels, and occasionally brain imaging are helpful. Psychological testing can clarify questions about intellectual level, learning impairments, brain damage, and personality structure (see Chapter 13). Table 28–5 lists common psychological tests administered to children.

There are several instruments designed for use by parents or teachers to describe their children, and there are also numerous instruments used clinically but more often in research to examine specific symptoms in children. Table 28–6 lists some of the commonly used clinical measures.

Table 28–5. Common psychological tests for children.

Intelligence tests
Bayley Scales of Infant Development (2nd) for 1 month–
$3^1/2$ years
Wechsler Preschool and Primary Scale of
Intelligence–revised (WPPSI–R) for 4–6 years
Wechsler Intelligence Scale for Children–III (WISC–III)
Stanford-Binet for 2 years–adult
Leiter International Performance Scale for 2–13 years
(does not require verbal language)
Peabody Picture Vocabulary Test–revised (PPVT–R) for
4 years–adult
(only measures receptive vocabulary)
Raven's Coloured Progressive Matrices for 5–11 years
(test of nonverbal reasoning)

Neuropsychological tests
Visual-Motor Integration assessed by copying figures
Bender Visual Motor Gestalt, Beery Visual Motor
Integration
*Batteries of tests for the detection of suspected brain
damage*
Reitan-Indiana test battery, Halstead-Reitan test battery,
Luria-Nebraska neuropsychologic battery

Academic achievement tests
Tests for reading, math, spelling, and written language
achievement such as
Woodcock-Johnson, Wide Range Achievement Test (WRAT),
Stanford Achievement Test, Wechsler Individual
Achievement Test (WIAT)

Personality assessment
Children's Apperception Test (CAT)
Rorschach inkblots
Sentence completion
Draw-a-person (DAP)
Personality Inventory for Children (PIC)

Adaptation
Vineland Adaptive Behavior Scales
(Questionnaires to assess daily living skills,
communication and socialization)

Table 28–6. Common checklists, rating scales,
and screening tests for children.

Child Behavior Checklist (CBCL)
Parent report form that asks about the child's usual
activities and relationships, and has a 113-item
symptom checklist

**Conner's Parent Questionnaire/Conner's Teacher
Rating Scale**
Short rating scale inquiring about presence and severity of
symptoms of Attention-Deficit Hyperactivity Disorder.
Although not diagnostic, it can be used in assessment,
and to follow effectiveness of treatment

Denver Developmental Screening Test
Used frequently by pediatricians, this test includes
simple ways to test a 1-month-old to 5-year-old child's
development in language, gross motor, fine motor, and
personal-social areas. Requires special items (wooden
blocks, specific pictures, etc.)

a combined type (most frequent), a predominantly in-attentive type, and a predominantly hyperactive-impulsive type. This most recent diagnostic terminology reflects current thinking about the possible heterogeneity of this disorder (Table 28–7).

Clinically, these children are brought to the doctor when their parents or teachers complain that they are hard to discipline, do not follow directions, seem to dawdle over the simplest tasks, leave projects and chores incomplete, forget to bring homework assignments and school notices home, and then forget to bring homework back to class. They may impulsively touch or bump into other children, dash into the street, or be unable to wait for their turn in a game. When motoric overactivity is present the child will fidget, squirm, and be "all over the place." Often social problems with peers, negative relations with family members, poor school achievement, and diminished self-esteem are the result of the core problems in attention, distractibility, impulsivity, and overactivity.

Although the symptoms must have been present before age 7 for the diagnosis to be made, the disorder is frequently not noticed until the child enters school, perhaps because school requires more controlled, directed behavior and because teachers observe the child acting differently from other same-age peers. However, with increased media focus on ADHD, and with more children being in school-like settings at an earlier age, some clinicians are seeing an increase in referrals of younger children for evaluation of ADHD-like symptoms. For severely affected preschoolers, the diagnosis may not be difficult, but in less obvious cases, parents may resist believing the child has any problems or may be convinced the child will grow out of it. Conversely, some referrals may be the result of parental intolerance for normative preschool exuberance.

In the evaluating physician's office, the child may or may not appear squirmy, noisy, distractible, or inattentive. Because a medical examining room is

CHILD PSYCHOPATHOLOGY

ATTENTION-DEFICIT/HYPERACTIVITY DISORDER

Symptoms & Signs

For over 50 years physicians have been evaluating and treating children who show various combinations of **motoric overactivity, impulsivity, distractibility, and inattentiveness.** During that time, the terminology describing these children has changed, reflecting the shifting ideas about etiology and about the relationship of the symptoms of overactivity to the symptoms of inattentiveness. Called at different times minimal brain damage, minimal brain dysfunction, hyperactive child syndrome, hyperactive reaction of childhood, and attention-deficit disorder with or without hyperactivity, the syndrome is now known as attention-deficit/hyperactivity disorder (ADHD). In *DSM-IV*, ADHD is divided into three subtypes:

Table 28–7. *DSM-IV* diagnostic criteria for attention-deficit/hyperactivity disorder.

A. Either (1) or (2):
   (1) *inattention:* six (or more) of the following symptoms of inattention have persisted for at least 6 months to a degree that is maladaptive and inconsistent with developmental level: (a) often fails to give close attention to details or makes careless mistakes in schoolwork, work, or other activities, (b) often has difficulty sustaining attention in tasks or play activities, (c) often does not seem to listen when spoken to directly, (d) often does not follow through on instructions and fails to finish schoolwork, chores, or duties in the workplace (not due to oppositional behavior or failure to understand instructions), (e) often has difficulty organizing tasks and activities, (f) often avoids, dislikes, or is reluctant to engage in tasks that require sustained mental effort (such as schoolwork or homework), (g) often loses things necessary for tasks or activities (eg, toys, school assignments, pencils, books, or tools), (h) is often easily distracted by extraneous stimuli, (i) is often forgetful in daily activities; (2) *hyperactivity-impulsivity:* six (or more) of the following symptoms of hyperactivity-impulsivity have persisted for at least 6 months to a degree that is maladaptive and inconsistent with developmental level:

Hyperactivity
(a) often fidgets with hands or feet or squirms in seat, (b) often leaves seat in classroom or in other situations in which remaining seated is expected, (c) often runs about or climbs excessively in situations in which it is inappropriate (in adolescents or adults, may be limited to subjective feelings of restlessness), (d) often has difficulty playing or engaging in leisure activities quietly, (e) is often "on the go" or often acts as if "driven by a motor," (f) often talks excessively

Impulsivity
(g) often blurts out answers before questions have been completed, (h) often has difficulty awaiting turn, (i) often interrupts or intrudes on others (eg, butts into conversations or games)

B. Some hyperactive-impulsive or inattentive symptoms that caused impairment were present before age 7 years.

C. Some impairment from the symptoms is present in two or more settings (eg, at school [or work] and at home).

D. There must be clear evidence of clinically significant impairment in social, academic, or occupational functioning.

E. The symptoms do not occur exclusively during the course of a pervasive developmental disorder, schizophrenia, or other psychotic disorder and are not better accounted for by another mental disorder (eg, mood disorder, anxiety disorder, dissociative disorder, or a personality disorder).

usually quiet, with few distractions, the child is less apt to exhibit the problem behaviors there than in a noisy classroom surrounded by other children.

Differential Diagnosis

Attention-deficit/hyperactivity disorder is a clinical diagnosis based on the family's description of the child's behavior, the school report, the clinician's observation, and, at times, comprehensive testing. There are no specific tests for ADHD. However, Conner's Parent Questionnaire and Teacher Rating Scale can help elicit a quantitative assessment of the specific ways the behaviors may show up.

Various types of continuous performance tests (CPTs) assess the child's ability to pay attention to routine, uninteresting stimuli, and components of many psychological tests (eg, trail making, mazes) assess attentional abilities.

Differential diagnosis includes hearing problems, impaired vision, poor nutrition, language-processing problems, thyroid dysfunction, pinworms, and adjustment disorder; ADHD must also be differentiated from several conditions that can be present concurrently, such as learning disorder, conduct disorder, oppositional defiant disorder, anxiety disorder, and mood disorder.

Epidemiology

This disorder is more common in boys than in girls, can be found in all socioeconomic groups, and has a prevalence of around 3–5% in school-aged children. Concurrent problems are frequent, and around two-thirds of ADHD children have another psychiatric diagnosis. These include conduct disorder (most common), learning disorder, oppositional defiant disorder, and mood and anxiety disorders. The etiology is not clear, although there appears to be an increased family incidence in first-degree relatives. Some other causative factors that have been considered include prenatal or perinatal insult, prenatal drug and alcohol exposure, and lead poisoning. Contrary to a recent popular theory, food additives and sugar are not found to cause ADHD in most children.

Etiology

Investigations into the biological factors involved in ADHD have focused on dopamine and noradrenergic systems, and when aggression coexists, on serotonin as well. Findings from brain-imaging studies have been variable. In a study that examined parents of children with ADHD who self-reported ADHD symptoms when they (the parents) were children, positron-emission tomographic scans administered during attention-requiring tasks revealed decreased glucose metabolism in the frontal and prefrontal cortex.

Treatment & Prognosis

Treating the child with ADHD requires a multimodal approach. Psychopharmacological treatment with psychostimulants (methylphenidate, dextroamphetamine, and pemoline) is widely used and is effective in up to 90% of ADHD children. Other medications used in clinical practice include some antidepressants (imipramine, desipramine, and bupropion) and clonidine. The purpose of medication should be explained to both parent and child, and its effectiveness should be monitored by home and school reports. Medication alone is rarely sufficient, since parents will need counseling on methods of managing their child's behaviors and breaking the frequent patterns of dysfunctional interactions that have evolved over the years the child was untreated. A variety of behavioral management techniques have been used with success, such as contingent reinforcement, time-outs, and daily reports from school to parents. Teachers and parents may need information about optimizing nondistracting environments for schoolwork and homework. Children also benefit from counseling to address issues of decreased self-esteem, poor peer relations, and expectation of failure. Presently multicenter studies are in progress to assess the efficacy of various combinations of therapeutic modalities.

The prognosis for children with ADHD is controversial. It was previously thought that children outgrew their symptoms in adolescence, and it was possible to stop medications as the child got older. Recently there has been increasing focus on adolescents and adults treated as children who continue to show some or all of the symptoms of ADHD on follow-up. In addition, adults are being identified who were untreated as children but manifest symptoms of impulsivity and poor attention, sometimes with coexistent antisocial personality disorder and substance abuse.

Illustrative Case:
ADHD—Hyperactive-Impulsive Type

A 7-year-old boy was referred by his first grade teacher because of behavioral problems in the classroom. Her note said "He's up when all the other kids are up, but he's up all the rest of the time too." In a phone conference she described him as a "wiggle worm" who was either squirming in his seat or running around the classroom during assignments. She also described his problems with classmates, who resented his rambunctious behavior during recess. His parents said that he had always been a very active child at home but were surprised at the teacher's complaint because they thought he would settle down once he started school. They were concerned about his impulsivity and noted that he had almost been hit by a car when he darted across a street trying to reach a friend on the other side.

Illustrative Case: ADHD—Inattentive Type

An 8-year-old girl, the only child of an intact middle-class family, was brought to the child psychiatry outpatient clinic at the medical center because she was doing very poorly in second grade, and the school was considering having her repeat the year. As part of the standard assessment package, the teacher and parents had each been asked to complete the Conner's Teacher Rating Scale and Parent Questionnaire, respectively. They had rated many behaviors associated with ADHD as present "pretty much" or "very much."

The parents, who both worked, described getting ready to leave for school each morning as "chaos" because their child was constantly losing or forgetting her school books, mittens, or teacher's notices, and no one would realize the item was gone until the last minute. Similarly, evenings were unpleasant because their daughter, who was supposed to do her homework after school at a baby sitter's home, never got it done despite multiple reminders. The stress of coping with these problems had begun to have a negative impact on their marital relationship. Intelligence testing done at the clinic showed full-scale IQ in the high average range, with little difference between verbal and performance IQ. The testing psychologist did note that it was constantly necessary to redirect the child to the testing materials and wondered whether the score would have been higher if attentional problems had not been present.

The family agreed to a trial of methylphenidate. A dose of 5 mg at breakfast and at lunchtime resulted in a marked increase in the child's ability to sustain attention. The teacher remarked to the father, "It's as if her twin sister has shown up in class." Encouraged by the good response to medication, the parents agreed to family counseling.

CONDUCT DISORDER

Symptoms & Signs

Children with conduct disorder (CD) do not just misbehave. Rather, they show behaviors that are closer to delinquent or predelinquent patterns. They violate the norms and rules of society or interfere with the basic rights of others in a repetitive and persistent way. Children with CD are often diagnosed as having antisocial personality disorder in adulthood, and existence of CD before age 15 is a prerequisite for the diagnosis of antisocial personality disorder. The *DSM-IV* criteria are very specific (see Table 28–8) and include physical fighting, physical cruelty to people and/or animals, using a weapon, threatening others, stealing or destroying property, setting fires, forced sexual activity, chronic lying ("conning" people), running away or staying away from home overnight, truancy, or breaking and entering. The diagnosis is modified by specifying severity and early or late onset. Children with early onset are more often aggressive boys and have a worse prognosis.

Comorbidity is common for CD, with coexisting conditions including ADHD, learning disorders, substance abuse, depression, and neurological vulnerabilities. Children with CD are at increased risk for suicide attempts, even in the absence of depression. Backgrounds of these children may reflect neglect, abusive or emotionally depriving parenting, social deviance, parental psychopathology, and parental substance abuse.

Clinically children with CD are often brought to

Table 28–8. *DSM-IV* diagnostic criteria for conduct disorder.

A. A repetitive and persistent pattern of behavior in which the basic rights of others or major age-appropriate societal norms or rules are violated, as manifested by the presence of three (or more) of the following criteria in the past 12 months, with at least one criterion present in the past 6 months:

Aggression to people and animals
(1) often bullies, threatens, or intimidates others, (2) often initiates physical fights, (3) has used a weapon that can cause serious physical harm to others (eg, a bat, brick, broken bottle, knife, gun), (4) has been physically cruel to people, (5) has been physically cruel to animals, (6) has stolen while confronting a victim (eg, mugging, purse snatching, extortion, armed robbery), (7) has forced someone into sexual activity

Destruction of property
(8) has deliberately engaged in fire setting with the intention of causing serious damage, (9) has deliberately destroyed property (other than by fire setting)

Deceitfulness or theft
(10) has broken into someone else's house, building, or car, (11) often lies to obtain goods or favors or to avoid obligations (ie, "cons" others), (12) has stolen items of nontrivial value without confronting a victim (eg, shoplifting, but without breaking and entering; forgery)

Serious violations of rules
(13) often stays out at night despite parental prohibitions, beginning before age 13 years, (14) has run away from home overnight at least twice while living in parental or parental surrogate home (or once without returning for a lengthy period), (15) is often truant from school, beginning before age 13 years

B. The disturbance in behavior causes clinically significant impairment in social, academic, or occupational functioning.

C. If the individual is age 18 years or older, criteria are not met for Antisocial Personality Disorder.

Specify type based on age at onset:
Childhood-Onset Type: onset of at least one criterion characteristic of Conduct Disorder prior to age 10 years
Adolescent-Onset Type: absence of any criteria characteristic of Conduct Disorder prior to age 10 years

Specify severity:
Mild: few if any conduct problems in excess of those required to make the diagnosis **and** conduct problems cause only minor harm to others
Moderate: number of conduct problems and effect on others intermediate between "mild" and "severe"
Severe: many conduct problems in excess of those required to make the diagnosis **or** conduct problems cause considerable harm to others

medical attention because others complain about their behavior. They will frequently state that they did not do what they are accused of and that other people are impinging on their rights rather than vice versa. Students will often say that their teachers are against them and neglect to describe their own contributions to the situation. A medical student, evaluating a 9-year-old boy, was convinced that one teacher was unfairly picking on the child and was surprised to receive reports documenting the child's provocative, aggressive behavior to students, multiple teachers, and family members.

Conduct-disordered children can be particularly difficult to interview because of such distorted explanations as well as their attempts to "con" people, their bravado and "tough" exterior, and their unwillingness to let down their guard. It requires perseverance and an open mind to see beyond their defensive, sometimes "off-putting" stance.

Often the home life of these children has been chaotic. Foster placement is not uncommon, but many times families are intact. Here, too, perseverance is needed to ascertain whether potentially treatable dysfunctional family patterns exist, either contributing to or resulting from the child's disturbance.

Epidemiology

The disorder is more common in boys (9%) than in girls (2%), although the addition of two behaviors in *DSM-IV* not found in *DSM-III-R* may increase the diagnostic frequency in girls ("often bullies, threatens or intimidates others" and "often stays out at night despite parental prohibitions").

Because there are no age limits in this diagnosis, a 4-year-old child who lies, fights, hits other children, sets fires, and destroys objects around the house qualifies for the diagnosis, just as would a 15-year-old adolescent who rapes, commits armed robbery, and beats up people. This diagnosis obviously encompasses a wide range of severity.

Treatment

Treatment for the child with CD needs to be multifaceted, with first consideration given to diagnosing associated, potentially treatable conditions, both common (eg, depression) and less common (seizure disorders or psychotic thought disorders). Educational intervention for learning disabilities and social intervention or out-of-home placement for children in obviously abusive or negligent environments are important. Interventions with the family include traditional family therapy, looking at ways in which the child may be "acting out" family problems, and parent effectiveness programs that attempt to increase parenting skills.

An interesting area of work with aggressive children draws from observations in social cognition that these children see hostile intentionality in others more frequently than do nonaggressive children. Aggressive children also have limited repertoires of social responses in both actual and hypothetical situations and are limited in considering the consequences of their actions. Social skills training groups can help these children correctly differentiate a playmate's accidental bump in the playground from an intentional punch and also help them develop alternatives to aggressive responses.

The most effective intervention in CD is called

multisystemic treatment (MST), an intensive, family-focused, home-based service. The primary objective is to assist both parents and community organizations in developing skills for intervening with risk factors for antisocial behavior in children with CD. Randomized clinical trials in three settings have established the efficacy of MST in reducing adolescent behavior problems and improving family functioning (Henggeler et al, 1998).

Illustrative Case: Conduct Disorder

A 10-year-old boy was brought to the pediatric psychiatry clinic by his tired-looking grandmother who had been raising him and his younger sister since his mother had died of a drug overdose 5 years before. The grandmother detailed a long history of problems managing the child, calling him "a real fighter, a mean kid," who never liked school, did poorly, and had been frequently truant. The present visit was precipitated by an incident at school in which he had robbed a younger boy of a leather jacket, threatening to beat him up. The grandmother knew little of his earliest history but believed his mother had been "on the street" when he was young. The child had been in and out of foster homes, as his mother attempted to overcome her substance abuse problems, which may have been present during her pregnancy.

The boy was defiant and sullen, appearing angry about having to be in the clinic. He dismissed questions about the school problems as a "big fuss about nothing" and said the accusation about the jacket was false. He refused to discuss any of his feelings or to play with games or toys, but he did agree to draw a picture of his family, which showed his grandmother, sister, himself, and his dead mother.

School records showed a recently diagnosed learning disorder with poor reading skills, but the child's truancy had interfered with efforts at remediation.

AUTISTIC DISORDER

Symptoms & Signs

Autism, a kind of pervasive developmental disorder, is one of the most fascinating and puzzling of the childhood psychiatric disorders. Despite its relative rarity (prevalence 4 per 10,000), it continues to intrigue investigators and clinicians alike. What causes these children, who may appear physically normal and often come from loving supportive families, to behave so oddly?

The hallmarks of the syndrome, first described by Leo Kanner in 1943, are very early-appearing impairments in three areas: social interaction, communication, and repertoire of interests and activities (Table 28–9).

Qualitatively and quantitatively **impaired social interaction** is manifested by marked uninvolvement

Table 28–9. *DSM-IV* diagnostic criteria for autistic disorder.

A. A total of six (or more) items from (1), (2), and (3), with at least two from (1), and one each from (2) and (3):

(1) qualitative impairment in social interaction, as manifested by at least two of the following: (a) marked impairment in the use of multiple nonverbal behaviors such as eye-to-eye gaze, facial expression, body postures, and gestures to regulate social interaction, (b) failure to develop peer relationships appropriate to developmental level, (c) a lack of spontaneous seeking to share enjoyment, interests, or achievements with other people (eg, by a lack of showing, bringing, or pointing out objects of interest), (d) lack of social or emotional reciprocity

(2) qualitative impairments in communication as manifested by at least one of the following: (a) delay in, or total lack of, the development of spoken language (not accompanied by an attempt to compensate through alternative modes of communication such as gesture or mime), (b) in individuals with adequate speech, marked impairment in the ability to initiate or sustain a conversation with others, (c) stereotyped and repetitive use of language or idiosyncratic language, (d) lack of varied, spontaneous make-believe play or social imitative play appropriate to developmental level

(3) restricted repetitive and stereotyped patterns of behavior, interests, and activities, as manifested by at least one of the following: (a) encompassing preoccupation with one or more stereotyped and restricted patterns of interest that is abnormal either in intensity or focus, (b) apparently inflexible adherence to specific, nonfunctional routines or rituals, (c) stereotyped and repetitive motor mannerisms (eg, hand or finger flapping or twisting, or complex whole-body movements), (d) persistent preoccupation with parts of objects

B. Delays or abnormal functioning in at least one of the following areas, with onset prior to age 3 years: (1) social interaction, (2) language as used in social communication, or (3) symbolic or imaginative play.

C. The disturbance is not better accounted for by Rett's disorder or childhood disintegrative disorder.

with people, decreased eye contact, strange use of facial expressions or gestures in social situations, a tendency to treat people as inanimate objects, relating to parts of a person (eg, their hands to get something) but not the whole person, limited pleasure in social interactions, little social or emotional reciprocity, little expression of empathy, and failure to make friends. Parents may say "he's different, not as attached to me as my other children," or "he just doesn't get involved with people," and preschool teachers may note an obliviousness to other children in a play group, punctuated by temper tantrums for seemingly inexplicable reasons.

Communication impairments show up in the most severe cases as a lack of spoken language or severe delay in language acquisition. In contrast to hearing-impaired or purely language-impaired children, autistic children have few compensatory gestures or sounds and show little communicative intent.

When spoken language does develop, it may be repetitive and idiosyncratic, with echolalia (seemingly senseless repetition of phrases or parts of phrases), pronoun reversal (as in "you want juice" when the child is thirsty), unusual prosody (inflection or "intonation" of language), or unusual intensity (loud or soft). Sometimes parents will say their child can speak normally, but on closer questioning the speech will be found to consist of unusual use of phrases ("Thank you" to indicate a request for an item) or repetition of advertising slogans or song fragments. In autistic children with better linguistic functioning, language may be pedantic or literal. The pragmatic function of verbal interchange to sustain and advance communication is flawed, and problems with contingent discourse increase relative to age compared to normal or Down syndrome children of similar linguistic abilities. Symbolic communication via make-believe play and social imitation play (tea parties, doll play, toy tools) is often deficient for the child's developmental age. Toys are used more for their sensorimotor qualities than their pretend aspects (eg, banging wooden trucks together or just spinning their wheels, rather than using them as vehicles; rubbing soft dolls rather than attempting to feed or dress them).

Restricted repertoire of behaviors and interests may be present as insistence on sameness (eg, foods must be eaten in a certain order, the route from home to school must not be altered), intense preoccupation with limited areas of knowledge (eg, list of presidents, train schedules, meteorology), stereotyped motor mannerisms (eg, hand flapping, twirling), or persistent preoccupation with parts of an object. *DSM-IV* diagnostic criteria for autistic disorder require that symptoms be present before age 3. Some children may not come to medical attention until after that age, but careful retrospective history, including family videotapes when available, will show the earlier abnormalities. By the time the child reaches school age, although oddities in language and social relations may persist, the major presenting problems are usually more behavioral.

Differential Diagnosis

Differential diagnosis of autistic disorders includes hearing or vision deficits, expressive and mixed receptive-expressive language disorders, mental retardation without autism, and other types of pervasive developmental disorders such as Rett's disorder, childhood disintegrative disorder, and Asperger's disorder.

Etiology

In contrast to earlier explanations that considered autism to be the result of cold, unemotional mothering, contemporary psychiatrists believe autism has biological causes. Evidence for this comes from several sources. The concordance rate for autism in monozygotic twins is much higher than that for dizygotic twins. Families with one autistic child are at a somewhat higher risk for a second, and nonautistic siblings of autistic children are at increased risk for impaired communication. About 75% of children with autism are also mentally retarded, and 25% develop seizures by later childhood and adolescence. Some of the medical diseases known to have neurological effects found in some children with autism include tuberous sclerosis, fragile X syndrome, and congenital rubella. Brain imaging, EEG, and neurochemical studies of autistic children are being actively conducted, and although abnormalities have been found, no specific etiology is known. Recent psychological studies have focused on the deficits underlying the pervasive social impairment, and some have shown that autistic children lack the ability to attribute mental states to others, ie, they lack what is called a theory of mind.

Treatment

Because children with autistic disorder cover a spectrum of severities, different treatment interventions are required. There are some general principles that apply to all. First, it should be determined whether the child has other medical conditions known to be associated with autism. This may help in ascertaining the future risk to the family of having other autistic children and may indicate potential problems that may develop in the child, such as the risk for seizures in tuberous sclerosis. Second, the family should be counseled about the nature of the condition. Several common myths about autism may need to be clarified.

1. Autism is not schizophrenia and is not characterized by hallucinations and delusions.
2. Autistic children are neither all superintelligent "idiot savants," with unusual isolated powers such as calendar calculation or musical talents (although there are rare instances of such abilities), nor are they all mentally retarded (although approximately three-fourths are).
3. Autism is not caused by bad parenting.
4. Children with autism can neither *always* function independently nor *never* function independently in adulthood. Prognosis depends on the degree of impairment, with better language development and higher intelligence being good prognostic signs. Still, most autistic people will eventually require some degree of supervised living arrangements.
5. Intensive, insight-oriented psychotherapy is not an appropriate treatment for autistic children, but supportive interventions for child and family may be helpful.

Subsequent treatment efforts should be directed at helping the family obtain appropriate school placement with emphasis on maximizing language and social functioning. Starting in the preschool years, such sustained intervention has been shown to increase adaptive functioning. Counseling can teach behavior management techniques and modifications shown to be particularly useful for these children. Parent groups can help families negotiate administrative hurdles and offer emotional support and practical suggestions. Psychopharmacological agents may have a place in the relief of some symptoms such as aggression, stereotypies, low frustration tolerance, and self-injurious behaviors.

Illustrative Case: Autistic Disorder

A 4-year-old boy was brought for evaluation because of delayed language development. Unlike his older brother, who had spoken full narratives when he was 4, the patient said only a few isolated words spontaneously. However, at times, his mother thought he would repeat sentences from commercial jingles he heard on television. His parents said that compared to his sibling, he was more "withdrawn" and seemed neither to relate to his brother nor to play with other children. Rather, he amused himself by playing with crayons, often lining them up in long rows but rarely coloring with them. He loved puzzles and could complete complicated ones that baffled his sibling. He would sometimes have temper tantrums, which seemed to be caused by his mother's attempts to rearrange objects in the home, but it was difficult for her to be certain of the cause of the tantrums because of her son's lack of communication. After describing her son's problems, she said quietly and sadly, "I think I've known something was wrong from the beginning. He isn't like other children. He doesn't care about people."

On examination, the child had diminished eye contact with all adults in the room and appeared preoccupied with a twirling top he had found in the waiting room. He seemed to react to sound but was uninterested in engaging in any play with the examiner. Physical examination was grossly normal although the child would not cooperate with some of the tasks on the Denver Developmental Screen, preferring to bang the wooden cubes together most of the time.

The child was referred for audiologic evaluation, which was normal, then for psychometric testing to assess the possibility of concurrent mental retardation. The psychologist chose to administer a Leiter test for intelligence, since it did not require the use of verbal language abilities, and a Vineland Adaptive Behavior Scale to assess his adaptive level of functioning apart from his intelligence level. The Leiter test showed low normal intelligence, but adaptive functioning on the Vineland Scale was much below normal.

SEPARATION ANXIETY DISORDER

Symptoms & Signs

Children with separation anxiety disorder do not want to be away from the people to whom they are most attached—usually their parents and most frequently their mother. The essential feature of this disorder is excessive and developmentally inappropriate anxiety aroused by real or anticipated separations from home or from major attachment figures, beginning before age 18 (Table 28–10).

All children go through a stage of developmentally expected separation anxiety during infancy, which may extend, in an attenuated form, up to 4 or 5 years. A 1-year-old child's protest at separation from a parent is thought to represent the normal expression of attachment. However, most children gradually become comfortable with being away from their families. Separation anxiety disorder is the persistence or return of separation fears after a child would be expected to have outgrown them. The symptoms must be present for at least 4 weeks, so that brief periods of homesickness when first attending camp or a few days of increased clinginess on entering first grade

Table 28–10. *DSM-IV* diagnostic criteria for separation anxiety disorder.

A. Developmentally inappropriate and excessive anxiety concerning separation from home or from those to whom the individual is attached, as evidenced by three (or more) of the following:

(1) recurrent excessive distress when separation from home or major attachment figures occurs or is anticipated, (2) persistent and excessive worry about losing, or about possible harm befalling, major attachment figures, (3) persistent and excessive worry that an untoward event will lead to separation from a major attachment figure (eg, getting lost or being kidnapped), (4) persistent reluctance or refusal to go to school or elsewhere because of fear of separation, (5) persistently and excessively fearful or reluctant to be alone or without major attachment figures at home or without significant adults in other settings, (6) persistent reluctance or refusal to go to sleep without being near a major attachment figure or to sleep away from home, (7) repeated nightmares involving the theme of separation, (8) repeated complaints of physical symptoms (such as headaches, stomach aches, nausea, or vomiting) when separation from major attachment figures occurs or is anticipated.

B. The duration of the disturbance is at least 4 weeks.

C. The onset is before age 18 years.

D. The disturbance causes clinically significant distress or impairment in social, academic (occupational), or other important areas of functioning.

E. The disturbance does not occur exclusively during the course of a pervasive developmental disorder, schizophrenia, or other psychotic disorder, and, in adolescents and adults, is not better accounted for by panic disorder with agoraphobia.

Specify if:
Early Onset: if onset occurs before age 6 years

are not sufficient for the diagnosis. The prognosis is better when the disorder appears in a younger child, closer to the age at which normal separation worries would be expected. Separation anxiety disorder in an adolescent has a worse prognosis.

Typically, children want to stay home or stay close to a parent, resisting sleeping away from home or going to school, and may have tantrums if forced to separate against their will. Often they will be preoccupied by worries about harm that may befall their parents or by concerns about themselves, such as being lost or kidnapped. At night the child may have trouble falling asleep, insist on sleeping in the parent's room or bed, and have nightmares about being separated. Physical symptoms such as headaches, stomachaches, palpitations, and dizzy spells may occur at times of real or anticipated separation (eg, Monday morning after a weekend at home). The usual problems that bring these children to medical attention are either the physical symptoms or the refusal to attend school, which are also the most common symptoms manifested in adolescents.

Although 75–80% of children who refuse to attend school may manifest separation anxiety disorder, the two are not synonymous. Other reasons children do not want to go to school include concern over poor academic performance, apprehension about being teased or bullied by their peers, or fear of a particular teacher. In some urban settings schools have become dangerous armed battlegrounds, and fear about physical well-being may be realistic. Children with enuresis or encopresis may be embarrassed to be with their peers. Children who have been sexually or physically abused around a school setting may be reluctant to return. Depressed children may not have enough energy or motivation to go to school, and depression is a common comorbid condition with separation anxiety disorder. Children with posttraumatic stress disorder or psychotic disorders may feel unable to leave home, and conduct-disordered children are frequently truant. Occasionally, a child who does not attend school is actually being kept at home to assist with chores or has a family that is too chaotic to prepare the child for school attendance.

Epidemiology

Anxiety disorders comprise some of the most common psychiatric disorders in children and adolescents, and separation anxiety disorder is the most common childhood anxiety disorder in nonreferred prepubertal children, although somewhat less frequent in adolescents. It is one of the few childhood disorders found equally or slightly more frequently in girls than in boys.

Comorbid conditions include depressive disorders and other anxiety disorders. Family histories may show increased rates of other anxiety disorders, agoraphobia, panic disorder, depression, or alcoholism.

Families of children with separation anxiety disor-

der have increased rates of other disorders, including agoraphobia, panic disorder, depression, and alcoholism. Separation anxiety disorder often develops in the context of a major life stress occurring in the family, such as illness, change of residence, or divorce, which will impact all family members.

Treatment

Treatment of refusal to attend school depends on carefully determining the cause and then treating it appropriately. In adolescents, it is particularly important to look for depression or psychotic thought processes. When separation anxiety disorder is present, the family should be enlisted to return the child to school as soon as possible. Engaging the family may be difficult. As noted, other mental disorders are common in family members. In addition, the mother-child relationship may be characterized by the mother's own general anxieties or specific worries about being separated from her child. Therefore, family therapy or counseling for the parent may be required in order to enable the family to carry out the recommendations about school reentry, and to change the underlying dynamics that may have contributed to the problem. Behavioral treatments, both classical and operant conditioning, cognitive therapy, and systematic desensitization have all proved effective in small numbers of cases.

Pharmacological treatment with antidepressants may be helpful for some children, although that is now being reevaluated. In instances in which the problems persist despite behavioral, supportive, family, and pharmacological treatment, hospitalization may be indicated.

Illustrative Case:
Separation Anxiety Disorder

A 7-year-old girl was brought by her parents because she had not attended school for the past 3 months. The problem had started after Christmas vacation, when she began to ask her parents whether she could sleep in their room because hers was "too cold." She then began to want continually to be in the same room as her mother, who described her daughter as "sticking to me like a shadow." When vacation was over, the child begged to stay home, saying she already knew how to read. When her parents initially rejected her request and insisted she attend school, she was sent home 3 days in a row because of stomachaches. Once she reached home, the stomachaches disappeared. The mother, who had not liked school herself, justified keeping her daughter home by agreeing that the child was a good reader, so perhaps she did not need to attend the rest of first grade. Although she had not mentioned it to her parents, the girl confided to the examiner that she worried a lot about kidnappers, who would grab children as they walked from school to home. She had not read or seen newspaper articles about any kidnapping but recalled a Disney movie in which an evil lady was trying to kidnap a dog.

DEPRESSION

Symptoms & Signs

Everyone has seen children who cry and are sad, but the existence of true depression as a syndrome in children was debated for many years. Early work by Spitz in the 1940s described a condition he called anaclitic depression in institutionalized infants deprived of contact with their mothers. The babies appeared sad, withdrawn, listless, and underactive, with feeding and sleeping problems. In the 1960s, Bowlby described the sequential reactions of children to the loss of their primary caretakers as protest that was followed by despair and then detachment. By the 1980s there was increased consensus that depression in children not only existed but was not rare. (Prevalence in school-aged children is now thought to be almost 2% and in adolescents almost 4–8%.) Psychiatrists saw many of these children and noted their impaired functioning.

Since publication of *DSM-III,* childhood depression has been diagnosed using the same criteria as those used in adults with a few minor modifications (eg, mood may be either depressed or irritable, failure to make expected weight gain rather than weight loss, and for dysthymic disorders, duration of symptoms may be shortened to 1 year rather than 2). (Tables in Chapter 20 present *DSM-IV* criteria for mood disorders.)

Natural History

Depressed preschoolers and school-aged children may look sad, complain of headaches or stomachaches, have sleep problems and separation anxiety, do poorly in school, and show psychomotor agitation and impaired concentration (which must be distinguished from ADHD). They may show impaired self-image, describing themselves as "stupid" and "no good," and may be unwilling to attempt tasks such as drawing or catching a ball, saying "I can't do that." In young children immature linguistic and cognitive capacities may make it difficult for them to describe sad, worthless, or guilty feelings or conceptualizations about death or suicide. Children may be hesitant to discuss these feelings with their parents. Parents, unable or unwilling to acknowledge the depth of their child's despair, may never ask the more difficult questions. Even when parents report no depression or suicidality in their child, assessment should be made directly through both questions and nonverbal play techniques with the child.

In adolescents, depression may present more as it does in adults. Depressed appearance and somatic complaints are less frequent than in younger children, but loss of pleasure in activities, hopelessness, psychomotor retardation, sleeping disturbances (often hypersomnia), weight changes, and drug use are more common. Withdrawal from family can be mistaken for age-appropriate quest for autonomy, but withdrawal from parents, immersion in fantasy, fascination with suicide, or confiding to a peer about self-destructive thoughts or plans should precipitate medical consultation.

A major depressive episode in either children or adolescents should raise suspicion of an onset of bipolar disorder, particularly when a family history of the disorder exists. This possibility should also be kept in mind during the follow-up period.

Epidemiology

Suicidal ideation, attempts, and completion also occur in children and adolescents. Suicidality is associated with depression, but also occurs in children with conduct disorders and substance use disorders, perhaps in relation to defects in impulse control. In a study of children 8–13 years old from a child psychiatry outpatient clinic, 58% had suicidal ideation and 9% had attempted suicide. Although depressed children were most likely to have suicidal ideation or attempts, 39% of the children with nonaffective disorders also had suicidal ideation. Methods used by children to attempt suicide include substance ingestion (most common), stabbing or cutting, running in front of vehicles, jumping from buildings, gas inhalation, asphyxiation by hanging, and gun shots. Some suicide attempts may be mistaken for accidents.

Differential Diagnosis

Evaluation of depressed children should include medical evaluation for organic causes of depressive symptoms and family history of depressive or bipolar disorders or schizophrenic disorders. Children with nonaffective mental disorders may show some of the characteristics of depression. For example, children with ADHD and learning disorders may be demoralized, have trouble concentrating, and be unhappy. Also preliminary assessment of current psychopathology in the parents is informative, particularly depression or psychological reactions to stressors such as divorce or death of a family member.

Treatment

Treatment of depressed children and adolescents combines individual psychotherapy, family counseling or therapy, and in some cases medication. Psychotherapy is usually the initial treatment. However, if the depression does not respond, if symptoms are severe, or if there is evidence of bipolar or psychotic features, antidepressants are indicated. Selective serotonin reuptake inhibitors (SSRIs) are most effective and have the safest side effect profile. Whenever suicidal ideation or attempts are present, the first treatment decision is whether the child is safe and whether hospitalization may be necessary.

CHILD MALTREATMENT

INTRODUCTION

Child abuse has been described since biblical times. Through the ages the belief that children were the property of their parents enabled unspeakable acts of brutality, exploitation, and mutilation against children to go unpunished. Throughout history, the most frequent act of violence against children, infanticide, was tolerated by society and even accepted under the guise of population control, appeasing the gods, or simply getting rid of an unwanted child. Until the early 1900s, there were no requirements in this country to educate children, there were no laws preventing children from being enlisted in the work force, and there were no legal constraints or social pressures to raise children without inflicting serious physical injury on them.

In the United States, children's rights have evolved over time in much the same way as the rights of other minority groups. The 1962 landmark paper of Dr. C. Henry Kempe, "The Battered-Child Syndrome," established the groundwork for the current approach to child abuse in this country. The article created an awareness within the medical community of child battering and ultimately played a pivotal role in the enactment of the 1974 federal Child Abuse Protection and Treatment Act (CAPTA), Public Law 93-247. As a result of CAPTA, all 50 states have developed laws that mandate professional reporting in cases of suspected or identified child abuse and neglect. State statutes define penalties for failing to report suspected child abuse and grant professionals immunity when they report in good faith. Most state statutes specify that this reporting requirement supersedes all claims of professional-client privilege. Moreover, when children are abused their rights supersede those of their abusive parents.

STATISTICS

Child abuse occurs at all strata of society. According to the Third National Incidence Study of Child Abuse and Neglect (NIS-3), under the harm standard 1,553,800 (23.1 per 1000) children were victims of maltreatment in 1993. To be counted under this standard the child must have suffered demonstrable harm at the hands of the caretaker. After the endangerment standard was added to include maltreated children in danger of being harmed, the national total of abused and neglected children was 2,815,600 (41.9 per 1000). Both rates were considerably higher than the 1986 and 1980 data reported in the NIS-2 and NIS-1 studies, respectively. In the NIS-2 report, 931,000 (14.8 per 1000) children and in the NIS-1 report, 625,000 (9.8 per 1000) children were reported to have been abused nationally. The NIS-3 study reported 381,700 (5.7 per 1000) children physically abused under the harm standard, 217,700 (3.2 per 1000) children sexually abused, 204,500 (3.0 per 1000) children emotionally abused, and 879,000 (13.1 per 1000) children neglected. The number of children reported in all categories in 1993 was substantially higher than the numbers reported in 1986 and 1980.

DEFINITION

Child abuse is defined by the civil laws of each of the 50 states as nonaccidental serious physical injury, sexual exploitation or misuse, neglect, or serious mental injury of a child less than 18 years of age, as a result of acts of commission or omission by a parent, guardian, or caretaker of the child.

Child abuse is commonly classified into four categories: physical abuse, sexual abuse, neglect, and mental or emotional abuse.

Physical abuse refers to serious bodily injury through excessive force inflicted from beating, biting, burning, kicking, or otherwise harming a child. Such injury might result in welts, bruises, lacerations, fractures, or burns, which might be mild in extent or could result in death. Serious bodily injury causes the child severe pain, impairs the child's functioning temporarily or permanently, or is part of a pattern of separate injuries to the child.

Sexual abuse of children includes exposure of a child to sexual acts or materials, fondling, intercourse, incest, rape, sodomy, exhibitionism, the use of a child in the sexual gratification of an adult, and the use of a child in the production of pornography.

Neglect is the result of failure to provide for the basic needs of the child, including food, clothing, nurturing care, education, and medical care. It includes prolonged or repeated lack of supervision. Such acts of omission endanger the child's life or development or impair physical functioning. Neglect is the most common of the reported abuses and is possibly the most life-threatening.

Emotional abuse is coercive, demeaning behavior toward a child by a parent or caretaker that interferes with the child's normal social or psychological development.

PHYSICAL ABUSE

The diagnosis of physical abuse of children relies heavily on physical evidence, particularly when children are too young, too frightened, or too intimidated by the threats of perpetrators to state what happened. Physical signs of injury inflicted may include multiple skin lesions in different stages of healing, injuries in the shape or pattern of the object used to strike, and injuries that are inconsistent with the history given by the caretaker of the child. The "battered-child syndrome" described children usually under the age of 3 years who had signs of multiple episodes of trauma including subdural hematomas, fractures, and bruises in various stages of healing often in combination with failure to grow and chronic malnutrition. "Shaken baby syndrome," described most often in children under the age of 2 years, is the result of violent back and forth shaking while the child is held by the arms or torso. The violent shaking alone can result in brain injury, including contusions, subdural and subarachnoid bleeding, retinal hemorrhages, long bone and rib fractures, and spinal injuries. Shaken baby syndrome is responsible for 50% of deaths in children due to nonaccidental trauma.

The widespread prevalence of physical abuse and the numerous problems that result have been the subject of much research and debate. Much of the early research focused on the short-term effects of physical abuse on childhood behavior. Some of the potential consequences of physical abuse are lower scores on measures of intellectual functioning and academic achievement, withdrawn or aggressive behaviors, disrupted peer and adult relationships, and psychological problems such as hopelessness, low self-esteem, and depression. There is also evidence that early maltreatment has negative effects on social cognitive development, that is, how children construct, interpret, and structure their social world, how they interpret the emotions of others, and how they justify their own behavior and moral judgments.

SEXUAL ABUSE

As in other forms of child abuse, the actual incidence of sexual abuse is unknown. The 1996 National Incidence Survey conducted by the federal government found that girls are abused three times more often than boys. Retrospective survey data vary but support the long held notion that at least 20% of American women and 5–16% of American men experienced some form of sexual abuse as children. In general, children are abused by adults known to them or to their families. Studies addressing this question show that between 10% and 30% of offenders are strangers to the victimized child.

Sexual abuse can involve multiple, increasingly invasive episodes over time. Disclosures are often delayed and unconvincing. Corroborating evidence of abuse such as medical findings or credible eyewitnesses are less frequent than not. Young children lack the cognitive skills to accurately date or state the number of abusive events and to describe what happened precisely. There are spoken or implicit threats by the perpetrator or family members if the child does not remain silent. And when abuse is disclosed, the family may be thrown into chaos, as a result of separation, financial stress, and emotional turmoil. Under this pressure, it is common for children to recant reports of abuse.

Since the recognition in the 1980s of sexual abuse of children as a significant clinical entity, there has been growing interest in the impact of early sexual abuse on the child's subsequent behavior and psychopathology. A wide range of symptoms have been observed in sexually abused children, including posttraumatic stress disorder, sexualized behavior, anxiety, depression, withdrawn behavior, aggression, somatic complaints, and school problems. Among teenagers who were sexually abused as children, a variety of negative outcomes have been identified including more verbal altercations with parents, multiple sexual partners, engaging in sexual activity at an earlier age, no use of birth control, depression, suicidal thoughts, episodes of running away, and low self-esteem.

ETIOLOGY OF CHILD ABUSE & NEGLECT

Although research into the causes of child abuse and neglect often focuses on single etiologic agents, it is increasingly acknowledged that there are many, diverse contributing factors. Studies have been conducted on characteristics of abusive parents and child victims, family and social factors, culturally determined parenting beliefs and practices, life events and the perception of stress, and perceived or actual lack of social supports. Young maternal age, lack of maternal education, and maternal depression are acknowledged preexisting parent-related risk factors of child abuse. Parents who were mistreated or rejected by their parents or who abuse alcohol and drugs are at high risk for abusing and neglecting their children. A 1993 study by the U.S. Department of Health and Human Services found that children in families in which alcohol is abused were nearly four times more likely to be maltreated overall, five times more likely to be physically abused, and 10 times more likely to be emotionally neglected than children in families in which alcohol is not abused. Other studies suggest that an estimated 50–80% of all cases of child abuse substantiated by child protective services involve some degree of substance abuse by the child's parents. Premature birth and the child's temperament also have been cited as risk factors of abuse, although the results of research studying these factors are less clear. Large family size, poverty, unemployment, the type of neighborhood in which the family lives, underuse of neighborhood support services, and decreased numbers of social exchanges among neighbors (social isolation) are identified factors contributing to child abuse. Culturally determined beliefs with respect to corporal punishment and discipline, aberrant parenting skills, and the use of violence by the previous generation all predispose to child abuse.

CHILDHOOD ATTACHMENT & ABUSE

Attachment is the propensity for humans to develop strong bonds of affection to particular individuals (see Chapter 4). A basic tenet of attachment theory is that the quality of early attachment becomes a prototype for other relationships throughout life. Longitudinal studies have supported the notion that attachment style remains stable over time and that early secure attachment provides psychological supports and benefits over the course of a child's development. There is considerable evidence that children who are maltreated, in comparison to those who are not, are more likely to exhibit a variety of psychological problems, including lack of empathy, hostility, antisocial behavior, impulsivity, passivity, and helplessness, which impact negatively on the quality of later relationships.

NEGLECT & FAILURE TO THRIVE

Abuse and neglect may have adverse effects on the growth of children. The symptom complex called **failure to thrive** is used to describe children who are not growing according to expected norms. The child may have absolute growth deficiency, that is growth less than two standard deviations below the mean weight or height expected for age, or may present with a sudden shift in a previous growth pattern to one far below that of the standard growth curve.

Until the latter half of the twentieth century, it was believed that all growth failure was the result of organic causes. It is now understood that environmental factors can result in disorders of growth. Studies in the 1980s separated failure to thrive with respect to physical (organic) and environmental (nonorganic) etiologies. Some identified family factors that predispose to nonorganic failure to thrive include lack of information about parenting, lack of family resources necessary to provide appropriate child care (including food, money, housing, and health care), and parental dysfunction as a result of depression, substance abuse, and mental incapacity.

Child-related factors contributing to failure to thrive are the difficult or difficult-to-feed child and the child with minor organic problems. Parent-child interactional problems include the unwanted child, failure of parent-child bonding, and the overinvolved or enmeshed parent. Finally, isolated families with no support or family dissolution can lead to nonorganic failure to thrive. In a study of 2067 socioeconomically disadvantaged inner city children by Skuse et al (1992), those identified as nonorganic failure to thrive (NOFT) were at six times increased risk for

subsequent abuse and neglect than those who had not failed to thrive. In addition to overall blunting of body size with near normal weight for height ratios, biological rhythms of sleep and appetite as well as self-regulation were disturbed. Children awaken frequently throughout the night, wandering in search of food, their appetites insatiable. Self-regulation is impaired including lack of control of urination and defecation. Disorders of bowel and bladder function sometimes take on an aggressive quality beyond simple encopresis and enuresis. Children may deliberately urinate over the belongings of others, conceal feces, and display soiled clothes in public places. Receptive and expressive language are often impaired and attention span is brief. Social relationships are impaired; these children are disliked by almost everyone they encounter. They often suffer from depression and low self-esteem. When removed from the neglectful environment, all symptoms and signs reverse, including their growth, measures of intelligence, school performance, and bizarre behavioral features.

Illustrative Case: Failure to Thrive

A 26-month-old boy was followed regularly by his pediatrician. He had been growing along the 25th percentile for children in his age range. At the age of 13 months he stopped gaining weight entirely. Medical evaluation for organic or physical causes of growth failure was negative. In carefully reviewing the family history, the boy's mother acknowledged that the father had left the household when the child was 13 months old. Investigation of the household by child protective services revealed that the home was chaotic, there was little food available, and that the older children had stopped going to school. Services were put into place to help the mother to cope with her loss, to treat her depression, and to organize the household.

MUNCHAUSEN SYNDROME BY PROXY

Munchausen syndrome by proxy, an example of physical and emotional abuse, was first described in 1977 by Meadow (see Chapter 27). In this syndrome, the parent, most often the mother, fabricates illness in her child or children, seeks medical attention for the child, and denies any knowledge of the cause of the disorder. The child is repeatedly brought to doctors for treatment and the offending parent cooperates fully with efforts to evaluate the problem. The diagnosis of the disorder is often confirmed when the child is separated from the perpetrating parent and all symptoms and signs of illness disappear.

EVALUATION OF THE ABUSED CHILD

Evaluations of child abuse are indicated when children present with histories of abuse or neglect, signs or symptoms of inflicted physical injury, sexual abuse, sexually acting out behaviors, unusual knowledge of sexual matters, evidence of inadequate guardianship or care, or emotional maltreatment such as might result from exposure to domestic violence.

It is most desirable that evaluations of abuse be carried out by a designated multidisciplinary team of professionals with training and expertise in the field. Teams certified as Child Advocacy Centers are qualified to carry out multidisciplinary evaluations of child abuse with compassion and sensitivity, thereby minimizing trauma to children and families. Ideally such teams should consist of medical, social service, law enforcement, mental health, child protective, and legal professionals. The team should collectively have expertise in techniques of forensic interview and physical examination and should be able to intervene on behalf of the child and family in crisis. Child abuse often creates medical problems for children, but always has social, legal, and psychological implications. Initial evaluations of child abuse, which take place in an Emergency Department, should be followed up when possible by specialized, multidisciplinary teams.

The clinical assessment of children who are victims of abuse and neglect has several basic elements: the previsit gathering of all background information, the interview of the accompanying caretaker or adult, the psychosocial assessment of the victimized child, the forensic interview of the child, when appropriate to the child's cognitive abilities and emotional state (conducted with a nonabusing parent to minimize trauma to the child), the medical evaluation, the collection of forensic evidence as indicated, the collection of cultures and blood specimens, detailed and objective documentation of the visit including the diagnosis and plan, the referral for treatment, and the follow-up plan.

Referrals & Previsit Gathering of Information

Children who have been removed from abusive homes may, in the safety of their new home, give delayed disclosure of abuse. Others may be referred when separated parents suspect each other of abuse. Children may present at school with injuries or histories of child abuse. Schools or mental health agencies may request evaluation of children with disclosures or behaviors suggesting abuse.

The previsit gathering of information is particularly important when children have been in the foster care system, have had previous evaluations of child abuse, or have had preexisting physical, behavioral, or mental conditions.

The Interview of the Accompanying Adult

When possible, the adult accompanying a child to an evaluation should not be a stranger to the child and should not be the suspected abuser. A trusted adult will be important to the evaluation process, par-

ticularly the medical assessment. The adult should be prepared with as much information as possible about the reason for referral as well as the past medical and other history to assist the team in making an informed decision and appropriate recommendations to ensure the child's safety and well being.

The Interview of the Child

In the case of the school-aged child the evaluation may include a lengthy and detailed forensic interview by a social worker or other professional trained in the techniques of the nonleading interview. To reduce the trauma of repeated interviews, the forensic interview should be conducted by one professional, while other involved professionals listen and observe behind a one-way mirror. The joint interview should have the full consent of the child and the guardian.

Medical Evaluation

The medical evaluation includes a general health history, weight, height, and blood pressure, and a head-to-toe examination. The assessment for child abuse and neglect should include the detailed documentation of physical findings, including skin lesions, bony deformities, external anogenital findings for evidence of past and recent trauma, and neurological and developmental assessment. Injuries resulting from physical abuse are documented by photographs. In the case of sexual abuse, colposcopy photographs are taken of the external anogenital area. Cultures and blood tests are collected when appropriate to the history or medical findings. Following the assessment phase, the team convenes to discuss the findings in the case and to determine the recommendations to ensure the safety of the child and the most appropriate treatment. The proper, detailed recording of findings is a critical component of the evaluation. The record is a legal document that may be subpoenaed in civil court child protective proceedings and in the criminal prosecution of alleged perpetrators.

DOMESTIC VIOLENCE & CHILD ABUSE

Child abuse often accompanies other forms of interfamily violence, including spousal abuse and violence among siblings. Children may be threatened and victimized as a way of controlling and punishing the adult victim of domestic violence. Episodes of spousal abuse may expand to include children, particularly when children purposely try to intercede or are accidental victims. Even when children are not directly attacked, they can experience serious emotional damage as a result of living in a violent household. Moreover, there is considerable concern that children come to believe that the violent behaviors they witness are acceptable. It is estimated that physical abuse and sexual abuse of children coexist with domestic violence in 30–50% of cases.

TREATMENT & INTERVENTION

Just as there is no identified single cause or simple model explaining why child abuse occurs, there is no simple model for successful treatment. One large study by Cohn and Daro (1987) found that one-third of families continued to abuse or neglect their children during treatment. In the same study one-half of families were considered no less likely to engage in abuse once treatment had ended. Successful intervention in child abuse must include strategies to improve the environment in which a child is raised and reduce caregiver stress in ways that support the development of the child. An example of a parental risk factor can be seen in the attitude a parent may have toward a crying child. In the high-risk environment, the parent sees the crying child as bad. The parent who sees the same crying child as upset might be at lower risk for abusing the child. Many child abuse prevention programs focus on skills needed by parents to improve their relationships with children at all stages of development. These programs also stress basic family skills, such as planning and preparing a meal, budgeting income, enhancing communication, improving self esteem, relaxation techniques, and identifying and using family and outside supports. Parents with alcohol and substance abuse problems are directed to therapeutic programs and those with depression are directed toward appropriate therapy.

CONCLUSIONS

Child abuse can be viewed as a condition resulting from family dysfunction. Recognition of this devastating societal problem is assigned to professionals who are trained to recognize the signs and symptoms of abuse in children and families. The goal of child abuse intervention is first and foremost to protect the child from further harm. To help children begin the road to recovery and to avoid significant negative sequelae of abuse takes the coordinated efforts of multidisciplinary evaluation and crisis intervention teams, comprised of medical, social service, child welfare, mental health, law enforcement, and legal professionals. Ongoing education of professionals and the public about the signs and symptoms of abuse is essential in ensuring that abused children who are identified in schools, in camps, in medical settings, or in therapy can be directed quickly to a safe setting.

There are systems in place to reduce the trauma of disclosure of child abuse. As improved research methodology enhances our understanding of the short- and long-term sequelae of child abuse, it will become possible to anticipate long-term behavioral and psychological problems resulting from abuse and to intervene effectively to prevent them. The ultimate goal, prevention of abuse, will result from our ever-increasing understanding of the problem.

MENTAL RETARDATION*

The American Association on Mental Deficiency defined mental retardation as "significantly subaverage intellectual functioning originating during the developmental period, accompanied by impairment in one or more of the following: maturation, learning, or social adjustment."

In 1992 the definition was changed to indicate that the impaired intellectual functioning had to exist concurrently with significant limitations in adaptive functioning in at least two of the following areas: communication, self-care, home living, social skills, community use, self-direction, health and safety, functional academics, leisure, and work, with onset before 18 years of age.

The prevalence of mental retardation in developed countries ranges from 1% to 3%. The incidence of emotional disorders in mentally retarded individuals is also very high, with various studies in the 1990s reporting ranges from 10% to 60%. It is usually an emotional problem or a difficulty in adjustment that brings people with mental retardation to the attention of society. For the vast majority of these individuals (the 85% who are mildly retarded and educable), difficulties begin during the school years. With adequate instruction in a supportive environment, these people can function in the general population and find a suitable vocation.

Diagnosis

The presenting symptoms in individuals with mental retardation are generally problems in adaptive function or personal independence. Independent functioning is less than expected for their age group in their community. People with mental retardation come to professional attention because of their behavior rather than their low IQ test result.

General intellectual functioning is measured by the intelligence quotient (IQ) (see Figure 28–1) using a standardized test such as the Wechsler Intelligence Scale for Children–III (WISC–III), Stanford-Binet, Kaufman Assessment Battery for Children, or the Wechsler Adult Intelligence Scale–Revised (WAIS–R) (see Chapter 13).

An IQ of 70 or below (two standard deviations below the mean) is considered significantly subaverage. Generally, there is a measurement error of about 5 points. The choice of test should consider the language and culture of the individual being tested. Other factors that may limit test performance are

---

* Included in this section is material contributed by Louis M. Flohr, MD, and Irving Philips, MD.

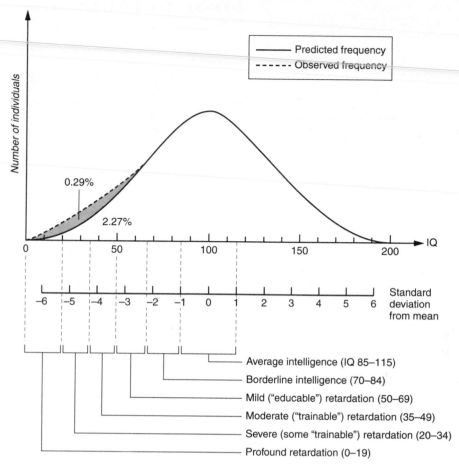

Figure 28–1. Distribution and classification of mental retardation. The shaded area denotes an increased incidence of 0.29% over the predicted frequency, resulting from organic causes of mental retardation. (Modified and reproduced, with permission, from Moser HW, Wold PA: The nosology of mental retardation: Including the report of a survey of 1378 mentally retarded individuals at the Walter E. Fernald State School. In: *Nervous System*. Bergsma D [editor]. Part 6 of: The Second Conference on the Clinical Delineation of Birth Defects. Williams & Wilkins for the National Foundation–March of Dimes, Birth Defects Original Article Series 1971;7:117.)

communication deficits and motor and sensory handicaps.

Scales have also been developed to measure adaptive function such as the Vineland Adaptive Behavior Scales or the American Association on Mental Retardation Adaptive Behavior Scale. In the Vineland Adaptive Behavior Scale, a composite score of daily living skills, communication, socialization, and motor skills is correlated with the expected skills for the person's age.

Adaptive function can be influenced by personality, education, vocational opportunities, medical conditions, and mental disorders. Problems with adaptation may be improved with remedial efforts while IQ is more likely to be stable.

Classification

DSM-IV describes four levels of severity (Table 28–11) of mental retardation: mild (IQ 70 to 55–50), moderate (IQ 55–50 to 40–35), severe (IQ 40–35 to 25–20), and profound (IQ below 25–20). Characteristics of levels of severity of mental retardation by age group are given in Table 28–12.

Mental Retardation, Severity Unspecified describes a condition in which there is strong presumption of Mental Retardation, but the individual cannot be tested by standard tests because, for example, the person is too impaired or uncooperative. Borderline Intellectual Functioning (IQ 71–84) is an IQ range higher than for Mental Retardation (an IQ of 70 or below). However, considering a measurement error of

Table 28–11. *DSM-IV* diagnostic criteria for mental retardation.

A. Significantly subaverage intellectual functioning: an IQ of approximately 70 or below on an individually administered IQ test (for infants, a clinical judgment of significantly subaverage intellectual functioning).

B. Concurrent deficits or impairments in present adaptive functioning (ie, the person's effectiveness in meeting the standards expected for his or her age by his or her cultural group) in at least two of the following areas: communication, self-care, home living, social/interpersonal skills, use of community resources, self-direction, functional academic skills, work, leisure, health, and safety.

C. The onset is before age 18 years.

Code based on degree of severity reflecting level of intellectual impairment:

Mild Mental Retardation:	IQ level 50–55 to approximately 70
Moderate Mental Retardation:	IQ level 35–40 to 50–55
Severe Mental Retardation:	IQ level 20–25 to 35–40
Profound Mental Retardation:	IQ level below 20 or 25

Mental Retardation, Severity Unspecified: when there is strong presumption of Mental Retardation but the person's intelligence is untestable by standard tests

approximately 5 points for IQ tests, a person with an IQ of 70–75 and significant deficits in adaptive function may meet the criteria for Mental Retardation.

The American Association of Mental Retardation classifies mental retardation on the basis of levels of support needed (intermittent, limited, extensive, and pervasive). Another educational classification was designed for school and class placement (educable, trainable, severe, and profound/custodial).

Illustrative Case: Mild Mental Retardation

When a 6-year-old well-adjusted boy was noted to have learning difficulties by his teacher, she re- quested evaluation and consultation from the school Child Study Team. Testing indicated that he had an IQ in the range of 63–69. His teacher continued to give him individually paced instruction in her class as suggested by the Individualized Education Program (IEP) developed by the Child Study Team. A similar approach, with individual tutoring as needed, was followed when he reached high school. The placid boy enjoyed participation on the track team and was accepted by his peers. His family encouraged his interest in fishing, and at age 16, he began to learn about commercial fishing at a local firm. When he was subsequently hired by the firm, he told his family, "I may never make it to manager, but I'll always make a decent living." He later married and had two children.

Illustrative Case: Moderate Mental Retardation

The neighbors of a teenager (age 14) with moderate mental retardation complained that he frightened their young daughter by asking her questions at the bus stop. The boy's parents were afraid that the next time this happened the police would be called. They sought help from a child psychiatrist.

The history revealed that the boy was born with microcephaly after 8 months of gestation. He required assistance with breathing for 2 weeks in the neonatal intensive care unit. During infancy, he had multiple hospitalizations for respiratory problems. Between the ages of 2½ and 8 years, he attended a day school for children with mental retardation. From there, he went to public school and attended special education classes, which he was still doing at the time of the evaluation.

Initial assessment showed a boy with odd-sounding nasal speech. When he felt anxious, he touched people's faces and clothes, asked many questions, and fidgeted. When he relaxed, he could sit still for

Table 28–12. Characteristics of levels of severity of mental retardation by age group.[a]

Degree of Severity	Percentage of All with Mental Retardation	Early Childhood	Elementary School and Adolescence	Adult
Profound below 20–25	1–2%	Considerable impairments in functioning	Possible speech and motor development	Sheltered setting
Severe 20–25 to 35–40	3–4%	Little or no communicative speech	May learn to talk, basic self-care skills	May perform simple tasks in sheltered setting, group home, or family
Moderate 35–40 to 50–55 (trainable)	10%	Can communicate or talk	Can learn up to second grade skills, independent travel in familiar places, can profit from vocational training	Sheltered workshop or general workforce under supervision
Mild 50–55 to 70 (educable)	85%	Often not distinguishable from normal, minimal motor delay	By late teens can acquire sixth grade skills	Can live in the community with supports

[a] Adapted by *DSM-IV.*

longer periods. The parents reported that his anxiety level and inappropriate behavior had increased since puberty. They expressed their own worries about his sexual maturity and immature coping abilities: "What if he masturbates in public? What if he tries to kiss a little girl? How can we explain to him what he should and should not do?" The parents agreed to counseling for themselves and social skills training for their son to help them cope with this new period of adjustment. The boy continued in school and lived at home until he was 19 years old. He then moved to a group home for young adults with developmental disabilities in a suburb of his hometown.

Etiology

Multiple mechanisms have been implicated as causative factors in mental retardation, including genetic conditions (Table 28–13), infections occurring in the mother during pregnancy (Table 28–14), prenatal exposure to toxins, perinatal injury and prematurity, and metabolic disorders (Table 28–15), central nervous system trauma, hypoxia, and environmental factors. A likely cause can be determined in about two-thirds of individuals with mental retardation and is more often identified in the most severely affected.

Table 28–13. Selected genetic syndromes associated with mental retardation.

Trisomy 18	
Trisomy 13	
Partial trisomy 14	
Trisomy 21 (Down)	
Lesch-Nyhan syndrome	X-linked
Lowe's (oculocerebrorenal)	X-linked recessive
Menkes	X-linked recessive
Rett's syndrome	X-linked
Fragile X	X-linked
Incontinentia pigmenti	X-linked dominant?
Seckel	Autosomal recessive
Sjögren-Larsson	Autosomal recessive
Smith-Lemli-Opitz	Autosomal recessive
Cockayne's	Autosomal recessive
Cohen	Autosomal recessive?
Dubowitz	Autosomal recessive
Laurence Moon Biedl	Autosomal recessive
Alpert's (acrocephalosyndactyly)	Autosomal dominant
Neurofibromatosis	Autosomal dominant
Tuberous sclerosis	Autosomal dominant
Williams	Microdeletion chromosome 7
Wolf Hirschhorn syndrome	Deletion of 4p
Cri-du-chat	Partial deletion of chromosome 5
Prader-Willi	Deletion in q11–q12 region of chromosome 15 (paternal)
Angelman syndrome	Deletion in q11–q12 region of chromosome 15 (maternal)

Table 28–14. Maternal infections during pregnancy associated with mental retardation in offspring.

Cytomegalic inclusion disease
Herpes simplex
Human immunodeficiency virus (HIV)
Rubella (German measles)
Syphilis
Toxoplasmosis

Common Conditions Associated with Mental Retardation

The most common causes of mental retardation are Down syndrome, fragile X syndrome, and fetal alcohol syndrome. Diagnosis of a rare syndrome for a child is useful to provide recognition of treatable occult congenital anomalies or later development of rare medical problems associated with the syndrome.

A. Down Syndrome: Down syndrome was first described as "mongolism" in 1866. The incidence is one in 650 births, and about 10% of institutionalized retarded patients have Down syndrome.

Three distinct chromosomal types of Down syndrome have been identified. (1) The best-known type, trisomy 21 (nearly 95% of cases), results when nondisjunction of chromosomes 21 occurs during meiosis. The complete descendant cell line has three chromosomes 21, or a total of 47 chromosomes in each cell of the body. The incidence is directly related to maternal age (and, according to some research, paternal age). The risk of giving birth to an

Table 28–15. Inborn errors of metabolism associated with mental retardation.

Amino acid
  Homocystinuria
  Maple syrup urine disease
  Methylmalonic acidemia
  Nonketotic hyperglycinemia
  Phenylketonuria
  Propionic acidemia
  Tyrosinosis
  Urea cycle disorders
Lipid
  Farber's lipogranulomatosis
  Generalized gangliosidosis
  Infantile Gaucher's disease
  Krabbe's disease
  Metachromatic leukodystrophy
  Niemann-Pick disease
  Tay-Sachs disease
Mucopolysaccharide
  Hurler's syndrome MPS I
  Hunter's disease II
  Maroteaux-Lamy syndrome VI
  Sanfilippo's syndrome III
Other
  Galactosemia
  Fucosidosis
  I-cell disease
  Lesch-Nyhan syndrome
  Mannosidosis
  Wilson's hepatolenticular degeneration

infant with trisomy 21 is less than 0.2% in women under 35 years of age, about 0.9% in those 35–40 years, 1.4% in those 40–45 years, and 2.5% in those over 45. (2) The second major form, the translocation type, is caused by fusion of two chromosomes, usually 21 and 15. The total number of chromosomes is 46 because the extra chromosome (or part of one) is fused to another. The abnormal chromosome can be found in an otherwise unaffected father, mother, or sibling. This type occurs at any maternal age, it is heritable, and once it is present, subsequent pregnancies of the same parents are theoretically at an increased risk. For this reason, the parents of any child with Down syndrome should be given genetic counseling. (3) Mosaicism, the least frequent type of Down syndrome, is caused by nondisjunction of chromosome 21 after fertilization during any of the early mitoses, which results in a "mosaic" of both normal and trisomic cell lines.

Down syndrome has been extensively studied. Mental retardation, its cardinal feature, can be present to any degree from profound retardation (IQ below 20) to borderline normal intelligence (IQ of 71–84). When the IQ scores of patients with Down syndrome are plotted on a graph, the scores form a normal distribution curve between 0 and 100, with the mean at the high end of the moderately retarded range (IQ of 35–49). Thus, although the characteristic clinical features of the syndrome (see below) make it easily diagnosable at birth, the future intellectual and social functioning of the child cannot be predicted with certainty at that time. Appropriate medical support and immediate enrollment of the parents and child in an infant development program are recommended to ensure optimal early development.

Although the full description of Down syndrome includes over 100 features and numerous medical complications, it should be emphasized that only some of the features will be seen in any one individual and that the physician's approach to a given family must strike a properly informed note, neither too pessimistic nor too optimistic. Besides the chromosome findings and some degree of retardation, characteristic features include epicanthal folds, oblique palpebral fissures, high cheekbones (hence the term "mongolism"), a large and protruding tongue, microcephaly, anteroposterior flattening of the skull, broad and thick hands, shortened and rounded small ears, and hypotonic musculature. Many patients have a single transverse palmar ("simian") crease that was originally thought to be pathognomonic of the syndrome but is seen in many other retardation syndromes and in nonretarded people as well.

Patients with Down syndrome are more susceptible to infections in childhood, have a 30–50% incidence of congenital heart defects, and have an increased incidence of cataracts, diabetes mellitus, seizures, thyroid disorders, leukemia, cervical spine instability, and gastrointestinal malformations. They also have a very high rate of developing dementia after age 40.

B. Fragile X Syndrome: Fragile X syndrome (named for an unstable constriction on the long arm of the X chromosome in cells cultured in media depleted of thymidine and folate) is a very common hereditary cause of mental retardation. The gene *FMR-1* contains a trinucleotide repeat of a cytosine–guanine–guanine residue (CGG). Normally there are 5–50 repeats of CGG and these are transmitted in a stable fashion to offspring. When there are 50–500 repeats there is no expression of the gene, but the repeat sequence expands in transmission to offspring (dynamic mutation). The repeats may expand up to 3000 in number and are associated with mental retardation. Fragile X has the property of anticipation (the disorder is more severely expressed in successive generations) and unaffected women in the same family have different risks of having a son with fragile X mental retardation since risk rises with the size of the repeat. Clinical characteristics include a long face with midfacial hypoplasia, large ears, large testes, and hyperextensible joints. Behavioral problems include learning disabilities, language impairment, attention deficit hyperactivity disorder, and autistic behaviors.

C. Fetal Alcohol Syndrome: First described in 1973, fetal alcohol syndrome, a frequent cause of mental retardation, is due to maternal use of alcohol during pregnancy. Although what if any dose of alcohol is safe for a fetus has not been determined, women with chronic alcohol use are at high risk for having offspring with a characteristic set of abnormalities. Clinical features include pre- and postnatal growth failure, cardiac abnormalities, and microcephaly. As head/face growth may reflect brain development, midface abnormalities such as maxillary hypoplasia and short palpebral fissures can be found. Hyperactivity, language disorders, eating disorders, stereotyped movements, anxiety, and depression may be found at increased rates in affected children.

Genetic Counseling & Prenatal Diagnosis

In prenatal genetic diagnosis, techniques such as amniocentesis, chorionic villus biopsy, and ultrasonography are performed to determine whether the fetus is affected by genetic diseases for which it is thought to be at risk. Chorionic villus biopsy can be performed in the first trimester, but is slightly more risky than amniocentesis, which is performed later. In amniocentesis, about 15 mL of amniotic fluid is removed from the uterus after a local anesthetic is applied to the site of needle insertion. The procedure takes about 10 minutes. Most centers recommend that women under age 35 (some say under age 37) should not have amniocentesis unless a possibility of genetic disease is disclosed by genetic counseling. The procedure is performed between weeks 15 and 18 of gestation, but results may not be available until up to 4 weeks later. Test results are negative in 95% of women over age 35. About 100 biochemical disorders and a large number of chromosomal problems are detectable.

Fetal visualization and biopsy are becoming increasingly useful for the detection of fetal abnormalities that are not associated with biochemical or chromosomal disorders. Ultrasonography makes it possible to detect physical anomalies and intrauterine growth problems and to determine gestational age. Fetoscopy permits direct visualization of the fetus and also makes it possible to sample fetal blood to detect hemoglobinopathies.

Treatment

Treatment for individuals with mental retardation is multidisciplinary, including educational, speech and language, medical, vocational, and behavioral interventions.

Special Education programs for the child are an integral part of treatment and should include academic skills, social skills, and vocational training. Children whose mental retardation is mild may master sixth grade academic skills and may develop sufficient social and vocational skills to permit partial or full independence. Children whose mental retardation is moderate may master up to second grade skills and may learn vocational skills that permit competitive employment with support. The severely to profoundly retarded child can establish self-care routines and

sometimes recognition of "survival" words ("help," "hot") (see Table 28–12). Universal public education for all retarded children became available in the 1970s as a result of parental pressure, lawsuits, and federal laws (see Table 28–16).

Psychotherapy may be helpful for the child with mental retardation. The therapist usually takes an active role and uses concrete interventions, paying particular attention to the developmental level of the patient. Behavioral therapy may improve adaptive behavior by using reinforcement and suppress maladaptive behavior. Cognitive therapy may be helpful for depression. Relaxation therapy may help reduce or control anxiety.

Pharmacological treatment of their psychiatric disorders may enable individuals with mental retardation to make more effective use of special education, social skills training, and other programs. Target problems (and their treatments) might include attention-deficit hyperactivity disorder (stimulants, such as methylphenidate), stereotypic movements (antipsychotic drugs), aggression and rage (β-blockers, buspirone, antipsychotic drugs), and self-injurious behavior (naltrexone, lithium, anticonvulsants).

Education for the family may address methods of enhancing competence of the child while maintaining realistic expectations. Parents may benefit from counseling or therapy to address their feelings of sadness, guilt, anger, and frustration regarding their family member's disorder and future.

Table 28–16. Major court decisions and laws regarding mental retardation.

Brown v. Board of Education, 1954	A separate educational system does not provide equal opportunity (race)
Public Law 88-164 The Mental Retardation Facilities and Community and Mental Health Centers Construction Act of 1963	Funds for university-affiliated facilities, mental retardation research centers, and community facilities
Wolf v. State of Utah, 1969	Children in Utah have a right to public education regardless of retardation
Wyatt v. Stickney, 1972	Minimum standards for medical care and privacy, prohibited aversive procedures, excessive use of psychopharmacology, least restrictive conditions
Donaldson v. O'Connor, 1975	Right to treatment, to remain in community if safe
New York Association for Retarded Children v. Rockefeller, 1972	Minimum standards of care
Souter v. Brennan, 1973	Prohibited unpaid labor
Public Law 94-142, 1975 Education for All Handicapped Children Act	Right to appropriate education
Public Law 95-602, 1978 Rehabilitative, Comprehensive Services, and Developmental Disabilities Act	Definition of developmental disabilities based on functional impairments
Wyatt v. Aderholt, 1982	Restrictions on sterilization
Youngberg v. Romeo, 1982	Constitutional rights for those confined in state institutions (safety, undue restraint, training)
Pennhurst v. Halderman, 1984	Least restrictive setting
Public Law 99-457	Benefits to children under 3 years of age
Social Security Amendments 1972 to 1990	Federal support for mental retardation facilities focusing on rehabilitation, Supplemental Security Income (SSI), community focus on help in home setting

REFERENCES & SUGGESTED READINGS

Ambrosini PJ, Bianchi MD, Rabinovich H, Elia J: Antidepressant treatments in children and adolescents. I. Affective disorders. J Am Acad Child Adolesc Psychiatry 1993;32:1.

American Association on Mental Deficiency: *Manual on Terminology and Classification in Mental Retardation.* Grossman H (editor). American Association on Mental Deficiency, 1977.

American Psychiatric Association: *Diagnostic and Statistical Manual of Mental Disorders,* 4th ed. (*DSM-IV*). American Psychiatric Association, 1994.

Bernstein GA, Borchardt CM: Anxiety disorders of childhood and adolescence. A critical review. J Am Acad Child Adolesc Psychiatry 1991;30:519.

Birmaher B, Brent D, and the Workgroup on Quality Issues: Practice parameters for the assessment and treatment of children and adolescents with depressive disorders. J Am Acad Child Adolesc Psychiatry 1998;37(Suppl):63S.

Child Welfare League of America: Highlights of Questions from the Working Paper on Chemical Dependency. Washington, DC, 1989.

Cohen DJ, Pauls D, Volkmar FR: Recent research in autism. Child Adolesc Psychiatr Clin North Am 1994;3:161.

Cohn AH, Daro D: Is treatment too late: What 10 years of evaluative research tells us. Child Abuse Negl 1987; 11:433.

Henggeler SW et al: *Multisystemic Treatment of Antisocial Behavior in Children and Adolescents.* Guilford, 1998.

Kanner L: *Childhood Psychosis: Initial Studies and New Insights.* Winston/Wiley, 1973.

Kempe CH et al: The battered-child syndrome. JAMA 1962;181:17.

King BH et al: Mental retardation: A review of the past 10 years. Part I. J Am Acad Child Adolesc Psychiatry 1997; 36:1656.

Kovacs M, Goldston D, Gatsonis C: Suicidal behaviors and childhood onset depressive disorders: A longitudinal investigation. J Am Acad Child Adolesc Psychiatry 1993; 32:8.

Ludwig S: Defining child abuse: Clinical mandate—evolving concepts. In: *Child Abuse, A Medical Reference.* Ludwig S, Kornberg AE (editors). Churchill Livingstone, 1992.

Meadow R: Munchhausen syndrome by proxy. The hinterland of child abuse. Lancet 1977;ii:343.

Quiggle NL et al: Social information processing in aggressive and depressed children. Child Dev 1992;63:1305.

Rutter M et al: Isle of Wight studies, 1964–1974. Psychol Med 1976;6:313.

Sedlak AJ, Broadhurst DD: *The Third National Incidence Study of Child Abuse and Neglect (NIS-3).* U.S. Department of Health and Human Services, Administration for Children and Families, Administration on Children, Youth and Families, National Center on Child Abuse and Neglect, 1996.

Sharma V, Matier K, Halperin J: Disruptive behavior disorders, assessment and differential diagnosis. Child Adolesc Psychiatr Clin North Am 1994;3:253.

Skuse D, Wolke D, Reilly S: Failure to thrive. Clinical and developmental aspects. In: *Child and Youth Psychiatry. European Perspectives,* Vol. II: *Developmental Psychopathology.* Remschmidt H, Schmidt M (editors). Hans Huber, 1992.

Sroufe LA: The role of infant-caregiver attachment in development. In: *Clinical Implications of Attachment.* Belsky J, Nezworski T (editors). Erlbaum, 1988.

State MW, King BH, Dykens E: Mental Retardation: A review of the past 10 years. Part II. J Am Acad Child Adolesc Psychiatry 1997;36:1664.

Steinhauer PD, Rae-Grant Q: *Psychological Problems of the Child in the Family.* Basic Books, 1983.

Styron T, Janoff-Bulman R: Childhood attachment and abuse: Long-term effects on adult attachment, depression, and conflict resolution. Child Abuse Negl 1997; 21:1015.

U.S. Department of Health and Human Services, National Center on Child Abuse and Neglect: *A Report on Child Maltreatment in Alcohol Abusing Families.* Government Printing Office, 1993.

Volk A: The pre-history of child psychiatry. Br J Psychiatry 1964;110:754.

Volkmar FR, Cohen DJ: Autism: Current concepts. Child Adolesc Psychiatr Clin North Am 1994;3:43.

Wiener JM: *Textbook of Child and Adolescent Psychiatry.* American Psychiatric Press, 1997.

Zametkin AJ et al: Cerebral glucose metabolism in adults with hyperactivity of childhood onset. N Engl J Med 1990;323:1361.

Section IV.
Treatment Modalities

Introduction to Psychiatric Treatment

29

Beth Goldman, MD, MPH, & Howard H. Goldman, MD, MPH, PhD

As the preceding chapters have attempted to show, a multifactorial approach is necessary to explain the etiology and pathogenesis of psychiatric illness. Similarly, the most useful treatment approaches are developed within the framework of the biopsychosocial model (see Chapters 1–3).

Psychiatric treatment may comprise one or many modalities and may be rendered in a number of settings depending on both the needs and the circumstances—physical, economic, geographic—of each individual patient. Weekly outpatient behavior modification treatment would be appropriate for an otherwise happy and successful advertising executive who wishes to be cured of fear of flying, whereas involuntary inpatient treatment along with pharmacotherapy and, later, social service interventions would be mandatory for the psychotic, assaultive mayor of Wino Park (Chapters 9 and 14). Furthermore, different treatment approaches may be useful at different times over the course of any individual patient's illness. For example, a young person undergoing a major depressive episode may not be able to respond to or tolerate exploratory psychotherapy without prior antidepressant drug therapy and supportive treatment. In this chapter, the settings in which mental illness may be treated are described as well as the individuals who deliver such treatment. In Chapters 30–41, the actual treatment techniques and their advantages and disadvantages are discussed.

SETTINGS IN WHICH MENTAL HEALTH CARE MAY BE OFFERED

Mental health services are traditionally delivered in hospitals, outpatient office settings, day treatment programs, and emergency rooms. In some cases, psychiatrists and other mental health professionals may work with, and in, other agencies such as penal institutions, law courts, schools at all levels, places of employment, and even in the patient's home.

Individuals requiring or requesting treatment may present in a variety of ways at a number of different "entry points" into the mental health care delivery system. New patients may present at the private offices of general physicians or specialists, mental health professionals, community-based crisis intervention centers, community mental health centers, or hospital emergency rooms. Specially trained professionals at these sites evaluate the current status and needs of each individual patient and make recommendations or referrals for further treatment. When patients are dangerous to themselves or others or are unable to care for themselves and do not understand their need for treatment, such a recommendation may be made mandatory by court order.

Inpatient Settings

Psychiatric hospitalization may be necessary for a variety of patients who cannot be treated effectively or safely as outpatients. Some patients require specialized diagnostic procedures (eg, for close observation of symptoms, specialized endocrine or sleep studies) that can be performed safely and properly only in a hospital; others may require almost constant nursing attention (eg, physically ill patients who develop dangerous side effects to medications, agitated patients who require seclusion) that can be provided only on an inpatient basis. Psychiatric patients are also admitted for their own protection or the protection of others, as in the case of suicidal or homicidal patients or patients who are so disorganized, depressed, or demented that they cannot care for themselves. Such patients are observed closely, protected, restricted, and confined and are usually treated for the specific mental disorder underlying their behavior. In some cases, individuals accused of criminal activity are admitted to a hospital for forensic psychiatric evaluation of criminal responsibility or competence to stand trial (Chapter 40). Hospitals may also be used inappropriately and unnecessarily when less intensive services would suffice, and some patients may even "manipulate the system" to obtain admission (eg, the homeless individual who uses the hospital as a shelter or the individual with antisocial personality disorder who is in trouble on the streets and "escapes" into the psychiatric unit).

Hospital settings offer a wide variety of treatment options, including medical treatment; group, individual, and family psychotherapy; social worker services; and occupational and recreational activity therapies. Ideally, the treatment plan is tailored to meet the medical, social, and psychological needs of each individual patient.

In the United States, inpatient psychiatric care may be delivered in state and county mental hospitals, private mental hospitals, general hospitals (often in specialized psychiatric units), Veterans Administration hospitals, and military hospitals. Improvements in the efficacy of somatic treatments (Chapter 30) that resulted in shortening the period of acute symptoms in many patients shifted the emphasis from long-term to short-term care and away from reliance on state and county hospital systems. Furthermore, since hospitalization can lead to stigmatization, loss of self-esteem, dependency, and regressed behavior, the trend is toward minimizing hospital stays and utilizing less restrictive treatment settings (eg, day treatment) in innovative and more intensive ways. Progress in this area is encouraged by governmental agencies (Medicaid and Medicare) and private third-party payers (eg, Blue Cross), who are reluctant to pay for inpatient services for any but the sickest of patients. Current managed care practices have encouraged the trend away from hospital admissions, favoring less expensive services provided in lieu of hospital days.

Outpatient Care

Outpatient services are provided in freestanding clinics, clinics attached to hospitals, community mental health centers (CMHCs), and private offices. Almost unknown in the nineteenth and early twentieth centuries, outpatient services now account for the majority of psychiatric utilization. In the 1950s the split between outpatient and inpatient care was approximately 25%/75%. Today, that ratio has been reversed.

Outpatient treatment is appropriate for patients with a wide variety of psychiatric illnesses varying from problems of living and adjustment disorders to those with psychotic and mood disorders. As alluded to above, the trend over the past 30–40 years has been to move away from inpatient care toward outpatient treatment. Traditionally, outpatient care has consisted of seeing a therapist in group or individual treatment for no more than 1 or 2 hours a week. Although many people who function well at home and at work benefit from such limited treatment, there are many others with more severe mental disorders who need a more intense level of care but who do not require 24-hour supervision as is provided in a traditional inpatient setting.

In the past—prior to the era of managed care—many patients who could not function within the limited framework of traditional outpatient treatment were hospitalized: (1) it was often easier to hospitalize a patient than to provide the complex and time-consuming kind of support that an outpatient in crisis may require; (2) third-party payers often paid for inpatient care more readily than intense outpatient care; and (3) few resources had been developed to provide intermediate alternatives to the choice between traditional outpatient and costly and restrictive inpatient care.

However, as managed care companies limit payment for inpatient treatment to only the sickest patients, innovations in outpatient care are developing. Less seriously impaired individuals may be seen in **intensive outpatient treatment,** where contact with the patient is "titrated" to the patient's condition. Patients who are more impaired may be treated in a **partial hospital** setting.

Partial Hospitalization

In partial hospitalization programs, patients receive much the same range of services provided in traditional inpatient settings but are, in most cases, allowed to go home at night. (Rarely, patients work or study by day but stay at the hospital at night.) Such care may be offered to hospitalized patients to help them readjust to life outside the hospital or to fairly ill patients who need supervision but who can safely be at home nights and weekends. This form of treatment is much less expensive than full-time hospitalization.

Chronically ill patients sometimes receive similar care in "day treatment" and "psychiatric rehabilitation" programs designed to provide structure, training in social skills, vocational training, and other treatment over longer periods of time.

Residential Treatment Programs

Residential treatment programs (often called three-quarter way or halfway houses) offer treatment in structured nonhospital settings. Some offer graduated services ranging from completely supervised homes with 24-hour supervision and a full range of structured activities and treatments to less supervised arrangements (eg, an apartment shared by two patients) in which patients combine treatment with other activities such as volunteer or paid work. Such facilities slowly move the patient in the direction of semi-independent or fully independent living.

Residential self-help communities are usually sponsored by nongovernmental agencies for the purpose of helping individuals with some specific difficulty, often chemical dependency. Examples include Oxford House and the Salvation Army (both created for persons with drug and alcohol problems). Residents in these communities often maintain ties with the community after leaving the residence.

Substitute homes provide shelter and limited treatment to patients who either do not require or would not benefit from other kinds of residential treatment programs. Persons living in such homes often are unable to live alone and unsupervised and have either no family support or families who cannot continue to provide care (eg, because of disruptive behavior or burnout). Treatment is usually confined to supervision of activities of daily living, medication, informal counseling (usually provided by a layperson who manages the home), and sometimes transportation to therapists' offices or in-house medication management provided by a psychiatrist on contract to the home. Examples include adult foster care homes, board and care homes, family care homes, and mental hygiene homes. There is increasing reliance on "supported housing," typically apartments scattered throughout a community with no live-in staff but supportive services as required.

Other examples of substitute housing include "crash pads" for people withdrawing from drugs or in crisis and in need of a safe place. Similarly, temporary shelters for abused women and even the homeless may be regarded as part of the mental health care system.

Emergency & Crisis Intervention

Crisis intervention services are offered by hospital and nonhospital facilities and provide episodic acute intervention in life-threatening or extreme circumstances involving patients with mental illness or others in crisis. In such settings, including private homes, patients are evaluated—sometimes over several hours—and, when feasible, attempts are made to help resolve the crisis. In many cases, these facilities serve as entry points into the mental health system whereby patients may be referred for further inpatient or outpatient care. In some crisis intervention settings, a patient may be seen frequently (eg, daily) on a short-term basis until the crisis has subsided. Crisis intervention settings use medical and psychosocial techniques; specific treatment methods are discussed in Chapters 39 and 41.

Also important are services such as suicide and drug prevention hotlines that offer telephone support and refer patients in crisis.

Community Outreach Services

In some communities, mental health professionals provide services to patients where they live and congregate. These **community outreach services** are utilized most commonly within the **community mental health** system, and are targeted to improve care for the chronically mentally ill. The best studied of these are assertive community treatment (ACT) teams. Services may include home visits to assess living conditions, improve medication compliance, and provide support. Mobile teams may identify and offer services to patients on the streets and other public places. Although such services are expensive, they have been shown to improve health status and reduce the use of hospital services.

Social Support Services

Social support services are offered by most mental health and community social service agencies to bolster the patient's natural support system (eg, family, church, neighborhood) or to provide a substitute system if natural supports are lacking. The effect of these services may be to alter the acute course of illness to prevent chronicity.

Nonresidential self-help organizations are the "outpatient" parallel to the residential self-help services described above and are often founded by individuals who have survived a problem and have banded together to help others who have had similar life experiences. Examples are Alcoholics Anonymous, Narcotics Anonymous, Schizophrenics Anonymous, Recovery, the Manic Depressive/Depressive Association, colostomy clubs, the Epilepsy Society, and burn recovery groups. A new "recovery movement" emphasizes the potential for patients to be "well" and integrated into their communities. This optimism counters decades of stigma and pessimism.

Miscellaneous agencies provide services, counseling, and assistance to a variety of individuals in need. Although not formally part of the mental health care system, these organizations often provide enough psychosocial assistance to prevent or avert crises. Examples include the Visiting Nurse Association, Homemakers Services, Big Brothers, Planned Parenthood, Traveler's Aid, and consumer credit agencies.

MENTAL HEALTH PROFESSIONALS

There are many different kinds of professional mental health care providers. Most have certain skills in common and provide similar services (eg, psychotherapy). Some have areas of specialized training and practice.

Psychiatrists are physicians—doctors of medicine or osteopathy—who have completed a 4-year residency training program in general psychiatry. Psychiatrists are trained to apply both biomedical and psychosocial diagnostic and therapeutic skills to the management of patients with physical and mental disorders. They are trained in techniques of psychotherapy and are skilled at both diagnosis and psychosocial formulation (psychodynamic, behavioral, or both). They are the only members of the mental health care team trained and licensed to prescribe medication and (along with nurses) to perform complete physical examinations. Subspecialties in psychiatry are discussed in specific chapters (eg, psychoanalysis in Chapter 31, geriatric psychiatry in Chapter 38, hospital consultation psychiatry in Chapter 39, and forensic psychiatry in Chapter 40).

Clinical psychologists are mental health professionals with doctorates (PhD, EdD, PsyD, DMH) or master's degrees who may be licensed as independent practitioners in psychotherapy and psychological assessment; some master's-level professionals have licenses restricting their practice to marriage and family counseling. These professionals attend graduate schools and have clinical placements and internships in which they learn psychotherapy, diagnosis, and psychological testing under supervision. When licensed, they may diagnose and treat patients with mental disorders. Psychologists often have specialized training in administering psychological tests and performing behavior and cognitive therapies. They also have more extensive research training than most physicians. As with physicians, the services of psychologists are now being reimbursed by insurance. In addition, psychologists are beginning to gain admitting privileges to some hospital inpatient services, permitting them to admit a patient jointly with a physician.

Clinical social workers are doctoral (DSW, PhD) or (more frequently) master's-level (MSW, MSSW) psychotherapists, caseworkers, and marriage, family, and child therapists trained in accredited schools of social work and social welfare and accredited by the National Association of Social Work as having completed a specified program of supervised clinical training. They are licensed by many states as independent practitioners, and increasingly they are being reimbursed by health insurance payers. Social workers are skilled at psychosocial therapies, are knowledgeable about community and social welfare resources, and have a special interest in families.

Clinical nurse specialists are registered nurses who may take special training in psychiatric nursing. They may be licensed as independent practitioners, but more often work in organized ambulatory health care settings and in hospitals. Nurses have special skills in the biomedical as well as the psychosocial aspects of mental health care.

Occupational, activities, and recreational/expressive therapists are registered practitioners from a variety of educational backgrounds with specialized training in using art, music, dance, drama, play, and vocational activities to help patients express their feelings and thoughts, learn new behavior, and develop or recover emotionally and socially valuable skills.

Pastoral counselors are clergy with specialized training in counseling patients with emotional disorders.

Case managers are individuals with diverse training and experience who provide advocacy and support to patients, usually outside of an office setting. They often link patients with needed services, but they may also provide direct support and counseling themselves.

Other mental health care providers include **clinical sociologists, clinical pharmacists,** and specialists in other related clinical disciplines who have developed clinical skills related to their core academic or professional training and apply them in clinical settings.

Psychoanalysts are graduates of psychoanalytic institutes, including Freudian, neo-Freudian, and Jungian training centers, who have completed a course of study, a personal analysis, and supervised training analyses (see Chapter 31). Although most are psychiatrists, other professionals have been trained as lay analysts. Training takes many additional years after completion of other professional mental health training.

Multidisciplinary teams of mental health professionals function in psychiatric and general hospital and ambulatory settings. The **inpatient team** has a traditional hierarchy and division of labor, with the psychiatrist leading the team; the nurse managing day-to-day ward activities and medications and monitoring patients; the psychologist performing psychological tests or leading patient therapy groups; the social worker finding a place for the patient to go on discharge, arranging for the financing of hospital and posthospital care, and often performing family therapy; and the occupational therapist organizing activities for the patient during the hospital stay. This traditional organization is still the mode, although in some settings the inpatient team has evolved with less differentiated functions and roles—and a less hierarchical organization.

The **outpatient team** tends to be less hierarchical, though certain functions are still performed by different disciplines (eg, psychiatrists manage medication and psychologists give tests and conduct behavior treatments). The functions of members of the **consultation/liaison team** are partly differentiated, as described in Chapter 39.

REFERENCES & SUGGESTED READINGS

Bubrich N, Teeson M: Impact of a psychiatric outreach service for homeless persons with schizophrenia. Psychiatr Serv 1996;47:644.

Center for Mental Health Services and National Institute of Mental Health: *Mental Health, United States, 1996.* Manderscheid RW, Sonnenschein MA, eds. DHHS Pub No (SMA) 96-3098. Supt of DOCS, US Government Printing Office. 1996.

DeHart M et al: Partial hospitalization at night: The Brussels Nighthospital. Psychiatr Serv 1996;47:527.

Karasu TB: *Treatment of Psychiatric Disorders.* American Psychiatric Association, 1989.

Lamb HR (ed): *Outcomes Assessment in Mental Health Treatment: A Compendium of Articles from Psychiatric Services.* American Psychiatric Association, 1998.

Lehman A: Public health policy, community services, and outcomes for patients with schizophrenia. Psychiatr Clin North Am 1998;21:221.

Mechanic D et al: Changing patterns of psychiatric inpatient care: 1988–1994. Arch Gen Psychiatry 1998;55:785.

Nickels M, McIntyre J: A model for psychiatric services in primary care settings. Psychiatr Serv 1996;47:522.

Ridgley MS et al: Characteristics and activities of care managers in the RWJ Foundation program on chronic mental illness. Psychiatr Serv 1996;46:737.

Rochefort DA (ed): *Handbook on Mental Health Policy in the US*. Greenwood Press, 1989.

Rosenheck RA, Neale MJ: Cost effectiveness of intensive psychiatric community care for high users of inpatient services. Arch Gen Psychiatry 1998;55:459.

30

Somatic Therapies

Beth Goldman, MD, MPH, & Glenn C. Davis, MD

Before World War II, the somatic treatment of psychiatric disorders consisted largely of "tranquilization," ie, sedating patients or restraining their actions. During the 1950s and 1960s, tricyclic antidepressants, monoamine oxidase inhibitors, and phenothiazine antipsychotics were developed. These agents provided more than tranquilization, they provided relief of specific symptoms.

The following sections on psychopharmacology are organized according to the treatment of five groups of syndromes: depression, mania, psychosis, anxiety (including anxiety disorders), and insomnia. The chapter concludes with a general introduction to electroconvulsive therapy and some brief comments on psychosurgery.

I. PHARMACOLOGICAL THERAPIES

In the sections that follow, each group encompasses several *Diagnostic and Statistical Manual of Mental Disorders,* 4th edition (*DSM-IV*) diagnostic entities, which vary in their responses to somatic treatments. The pharmacological agents are reviewed, including indications and side effects. Clinical strategies, including drug selection, initiation of treatment, increasing dosage, determination of duration of treatment, and maintenance management, are discussed. Illustrative cases are presented when considered to be useful.

INTRODUCTION TO RATIONAL PHARMACOLOGICAL THERAPEUTICS

TARGET SYMPTOMS & DIAGNOSIS

A common reason for treatment failure in any field of medicine is that an inaccurate diagnosis is made, and, as a result, an inappropriate treatment plan is devised. *DSM-IV* lists the current defining symptoms for psychiatric disorders (the diagnostic criteria). **Defining symptoms** are symptoms that serve to iden-

tify distinct syndromes. Their purpose is differential diagnosis. When defining symptoms are effective in the differential diagnosis of a syndrome, the criteria are said to have discriminant validity. It is essential to learn the *DSM-IV* syndromes, but it is equally essential to understand that defining symptoms do not specify all of the symptoms that may be part of a given syndrome.

Target symptoms are symptoms that respond to treatment. Observation of improvement in target symptoms permits the clinician to monitor overall improvement in the patient. Many diagnostic entities involve symptoms that do not remit with pharmacological treatment, and these must be recognized and addressed in the course of treatment.

After a drug has been chosen for treatment, it is essential to proceed by a series of steps to determine whether the drug has been therapeutically effective. Drug therapy is commonly discontinued without adequate trial, either because the dose is too low or because not enough time has passed to determine if the drug has been effective. Conversely, it is not uncommon for drug treatment to be initiated and then maintained for months or years with no attempt to determine whether the medication is effective; a significant part of the practice of clinical psychopharmacologists consists of discontinuing medications started and maintained by other physicians that have no demonstrable benefit to the patient. In fact, in some cases the drug may have contributed to the patient's symptoms, in which case the patient improves following its discontinuation.

When altering a patient's medication regimen, it is important to do so in a rational, stepwise fashion, changing only one medication at a time, so that it is possible to determine which drug may have led to improvement or worsening of symptoms or to undesirable side effects.

COMPLIANCE, "THERAPEUTIC ALLIANCE," & INFORMED CONSENT

Even the most effective drug is worthless if the patient does not take it as prescribed. Whenever possible, the development of a caring doctor-patient relationship should precede the prescription of a drug. There must be an understanding that the doctor and

SOMATIC THERAPIES / **429**

the patient will work together to help relieve the patient's distress. The physician must be able to listen to and respect the patient, and the patient must be able to trust the physician. This is often called the "therapeutic alliance." Within the relationship, the physician must be able to address the patient's concerns and fears about having to take psychotropic medication (eg, becoming addicted, being a "weak person"). Patients are less likely to discontinue taking a drug if, before starting the medication, they are informed about the side effects of the drug and are given a realistic account of what to expect while taking it (eg, understanding that the drug will not "work" right away). This procedure is part of the process of informed consent, in which the patient is told of, or is given a written description of, the drug's side effects, the potential risks and benefits of taking the proposed medication, as well as of alternative treatments. Informed consent must be obtained before any psychotropic drug is prescribed and must be clearly documented.

PHARMACOTHERAPY OF DEPRESSION

AGENTS & CLASSES OF AGENTS

Between the 1950s and the late 1980s two classes of drugs dominated the pharmacological treatment of depression, the heterocyclic antidepressants and the monoamine oxidase inhibitors. Although other antidepressants were introduced in the 1960s and 1970s, by the late 1980s and early 1990s a third group of drugs, the selective serotonin reuptake inhibitors (SSRIs), emerged and became prominent. In addition, a variety of "other antidepressants," each with a different mechanism of action, have emerged since the introduction of SSRIs (Table 30–1). Agents such as lithium, anticonvulsants, antipsychotics, and thyroid hormone may be used alone or as adjuncts to antidepressants in patients who are refractory to treatment. Depressive syndromes vary in their response to these agents. Antidepressants are generally equally effective in treating major depression; however, individual patients may respond to one agent better than they do to another. Depressive syndromes defined in *DSM-IV* include major depressive disorder, dysthymic disorder, mood disorder due to a general medical condition (depressed), adjustment disorder (with depressed mood), bipolar disorder (depressed), and cyclothymic disorder. Although each of these diagnoses is an indication for antidepressant therapy and each depressive syndrome responds to antidepressants variably in different patients, the focus of the pharmacotherapy of depression is on the target symptoms.

Table 30–1. Antidepressants.

	Usual Therapeutic Dosage (mg/d)
Selective serotonin reuptake inhibitors	
Fluoxetine	10–80
Fluvoxamine	100–300
Sertraline	50–200
Paroxetine	10–50
Citalopram	20–40
Nefazodone	300–600
Heterocyclic antidepressants	
Imipramine	150–300
Amitriptyline	150–300
Desipramine	150–300
Nortriptyline	50–150
Doxepin	150–300
Protriptyline	15–60
Trimipramine	150–300
Clomipramine	75–400
Maprotiline	150–200
Monoamine oxidase inhibitors	
Phenelzine	45–90
Tranylcypromine	30–50
Miscellaneous	
Amoxapine	150–450
Trazodone	150–300
Bupropion	200–450
Venlafaxine	75–375
Mirtazapine	15–45

INDICATIONS

1. TARGET SYMPTOMS & SYNDROMES

The target groupings for depressive disorders are neurovegetative, psychomotor, mood, cognitive, psychotic, and secondary symptoms associated with social impairment.

The neurovegetative symptoms of impaired sleep, appetite, sexual drive, and altered diurnal rhythm are among the first symptoms to respond to treatment—often within 10 days to 2 weeks, but at times not for 3–4 weeks. When sleep improves in the first few days of treatment, it is usually a result of the concurrent use of sedatives or sedating antidepressants and should not be mistaken for improvement in sleep, which will occur from specific antidepressant effects.

Psychomotor symptoms may be either increased (agitation) or decreased (retardation) in depression. Both behaviors will improve, and generally over the same interval as neurovegetative features—usually 3–4 weeks after starting treatment or 7–14 days after achieving an appropriate dosage level. Social withdrawal is frequently mistaken for psychomotor retardation. As the patient improves clinically, psychomotor behavior will normalize, though the patient may remain withdrawn. Psychomotor behavior can be monitored in the clinical interview or by the nursing staff, observing the patient's facial and hand gestures and total activity level.

Ironically, mood improvement lags behind recovery of neurovegetative and psychomotor functions. The first indication of mood improvement may be transition of the persistent or predominant mood to another mood state. A common occurrence is a shift from a profound and pervasive depressive mood to irritability or anger. It is important to recognize that the diagnosis of depression does not require the presence of depressive mood; other mood states may predominate in depression, such as irritability, dysphoria, or anger.

Concentration, attention, memory, and learning are important cognitive skills that are impaired in depression. This group of target symptoms tends to improve with mood. Depressed thought lags significantly behind other aspects of depression. Guilt, distorted cognition, and rumination persist long after mood has begun to improve. Depressive ideation is the expression in thought of the disturbance in drive and cognitive skills that comprises depression. Its recovery depends on social and individual factors as much as on improvement in the depressive process.

Psychotic symptoms in depression improve slowly, although concurrent use of neuroleptics results in a prompt reduction in agitation. Depressive delusions and hallucinations improve over many weeks.

Although social impairment is not a biological feature of depression, it is listed as a target symptom in order to maintain practitioner awareness that rehabilitation and improved morale should be part of the treatment plan (see Chapter 20).

2. SPECIFIC DISORDERS

Major Depressive Episodes

In uncomplicated depressive episodes meeting the criteria for major depression, antidepressants should bring about a remission in 65–75% of patients. "Uncomplicated" has the following implications: a first episode, a recurrent episode in a well-treated recurrent disorder, no comorbid conditions such as drug or alcohol dependence, and good compliance with treatment. Unfortunately, many presentations of depression are complicated by substance abuse, comorbidity, and social disadvantage—complications that delay response and result in incomplete resolution of symptoms and compliance difficulties that challenge the clinician's ability to assist the patient. Nevertheless, the clinician should expect the entire syndrome of an uncomplicated major depressive episode to remit with effective treatment over the course of several months. The primary symptoms of depression remit sooner. Social impairment and demoralization caused by the disorder often persist and appear as "residual symptoms."

Dysthymic Disorder

DSM-IV defines dysthymic disorder as a chronic depressive syndrome, with symptoms present for about 2 years. Although symptom criteria may appear to be less rigid than those of major depression, patients with this syndrome are usually quite impaired. There are few studies documenting the percentage of patients with dysthymic disorder who respond to antidepressants, but there is general agreement that the recovery rate is somewhat lower than that of major depression. However, there is some evidence that patients with dysthymic disorder may respond to SSRIs better than to heterocyclic antidepressants. The study of dysthymia is further complicated by the fact that many—perhaps most—patients with dysthymia have a lifetime history of major depressive episodes. A trial of an antidepressant is standard practice.

Secondary Mood Disorder

Depressive syndromes secondary to organic causes do not have a predictable response rate to antidepressants. Selected disorders such as hypothyroid-induced depressive states respond very well to treatment (eg, thyroid replacement and antidepressants), although they respond more readily to electroconvulsive therapy. Depressive syndromes associated with brain injury may also respond to medication.

Adjustment Disorder

Depressive symptoms associated with adjustment reactions do not respond to antidepressants. When depressive symptoms following a stressor meet the criteria for major depression, the diagnosis of major depression supersedes (hierarchically) the diagnosis of adjustment disorder with depressive mood, and standard antidepressant treatment should be initiated.

Bipolar Disorder

A depressive episode in a patient with bipolar disorder will respond to standard antidepressant treatment. Nevertheless, a clear understanding of the natural history of bipolar disorder and its treatment is necessary to treat a depressive episode and manage the underlying vulnerability to recurrent depressive and manic episodes. Furthermore, antidepressants have the potential for precipitating manic or hypomanic episodes in bipolar patients. The diagnosis of bipolar disorder, depressed episode requires knowledge of the use of lithium and other mood stabilizers in bipolar disorder and of the difficulties of treating depression in a patient taking mood stabilizers.

Cyclothymic Disorder

Cyclothymic disorder is an attenuated version of bipolar disorder and may be treated with mood stabilizers and/or antidepressants. Often no treatment is required because the episodes are brief and tolerable. Furthermore, cyclothymic individuals frequently reject treatment (as do people suffering from bipolar disorder) because mood stabilizers may block the hypomanias (which are "liked" by the patient). Few cyclothymic patients seek treatment or accept it when offered. A patient with bipolar II (a designation reserved for patients with major depression and hypomania) will often seek treatment because the depressive episodes are disabling.

DRUG CHOICE

Following accurate diagnosis and identification of target symptoms in the depressed patient, the next step in rational pharmacotherapy is selection of the proper antidepressant. Table 30–1 lists antidepressants in common use. Within the last decade, a number of antidepressants, such as fluoxetine, clomipramine, bupropion, sertraline, paroxetine, venlafaxine, fluvoxamine, nafazodone, and mirtazapine, have been approved for use. Another drug, citalopram, has recently been approved by the Food and Drug Administration (FDA). The SSRIs have profoundly altered clinical practice. Beginning with fluoxetine, the SSRIs have emerged as the most frequently used first-choice antidepressants. The ranges of daily dosage for the more commonly used SSRIs are included in Table 30–1.

Several principles guide the choice of pharmacological agent. It is important to obtain a history of the patient's prior responses to specific agents, including both efficacy and adverse reactions. If a particular drug worked in a prior depressive episode and did not cause problems, it is wise to use it again. If a member of the patient's family had a positive response to a particular drug, that drug should be considered for the patient as well. If there is no prior history of treatment, it is necessary to match the patient's clinical condition with the drug and proceed somewhat empirically.

1. SELECTIVE SEROTONIN REUPTAKE INHIBITORS

Efficacy

No one class of antidepressant drugs has been found to be more effective than another in the treatment of "classic" major depression. Most claims for differential efficacy are limited to alternative classifications of depression, such as "atypical depressions," which may respond better to monoamine oxidase inhibitors (see below).

Compliance

The major cause of failure in the treatment of depression is lack of compliance. Patients often do not take antidepressants because of a failure in patient education. The patient should understand the symp-

toms of depression, the expected side effects of medication, the risks of no treatment, and the expected time course for improvement. Lack of compliance often results from failure to develop a therapeutic alliance.

The SSRIs, which act by inhibiting the reuptake of serotonin from the synaptic cleft to the presynaptic neuron, are widely prescribed both by psychiatrists and by primary care physicians. They have proven efficacy in major depressive disorder, as well as some anxiety disorders (see below). Their extensive use relates to both their wide range of effectiveness and their ease of administration. The popularity of the book *Listening to Prozac* (Kramer, 1993) has added to the general reputation of fluoxetine (and by implication other SSRIs) for a wide range of effects.

The SSRIs may be given in a single daily dose (usually in the morning), a fact that has resulted in good compliance in many patients for whom multiple daily dosing is a problem. Up to 75% of patients may respond to an initial (low) dose, another feature of SSRIs (particularly fluoxetine) that leads to good compliance. Patients generally do not like escalating doses such as are necessary with tricyclic antidepressants: "You started me on one pill and now I'm taking six; it's too much." The enhanced psychomotor activity of SSRIs is particularly uncomfortable. Sexual dysfunction and weight gain may also interfere with long-term compliance.

Adverse Effects

Most patients will experience at least some adverse effects when starting on a drug. The particular spectrum of adverse effects in one class of antidepressants may limit their use. The SSRIs generally have a low risk of unpleasant anticholinergic adverse effects, a common problem with tricyclic antidepressants and monoamine oxidase inhibitors. In addition they are not associated with the risk of fatal cardiac arrhythmias common in overdose of heterocyclic antidepressants. On the other hand, the central nervous system (CNS) and extrapyramidal effects of insomnia, psychomotor agitation, tremor, and headache tend to be more common than with tricyclic antidepressants, as are gastrointestinal symptoms of nausea and diarrhea. Use of SSRIs can result in a "serotonin syndrome," comprised of palpitations, agitation, muscle twitching, and even delirium. Decrease of libido and/or difficulty achieving orgasm are commonly reported with SSRIs and weight gain can occur with long-term use.

Table 30–2 lists the common adverse side effects of antidepressants, which vary in their profiles. It is important to consult textbooks on psychopharmacology—as well as package inserts—whenever there is a question of drug-drug interaction.

Physicians must listen carefully to patients' complaints. After years of prescribing drugs, it is easy for the physician to dismiss a new complaint as unrelated

Table 30–2. Adverse effects of antidepressants.

Mechanism	Side Effect
Anticholinergic	Dry mouth, blurry vision, urinary retention, constipation, toxic confusional state, tachycardia
Antihistaminic	Sedation
Adrenergic/autonomic	Excitement, tremor, palpitations, cardiac arrythmias, orthostatic hypotension, hypertensive crisis (cheese effect)
Serotonergic	Sedation, restlessness, sexual dysfunction
Unknown	Weight gain

to the medication. For example, a patient taking nortriptyline reports tinnitus; although it is tempting to regard the complaint as hypochondriacal or as a somatic preoccupation, tinnitus is, in fact, listed as an infrequent possible side effect of nortriptyline (ironically, nortriptyline is also used to treat tinnitus). In this case the tinnitus was dose related and disappeared following reduction of the dose.

The presence of concurrent medical illness also affects the choice of antidepressant. For example, liver disease may cause the clinician to select a drug excreted by the kidney or at least to initiate treatment at low doses and delay dosage increases.

Finally, it is possible to take advantage of some of a drug's side effects when selecting the most appropriate agent. For example, a sedating drug such as doxepin may be chosen when treating a depressed patient with insomnia, because the patient may initially be motivated to take it for its hypnotic effect. In contrast, a patient with severe psychomotor retardation may do better on a more stimulating drug such as bupropion.

2. HETEROCYCLIC ANTIDEPRESSANTS

Efficacy

Until the emergence of the SSRIs in the late 1980s, the heterocyclic antidepressants were the agents most frequently used to treat major depressive disorder. They work by increasing the level of monoamines in the synapse and remain as effective as SSRIs and other antidepressants, but are limited by their side effect profiles.

Compliance

Compliance is probably more of a problem with heterocyclic antidepressants than with SSRIs because they have more unpleasant side effects and because they must be started at a low dose and "titrated upward." Many patients are bothered by the antihistaminic, anticholinergic, and cardiovascular side effects of heterocyclic antidepressants and, because they provide little immediate symptom relief other than, perhaps, for insomnia, patients are prone to be-

come discouraged and discontinue them. It is these patients that require a good therapeutic alliance along with frequent initial visits if treatment is to be successful. Starting patients at fairly low bedtime doses and adjusting the dose upward slowly as well as clearly informing patients of expected side effects may help improve compliance.

Adverse Effects

Anticholinergic side effects limit the use of heterocyclic antidepressants in asthma and closed-angle glaucoma. They also can increase heart rate. This class of agents should be avoided or used very carefully in patients with cardiac conduction delay. The risk of orthostatic hypotension should be considered carefully before prescribing these agents for patients at risk for falls. Because some of these agents have strong antihistaminic effects, they can be quite sedating. Finally, because fatal cardiac arrhythmias occur with overdose, suicidal patients should not be given access to potentially fatal doses of heterocyclic antidepressants. A common clinical problem is the treatment of depressed patients with cardiac arrhythmias or congestive heart failure. The SSRIs and bupropion are thought to impose lower risks in patients with compromised cardiovascular systems.

3. MONOAMINE OXIDASE INHIBITORS

Efficacy

Monoamine oxidase inhibitors (MAOIs) are often selected to treat "atypical depression," which is characterized by hypersomnia, hyperphagia, somatic complaints, and dysphoria. The MAOIs may also be more effective in treating the depressed episodes of bipolar patients. They are also used as a second-line drug when treatment has been started with heterocyclic or SSRI drugs but has failed.

Compliance

Because these drugs may lead to serious consequences when combined with certain foods and pharmacological agents (see below), it is important to assess the patient's ability to understand and comply with dietary and other restrictions. They should not be used, for example, by alcoholic patients who cannot remain abstinent.

Adverse Effects

MAOIs were probably underutilized in the 1970s because of clinicians' fears about the adverse effects. They share some adverse effects with heterocyclic antidepressants, including orthostatic hypotension, sedation, urinary hesitancy, constipation, dry mouth, and weight gain. Specific effects of MAOIs include insomnia and daytime stimulation, hypertensive crises (related to interactions with medications and selected foods), muscle cramps, myoclonic twitches, and hyperpyrexic reactions. The spectrum of foods to be avoided is broad and includes beer and red wine, aged cheeses, fava beans, yeast, smoked meats, and liver. All sympathomimetic amines need to be avoided. Particularly apt to cause problems are over-the-counter cold remedies such as pseudoephedrine because the patient believes drugs that can be purchased without prescription are "weak" or harmless.

Other prescription drugs such as meperidine and fluoxetine have been implicated in patient fatalities when combined with MAOIs. Patients must be carefully educated about the risk of hypertensive crisis, which is potentially fatal, and given lists of foods and medications to avoid. Some clinicians suggest that patients receiving these drugs be instructed to wear Medic-Alert bracelets so that potentially fatal drug interactions can be avoided in unconscious patients.

4. OTHER ANTIDEPRESSANTS

Five antidepressants currently available in the United States do not fit into the above categories: amoxapine, bupropion hydrochloride, venlafaxine hydrochloride, nafazodone hydrochloride, and mirtazapine.

Amoxapine was introduced in the United States in 1980. It is structurally similar to the antipsychotic drug loxapine and, thus, can cause extrapyramidal side effects (see antipsychotics, below). It is rarely used today.

Bupropion was introduced to the American market but was rapidly withdrawn because of concern about seizure potential. It was reintroduced in 1989 and has proven to be an effective and useful agent that does not tend to cause sexual dysfunction. It acts on dopamine and norepinephrine and is, thus, quite activating. The drug may also be useful for the treatment of attention deficit disorder and is FDA approved as a smoking cessation aid.

The FDA approved venlafaxine, which inhibits the reuptake of serotonin and norepinephrine, in 1994. Some studies suggest that this drug has a faster onset of action than other antidepressants and may have some utility in treating treatment resistant patients. Unlike the SSRIs, drug/drug interactions are not as much a problem with venlafaxine.

Nefazodone, which appeared in 1995, has a relatively complex mechanism of action. It inhibits the reuptake of serotonin and norepinephrine presynaptically while antagonizing type 2A serotonin receptors postsynaptically. It is more sedating than SSRIs and much less likely to cause sexual dysfunction than most other antidepressants.

Mirtazapine, a relatively new antidepressant on the market, selectively blocks presynaptic α_2-adrenergic receptors and also antagonizes 5-hydroxytryptamine

(5-HT2, 5-HT3) and H1 receptors. Orthostatic hypotension may limit its use in some patients.

Carbamazepine, lithium, valproate, lamotrigine, and gabapentin are listed in Table 30-3 under the heading "mood stabilizers." These drugs may not be effective when used alone to treat a depressed episode, but they may be used in combination with an antidepressant to potentiate its effects. They may also be used to prevent recurrent episodes of depression. They will be discussed in greater detail below in the section on mania.

THERAPEUTIC STRATEGIES

1. SELECTIVE SEROTONIN REUPTAKE INHIBITORS

In some ways, SSRIs are easier to prescribe than heterocyclic antidepressants and MAOIs because of their more benign side effect profile. Since many people tolerate them so well the majority of patients can be started on a dose that is likely to be therapeutic (eg, 20 mg of fluoxetine). However, it may be necessary to start with 5 mg, particularly in geriatric patients. There is risk of accumulation of drug because of the long half-life of SSRIs. Many patients may be managed on an every-other-day dose. If a patient has not responded after 4 weeks at the expected therapeutic dose, for example 20 mg in the case of fluoxetine, the dose may be increased. It is unlikely that the patient will respond to further increases if there has been no response after an additional 2 weeks of treatment.

This class of drugs has turned out to be more complex to use than originally thought as we have found out more about their effect on the hepatic microsomal P450 enzymes. Clinicians must be aware that SSRIs may profoundly affect the levels of other drugs. For example, fluoxetine inhibits the metabolism of tricyclic antidepressants, so, if both drugs are used together, the dose of the tricyclic must be very low. In addition, potentially fatal interactions, such as the combined use of SSRIs and MAOIs, should be kept in mind when these agents are prescribed.

Table 30–3. Mood stabilizers.

	Usual Therapeutic Dosage (mg/d)
Carbamazepine	600–1200
Lithium carbonate	600–2400
Valproic acid	750–3000
Lamotrigine[a]	50–200
Gabapentin[a]	900–1800

[a] Less well studied, off label use.

There is no standard pretreatment workup for SSRIs, but as with the prescription of other psychotropic medications, a careful medical and medication history is essential. Caution should be used in switching between SSRIs and other antidepressants and in combining SSRIs with over-the-counter drugs such as pseudoephedrine; lower doses should be used in patients with renal and hepatic disease.

The SSRIs are generally administered in the morning, reducing the likelihood that peak blood level will occur at night, a phenomenon that may cause unpleasant arousal and sleep difficulties.

Blood levels are not routinely available, nor is there consensus on a therapeutic range.

Treatment Failure

Common causes of treatment failure include compliance problems, the inability to achieve an adequate dose of medication, and failure to maintain the patient on an adequate dose for a long enough time. Sometimes the patient has improved but the physician or patient fails to recognize the improvement. Some patients who initially present with apparently depressive symptoms actually have character disorders that may not respond well or reliably to pharmacologic treatment (see Chapter 24). Depressed patients may be so socially impaired that their behavior and self-report fail to improve even as the biological aspects of the depression remit. Furthermore, concurrent medical problems and psychiatric comorbidity may make assessment difficult. Patients suffering from a major depressive episode who also have borderline personality disorder are particularly difficult to assess because their volatile affects and acting-out behavior may continue.

Of course some depressed patients actually fail to respond to an adequate therapeutic trial. This may occur in an uncomplicated first presentation of depression up to 25% of the time. In recurrent depressive illness or in depression with psychiatric or medical comorbidity, treatment failure occurs more frequently. "Refractory depressions" are defined by failure to respond to two complete antidepressant trials. Because many of the antidepressants are thought to work through similar mechanisms, an agent that differs in its spectrum of neurotransmitter actions should be selected for the second trial. For example, if fluoxetine (a serotonergic agent) was used in the initial trial, desipramine (a drug that affects noradrenergic systems) might serve as the next drug tried. Other treatment strategies, such as giving combinations of agents, are beyond the scope of this chapter. Finally, electroconvulsive therapy (ECT) may be warranted. It is the most effective treatment, with a 90% success rate for major depressive disorder, and should always be considered after failure of drug therapy.

Failure of a trial of treatment should always cause the physician to reconsider the initial diagnosis.

Maintenance & Prophylaxis

It is generally believed that full treatment doses should continue for 9 months to 1 year. The earlier practice of reducing the dose after 6 months and maintaining the patient on a "maintenance dose" is no longer considered helpful. When the decision is made to discontinue the medication, the dose should be tapered.

There is debate about whether a patient should remain on antidepressants for more than 1 year, although a consensus is developing that patients should be treated for as long as the drug is well tolerated. Antidepressants do prevent recurrences, and the decision to maintain a patient on antidepressants for longer than a year is usually made because the patient suffers frequent recurrences, because the symptoms recur during the process of dose tapering, or because there are severe morbidity or mortality risks without treatment.

2. HETEROCYCLIC ANTIDEPRESSANTS

Desipramine is used as a prototype of the heterocyclic antidepressants to illustrate a treatment approach. The therapeutic strategy will remain the same for most heterocyclic antidepressants, although the dosing schedules may not, since all heterocyclic antidepressants are not equipotent.

Pretreatment Workup

Workup before initiating antidepressants is done mainly to rule out organic causes of depression. In patients over 45 years of age or with histories of cardiac disease, an electrocardiogram (EKG) is recommended. Other baseline tests, such as complete blood counts or liver function tests, are usually not necessary.

Initiating Treatment

It is essential at the outset to educate the patient about the antidepressant being recommended. A drug should be given only after it is clear that compliance can be anticipated. If the patient has never taken an antidepressant before, it is prudent to give a test dose the first night. A healthy young patient may be given 25–50 mg of desipramine, whereas a geriatric patient might be given 10–25 mg. The patient should be told what to expect and to call if there are unexpected adverse effects or if additional questions need to be answered.

Dose Increments

Although individual patients may improve on low doses of antidepressants, most will not improve unless a dose of at least 150 mg/d of desipramine is achieved. An initial goal, then, is to achieve a dosage of 150 mg daily as quickly and safely as possible without affecting compliance. There are many schedules for dose increases. For example, addition of 25 mg every other day or 50 mg every 3 or 4 days may be well tolerated in young healthy patients. Once 150 mg/d is achieved, a 7- to 14-day period can be used to monitor target symptoms. If no improvement occurs, the dose may be increased (for example) by 50 mg a week. The upper limit of desipramine dosage is generally 300 mg/d unless serum levels still fall well below the upper limit of the therapeutic range at that dose. It is important to emphasize that the major skills to be mastered are not pharmacological, but rather skills that assist the patient in tolerating benign side effects and inculcate appropriate expectations for improvement. Because heterocyclic antidepressants remain in common use today, it is important to learn this careful, timed, stepwise process.

Duration

A key reason for failure in treatment is the failure to treat for an adequate length of time. A 7- to 14-day trial at each dosage increment is adequate. When either the maximum dose (eg, 300 mg/d of desipramine) or a dose that cannot be raised further because of adverse effects is achieved, a 2- to 4-week period should elapse before the antidepressant trial is terminated. When adverse effects are benign (eg, dry mouth), further education about treatment and drug side effects is necessary before the drug is abandoned.

Blood Levels

Although serum levels are measurable for all antidepressants, at least on a research basis, levels of tricyclic antidepressants are commonly the only measures available in most hospitals. A number of problems exist in regard to serum levels of drugs. Few drugs have established therapeutic ranges. Antidepressants have many metabolites, several of which may have therapeutic effects. Among the tertiary tricyclic antidepressants (amitriptyline and imipramine), both the parent tertiary and the derivative secondary amine (nortriptyline and desipramine, respectively) are, by convention, added together to form one serum level. Even with established therapeutic ranges, the information has limited utility. For example, for desipramine, the therapeutic range is 150–300 ng/mL. If the serum level is below 150 ng/mL, it is clear that the dose should be raised. If the level is above 300 ng/mL, the dose should be decreased (toxic levels usually exceed 500 ng/mL). When the serum level lies within the therapeutic range and the patient has been on the antidepressant for 2–3 weeks without benefit, the dose may be increased if the level is not already at the high end of the therapeutic range. Thus, a dose within the therapeutic range that fails to produce an antidepressant effect does not indicate failure of the trial. The trial should proceed until the upper limits of the dose (in this case, 300 mg/d) have been achieved or until the serum level exceeds the usual therapeutic levels. In general, serum levels are measured toward the end of a clinical trial when no improvement has occurred. They are obtained more frequently in high-risk individuals such as the aged.

3. MONOAMINE OXIDASE INHIBITORS

The strategy for initiating and titrating dosage with MAOIs is similar to that for the heterocyclic antidepressants, although dosage increments are usually smaller. The physician must check the patient for orthostatic hypotension and continually reinforce the need for maintaining the tyramine-free diet and drug restrictions (many patients begin to "cheat" after successfully negotiating a glass of red wine or a slice of pizza, for example).

A different approach is used for monitoring the dose of MAOIs, although few hospitals have the appropriate assay available, ie, measurement of "percent inhibition." Several studies have demonstrated that monoamine oxidase must be inhibited 85% to achieve therapeutic results. Platelets contain monoamine oxidase and can be used to assay inhibition. A baseline sample of blood is drawn, and platelets are separated and tested with a monoamine oxidase substrate to determine its converting activity. After the patient has been on the inhibitor, platelets are again obtained and tested for monoamine oxidase activity. This later activity is compared with baseline, producing the measure "percent inhibition" (the dose is raised if monoamine oxidase activity is inhibited less than 85% over baseline). A target dose of 1 mg/kg is commonly used.

4. OTHER ANTIDEPRESSANTS

As with the SSRIs, no special pretreatment workup, other than to rule out organic causes of depression, is indicated and blood levels are not generally available for the "other" antidepressants.

In patients being considered for bupropion, the history should cover past and present seizure activity as well as factors that may predispose the patient to seizure activity. Venlafaxine may have some advantage over other agents because of its minimal risk of drug-drug interactions.

Lithium and anticonvulsants may be used either as an adjunct to antidepressants in treatment-resistant patients or, in cases of frequent recurrent depression or atypical bipolar disorder, to prevent recurrences.

CASE STUDY: MAJOR DEPRESSIVE EPISODE

Mr M was referred by his primary care physician for assessment and treatment of depression. He had recently been involved in a boating accident in which he was severely burned over his lower extremities.

After discharge from the hospital, he began to flounder in his work as an attorney in solo practice. His physician was concerned that he had developed depression.

Assessment of the patient showed a clearly depressive mood, terminal insomnia, loss of concentration, decreased appetite, a 12-lb weight loss, inability to work productively, and ruminations about his accident. He had passing thoughts of suicide and feelings of being overwhelmed.

Mr M was divorced, and his teenage son lived in his home. Furthermore, he had a strong family history of depression and, to make matters worse, a gun collection.

The psychiatrist judged Mr M to be suffering from major depression and was able to identify target symptoms for the early phase of treatment (sleep and appetite disturbance and some psychomotor retardation). After discussion of the various treatment alternatives, his living at home, and his gun collection, Mr M agreed to the following plan.

1. Initiate fluoxetine, 10 mg in the morning, to be increased to 20 mg within 1 week.
2. Mr M's son to stay with his mother.
3. Mr M to move in with his parents for a brief time.
4. Mr M's brother to padlock the gun locker and keep the key. (The doctor is to contact the brother and secure his agreement.)
5. Mr M to return in 1 week for reevaluation and to call in several days about drug effects.

Mr M called 2 days later and reported "feeling wired" and no improvement. Otherwise, he was tolerating the fluoxetine well. On reevaluation in 1 week, he was still tolerating the medication, now at a dosage of 20 mg in the morning, and no longer felt agitated. He was seen weekly for 5 weeks. In the third week, his sleep and appetite began to improve. He began to be able to work at the office a few hours a day during the fourth week and returned to his home, but still felt that his concentration was impaired and that his energy level was still diminished. The dose was increased to 30 mg a day. By the sixth week, he recognized clear improvement in mood and energy and had his son return home. Mr M continued seeing the psychiatrist and taking fluoxetine for about a year after returning to work.

PHARMACOTHERAPY OF MANIA

AGENTS & CLASSES OF AGENTS

Lithium is the standard treatment for manic episodes and is usually the first-line agent unless there has been documented treatment failure or the drug is medically contraindicated. It may be effective in the treatment of as many as 95% of acute manias. Now that valproic acid (an anticonvulsant) has been approved by the FDA for the treatment of mania, it is becoming more commonly used outside of research and academic settings. Carbamazepine is also used. Calcium channel blockers have also been tried with variable results. Other agents, such as benzodiazepines, may also be used for sedation early in treatment along with lithium or an anticonvulsant to help manage the patient, as lithium and anticonvulsants do not have immediate antimanic effects.

Before the introduction of lithium in the United States in 1970, neuroleptics were used to control the symptoms of mania and are still used in combination with lithium and/or anticonvulsants in "psychotic" or "tertiary" mania. In this chapter, the discussion will focus on lithium. Anticonvulsants will be taken up at the end of this section.

INDICATIONS

1. TARGET SYMPTOMS & SYNDROMES

The symptoms of mania likely to respond first are increased psychomotor activity, pressured speech, and lack of sleep, followed by improvement in the patient's expansive mood, grandiosity, and intrusiveness. In some patients, affective symptoms may include irritability and hostility in place of expansiveness, or mood may be labile and shift from day to day or from hour to hour. Symptoms relating to disorganization of the form of thought (eg, flight of ideas, loosening of association) are more likely to respond to lithium than delusional content, such as paranoia. Target symptoms often do not begin to abate until 1–2 weeks after initiating treatment and may diminish slowly over time. Lithium alone is often not effective in treating psychotic manic symptoms such as delusions and hallucinations (see Chapter 20).

2. SPECIFIC DISORDERS

Lithium may be used to treat an acute manic episode and to prevent recurrences of mania. As mentioned above, it is also used in some cases in the treatment and prevention of depression, particularly when a patient is judged to have an "atypical" bipolar disorder (bipolar II) with brief hypomanic episodes preceding depressive periods. (See more about this below, under anticonvulsants.) Lithium may also be considered in treating patients with hypomanic or cyclothymic disorders, although in these cases the decision to treat must balance the socioeconomic risks of the illness against the side effects of the drug.

Compliance

Voluntary discontinuance of lithium is a common problem in patients suffering from manic-depressive illness and is often a function of the presence of grandiose-euphoric manias. Patients have difficulty understanding that the "highs" are part of their illness, and even when they do, they may not wish to give up the mania. Bipolar patients with a predominance of depressive over manic episodes or those who have dysphoric, irritable, and paranoid manias tend to be more compliant, since they have generally suffered adverse consequences of mania. Side effects may also limit patients' willingness to take lithium, particularly if tremor develops.

Adverse Effects

Adverse effects of lithium include dry mouth, thirst, urinary frequency, tremor, and gastrointestinal distress, which may include nausea, vomiting, and diarrhea. Nontoxic goiter can occur in patients receiving chronic lithium therapy. Hypothyroid states may develop during treatment as well. Rarely, nephrogenic diabetes insipidus may develop. Serious lithium toxicity usually occurs at serum levels over 1.5 mEq/L and includes drowsiness, slurred speech, blurred vision, hyperactive deep tendon reflexes, ataxia, cardiac arrhythmias, and seizures. Completed suicide can occur with a lithium overdose, although it is more likely when combined with other drugs.

Several medical conditions may make the management of bipolar disease difficult, particularly hypertension requiring the use of diuretics, because patients require less lithium and must be followed more closely if treated with both lithium and diuretics. Other conditions or drugs that influence salt and water balance may also pose difficulties for management with lithium.

THERAPEUTIC STRATEGIES

Pretreatment Workup

The patient should have had a complete physical examination within 6 months before treatment is started. It is also customary to check renal function and serum electrolytes and to assess thyroid function as a baseline for subsequent monitoring of function during chronic treatment with lithium. The clinician should be certain that women of childbearing age are not pregnant, and they should be warned not to become pregnant. An EKG may be obtained to rule out arrhythmias that may be exacerbated by lithium treatment.

Initiating Treatment

Lithium carbonate may be initiated at a dosage of 300 mg two or three times daily in young healthy adults. Most patients will require between 900 and 1800 mg/d to achieve therapeutic lithium levels. Large patients or those who have more severe symptoms may require higher doses; frail elderly patients or patients who receive diuretics or who have compromised renal function may need lower doses.

Dose Increments

Three to 5 days after initiation of treatment a lithium level should be obtained in the early morning, prior to the first dose. The dose should be increased by 300 mg if the level is below 0.8 mEq/L. Lithium levels should be measured frequently early in the course of management and less often once stable therapeutic levels have been achieved. Generally, the therapeutic range for lithium is considered to be 0.8–1.2 mEq/L, and achieving this level may require lithium doses up to 2400 mg/d.

Duration

It may take 3–5 days to achieve a steady state for any lithium dose. Once a therapeutic level has been achieved, it takes 1–2 weeks for improvement in target symptoms. If no improvement has occurred by that time, the dose can be increased as long as the lithium level does not exceed the therapeutic range.

Blood Levels

Blood levels are an important part of monitoring lithium treatment. The sample should always be drawn as close to 12 hours after a lithium dose as possible, which usually means before the morning dose. Once stabilized on a therapeutic dose, patients being maintained on lithium should have their levels checked about every 4 months or whenever their water or electrolyte status changes (eg, when diuretics are initiated, when sweating more).

Treatment Failure

Few manic patients will fail to recover on therapeutic lithium trials. In the treatment failures, neuroleptics or anticonvulsants may be added to the regimen. Electroconvulsive therapy (ECT) may be tried to "break" a manic episode, but this procedure may also precipitate mania. Occasionally, the diagnosis of mania is incorrect. Early in the course of illness, intoxication (eg, with stimulants), disorganized anxious states, schizophrenia, and other causes of psychosis may be mistaken for mania. Most of these conditions will improve over time without intervention. Chronic manic-like syndromes can be caused by metabolic or endocrinological disorders.

A key cause of treatment failure is rapid-cycling manic-depressive illness. Rapid cycling (conventionally defined as three or more episodes per year) is difficult to treat and may be exacerbated by lithium and by heterocyclic antidepressants. Rapid cycling bipolar illness and bipolar II disorder are now conventionally treated with anticonvulsants (see below).

Maintenance & Prophylaxis

Once the manic episode has abated, the patient's lithium requirement often decreases. In most cases, patients should also be kept on a maintenance dose of lithium to prevent recurrences. This is particularly true of patients whose manic episodes result in significant destructive behavior. There is recent evidence that patients who discontinue their lithium may eventually fail to respond to it again when they become manic.

Patients receiving maintenance doses of lithium should continue to have lithium levels, thyroid function, serum electrolytes, and renal function monitored periodically.

Anticonvulsants

Two anticonvulsants, carbamazepine and valproate, are now commonly used to treat bipolar illness. As mentioned above, they are utilized when lithium cannot be tolerated or has failed in the treatment of "classic" mania. In addition, these agents have been shown to be more effective than lithium for the treatment of bipolar II disorder, rapid-cycling bipolar disorder, and mixed states.

Both of these drugs may cause sedation, nausea, and dizziness initially. Like lithium, doses are titrated upward and levels are checked frequently until the patient is within the therapeutic range. Because carbamazepine stimulates its own hepatic metabolism, the dose requirement is likely to increase after the patient has been apparently stabilized.

Carbamazepine has been associated with decreases in the white blood cell count, so the complete blood count (CBC) must be checked frequently when initiating treatment. Both agents may also cause elevations in transaminases, so liver function should also be monitored.

Compliance with these agents may be limited by sedation, ataxia, and nausea initially. Other side effects, such as rash and changes in the white blood cell count and liver function, may necessitate a permanent or temporary discontinuation of these drugs. In the long term, valproic acid is associated with significant weight gain in some patients, as well as changes in hair texture, which may create compliance problems.

Two other anticonvulsants, gabapentin and lamotrigine, are also being used in some research settings for the treatment of rapid cycling disorder or mixed states. Lamotrigine appears to have significant antidepressant activity but is associated with Stevens-Johnson syndrome. Gabapentin seems to have fewer side effects than lamotrigine.

CASE STUDY

Please see the Mayor of Wino Park in Chapter 14 for a description of the treatment of a patient with severe mania.

PHARMACOTHERAPY OF PSYCHOSIS

AGENTS & CLASSES OF AGENTS

Over the centuries, sedation has been virtually the only method of treatment of psychosis, anxiety, and depression. Alcohol, bromides, opium, or, in the earlier part of this century, barbiturates have all been used to "calm" psychotic patients. Wet packing, restraints, and other nonpharmacologic treatments have been routinely used as well.

In 1952, chlorpromazine was used to protect the body from its own autonomic compensatory reactions during surgery. It was soon discovered incidentally to have a beneficial effect on psychotic patients who happened to receive the drug and thus was extended from anesthesiology to psychiatry. This drug and others like it were the first therapeutic agents to exhibit a specific antipsychotic action (rather than merely sedating effects). They are known as neuroleptics, antipsychotic drugs, or sometimes, inappropriately, "major tranquilizers." Almost all effective neuroleptics act on dopamine neurotransmission, blocking dopamine receptors. For ease of discussion, those antipsychotic drugs released prior to 1990 will be described as "typical antipsychotics" and those released after 1990 will be called "atypical antipsychotics." This distinction is made because the atypical antipsychotics, being much more specific to dopamine receptor subtypes, have a much more favorable side effect profile (and probably a wider range of symptom control) than the older, typical agents.

There are five classes of typical neuroleptics (Table 30–4), including phenothiazines (aliphatic, piperidine, and piperazine types), thioxanthines, butyrophenones, indoleamines, and dibenzoxazepines. Atypical neuroleptics are classed as dibenzodiazepines, benzisoxazoles, and dibenzothiazepines. All neuroleptics are theoretically equally effective antipsychotic agents with respect to the so called "positive symptoms" of schizophrenia such as hallucinations and delusions. Patients who fail to respond to a drug from one class may respond to one from another. In addition, the atypical agents are felt to have some efficacy in treating the "negative" symptoms of schizophrenia.

INDICATIONS

Neuroleptics are effective in treating psychotic symptoms that may be seen in schizophrenia, brief reactive psychosis, schizophreniform disorder, affective illness (manic and depressed), and organic mental disorders. They are less effective in treating delu-

Table 30–4. Neuroleptics.

	Chlorpromazine Equivalence	Common Dosage (mg/d)
Typical neuroleptics		
Phenothiazines		
Chlorpromazine	1	100–1000
Thioridazine	1	100–800
Mesoridazine	2	50–400
Trifluoperazine	36	5–60
Perphenazine	11	8–64
Fluphenazine	85	2–60
Thioxanthenes		
Thiothixine	19	2–120
Chlorprothixene	2	100–600
Butyrophenones		
Haloperidol	62	2–30
Dibenzoxazepines		
Loxapine	7	20–160
Dihydroindolone		
Molindone	10	20–200
Depot		
Fluphenazine decanoate		12.25–25/month
Haloperidol decanoate		50–100/month
Atypical neuroleptics		
Dibenzodiazepine		
Clozapine	2	300–900
Olanzapine	—	5–10
Benzisoxazole		
Risperidone	—	2–6
Dibenzothiazepine		
Quetiapine	—	300–700

[a] —, not established.

sional disorders and have a limited place in the treatment of severe anxiety and borderline states.

1. TARGET SYMPTOMS & SYNDROMES

Neuroleptics have pharmacological effects that lead to remission of some psychotic symptoms and attenuation of other associated symptoms. Since the effects of neuroleptics are not "disorder specific" but rather "symptom specific," leading either to remission or attenuation of symptoms, knowledge of the target symptoms is essential. Psychotic disorders are associated with disturbances of arousal, affect, thought (both formal thought disorder and content disorder), psychomotor activity, and social adjustment.

Symptoms of arousal include agitation, anxiety, confusion, disorientation, insomnia, excitement, and vigilance. These symptoms are the first to improve after initiation of neuroleptics—within hours at the earliest but routinely in 3–5 days.

Affective symptoms often overlap with arousal. Reduction in arousal secondarily reduces affects as well. Common affective symptoms associated with psychosis include aggressiveness, anxiety, depression, grandiosity, hostility, irritability, negativism, and suicidal tendencies. Affects improve, after the initial effect of reduced arousal, over 1–3 weeks of treatment. The depression, which is often secondary, is less likely to respond than some other affective symptoms.

Formal thought disorder may be divided into fluent or "positive" symptoms (loosening of associations, flight of ideas, pressure of speech and thought, and circumstantiality) and nonfluent or "negative" symptoms (poverty of content of thought, blocking, and uncommunicativeness). Fluent thought disorder often dramatically improves following reduction in arousal and affect, often leaving some residual speech or communicative problem. Nonfluent negative symptoms do not tend to improve as dramatically and are frequently present after the resolution of other target symptoms. As mentioned above, however, these symptoms are more likely to respond to atypical antipsychotics.

Disturbances in content of thought include delusions, hallucinations, feelings of unreality, and paranoid or bizarre ideation. Neuroleptics are effective when these symptoms are acute or subacute but less effective when they are chronic. In the case of an acute disturbance, reduction in paranoia and delusional content may be seen within a few days to a week.

General motor and psychomotor behaviors are altered in psychosis. Catatonia, waxy flexibility, retardation, and hyperactivity can be observed. Psychomotor symptoms include peculiar mannerisms and facial grimaces and stereotypical behavior. These motor symptoms may improve slowly (over several weeks), but increased motor behavior associated with agitation will respond more promptly. Because typical neuroleptics have profound extrapyramidal side effects, ongoing assessment of motor behavior is important to detect akathisia and pseudoparkinsonism. It is important not to mistake these extrapyramidal syndromes for a continuation of psychotic motor behaviors.

As with depression, many symptoms experienced by schizophrenic patients are not specifically treated with neuroleptics. Defective judgment, social withdrawal, and deterioration of social habits fall into this class of symptoms. Poor rapport, lack of insight, and inappropriateness of affect may be primary symptoms of schizophrenia, but remain largely untreatable with medication. However, some of these symptoms may respond in part to newer agents and/or supportive psychotherapy and social skills training.

2. SPECIFIC DISORDERS

Schizophrenia

Schizophrenia is subdivided into catatonic, disorganized, paranoid, undifferentiated, and residual types. Neuroleptics are effective in treating the acute exacerbations of any subtype of the schizophrenias. Acute symptoms, such as those seen in a fluent thought disorder and the thought content problems of hallucinations and delusions, respond well. Typical neuroleptics are less effective than atypical neuroleptics in treating residual symptoms, particularly nonfluent formal thought disorder, poverty of speech, poverty of content of speech, blocking, and negativism (the so-called negative symptoms of schizophrenia).

Neuroleptics also are effective in the prophylaxis of acute schizophrenic relapses. Placebo substitution studies clearly demonstrate fewer recurrences in groups continuing to receive neuroleptics compared to those switched to placebo.

Delusional Disorders

Neuroleptics are not very effective in delusional disorders. This disorder, with onset in the middle years of life, has no known effective pharmacotherapy, although most psychiatrists will conduct a treatment trial in hope of a response.

Brief Reactive Psychosis & Schizophreniform Disorder

Neuroleptics are usually quite effective in reducing the acute psychotic symptoms associated with either brief reactive psychosis or schizophreniform disorder. Many clinicians withhold pharmacotherapy for a few days to see if hospitalization and withdrawal from a stressful environment will ameliorate symp-

toms. When neuroleptics are used, their prompt withdrawal is usually accomplished days or weeks after recovery. Many individuals with schizophreniform disorders go on to develop schizophrenia, in which case guidelines for the management of schizophrenia are in order.

Affective Illness

The neuroleptics are used in depressive disorders in the management of psychosis. Treatment is often initiated with a neuroleptic and continued with addition of an antidepressant, although some physicians initiate both concurrently. In either case, the neuroleptic should be withdrawn after weeks to months as long as psychotic symptoms have remitted. Psychotic symptoms in depression—particularly delusions of self-deprecation and self-accusation—may respond to antidepressants alone, but frank hallucinosis usually requires neuroleptics.

A similar case can be made for psychotic mania. Neuroleptics are used in combination with mood stabilizers for a brief period to reduce arousal and psychotic symptoms. Since no parenteral forms of mood stabilizers are available, neuroleptics alone are often used until the patient is willing to take oral medications.

Anxiety Disorders

Neuroleptics are rarely indicated in anxiety disorders, although psychoses may be misdiagnosed as anxiety. Occasionally, arousal is so uncontrolled (eg, in a severe chronic case of posttraumatic stress disorder) that anxiolytics are ineffective and a brief course of neuroleptics may be indicated. Neuroleptics are sometimes used briefly to reduce arousal and affective intensity in patients with borderline personality disorder.

Organic Mental Disorders

Psychotic symptoms are often present in a wide variety of brain and systemic disorders. Inflammatory, allergic, endocrine, or infectious diseases involving the brain and degenerative disorders such as Alzheimer's, Huntington's, or Parkinson's disease can present with psychotic symptoms. Symptomatic improvement can often be achieved using low doses of neuroleptics in psychoses of known organic origin. Consultation-liaison services in hospitals are heavy prescribers of low-dose neuroleptics in dementia and delirium presenting with psychotic symptoms and behavior management problems.

DRUG CHOICE

Efficacy

Although neuroleptics have major differences in potency, all typical neuroleptics appear to have equal efficacy for "positive symptoms." Fluphenazine and haloperidol are among the most potent neuroleptics; among the least potent (milligram for milligram) are chlorpromazine, thioridazine, and clozapine. As a general rule, the more potent drugs have fewer non-specific adverse effects such as sedation, hypotension, and anticholinergic effects than the low-potency drugs. However, high-potency drugs cause more extrapyramidal side effects than low-potency ones. Unless other factors intervene, it is reasonable to select a high-potency neuroleptic.

Factors that might influence this decision include the need for sedating effects (chlorpromazine, thioridazine); sensitivity to extrapyramidal effects, requiring very low doses at initiation of treatment; and patient preferences based on prior experience with the drugs. In general, a history of good response to a particular neuroleptic should prompt the clinician to use that agent again for that patient.

Clozapine and the other "atypical" neuroleptics have a somewhat different spectrum of side effects and a potential for effectiveness in schizophrenia refractory to other treatment. The risk of agranulocytosis limits the use of clozapine to patients who have failed to improve on two neuroleptics. Initially, CBCs had to be performed on a weekly basis, making the administration of clozapine expensive and cumbersome. This requirement has since been relaxed to some extent. Because clozapine has little effect on the extrapyramidal system, it is also useful in the treatment of psychotic schizophrenic patients with tardive dyskinesia. Clozapine has also been used in the treatment of psychosis in patients with Parkinson's disease, where extrapyramidal effects of neuroleptics pose a significant management problem.

The new drugs risperidone, olanzapine, and quetiapine provide an acceptable alternative to the older antipsychotics for the treatment of schizophrenia since, like clozapine, they enhance serotonin function. Also like clozapine, they are probably helpful in treating both "negative" symptoms as well as secondary affective symptoms (secondary depression). They are less likely to cause extrapyramidal syndromes than the high-potency typical antipsychotics, although risperidone, particularly in doses greater than 6 mg/d, still carries some risk. Unlike clozapine, these agents do not appear to have the risk of agranulocytosis. These drugs are rapidly becoming first-line agents for psychotic syndromes. In settings in which cost is a factor, however, the traditional neuroleptics are still often tried first.

Compliance

Failure to take neuroleptics consistently is the major reason for readmission of schizophrenic patients in acute episodes. Patients do not like neuroleptic medication because it slows thinking and affects motor performance ("It feels like a mental straitjacket"). (One young patient dissolved his medication in his parents' coffee in the morning "so they will know

how it feels.") Uncomfortable subjective effects of neuroleptics are corroborated by normal volunteers. Education of the patient and family is essential.

Long-acting parenteral neuroleptics were developed to ease administration and improve compliance. Two such neuroleptics are available in the United States: fluphenazine decanoate and haloperidol decanoate. Both drugs may be effective for 1–4 weeks after injection. Some degree of compliance is still necessary, since the patient must appear at a treatment facility to receive the next injection. There is some additional risk of neuroleptic malignant syndrome with long-acting agents, presumably because the drug cannot be promptly discontinued on emergence of the syndrome.

Adverse Effects

See Table 30–5 for a list of common adverse effects.

A. Pharmacotherapy of Extrapyramidal Syndromes: With the use of high-potency typical neuroleptics, adverse effects consist largely of extrapyramidal syndromes, the most common of which are acute dystonia, akathisia, and pseudoparkinsonism. The risk of extrapyramidal syndromes is much lower with the atypical agents, although not absent. Anticholinergic agents (Table 30–6) and switching to an agent that is less likely to cause extrapyramidal syndromes are the most common means of managing these conditions.

Acute dystonic reactions associated with neuroleptics include muscle spasms in the neck, oral, facial, buccal, and lingual regions. A typical reaction may be torticollis. Acute dystonias, the only extrapyramidal syndromes with a higher incidence in the young than the old, usually occur within a day after starting therapy or after a dose increase. Oral, intramuscular, and intravenous anticholinergic agents are effective in eliminating the symptoms. Intramuscular or intravenous therapy is recommended initially because the symptoms are extremely disturbing. Diphenhydramine, 50 mg intramuscularly or intravenously, is given, followed by 50 mg orally every 4 hours for several doses. Benztropine and biperiden may be

Table 30–5. Adverse effects of neuroleptics.

Anticholinergic effects	Dry mouth, difficulty urinating, constipation, blurred vision, toxic-confusional states
α-Adrenergic blockade	Orthostatic hypotension, impotence, failure to ejaculate
Dopaminergic blockade	Extrapyramidal syndromes, galactorrhea, amenorrhea, impotence, tardive dyskinesia, weight gain
Antihistaminic effects	Sedation
Hematologic	Agranulocytosis (clozapine primarily)

Table 30–6. Anticholinergic agents.

	Dosage Ranges (mg/d)
Benztropine	1–6
Biperiden	2–8
Diphenhydramine	50–300
Trihexyphenidyl	4–15
Procyclidine	10–20

used as well. When a dystonic reaction occurs, the patient usually wishes to discontinue the drug. Therefore, it is important to recognize the patient's vulnerability to dystonias so that therapy can be started with low doses and increased by small increments. If anticholinergics are continued for a few days and the neuroleptic is continued or reduced in dose, dystonic symptoms rarely return. Some clinicians (controversially) start all young patients on a "prophylactic" dose of anticholinergic agent. It is common for patients to state that they are "allergic" to haloperidol (for instance) because they once had an acute dystonic reaction.

The extrapyramidal movement disorder called akathisia is composed of purposeless movements, usually of the lower extremities, and a subjective feeling of restlessness. The subjective restless feeling is quite uncomfortable, often worse than the motor restlessness. Akathisias are treated with anticholinergic agents. Both akathisias and pseudoparkinsonism usually occur after 2 weeks of neuroleptic treatment. The dose of neuroleptic usually must be decreased in addition to adding an anticholinergic.

Neuroleptic-induced pseudoparkinsonian syndrome closely resembles Parkinson's disease: cogwheeling movements, pill-rolling tremors, gait disturbances, and flat facies may all be present. Pseudoparkinsonism is usually treated by a 2-week course of anticholinergic medication. After discontinuing the anticholinergic drug, careful monitoring for the return of extrapyramidal symptoms is important. In general, symptoms do not return. Few psychopharmacologists support continuous treatment with anticholinergics unless repeated efforts to discontinue the drug have resulted in the resurgence of unwanted side effects.

The development of extrapyramidal side effects may be an indication that the patient is at increased risk of developing tardive dyskinesia later in life, a syndrome that may develop as a side effect of ongoing therapy. Tardive dyskinesia is an involuntary movement disorder that consists of irregular choreiform or athetoid movements (or both). Patients taking typical neuroleptics develop the disorder at a rate of 2–4% per year over the first 7 years of exposure. Elderly women are at greater risk. Dystonias range from darting tongue movements and mouth puckerings to trunk twisting, pelvic thrusting, and grunting. Needless to say, the disorder can be quite crippling socially.

Details of the treatment of tardive dyskinesia are beyond the scope of this chapter. Early recognition is essential, since drug discontinuation will lead to disappearance of symptoms in one-third of patients and attenuation of symptoms in another third. Unfortunately, there is no effective or standard treatment for tardive dyskinesia, although vitamin E, calcium channel blockers, and benzodiazepines have been used with minimal success. Patients may be switched to an atypical neuroleptic. The presence of tardive dyskinesia in patients with repeated acute psychotic episodes poses a major clinical challenge.

B. Concurrent Medical Illness: Few medical conditions act as contraindications to neuroleptics in the treatment of psychosis. A number of illnesses (eg, liver disease) may affect the selection of drug dose and the frequency of visits and medical monitoring. Low-potency neuroleptics should be avoided or used with caution in elderly patients. Doses should be kept low and patients should be monitored carefully for hypotension and anticholinergic symptoms, including delirium.

THERAPEUTIC STRATEGIES

The primary use of neuroleptics is the control of acute psychotic symptoms. Clinical guidelines for their use in conditions other than schizophrenia are not described and should not be assumed to be identical. In particular, in other conditions such as psychotic depression or mania, the neuroleptic dose is often much lower, and the duration of use briefer, than in the treatment of psychotic exacerbations of schizophrenia.

Initiating Therapy

The first step before initiating therapy in an acute psychotic episode is a review of prior treatment. Successful treatment of a previous episode serves as a guideline for the choice of neuroleptic and its ideal dose. The goal of pharmacotherapy with neuroleptics is to use the lowest effective dose. Because the dosage range is broad, prior experience with the patient's requirement will shorten the acute treatment course. For illustrative purposes, initiation of haloperidol will be described. Other neuroleptics are used similarly, with dosages adjusted to account for differences in potency.

In a first psychotic episode, 5 mg of haloperidol twice daily may not only initiate treatment but may be an adequate maintenance dose. Most psychotic patients will respond to a total daily dose of 5–15 mg haloperidol or its equivalent in another neuroleptic.

Dose Increments

If after 2–5 days the patient shows no improvement in symptoms of arousal, such as excitement, increase the dose by 2 mg. (If an "as needed" dosage has been prescribed, add an amount equal to the average dose employed.)

Duration

There is a great temptation to increase the dose unnecessarily because of lack of patience. The effects of neuroleptics take time—even the effects on arousal may take a week, and hallucinations and delusions take much longer than that. Hallucinations may not be reported but may be elicited on specific inquiry for up to 2 weeks or more. Delusional material may take even longer to subside. Distorted thoughts may remain even after the persisting delusions have disappeared. Patience is essential. When treatment necessitates hospitalization, the use of high doses often serves a ward staff's need to achieve control on the unit rather than the patient's need for appropriate symptomatic treatment.

Blood Levels

In general, assays for neuroleptics are not available, and when they are available guidelines for their use in dosing patients lack proof of validity.

Treatment Failure

Acute psychotic episodes usually respond to neuroleptics when the drug can be tolerated in appropriate doses. Chronic psychotic symptoms are not, in general, as likely to disappear, although some researchers feel that the atypical antipsychotics have a direct effect on negative symptoms. Since both hallucinations and delusions may become chronic, it is often difficult to predict whether neuroleptics will be effective in a patient with chronic symptoms. One target symptom group that is useful in predicting treatment response is arousal (agitation, anxiety, confusion, disorientation, insomnia, excitement, and vigilance). When the presentation includes significantly increased arousal and the recent or subacute onset of hallucinations and delusions, there is a high probability of remission of all psychotic symptoms. When hallucinations and delusions have a long history, or when little arousal is present, there is far less likelihood of improvement on neuroleptics.

The introduction of atypical neuroleptics has provided useful new treatments for refractory schizophrenia and for schizophrenics with tardive dyskinesia.

CASE STUDY: ACUTE PSYCHOTIC EPISODE

John S was brought to the emergency room in the morning by his father and mother. He had returned from college unexpectedly several days earlier. The family was angry at first, then puzzled and worried. John had been an A student in high school and had been accepted at prestigious colleges, but decided instead to attend a state university close to home. According to the parents, he had behaved in bizarre ways over the last several days. John himself reported that a number of people, including his college roommate, had a plan to kill him. He had been up all night and had become very upset when questioned by his parents about his ideas. With enormous effort, his father had convinced John to come with him to the hospital.

On examination by the emergency room physician, John was found to be in good health. A drug screen was negative for evidence of "street drugs" that might cause psychosis. The physician found John to be paranoid, hypervigilant, and delusional, with his thinking confused and circumstantial. The physician observed behavior that he took to represent evidence that John was hearing voices. History provided by John's father suggested that his symptoms had developed over a 6-week period.

The psychiatrist on call confirmed the emergency room physician's findings, also determining that John had few friends in high school and a history of mild obsessive-compulsive behaviors. The psychiatrist recommended hospitalization. John at first rejected the recommendation, but his father ultimately convinced him to enter the hospital voluntarily.

On admission, a diagnosis of presumed schizophreniform disorder was confirmed after careful evaluation for affective illness such as mania. An atypical antipsychotic was prescribed. John not only remained in his room most of the first 3 days but barricaded the door the first night. The nursing staff felt he was little improved by day 3, and the psychiatry staff felt he was slightly less aroused. Both felt his psychomotor behavior was reduced. John still demonstrated some speech interruption that appeared to be related to auditory hallucinations, although he denied hearing voices. His dose was increased on the evening of the third day. John began to interact with the staff by the sixth day. He became less irritated and less seclusive.

John was discharged to home care after 14 days. On discharge, he still had paranoid ideation, but it was less firmly held and subject to doubt. He was far less aroused and able to talk about school, career goals, and his hospitalization. He agreed to cooperate in a specialized day treatment program (described further in Chapter 29).

PHARMACOTHERAPY OF ANXIETY & ANXIETY DISORDERS

AGENTS & CLASSES OF AGENTS

The *DSM-IV* anxiety disorders include a wide spectrum of different syndromes, for which a variety of different drugs are used. As we have come to learn more about these specific disorders it has become clear that they are distinct and different illnesses, each of which frequently responds to a different type of drug. Agents that have already been discussed, such as antidepressants, are now thought to be specifically effective for syndromes such as panic disorder and obsessive-compulsive disorder. For this discussion, the term "anxiolytic" is reserved for other agents that have been used for their more general sedating qualities and/or specific "antianxiety" properties (such as action on γ-aminobutyric acid receptors).

For the past several decades the most popular class of anxiolytic compounds has been the benzodiazepines. These drugs have virtually replaced all other anxiolytics because of their specificity, potency, and safety. Buspirone, a nonbenzodiazepine compound, is marketed for the treatment of generalized anxiety disorder and has little potential for abuse. Antihistaminics are still used as anxiolytics, although their effects are primarily sedative. Barbiturates and their congeners, anxiolytics of choice in past decades, have fallen into disfavor because they produce dependency and tolerance and are dangerous in overdose. There is rarely any reason to depart from the use of benzodiazepines or buspirone in the treatment of symptomatic anxiety per se. (See Table 30–7 for a list of anxiolytics and their dosage ranges.)

INDICATIONS

1. TARGET SYMPTOMS & SYNDROMES

Anxiety may be manifested as an internal subjective experience characterized by apprehensive expectation or worry as well as in symptoms of motor tension, autonomic hyperactivity, and vigilance (ie, arousal). All anxiety-dependent symptoms respond to anxiolytics. When anxiolytics are effective, all symptoms improve over the same time course, and usually immediately. Although diazepam and chlordiazepoxide were introduced for the treatment of anxiety in the 1960s, the use of anxiolytics to treat specific anxiety disorders had to await developments in the classification of disorders. Donald Klein and others in the early 1970s recommended separating panic and panic with agoraphobia from other anxiety conditions on the basis of their pharmacological responses to heterocyclic antidepressants and MAOIs. In 1980, *DSM-III* reclassified neurotic disorders as anxiety disorders according to specific criteria. In doing so, *DSM-III* and, subsequently, *DSM-IV* improved the prediction of treatment response to drugs and to behavioral interventions (see Chapter 21).

2. SPECIFIC DISORDERS

Generalized Anxiety Disorder

Generalized anxiety disorder (GAD) shares many features of dysthymic disorder, such as chronicity and comorbidity with major depression. Patients meeting criteria for GAD respond to benzodiazepine anxiolytics, or sometimes buspirone, with a reduction in symptoms. Symptoms usually return when the drug is discontinued. Even with treatment, patients with GAD may not evidence functional improvement (indicated by enhanced productivity or sociability).

Panic Disorder & Agoraphobia

There are four pharmacological approaches to the therapy of panic disorder, but data as yet fail to support one over the others. The major chemotherapeutic approaches to panic disorder include heterocyclic antidepressants (eg, imipramine), SSRIs (eg, fluoxetine), MAOIs (eg, phenelzine), and benzodiazepines (eg, alprazolam). Nonpharmacological approaches include behavior therapy (exposure) and cognitive therapy. With effective treatment, the frequency and intensity of panic episodes are reduced or eliminated. Anticipatory anxiety usually improves after effective treatment of panic. Although there is controversy over whether agoraphobia exists in the absence of panic disorder, most psychopharmacologists believe that both groups of syndromes respond to appropriate treatment. Investigators have suggested recently that drug therapies are effective in treating the panic symptoms but that behavior therapies are more effective in treating phobic avoidance and agoraphobia. Although we emphasize the pharmacological treatment of panic disorders in this chapter, attention to behavioral and cognitive therapy is warranted.

Target symptoms for panic attacks include the subjective inner experience ("I'm going to die," "I'm

Table 30–7. Anxiolytics.

	Dosage Range (mg/d)
Benzodiazepines	
Chlordiazepoxide	15–200
Diazepam	4–40
Chlorazepate	15–60
Halazepam	60–160
Parzepam	20–60
Lorazepam	1–6
Oxazepam	45–120
Alprazolam	1–6
Estazolam	0.5–2.0
Clonazepam	0.25–3.0
Barbiturates	
Amobarbital	60–150
Pentobarbital	90–120
Phenobarbital	30–120
β-Blockers	
Propranolol	60–240
Atenolol	50–100
Antihistamines	
Hydroxyzine	75–400
Diphenhydramine	50–300
Azaspirodecanedione	
Buspirone	15–60

having a heart attack," "I'm going crazy") and symptoms of autonomic stimulation (tachycardia, tachypnea, tremor, shortness of breath, etc). Benzodiazepines such as alprazolam have the advantage of prompt reduction in anxiety (with panic attacks requiring several weeks to respond). Heterocyclic antidepressants, SSRIs, and MAOIs are effective in reducing panic attacks, but with these drugs there is a latency period of several weeks from the establishment of a therapeutic dose, and they have little to no direct effect on anticipatory anxiety. Alprazolam is usually effective in doses of 3–9 mg/d, imipramine in doses of 100–250 mg/d, fluoxetine in doses of 10–40 mg/d, and phenelzine in doses of 30–60 mg/d. Dose escalation of heterocyclic antidepressants, SSRIs, and MAOIs should follow the principles discussed in the section on depression. However, it is thought that lower doses are required to treat panic disorder than to treat major depression. Furthermore, patients with panic disorder are often prone to develop agitation and may need to be introduced to these drugs more slowly.

Simple & Social Phobia

The current treatment of choice for simple phobia is exposure, a form of behavior therapy. Some simple phobias may be "agoraphobia-like," in that the patient remains house-bound for fear of encountering the feared situation. In such a case the standard treatment for agoraphobia may be attempted.

Social phobia may be divided into two types, circumscribed and generalized, which require different pharmacological approaches. The standard treatment for circumscribed social phobia, such as stage fright, has been the use of β-blockers (eg, propranolol, 80–120 mg) to reduce autonomic arousal prior to social exposure such as a lecture. Benzodiazepines may also be used, but they present the risk of impairing performance and cognition. SSRIs and MAOIs have been used successfully to treat generalized social phobia.

Obsessive-Compulsive Disorder

It appears clear that obsessive-compulsive disorder (OCD) is a distinct biological illness. The heterocyclic agent clomipramine and SSRIs such as fluoxetine and fluvoxamine are used as drugs of choice. Because of the profile of adverse effects of clomipramine, SSRIs are frequently used first, even though clomipramine may be somewhat more effective. Other heterocyclic antidepressants and benzodiazepines have been of negligible benefit.

Both obsessional and compulsive symptoms improve with clomipramine treatment, usually after the first couple of weeks and continuing into the second month. About half of obsessive-compulsive patients experience moderate to marked improvement. It is helpful to inventory compulsive behaviors (such as checking rituals) and collect baseline information on

their frequency before starting medication in order to titrate the dose.

Clomipramine is a tricyclic antidepressant with potent serotonin agonist effects—adverse effects follow the pattern of other serotonergic drugs such as fluoxetine, including restlessness and sexual dysfunction. It also has the anticholinergic and cardiac side effects that are typical of other heterocyclic antidepressants. The initial dose is often 50 mg daily, increasing (as with the heterocyclic antidepressants) to 300 mg daily. The upper end of the dose range of the SSRIs is used in OCD, eg, up to 80 mg of fluoxetine (see Table 30–1).

Posttraumatic Stress Disorder

There is no specific pharmacotherapy for posttraumatic stress disorder. Symptomatic approaches are frequently used, targeting anxiety (benzodiazepines), depression (SSRIs or heterocyclic antidepressants), and sleep (again benzodiazepines). Heterocyclic agents appear to be useful only when the patient meets criteria for major depression. Anxiolytics frequently provide minimal benefit in high-arousal states. Patients often abuse alcohol or other substances to reduce arousal. MAOIs may be of assistance in attenuating flashbacks, but this effect has not been proven.

Organic Mental Disorders

The response of organic mental disorders with associated anxiety to benzodiazepines is highly variable. Empirical trials are frequently recommended, but careful assessment is required to determine if improvement has occurred. Benzodiazepines may produce disinhibition in some individuals with organic mental disorders.

DRUG CHOICE

1. BENZODIAZEPINES

Efficacy

The selection of a specific benzodiazepine is governed by its intended use. If the intent is to treat a brief episode of "high anxiety," a short- to medium-acting rapidly absorbed agent is selected (such as alprazolam or lorazepam). For continuous coverage of anxiety or for prophylaxis of panic disorder, longer-acting potent benzodiazepines may be more desirable (diazepam is a reasonable choice, although clonazepam has been used increasingly). One common problem is the prescription of short-acting benzodiazepines that "wear off" before the next dose, producing early abstinence or rebound anxiety and craving for the drug. This problem is alleviated by more frequent doses or by switching to a longer-acting benzodiazepine.

Compliance

For the most part, anxious patients like taking benzodiazepines, since the rapid anxiolytic action is quite reinforcing. In very anxious patients with only mild attenuation of symptoms, escalation of dose without the physician's knowledge may occur. Compliance with physician recommendations to discontinue benzodiazepine use can be a problem as well. Since physicians have very different approaches to the use of benzodiazepines, patients often feel trapped—eg, when referred to Dr Q, John S discovered that Dr Q disapproved of Dr T's use of clorazepate. John also felt accused of being an "addict."

The as needed use of anxiolytics may also provide difficulties in the management of anxiety. As needed use of benzodiazepines should be confined to individuals who require anxiolytics on a less than daily basis. For persistent anxiety states, daily as needed use may exacerbate the problem through rebound anxiety or failure to manage the symptoms adequately.

Adverse Effects

Benzodiazepines are safe and effective medications. Because sedation is the most common side effect, patients should be advised to be cautious (particularly initially) in tasks that require alertness (such as driving). Other less common side effects include dizziness, weakness, nausea, impaired performance of complex motor tasks, ataxia, and memory difficulties (anterograde amnesia).

Although benzodiazepines are far safer than barbiturates with regard to lethality, they can produce physical dependence. At therapeutic doses for anxiety, physical dependence does not generally present a serious abstinence problem. Nevertheless, at high doses, abrupt discontinuation can lead to serious consequences such as seizures—even status epilepticus.

Patients should be withdrawn slowly (eg, 10% a day) if withdrawal symptoms are to be avoided. Common withdrawal symptoms include anxiety, tremor, palpitations, sweating, nausea, and confusion. More commonly, patients report a recurrence of the anxiety for which the drug was initially prescribed.

2. OTHER DRUGS

Buspirone is a drug that appears to be more effective in theory than it does in practice. Researchers believe that it exerts its anxiolytic actions via the serotonin system. It is nonsedating and is not habit forming. Although research studies found it to be at least as effective for the treatment of generalized anxiety disorder as benzodiazepines, this does not appear to have been borne out in the long run. The drug does not appear to be as effective in patients who have already been exposed to benzodiazepines. The fact that buspirone takes 2 to 4 weeks to begin working (unlike the benzodiazepines, which take effect immediately) may account, in part, for its disappointing results.

β-Blockers such as propranolol are successful in managing generalized anxiety in patients who are "tuned in to their bodies," eg, those who are particularly aware of their pulse rate. Since β-blockers slow the heart rate, such individuals are reassured, and subjective anxiety may subside. For most anxious individuals, however, the internal subjective experience of anxiety is the central symptom, and for such patients β-blockers tend to be ineffective.

Antihistamines are often used in elderly patients or in patients with chronic drug misuse or dependency problems. Unfortunately, they are more sedating than anxiolytic.

Neuroleptics are occasionally used to reduce "high anxiety" but do so less specifically through reducing arousal. Since neuroleptics have undesirable adverse effects, lack specificity, and are associated with long-term risks of tardive dyskinesia, they are not commonly used even in severe anxiety.

Barbiturates are rarely used for the treatment of anxiety.

THERAPEUTIC STRATEGIES

1. BENZODIAZEPINES

Pretreatment Workup & Contraindications

There are few, if any, absolute medical contraindications for benzodiazepines—they may be used safely in most medical conditions and in combination with most medications. In patients with chronic obstructive pulmonary disease, caution should be used as high doses of these agents tend to depress respiration. Hypersensitivity to benzodiazepines and a history of paradoxical excitement are two of the rare contraindications. No routine laboratory studies are required prior to initiating treatment.

Initiating Treatment

The initial dose of an anxiolytic is often the therapeutic dose as well. Except for panic disorder and agoraphobia, there is little need to escalate the initial dose gradually as is done with the antidepressants and neuroleptics to achieve satisfactory therapeutic results.

Dose Increments

Initial daily doses are generally increased by 50–100% if the first dose is ineffective—eg, alprazolam, 0.25 mg four times daily, may be increased to 0.5 mg four times daily after 3–5 days and then, if necessary, to 1 mg four times daily—a stiff dose for general symptoms of anxiety but still less than may be needed in panic disorder.

Duration

The duration of treatment is perhaps the major area of disagreement among physicians. Chronic management with benzodiazepines is generally accepted in specific disorders such as panic disorder and agoraphobia, when discontinuance is followed by recurrence of symptoms. More controversial is the chronic use of benzodiazepines in the management of generalized anxiety disorder and "common anxiety." In cases in which anxiety can be shown to disrupt occupational, social, or family functioning, and if adequate functioning is restored with use of the drugs, and discontinuance is followed by return of dysfunction, the chronic use of these agents seems justified.

Blood Levels

Therapeutic levels of benzodiazepines have been established in research settings but are not generally available. Even if they were, they would not be cost effective, since appropriate doses can be determined quickly and safely.

Treatment Failure

Anxiolytics are highly effective in reducing anxiety but rarely eliminate all anxiety. Thus, "treatment failure" with benzodiazepines usually means absence of an adequate anxiolytic response. When high doses are not effective, careful reassessment of the diagnosis is called for. A masked psychotic state may be present and may require use of neuroleptics.

PHARMACOTHERAPY OF INSOMNIA

Insomnia has many causes. In this section, the term denotes the complaint of trouble falling asleep, sleep continuity interruption, poor sleep quality, or decreased total sleep time that has no cause that may be more specifically treated, eg, major depression. Primary insomnia may be diagnosed when such disturbances occur more than three times a week for at least 1 month and result in daytime fatigue or impaired daytime functioning.

Insomnia is a common complaint in general medical practice. It is usually not caused by a primary psychiatric disorder or other specific sleep disorder. "Ordinary" insomnia may result from anxiety, stress at work or at home, or even poor "sleep hygiene," ie, bad sleep habits. The physician's first task is to determine whether there may be a specific psychiatric or medical cause for insomnia. In the absence of a primary cause, the decision as to whether to prescribe hypnotics must be made. Other management strategies may be more appropriate, such as behavioral instruction or even encouraging the patient to "live with the problem."

AGENTS & CLASSES OF AGENTS

The most important class of sedative-hypnotics is the benzodiazepines. As discussed in the section on pharmacotherapy of anxiety and anxiety disorders, any benzodiazepine may be used as a sedative-hypnotic in the proper dose. Nevertheless, pharmaceutical companies have marketed specific benzodiazepines as sedative-hypnotics and, by their dosage formulations (milligrams of drug per tablet or capsule), have made them more convenient to use as hypnotics rather than anxiolytics, eg, flurazepam rather than diazepam for sleep (Table 30–8).

INDICATIONS

Physicians differ widely in their opinions about the use of sleep-inducing medications. Some guard against abuse and dependency by rarely prescribing sedatives except in hospital settings, whereas others offer them liberally on patient request, often over a period of years. Most physicians would agree that severe insomnia (eg, primary insomnia) that interferes with daily functioning and that can be anticipated to be of brief duration is a good indication for pharmacotherapy. Furthermore, most physicians would agree that the chronic prescription of sedative-hypnotics over months or years is not appropriate. In the prescription of anxiolytics and sedative-hypnotics, physicians are often at odds with the wishes of their patients. The best guide to appropriate prescription is (1) an understanding of the causes of insomnia, eg, in terms of acute stressors or personality factors, (2) good patient education about the risks and benefits of sedatives, and (3) monitoring, as objectively as pos-

Table 30–8. Sedative-hypnotics.

	Dosage Range (mg/d)
Benzodiazepines	
Flurazepam	15–30
Temazepam	15–30
Triazolam	0.125–0.5
Quazepam	7.5–15
Lorazepam	2–4
Barbiturates	
Secobarbital[a]	100
Phenobarbital[a]	100–120
Pentobarbital[a]	100
Amobarbital[a]	100–200
Miscellaneous	
Chloral hydrate[a]	500–1000
Ethchlorvynol[a]	500–1000
Zolpidem	5–10
Antihistamines	
Diphenhydramine	50–150
Hydroxyzine	10–400
Doxylamine	25–150

[a] Not generally recommended for insomnia.

sible, of improved functioning brought about by the use of sedatives. In most instances, daily use of sedative-hypnotics should not continue for longer than several weeks.

The diagnosis and treatment of specific sleep disorders are beyond the scope of this chapter. Sleep symptoms (not associated with specific syndromes) are generally reported by patients as "trouble falling asleep," "wakefulness," or "not getting enough sleep." Identification of the specific sleep complaint is important, since "trouble falling asleep" (initial insomnia) may suggest the use of a short-acting benzodiazepine such as triazolam, whereas a patient with multiple awakenings (sleep continuity disorder) may require a longer-acting sedative such as flurazepam.

DRUG CHOICE

1. BENZODIAZEPINES

Efficacy

All drugs in the benzodiazepine class appear to be equally effective as sedative-hypnotics if the proper dose is selected. The major differences lie in their pharmacokinetic properties. Selection of a specific benzodiazepine is usually based on the type of insomnia (initial or terminal insomnia and continuity problems), the side effect profile, and patient preference.

Compliance

Compliance with the use of sedative-hypnotics is rarely a problem. Patients complaining of insomnia are generally seeking chemical assistance in producing or maintaining sleep. On the other hand, patients may escalate the dose of sedative without the knowledge of the physician. Assisting a patient in giving up sedative-hypnotics is often a problem. The patient should understand that discontinuing medication will often result in rebound insomnia that is mistaken for ordinary insomnia. Return of insomnia may reinforce the patient's conviction that sedative-hypnotics are necessary for comfortable functioning during the day.

Adverse Effects

The adverse effects of benzodiazepines are discussed in the section on anxiolytics. Patients using sedatives most frequently complain of daytime grogginess. This can often be avoided by using a shorter-acting drug or by taking the nighttime dose earlier in the evening.

2. OTHER SEDATIVE-HYPNOTICS

Zolpidem is structurally related to benzodiazepines but is more selective, thus having little anticonvulsant and muscle relaxant activity. It is marketed as being less likely to cause rebound insomnia and/or tolerance than benzodiazepines, but is not free of such risks and other benzodiazepine-like side effects.

Barbiturates and antihistamines are still commonly used for sedation—barbiturates in hospital settings and antihistamines for elderly persons or those with a history of substance abuse. Many physicians use sedating heterocyclic antidepressants. Since the second-choice drugs have other chemical and psychotropic effects, their use is discouraged.

THERAPEUTIC STRATEGIES

"Common insomnia" is generally reported as trouble falling asleep (long sleep latency) or multiple awakenings (sleep continuity disorder). In general, early morning awakening (terminal insomnia) is associated with major depression.

Pharmacological treatment of insomnia should be confined to several weeks. When symptoms persist and the patient appears to have reduced total sleep time even when taking a sedative-hypnotic such as flurazepam, referral to a sleep disorder center may be indicated. Attention to appropriate sleep hygiene is an important aspect of the assessment and treatment of insomnia. Does the patient nap during the day? Toss and turn in bed? Snack before bedtime? Patients are instructed not to nap, to get out of bed to work or read until sleepy, and to refrain from snacking. The more obvious approach of understanding and mastering anxiety, conflicts, and life challenges that precipitate insomnia should not be overlooked. Patients need to understand the goals of the use of sedative-hypnotics—usually brief assistance with trouble falling asleep or awakening.

II. OTHER SOMATIC TREATMENTS

ELECTROCONVULSIVE THERAPY

Historical Overview

The historical origins of electroconvulsive therapy (ECT) date back to the late nineteenth and early twentieth centuries, when scientists began to examine the phenomenology of mental disorders and to investigate the nature of brain dysfunction. Two important and unrelated ideas converged to result in ECT. During the 1920s, researchers counting heads in French "lunatic asylums" noted a low prevalence of epilepsy in schizophrenic patients. This finding led Marchand to hypothesize a biological antagonism between epilepsy and psychosis. The idea that one disease could be used to treat another was exemplified by von Jauregg, who treated tertiary syphilis by giving patients malaria. The confluence of these two ideas led von Meduna to induce seizures in schizophrenic patients (first by injecting oil of camphor and later with pentylenetetrazole). At about the same time, Sakel achieved a similar result by inducing insulin coma in psychotic patients, although the seizure resulting from the hypoglycemic state was at first considered to be an undesirable by-product of the procedure rather than its therapeutic basis.

In 1938, Cerletti and Bini performed the first procedure in which an electrical current was passed directly through the brain, resulting in a generalized tonic-clonic seizure. The patient, who was found wandering around the train station in Rome, recovered from his psychotic episode after 11 treatments and was discharged within a few months. After the success of this treatment was publicized, it rapidly replaced other forms of seizure induction because it is easier to control than seizures induced with injected substances and was demonstrably safer.

Initially, ECT was performed with the patient alert and awake. The procedure was both frightening and associated with complications resulting from the often violent tonic-clonic convulsions. In addition, the procedure was at first often used indiscriminately, since there were few alternatives for treating severely depressed psychotic or violent patients. The procedure has been portrayed as a tool used by sadistic psychiatrists to punish "difficult" patients (eg, *One Flew Over the Cuckoo's Nest*). Hence, the procedure fell into disfavor, particularly as effective antidepressant and neuroleptic medications were introduced.

Today, ECT is enjoying a resurgence of popularity. The technique has been greatly modified since the early days. The patient is paralyzed to prevent the peripheral manifestations of the seizure, and anesthesia (sleep) is induced so that the patient is not conscious of the frightening sensations of being paralyzed and having a seizure. Modern techniques have significantly reduced morbidity and mortality as well, allowing ECT to regain its place as a respected and legitimate method of treatment for selected patients with serious psychiatric disturbances.

Indications

Electroconvulsive therapy is used today as a first-line treatment for patients who need rapid resolution of life-threatening symptoms, who cannot tolerate the medical risks of other treatments, or who have a history of poor response to other treatments. It is considered to be effective treatment for major depression with or without psychotic features, for bipolar illness (both depressed and manic phases), and for catatonic schizophrenia. It should be considered also in cases of schizophrenia with strong affective symptomatology. It is not considered effective for other forms of schizophrenia, although it is sometimes used for this purpose in highly treatment-resistant patients.

There is controversy surrounding the use of ECT for some other conditions for which its efficacy is considered merely suggestive. These include delirium, severe organic affective/psychotic syndromes, and several medical conditions, including Parkinson's disease and catatonia secondary to organic causes.

Efficacy

Electroconvulsive therapy is more effective than antidepressants alone for the treatment of major depression with psychotic features and is as effective as the combination of antidepressants and neuroleptics. In one study, ECT was effective in most cases in which drug treatment failed. As a rule, bilateral ECT is more effective than unilateral ECT (80–85% versus 90–95%). However, because there is some evidence that bilateral ECT imposes a higher risk of memory impairment, bilateral ECT is commonly reserved for patients who have failed unilateral ECT or for those in whom rapid resolution of symptoms is of paramount importance.

Contraindications

Although there are no absolute contraindications to ECT, the procedure is usually not undertaken in the presence of increased intracranial pressure. Patients with a recent history of myocardial infarction, recent intracerebral hemorrhage, bleeding or unstable vascular aneurysm, retinal detachment, pheochromocytoma, or untreated glaucoma and those who have an American Society of Anesthesiologists (ASA) anesthetic risk of 4 have been treated with ECT but require special care and expertise.

Adverse Effects

Many patients experience some degree of confusion following ECT, which is to be expected given the normal occurrence of confusion in the postictal state. In patients who remain confused for a day or two following each treatment, it is often advisable to give two rather than three treatments per week. Electroconvulsive therapy has also been associated with long-term memory deficits, which are usually characterized by little or no memory of the period of hospitalization and, in some cases, events just before and just after hospitalization. Fewer than 1% of patients complain of amnesia 6 months after the treatment.

Because both pulse and blood pressure rise significantly during the seizure, patients with cardiac dysfunction are at higher risk for untoward events such as ischemia or arrhythmia. The anesthesiologist often uses medications to control pulse and blood pressure during the procedure. Occasionally, a patient may experience a prolonged (usually defined as longer than 2 minutes) seizure or a "late" seizure (which may in fact simply be a prolonged seizure masked by the barbiturate the patient has received). An occasional patient may experience prolonged apnea or laryngospasm.

Other side effects include burns from poor contact with the electrode, loose or broken teeth, and peripheral nerve palsy. Most patients experience some anxiety and apprehension, particularly early in the course of treatment. Headache, muscle aches, and a vague sense of confusion for a few hours after the treatment are common.

Morbidity & Mortality

Studies indicate that about one in 1300 to 1400 patients may experience significant adverse effects from ECT. The risk of death is 4.5 per 100,000 treatments.

Mechanism

Although it is clear that central nervous system seizure discharge is required for ECT to be effective, we do not understand the underlying neurophysiological or neurochemical mechanisms. Electroconvulsive therapy has many central nervous system effects, causing changes in the electroencephalogram (EEG), hypothalamic hormone secretion, calcium metabolism, biogenic amine levels, and receptor sensitivity. The amnesia precipitated by ECT may itself contribute to the improvement. Further research on the effects of ECT may clarify the neurochemical mechanisms that underlie affective disorders.

Technique

When ECT is being considered, it is important to be sure that both the patient and the patient's family understand its risks and benefits and concur with the decision to provide treatment in this way. It may be necessary to explain the procedure several times to the patient, who may have some cognitive impairment as a result of the illness. A thorough medical evaluation is then done to determine if the patient may need pretreatment of any kind or special care during the treatment. Of course, informed consent is required.

Treatments are commonly done in the morning, usually three times a week. The patient has nothing to eat or drink after midnight before each treatment. An intravenous line is started, and atropine or a similar agent is administered. The electrode sites are carefully cleaned, and once the electrodes are placed on the patient's scalp, the machine is tested to make certain that the circuit is complete. At this point, the patient is usually oxygenated with an Ambu bag and then given a short-acting barbiturate intravenously to induce light sleep. When the patient is asleep, a bite block is inserted to protect the teeth, and succinylcholine is administered. When paralysis is confirmed (eg, by testing with a nerve stimulator, looking for termination of fasciculations, or testing plantar response), the electrical stimulus is applied. During this process, the patient is carefully monitored. Pulse and blood pressure are checked before the procedure, af-

ter anesthesia, during the seizure, and periodically during and after recovery. Since many ECT machines have a built-in EEG monitor, the seizure itself may be directly monitored. If no EEG is available, seizure duration is monitored by inflating a blood pressure cuff on one leg (usually at the midcalf level) after the patient is asleep and before the succinylcholine is given. The seizure can then be timed by watching the tonic-clonic movements in the unparalyzed limb. If the clinician is satisfied that an adequate seizure has been obtained, the patient is monitored carefully until alert. If the seizure was not adequate, a second stimulus, usually of greater duration or intensity, may be delivered. After initial recovery (eg, in the recovery room or ECT suite), the patient's vital signs and cognitive status are monitored on the ward for several hours. It is also good practice to watch for persistent signs of organicity (eg, disorientation, confusion). When this occurs, the treatments are often administered less frequently or even discontinued. Most depressed patients receive between 9 and 12 treatments. Manic patients often respond to only one or two, but schizophrenic patients may receive 15 or more treatments. Currently, most clinicians deliver just enough stimulus at each treatment to obtain an adequate seizure (that is, the stimulus just exceeds the seizure threshold). However, a recent study indicates that increasing the stimulus intensity to 2.5 times the seizure threshold may increase the efficacy of both unilateral and bilateral ECT. Some clinicians deliver several stimuli in one treatment session (multiple monitored ECT). This procedure may lead to more severe cognitive impairment.

In most cases, patients start receiving antidepressant medication after the completion of treatment in order to prevent relapse. In some cases, periodic maintenance courses of one or two ECT treatments every several months, as indicated by the historical pattern of response, are recommended to prevent relapse and are conducted on an outpatient basis.

PSYCHOSURGERY

Once a fairly common procedure, psychosurgery for mental disorders has declined precipitously over the last three decades to the point at which it is almost never used today. Most "psychosurgery" these days is done on patients with epilepsy and involves ablation of the presumed epileptic focus. Most remaining psychosurgery utilizes stereotactic techniques to localize small key areas of the brain. The anatomic target is chosen selectively based on symptoms. For example, cingulectomy has been used to treat patients with severe chronic pain with depression and addiction, and internal capsulotomy has been shown to be effective in patients with severe obsessive-compulsive disorder who are extraordinarily impaired (eg, hospitalized more than 10 years) and have not responded to behavior therapy or pharmacotherapy. Severe chronic recurrent depressions have been treated with innominotomy, and posteromedial hypothalamotomy has been used in patients with restless, aggressive, and destructive behavior.

Unlike the psychosurgery done earlier in the century that involved larger and less selective areas of the brain—often leaving patients with extensive behavioral morbidity—modern techniques usually cause little or no personality change. However, clinicians recommending psychosurgery must scrupulously guard the rights of patients. Patients and their families should fully understand the risks and potential benefits.

REFERENCES & SUGGESTED READINGS

Abrams R: *Electroconvulsive Therapy.* Oxford University Press, 1988.

Andreasen NC: Improvement of negative symptoms: concepts, definition and assessment. Int Clin Psychopharmacol 1997;12(Suppl 2):57.

APA Task Force on ECT: The practice of ECT: Recommendation for treatment, training and privileging. Convuls Ther 1990;6:85.

Aronson T, Shukla SL: Long-term continuation antidepressant treatment: A comparison study. J Clin Psychiatry 1989;50:285.

Bouckoms AJ: Ethics of psychosurgery. Acta Neurochir 1988;44:173.

Brar JS et al: The effects of clozapine on negative symptoms in patients with schizophrenia with minimal positive symptoms. Ann Clin Psychiatry 1997;9:227.

Breier A et al: Effects of clozapine on positive and negative symptoms in outpatients with schizophrenia. Am J Psychiatry 1994;151:20.

Calabrase JR et al: A medication algorithm for treatment of bipolar rapid cycling? J Clin Psychiatry 1995;56(Suppl 3):11.

Cardoso F et al: Dystonia and dyskinesia. Psychiatr Clin North Am 1997;20:521.

Claghorn JL et al: Paroxetine versus placebo: A double-blind comparison in depressed patients. J Clin Psychiatry 1992;53:434.

Cohen LS et al: Psychotropic drug use during pregnancy: weighing the risks. J Clin Psychiatry 1998;59(Suppl 2):18.

Conley R et al: Olanzapine compared with chlorpromazine in the treatment of resistant schizophrenia. Am J Psychiatry 1998;155:914.

Coryell J et al: Lithium discontinuation and subsequent effectiveness. Am J Psychiatry 1998;155:895.

Coryell W: The treatment of psychotic depression. J Clin Psychiatry 1998;59(Suppl 1):22.

Cramer JA et al: Compliance with medication regimens for mental and physical disorders. Psychiatr Serv 1998;49:196.

Davis JM et al: Dose response of prophylactic antipsychotics. J Clin Psychiatry 1993;54(3, Suppl):24.

Dubovsky SL: Generalized anxiety disorder: New concepts and psychopharmacologic therapies. J Clin Psychiatry 1990;51(Suppl):3.

Dunner D et al: Venlafaxine in dysthymic disorder. J Clin Psychiatry 1997;58:528.

Fatemi SH et al: Lamotrigine in rapid cycling bipolar disorder. J Clin Psychiatry 1997:58:522.

Fink M (editor): ECT in the high risk patient. Convuls Ther 1989;5(1) [entire issue].

Frank E: Enhancing patient outcomes: Treatment adherence. J Clin Psychiatry 1997;58(Suppl 1):16.

Frank E et al: Three-year outcomes for maintenance therapies in recurrent depression. Arch Gen Psychiatry 1990;47:1090.

Freeman TW et al: A double-blind comparison of valproate and lithium in the treatment of acute mania. Am J Psychiatry 1992;149:108.

Gelenberg AJ, Bassuk E: *The Practitioner's Guide to Psychoactive Drugs,* 4th edition. Plenum Medical Book Company, 1997.

Goodman WK et al: Biological approaches to treatment-resistant obsessive compulsive disorder. J Clin Psychiatry 1993;54(6, Suppl):16.

Goodwin FK, Jamison KR: *Manic-Depressive Illness.* Oxford University Press, 1990.

Greden JF: Antidepressant maintenance medications: When to discontinue and how to stop. J Clin Psychiatry 1993;54(8, Suppl):39.

Greenblatt DJ, Harmatz JS, Shader RI: Plasma alprazolam concentrations relation to efficacy and side effects in the treatment of panic disorder. Arch Gen Psychiatry 1993;50:715.

Hale AS: Olanzapine. Br J Hosp Med 1997;58:442.

Jenicak, PG: Verapamil for the treatment of acute mania: A double blind placebo controlled trial. Am J Psychiatry 1998;155:972.

Jenike M et al: Open trial of fluoxetine in obsessive-compulsive disorder. Am J Psychiatry 1989;146:909.

Joffe RT et al: A placebo-controlled comparison of lithium and triiodothyronine augmentation of tricyclic antidepressants in unipolar refractory depression. Arch Gen Psychiatry 1993;50:387.

Kane J, Honigfeld G, Singer J, Meltzer H: Clozapine for the treatment-resistant schizophrenic. Arch Gen Psychiatry 1988;45:789.

Keck P et al: Time course of antipsychotic effects of neuroleptic drugs. Am J Psychiatry 1989;146:1289.

Keck PE Jr et al: Anticonvulsants and antipsychotics in the treatment of bipolar disorder. J Clin Psychiatry 1998;59 (Suppl 6):74.

Keller M (editor): Mood disorders. Psychiatr Clin North Am 1996;19 [entire issue].

Keller M (editor): New uses for antidepressants. J Clin Psychiatry 1997;58(Suppl 14)[entire issue].

Kramer P: *Listening to Prozac.* Viking Penguin, 1993.

Kulin NA et al: Pregnancy outcome following maternal use of the new selective serotonin reuptake inhibitors. JAMA 1998;279:609.

Kupfer DJ, Carpenter LL, Frank E: Possible role of antidepressants in precipitating mania and hypomania in recurrent depression. Am J Psychiatry 1988;145:804.

Kupfer DJ et al: Five-year outcome for maintenance therapies in recurrent depression. Arch Gen Psychiatry 1993;49:769.

Latinen LV: Psychosurgery today. Acta Neurochir 1988;44(Suppl):158.

Leonard BE: The comparative pharmacology of new antidepressants. J Clin Psychiatry 1993;54(8, Suppl):3.

Leonard HL: New developments in the treatment of obsessive-compulsive disorder. J Clin Psychiatry 1997;58 (Suppl 4):39.

Littrell KH et al: Marked reduction of tardive dyskinesia with clozapine. Arch Gen Psychiatry 1998;53:279.

Marks IM: *Fears, Phobias, and Rituals.* Oxford University Press, 1987.

Mavissakalian M, Perel J: Imipramine dose-response relationship in panic disorder with agoraphobia. Arch Gen Psychiatry 1989;46:127.

McElvoy S et al: Valproate in the treatment of rapid-cycling bipolar disorder. J Clin Psychopharmacol 1988;8:275.

McGrath PJ et al: A double-blind crossover trial of imipramine and phenelzine for outpatients with treatment-refractory depression. Am J Psychiatry 1993;150: 118.

Mortimer AM: Cognitive function in schizophrenia—do neuroleptics make a difference? Pharmacol Biochem Behav 1997;56:789.

Mukherjee S, Sackeim HA, Schnur DB: Electroconvulsive therapy of acute manic episodes: A review of 50 years' experience. Am J Psychiatry 1994;151:169.

Nelson JC: Combined treatment strategies in psychiatry. J Clin Psychiatry 1993;54(9, Suppl):42.

Orloff LM et al: Long-term follow-up of 85 patients with obsessive-compulsive disorder. Am J Psychiatry 1994; 151:441.

Peselow ED, Sanfilipo MP, Difiglia C, Fieve RR: Melancholic/endogenous depression and response to somatic treatment and placebo. Am J Psychiatry 1992;149:1324.

Pollack M, Otto M (editors): Anxiety disorders: Longitudinal course and treatment. Psychiatr Clin North Am 1995;18 [entire issue].

Post RM et al: Lithium-discontinuation-induced refractoriness: Preliminary observations. Am J Psychiatry 1992; 149:1727.

Post RM et al: Algorithm for bipolar mania. Mod Probl Pharmacopsychiatry 1997;25:114.

Preskorn SH: Tricyclic antidepressants: The whys and hows of therapeutic drug monitoring. J Clin Psychiatry 1989;50:34.

Rabheru K et al: A review of continuation and maintenance electroconvulsive therapy. Can J Psychiatry 1997;42:476.

Reimherr F et al: Optimal length of continuation therapy in depression: A prospective assessment during long term fluoxetine treatment. Am J Psychiatry 1998;155:1247.

Reynolds GP: What is an atypical antipsychotic? J Psychopharmacol 1997;11:195.

Rickels K et al: Antidepressants for the treatment of generalized anxiety disorder: A placebo-controlled comparison of imipramine, trazodone, and diazepam. Arch Gen Psychiatry 1993;50:884.

Sackeim HA et al: Effects of stimulus intensity and electrode placement on the efficacy and cognitive effects of electroconvulsive therapy. N Engl J Med 1993;328:839.

Sharma T et al: The cognitive efficacy of atypical antipsychotics in schizophrenia. J Clin Psychopharmacol 1998; 18(Suppl 1):125.

Shebak S, Cameron A, Levander S: Clonazepam and imipramine in the treatment of panic attacks: A double-blind comparison of efficacy and side effects. J Clin Psychiatry 1990;51(Suppl):14.

Smith TE et al: Standards of care and clinical algorithms for treating schizophrenia. Psychiatr Clin North Am 1998; 21:203.

Swartz CM: Neuroendocrine effects of electroconvulsive therapy (ECT). Psychopharmacol Bull 1997;33:265.

Tancer ME et al: Role of serotonin drugs in the treatment of social phobia. J Clin Psychiatry 1997;58(Suppl 5):50.

van Ameringen, Mancini C, Streiner DL: Fluoxetine efficacy in social phobia. J Clin Psychiatry 1993;54:27.

Wehr TA et al: Rapid cycling affective disorder: Contributing factors and treatment responses in 51 patients. Am J Psychiatry 1988;145:179.

Zito JM: Pharmacoeconomics of the new antipsychotics for treatment of schizophrenia. Psych Clin North Am 1998; 21:181.

Psychoanalysis & Long-Term Dynamic Psychotherapy*

31

Robert S. Wallerstein, MD, & Mitchell D. Wilson, MD

Sigmund Freud said that psychoanalysis was three things:

1. A theory of how the mind works. Psychoanalysis attempts to understand and explain the normal and the abnormal functioning of the human mind at all ages. Many of the central psychoanalytic concepts—the unconscious, psychic determinism, infantile sexuality and the theory of drives, the Oedipus complex, ambivalence, anxiety, the defense mechanisms, psychic conflict, the structure of the mind or of the psychic apparatus—form a body of scientific knowledge that has now become part of our intellectual heritage (see Chapter 2). In 1947, Ernst Kris summarized psychoanalysis as a theory of the mind most tersely: Psychoanalysis is

> nothing but human behavior considered from the standpoint of conflict. It is the picture of the mind divided against itself with attendant anxiety and other dysphoric affects, with adaptive and maladaptive defensive and coping strategies, and with symptomatic behaviors when the defenses fail.

However, psychoanalysis is more than a theory of the mind and behavior.

2. An investigative or research method. The technique of free association by the patient (analysand) makes it possible for the analyst to gain access to the data and processes of mental life, conscious or otherwise and rational or not. The data thus retrieved are rendered coherent and intelligible according to the theory of psychoanalysis. As Otto Fenichel said in 1941, it is the phenomenal data of psychoanalysis that may be irrational; the method and the theory are rational.

3. A specific form of therapy of mental illness. Psychoanalysis uses free association to obtain data in the form of thoughts, feelings, memories, fantasies, and dreams and then proceeds to order and comprehend the data within the framework of psychoanalytic theory. Through interpretation of psychic data,

leading to insight and "working through," the treatment process is carried progressively forward.

Dynamic psychotherapy—also called psychodynamic therapy, psychoanalytic psychotherapy, or psychoanalytically oriented psychotherapy—is intensive psychological therapy based on psychoanalytic theory but without the specific technique of free association. A variety of techniques are employed, including interpretation, to treat patients not considered suitable candidates for psychoanalysis.

Both psychoanalysis and the psychoanalytic psychotherapies described in this chapter are "open ended," ie, protracted therapies that may continue for many years. At the start of therapy, the analyst, or therapist, and the analysand, or patient, agree to explore the patient's psychological problems for whatever period of time is necessary to achieve an acceptable result. This is in contrast to short-term or brief (time-limited) psychotherapy (described in Chapter 32), which usually consists of 12 or 20 weekly or twice-weekly sessions of 50 minutes each. The critical distinction between psychoanalysis and short-term therapy is not the difference in duration, important as that is, but the fact that time-limited psychotherapy is not open ended; from the first session the patient is conscious of the agreed termination date and knows that what has to be done must be achieved by that date. One consequence is that the patient may be tempted, consciously or not, to withhold painful areas from therapeutic scrutiny—to be "saved by the bell," as it were. If open-ended therapy is to be completed successfully, whatever is not talked about now or next week will come out later, because treatment continues until all of the relevant psychological issues and problems are explored and resolved to the extent possible, however long it takes. Long-term and open-ended therapy is thus much more than an extended form of short-term (time-limited) therapy; they differ in very significant ways.

PSYCHOANALYSIS

Psychoanalysis is a process of examination in continuity of the internal working of the mind on a day-to-day basis. On each successive day, the analyst and

---

* This chapter is an edited version of a more comprehensive and detailed treatment of the subject matter that was prepared by Dr Wallerstein. The editor is grateful for permission to adapt it for *Review of General Psychiatry.*—HHG.

the patient can start where they left off and go from there. Ideally, this process would go forward 7 days a week for an hour each day. (This became the "50-minute hour" to allow time for analysts to order their thoughts, make notes, and get ready for the next patient.) However, to free weekends, the analytic work week, in practice, is the traditional five working days, and Freud often complained of the "Monday crust"— the sealing over of open mental surfaces during the weekend, so that the first task on Monday would be to reestablish the continuity of daily exploration. Because of the limited availability of qualified analysts and the need to accommodate more patients, analyses are now often conducted 4 days a week. Most analysts do not consider fewer than 4 days a week proper psychoanalysis, because the vital element of continuity does not survive longer or more frequent interruptions. Ideally, each session is scheduled at the same time each day so that the analysis can blend into the rhythm of the patient's life.

In classical psychoanalysis, the patient is recumbent on a couch with the analyst behind and out of the patient's line of vision. Intrusions, such as telephone calls, are avoided except in emergencies. The patient tries to say whatever comes to mind, no matter how seemingly remote, irrelevant, trivial, repugnant, anxiety provoking, or shameful (the "fundamental rule"). The patient agrees to refrain from motor activity so that all available energy can be channeled into the effort to verbalize mental content. The analyst decides when and how to interject questions and comments; no attempt is made to sustain a conversational dialogue. The analyst must unswervingly focus attention on the effort to track the shifting subject matter of the patient's discourse and keep personal concerns, prejudices, values, and judgments out of the analytic field. The purpose is to gain and maintain full access to the contents of the patient's mind, conscious and unconscious, now and in the remote past, and even to infancy if that can be achieved. Dreams, fantasies, wishes, fears, thoughts, and feelings of all kinds are discussed in the analysis. What is experienced by people practicing or undergoing psychotherapy is that "one thing leads to another." The patient focuses on his or her mental processes and free associates in what is apparently a random manner. The analyst apprehends what the patient verbalizes by a counterpart process of "free-floating attention" without preconceptions about what is important or what the relationships are between various items of content.

It is within this "regressive" analytic process that the patient's mental life, including its conflictual matter, slowly begins to emerge around the analyst. Long-forgotten (repressed) feelings, traumas, and reaction patterns, along with active or discarded defensive or adaptive strategies, all eventually "come out again" in the interaction with the analyst, and what results is called the **transference.** The psychic past is reenacted in the analytic present. It is recognized and interpreted via the inappropriateness of the patient's present (transference) reactions and feelings to the reality of the ongoing interaction with the analyst. The complete revival of the past in the present is called the "regressive transference neurosis." Through the systematic interpretation of these complex transference phenomena, unresolved problems from the past are reworked, more adaptive solutions are found, and maladaptive, neurotic solutions are discarded. In the course of analysis, patients "rewrite" their autobiographies and along the way shed the neurotic symptoms and the problems that first brought them to treatment.

Success in psychoanalysis relies essentially on skillful interpretation leading to enlarging insights. The analyst helps the patient see connections between unconscious wishes and beliefs and conscious speech and behavior. Slowly, patients begin to understand their own mental scheme of things. Symbolic meanings and mental connections begin to take on plausible configurations that "make sense." The insights gained are then "worked through" repeatedly as they reappear in other contexts as long as the analysis continues.

In a classic 1954 paper, Edward Bibring described five essential psychotherapeutic techniques: abreaction (catharsis), suggestion, manipulation, clarification, and interpretation. Different combinations of these techniques characterize the different psychoanalytically based psychotherapies. Within psychoanalysis proper, interpretation is the central technique, and the others are deployed only to enhance interpretation. There is a vast literature on the nature of interpretation: the issues of tact and timing in making interpretations; what makes interpretations "mutative" (ie, able to effect change); the special nature of interpretations of the transference relationship; interpretations in the here and now as opposed to reconstructive interpretations of past (including infantile) matter; and the role of interpretation and insight in relation to behavioral change. This essentially is what is involved in the proper conduct of psychoanalysis.

Indications & Contraindications

Of patients who come for psychiatric evaluation, psychoanalysis has been called the treatment of choice for that narrow middle group that is sick enough to need it and well enough to tolerate it (Gill, 1951). Most psychiatric patients have symptoms or problems in living that can be resolved to their satisfaction with therapies that are less intensive or less prolonged than analysis (including expressive and supportive psychotherapies and crisis-oriented and brief dynamic therapies). Patients with acute reactive illnesses, situational maladjustments, and various circumscribed symptom-neurotic and character-neurotic states do not need the thoroughgoing life and character reconstruction that psychoanalysis offers. Other patients whose illnesses are severe enough to require psychoactive drug management cannot always tolerate the anxiety-provoking stresses of psychoanalysis. For patients with fragile or vulnerable "ego strength" (including a tenuous hold on reality), psychoanalysis can be psychologically disorganizing, with dangers of regressive, even psychotic swings, severe acting out, flight from treatment, or suicidal pressures. Such patients, including borderline and narcissistic patients, those with character, addictive, or severe sexual disorders, those with character neuroses, and even some with severe and refractory symptom neuroses, are often deemed too ill for psychoanalysis and need to be treated by other dynamic (more supportive) psychotherapies.

There is controversy within the field between those who advocate "narrowing" and those who advocate "widening" the scope of indications for psychoanalysis. From the perspective of a proponent of "narrowing," only about 5% of patients who come for psychiatric evaluation and treatment are suitable candidates for psychoanalysis. These are patients with classical symptom neuroses and moderate character neuroses set within the context of a "strong ego organization"—ie, they are not only amenable to psychoanalysis but are able to tolerate it as well.

Benefits

Given the limited role of psychoanalysis in the treatment of neurotic disorders, it is proper to question both its social value and its scientific importance. Psychoanalysis is valuable and important in three areas: research, education, and treatment. As a research investigative technique, psychoanalysis affords access to the innermost workings of the mind and to knowledge of psychological development, character formation, and normal and abnormal mental processes. Knowledge about mental functioning derived from psychoanalytic research forms the basis of the theory of psychoanalysis as a comprehensive theory of the mind. From this theory have evolved the specific therapeutic applications of both psychoanalysis and the psychoanalytically based dynamic psychotherapies.

As an educational tool, the personal analysis of the therapist—required for those who seek certification as psychoanalytic practitioners and often sought by those who seek enhanced professional effectiveness as dynamic psychotherapists—is necessary to provide successive generations of clinicians best qualified to offer these therapeutic resources to patients who need them.

As specific treatment for that small number of patients for whom it is indicated, psychoanalysis offers the best hope—not always realized—for the thoroughgoing resolution of neurotic problems and for fundamental character reconstruction. Since individuals in analysis are often in positions of responsibility, making decisions that affect others, the social value of the technique is apparent.

Limitations

Those who would widen the scope of indications for psychoanalysis believe that because the therapeutic goal of psychoanalysis is fundamental personality reorganization, the results, when successful, are more complete and enduring than can be achieved with less ambitious forms of therapy. Over the years, psychoanalysis has therefore been extended and modified to treat broader categories of patients, including children and adolescents (Melanie Klein, Anna Freud)—an extension that has by now become the established discipline of child and adolescent analysis—groups (Henry Ezriel, S.R. Slavson), delinquents (August Aichhom), patients with psychosomatic disorders (Franz Alexander and many others), overtly psychotic patients (Harry Stack Sullivan, Frieda Fromm-Reichmann), narcissistic characters (Heinz Kohut and others), and patients with borderline personality disorders (Otto Kernberg). The movement to extend the indications for analysis to more kinds of mental disorders was reviewed by Leo Stone in 1954 in a widely cited article on the widening scope of psychoanalysis. Anna Freud (1954), in discussing that paper, undertook to spearhead the opposing trend toward narrowing the indications for analysis back to classically neurotic adults and children. Glover in 1954 divided patients for whom psychoanalysis might be the treatment of choice into three categories: the ideally suitable, the moderately suitable, and those for whom psychoanalysis was the last hope albeit a forlorn one. The patients in the third category had severe personality disorders and were to be offered analysis as a "heroic measure" (this was in the days before adjunctive pharmacotherapy was available). The concept of intensive psychoanalytic treatment for patients much sicker than those usually seen in outpatient practice was a major rationale for the psychoanalytic sanatorium (such as the Menninger Foundation), where treatment could be conducted in a protected milieu with total life management.

PSYCHODYNAMIC PSYCHOTHERAPY

The psychoanalytically based dynamic psychotherapies are available for that much larger population of psychiatric patients who are not candidates for psychoanalysis proper. Psychodynamic psychotherapy, created in the United States, is now practiced worldwide. It was developed between World Wars I and II and refined as a coherent body of theory and technique in the decade after World War II, when psychoanalytic theory became the dominant psychological perspective of psychiatrists in the United States. The dynamic psychotherapies arose in pragmatic response to the treatment needs of the vast majority of patients who were not suitable candidates for psychoanalysis proper.

The dynamic psychoanalytically based psychotherapies have been divided conceptually into two types: expressive and supportive. The treatment aim of the **expressive** type is to uncover (or make conscious) psychological conflict through analysis of the patient's defenses and resistances and, in this way, to resolve conflict through interpretation, insight, and change motivated by insight; the treatment aim of the **supportive** type is to diminish the force of external (situational) or internal (instinctual, drive-related) pressures by a variety of ego-strengthening techniques. Supportive therapies thus increase the patient's capacity to suppress mentally painful conflict and its dysphoric or symptomatic expression, thereby effecting behavioral change and symptomatic relief through means other than interpretation and insight.

As useful as this expressive-supportive division is for heuristic, prescriptive, and prognostic purposes, it is also a misleading oversimplification. All psychiatric treatment that helps patients is supportive, even when most uncompromisingly expressive, as in psychoanalysis. What could be more supportive than an open-ended psychoanalysis offered daily for as long as necessary, in which the patient is encouraged to express any kind or amount of verbal content, with the entire enterprise consisting of two people whose energies and intellect are focused exclusively on the problems and concerns of the one? Or, as Herbert Schlesinger (1969) has reminded us, any treatment, no matter how supportive in the sense of strengthening defenses and suppressing unwanted conflict and symptom expression, must also be expressive of some aspect of the patient's concerns. The important question, according to Schlesinger, is not expressive versus supportive but rather *expressive of what?*—and when, and how, in regard to the patient's mental and emotional life—and *supportive of what?*—and when, and how, in regard to that same mental and emotional life. Indeed, in every therapeutic decision to foster the expression of some aspect of mental conflict and distress in whatever way, there is a tacit decision to avoid (ie, suppress) some other aspect of mental conflict and distress.

Whatever one thinks of these arguments, at the practical level of ongoing psychotherapy there has always been a useful distinction between therapeutic interventions that have a preponderantly expressive effect and those that have a preponderantly supportive effect. Paul Dewald in his 1964 book has presented in a systematic way every aspect of the psychotherapeutic process: (1) the beginning of the process and the establishment of the therapeutic situation and the "therapeutic contract"; (2) the patient's role and activity and (3) the therapist's role and activity in the therapeutic process; (4) the handling of the transference; (5) the handling of manifestations of re-

sistance, regression, and psychic conflict; (6) the role of insight and working through in bringing about change; (7) the emotional involvements of the therapist (the "countertransference"); (8) the adjuvant role of psychoactive drugs; and (9) the process of natural termination. All of the foregoing are discussed by Dewald from the contrasting perspectives of expressive and supportive psychotherapeutic approaches.

Techniques & Patient Selection

The dynamic psychotherapies, expressive or supportive, are quite similar to each other in procedural form and greatly different from the formal structure of the psychoanalytic interview. In psychoanalysis the patient does most of the talking while the analyst chooses when and how to intervene; in psychotherapy the format is more like a conversation: the patient sits in a chair facing the therapist, with the expectation of feedback and reciprocal exchange. In psychoanalysis the patient tries to say everything that comes to mind without editorial revision or censorship; in psychotherapy the patient agrees to present problems and distress for consideration only to the extent that he or she is able and willing. No "fundamental rule" is violated by a decision to withhold specific items of mental content, either temporarily or permanently.

The frequency of weekly sessions with the therapist is more flexible in psychotherapy, ranging from one to three or four sessions a week, with once or twice a week most common. Unless some form of time-limited therapy is elected, the duration is open ended, as with psychoanalysis. Although in practice psychotherapy is usually briefer in duration than psychoanalysis (1–2 years versus 3–5 years), it can continue for just as long and may even (unlike psychoanalysis) continue for the life of the patient. Such "therapeutic lifers" have consciously undertaken, out of need, to continue a supportive relationship with the therapist similar to the lifelong medical maintenance regimens required by diabetic patients, cardiac patients, and others with chronic and incurable but manageable disorders. In terms of total time spent in therapy, the dynamic psychotherapies usually consume 50–200 hours, in contrast to 600–1000 hours in analysis. The treatment hour is usually 50 minutes, but in some sustained, essentially supportive psychotherapies, particularly with schizoid individuals and others fearful of interpersonal intimacy, sessions are in some instances curtailed to no more than 30 minutes each. In both expressive and supportive therapies, at times of acute crisis or emergency, sessions may be extended as long as necessary—up to 2 hours or more. Occasionally in the psychotherapies, emergency weekend or evening sessions are held. Supportive treatment sessions may be scheduled less frequently than once a week, and the time may come—if the patient is seeing the therapist only once a month—when the sessions should be characterized as follow-up visits or "reporting in" rather than a continuing psychotherapeutic process.

In the psychotherapies (again in contrast to psychoanalysis), there is greater use of adjuvant drug management, coordination of care with the patient's family physician, telephone contacts, and involvement of third parties (family, employers, teachers, etc). All of these extra-session activities are more frequent the more supportive and the less expressive the particular psychotherapy is intended to be. Within this overall common structure, then, how do the technical interventions differ between the more expressive and the more supportive psychotherapies?

A. Expressive Psychotherapy: Essentially, in expressive psychotherapy, the patient is free to bring up problems and anxieties in his or her own way, the therapeutic emphasis is on interpretation and insight, and the objective is to bring about beneficial change by resolution of as much psychic conflict as possible. This is accomplished by uncovering unconscious conflicts and, through understanding, achieving mastery. These are to some extent the techniques of psychoanalysis but without free association, dream analysis, or deep discovery of infantile sources of current pain.

Expressive psychotherapy is the treatment of choice for persons with enough ego strength, intelligence, and anxiety tolerance to participate in therapy and with serious but relatively circumscribed neurotic conflicts and symptoms—ie, individuals who need help but not the greater commitment implied by a decision to enter analysis. If such patients will assume responsibility for their character traits and their problems in living and are willing to look introspectively at the irrational aspects of their interpersonal relationships, significant help and change can be effected without the full-scale reconstructive effort required to uncover the infantile developmental roots of the neurotic personality development. For example, the issue is whether a patient with severe marital problems can be helped to resolve the problems without the need to recreate the earlier prototype, the infantile conflicts with the mother, repressed behind the childhood amnesia. In psychoanalysis, the aim is to pursue conflicts back to their infantile roots so they can be carefully analyzed; in analytically oriented expressive psychotherapy the aim is to recognize (and only partially to analyze) those same conflicts and use that recognition in therapy. Insight is achieved, but only to the "depth" of the problem being addressed—it never penetrates to the unconscious infantile origins of the patient's original conflicts.

Expressive therapy is indicated for patients with problems similar to those treated in psychoanalysis—patients with classical symptom neuroses (dysthymic disorder, anxiety disorders) and with the character neuroses (personality disorders). **Character neuroses** that cause problems in living (eg, rigidly compulsive or chronically depressive characters) and **symptom neuroses** (eg, characterized by irrational compulsions or bouts of depression) can at times blend into each other, or one may give way to the other.

The distinction between those who need psychoanalysis and those who can be treated by less intensive therapy is well illustrated by the example of psychotherapeutic work with a patient suffering from posttraumatic stress disorder (see Chapter 21). The therapeutic work would be limited to a defined sector of the individual's life and problems and directed toward the stresses precipitating the breakdown and enough of their underlying causes to permit resolution of the current conflict. Thus, in the case of the survivor of an accident, grief-stricken over the death of a companion and feeling guilty for having luckily survived, the events surrounding the death, ambivalent (love? hate?) feelings about the companion, and perhaps even a parallel between the adult friendship and conflictual sibling relationships of childhood might all come within the scope of the expressive therapeutic work. Therapy in this example probably would not explore earlier conflicts in the infantile relationship with the parents.

However, expressive psychotherapy need not be confined to a specific area of difficulty. It could include concern with characterological problems and symptoms and their maladaptive roles in the patient's life, but with the object of working only at the level of the individual's willingness and capacity to assume responsibility for their modification in the present without the need for the concomitant uncovering of their infantile roots in the past. Such treatment can be long term and can undertake to explore and modify the entire range of the patient's life adjustments, attitudes, and reactions.

In expressive psychotherapy conflict resolution and symptomatic relief are made possible by the relative "autonomy" of the present-day neurotic problem from its earlier infantile prototype, though clearly a developmental line can be traced from one to the other. Success depends on the ability of the patient and therapist to resolve the conflict in the "here and now," without the necessity of exploring its roots in infancy or its development from earlier neurotic relationships. Because such relative autonomy of conflict is common, there is a very large population of psychoneurotic patients who can use expressive dynamic psychotherapy. Because it is accepted dogma among psychiatrists that expressive (uncovering, interpretive) treatment is "better" because presumably it leads to changes that are more stable and more able to withstand adverse environmental pressures, the therapeutic tendency is fostered among practitioners of dynamic psychotherapy to—in the words of a popular training aphorism—"be as expressive as you can be and as supportive as you have to be."

B. Supportive Psychotherapy: It is easier to agree on and expound the indications for expressive psychotherapy than to explain when supportive psychotherapy is called for and how it should be managed. Expressive psychotherapy is similar to foreshortened analysis, and most interested people understand something about analysis, even if they do not agree on when it should be used. Supportive psychotherapy, on the other hand, employs all manner of techniques and can be used in the management of all classes of patients not candidates for analysis or expressive psychotherapy.

In its early days psychoanalysis was acclaimed as the first successful scientific psychotherapy, in contrast to all preexisting therapies, which were viewed only as different types of suggestion therapy and therefore inherently unpredictable and unstable. Hypnosis was the prototype of such suggestive therapies. This view was expressed by Freud many times and was emphasized forcefully by Edward Glover in 1931. As employed by nonanalytically trained practitioners, supportive psychotherapy often involves heavy doses of common-sense reassurance, to the extent that this, along with suggestion, came to be considered characteristic of the supportive approach. This perception is misleading and oversimplified. Explicit reassurance is seldom comforting to patients with problems severe enough to bring them to a therapist and the effort to give reassurance may only convince the patient that the therapist simply does not understand the nature of the difficulty or does not want to hear about it.

What, then, does supportive therapy actually consist of? One of the earliest efforts to explain supportive psychotherapy was made by Merton Gill (1951), who identified three kinds of interventions that he felt "strengthened the defenses," in contrast with expressive approaches that undertook to uncover and interpret defenses as a step toward eventual integration. These explicitly supportive interventions are (1) to consistently encourage adaptive (and discourage maladaptive) combinations of impulse and defense expression, both behaviorally and symptomatically; (2) to deliberately refrain from interpreting defenses and character configurations, no matter how rigid or maladaptive, that are deemed essential to maintain functioning; and (3) to partially uncover some aspect of neurotic conflict (eg, within a troubled marriage or work situation) in an effort to reduce inner conflict that might be creating unwanted symptoms (eg, anxiety, depression, phobic avoidances). In this way the balance of psychic forces is altered, rendering repression of the core of neurotic conflict easier to accomplish. An example would be not exploring in detail how the origin of a troubled marital or work situation relates to earlier ingrained patterns of interpersonal difficulty.

Differentiating the five therapeutic techniques listed by Bibring—abreaction, suggestion, manipulation, clarification, and interpretation—it can be said that psychoanalysis uses mostly interpretation, with other techniques employed only when necessary to facili-

tate and enhance it; expressive psychotherapy uses interpretation to a large extent but also uses clarification as well as the other techniques; and supportive psychotherapy uses all five techniques in whatever proportions seem to be called for by the specific needs of the patient.

Techniques of Supportive Psychotherapy

The principal therapeutic ingredient of supportive psychotherapy is the evocation and firm establishment of a positive dependent emotional attachment to the therapist. Within this bond, the patient's emotional needs and wishes are allowed to achieve varying degrees of overt or covert (symbolic) gratification. In supportive therapy, the meanings and sources of the bond between the patient and the therapist are for the most part not interpreted or "analyzed."

This dependent emotional attachment seems, in turn, to be an essential precondition to the proper functioning of various other supportive mechanisms. It is also the basis of the so-called "transference cure," the willingness and capacity of the patient to reach therapeutic goals, change behavior and modes of living, and give up symptoms "for the therapist" as the quid pro quo for the emotional gratifications received within the benevolent dependent attachment. On this base, then, other supportive devices are employed as indicated by the clinical needs of particular patients. If the dependent need for continued emotional gratification cannot be transferred (see below) or somehow either terminated or made therapeutically sustaining, it can be incorporated into a continuing and even an unending therapeutic relationship.

These chronic maintenance supportive therapies may be employed over long periods in the management of vulnerable patients whose hold on reality is tenuous. Patients with comparable dependent tendencies but greater psychological resources (eg, a greater capacity to identify with the therapist) are often able to terminate treatment, perhaps after a period of "weaning" as first advocated by Alexander and French (1946). These are patients who can identify successfully with the therapist and the therapist's approach toward and mastery of conflict pressures and who thus can learn to go forward on their own.

Intermediate between those patients who can be helped to achieve reasonable psychological autonomy by identification with the therapist and those for whom continued (perhaps lifelong) therapy is necessary are those whose attachments and the emotional gratifications derived therefrom can be "transferred" within the patient's now-improved life situation. The transfer is usually made to the spouse, and the success of transfer depends not only on the effectiveness of the psychotherapeutic work within ongoing treatment but also on the capacity and willingness of the spouse (or other significant person) to carry the transferred emotional burden indefinitely. Obviously, some patients will be more fortunate than others in the matter of availability of someone willing and able to accept such a burden.

Another useful supportive mechanism is to foster the displacement of the patient's neurotic behavior into the therapeutic relationship so that its ill effects can be ameliorated in "real life." A typical example would be to encourage an unduly dependent and submissive patient to be more assertive outside treatment by allowing greater (covert) submissiveness to the therapist, which is experienced by the patient as requiring the altered (more assertive) external behaviors as the price of continuation of the dependent gratifications within the treatment. The success of this maneuver depends on life circumstance, the reinforcing positive feedback, and enhanced self-esteem. Beneficial change stabilizes when the new behaviors bring real reward and gratification rather than neurotically anticipated disaster.

What has just been described are varieties of the "transference cure," whereby the patient "does what the therapist wants" in exchange for the satisfaction of emotional needs. The "antitransference cure" occurs when the patient makes changes not "for the therapist" but "against the therapist," ie, in the face of what are perceived as the therapist's contrary expectations, usually as an act of triumph over the therapist in the overt or covert treatment struggle. Such "cures," of course, must somehow be buttressed against their potential instability by enduring, beneficial real-life consequences.

The **"corrective emotional experience"** is a concept Alexander and French invoked almost as the all-explanatory construct to elucidate the mechanism of action of supportive psychotherapy. Basically, this consists of deliberately responding to the patient's expressed emotional needs in a way that is different from what he or she has been led, by accumulated life experiences, to expect, with the effect of jarring entrenched patterns of neurotic (ultimately self-defeating) interactions. The concept can in a sense be applied to the entire range of supportive therapeutic techniques, since everything that goes on in psychotherapy is intended to function in some sense as a corrective emotional experience. However, the term is more useful if it is restricted to treatments whose central mechanism consists of interaction with a kindly, understanding, reality-oriented therapist able to absorb the patient's onslaughts and importunities in a spirit of benevolent neutrality without becoming entangled in the kind of interacting neurotic relationships the patient has used to maintain a life of suffering in the years before treatment was sought.

Reality testing and reeducation are related, but differ in subtle ways from the corrective emotional experience in the conduct of supportive psychotherapy. Reality testing and reeducation consist of helping patients with difficulties in this area distinguish internally derived expectations and fantasy from the external reality of the situation. Again, broadly speaking, they have a role in any type of psychotherapy, including psychoanalysis, but direct educational efforts by the therapist are more characteristic of psychotherapy when the therapeutic emphasis is in greater part supportive. The therapist gives advice, explains, and instructs the patient about what types of behavior are tolerable and expected in the community. The therapist must do this in a way that is perceived as nonjudgmental and, to the extent that the therapeutic intervention is coercive, that it is guided solely by the patient's well-being and best interests.

No purpose is served by trying to make a clear distinction between such educational activities and the steady provision of a corrective emotional experience. In both instances, the patient is taught the techniques of reality-oriented problem solving and reality-corrected emotional responses on the basis of the "borrowed strength" derived from psychological identification with the therapist in the role of helper and healer. Again, the stabilization of progress during and after treatment depends on positive reinforcement from the environment along with some measure of transfer of the attachments to the spouse or other stable life companion.

Another form of supportive psychotherapy involves the kind of life manipulation required by very ill patients who come to hospital, residential care, and day hospital settings—eg, the alcoholic, the drug addict, the acting-out or suicidal patient. In such cases, a major aspect of treatment involves the planned disengagement, temporarily or even at times permanently, from noxious life situations. For other patients, the opposite is true: success can be achieved only if psychotherapy is conducted while contact with the patient's accustomed environment is maintained. With these patients, if the usual interacting life situation cannot be properly maintained, for whatever reason, the chances for an optimal result diminish, at times sharply.

Still another helping mechanism that can play a major role in supportive psychotherapy is the "collusive bargain." The "bargain" the therapist makes with the patient is to exempt specific problems, symptoms, and areas of personality malfunction from therapeutic scrutiny—leaving more or less consequential islands of maintained psychopathology—in return for the patient's willingness to make substantial changes in other areas. This is similar to the "transference cure," in the sense that the patient makes changes "for the therapist" in return for a specific reward—the shielding from therapeutic interference of a particularly tenacious or rewarding symptom or behavior. The success of such a maneuver depends on the value of the symptom or behavior to the patient as well as the patient's ability to detach the symptom or behavior from other problems or symptoms, which patient and therapist can then address. For example, a homosexual patient with conflicts about professional achievement may decide with a therapist to discuss the professional life issues and to ignore or deemphasize the life-style issues. Since the symptom or behavior "allowed" to the patient in this compromise solution is experienced as at least in some ways rewarding or gratifying, these particular therapeutic outcomes have a built-in stability.

Another technique available to patients who need supportive therapy is transfer of the attachment or dependency either to fortunate life circumstances (eg, wealth or social or cultural advantage) or to alternative psychological supports. These may be selected by the patients, sometimes with the concurrence of the therapist. Alcoholics Anonymous and similar self-help groups are examples. In turning to external material or alternative psychological supports for continuing emotional dependencies and gratifications, patients can sometimes save a failing or stalled therapeutic situation, ie, they can stabilize even if they cannot always enhance their level of psychological functioning.

It should be clear from the foregoing that there are many ways in which psychotherapy can support and maintain improved psychological functioning and, additionally, that ways can be built in to maintain such improvement in a stable and enduring fashion. These techniques can be combined in various ways to meet the needs of specific patients: to form a basis for therapeutic "trades," to replace maladaptive impulse-defense configurations with more adaptive (healthy) ones, to decide what to talk about and explore, and to decide specifically what *not* to talk about. Success in these endeavors may improve the patient's life situation, may help in the transfer of emotional attachments or in undertaking or disengaging from ongoing life context, and may provide positive reinforcements that result in enhanced self-esteem and more comfortable and rewarding life experiences.

Given this great variety of techniques available for supportive psychotherapy, it should be obvious that a high degree of skill and extensive experience are required by the therapist. This is contrary to the common misconception that more skill in psychodynamics is required to conduct expressive psychotherapy and that the supportive psychotherapists dispense mostly common sense, good will, and kindly reassurance. Actually, neither kind of psychotherapy involves less knowledge or skill than the other, though supportive psychotherapy calls for greater flexibility and permits or even requires a wider deployment of "extras" in regard to the two-person treatment situation, such as the use of adjuvant psychoactive drug management, contacts with third parties (including other treating physicians), and telephone or other contacts with the patient outside of scheduled sessions.

Indications

Supportive psychotherapy is the treatment of choice for a more diverse range of patients than ex-pressive psychotherapy. It is indicated for some patients "not sick enough" for analysis and for the great majority of very ill patients considered too sick for analysis or *any* intensive expressive approach. The first category includes many patients who may be caught up in disruptive responses (anxiety, depressive affect, rage) to traumatic or otherwise disturbing situations—some grief reactions, acute anxiety states, adjustment disorders, etc. In some cases, expressive-interpretive activity is also indicated, but often there may be just a need to slow up, to take stock, to reassess the clinical situation and the therapeutic options, and to reintegrate, over time, to the best of one's coping or mastery potential. Supportive therapy in such cases usually is of shorter duration than expressive psychotherapy or psychoanalysis.

A larger category of patients for whom supportive psychotherapy is indicated consists of those much sicker individuals who require sustaining psychotherapeutic relationships, perhaps for life, and who respond slowly to the therapist's best efforts. Stability of psychological functioning at the best achievable level is often the modest therapeutic goal, though at times the hope for cure should be pursued because greater success is sometimes possible. This group includes most patients with psychosis or severe personality disorders, severe addictions, alcoholism, sexual disorders, and acting-out, delinquent, and antisocial characters. In almost all of these cases, some degree of expressive therapeutic work can usually be done, but with difficulty, because these patients have poor impulse control and low tolerance for anxiety and are vulnerable to regressive (psychotic or suicidal) swings in psychological functioning and integrity. The eruption of a florid psychotic state is a potential danger that often cannot be ignored. Attempts at "widening the scope" of expressive therapy (including psychoanalysis) in an effort to do something for these much sicker patients (see section on indications and contraindications for psychoanalysis) have met with poor results.

Recent Developments

In the past two decades psychoanalysts have recognized, increasingly, that the long-held distinctions between psychoanalysis, long-term psychodynamic psychotherapy, and some aspects of supportive psychotherapy are less clear than previously thought. Several trends in psychoanalytic thinking have contributed to this change. One important development was heralded by Greenberg and Mitchell's book, *Object Relations in Psychoanalytic Theory,* published in 1983. These authors emphasized that the central role the therapeutic relationship plays in the practice of psychoanalysis is relatively independent of the analyst's particular theoretical persuasion. By emphasizing the object relationship between analyst and patient (and the patient with historically important objects, such as parents and siblings), the therapeutic relationship is reconceptualized as an interpersonal interaction. Classical descriptions of the analyst as an objective observer outside of the field of observation have given way to a view of the analyst and patient working together and mutually influencing each other.

Another important work that propelled psychoanalytic thinking in a more interpersonal direction was *Analysis of Transference* by Merton Gill and Irwin Hoffman (1982). Through careful analysis of audio-taped psychotherapy sessions, it was shown that the analyst has a profound role in shaping the treatment process. Gill and Hoffman emphasized the importance of calling the attention of patients to their thoughts, feelings, and perception of the here and now of the interpersonal interaction between the analyst and patient (transference interpretation). They also showed that patients' perceptions of the analyst are not always (or even inherently) distorted perceptions or mere repetitions from patients' past. Hoffman (1983), in a subsequent paper, "The patient as interpreter of the analyst's experience," demonstrated the clinical importance of the analyst taking the patient's perceptions at face value, and not assuming the patient is distorting reality.

Finally, several psychoanalytic writers (including James McLaughlin, Judy Chused, Dale Boesky, Warren Poland, and Owen Renik) have called attention to **transference-countertransference enactments.** These enactments are interactions between analyst and patient that reveal important aspects of the conflicts and desires of the patient (and at times the analyst), which otherwise may have remained hidden. Rather than the classical picture of the analyst "sitting on the sidelines" watching the patient's mind work, the analyst is always engaged and involved in various forms of action and interaction with the patient. As Renik (1993) points out in an important paper, "Countertransference enactment and the psychoanalytic process," the analyst is often caught off guard by things said to or felt about a patient. The analyst at those points can understand only retrospectively what has occurred and what it means about the patient's conflicts. Instead of being considered a technical "mistake," enactments are seen as inevitable and necessary for the successful outcome of psychoanalysis or long-term dynamic psychotherapy.

In summary, relational factors in the outcome of psychoanalysis or psychotherapy are now given greater legitimacy. Support, a friendly attitude, tactful suggestions, humor, and more or less routine human reactions are now seen as important, and often essential, ingredients in a successful treatment. Analysts better appreciate their own involvement in the therapeutic relationship. Interpretation, previously thought to be the analyst's or therapist's main activity, is only one of several important clinical interventions, even in conventional psychoanalysis. The role of insight in therapeutic gain, previously thought to be the central factor in therapeutic success, is relegated to lesser status. These recent developments have been supported by the research of Wallerstein and colleagues in the Menninger Psychotherapy Research Project (Wallerstein, 1986). This research strongly suggested that distinctions between long-term, expressive psychotherapy and psychoanalysis were often difficult to discern. Supportive aspects of the therapeutic relationship were shown to be as important, and in some cases more important, than insight alone. For the patient the ultimate goal of psychoanalysis and long-term psychodynamic psychotherapy remains increased understanding of themselves and their conflicts; however, this self-understanding now takes place in the safety of a uniquely intimate and professional relationship between patient and therapist.

OTHER SCHOOLS & PARADIGMS

The discussion of psychotherapies in this chapter has been within the framework of psychoanalytic (psychodynamic) theories of mental functioning. Other kinds of psychotherapies have been developed within different theoretical models of how the mind works, such as the behavioral model based on a learning theory paradigm and the existentialist-humanist model based on a phenomenological-existentialist view of mental life and function. The therapies that derive from these schools differ radically in concept and in practice from those described in this chapter, and they are discussed elsewhere in this book.

REFERENCES & SUGGESTED READINGS

Alexander F, French TM: *Psychoanalytic Therapy: Principles and Applications.* Ronald Press, 1946.

Bibring E: Psychoanalysis and the dynamic psychotherapies. J Am Psychoanal Assoc 1954;2:745.

Dewald PA: *Psychotherapy: A Dynamic Approach.* Basic Books, 1964.

Fenichel O: *Problems of Psychoanalytic Technique.* Psychoanalytic Quarterly, 1941.

Freud A: The widening scope of indications for psychoanalysis [discussion]. J Am Psychoanal Assoc 1954;2:607.

Freud S: Lines of advance in psychoanalytic therapy (1918). In: *Standard Edition of the Complete Psychological Works of Sigmund Freud,* Vol 17. Hogarth Press, 1955.

Gill MM: Ego psychology and psychotherapy. Psychoanal Q 1951;20:62.

Gill MM, Hoffman IZ: *Analysis of Transference, Vol. II.* Psychological Issues, Monograph 54. International Universities Press, 1982.

Glover E: The therapeutic effect of inexact interpretation: A contribution to the theory of suggestion. Int J Psychoanal 1931;12:397.

Glover E: The indications for psychoanalysis. J Ment Sci 1954;100:393.

Greenberg JR, Mitchell SA: *Object Relations in Psychoanalytic Theory.* Harvard University Press, 1983.

Hoffman IZ: The patient as interpreter of the analyst's experience. Cont Psychoanal 1983;19:389.

Kris E: The nature of psychoanalytic propositions and their validation. In: *Freedom and Experience: Essays Presented to Horace Kallen.* Hook S, Konvitz MR (editors). Cornell University Press, 1947.

Renik OR: Countertransference enactment and the psychoanalytic process. In: *Psychic Structure and Psychic Change. Essays in Honor of Robert S. Wallerstein, MD.* Horowitz MJ, Kernberg OF, Weinshel EM (editors). International Universities Press, 1993.

Schlesinger HJ: Diagnosis and prescription for psychotherapy. Bull Menninger Clin 1969;33:269.

Stone L: The widening scope of indications for psychoanalysis. J Am Psychoanal Assoc 1954;2:567.

Wallerstein RS: *42 Lives in Treatment: A Study of Psychoanalysis and Psychotherapy.* Guilford Press, 1986.

Time-Limited Psychotherapy

32

Charles R. Marmar, MD

Historical Trends & Rationale for Brief Dynamic Psychotherapy

In the decades since Freud's original writings on the technique of psychoanalysis, the trend among practitioners working in the tradition of psychodynamic psychotherapy has been toward increasing length of treatment. Long-term treatments aim for both symptom resolution and fundamental changes in character structure such as capacities for intimacy and autonomy. Certain theoreticians have advocated briefer, more active, and more focused approaches to deal with carefully delineated areas of psychopathology. Ferenczi and Rank (1925) focused on the physical separation of the infant from the mother at the moment of birth and later the psychological emancipation of the child from the mother led to an emphasis on time-limited treatment, with a focus on the meanings of separation, a theoretical position reiterated in the contemporary work of James Mann (1973) (see below). Alexander and French developed new techniques for time-limited psychoanalysis. They emphasized the therapeutic potential of the corrective emotional experience, or the reexperiencing (under more favorable circumstances) of a traumatic emotional situation from the past. Alexander and French (1946) recommended that the therapist assume a particular role that might counteract the earlier trauma or interpersonal deficits. If, for example, a patient has repeatedly experienced painful relationships with critical, unappreciative, or abusive caretakers, the therapist might adopt a warm, empathic, and compassionate role to provide a compensatory experience.

Alexander's goal was to speed up the time course of psychoanalysis rather than to provide a specific set of technical guidelines for conducting brief, problem-focused dynamic psychotherapy. In contrast, contemporary schools of brief psychotherapy advocate a more restricted approach, with the focus on a single problem or at most on several interrelated conflicts that have been purposely chosen to the exclusion of other possible issues. The theoretical writings of French are relevant in this regard. It was French (1958) who introduced the term focal conflict, which he defined as a wish or intention that conflicts with the person's enduring expectations and values. The conflict renders the person incapable of meeting his or her expectations, and the result is frustration, with use of various emotional defenses and compromises. For example, a person might wish to function as a more separate, independent person but fears that to pursue such autonomous aims would hurt other important people, who would be left out; the person would then compromise by resentfully stifling these strivings toward independence. Choosing a specific focal conflict helps to organize the work in brief psychotherapy and focuses attention on an emotional problem of manageable proportions. Balint et al (1972) provide an excellent example of the technique for limiting the approach in brief treatment to a selected sector of the personality and guarding against diffusion of effort.

Features of Brief Dynamic Psychotherapy

A. Application of Psychoanalytic Principles: The principles of psychoanalytic psychotherapy are applied to the resolution of specific problems rather than to the entire range of personality functioning.

B. Selection Criteria: Specific selection criteria are designed to permit careful screening of prospective patients and selection of those for whom brief dynamic psychotherapy would be appropriate.

C. Primary Focus: A primary focus—typically a problem behavior or negative self-image that surfaces in the context of current difficulties in interpersonal relations—is chosen.

D. Therapeutic Alliance: Because of the time limits on brief psychotherapy, the therapist must actively seek ways to facilitate the rapid establishment of a therapeutic alliance. Such a partnership creates a safe environment in which the patient feels understood and views the therapist as empathic, respectful, and nonjudgmental, all of which help to deepen rapport. Within this alliance, patients ideally are willing to reveal thoughts and feelings, reflect on the nature of personal problems, and explore their own contributions to these problems. Foreman and Marmar (1985) and Safran and Muran (1998) describe approaches to identifying and repairing problems in the therapeutic alliance resulting in greater compliance and better outcomes.

E. Working Through: Treatment includes a phase of working through that concentrates on the resolution of the focal conflict. This phase usually includes an opportunity for the patient to express feelings and ideas about current stressful interpersonal experiences and to identify subjectively distorted meanings of these events. Distortion may take the form of exaggerated self-deprecation or identification of current negative feelings about the self with difficulties in earlier relationships. The patient's relationship with the therapist is clarified, and ways in which the patient repeats various aspects of the focal conflict in the relationship with the therapist are pointed out. When possible, the patient's distorted reactions to the therapist are linked to similar reactions in important current interpersonal relationships and to related patterns in earlier developmental sequences.

F. Termination: The meaning that termination of therapy holds for the patient is carefully considered in brief dynamic psychotherapy. Because of the short overall duration of treatment, the patient may perceive termination as an abrupt loss of a valued supportive relationship. Although both parties have agreed that treatment should be brief, the patient often feels rejected, and the same negative self-images that first brought the patient into treatment may be transiently intensified during termination. The loss of the therapist at termination is therefore another opportunity for the patient to master general problems in the area of separation and attachment.

Summary of Rationale & Features of Brief Dynamic Psychotherapy

Brief dynamic psychotherapy is indicated when a specific emotional problem can be identified and when the patient can rapidly form a trusting relationship with the therapist and tolerate exploration of that problem in a brief time frame. The goals of work are focused and more narrowly defined, as opposed to the more thorough but more diffusely defined longer-term dynamic therapies. Common to all brief therapies is a limited or fixed number of sessions, usually between 12 and 20 but sometimes extending to 30, although some flexibility exists in different approaches. The rationale for brief therapy is practical: Treatment seeks to be cost-effective and accessible to a broader segment of the population, since many people cannot make the commitment of time, money, and emotional energy required for more protracted treatment.

CONTEMPORARY SCHOOLS OF BRIEF DYNAMIC PSYCHOTHERAPY

David Malan & the British School

Beginning with the ground-breaking work of Balint et al (1972) in the development of focal psychotherapy and evolving further through the efforts of David Malan (1963, 1976) at the Tavistock Clinic in London, the British have made major contributions to the theory, practice, and research evaluation of time-limited dynamic psychotherapy. The technical guidelines advocated by Malan and his collaborators are discussed below.

Selection Criteria

For Malan, the initial selection process is a crucial first step. The pretreatment interview begins with a careful psychiatric history and mental status examination in order to exclude individuals with a current or past history of serious psychiatric disorders (eg, schizophrenia, mania, major depressive episodes), suicide attempts, severe childhood trauma, and long-standing complex family and marital problems. The second component of the evaluation is a psychodynamic history focused on current and past major interpersonal relationships, with a search for recurrent patterns of conflict. The patient's capacity to form an open, trusting relationship with the interviewer is evaluated as well as the patient's response to some initial tentative interpretations of recurring difficulties in interpersonal relationships. The extent to which the patient is motivated to engage in psychotherapy is also determined.

Duration & Focus of Treatment

Malan recommends that a fixed time limit be determined at the outset of treatment. Experienced therapists conduct treatments extending over an average of 18 sessions, whereas a time limit of 30 sessions is recommended for trainee therapists. Malan emphasizes work on the focal conflict in the context of important recurrent maladaptive patterns in relationships and points to two specific triangular configurations to be used in working on the focal conflict.

The first triangle consists of the patient's aim or intention, the subjectively perceived threat that makes expression of the aim dangerous, and the efforts to ward off anxiety through the use of specific defenses. For example, a patient may intend to be more open in expressing emotions in close relationships but feels that this would not gain the respect of others, who would feel that the patient was being too sentimental or emotionally out of control. The patient then tries to ward off the potential anxiety about the reactions of others by being intellectual and distant rather than emotional.

The second triangle is that of persons and involves the identification of recurrent patterns of relationships in three contexts: (1) the relationship with the therapist (the transference relationship), (2) the patient's relationships in current interpersonal situations outside of therapy, and (3) the real or imagined relationships (both past and present) with parental figures or siblings. To continue with the patient used in the previous example, the person who feels blocked in expression of emotion is likely to act in a controlled, intellectualized manner both with the therapist and in current emotional and occupational relationships; such a person is also likely to have originally developed this pattern in relating to parental figures.

Treatment

A. Order of Interpretive Work: Malan's technique consists of carefully timing the work to make the patient aware of the triangular structure of the recurrent relationship patterns. The technical competence of the therapist conducting brief dynamic psychotherapy is therefore in part determined by the ability to formulate such triangular patterns quickly and accurately and pace subsequent interpretations at a level of awareness that is tolerable for a specific patient. Malan's recommendations for the order of interpretive work in brief dynamic psychotherapy are as follows:

1. The nature of the focal conflict is communicated to the patient before extensive connections are made among past, current, and transference relationships.
2. In interpreting the focal conflict, the therapist discusses the patient's defensive avoidance of the expression of aims before undertaking an in-depth exploration of the aims themselves. For example, a patient who wants to be more direct in expressing anger but fears harming others in the process may be quiet and withdrawn when angry with friends. The therapist might point out that the patient became withdrawn in the same way after the therapist made a certain comment, and the therapist would then invite the patient to examine this behavior before directly asserting that the patient must be angry with the therapist.
3. The repetitive pattern of maladaptive interpersonal behavior is interpreted in its past, current, and transference aspects. The way in which this is done varies and depends on the patient's capacity to appreciate this pattern in different relationship contexts. Once it is clearly developed, the manifestation of the focal conflict in the patient's relationship with the therapist receives primary emphasis.
4. The analysis of the links between the way in which the patient relates to the therapist and the similar way in which the patient related to parental figures in the past is termed the parent-transference linking interpretation. Malan stresses the importance of this interpretation above all other possible interpretations that can be made in brief psychotherapy.

B. Termination Phase: The loss of the therapist at the termination of brief psychotherapy has meanings for the patient that are explored for possible linkages to unresolved meanings of earlier losses, usually of parental figures. The focal conflict is frequently reactivated or intensified during the termination phase, so that there is yet another opportunity to work through the focal conflict.

Peter Sifneos: Short-Term Anxiety-Provoking Psychotherapy

While Malan was formulating the technique of brief dynamic psychotherapy at the Tavistock Clinic, Peter Sifneos (1972) was articulating a similar approach based on his experience at Massachusetts General Hospital in Boston. Like Malan, Sifneos departed from the tradition of more supportive and anxiety-suppressive brief psychotherapies by advocating an exploratory, interpretive approach usually reserved for long-term psychoanalytic treatments. The objective of both theorists was to enable patients to make changes in their characters through resolution of certain key neurotic conflicts.

Selection Criteria

Sifneos's approach also emphasizes specific inclusion and exclusion criteria in order to select patients who can quickly engage in the therapeutic process and can tolerate the anxiety evoked by early and repeated interpretive work, in particular, frank examination of the transference reaction. Patients who are the most appropriate candidates for short-term anxiety-provoking psychotherapy have the following characteristics:

1. Above-average intelligence, as determined by the capacity for new learning.
2. A history of at least one mutual, give-and-take relationship, with implied shared intimacy, emotional involvement, trust, and the capacity for ambivalent feelings.
3. Ability to acknowledge and express a range of emotions, as directly observed in the patient's interaction with the evaluating therapist.
4. A circumscribed chief complaint related to a limited area of interpersonal functioning.
5. Motivation for change, which Sifneos regards as a multifaceted characteristic that includes the capacity and willingness to look for personal contributions to one's difficulties, an ability to appreciate that symptoms are psychological in origin, the capacity to provide an open and honest account of feelings, a willingness to be actively involved in the therapeutic relationship, and a willingness to experiment with new ways of functioning. Sifneos stresses the importance of realistic rather than magical expectations about changes arising from therapy as well as the patient's willingness to make reasonable sacrifices with regard to schedule arrangements and payment of fees.

Treatment

Sifneos's approach incorporates five phases, as described below.

A. First Phase (Patient-Therapist Encounter): A therapeutic alliance is formed through mobilization of the patient's initial positive feelings toward the therapist as well as early exploration of the patient's apprehensions regarding treatment. In this phase, the therapist also arrives at a tentative psychodynamic hypothesis about the relationship of current symptomatic disturbances to long-standing character problems that cause conflicts in interpersonal relationships. The focus of treatment—an emotional problem that the patient is motivated to solve and that has relevance for both current interpersonal difficulties as well as basic (core) neurotic conflicts—is also determined during the first phase.

B. Second Phase (Early Treatment): The therapist is careful to differentiate realistic goals from the patient's more immature wishes to be totally gratified in disavowing adult responsibility for dealing with problems. The therapist tactfully confronts the patient's idealized versions of what treatment will accomplish in order to encourage active problem solving and discourage the development of an overly dependent relationship.

C. Third Phase (Height of Treatment): In the third phase, the therapist relates the patient's past unresolved difficulties in interpersonal relationships to current emotional problems. As these patterns of conflict are explored, the patient frequently experiences moments of resistance (transference resistances) to the deeper understanding of these patterns, in part because of fearful expectations of the therapist's reactions or attitudes toward the patient.

These impediments to treatment are discussed so that the patient is allowed to see the irrational basis for these fears and so that exploration can then return to bolder elaboration of the focus. A cycle of events then typically occurs: Progress in understanding leads to resistance, followed first by interpretation of the fears underlying the resistance and then by further deepening of the work. The therapist asks anxiety-provoking questions in order to help the patient observe how he or she evades painful feelings as well as to demonstrate the reasons underlying this avoidance. Such confrontations may trigger the patient's anger toward the therapist, a response that is made more acceptable to the patient because of the prior establishment of a therapeutic alliance.

Sifneos has likened this emotional problem solving to the completion of a complex mathematical puzzle. He cautions against an overly intellectualized approach, however, and emphasizes that it is a learning experience that occurs within the context of an emotional exchange between the patient and the therapist.

D. Fourth Phase (Evidence of Change): In the fourth phase, the therapist determines when sufficient mastery and resolution of the problem have occurred, so that termination may be considered. The criteria for resolution include less anxiety during treatment sessions; relief of symptoms such as sleeplessness, phobias, or self-defeating behavior; adaptive changes in the interpersonal behavior associated with the focus; and evidence that the patient can be-

gin to relate what has been learned to new social contexts by making appropriate changes in behavior. For example, after successful therapy, a patient who has stifled expression of independent wishes and actions in the presence of parental figures and who has sought treatment because this behavior has been carried over into the marital relationship will be able to define and assert needs not only with the spouse but also with important figures in the workplace or in social relationships.

E. Fifth Phase (Termination): Sifneos proposes that the exact termination date not be set until appropriate change has been demonstrated in the target behavior. At that point, the therapist addresses the natural ambivalence the patient feels at the thought of separating from the therapist. The disappointment of separating from a recently acquired helpful figure is set against the more realistic background of the gains achieved in treatment. The patient is encouraged to extrapolate this new knowledge to future challenges. The therapist in turn also experiences a resistance to termination that must be addressed, because as the therapist experiences growing concern for the patient, there will be a deepening curiosity about the origin of the patient's difficulties as well as anxiety and guilt in acknowledging that treatment is ending but has failed to address certain psychopathological problems (specifically, those not related to the central focus). Therapists may have to struggle with the temptation to extend treatment. Sifneos believes that separation at termination is facilitated by a progressive, active, problem-solving posture on the part of the patient rather than a more regressive dependent attachment.

Habib Davanloo: Broad-Focused Short-Term Dynamic Psychotherapy

Habib Davanloo's (1979, 1980) work, which incorporates some theoretical concepts from both Malan and Sifneos, has broadened both the scope of problems that can be addressed in brief psychotherapy and the extent of the resolution hoped for in treatment.

Selection Criteria

In this approach, selection criteria in time-limited therapy have been expanded to include patients with long-standing severe characterological deficits (ie, personality disorders) that imply the existence of multiple interrelated conflicts that are not easily limited to a single focus. Davanloo considers neither severe problems nor long-standing difficulties as automatic criteria for excluding patients from treatment. Contrary to expectation, he reported some good outcomes in brief treatment of individuals with long-standing severe character problems and unexpected instances of poor outcome when mild character difficulties of more recent onset were the presenting complaint. Whereas Sifneos recommends his short-term anxiety-provoking psychotherapy for a rigorously selected 5–10% of psychiatric outpatients, Davanloo's broader selection criteria make it possible to treat about 30–35% of outpatients with psychiatric problems by broad-focused short-term therapy.

In 1979, Davanloo specified criteria for his approach to brief dynamic psychotherapy. These overlap the criteria of Malan and Sifneos (history of adequate interpersonal relationships, capacity to tolerate and express feelings, awareness that problems are psychological in origin, and response to the therapist's initial interpretations). Davanloo emphasizes the need to confront the patient's way of avoiding real feelings by including such defensive behavior as vagueness, passivity, denial, or withdrawal. Such repetitive confrontation is often irritating to patients, who are encouraged to express the frustration and resentment they feel about this process. The ability to express that anger and to begin recognizing the pattern of not expressing feelings under frustrating circumstances reflects qualities indicating that the patient is a suitable candidate for broad-focused short-term therapy.

Duration of Treatment

Davanloo recommends a flexible number of treatment sessions. For well-functioning patients with circumscribed problems, 5–15 face-to-face sessions lasting an hour each are usually sufficient to deal with the presenting problem. For adequately functioning patients with several presenting problems, 15–25 sessions are recommended; about 20–30 sessions are recommended for patients with long-standing severe personality problems.

Treatment

A. Early and Middle Phases: As in other brief dynamic psychotherapeutic approaches, the therapist assumes an active role and places high priority on the early and repeated interpretation of transference (ie, the ways in which the patient misperceives the therapist as a result of experiences in earlier relationships). For example, a patient with a harsh and critical mother was made to feel during her childhood that her anger toward her mother was not justified. The patient had therefore developed a pattern of suppressing her anger when frustrated and instead becoming moody and uncooperative, without clearly communicating what was upsetting her. Such a pattern is highly likely to recur during treatment, and when it does appear, the therapist will make the interpretation that the patient is feeling resentfully misunderstood, that she feels as though she is not justified in this anger, and that instead of expressing the feeling, she becomes moody and uncommunicative. After the pattern has been clarified, the therapist addresses the patient's unwarranted expectation that she will be punished for her behavior, and the patient

gradually comes to trust more open expression of her frustration. This active, interpretive approach is recommended by Davanloo both to accelerate the understanding and resolution of emotional problems and to prevent patients from becoming excessively dependent on the therapist. Instead, patients are encouraged to rely on their own coping capacities in preparation for the termination of treatment.

In treatments that are going well, the patient gains considerable understanding into these recurrent ways of avoiding the expression of emotions and usually begins to experiment with more open demonstration of feelings by about the eighth session. This increased communicativeness occurs not only in the treatment setting but also in the patient's relationships with other important persons in everyday life. At the same time, anxiety and depression are lessened, partly because the patient feels an upsurge in morale as a result of participating in a helpful treatment relationship and partly because the patient is able to negotiate more appropriately for satisfaction of needs in interpersonal conflicts. At this point, termination of therapy may be contemplated.

B. Termination Phase: Davanloo also recommends a flexible approach to the termination phase that takes into account the patient's level of functioning as well as the limited or extensive nature of the presenting problems. In well-functioning patients who are capable but hold themselves back in work and love relationships because of irrational fear of success, disengagement from treatment is uncomplicated, and patients do not ordinarily experience deep feelings of loss at termination. On the other hand, for those individuals who have sustained important losses in their lives, particularly during sensitive developmental periods in early childhood or adolescence, mourning the imminent departure of the therapist is an essential and helpful aspect of treatment. Because the patient knows when the relationship will end, there is an opportunity to explore the feelings about this loss, which stands in contrast to the more traumatic losses that occurred in earlier developmental periods. For patients with severe personality difficulties or those with multiple problems rather than a single focus, Davanloo recommends several additional sessions during the termination phase in order to help the patient negotiate a manageable separation.

James Mann: Time-Limited Psychotherapy

James Mann's (1973) unique approach to brief dynamic psychotherapy places major theoretical and technical emphasis on the meaning of time—ie, the patient's difficulty in accepting the finiteness of time, in mastering separations, and in ultimately accepting his or her own mortality. As a result, the selection of patients, the development of the focus in brief treatment, the approach to working through emotional problems, and the handling of the termination phase are organized along a common theme that addresses the meanings of time for the patient. The termination phase assumes paramount importance, because it provides a living model of loss, separation, and the time-limited nature of attachments.

In his theoretical discussion, Mann differentiates two ways in which people experience time: (1) Categorical, or adult, time is governed by a realistic understanding of the finite quality of time and is measured by the watch and the calendar; (2) existential, or child, time is governed by immature fantasies of timelessness and personal invincibility. Because the development of a mature appreciation of time is a challenge for everyone, particularly for people with a history of difficulty in early separation experiences (who are forever waiting for the loved one's return), a child's perception of time is never entirely set aside, even in the most mature adults. Both kinds of time may be used simultaneously to evaluate an experience. Stressful life events may alter a person's perception of time from a realistic, adult appreciation of its finiteness to a more childlike experience of time and functioning (regression with stress). Alternatively, the same individual may simultaneously reflect different levels of adaptation to the finiteness of time, as shown in successful time management in one sphere (being prompt for meetings) with an adherence to more immature perceptions of time in another area of functioning (failing to plan for retirement as a denial of aging).

Selection Criteria

Ideal candidates for Mann's brief dynamic psychotherapy are young adults in developmental transition, ie, those who are moving from the late stages of adolescence into young adulthood. The prototype is a college student struggling simultaneously to handle separation from parents and to establish autonomous social, occupational, and sexual identities. Mann's approach stresses that the patient must have the ability to tolerate the frustration of the time limits inherent in this type of therapy. Above-average intelligence, a criterion emphasized by Sifneos, is seen as helpful though not essential in Mann's approach. Mann has suggested that his approach, which is both short term and fixed in duration, may be appropriate for those with limited economic resources and educational background. Long-term exploratory psychotherapies are frequently both too costly and too ambiguously defined to serve the interests of this group of patients.

The exclusion criteria for Mann's time-limited approach include past or current psychotic disorders, serious alcohol or drug abuse, and borderline personality disorder. Patients with strong passive longings to be cared for, who are frequently reluctant to give up these feelings in favor of more independent behavior, are also excluded. Individuals with these problems frequently require long-term dynamic psychotherapy.

Duration & Focus of Treatment

Mann specifies a 12-session, once-weekly, time-limited treatment. The focus emerges after a process of gradual clarification, which may require several sessions, and the 12-session limit begins only after a focus has been mutually defined. Once the focus has been established, the time limit is fixed, and the date of termination is set in advance. If no workable focus can be specified during the preliminary interviews, the patient is referred for an appropriate alternative treatment.

Mann describes four basic conflicts that are a frequent focus in treatment: dependence versus independence, passivity versus activity, diminished versus adequate self-esteem, and unresolved versus resolved grief. Mann emphasizes the paramount importance of the elements of separation and individuation as they relate to the four central issues. For example, while activity-passivity struggles may involve anxiety about surpassing a rival, anxiety about aggressively dominating another, or anxiety about separating from a caretaker, Mann considers the latter to be the most important theme.

Treatment

A. Early Phase: Mann describes an initial "honeymoon" phase characterized by the patient's relief in feeling understood, particularly when the therapist is tactful in defining the problem that is the focus. The recommendation for brief rather than longer-term treatment stimulates hope for a rapid resolution of difficulties. The patient is intellectually aware of the time limit; at an emotional level, however, the patient often longs for an open-ended and idealized reparative relationship with the therapist that will compensate for earlier disappointments and frustrations in formative relationships.

B. Middle Phase: The therapist's inevitable failure to meet all of the patient's expectations in the first few hours of treatment leads to disillusionment, which ushers in the middle phase of treatment, frequently at about the sixth session. The original presenting symptoms may intensify, as Mann (1973) explains:

> The characteristic feature of any middle point is that one more step, however small, signifies the point of no return. In the instance of time-limited psychotherapy, the patient must go on to a conclusion that he does not wish to confront. The confrontation that he needs to avoid and that he will actively seek to avoid is the same one that he suffered earlier in his life; namely, separation without resolution from the meaningful, ambivalently experienced person. Time sense and reality are coconspirators in repeating an existential trauma in the patient.

C. Termination Phase: With the inevitable approach of termination, a deepening sense of pessimism and disillusionment usually (not always) dominates the eighth through the tenth sessions. The patient is more or less aware of the threat of termination and struggles to guard against the emotional pain of the loss of a valued relationship only recently established. With surprising frequency, the patient seems to forget the termination date and believes there are more sessions left than are actually remaining. The therapist points out the patient's incorrect perceptions of time in the context of brief dynamic treatment. The patient's negative feelings toward the therapist at this stage frequently recapitulate negative feelings toward frustrating figures in earlier life. The important difference is that while facing an agreed upon termination date, the patient now has an opportunity to experience and master the emotions related to separation from the therapist. In so doing, the patient develops a capacity to function more independently and deal more adaptively with the imperfect and time-limited nature of human experience. Feelings of anger at being abandoned, guilt for having angry feelings toward frustrating figures, sadness at the loss of a valued figure, and wishes for reunion can be examined in this phase.

Klerman & Weissman: Short-Term Interpersonal Psychotherapy

Klerman and Weissman have described a time-limited psychotherapeutic method specifically tailored to treat individuals with depression. The focus of this approach is on interpersonal behaviors that contribute to depressive states (Weissman and Klerman, 1973; Neu et al, 1978). In contrast to the brief dynamic psychotherapies, little attention is directed toward the exploration of unconscious conflicts or the repetition of unresolved parent-child problems in the patient's relationship with the therapist (ie, there is minimal transference interpretation). Treatment is time limited, averaging 14 sessions in one study. Weekly 50-minute sessions are provided for individuals with depression triggered and exacerbated by interpersonal problems.

Klerman and Weissman describe seven types of technical interventions. The first is nonjudgmental exploration, which is particularly relevant early in treatment and denotes the support and encouragement given to the patient to discuss problems openly. The therapist's availability, empathy, and nonjudgmental attitude are essential in facilitating the patient's self-disclosure.

Elicitation of material, a second technique, involves active probing for new information. Such probing is common during early treatment but may be indicated whenever a more complete understanding of past or current difficulties is indicated. Next is clarification, or rephrasing of the patient's comments to point out inconsistencies and make covert communications more overt.

Additional techniques include direct advice, in which the therapist guides the patient toward more adaptive interpersonal behavior to increase the chances that others will be warmly receptive of the patient rather than critical or distant. Decision analysis explores alternative courses of action in order to broaden the patient's understanding of the short- and long-range consequences of behavior toward others. Development of awareness is used to facilitate insight into the patient's interpersonal behavioral patterns and clarify ways in which the patient attempts to disavow or ignore these patterns.

This brief treatment approach is noteworthy both for its careful specification of treatment approaches in published manuals as well as for the attention paid to research on the effectiveness of the recommendations. Markowitz (1998) reviews efficacy research on interpersonal psychotherapy demonstrating utility for unipolar depression, eating disorders, and depression in human immunodeficiency virus (HIV)-positive men. The approach may be of particular interest to general practitioners and other nonpsychiatrist physicians, since extensive training in psychodynamic theory and technique is not required.

BRIEF DYNAMIC PSYCHOTHERAPY OF POSTTRAUMATIC STRESS DISORDER

Building on the general principles of brief dynamic psychotherapy, a specific model has been developed to address the psychological responses of individuals following natural and human-caused disasters (Horowitz, 1986; Marmar and Freeman, 1988; Marmar, 1991; Weiss and Marmar, 1993; Marmar et al, 1995). The treatment is appropriate for adults who meet criteria for posttraumatic stress disorder (PTSD) as a consequence of a single traumatic life event in adulthood, functioned adequately in work and love relations prior to the trauma, have social supports, are not currently abusing alcohol or drugs, do not have a concurrent anxiety, depressive, or other Axis I disorder, and are not currently suicidal or homicidal.

The treatment is a 12-session, once-weekly individual outpatient psychotherapy. The technique involves the rapid establishment of a therapeutic alliance, permission to tell the story of the traumatic event from start to end, encouragement to retell the story in the present tense with all the emotions and cognitions that occurred at the time of the traumatic event, and emphasis on retelling the story of the event repeatedly during the course of treatment to permit a reconstruction of all aspects of the trauma, particularly those elements that are subject to the patchy psychogenic amnesia typical of the memory of adults for traumatic events.

A psychodynamic focus is established on the problematic weak and strong self-concepts activated by the traumatic event. Typically these self-concepts focus on views of the self as terrified, helpless, and unable to reestablish a sense of the world as safe, predictable, and controllable. A disparate set of self-concepts, involving a view of the self as dangerous, omnipotent, and responsible for the traumatic event or its sequelae, may operate out of awareness, cause extreme feelings of guilt, and motivate self-defeating behavior in attempt to expiate the imagined harm caused to the self or others. The problematic weak and strong self-concepts triggered by the traumatic event may be intensified by the activation of latent self-concepts related to childhood or adolescent development. These earlier views of the self are ordinarily held out of awareness in adults whose success in work and love stabilizes a positive coherent view of self that is shattered in the aftermath of the adult traumatization.

The therapist aims to allow the patient to express the feelings related to the traumatic event by countering the patient's tendency to avoid discussion of the event and by modulating the level of emotional arousal to prevent the patient from being overwhelmed by traumatic affect. As in the more general forms of brief dynamic psychotherapy discussed above, interpretations of resistances to the expression of feelings generally precede an in-depth reconstruction of the trauma, emphasizing transference resistance interpretations that address the patient's reluctance to disclose the trauma because of fears of overwhelming the therapist. Countertransference issues that arise in the treatment of patients with PTSD include exaggerated therapist fears of harming the patient by confronting the trauma, horror and revulsion at hearing about the traumatic event, which may lead the therapist to conspire with the patient in phobic avoidance of the trauma, and aggressive urges toward the patient that result in part from the unconscious resonation in the therapist of sadistic themes related to the role of perpetrators in assaults, combat, and other human-caused disasters.

The termination phase of brief dynamic therapy for PTSD is often marked by temporary regression because of the anticipated loss of a recently acquired support. The loss of the therapist frequently triggers the same problematic weak and powerful self-concepts that were triggered by the traumatic event. This permits a direct, here-and-now transference exploration of these views of the self, allowing for a more thorough working through of the irrational meanings of the trauma.

EFFECTIVENESS OF BRIEF DYNAMIC PSYCHOTHERAPY

Despite the methodological difficulties encountered in assessing the outcome of various psychotherapies, major progress occurred in the 1970s. The most thorough research on the effectiveness of psychotherapy

has been conducted by Smith et al (1980), who reviewed and analyzed 375 studies. Since the average duration of treatment was 17 sessions, this report mainly considers the outcome of brief psychotherapy. In general, the average patient who received treatment was better off than 75% of those who either received no treatment or were on waiting lists for treatment and were used as controls. Effectiveness of treatment was assessed by several criteria, including improvement in symptoms, patient satisfaction, and decreased reliance on medication. The study indicated that the many different schools of psychotherapy were about equally helpful. Brief dynamic psychotherapy —along with brief behavioral, interpersonal, cognitive, and other approaches—is a treatment with well-documented effectiveness in relieving various psychological symptoms, as described above.

The relative effectiveness of brief dynamic psychotherapy compared to long-term dynamic treatments has not been extensively studied. Although the general question of brief versus long-term treatment in the different approaches has been reviewed by Butcher and Kolotkin (1979) and by Luborsky et al (1975), the former failed to find a strong correlation between the efficacy of different therapies and the length of treatment. The negative finding may be due in part to currently limited abilities to reliably evaluate the types of personality changes that are more likely to occur in long-term treatment. Changes in psychological symptoms and social functioning, on the other hand, are more easily determined. Definitive evaluation of the merits of brief versus long-term treatment awaits development of improved methods of assessing characterological change.

Brief dynamic psychotherapy for outpatients with moderate to severe psychiatric conditions has been shown to be effective in alleviating symptoms and improving social functioning. Barber and Ellman (1996) and Horowitz et al (1984) have found that brief therapy is effective in treating posttraumatic stress disorders. They have also discussed the modification of the techniques of brief dynamic psychotherapy for patients with different personality disorders. Weissman et al (1981) have studied the outcome of interpersonal psychotherapy and found that 14-session treatments have been effective in treating major depressive disorders. Very few negative effects of brief dynamic psychotherapy have been reported. Rather than becoming worse, patients for the most part either improve or (at worst) do not improve after brief dynamic psychotherapy. This method of treatment seems to be the most useful when a specific focus can be defined, when the problem is related to recent stressful life circumstances, and when the patient has the capacity to tolerate rapid engagement and confrontation, working through, and disengagement from the treatment process.

REFERENCES & SUGGESTED READINGS

Alexander F, French T: *Psychoanalytic Therapy: Principles and Applications.* Ronald Press, 1946.

Balint M, Ornstein PH, Balint E: *Focal Psychotherapy.* Lippincott, 1972.

Barber JP, Ellman J: Advances in short-term dynamic psychotherapy. Curr Opinion Psychiatry 1996;9:188.

Butcher NJ, Kolotkin RL: Evaluation of outcome in brief psychotherapy. Psychiatr Clin North Am 1979;2:157.

Davanloo H: Techniques of short-term psychotherapy. Psychiatr Clin North Am 1979;2:11.

Davanloo H (editor): *Short-Term Dynamic Therapy,* Vol. I. Jason Aronson, 1980.

Ferenczi S, Rank O: *The Development of Psychoanalysis.* Nervous and Mental Disease Publication Co., 1925.

Foreman S, Marmar CR: Therapist actions that address initially poor therapeutic alliances in psychotherapy. Amer J Psychiatry 1995;132:922.

French TM: *The Integrations of Behavior,* Vol. 3. University of Chicago Press, 1958.

Horowitz MJ: *Stress Response Syndromes,* 2nd ed. Jason Aronson, 1986.

Horowitz MJ et al: Brief psychotherapy of bereavement reactions: The relationship of process to outcome. Arch Gen Psychiatry 1984;41:438.

Horowitz MJ et al: *Personality Styles and Brief Psychotherapy.* Basic Books, 1984.

Luborsky L, Singer B, Luborsky L: Comparative studies of psychotherapies. Arch Gen Psychiatry 1975;32:995.

Malan DH: *A Study of Brief Psychotherapy.* Plenum, 1963.

Malan DH: *Frontiers of Brief Psychotherapy.* Plenum, 1976.

Mann J: *Time-Limited Psychotherapy.* Harvard University Press, 1973.

Markowitz JC: *Interpersonal Psychotherapy.* American Psychiatric Press, 1998.

Marmar CR: Brief psychotherapy of posttraumatic stress disorder. Psych Ann 1991;21:405.

Marmar CR, Freeman M: Brief dynamic psychotherapy of posttraumatic stress disorders: Management of narcissistic regression. J Traumatic Stress 1988;1:323.

Marmar CR, Weiss DS, Pynoos R: Dynamic psychotherapy of posttraumatic stress disorder. In: *Neurobiology and Clinical Consequences of Extreme Stress: From Normal Adaption to PTSD.* Friedman MJ, Charney DS, Deutchy K (editors). Raven, 1995.

Neu C, Prusoff B, Klerman G: Measuring the interventions used in short-term interpersonal psychotherapy of depression. Am J Orthopsychiatry 1978;48:629.

Safran JD, Muran JC: The therapeutic alliance in brief psychotherapy: General principles. In: *The Therapeutic Alliance in Brief Psychotherapy.* Safran JD, Muran JC (editors). American Psychological Association, 1998.

Sifneos PE: *Short-Term Psychotherapy and Emotional Crisis.* Harvard University Press, 1972.

Smith ML, Glass GV, Miller TI: *The Benefits of Psychotherapy.* Johns Hopkins University Press, 1980.

Weiss DS, Marmar CR: Teaching time-limited dynamic psychotherapy for posttraumatic stress disorder and pathological grief. Psychotherapy 1993;30:587.

Weissman M, Klerman G: Psychotherapy with depressed women: An empirical study of content themes and reflection. Br J Psychiatry 1973;123:55.

Weissman M et al: Depressed outpatients: Results one year after treatment with drugs and/or interpersonal psychotherapy. Arch Gen Psychiatry 1981;38:51.

33

Behavior Therapy & Cognitive Therapy

Hanna Levenson, PhD, Jacqueline B. Persons, PhD, & Kenneth S. Pope, PhD

INTRODUCTION

"This is the golden age of cognitive therapy. Its popularity among society and the professional community is growing by leaps and bounds" (Seligman, 1992, p ix). In a similar tone, Safran and Segal (1990) note that "these seem like good times for cognitive therapists. The cognitive revolution in psychotherapy . . . has become a mainstream psychotherapy tradition" (p 3). Data reveal that clinician interest in cognitive approaches has increased *600%* since 1973 (Norcross et al, 1989)! And in a survey of graduate and internship training directors in psychology, over half indicated that a cognitive-behavioral approach was their program's major theoretical orientation (Levenson and Evans, in press). Interest in cognitive-behavioral approaches has been spurred by the positive outcome that results from careful and replicable research, the increasing sophistication of the consumer–client–patient who demands effective treatment, and the increased emphasis on cost containment of managed health care.

Although there are many types of behavior and cognitive therapies, they have in common several elements that form an underlying core and theoretical rationale (see also Chapter 2). For this reason, the terms behavior therapy, cognitive therapy, and cognitive-behavioral therapy are viewed as roughly interchangeable. The approach of the behavior or cognitive therapist involves an implicit five-step procedure.

1. The individual is evaluated for "symptoms" of behavioral dysfunction, which may be noted by direct observation (eg, overeating, stuttering, crying), by the individual's verbalization of thoughts and feelings (eg, suicidal thoughts, depression), and by clinical measurements (eg, blood pressure, heart rate). The behavioral-cognitive therapist does not conceptualize a problem in terms of a psychiatric diagnosis (eg, schizophrenia), but instead defines it in terms of **specific behaviors** that affect the individual's functioning (eg, hallucinating in public).
2. The therapist and client, working collaboratively, determine the goals of the treatment. These often focus on specific behaviors to be changed, ie, **target behaviors.**

3. In addition to defining the problem in behavioral terms, the therapist develops a hypothesis about the underlying beliefs and/or environmental events that maintain or minimize these behaviors. Steps 1 and 3 are referred to as **developing a case formulation or conducting a behavioral analysis.** Careful documentation and quantification are of great importance in determining factors that influence or trigger the undesired behaviors and in evaluating the effectiveness of the interventions. Since clients are often unaware of sequences of events that lead to a specific type of behavior, direct observation of clients in their environments is sometimes a necessary part of behavioral analysis. Clients can often be trained in the skills of self-observation and in recording of events so that the behavioral analysis is more accurate. Data derived from the analysis are used by the therapist to formulate a clinical hypothesis (the case formulation) about what stimulates (precedes) and what maintains (reinforces) the undesired actions, thoughts, feelings, or physiological changes. Newer formulations also include proposals about the nature of the cognitions (beliefs, attitudes) that may underlie and play a causal role in problematic behaviors and symptoms.
4. Using methods supported by theories and findings from the literature, the clinician tests the hypothesis of cause and effect by altering the behavior, the underlying cognitions, or the environment (or all three) and observing the effects of the alteration on the client's dysfunctional actions, thoughts, and feelings.
5. From systematic observation and documentation of behavioral changes, the clinician either revises the hypothesis or continues with treatment until the goals of therapy are reached, ie, the target behaviors are changed. It is important to stress that behavior therapy is based on a way of thinking about people and problems and is not a set of techniques. Testing one hypothesis often leads to the development of another hypothesis, which in turn must be tested. Systematic data collecting, used to monitor the outcome of treatment, which can be conceptualized as a clinical experimental study with an

$N = 1$, is a central component of therapy (see Barlow et al, 1984).

Other Characteristics Shared by Behavior & Cognitive Therapies

In addition to sharing the empirical, scientific approach outlined above, behavior and cognitive therapies have other characteristics in common:

1. Therapy involves action as well as discussion. It is often directive, structured, and brief or time limited.
2. The client must be a responsible participant in the therapy and capable of achieving personal change.
3. The present (here and now) determinants of behavior are emphasized rather than the historic (then and there) determinants.
4. It is assumed that human behavior follows natural laws.
5. It is assumed that people's behavior reflects their adaptation to the environment and not necessarily underlying pathological disorders.
6. It is assumed that behavior can be changed directly without changing personality dynamics.
7. Paraprofessionals, lay people significant to the client, and even the clients themselves can carry out treatment.
8. The treatment often involves "homework." Only in rare instances is treatment confined to 1 or 2 hours a week with the therapist. Rehearsal, practice, and other activities are generally carried out by the client between sessions.

Historical Context

In his experiments on learned and unlearned (conditioned and unconditioned) behavior, Ivan Pavlov (1849–1936) trained dogs to salivate at the sound of a bell by repeatedly pairing a conditioned stimulus (bell) with an unconditioned stimulus (food powder) that naturally causes an unconditioned response (salivation). Similarly, John B. Watson (1878–1958) taught a 1-year-old boy to be afraid of a white rat by pairing the child's approach to the rat with a loud noise. The boy then generalized his fear to other white furry objects. This study suggested the process whereby phobias might develop and gave impetus to later work on aversive conditioning and counterconditioning.

For their research using **classical conditioning,** Pavlov and Watson are credited with beginning the systematic study of the effects of environment on behavior. **Operant** (instrumental) conditioning has also had a major effect on behavioral theory as applied to clinical problems. In the 1950s, behavioral modification began to attract attention, largely because of the work of B.F. Skinner (1904–1990). Skinner used operant conditioning principles—which hold that behavior is a function of its consequences (**rein-**

forcers)—to change the behaviors of psychotic patients who were in the wards of state hospitals. Techniques such as extinction and positive reinforcement, as well as programmatic efforts such as token economies (all described in subsequent sections), are examples of applied operant conditioning principles. Recent applications of operant principles to clinical problems include Linehan's (1993) dialectical behavior therapy for the treatment of borderline personality disorder. The therapist following Linehan's protocol conducts repeated behavioral analyses of problem behaviors (eg, self-destructive wrist cutting) in an attempt to develop hypotheses about the function of the problem behaviors.

Throughout the 1950s and 1960s, behavior modification focused on stimulus (S) and response (R), while factors mediating the stimulus-response (S-R) connection were largely ignored. However, with the accumulation of empirical clinical data, it soon became clear that the variance in how someone responded to a situation could not always be predicted by the stimulus that preceded it or the consequence that followed it.

To improve their ability to understand, predict, and control behavior, therapists and researchers (eg, Albert Bandura, Julian Rotter) began exploring cognitive variables such as expectancy (predictions of future happenings), attributions (inferred characteristics of people or events), and mental images (ideas). Whereas traditional behavior therapy focused on observable S-R connections, cognitive behavior therapy took into account the importance of mediating factors within the organism (S-O-R). Since the 1970s cognitive variables have been given a central role in the understanding of processes that influence behavior (eg, self-instruction, cognitive therapy for depression, imagery techniques).

Cognitive therapy—which is farther along the continuum from behavior therapy to cognitive behaviorism—focuses more on the individual's interpretations of internal and external events and views them as crucial in understanding behavior. The purely cognitive view holds that dysfunctional thoughts may be influenced by dealing with the individual's thoughts directly. Most cognitive-behavioral therapists now utilize principles from both the behavioral (Pavlovian, Skinnerian) and cognitive theories.

TECHNIQUES

Although the exact number of cognitive-behavioral intervention strategies is not known, it is estimated to be in the hundreds. Several approaches have been selected to illustrate various techniques, but by no means should these be considered all-inclusive or even representative of this quickly expanding field. Any attempt to classify these treatments into behavioral or cognitive categories is frustrating for all but the most naive, since the methods in the field have so intertwined behavioral and cognitive perspectives. However, the techniques have been presented in a progression from those relying more on observable behavior to those relying more on private and subjective cognitions.

Positive Reinforcement & Extinction

Reinforcement and extinction are discussed first, since they represent an early attempt to apply behavioral principles to treatment of seriously disturbed patients. It is a well-known learning principle that the probability a specific behavior will occur is increased when the behavior is followed by certain pleasurable consequences (reinforcers). For example, in a now classic study, it was demonstrated that certain verbal responses of a patient would be increased by an approving "mm-hm" from the therapist. When a behavior is no longer reinforced and is ignored, the probability of its occurring is decreased. For example, ignoring a patient's request for special treatment should lead to the elimination of these requests.

A clinical example from the literature will illustrate not only the effectiveness of positive reinforcement but also the care with which behavioral data are used for determining improvement:

39-year-old woman with a diagnosis of schizophrenia exhibited self-destructive behaviors such as burning herself and her clothing with cigarettes at a baseline rate of once a day. Because she liked to smoke (ie, would frequently indulge in this behavior), hospital staff members were instructed to inspect the patient for burns every hour and to give the patient half of a cigarette (reinforcer) and praise her for her appearance (secondary social reinforcer) if she were found to be burn-free. If she burned herself during the hour, she received no further cigarettes that day. Burns decreased from one a day to one approximately every 4 days (0.24 burns a day), and during the last 2 weeks of her hospitalization she remained burn-free.

Among the learning theory concepts that are important in applying positive reinforcement and extinction are the concepts of shaping, prompting, and modeling. Since it may take some time for a specific behavior (eg, speech in a mute patient) to be elicited, the desired behavior must be **shaped** by the therapist's reinforcing successive approximations of the wanted behavior (eg, progressively rewarding lip movement, then vocalizations, then isolated words, and finally sentences). Desired behaviors may also be **prompted** (eg, shaping the lips of the patient) or **modeled** (eg, saying words in front of the patient).

In institutional settings such as inpatient psychiatric wards or prisons, behaviors can be reinforced indirectly by issuing tokens (secondary reinforcers) that can be "traded in" for primary reinforcers or for other reinforcers such as watching television. This **token economy** approach is based on the premise

that dysfunctional behavior exists because it has been reinforced. Even professional staff members inadvertently reinforce undesired behavior by attending to (and thereby reinforcing) unwanted behavior such as head banging or delusional speech. Token economies represent an effort to provide an environment that systematically reinforces the desired behavior and extinguishes self-defeating dysfunctional activities.

Tokens (such as poker chips or points) offer several advantages over direct reinforcers: (1) They are readily available and can be handed over immediately after the desired behavior. (2) Tokens may be saved and redeemed later when the desire arises for goods or services, so that satiation is not a problem. (3) The number of tokens issued for a specific behavior may be increased or decreased depending on how consistently the new behaviors are evidenced.

The staff must be trained to recognize desired behavior, to administer tokens, and to ignore dysfunctional actions. They must consistently apply the reinforcement and extinction principles. One or two staff members who do not apply these principles reliably and readily can undermine the efforts of the others.

A study spanning a 6-year period including a postinstitutionalization follow-up indicated that 89% of the patients in a token economy unit had improved while on the ward, whereas improvement was seen in only 46% of patients receiving milieu therapy alone. Eighteen months following discharge, 92% of patients treated in the token economy unit and 71% of those treated in the milieu therapy unit were living in the community. A little-emphasized but important result of token economies is the improved morale and efficiency of the staff, who see progress and feel a sense of accomplishment with a difficult population.

Aversive Procedures

Much of our everyday behavior reflects avoidance of aversive consequences built into various components of our personal and institutional lives—disapproval from friends, failing grades, imprisonment, etc. The application of this principle to clinical problems is **aversive therapy.** Aversive procedures are useful clinically either when dysfunctional or inappropriate behavior is naturally reinforcing to the individual (eg, addictions, deviant sexual behavior) or when behavior is self-destructive and needs to be brought under control quickly.

There are three main aversive procedures: classical conditioning, punishment, and avoidance training. The aversive stimuli used clinically are numerous, but usually involve electric shock, chemicals, or vivid descriptions of noxious scenes.

In **classical conditioning** procedures, the stimuli leading to unwanted behavior (eg, sight and smell of one's favorite alcoholic beverage) are paired with a noxious stimulus (eg, shock). After the unconditioned stimulus (shock) is repeatedly associated with the conditioned stimulus (alcohol), patients develop the same feeling toward the alcohol as they feel toward the shock (fear). Since learned responses are more generalizable in lifelike settings, clinicians have had barlike settings constructed in inpatient alcohol units. Here patients are exposed to the sights, sounds, and smells of a bar, but these stimuli are paired with shocks. The goal of such treatment is avoidance of bars by the patients once they have been discharged.

In **punishment** procedures, a specific behavior (eg, drinking alcohol) is followed by a noxious stimulus or punishment. In the bar setting just described, punishment was used as a component of the treatment. Patients who had poured a favorite alcoholic beverage received a strong electric shock to the little finger (punishment) when they started to take the drink, The shock continued until the patient spit out the alcohol (**negative reinforcement** or **escape conditioning**). Thus, the patient was punished for undesired behavior (drinking) and then reinforced for desired behavior (spitting out the alcohol).

In **avoidance training** procedures, patients can escape the noxious stimulus if they avoid the undesired behavior. This is the theory behind the use of disulfiram. If the patient drinks even a small amount of alcohol while a dose of disulfiram is still in the body, severe nausea and vomiting will occur. The patient can avoid these unpleasant effects by not drinking (see Chapter 17).

The effectiveness of aversive principles for the treatment of self-destructive behaviors is well documented. For example, Lovaas and Simmons (1969) reported a case in which a 16-year-old mentally retarded girl bit her hands (and had previously bitten them to the extent that one finger had to be amputated), ripped her nails out with her teeth, and severely banged her head. Five 1-second shocks following these behaviors eliminated the problem.

In general, aversive techniques are most effective when used in conjunction with other forms of treatment and with procedures that reinforce the patient for desired behavior. When using aversive techniques, the clinician must always consider ethical factors and keep in mind that aversive techniques are more susceptible to abuse than other procedures.

Exposure

Modern exposure treatments had their origins in systematic desensitization, developed by Joseph Wolpe (1958). Wolpe, a psychiatrist trained in South Africa around the time of the second World War, noted that patients he treated for "war neurosis" using traditional psychoanalytically based methods did not appear to benefit much from treatment. His extensive readings, including Pavlov's writings, Jacobson's (1938) *Progressive Relaxation,* and others, led him to develop a new treatment for fears and phobias, which he named "systematic desensitization." In systematic desensitization, Wolpe developed a "hierarchy" or list of situations that were frightening to the patient, ordered from least to most fear-evoking. After training his patients to use Jacobson's relaxation methods, Wolpe systematically carried out brief pairings of relaxation and fear-evoking situations, beginning with the least-fear-evoking situations and moving gradually up to more frightening ones. During the pairings, the patient was instructed to use the relaxation strategies, then to imagine the fear-evoking stimulus briefly until the fear increased, then to relax again, then to imagine the fear-evoking situation again, and so on, over and over, with repeated pairings of fear-evoking images and relaxation, until the patient could imagine (and confront, in vivo, or "in real life") the fear-evoking cues without experiencing fear.

Wolpe's new method was quite effective, and he collected data on and published the results from a series of 210 cases effectively treated in this manner (Wolpe, 1958). Wolpe's view was that the therapy worked via the mechanism of "reciprocal inhibition," that is, the relaxation and the anxiety reciprocally inhibited one another to produce the therapeutic result. Later research did not support Wolpe's view that systematic desensitization was the therapeutic mechanism, and the current view is that systematic desensitization and a variety of methods derived later for treatment of fears and phobias are all effective because they involve therapeutic *exposure* to the feared situation.

Exposure treatment involves exposure of clients to the stimuli that evoke discomfort until they become accustomed to them. The types of procedures vary, ranging from those evoking little anxiety (as in the slow, graded, imagined process of desensitization) to those immersing the client in the feared situation (process of flooding).

Marks (1981) has done extensive work in both developing the theory and refining the clinical practice of exposure treatments. Based on past systematic research, he outlined the conditions most suitable for exposure therapy: agoraphobia, social phobias, illness phobias, simple ("specific") phobias, obsessive thoughts, compulsive rituals, obsessive-compulsive disorder, and types of sexual dysfunction (see Chapters 21 and 25).

For treatment of agoraphobia, Marks suggests choosing to work on simple but important activities at first. Initially, a reassuring person should accompany the agoraphobic person into the feared situations (eg, driving on a freeway). Exposure can then be attempted alone but at less anxiety-provoking times (eg, not at rush hour). Prolonged exposures (1–2 hours) seem to be more effective than short exposures. The client is required to record behaviors in a diary.

A married 40-year-old woman had been agoraphobic for 15 years. Lately, she had been unable to leave the house without her husband, fearing that if she went outside alone she would have a panic attack, would become overwhelmed and go crazy, screaming hysterically in the street, out of control, embarrassing and humiliating herself. She chose as her goal (target behavior) the ability to cross a busy street alone. Treatment began with crossing a street with the therapist. After they had done this several times, the therapist stood apart and then moved farther away as the client crossed the street. By the end of the first 1 1/2-hour treatment session, the woman was able to cross the street alone. She felt pleased with her accomplishment and much calmer. She was given homework assignments consisting of crossing streets near her home. By the end of the eighth treatment, the woman was crossing streets and shopping alone without anxiety.

In a theoretical paper, Foa and Kozak (1986) propose that all effective exposure treatments for fears and phobias are effective because they promote cognitive change by providing patients with information that contradicts the beliefs underlying their fears. Thus, the agoraphobic described above is anxious before treatment because of her belief that she will lose control. The exposure treatment teaches her that if she goes outside alone, the catastrophes she fears do not occur. Exposure treatments for panic disorder developed by David Barlow and his colleagues (Craske and Barlow, 1993) extend the treatment of panic and agoraphobia to include not just exposure to the external situations these patients fear, but also exposure ("interoceptive exposure") to the feared internal sensations (eg, dizziness, pounding heart rate). Exposure treatment for obsessive-compulsives includes both exposure to the situations these patients fear (eg, touching items the patient believes are contaminated) and blocking of the rituals (eg, hand washing) the patient typically uses to neutralize the fear; this treatment is called exposure and response prevention (see Riggs and Foa, 1993).

Exposure therapies for treatment of anxiety disorders have been studied extensively in randomized controlled trials. Results are impressive (see Barlow, 1993; DeRubeis and Crits-Christoph, 1998). In general terms, exposure treatments are consistently more effective than wait-list controls, and a few recent studies have shown them to be superior to alternative psychotherapies for treatment of anxiety disorders (see Barlow et al, 1989; Borkovec and Costello, 1993; Foa et al, 1991).

Self-Talk

Self-talk is widely used and appears to be the most thoroughly researched cognitive-behavioral intervention that addresses childhood difficulties focusing on problem behaviors, hyperactivity, and impulsivity (Kendall, 1991). It is common for children to repeat instructions to themselves as they attempt new tasks. For example, while crossing the street unaccompanied for the first time, a child may engage in a running monologue of the parents' instructions: "Stop at

the corner. Wait for the light to change from red to green, and make sure the 'walk' sign is on. Now look both ways to make sure no traffic is coming." These instructions may be repeated aloud, in a whisper, or silently. Adults too may attempt to learn new tasks in this way, eg, in taking up golf or tennis or assembling a bicycle.

People may be taught to use such self-talk—in the form of evaluative statements, suggestions, reminders of sequential steps, and encouragement—to help them relax, to improve performance of cognitive and physical activities, to increase motivation, and to become more aware and alert. Such self-talk is obviously related to the processes of covert modeling and cognitive therapy (see below).

Various techniques may be used for teaching self-talk in therapy, but the general approach is demonstrated by Meichenbaum's (1977) program of self-talk for children, which has been successful in treatment of problems related to hyperactivity, aggression, disruption, and cheating. There are five basic steps after the problem has been identified and the behavior to be learned has been defined: (1) The child observes as an adult model performs the behavior. While the child is watching, the model describes the behavior aloud. (2) The child performs the same task while the model gives instructions. (3) The child performs the task while giving instructions aloud. (4) The child whispers the instructions while performing the task. (5) The child performs the task without audible speech.

In using self-talk techniques, it is often important first to identify and modify the child's current maladaptive self-statements. To do this, the therapist helps the child to recognize critical self-references (eg, "I am so stupid, I can't do this homework"), monitor them, and then generate alternative self-statements that serve to encourage more adaptive coping (eg, less anxiety, hopelessness) (Francis and Beidel, 1995).

Cognitive Therapy

The underlying premise of cognitive therapy is that affect and behavior are largely functions of how people construe (structure) their world. According to one cognitive theory, everyone has "filters" through which the world is interpreted (eg, seeing the glass half-full versus seeing it half-empty). These constructs are called "schemas." When these constructs become distorted and dysfunctional, clients experience helplessness, anxiety, and depression. Aaron T. Beck, a psychiatrist at the University of Pennsylvania, developed cognitive therapy for depression when he noted, in his clinical work, the prominent stream of negative cognitions reported by depressed patients. The goals of cognitive therapy are (1) to make clients aware of their cognitive distortions and (2) to effect change through correction of these distortions. Common distortions (errors in information processing) that make people depressed include selective abstractions (missing the significance of a total situation by selecting a detail out of context), arbitrary inferences (jumping to a conclusion with missing or contradictory evidence), overgeneralizations (unjustified generalizations on the basis of one incident), and magnifications (exaggerating or elaborating on specifics). (See the writings of Beck et al [1979] for a detailed description of the therapy.)

The numerous strategies used in cognitive therapy are designed to help the client become aware of negative automatic thoughts (eg, "If I can't be perfect, then no one will love me"); to recognize connections among thoughts, mood, and behavior; and to replace distorted thoughts with more realistic interpretations.

The following discussions between patient and therapist are examples from Beck et al (1979):

P: The only way I could ever be happy is if I could be a great writer.
T: What level of writing would you have to reach?
P: I would have to be as good as [a specific poet].
T: Did this poet achieve great happiness?
P: No, I guess not. She killed herself.

A central component of the therapy is "homework." Patient and therapist work together to devise assignments the patient can do outside the therapy session to forward the work of the therapy. Often assignments include monitoring and recording emotions and situations associated with negative automatic thoughts (Table 33–1), behavioral experiments designed to test the accuracy of some of the client's negative beliefs, and activities designed to practice and strengthen newer, more adaptive beliefs.

Table 33–1. Example of a daily record of dysfunctional thoughts.

Date	Situation	Emotion(s)	Automatic Thought(s)	Rational Response	Outcome
	1. Describe actual event leading to unpleasant emotion or 2. Describe stream of thoughts, daydream, or recollection leading to unpleasant emotion	1. Specify sad/anxious, etc. 2. Rate degree of emotion, 1–100	1. Write automatic thought that preceded emotion 2. Rate belief in automatic thought, 0–100%	1. Write rational response to automatic thought 2. Rate belief in rational response, 0–100%	1. Rerate belief in automatic thought, 0–100% 2. Specify and rate subsequent emotion, 1–100
9/8	Received a letter from friend who was recently married	Guilty 60	"I should have gone to her wedding" 90%	It was inconvenient; she wouldn't be writing if she was angry about it 95%	10% Guilty 20
9/9	Was thinking of all the things I wanted to get done over the weekend	Anxious 40	"I'll never get all of this done. It's too much for me" 100%	I've done more than this before, and there is no law that says I have to get it all done 80%	25% Anxious 20
9/11	Made a mistake ordering supplies	Anxious 60	Pictured my boss yelling at me 100%	There is no evidence my boss will be angry; even if he is, I don't have to be upset 100%	0% Relieved 50
9/12	Pictured myself being depressed forever	Sad/anxious 90	"I'll never get better" 80%	I have gotten better in the past. Just because I think something is true doesn't make it true 80%	40% Sad/anxious 60
9/13	My date called and said he couldn't go out with me because he had to work	Sad 95	"He doesn't like me. NO ONE could ever like me" 90%	He asked me out for next weekend, so he must like me. He probably did have to work. Even if he didn't like me, it doesn't follow that "no one could ever like me" 90%	30% Sad 50

Source: Reproduced, with permission, from Beck et al: *Cognitive Therapy of Depression.* Guilford Press, 1979, p. 288.

Another central component of the therapy is the identification of recurrent or common themes, often stated as beliefs the person holds about him or herself or others, that make the person vulnerable to depression (see Persons, 1989):

T: Your automatic thought was, "Your children shouldn't fight and act up." And because they do, "I must be a rotten mother." Why shouldn't your children act up?

P: They shouldn't act up because . . . I am so nice to them.

T: What do you mean?

P: Well, if you're nice, bad things shouldn't happen to you. (At this point, the patient's eyes lit up.)

The therapy focuses explicitly on reducing depressive symptoms and accomplishing other concrete, here-and-now goals that the patient and therapist set collaboratively at the beginning of the therapy. The outcome of the therapy is monitored frequently, ideally weekly, and adjustments are made when the patient is not responding as expected. In contrast to the more traditional psychotherapies, in cognitive therapy the clinician is active and directive, and the focus is on "here and now" problems.

The efficacy of cognitive therapy for depression has been studied in numerous randomized controlled trials (for reviews of this literature, see the Agency for Health Care Policy and Research, 1993; see also DeRubeis and Crits-Christoph, 1998). Results show that cognitive therapy is as effective as antidepressant medications for treating depression. Studies comparing cognitive therapy with other psychotherapies have not shown cognitive therapy to be superior to other psychotherapies; however, it is important to remember that few psychotherapies for depression have been subjected to a randomized controlled trial. Some recent evidence indicates that severely depressed patients benefit most from combined psychotherapy and pharmacotherapy (Thase et al, 1997). Three or four studies (see DeRubeis and Crits-Christoph, 1998) report that patients treated with cognitive therapy relapse less often than patients treated with pharmacotherapy.

Positive Imagery

Singer (1974) pioneered the research, theory, and clinical applications of positive imagery. The idea is simple: engaging in positive imagery tends to elevate one's moods and affects, tends to increase enjoyment, and can decrease the frequency and intensity of potentially debilitating and self-defeating thoughts and feelings. The key idea is that imagery need not be explicitly related to one's difficulties or embody modeled "answers"; it just needs to be pleasant. This approach has been effective in the treatment of pain, anxiety, severe depression, and phobic behavior.

The client presented for psychotherapy with the following pattern of severe anxiety and depression: On awakening each morning, she began to worry about her job, finances, and children. By the time she got to work, she was a "nervous wreck." She often returned home early because of "sickness," and more recently she began missing days of work. Though exhausted at the end of day, she had trouble falling asleep. Anxious about her situation and concerned and sad about the way things were going, she tossed and turned all night.

The treatment plan for modifying various aspects of the client's experiences, habits, and situation included the use of positive imagery. Four times a day (upon awakening and before lunch, dinner, and going to bed), the client spent at least 15 minutes with her eyes closed, thinking of the most pleasant scenes she could imagine. According to her reports during subsequent weeks of therapy, the imagery varied widely and included scenes of vacations she had taken or would like to take, funny scenes, and sexual fantasies. Some imagery was far from realistic (eg, she pictured herself floating high above the clouds). She found that these positive scenes were helpful in "setting the tone" for her days and nights; breaking the momentum generated by her depressive, anxious, and obsessive thoughts; relearning what it felt like to enjoy herself; and freeing her from the depression of what she described as "those days when my worries seemed to snowball and come down and crush me."

MISCONCEPTIONS ABOUT BEHAVIOR-ORIENTED THERAPY

Popular misconceptions and concerns about the use of behavior-oriented therapies are listed and briefly described below.

1. *Behavior therapy is coercive, manipulative, and controlling.* Because behavioral techniques are often powerful, direct approaches to changing behavior, they are criticized for controlling the individual's behavior. Behavior therapists respond to this concern by pointing to the way in which the behavior therapist and patient work closely together as a collaborative team, the way in which the methods of the therapy are completely transparent ("out on the table," understood by both patient and therapist, not mysterious, understood only by the therapist), the way in which much of the therapy is self-directed (eg, homework done outside the session by the patient), and the way in which a central goal of the therapy is to empower patients by teaching them the skills needed to overcome or manage difficulties.

2. *Behavior therapy is superficial, and "symptom substitution" will occur.* Proponents of the theory that many undesired behaviors are symptoms of (or epiphenomena associated with) an underlying disease argue that if only symptoms are addressed, new symptoms will appear at a later date because the underlying problem (ie,

disease) has been left untreated. Extensive empirical data from published reports fail to support any indication of new symptoms occurring after the target behaviors have been removed. In fact, effective treatment of specific target behaviors has often resulted in improvement in other aspects of the clients' lives.

3. *Behavior therapists ignore feelings and treat humans as robots.* This criticism of behavior therapy derives in part from the way cognitive and behavior therapies emphasize the use of techniques and interventions to address clinical problems very directly—even aggressively—in contrast to more traditional therapies, which place greater emphasis on the patient-therapist relationship. Cognitive-behavioral therapists in recent years have begun to recognize the importance of the therapeutic relationship (see Persons, 1989; Safran and Segal, 1990). It is also important to remember that without a strong, trusting relationship with the therapist, patients in cognitive and behavior therapies are unlikely to be willing to carry out the technical interventions of the therapy. A good example of this is exposure therapy, which is frequently quite stressful and difficult for the patient. The effective behavior therapist knows how to use the power of a warm, strong, trusting therapeutic relationship to strengthen the therapy.

4. *Behavior therapy is limited to a narrow spectrum of disorders.* Disorders that seem particularly amenable to behavioral-cognitive psychotherapies are by no means limited to simple phobias but rather span a wide range of difficulties including unipolar depression (Beck et al, 1979), eating disorders (Compas et al, 1998), substance abuse (Beck et al, 1993), obsessive-compulsive disorder (Riggs and Foa, 1993; Steketee and Lam, 1993), marital difficulties (Baucom et al, 1998), panic disorder and agoraphobia (Craske and Barlow, 1993), personality disorders (Beck et al, 1990; Linehan, 1993), autism and other developmental disorders (McEachin et al, 1993), schizophrenia (Wong and Liberman, 1996), bipolar illness (Basco and Rush, 1996), sex offenders (Marshall and Eccles, 1996), trichotillomania (Stanley and Mouton, 1996), and insomnia (Morin et al, 1993). Cognitive-behavioral methods have also been applied to a growing range of patients, including the elderly (Thompson et al, 1987), children (Kendall, 1991), and inpatients (eg, Wright, 1987).

5. *Cognitive-behavior therapy denies the importance of resistance.* Perhaps because behavior therapy and cognitive therapy stood, in their early development, in such contrast to psychodynamic approaches that analyzed resistance, many therapists may have mistakenly assumed that behavioral and cognitive therapy ignored this phenomenon. However, because resistance is manifested in observable behavior and is reflected in client cognitions, behavior therapy and cognitive therapy have developed a variety of specific procedures for addressing resistance, which they often describe using the term "noncompliance." "Recommended strategies for forestalling client resistance include offering a clear rationale for treatment procedures, emphasizing the gradual nature of change, using Socratic dialogue and hypothesis-testing techniques, and conducting thorough task analyses of the patient's problems, skills, and goals that can guide the therapist in the selection of appropriate procedures and homework assignments" (Kendall et al, 1991).

6. *Behavioral-cognitive techniques are practiced only by psychologists and paraprofessionals, not by psychiatrists.* This statement has some validity, although several of the well-known pioneers in these fields are psychiatrists (Wolpe, Agras, Beck). Behavioral techniques can often be implemented by paraprofessionals and the clients themselves. This is seen by many as an advantage, since professional time can be devoted to developing treatment strategies and performing thorough behavioral analyses. Unfortunately, most residency programs for psychiatrists do not include training in basic behavioral science. This is a regrettable situation, since research in behavioral science has led to a number of specific treatment programs and has provided a method of approaching problems that has great clinical value. With the increasing importance of evidence-based approaches to treatment in psychiatry, training opportunities for psychiatrists in cognitive and behavior therapies are likely to increase.

RECENT TRENDS IN BEHAVIOR & COGNITIVE THERAPIES

Several trends have emerged:

1. *With the increase in emphasis on effective and cost-effective treatment, cognitive-behavioral methods will flourish.* Wilson and Agras (1992), in an article on the future of behavior therapy, state that the press for more efficient treatments will lead to an improvement in the dissemination of behavioral techniques. They note that "stripped-down versions" of behavior therapy via computers (eg, Burnett, 1989) are already under way. Treatment manuals describing detailed assessment and application of theory and technique are also predicted to increase (eg, Agras et al, 1989).

2. *New cognitive and behavior therapies will continue to be developed to address additional clinical problems.* Of growing interest to clinicians is the new field of behavioral medicine (see Chapter 36), which involves the use of behavioral and cognitive principles and techniques in the treatment of medical problems such as heart disease, obesity, irritable bowel syndrome, diabetes, cancer, and chronic pain (Compas et al, 1998). Cognitive and behavior therapists are also beginning to develop methods to treat the personality disorders (see Beck et al, 1990; Linehan, 1993). New developments in treatment for children include the application of cognitive and behavior therapies to the treatment of attention-deficit hyperactivity disorder, learning disabilities, depression, and childhood aggression.

3. *Application of cognitive and behavior therapies to heterogeneous, complex disorders and populations will receive increasing attention.* A recent important debate in the literature points to the fact that the randomized clinical trials typically used to demonstrate the efficacy of psychotherapies, including cognitive and behavior therapies, typically study homogeneous populations of patients with one or two disorders, not the heterogeneous samples of patients with multiple comorbidities typically seen in clinical practice (Persons & Silberschatz, 1998). To address this weakness, researchers will begin, and have begun, to study the efficacy of their methods with more complex patients and problems (cf. Linehan's [1993] work with borderline personality disorder). The study of more complex populations is likely to increase the importance of individualized case formulation, a method in which the clinician uses the theory to develop an idiosyncratic formulation of the case and then uses that formulation to guide treatment decisions as the therapy proceeds (see Persons, 1989).

4. *Although the effectiveness of cognitive therapy has been well documented, much is still unknown about how and why cognitive and behavioral therapy works.* Researchers in the field are working to learn more about the process whereby cognitive-behavioral therapies have achieved their results. For example, Castonguay (1992) found evidence for the importance of a common factor—the working alliance—as being the only significant predictor of both the reduction of depressive symptomatology and im-

provement in global functioning in a cognitive therapy.

5. *There will be more integration of cognitive-behavioral approaches with other systems of psychotherapy.* Beck and Haaga (1992), in a paper on the future of cognitive therapy, predicted that the movement toward psychotherapy integration will continue at an accelerated pace and that cognitive-behavioral techniques have much to contribute to future integrative therapies. The fact that most clinicians practicing today were not originally trained in the cognitive and behavior therapies, coupled with the increasing evidence of the effectiveness of these therapies, increases the pressure to find modes of integrating therapies.

6. *There is growing attention to strengthening the effectiveness of cognitive and behavior therapies.* Although cognitive and behavior therapies have been shown to be effective in the treatment of a number of clinical problems, not all patients can comply with the therapies or benefit from them. Thus, for example, the response rate to cognitive therapy for depression is typically about 60%, with 40% of patients failing to show a full response to the treatment. Thus, researchers are working hard to develop new, more effective therapies and to strengthen the therapies already in place.

7. *Cognitive and behavior therapists will devote increasing attention to dissemination of their methods.* Cognitive and behavior therapists are becoming increasingly aware of the fact that although data from randomized trials show many new cognitive and behavior therapies are quite effective, clinicians are slow to adopt these new methods. Increasingly, researchers and others are emphasizing the need to actively work to disseminate the new methods to consumers, clinicians, insurance companies, policymakers, and others. Laypersons have formed organizations such as the Anxiety Disorders Association of America and the Obsessive Compulsive Foundation, which educate their constituents about effective treatments for these disorders, many of which include the behavior and cognitive therapies described here. In addition, there is a growing number of self-help texts and workbooks employing cognitive-behavioral techniques that can be used alone or in conjunction with professional therapy (eg, Barlow and Craske, 1989; Bourne, 1990; Burns, 1980).

REFERENCES & SUGGESTED READINGS

Agency for Health Care Policy and Research, U. S. Public Health Service. *Clinical Practice Guideline Number 5. Depression in Primary Care: Volume 2. Treatment of Major Depression.* Rockville. Maryland, 1993.

Agras WS et al: Cognitive-behavioral and response-prevention treatments for bulimia nervosa. J Consult Clin Psychol 1989;57:215.

Bandura A: *Social Learning Theory.* Prentice-Hall, 1977.

Barber JP, Luborsky L: A psychodynamic view of simple phobias and prescriptive matching: A commentary. Psychotherapy 1991;28:469.

Barlow DH (editor): *Clinical Handbook of Psychological Disorders: A Step-by-Step Treatment Manual,* 2nd ed. Guilford, 1993.

Barlow DH, Craske M: *Mastery of Your Anxiety and Panic.* Graywind, 1989.

Barlow DH et al: Behavioral treatment of panic disorder. Behav Ther 1989;20:261.

Barlow DH, Hayes SC, Nelson RO: *The Scientist-Practitioner: Research and Accountability in Clinical and Educational Settings.* Pergamon, 1984.

Basco MR, Rush AJ: *Cognitive-Behavioral Therapy for Bipolar Disorder.* Guilford, 1996.

Baucom DH et al: Empirically supported couple and family interventions for marital distress and adult mental health problems. J Consult Clin Psychol 1998;66:53.

Beck AT: Is behavior therapy on course? Behav Psychother 1985;13:83.

Beck AT, Haaga DAF: The future of cognitive therapy. Psychotherapy 1992;29:34.

Beck AT et al: *Cognitive Therapy of Depression.* Guilford, 1979.

Beck AT et al: *Cognitive Therapy of Personality Disorders.* Guilford, 1990.

Beck AT et al: *Cognitive Therapy of Substance Abuse.* Guilford, 1993.

Blackburn IM et al: The efficacy of cognitive therapy in depression: A treatment trial using cognitive therapy and pharmacotherapy, each alone and in combination. Br J Psychiatry 1981;139:181.

Borkovec TD, Costello E: Efficacy of applied relaxation and cognitive-behavioral therapy in the treatment of generalized anxiety disorder. J Consult Clin Psychol 1993;61:611.

Bourne EJ: *The Anxiety and Phobia Workbook.* New Harbinger, 1990.

Burnett KF: Computers for assessment and intervention in psychiatry and psychology. Curr Opin Psychiatry 1989;2:780.

Burns DD: *Feeling Good: The New Mood Therapy.* Signet, 1980.

Campbell M et al: Psychopharmacology. In: *Handbook of Autism and Pervasive Developmental Disorders.* Cohen DJ, Donnellan AM (editors). Wiley, 1987.

Castonguay LG: Unique and common factors in cognitive therapy for depression. PhD Dissertation, State University of New York, Stony Brook, 1992.

Compas BE et al: Sampling of empirically supported psychological treatments from health psychology: Smoking, chronic pain, cancer, and bulimia nervosa. J Consult Psychol 1998;66:89.

Craske MG, Barlow DH: Panic disorder and agoraphobia. In: *Clinical Handbook of Psychological Disorders: A Step-by-Step Treatment Manual,* 2nd ed. Barlow DH (editor). Guilford, 1993.

DeRubeis RJ, Crits-Christoph P: Empirically supported individual and group psychological treatments for adult mental disorders. J Consult Clin Psychol 1998;66:37.

Epstein N, Baucom DH: Cognitive-behavioral marital therapy. In: *Comprehensive Handbook of Cognitive Therapy.* Freeman A et al (editors). Plenum, 1989.

Epstein N, Baucom DH, Rankin LA: Treatment of marital conflict: A cognitive-behavioral approach. Clin Psychol Rev 1993;13:45.

Fiske ST, Linville PW: What does the schema concept buy us? Pers Soc Psychol Bull 1980;6:543.

Foa EB, Kozak MJ: Emotional processing of fear: Exposure to corrective information. Psychol Bull 1986;99:20.

Foa EB et al: Treatment of posttraumatic stress disorder in rape victims: A comparison between cognitive-behavioral procedures and counseling. J Consult Clin Psychol 1991;59:715.

Francis G, Beidel D: Cognitive behavioral psychotherapy. In: *Anxiety Disorders in Children and Adolescents.* March JS (editor). Guilford, 1995.

Garner DM et al: Comparison of cognitive-behavioral and supportive-expressive therapy for bulimia nervosa. Am J Psychiatry 1993;150:37.

Gitlin B et al: Behavior therapy for panic disorder. J Nerve Ment Dis 1985;173:742.

Higgins ET: Self-discrepancy theory: What patterns of self beliefs cause people to suffer? Adv Exp Soc Psychol 1989;22:93.

Jacobson E: *Progressive Relaxation.* University of Chicago Press, 1938.

Kendall PC, Holloon S (editors): *Cognitive-Behavioral Interventions: Assessment Methods.* Academic Press, 1982.

Kendall PC: Toward a cognitive-behavioral model of child psychopathology and a critique of related interventions. J Abnorm Child Psychiatry 1985;13:357.

Kendall PC (editor): *Child and Adolescent Therapy: Cognitive Behavioral Procedures.* Guilford, 1991.

Kendall PC, Vitousek KB, Kane M: Thought and action in psychotherapy: Behavioral approaches. In: *The Clinical Psychology Handbook,* 2nd ed. Hersen M, Kazdin AE, Bellack AS (editors). Pergamon, 1991.

Klass ET: Guilt, shame and embarrassment: Cognitive-behavioral approaches. In: *Handbook of Social Anxiety.* Leitenberg H (editor). Plenum, 1990.

Lanyon RI, Lanyon BP: *Behavior Therapy: A Clinical Introduction.* Addison-Wesley, 1978.

Levenson H, Evans S: The current state of brief therapy training in APA-accredited graduate programs and internship programs. *Professional Psychology: Research and Practice,* in press.

Linehan MM: *Cognitive-Behavioral Treatment of Borderline Personality Disorder.* Guilford, 1993.

Lovaas OI, Simmons JQ: Manipulation of self-destruction in three retarded children. J Appl Behav Anal 1969;2:143.

Marks I: *Cure and Care of Neuroses.* Wiley, 1981.

Marshall WL, Eccles A: Cognitive-behavioral treatment of sex offenders. In: *Sourcebook of Psychological Treatment Manuals for Adult Disorders*. Van Hasselt VB, Hersen M (editors). Plenum, 1996.

McEachin JJ, Smith T, Lovaas OI: Long-term outcome for children with autism who received early intensive behavioral treatment. Am J Ment Retard 1993;97:359.

Meichenbaum D: *Cognitive-Behavior Modification: An Integrative Approach*. Plenum, 1977.

Morin CM et al: Cognitive-behavior therapy for late-life insomnia. J Consult Clin Psychol 1993;61:137.

Norcross JC, Prochaska JO, Gallagher KM: Clinical psychologists in the 1980s: Theory, research, and practice. Clin Psychol 1989;42:45.

Paul GL, Lentz RL: *Psychological Treatment of Chronic Mental Patients*. Harvard University Press, 1977.

Persons JB: *Cognitive Therapy in Practice: A Case Formulation Approach*. Norton, 1989.

Persons JB, Burns DD, Perloff JM: Predictors of dropout and outcome in cognitive therapy for depression in a private practice setting. Cognitive Ther Res 1989;12:557.

Persons JB, Silberschatz G: Are results of randomized controlled trials useful to psychotherapists? J Consult Clin Psychol 1998;66:126.

Pilkonis PA et al: Course of depressive symptoms over follow-up: Findings from the National Institute of Mental Health treatment of depression collaborative research program. Arch Gen Psychiatry 1992;49:782.

Riggs DS, Foa E: Obsessive compulsive disorder. In: *Clinical Handbook of Psychological Disorders: A Step-by-Step Treatment Manual*, 2nd ed. Barlow DH (editor). Guilford, 1993.

Safran JD, Segal ZV: *Interpersonal Process in Cognitive Therapy*. Basic Books, 1990.

Seligman MEP: Foreword. In: *Comprehensive Casebook of Cognitive Therapy*. Freeman A, Dattilio FM (editors). Plenum, 1992.

Singer JL: *Imagery and Daydream Methods in Psychotherapy and Behavior Modification*. Academic Press, 1974.

Smith D: Trends in counselling and psychotherapy. Am Psychol 1982;37:802.

Sokol L et al: Cognitive therapy of panic disorder: A nonpharmacological alternative. J Nerv Ment Dis 1989;177:711.

Stanley MA, Mouton SG: Trichotillomania treatment manual. In: *Sourcebook of Psychological Treatment Manuals for Adult Disorders*. Van Hasselt VB, Hersen M (editors). Plenum, 1996.

Steketee G, Lam J: Obsessive-compulsive disorder. In: *Handbook of Effective Psychotherapy*. Giles TR (editor). Plenum, 1993.

Thase ME et al: Treatment of major depression with psychotherapy or psychotherapy-pharmacotherapy combinations. Arch Gen Psychol 1997;54:1009.

Thompson LW, Gallagher D, Breckenridge JS: Comparative effectiveness of psychotherapies for depressed elders. J Consult Clin Psychol 1987;55:385.

Turkat ID, Maisto SA: Personality disorders: Application of the experimental method to the formulation and modification of personality disorders. In: *Clinical Handbook of Psychological Disorders*. Barlow DH (editor). Guilford, 1985.

Turner S, Calhoun KS, Adams HE: *Handbook of Clinical Behavior Therapy*. Wiley, 1981.

Wilson GT, Agras WS: The future of behavior therapy. Psychotherapy 1992;29:39.

Wolpe J: *Psychotherapy by Reciprocal Inhibition*. Stanford University Press, 1958.

Wong SE, Liberman RP: Biobehavioral treatment and rehabilitation for persons with schizophrenia. In: *Sourcebook of Psychological Treatment Manuals for Adult Disorders*. Van Hasselt VB, Hersen M (editors). Plenum, 1996.

Wright JH: Cognitive therapy and medication as combined treatment. In: *Cognitive Therapy: Applications in Psychiatric and Medical Settings*. Freeman A, Greenwood V (editors). Human Sciences Press, 1987.

Group Psychotherapy

34

Nick Kanas, MD

Group psychotherapy is a form of treatment in which beneficial changes in emotionally disturbed patients occur as a result of their interactions with other patients and at least one trained professional therapist in a group setting. Therapeutic results include both relief of symptoms and resolution of intrapsychic and interpersonal problems. The therapist's tools are clinical experience and applied theories of individual psychodynamics and interpersonal systems.

HISTORY OF GROUP PSYCHOTHERAPY

The first psychotherapy group was described in 1907 by Joseph Pratt, a Boston internist, who developed a group method of educating and improving the morale of patients with tuberculosis. Around 1910, Jacob Moreno in Europe began using theatrical techniques to have patients "act out" problem situations in a group setting; this later became known as psychodrama. In the late 1920s and early 1930s, a number of psychiatrists began applying psychoanalytic theory to groups, emphasizing issues of transference, free association, and recapitulation of family problems.

During the late 1930s and early 1940s, Kurt Lewin began emphasizing the importance of group member interactions and introduced the notion of group dynamics, a phenomenon describing actions in a group as being more than the sum of individual interactions. The need to train more therapists in the theory of group dynamics became obvious after World War II, when large numbers of veterans requiring psychiatric assistance began to overburden the personnel resources of the mental health system. Programs to train therapists using Lewin's concepts were established at the National Training Laboratories in Maine and at the Tavistock Clinic in England, where the work of Bion and Ezriel led to the "group-as-a-whole" approach to treatment.

During the ensuing 30 years, numerous approaches to group psychotherapy were introduced, including transactional analysis, and gestalt (which now are often combined in redecision therapy), interpersonal, existential, and behavioral approaches. Currently, techniques borrowed from a number of theoretical schools are being consolidated to devise new responses to the specific needs of patients. Managed care pressures are encouraging therapists to develop groups that are cost effective and short term.

EFFECTIVENESS OF GROUP PSYCHOTHERAPY

Clinical experience and anecdotal evidence support the view that group psychotherapy is effective treatment for properly selected categories of patients. Successes have been reported in both inpatient and outpatient settings with both psychotic and nonpsychotic patients. A number of theoretical approaches to group psychotherapy have been advocated.

Evidence from controlled studies also attests to the usefulness of group psychotherapy. A number of reviews have concluded that group psychotherapy is effective for patients with personality and anxiety disorders; substance-related disorders; schizophrenia; depressive and stable bipolar disorders; and medical illnesses, including asthma, myocardial infarction, obesity, chronic pain, and ulcers. Group psychotherapy has been found to be as effective as or even more effective than individual psychotherapy in studies directly comparing the two methods.

INDICATIONS & CONTRAINDICATIONS FOR GROUP PSYCHOTHERAPY

In organizing a psychotherapy group, the therapist must take into account both diagnostic and individual psychodynamic factors.

Diagnostic Factors

A. Indications for Psychotherapy in Heterogeneous Groups: Table 34–1 shows disorders for which treatment in a heterogeneous group (ie, consisting of a variety of psychiatric disorders) is most appropriate. In such groups, the diversity of problems and issues allows for maximal interaction and breadth of discussion. In establishing the group, the therapist should consider whether one patient will be perceived as "too different" by the others, since this may result in scapegoating and rejection. For example, an elderly woman in a group of young adults might be rejected by the other members even though

Table 34–1. Indications and contraindications for group psychotherapy, based on diagnostic considerations.

Indications
Most personality disorders[a]
Most anxiety disorders[a]
Somatoform disorders[a]
Substance-related disorders[b]
Schizophrenia and related psychotic disorders[b]
Stable bipolar disorders[b]
Posttraumatic stress disorder[b]
Eating disorders[b]
Medical illness[b]
Depressive disorders[c]
Adjustment disorders[c]

Contraindications
Acute manic episode
Antisocial personality disorder

Questionable[d]
Schizoid personality disorder[a]
Paranoid personality disorder[a]
Cognitive disorders[a]
Sleep disorders[a]
Dissociative disorders[a]
Factitious disorders[a]
Sexual and gender identity disorders[c]

[a] Therapy in heterogeneous groups (ie, groups of patients with different disorders) is recommended.
[b] Therapy in homogeneous groups (ie, groups of patients with same disorder) is recommended.
[c] The type of group (heterogeneous or homogeneous) depends on the individual case.
[d] The decision about the appropriateness of group psychotherapy is based on factors such as the patient's degree of impairment and desire for treatment and on individual psychodynamic factors.

she is in the group to work on issues unrelated to aging. If at least two elderly patients are in the group, the tendency to scapegoat would be lessened.

Group psychotherapy with heterogeneous groups is particularly beneficial for patients with most personality and anxiety disorders. Patients with personality disorders tend to blame others for their maladaptive interactions and lack insight into their own role in provoking interpersonal strife. Since they do not have significant degrees of anxiety or other symptoms, they are only weakly motivated to change and often come to treatment at the urging of a spouse, employer, or primary-care physician. The group psychotherapy setting is an environment in which such patients can display and then be confronted with their maladaptive interactions. At the same time, other group members can offer support and reinforcement for positive changes, and this "reward" encourages them to remain in treatment.

In contrast to patients with personality disorders, patients with anxiety disorders often have a number of symptoms, such as phobias and compulsive behavior, and perceive their difficulties as coming from within. For these reasons, anxious patients do well in individual psychotherapy, although many also benefit from group psychotherapy. Such patients use the

group to gain insight into the cause of their problems and to understand the effects their symptoms may have on other people.

Other patients benefiting from heterogeneous group psychotherapy include those with somatoform disorders. Such patients do well in supportive group settings, in which the impact of their symptoms on others can be explored. In some cases they may also gain insight into the causes of their problems.

B. Indications for Psychotherapy in Homogeneous Groups: Table 34–1 shows disorders for which a homogeneous group format is more appropriate. All of the patients have a similar problem, and the group is oriented toward addressing that problem. Homogeneous psychotherapy groups differ from support groups involving interaction with people who share some common problem in that the approach is more insight oriented and the leader is professionally trained. For example, a psychotherapy group made up of alcoholics differs from a meeting of Alcoholics Anonymous in that patients in psychotherapy not only gain support and encouragement for sobriety but also focus on problems related to their alcoholism, such as intrapsychic conflict and maladaptive interpersonal relationships. Although more limited in scope than their heterogeneous counterparts, homogeneous groups quickly become cohesive and allow for greater depth in exploring a particular set of problems.

Group psychotherapy in a homogeneous group is the treatment of choice for patients with substance-related disorders. By orienting these groups around the addiction problem, several issues that affect the patients in similar ways may be discussed. Such groups are particularly useful for confronting patients who deny having the diagnosed problem. For example, group psychotherapy of alcoholics should emphasize abstinence as the treatment goal and deal specifically with members' denial. The predisposing causes of alcoholism should be explored only after its manifold sequelae are thoroughly discussed. At all times, confrontation and frank discussion should be tempered with support, advice, and reinforcement of positive changes.

Although a few stable schizophrenics can be treated in heterogeneous groups, most schizophrenics do better in homogeneous groups. In heterogeneous groups consisting of both psychotic and nonpsychotic patients, it is difficult to create a group environment meeting the needs of both populations. For example, the use of uncovering techniques may help a nonpsychotic patient, but self-disclosure may produce intolerable anxiety in a schizophrenic patient. Conversely, education and reality testing may help a psychotic patient but be experienced as unbearably boring by a less disturbed group member. Schizophrenics do well in homogeneous groups emphasizing controlled expression of emotions, reality testing, and socialization and contact with others.

Homogeneous groups are beneficial for patients suffering from chronic pain and illness such as asthma, myocardial infarction, and cancer. In such groups, themes involving disfigurement or loss of function, the responses of loved ones, and the fear of death can be raised and dealt with in a supportive, caring manner.

For treatment of some conditions, such as depressive or adjustment disorders, either homogeneous or heterogeneous group psychotherapy may be indicated. The choice in specific cases depends on the nature and severity of the problem, the availability of other patients with a similar problem to participate in a group, and the desires of the leader to form a specialized group that is oriented toward a single issue.

C. Contraindications to Group Psychotherapy: Group psychotherapy is not for everyone. Overstimulation in the group environment causes patients with acute manic episodes to become more hyperactive and pressured, although recent evidence suggests that patients with stable bipolar disorders do well in homogeneous groups. Patients with severe antisocial personality disorders who are more interested in manipulating others than in improving their interpersonal relationships usually hinder group progress.

D. Questionable Indications for Group Psychotherapy: Table 34–1 lists several disorders for which group psychotherapy is "questionably" indicated. The decision about whether group psychotherapy is indicated depends on factors such as the degree of impairment, desire for treatment, and individual psychodynamic factors.

Individual Psychodynamic Factors

Along with general diagnostic considerations, individual psychodynamic factors must also be assessed in pondering referral for group psychotherapy. Since intrapsychic conflicts influence and are influenced by interpersonal relationships, it is helpful if patients can view their problems in terms of difficulties experienced in relationships with others. Some therapists view this capacity as a criterion of the potential for gaining insight and making progress in group psychotherapy.

The process of uncovering unconscious conflicts can provoke strong feelings. For some patients, transference feelings evoked in a group setting are more intense than those that arise in individual therapy; for others, the group setting is more tolerable because transference feelings can be distributed among other group members in addition to the therapist. Patients with problems resulting from unconscious conflicts may benefit from group psychotherapy, particularly if they are unable to tolerate transference feelings evoked in individual psychotherapy.

Group psychotherapy is particularly useful for patients whose psychodynamic problems lead to maladaptive interpersonal relationships, since these inter-actions can be observed and explored in the group. For example, authority or dependency conflicts may be observed in the way some group members relate to each other or to the group leader.

Extremely manipulative patients, inveterate malingerers, and those who are socially deviant or engage in extreme acting-out behavior do not do well in group psychotherapy except in controlled settings. Patients must have some ability to relate to others and tolerate individual differences. For this reason, patients with schizoid or paranoid personality disorder often do poorly in the group setting. Group psychotherapy patients need adequate impulse control so they can tolerate confrontation with other group members. Patients with severe cognitive disorders may become confused or anxious in group psychotherapy. Finally, patients in acute distress who are unable to tolerate the process of assimilation as new members usually do better in individual psychotherapy, where their needs can be tended to more quickly and specifically.

PRACTICAL CONSIDERATIONS IN ESTABLISHING & LEADING THE GROUP

In setting up a psychotherapy group, the therapist should take into account its setting and purpose, the types of patients to be included, what their treatment goals will probably be, and whether they have complementary personality characteristics.

Numbers of Patients; Age Ranges

Most groups have 6–12 patients, with eight often considered the optimal number. Having four or fewer patients inhibits free expression because members are afraid to disagree lest someone drop out, which would mean that the sessions would have to be discontinued. With more than 12, there is too little time for each patient. Inpatient groups tend to be **open,** which means that new patients are admitted to the group as others are discharged. Outpatient groups may be open or closed. In **closed** groups, the makeup stays the same for long periods without addition of new members.

The age range of patients in most groups is 20–60 years, with adolescent and geriatric patients often being treated in homogeneous groups formed specifically for the purpose of dealing with their problems. Some therapists advocate separate groups for young (20–40 years) and middle-aged (40–60 years) adults.

Preparatory Sessions for Patients Entering the Group

Most therapists advocate preparatory sessions for prospective group members. A variety of formats for these sessions can be used, ranging from a brief one-to-one discussion with the therapist to participation in a minigroup in which patients sample the group experience by undergoing a number of structured exercises. Preparation reduces the patient's anxiety over what to expect, establishes a working alliance between therapist and patient, and allows the therapist to observe the patient's reactions in a structured interpersonal setting. Careful preparation significantly reduces the number of dropouts and improves attendance at the sessions. A combined factual-experiential approach is more effective than just providing factual information about "what group psychotherapy is all about."

Whether or not a patient goes through a preparatory phase, the therapist should have some indication of how the patient interacts with others. One way to find out is to ask about the patient's experience with other kinds of groups (at church, at the office, etc). A more direct approach would be to draw the patient's attention to the process of interaction during the interview. The patient's response—particularly the degree of defensiveness or interest in this novel way of looking at behavior—will serve as a clue to his or her later behavior in the group.

Ground Rules

Ground rules regarding timely attendance, payment of fees, notification of planned absences, and discussion of issues before making major life changes are important aspects of the group. Patients will sometimes violate these rules for psychodynamic and interpersonal reasons. The therapist should monitor such behavior and not hesitate to bring it up in the group for general discussion.

A patient who becomes threatening or disruptive may have to be temporarily excluded from the group. The reasons should be explained to the patient and discussed with the other members. When stable and in control again, the patient may reenter the group.

Frequency & Duration of Therapy

Most psychotherapy groups meet once or twice a week, although inpatient groups and psychodynamically oriented outpatient groups may meet three to five times a week. A typical session lasts 1–2 hours.

The duration of therapy in inpatient groups is influenced by the average length of hospitalization, which is less than a month in most acute care units. For this reason, inpatient groups are usually characterized by rapid turnover. Outpatient groups tend to be longer term, with some patients remaining in the group months to years, depending on their problems and treatment goals. Briefer, time-limited outpatient groups (lasting 1–4 months) generally emphasize the establishment of realistic, limited treatment goals—eg, the resolution of current problems rather than the uncovering of unconscious conflicts—and the use of didactic and supportive techniques. In these groups, therapists tend to take an active role, encouraging patient responsibility and focusing on practical issues.

Careful patient selection and pretraining are critical for the success of therapy in short-term groups.

Number of Therapists

Managed care and pressures to be cost effective frequently allow for no more than one therapist per group. However, some groups use a **co-therapy model,** in which two therapists are present. Both therapists should have roughly equal training and experience so that one will not be perceived as "junior" and be scapegoated by the group. Since sessions may be disrupted or made ineffective by competition or by theoretical or technical differences of opinion between therapists, co-therapists should work to maintain a good relationship. Male-female co-therapy teams are effective in encouraging discussion of parental, gender, and sexual themes.

Advantages of co-therapy include enhanced objectivity in assessment of patients, resulting from discussion between the therapists after group sessions; the potential for increased transference feelings in the group; continuity of the group when one therapist goes on vacation or becomes ill; and better control of the group in times of crisis (eg, admission of a hostile, disruptive patient).

Combined Individual & Group Psychotherapy

Some patients undergo both individual and group psychotherapy at the same time. In some cases, the therapist is the same in both settings; in other cases, the patient has one therapist for group psychotherapy and a different one for individual psychotherapy. Most therapists prefer the former, since the patient can be managed without the need for time-consuming and perhaps conflictual communication with another therapist. Some group patients not receiving combined therapy resent another member's private access to the therapist; however, this competitive issue can usually be dealt with in the group.

Adding group psychotherapy for patients in individual psychotherapy is recommended if the patient does not make adequate progress in the one-to-one situation and if it appears that the group setting would allow the patient to experiment with new ways of relating to others. The challenge and stimulation of group interaction can uncover problems in personality function while at the same time providing relief from a one-to-one treatment focus.

Adding individual psychotherapy for patients in group psychotherapy is recommended if the patient has difficulty sharing problems in a group setting, if the patient wants to intensify efforts to resolve a particular problem or conflict, or if it is felt that a sudden crisis or stressful event in the patient's life can be dealt with more quickly and effectively in individual treatment.

Problems of resistance or countertransference arising in one treatment setting should be dealt with in that setting; the issue should not be avoided by recommending both individual and group psychotherapy. If there is a danger that the dissonance resulting from two treatment approaches might overrun fragile defenses, combined treatment should not be used.

Format of Sessions

Most psychotherapy groups are **discussion oriented.** Patients are expected to talk about problems and other significant aspects of their personal lives. They are encouraged to divulge feelings, be open and honest, and listen to issues involving other patients. Some issues directed toward the therapist may be referred back to the group, with the therapist asking what the members think about that issue. To stimulate discussion, the therapist may utilize a technique called the "go-around," in which each patient is asked in turn to express his or her thoughts about the issue at hand. In other group psychotherapy approaches, a lecture format may be used during part of the session, with interpersonal and intrapsychic issues diagrammed on a blackboard. Videotape playback is also used in some group settings to stimulate discussion.

Some psychotherapy groups are more **action oriented.** In psychodrama, patients are asked to assume roles (spouses, parents, etc) in acting out a specific problem. In some behavioral approaches, patients practice techniques aimed at resolution of symptoms, such as systematic desensitization (see Chapter 33). Groups focusing on cognitive and behavioral techniques have been used successfully with patients suffering from anxiety and depressive disorders. In activity groups such as music or art therapy groups, patients meet to engage in activities that serve as a basis for intrapsychic and interpersonal learning.

GROUP DYNAMICS

When people come together in groups for any purpose, forces are set in motion that affect each member. Such forces are a feature of collective human behavior and go beyond the dynamics of dyadic (in pairs) interactions. For example, a normally nonviolent, law-abiding person may commit arson and other violent crimes in the context of a mob.

The therapist must be aware of the collective forces operating in a psychotherapy group at any given moment. Since the group environment exerts strong pressures on the members, the results may be negative as well as positive. The therapist's role is to maximize the therapeutic potential of the group environment for each individual. For example, in group settings where open and honest interactions occur, the members gradually learn the importance of free exchange of ideas and feelings and can apply these principles in their daily lives. If feelings are kept bottled up during group sessions and the therapist does not encourage their expression, group work will be unproductive, and patients will be less inclined to express themselves openly in daily life.

Each individual in the group is affected by his or her perceptions of what other members think and feel about various issues. In psychotherapy groups, many (perhaps all) patients often have the same perception, which can be called a **group norm.** Group norms exert powerful predictive forces (pressure to conform) on the actions of individual members. If an individual's view of what is normative in a group is not in accord with reality, the discrepancy provides clues to psychodynamic and psychopathological factors affecting that member. For example, a withdrawn, paranoid patient might perceive the group setting as hostile and nonsupportive even though most of the other members see it as a place in which they can express their concerns in a friendly environment. Such discrepancies alert the therapist to important issues of individual and group dynamics, issues that become "grist for the therapeutic mill."

The therapist may sometimes wish to comment on a significant characteristic of the group, such as its avoidance of a specific topic. For example, a group member makes a suicidal gesture; in the next group session it would not be unusual for members to avoid this topic, talking about emotionally bland or trivial matters or behaving in a pressured, anxious manner. This resistance can be overcome by a simple comment: "Many of you seem anxious today. I wonder if John's overdose has something to do with that." In most instances, the patients will then begin to discuss their feelings (anger, sadness, guilt). Such **process comments** are usually intended to provide opportunities for insight into psychodynamic or interpersonal issues or to dispel group resistance to a topic.

PHASES OF GROUP DEVELOPMENT

The group environment is affected by several factors, including the personalities of group members; the style and therapeutic stance of the therapist; the physical setting, ie, whether inpatient or outpatient; and, perhaps most importantly, the phase of group development. A developmental sequence of phases can be observed to occur in all groups but is most obvious in long-term, closed outpatient groups. Progress from one phase to another is dependent on successful resolution of issues involving the previous phase. Group development may cease to progress if this resolution does not occur.

Although numerous phases have been described, most conceptual models portray four main phases of group development. The **first phase** is characterized by hesitant participation and the establishment of initial group norms; the members depend on the therapist for guidance and approval. During this phase, the members should be able to perceive some common purpose in being there and declare their individual goals, while the therapist works in a quiet way to encourage the establishment of bonds between members. The **second phase** is characterized by conflict, dominance, and the establishment of a hierarchy ("pecking order") among the patients. The therapist is often seen as an appropriate focus of rebellion, and fantasies may be entertained of excluding the therapist from the group. Several patients may band together to attack verbally or exclude a particular patient from their discussions, thereby identifying that patient as the group scapegoat. An important task of the leader is to help the group deal constructively with these aggressive tendencies. In the **third phase,** true group cohesiveness is established along with a sense of intimacy, mutual affection, and need for each other. Overdependence or rebellion against the therapist has been worked through, and the therapist is reintegrated with the group. Much productive group work can be accomplished in the third phase. The **fourth phase** occurs when the group terminates. It may last for several sessions as the members say good-bye, review their progress, and prepare for life without the group.

THERAPEUTIC FACTORS

The benefits of group psychotherapy may be enhanced by the therapist's recognition of factors that contribute to improvement in a patient's condition. In his classical work, Yalom has described a method of studying some of these therapeutic factors, which include altruism, cohesiveness, universality, interpersonal learning (both input and output), guidance, catharsis, identification, family reenactment, self-understanding, installation of hope, and existential factors. At the time of discharge, patients are given 60 statements describing these 12 potentially helpful attributes of their experience in group psychotherapy and are asked to rank the statements from most to least helpful. The ranking of statements is then used to create a similar ranking of the 12 therapeutic factors. Psychiatric outpatients tend to value their group experience for (1) giving them feedback on interpersonal behavior, (2) allowing them an opportunity to vent repressed feelings, (3) giving them a sense of acceptance by other people, and (4) helping them discover unconscious motivations for what they do. In contrast, psychiatric inpatients tend to value their group experience for (1) giving them feelings of optimism through watching other patients improve and leave the hospital, (2) giving them a sense of acceptance by other people, (3) improving self-esteem through their ability to help others, and (4) allowing them to feel less isolated. It is apparent that what is considered therapeutic in a group may vary depending on the type of patient in the group, the group setting, and the length of stay. The therapist should keep these issues in mind and make appropriate use of the therapeutic factors that are most suited to the patients' needs.

TYPES OF PSYCHOTHERAPY GROUPS

Psychotherapy groups can be categorized in a number of ways: inpatient versus outpatient, experiential versus didactic, supportive versus uncovering, affective versus cognitive, etc. Table 34–2 categorizes a number of psychotherapy groups in terms of their theoretical orientation. The therapeutic goals of most of these groups are relief of symptoms and resolution of intrapsychic and interpersonal problems. However, these goals are achieved in different ways.

Table 34–2. Types of psychotherapy groups.

Theoretical Orientation of Group	Major Goals	Importance of Patient-Therapist Transference Interpretations	Importance of Group Member Interactions	Importance of Here-and-Now Emphasis	Further Reading
Psychodynamic	Resolution of intrapsychic problems	Extremely important	Moderately important	Moderately important	Rutan (1992)
Interpersonal	Resolution of intrapsychic and interpersonal problems	Minimally important	Extremely important	Extremely important	Leszcz (1992)
Redecision	Resolution of intrapsychic problems	Minimally important	Minimally important	Extremely important	Gladfelter (1992)
Psychodrama	Resolution of intrapsychic and interpersonal problems	Minimally important	Moderately important	Extremely important	Kipper (1992)
Existential	Awareness of basic problems affecting existence	Minimally important	Extremely important	Extremely important	Mullan (1992)
Behavioral	Resolution of symptoms	Minimally important	Moderately important	Moderately important	Ellis (1992)

In some groups, the projection of unconscious conflicts onto the therapist is seen as crucial, and transference interpretations are viewed as major therapeutic interventions. In other groups, patient interactions are seen as prominent group activities, since they stimulate the discussion of interpersonal issues through which patients learn more about their behavior outside of the group. The focus of some groups is on activities that occur in the group itself (**here-and-now approach**), whereas other groups emphasize past events and activities that occurred outside the group (**there-and-then approach**). Many psychotherapy groups use a combination of theoretical principles borrowed from several of the schools represented in Table 34–2. When used in an appropriate and clinically relevant manner, this eclectic approach provides the therapist with a number of techniques to meet the needs of patients.

Issues and conflicts addressed in group psychotherapy may be categorized as affecting the entire group (**group-as-a-whole approach**) or affecting an individual or part of the group. Particularly in early group sessions—when members may display similar affects, such as depression or helplessness, together with an attitude of dependency on the leader—the focus may be on issues and events that affect the group as a whole. As the group develops, and as more differentiated and individualized responses and reactions occur, it may be necessary to intervene at the level of the individual or discuss interactions between several individuals. Theoretical approaches must be flexible enough to account for such developmental factors, and techniques should include both group- and individual-level interventions.

SUMMARY

Group psychotherapy is an established method of treatment in which patients may achieve relief of symptoms and resolution of intrapsychic and interpersonal problems as a result of interactions with other patients and the therapist, both in inpatient and in outpatient settings. Diagnostic considerations and individual psychodynamic factors should be taken into account in referring patients to a suitable group, and there are few absolute contraindications. Therapy groups may be heterogeneous (mixed disorders) or homogeneous (same disorder), open or closed. Adequate preparation of patients for group psychotherapy reduces the number of dropouts. Groups using a co-therapist team approach offer several advantages over groups with just one therapist. Some patients benefit from being treated both individually and in a group during the same period.

Group therapists must be aware of issues involving individual psychodynamics, group dynamics, group development, and specific therapeutic factors relevant to the group. Most therapists use a combination of theoretical principles and techniques in constructing psychotherapy groups that best meet the needs of their patients.

REFERENCES & SUGGESTED READINGS

Ellis A: Group rational-emotive and cognitive-behavioral therapy. Int J Group Psychother 1992;42:63.

Gladfelter J: Redecision therapy. Int J Group Psychother 1992;42:319.

Kanas N: Group psychotherapy with bipolar patients: A review and synthesis. Int J Group Psychother 1993;43:321.

Kanas N: *Group Therapy for Schizophrenic Patients.* American Psychiatric Press, 1996.

Kaplan HI, Sadock BJ (editors): *Comprehensive Group Psychotherapy,* 3rd ed. Williams & Wilkins, 1993.

Kapur R, Miller K, Mitchell G: Therapeutic factors within in-patient and out-patient psychotherapy groups. Br J Psychiatry 1988;152:229.

Kipper DA: Psychodrama: Group psychotherapy through role playing. Int J Group Psychother 1992;42:495.

Leszcz M: The interpersonal approach to group psychotherapy. Int J Group Psychother 1992;42:37.

Leszcz M: Introduction to special issue on group psychotherapy for the medically ill. Int J Group Psychother 1998; 48:137.

Mullan H: "Existential" therapists and their group therapy practices. Int J Group Psychother 1992;42:453.

Piper WE, Joyce AS: A consideration of factors influencing the utilization of time-limited, short-term group therapy. Int J Group Psychother 1996;46:311.

Rutan JS: Psychodynamic group psychotherapy. Int J Group Psychother 1992;42:19.

Steenbarger BN, Budman SH: Group psychotherapy and managed behavioral health care: Current trends and future challenges. Int J Group Psychother 1996;46:297.

Tillitski CJ: A meta-analysis of estimated effect sizes for group versus individual versus control treatments. Int J Group Psychother 1990;40:215.

Vandervoort DJ, Fuhriman A: The efficacy of group therapy for depression: A review of the literature. Small Group Res 1991;22:320.

Vinogradov S, Yalom ID: *A Concise Guide to Group Psychotherapy.* American Psychiatric Press, 1989.

Yalom ID: *The Theory and Practice of Group Psychotherapy.* Basic Books, 1970.

35

Family & Marital Therapy

Rodney J. Shapiro, PhD

Contemporary family therapy offers an array of seemingly contradictory theories and practices, but some basic assumptions clearly distinguish family therapy from other psychotherapeutic approaches. A fundamental assumption common to all models of family therapy is that disturbed psychological functioning is not limited to a single individual but reflects disturbed interactions between persons who have significant relationships with each other. The family is the primary context in which important relationships develop and endure.

Family therapists are not primarily concerned with the origins of dysfunction, which are regarded as hypothetical and not amenable to change through psychotherapy. The emphasis instead is on the present and on the patterns of family interaction that sustain existing problems. The therapist can evaluate problems and design interventions on the basis of data provided by family members or observable in the treatment setting. The goal of family therapy is not to change the individual but to set right the system of relationships in which the individual is involved. This may then result in change in one or more family members.

ORIGINS & DEVELOPMENT OF FAMILY THERAPY

Research Contributions

Family therapy is a relatively recent development in the history of psychiatry. The primary concepts grew out of research conducted during the 1950s and 1960s that explored the families of schizophrenic adolescents and young adults. Murray Bowen is generally regarded as a dominant figure in the history of family therapy. His studies led him to view families as systems that facilitate or impede individual ego differentiation. A central premise, for Bowen, was that there is a direct relationship between differentiation of self and psychological dysfunction. Another major component of his work was his multigenerational model of family dynamics. He noted that problems unresolved in one generation tend to be transmitted through succeeding generations. Bowen's ideas were translated into a distinctive treatment approach that continues to attract a strong following.

Wynne and his coworkers generated a series of important studies on schizophrenia. Their rigorously designed research demonstrated an association between thought disorder in schizophrenics and patterns of deviant communication in their parents. Family therapists have long recognized the clinical relevance of these findings. Therapists who work with families of psychotics continue to regard clear and unambiguous communication as an essential goal for symptomatic improvement.

In the early 1950s, the anthropologist Gregory Bateson assembled a research team that included Jay Haley, Don Jackson, and John Weakland, future leaders in the field of family therapy. This creative group broke with existing models of psychopathology by basing their work on the assumption that all behavior (even symptoms) can be defined as communication. They explored patterns of communication in families, and their "double-bind" theory attracted considerable attention when it was first published in 1956. They postulated that schizophrenics are often beset by contradictory messages from parents that are impossible to ignore and yet cannot be responded to in any rational manner. The implication of this theory was that double-binding communication plays a role in the etiology of psychosis, but this idea was subsequently modified as it became evident that the double bind is not confined to schizophrenic family functioning and has no causal relationship with the development of psychosis. However, this group's studies on communication have greatly influenced the concepts and practices of family therapy.

Don Jackson took the lead in formulating clinical applications of the group's studies of communication, and his ideas continue to be fundamentally important for family therapists. He formulated the concept of "family homeostasis" to describe how interacting roles and behaviors tend toward maintaining the family system in a state of equilibrium. Patterned sequences of communication (feedback loops) ensure that parameters of permissible change are not breached. Dysfunctional families are particularly rigid and resistant to change. For example, freedom of expression may not be permitted even when it could be adaptive. Healthier families can tolerate greater degrees of change, sometimes even resulting in a new homeostatic system.

Systems Theory & Cybernetics

General systems theory does not conform to the precise criteria of a scientific theory in that it lacks specificity and has not been validated with objective testing. In the strictest sense it is not a theory as much as it is a point of view, a way of understanding that became accepted in many of the natural sciences during the 1950s. Until this time, the focus in biology and psychology was on the individual organism. The environment was regarded as something "outside there" that exerted influence and elicited reactions. As biologists began to observe animals in their natural habitat, and social scientists studied small-group behavior, a shift in understanding occurred. The individual organism is inseparable from the environment. One cannot be understood without the other. They comprise an interacting whole, a system. The notion of a single unit, out of context, is an artificial construct. The human organism is a complex biological and psychological open system in constant interaction with the environment. This perspective was adopted as the cornerstone of what became known as family systems theory.

A particular aspect of systems theory, known as the cybernetic model, explains the mechanics of self-regulating systems (such as homeostatic biological processes). This model was adopted by family therapists to explain how interactional patterns in families are regulated by communication transmitted through recurring feedback loops. The cybernetic principle demonstrates a fundamental tenet of family therapy known as circular causality. Traditional theories of psychology are based on linear causality, ie, a temporal sequence of cause leading to effect: A > B, B > C, C > D, etc. To understand a patient's current behavior, the therapist explores a chain of past events stemming from the original cause. The key assumption in family therapy is that problems or symptoms are maintained and reinforced by interactional patterns of communication. The past is deemphasized, and the focus is on the present for understanding and treatment of psychological problems.

Clinical Innovators

The first generation of practicing family therapists came to prominence in the early 1960s. Nathan Ackerman and Virginia Satir were among the first to adapt psychodynamic principles of individual therapy to treatment of the family unit. They were celebrated for their imaginative formulations and clinical skills. Their techniques for establishing rapport and overcoming resistance have been incorporated into mainstream family therapy. Carl Whitaker stands out as a uniquely innovative clinician whose ideas continue to influence the practice of family therapy, particularly in terms of integrating intrapsychic and interactional dynamics. A point he emphasized is the tendency for the therapist to become a target for family projections. To prevent this the therapist must rely on subjective cues (warning signs) to avoid acting out the unconscious wishes of the family. The importance of therapist self-awareness remains a guiding principle of psychodynamic family therapy.

PRIMARY MODELS OF FAMILY THERAPY

The initial schism in the field of family therapy occurred over the acceptance or rejection of psychoanalytic theory. Although many of the originators of family therapy were trained in psychoanalysis and some retained their psychodynamic views, the majority renounced psychoanalysis as incompatible with family therapy.

The movement away from psychoanalysis steadily gained momentum, with the result that the currently dominant models of family therapy reflect an almost complete break with psychoanalytic theory and practice. Interpretation has little or no place in contemporary family therapy, insight is regarded as irrelevant for change, and the subjective states of client and therapist are largely ignored; the emphasis is on actual behavior and active treatment interventions. However, recently emerging developments in the field now include some reconsideration of the relevance of subjective states and the influence of past experience.

Structural Family Therapy

Salvador Minuchin developed his model of structural family therapy during the 1960s and 1970s and, until very recently, it was the most influential and widely practiced form of family therapy. Central to Minuchin's work is the concept of the family as a structural organization established by the hierarchic arrangement of relationships and the boundaries between family subgroups and members. In a well-functioning family, there is a clear hierarchical differentiation between the parents, who have executive functions, and the children, who have some input but much less power in decision making. The boundaries in a healthy family separate the parents from the children but allow sufficient interaction between the subgroups to maximize closeness and cooperation.

In dysfunctional families, there may be lopsided or chaotic hierarchical arrangements. For example, one parent may have excessive power, with the other parent powerless; or a particular child may have inordinate power, with the parental coalition weak or nonexistent. Such families are likely to experience major problems in rearing and attempting to discipline their children. In dysfunctional families, boundaries between the subgroups tend to be either too rigid or too weak. When boundaries are extremely rigid, eg, between parents and children, the subgroups withdraw from each other, there is no feeling of family closeness and involvement, and the children are at risk of becoming delinquent or running away. When boundaries between subgroups are weak, families are said to be "enmeshed." In these families, emotional dependence is so pervasive that family members may fail to achieve sufficient autonomy and differentiation to function successfully.

The goal of structural therapy is to modify the hierarchic relationships and boundaries so as to promote healthier functioning, eg, in a family in which the parental alliance is weak and one parent is overly involved with a child, treatment strategies are designed to form a parental subgroup that is separated from the child.

Impressive results have been reported from the application of structural family therapy to the study and treatment of children suffering from psychosomatic disorders. Examination of the family systems of children with certain psychosomatic disorders reveals a characteristic pattern of personal dynamics: excessive emotional involvement of family members (enmeshment), overprotectiveness, rigidity of coping mechanisms, and ineffectiveness in resolving conflicts. A key finding is that children with certain psychosomatic illnesses are inappropriately involved with the conflicts of their parents. A typical sequence of interactions recurs in these families. Conflict in the parental unit triggers stress and symptoms in the child; the child's symptoms become a focus of concern for the parents; and the conflict between the parents is temporarily diverted by the symptoms of the child, which are both a reaction to stress and a temporary solution to stress. Family therapy is effective in breaking this cycle of interaction and bringing about improvement of symptoms.

Minuchin's considerable influence has been somewhat eroded in recent years by feminist criticism. His model of healthy family functioning, based on traditional roles of hierarchical power and gender, has been under attack as outmoded, sexist, and rigid. Future modifications of his work should address these concerns, but even his critics accept the validity of his core conceptualization of the family as a dynamic structure that functions most effectively with appropriate role differentiation and boundaries.

Strategic Family Therapy

Strategic family therapy was developed during the 1960s and 1970s, and though somewhat modified, retains great influence in the practice of contemporary family therapy. The emphasis is on effective methods of promoting rapid change in families by defining a problem and devising an appropriate strategy for solving it. Methods of interviewing have been developed to rapidly pinpoint key problem areas in families. The patterns of interactions that reinforce and sustain these problems and that keep a family "stuck" are identified. A strategy is then designed to modify the interactional patterns and hence change the problem.

There are significant differences among the various models of strategic therapy. The best-known approaches are the brief therapy methods of Watzlawick and his colleagues at the Mental Research Institute in Palo Alto, California and the inventive problem-solving techniques of Jay Haley and Chloe Madanes. Selvini Palazzoli headed a group of psychoanalysts in

formulating a model of strategic therapy that grew out of their intensive work with anorexic and psychotic adolescents. The ideas of this group dominated the family therapy field throughout the 1980s. Their methodology for understanding and overcoming resistance is still utilized in some form by most family therapists. The use of a therapy team was popularized by this group. While one or two therapists interview a family, several more therapists observe from behind a one-way mirror. The observing team may phone in suggestions or consult with the therapists during or after the session. The entire therapy team may confer following a session (while the family waits), and a written pronouncement or prescription is then read to the family. The statements are designed to unbalance family defenses by reformulating some basic assumptions. For example, a demanding wife might be described as "trying to help her husband improve himself"; a passive compliant husband might be described as "sensitive and caring in not expressing angry feelings that could hurt his wife."

Treatment methods used in strategic family therapy often take the form of directives given to the family that require family members to do something, either during the session or at home. An intervention may involve a minor change in only one family member, since strategic therapists believe that a change in any one part of the system will result in a change in the whole system. These directives may be straightforward or paradoxical.

If families appear to be reasonably compliant and likely to cooperate, the directives are usually straightforward. A simple example is that of a wife anxious about an impending job interview. The therapist realized that this anxiety was in part related to the wife's awareness of her husband's resistance to her taking a job outside the home. The directive given to this couple was for the husband to apply his considerable experience in the business world to the task of teaching his wife how to handle the job interview. This directive endorsed the power of the husband by putting him in charge of the symptom, and he successfully helped his wife prepare for and participate in the interview. This simple measure had in fact altered the relationship between the couple, so that the symptom was no longer "necessary."

When families are less compliant and oppose the therapist, paradoxical techniques are often successful. The idea of paradoxical therapy is based on the notion that resistant families have an interest in opposing change of any kind, from any source. The therapist therefore suggests a directive that if contradicted by the family would paradoxically lead to positive change. A common example of such an intervention is a therapist patiently advising a family that has resisted previous therapists not to change, that in fact change might be harmful. To defeat this new therapist, the family must actually change. Although this scenario seems simple, implementing it actually requires a high degree of therapeutic skill. Should the process of change continue, the therapist gradually accepts and supports the process; and with lessened resistance, the movement toward positive changes becomes self-sustaining.

Strategic treatment methods may offer dramatic results, and therein lies both their strength and their weakness. When family systems are rigid and unyielding, paradoxical methods can often alter the entrenched equilibrium of the system. On the other hand, this dramatic type of intervention may hold a seductive fascination for therapists who are somewhat manipulative and impatient with the more difficult and time-consuming processes usually necessary in psychotherapy.

Solution-Focused Therapy

The most current variant of strategic therapy is known as solution-focused therapy. Developed by Steve de Shazer and his colleagues, it shares the fundamental assumptions of strategic therapy, namely, minimizing personal history and subjective experience and focusing primarily on brief methods for solving presenting problems. However, de Shazer's model differs from existing strategic therapies in one important respect. Strategic therapists customarily place great importance on highlighting the primary problems presented by clients. This leads to an examination of how and why their efforts have resulted in repeated failure. The therapist then offers a totally different strategy in order to solve the problems presented. The implication of this approach is that the individual or family does not know what to do and that the therapist is the expert who can provide the right solution.

In solution-focused therapy the problems presented are not dwelt on at length so as not to slant the therapy process toward failure. Rather, the emphasis is on encouraging family members to talk about whatever they have done that was in any way helpful in dealing with their problems. The therapist helps them select and develop those solutions that seem most promising. The underlying premise of this approach is that self-doubt and pessimism prevent clients from recognizing the solutions that are right for them. Instead of dwelling on past failures or present difficulties, they are urged to face the future with a new awareness of how best to tackle the problems as they recur. A primary assumption of this approach is that people are intrinsically motivated to improve themselves. Traditional concepts of resistance or ambivalence about change are rejected and viewed as obstructive to treatment. Solution-focused therapy is particularly appealing to therapists who want to practice brief therapy, but are uncomfortable with the dictatorial methods advocated by the major schools of strategic therapy. The collaborative therapist-client relationship is more likely to promote positive rapport, and it offers clear and straightforward guidelines for achieving desirable changes. Critics regard the model as conceptually naive and simplistic, and unproven as a treatment modality.

Psychodynamic Family Therapy

The current state of family therapy represents a radical departure from traditional psychodynamic therapy. Nevertheless, a growing minority of theorists continue to believe that an integration of intrapsychic concepts and family therapy is possible. The general consensus is that mainstream psychoanalysis is not compatible with family therapy, but as Scharff and others have shown, object relations theory does hold some promise for bridging the gap between the individual and the family. Concepts such as introjection, splitting, and projective identification help us understand more about the unconscious determinants of mate selection and the process whereby one person in a system may be acting out the projections of other family members.

A theoretical synthesis of psychodynamic and systems theory has yet to be formulated, but this does not mean that the therapist cannot draw from both approaches in clinical work with families. The broad view is to regard psychodynamic theory and family systems theory as two different dimensions of the same phenomenon in that both yield data that contribute to an overall understanding of family dysfunction. The psychodynamic orientation permits in-depth examination of the motivation and subjective experience of each family member, whereas the interactional perspective provides information about the person's social context as a source of determining individual behavior. It is no coincidence that most of the master clinicians in family therapy had extensive training and experience in psychodynamic therapies, which did much to shape their clinical understanding and skills.

Cognitive-Behavioral Family Therapy

Cognitive-behavioral therapy is not a model of family therapy, but mention must be made of the increasing utilization of behavioral techniques in clinical work with couples and families. This approach is grounded in social learning theory, behavior modification, and cognitive therapy. Basically it is employed as a means of reinforcing specific desirable behaviors and eliminating undesirable behaviors. For some years it has been used successfully in improving parenting skills. A current trend in couple therapy is to use these methods for improving communication skills, enhancing sexual performance, and defusing cycles of anger and violence.

CHARACTERISTICS OF FAMILY THERAPY

As a conceptual model, family therapy can be distinguished from other forms of psychotherapy. This distinction also holds true at the level of clinical application. Despite obvious differences among practitioners of family therapy, there are principles of treatment to which most subscribe. For this reason in some basic respects family therapy includes therapeutic practices that vary radically from those used by individual or group therapists.

Comparison with Individual & Group Therapy

For many years, individual therapy was the principal mode in which psychotherapy has been conducted, and the essential characteristics of individual psychodynamic therapy continue to reflect psychoanalytic tradition. The therapist works with one person who presents with a self-recognized problem or who is identified by others as having a problem. If deemed suitable for psychodynamic therapy, the patient is expected to freely verbalize thoughts and feelings. Significant events from the past are revived and reexamined. The therapist's role is that of listener endeavoring to understand the implications of these reports. The patient is guided toward greater self-awareness as a prerequisite to changes in behavior and symptoms. A growing number of therapists minimize or refute psychoanalytic theory, but they maintain their belief in historical causality and continue to formulate psychological problems in terms of internal mental processes. The goal of treatment is to modify the subjective experiences of the individual patient through verbal interaction to produce symptomatic, behavioral, or personality change.

These conditions rarely occur in family therapy, where participation by one or more family members is usually required. The therapist is interested in the objective reality of family relationships; individual dynamics, defenses, and symptoms are translated into interactional terms. Because family therapists are primarily concerned with observable behavior, they are alert to nonverbal cues and communication sequences. Current functioning is the major focus in family therapy. The goal of individual therapy is to change the individual, whereas the family therapist strives to bring about change in the family's system of relationships.

On initial observation, family therapy may seem like group therapy applied to a group of family members. The only points of similarity, however, are that both group and family therapy require participation by more than one person and both are concerned in varying degrees with interpersonal relationships. The distinction between the aims of individual therapy (changing the individual patient) and family therapy (changing the system of relationships) applies to the comparison of group therapy and family therapy as well. Group therapy is also designed to produce change in the individual patient. Interpersonal relationships among group members do provide significant material for group therapy, but only in terms of highlighting the problems of individual participants.

There are other less apparent but highly significant differences between group and family therapy. The participants in group therapy are usually strangers to begin with; they may be urged not to see one another socially between sessions; and they may have no expectation of continuing contacts with one another beyond the life of the group. These conditions facilitate self-disclosure and confrontation, since there is no inhibiting concern that future relationships will be impaired. Furthermore, all members of the group admit to having problems; they are all "in the same boat." Their shared identity as patients also provides assurance of acceptance and encourages self-revelation.

Families, on the other hand, are bound by historical continuity, and this creates a treatment situation radically different from that of group therapy. Family members are linked by a common past, have ongoing contact, and anticipate continuing involvement in the future. Concerns about impairing relationships may severely inhibit openness and confrontation. Family members are sometimes motivated to participate in therapy because they feel they can help the person who has been identified as the patient, the one who is "sick." The relatives usually resist being labeled as patients and may deny or be unaware of the impact that their own behavior or problems have on the identified patient. These conditions make for greater resistance than is found in group therapy. A climate of support and acceptance is also less likely in family settings. Family members are all too aware of each other's faults, and criticism and even scapegoating are typical aspects of family life.

Families are generally more resistant to treatment at the outset than are patients seeking individual or group therapy. This initial obstacle poses an immediate challenge to the family therapist. It may take considerable skill to neutralize resistance and establish positive relationships with family members so that therapy can proceed. On the other hand, family members are bound by deeply entrenched loyalties and obligations, and this common bond provides a powerful incentive for mutual involvement in therapy. In contrast, group therapy members experience transient relationships and less profound emotional involvement with one another.

Another difference between group and family therapy that has important clinical implications is that the therapist in the family group is literally outnumbered. Family members often share rigidly held beliefs and attitudes, and the therapist, as the representative of an alternative perspective, may not have sufficient power to influence the group. This situation is a special problem in psychotic families, which are characteristically impervious to messages from outside sources. Participants in group therapy—even if all of them are psychotic—do not share a history of common beliefs, and the group therapist often finds allies among the group members who may help influence the ideas and behavior of any one patient.

Indications & Contraindications for Family Therapy

Most family therapists contend that family therapy is indicated for all problems affecting family relationships. Contraindications can involve practical obstacles, such as geographic distance that prevents attendance of family members at meetings, older patients who may have outlived their families, and adult immigrants who may have no family ties in their adopted country.

There are also some clinical conditions that make family therapy inadvisable. It may be unwise to initiate family therapy if one member is in the throes of a psychotic episode. A paranoid individual may have such a hostile relationship with the family that attempts to bring all members together for meetings are doomed to failure. Family therapy is generally inadvisable when the irrevocable breakup of a family has already occurred, eg, if one spouse has decided on marital separation, it may simply postpone the painful process if both partners meet at the insistence of a therapist.

Obviously, these contraindications apply to only a small percentage of the cases that typically come to the attention of practitioners of family therapy. For the great majority of patients, the inclusion of family members enriches the data source for a thorough assessment, and participation of the family can often expedite the treatment process. Although family therapy is helpful for most problems, there are two problem areas for which family therapy is definitely the treatment of choice. Family therapists are unanimous in endorsing the value of their approach for problems of children and adolescents and for marital conflict. These areas deserve more detailed consideration.

FAMILY THERAPY FOR CHILDREN & ADOLESCENTS

In the case of children, there are two overwhelming arguments in favor of family therapy rather than individual therapy. First, it is assumed that problems of children always indicate family dysfunction; individual therapy for the child ignores the family's problems. Second, any therapeutic success from individual therapy with the child would be short-lived unless the dysfunctional family system was also treated. In fact, the family may well resist changes that seem incompatible with the needs of the parents and the other children. It is not uncommon for parents to undermine or terminate therapy at a point when the child is manifesting signs of healthier attitudes and behavior.

Some individual therapists object to family therapy for adolescents. They believe it impedes the adoles-

cent's strivings for independence and argue that adolescents need confidentiality to talk freely about sex and other personal matters. Family therapists reply that adolescents with problems have failed to develop independence precisely because their families have difficulty permitting or encouraging this phase of development. The therapist must help the entire family adjust to the increasing independence of one or more of its members. As the family learns to cope with the separation and individuation of the offspring, additional psychotherapy can be helpful for the adolescent, who is now free to deal with problems in the world away from home. A combination of family therapy and individual or group therapy is usually most effective for adolescents.

Younger children should always be seen separately from their parents for at least one evaluation session. This ensures that they have the privacy and protection to report events and express feelings that might otherwise remain suppressed. In cases of known or suspected abuse, separate evaluation meetings for the child are essential. Children often do well with individual play and verbal therapy in addition to their involvement in family therapy.

The concept of triangulation has special relevance when working with problems of children. The difficult or symptomatic child is often that child who is most involved with the parents and thereby represents the third member of a triangle. The role may be identified with concern (the child as identified patient) or with negative attributions (the child as behavioral problem). How and why a particular child becomes involved in a triangle is an important question for the diagnostician, and attempting to modify or undo this dynamic is the task of the family therapist.

Illustrative Case

A couple requested help because their 7-year-old son, an only child, had developed school phobia. A thorough evaluation revealed that the child's presenting problem was an interpersonal relationship problem involving all family members. The mother, an extremely anxious and dependent woman, had always looked to her husband for direction and support. When they met, he was insecure, but he compensated by asserting strong control in the relationship and by encouraging his wife's dependence. Over several years, however, the husband became increasingly successful in business, and as he developed greater self-confidence, he began to perceive his wife as undesirably weak and demanding. When the wife realized that her husband was becoming more distant emotionally, she became even more anxious and dependent. This caused the husband to become even more distant and preoccupied with work, so that the wife's anxiety in turn increased.

The birth of the child was welcomed by both parties. The wife looked to the child for the support her husband failed to provide. The husband hoped that his son would serve as his surrogate for his wife's attentions and thus free him from her demands and alleviate his guilt about his withdrawal from her. As the child grew, he learned to tolerate his father's lack of involvement, since it seemed to ensure the continuing attention of his doting mother.

This pattern of interaction stabilized over a number of years until an unavoidable developmental shift disrupted the family's equilibrium. At age 6 years, the son began to attend primary school. The start of formal schooling represented the first major separation for mother and son. The family had worked actively to minimize the son's earlier attendance at nursery school and kindergarten, but such avoidance was no longer possible. On most mornings before school, the child complained about various ailments and "upset" feelings. More often than not, the parents permitted him to stay home. Extensive medical investigations ruled out any organic basis for the symptoms.

The parents grew increasingly distressed and felt great conflict about the situation. On the one hand, the child's symptoms helped to stabilize the marital relationship, and both parents now felt threatened by the possibility of a disruption of the status quo. On the other hand, the parents were genuinely concerned about the consequences of their son's missed days of school. Periodically, and with much ambivalence, they would urge the boy to go to school, but this simply heightened his anxiety and precipitated his symptoms. A conference with a pediatrician led to the referral for family therapy.

The goals of treatment were to facilitate a collaborative relationship between the parents, encourage a closer bond between father and son, help the mother achieve greater independence and autonomy, and firmly but benignly reinforce the son's school attendance as an important step toward appropriate separation from his parents. The family responded well to therapy, and these goals were realized to their satisfaction.

MARITAL & COUPLES THERAPY

The variety of family life-styles in our culture requires a broader focus that encompasses more than conventional marriage. Accordingly, the term "marital therapy" is here defined as the treatment of any unit of two adults who consider themselves a couple by reason of cohabitation or mutual commitment.

The conceptual basis of marital therapy is strongly identified with family systems theory. Marital therapy can best be distinguished from family therapy on the basis of the unit of treatment. It is confined to one generation (the adult dyad), whereas family therapy encompasses two generations (parents and children) and sometimes three (grandparents). All family therapists include marital therapy as part of their work, but not all marital therapists work with families. Marital therapy is clearly indicated when presenting problems primarily involve the marital relationship. Treatment disposition is less clear when the presenting problems are a mix of individual and marital concerns or when marital issues surface early in the course of individual therapy. The decision on whether to implement couples therapy is usually based on the therapist's assessment of the causes and the relative significance of each problem.

Most clinicians now recognize the effectiveness of involving the partner in cases of sexual dysfunction. There has been growing recognition that sexual dysfunction is best understood as one significant component of a complex interpersonal system. In practical terms, treatment of a sexual problem must take into consideration the couple's overall relationship. A knowledge of family systems theory and mastery of techniques of marital therapy are essential components of training for sex therapists.

Family and marital therapy have demonstrated value as adjunctive treatments for alcoholism, and to a lesser extent for drug abuse. Several studies have produced important insights into the marital system of alcoholics and drug abusers. The spouse of the substance abuser may inadvertently play a role that reinforces addictive behaviors. No matter what treatment program is utilized, compliance with treatment and a successful outcome are less likely without involvement of the spouse, particularly in the initial stage of recovery. Substance abuse is a multifaceted problem, and most family therapists recommend a combination of individual and marital therapy as well as consistent participation in twelve-step programs such as Alcoholics Anonymous.

A serious problem often related to substance abuse is domestic violence. Conventional treatment methods have focused on the victims of abuse (women, children, the elderly). Male perpetrators are regarded as unmotivated to change and resistant to treatment, and the standard approach is to coerce them into treatment by means of court orders or the threat of legal recourse. Treatment for the male is usually individual therapy or participation in a group for male batterers. When the batterers are willing to enter treatment, a combination of individual or group and couples therapy may be the most effective approach.

The problem of spousal abuse has sparked controversy in the family therapy field. Can we explain spousal abuse in interactional terms? Adherence to the interactional model would imply that a physical attack is a reaction to the behavior of the spouse. Some family therapists have understandably taken strong exception to this explanation. This issue is highly significant and is discussed more fully in the section on the feminist perspective in family therapy.

The role of the therapist when working with couples is more difficult and complex than it is when working with individuals or even entire families. In individual therapy, the therapist strives to achieve a collaborative and mutually positive relationship with one person. In therapy with families, some members may dislike or attack the therapist, but others will provide support and protection. With couples, however, the challenge is to establish a positive alliance with *each* partner within a context often marked by accusations, blaming, and attempts to manipulate the therapist into taking one side or the other.

A therapist who attempts to maintain strict neutrality (along the lines of traditional psychoanalytic psychotherapy) may lose the cooperation of both partners, since they are likely to ascribe the therapist's neutrality to a lack of interest or concern. The marital therapist must constantly change sides, but in a way that neither antagonizes one partner to the point of leaving nor establishes a one-sided alliance with the other. The goal is not to maintain neutrality but to be able to side with each partner individually at different points in the therapy.

The tendency to assume positions of right and wrong is the most common risk in therapy with couples. The therapist must resist being drawn into arguments. A solid grounding in family systems theory is the therapist's best deterrent, since it is usually clear that there is neither a right nor a wrong answer when a couple's disputes are explored from an interactional point of view. Partners who adopt polarized positions are said to have become snared in a repetitive sequence of interactions and are unable to experience or choose alternative ways of responding. This is shown in the following case, which also demonstrates how a seemingly simple dispute can mask complex interpersonal dynamics.

Illustrative Case

A major source of conflict for a couple was the husband's apparent unwillingness to find secure employment. The wife came from a wealthy family and received a monthly allowance from her parents. The wife periodically became furious at her husband for his "laziness" in not finding "significant" work. He spent most of his time caring for their children at home and engaging in charity and volunteer work. He protested that they did not need the extra income and that he was unable to find suitable work in any case. The more the wife pressured him, the less the husband did to change the situation. At one point the wife turned to the therapist in sheer exasperation and asked, "Don't you think a grown man should have a steady job?"

The therapist's initial reaction was to agree with the wife that it was "wrong" for the husband to resist employment and that he was clearly exploiting her. The therapist refrained from expressing an opinion, however, and sought to understand more about the interactional dynamics of the dispute. It became clear that whenever the husband did make genuine efforts to find a job, tentative as these were, the wife did not

support him and in fact put obstacles in his way; she was unconsciously resisting his possible employment. The dispute about work masked some underlying issues that could not easily be reduced to a matter of simple right or wrong. The wife had great difficulty expressing warmth and affection for either her husband or her children. The husband protected her from her deficiencies in parenting by taking care of the children during the day. One of the stabilizing influences in the marriage was the wife's certainty that her husband would never abandon her. He was a dependent and rather masochistic partner and seemed to put up with a good deal of verbal abuse. His refusal to work also enabled his wife to remain dependent on her parents, who were sympathetic to her plight and provided emotional and financial support.

Avoiding employment served as a defense mechanism for the husband as well. He related to his wife as if she were a scolding mother. His dependency needs were met by knowing that his wife seemed to need him as much as he needed her. Despite their bitter arguments, he sensed that she actually tolerated his lack of employment. His immaturity and poor self-esteem made him feel safer with children than with adults, and he looked to his children for closeness and acceptance. Having always led a sheltered life, he had profound fears of testing himself in the everyday world and subconsciously protected his self-esteem by assuring himself that he was too good for most of the jobs that were available.

Attributes & Values of the Therapist

The personal attributes and values of the therapist can play a determining role in establishing a therapeutic relationship with couples and in effecting a successful outcome in treatment. The therapist's age, gender, sexual orientation, marital status, and cultural background may be significant in particular situations. A marked discrepancy in age is often a problem; couples may feel inhibited and awkward with therapists who are much younger or older than themselves, and therapists are more likely to experience countertransference reactions in such circumstances. Gender is also a significant consideration in couples therapy. If the therapist is male, the husband may see him as a competitor, whereas the wife may feel that he is incapable of understanding her. If the therapist is female, the wife may view her as a competitor, whereas the husband may believe that she is biased against men. Ethnic and cultural differences between therapist and clients may also prove detrimental to treatment, particularly if these differences are unacknowledged or not discussed.

Nontraditional Couple Systems

The work of contemporary marital therapists is by no means limited to couples who meet the legal definition of marriage. A high divorce rate and resistance to traditional marriage are creating considerable numbers of single adults and parents, unmarried co-habitants, and people who marry more than once. Rapidly changing social and moral values are reflected in greater tolerance for alternative life-styles and reformulations about what constitutes "normal" family functioning. The domain of the marital therapist includes a high proportion of unmarried couples and remarriage families. Training in work with gay and lesbian couples is now a prerequisite for all marital therapists. So called "nontraditional" couple systems are very much part of the norm. Assumptions that have long prevailed in marriage counseling are being revised in favor of a broader and less judgmental perspective. This has led to innovative and flexible approaches to assessment and treatment.

A related development in marital and family therapy has been fueled by the reality of the ethnic and cultural diversity that constitutes modern society. Traditional therapy, generated by and for a relatively homogeneous white American middle-class, was based on beliefs and values that are often inapplicable to much of the population. This realization is underscored by a number of recent studies. Best known is the work of McGoldrick, who has provided an analysis of the characteristics of the family systems representing the major ethnic groups in the United States. Knowledge of this work is indispensable for the enlightened couple and family therapist.

Couples considering or going through separation often look to marital therapists for help. When one or both partners are considering separation, the marital therapist can provide a safe and productive environment for working through this difficult life event. If a separation has already been effected, it may be unwise to insist on conjoint treatment. Couples who are moving irrevocably toward permanent separation need to maintain appropriate distance, not enforced closeness. One exception to this recommendation is the couple who mutually accepts the reality of separation and wishes to use couples therapy as an aid in working through the separation process. The term "divorce therapy" has been coined to describe this process of working through a dissolution of marriage. Therapy for couples contemplating or in the midst of separation and divorce may be particularly helpful when children are involved.

CURRENT TRENDS IN FAMILY THERAPY

Constructivism

A growing number of theorists are challenging and revising the theoretical and clinical assumptions of family therapy. The general thrust of these criticisms is that the prevailing concepts are too mechanistic and reductionist, and that clinical practice has become overly concerned with techniques and quick solutions.

The role and function of the therapist are the primary concern of the revisionists. Family therapists usually perceive their role to be that of a "technician" who objectively assesses and corrects malfunctions in an external system (the family). The idea of the therapist as objective observer, separate from what is observed, is an implicit assumption in family therapy.

Critics of this view have adopted the constructivist position that the outside world is not separable from the observer. External "reality" is a synthesis of subjective preconceptions and what actually is out there. Constructivism derives from a long tradition of speculations in western philosophy concerning the nature of reality. Renewed interest in constructivism is evident in postmodernist literature and art, but the impetus for adapting it to systems theory has come from research studies in biology, cognition, and linguistics that demonstrate that the brain mediates and transmutes perceptions of the outer world. The compelling conclusion is that there is no way to "know" what reality is.

Research on neural and cognitive functioning has increased our knowledge of the individual, but these findings are too restrictive for direct application to the complexities of social behavior. Social construction theory, developed by social psychologists, does supply the link from individual to interpersonal, and this theory has definite relevance for family therapy. Social construction theory maintains that our beliefs about the outside world are constructed through social interchange. We learn from exchanging information. The implication is that there are no objective facts; we hold to beliefs, attitudes, and opinions inculcated by past interactions and modified or reinforced by current and future interactions. Our knowledge of the world (and ourselves) is essentially a complicated set of "stories" that is kept private by the individual or shared with small groups (eg, the family) and large groups (eg, society).

The Use of Narrative

The constructivist influence has produced some new directions in family therapy. One idea that has gained widespread acceptance is that the therapist must strive for greater self-awareness, resist premature conclusions, and attend empathically to what the family reveals. The role of the therapist is now one of catalyst rather than director. The emphasis on listening and empathy may seem like a reversion to the traditional psychodynamic position, but the major difference is that, unlike the family therapist, the psychodynamic therapist has a preconceived theory that determines both what is attended to and what conclusions may be drawn from what is heard.

The idea of listening with an open mind leads naturally to the notion that each family has its own unique stories to tell and that these stories change over time. The family can be viewed as a constantly changing linguistic system rather than as a predictable homeostatic system. This conceptual shift has led to a revised view of the nature of psychological problems. A core assumption in family therapy is that problems tend to maintain family equilibrium (homeostasis). The narrative view is that problems, however they develop, are impediments to family functioning. In practice this reformulation moves from an implicitly critical attitude ("families need their problems") to one of complete acceptance and empathy.

The utilization of narrative to effect change is gaining rapid acceptance among family therapists. Michael White developed an approach that transforms the way in which a family experiences their problems. Instead of assuming that a problem is something inside an individual, he asks the family to consider it as something external. He then engages with the family to examine this "outside" problem thoroughly and to devise solutions. The problem is labeled as an entity to make it tangible, something that can be pinned down and overcome. Psychiatric labels are shunned as implicitly derogatory explanations that reinforce helplessness (internalized disease). The family and therapist create a name that captures the experiential quality of the problem. Humor enhances the creativity of the exercise, as in the case of an encopretic child whose family talked about how the "sneaky poo" affected their lives.

Labeling and externalizing a problem diminish shame and absolve both patient and family of guilt. Energy that might be bound up in defensiveness is released for constructive purposes. The family and therapist engage in narrative creative problem solving. As in the work of de Shazer, described earlier, the therapy then becomes solution focused rather than problem focused. The narrative therapist rarely instructs or interprets; the preferred mode of communication is in the form of enquiry. Typical questions would be: When did this problem come into your life? How has it affected your life? If you were to give this problem a name, what would it be? Has it affected others in your life? Can you remember a time when you challenged the problem?

The use of narration has particular relevance for the practice of direct team observation. As previously described, the use of a team that observes and gives feedback and directions to a therapist is common in family therapy. The constructivist influence has led to recent modifications of this procedure. After observing part of a session, the team is invited to join the therapist and family. Without prior discussion, the team members then spontaneously reflect their subjective impressions of the family, their problems, and the interview. The reflections usually highlight strengths and positive attributes. The family is then invited to reflect in turn on *their* reactions to what they heard. A "conversation" ensues. The therapist and colleagues do not assume roles of authority. They collaborate with the family members as equals, with the goal of achieving mutual understanding. This process often produces radically new and help-ful transformations of problems and solutions. The reflective team represents narrative therapy in its purest form.

Narrative therapy seems to hold promise as a new approach in dealing with challenging or seemingly intractable problems. The concept of narration is attracting the attention of therapists who have not previously been drawn to family therapy. The practice of narrative therapy requires a mastery of specific sequential protocols of enquiry, and acquiring such proficiency takes intensive training and considerable experience.

The Feminist Perspective

A uniform model of healthy family functioning is important in family therapy because it provides directions for interventions and goals for treatment. Until recently family therapists have by and large subscribed to the societal ideal of the intact family with clear roles based on gender and age. The parents have distinct roles (father as breadwinner and primary authority; mother as supportive and nurturing), and they cooperate in establishing and implementing rules and regulations for the children.

Deviations in these parental roles are believed to be instrumental in creating and maintaining dysfunction. This view has been strongly endorsed in structural, strategic, and psychodynamic family therapy. The most frequently cited deviant pattern is that of an overly involved mother and a minimally involved or absent father. In structural and strategic therapy clinical interventions and strategies are devised to correct this imbalance by reducing the mother's involvement and increasing the father's involvement. When a father is not available, the female single parent is often encouraged to enlist the aid of an adult male partner, family member, or friend to serve as a "father figure."

This perspective has been challenged in recent years by social scientists and feminist practitioners. They point out that the healthy family model (proposed above) is an historical product representing the patriarchal bias of western society. For centuries, males had a legally enforced birthright of dominance in all areas of life. Females were socialized to accept subordination to males and conditioned to believe that child rearing is more important than education or career advancement. The advent of industrialization amplified this distinction as males were compelled to spend most of their days in employment outside the home. Fathers had to reduce their emotional involvement in the family to survive economically, and mothers increased their investment in the family to compensate for this loss. Economic progress has accelerated the transformation of the family in western society. A consumer-based society requires constant increases in income to match or exceed expenditures. The norm is now the dual income family with more equitable sharing of domestic responsibilities. Education and career opportunities are now regarded as indispensable rights for women. Progress in gaining economic power has galvanized women to seek redress of inequities in other spheres of modern life.

The traditional family has come under siege. New roles have become necessary to preserve family functioning. Discrepancies in power must give way to more flexible and egalitarian marital partnerships, and children have to adjust accordingly. Many couples have been unable to cope with the inevitable struggles, and with the weakening of social taboos, divorce has become an increasingly acceptable solution. High rates of divorce have dramatically increased the number of single-parent family units. The great majority of these are headed by women, with the result that the overinvolvement of mothers and lack of involvement by fathers is now commonplace.

Feminist clinicians understandably protest the pathologizing of these roles by family therapists. New models of therapy are required for nontraditional family systems. The goal of the therapist is to help the family function adaptively when one parent is peripheral or absent. Power and hierarchy can be minimized, and shared responsibility and participation emphasized in these families. The centrality of the mother's role should be understood and supported. Rather than focusing on the "overinvolvement" of the mother, the therapist would be more constructive in addressing and eliciting the participation of the uninvolved father.

The constructivist influence is also apparent in the model of therapy advocated by feminist clinicians. The process of therapy is characterized by openness and empathic dialogue. The therapist initiates a discussion of traditionally prescribed sex roles and, when necessary, helps the family relinquish its reliance on hierarchic power. Facilitating individual autonomy and affiliation empowers all family members. Flexibility and cooperation result in improved family functioning.

The most trenchant and controversial criticism raised by feminists has to do with the role of personal responsibility and accountability in human behavior. The cybernetic model of family therapy depicts behavior as interactional. Subjective motivation has no place in this model. Individual behavior is reactive. The advantage of this perspective is that it allows for objective assessment (observing the interactional patterns of families) and it avoids blaming and pejorative clinical labeling (we do what we do because of what is done to us).

Feminist therapists object that this paradigm fails to recognize the role of volition in human behavior. In most circumstances we can choose to act or not to act, and this is particularly relevant when our behavior may be injurious to others. The problem of violence against women and children has generated the most heated debates about this issue. The cybernetic model, if applied scrupulously, would consider a violent act to be a response to some behavior. The feminist objection is not only that the man is exculpated from blame or responsibility but that the woman is viewed as eliciting (provoking) the violence. Adhering to the cybernetic model, when applied to this context, reflects what the feminists regard as the male bias that has informed family therapy since its inception. In terms of clinical procedure, they argue convincingly that therapy in cases of spousal abuse should not be based on the cybernetic model. In effect, this means that couples therapy is usually inadvisable. Separate therapy for the wife should be designed to reinforce her self-esteem, autonomy, and assertiveness. Whether by legal coercion or through therapy, the male offender should be encouraged to recognize and accept responsibility for his actions.

CONCLUSIONS

The practice of contemporary psychiatry reflects a movement away from long-term psychodynamic therapy and toward a greater concentration on brief methods of psychotherapy and medication. This shift toward pragmatic and focused treatment is compatible with the goals of family therapy and has resulted in increased cooperation between practitioners of individual-based therapy and family therapists. It is important to recognize that family systems theory remains somewhat at odds with the dominant conceptual models of psychiatry and psychology. The interactional perspective is not congruent with linear causality as reflected in the emphasis on specific "causes" and diagnostic labeling that characterizes mainstream psychiatry. Although there is not yet a theoretical synthesis that will accommodate these divergent paradigms, some movement toward this goal is already apparent. Modifications in strategic therapy, the popularity of narrative therapy, and the impact of feminist thinking grew out of dissatisfaction with the rigidity of the cybernetic interactional perspective that has until recently dominated family therapy. The newer models of therapy are conceptually and clinically relevant for working with individual patients. We seem to be moving toward a theoretical integration of the systems of the family and the individual, and future forms of therapy will probably be more inclusive than exclusive.

Although family therapy is in a state of transition, it is clearly a valid type of psychotherapy whose clinical effectiveness has been amply documented in several reviews. The systems theory perspective has introduced a critical new dimension in revealing the interplay of family interaction and disturbed psychological processes. The development of new family therapy techniques is influencing the practice of psychotherapy as a whole. A considerable body of research evidence, accumulated since the early 1980s, attests to the efficacy of family therapy in the treatment of psychotic and affective illnesses that do not respond to traditional psychotherapeutic approaches, eg, the management of patients with schizophrenia. Studies have shown that such patients living in highly conflictual family situations are prone to frequent relapses despite carefully monitored drug therapy. Ensuring that the families of patients with schizophrenia participate in psychoeducation and supportive therapy significantly reduces the frequency of psychotic episodes and the need for rehospitalization. Recent research indicates that the same structured model of family education and support significantly reduces the relapse rate even in low conflict families.

Involvement of the family—particularly the spouse —has been shown to increase treatment compliance in cases of serious or chronic medical illness signifi-

cantly. Evidence also suggests that family therapy is frequently effective as part of an overall treatment approach in dealing with complex social and psychological problems such as substance abuse, domestic violence, sexual molestation, and delinquency.

The widespread applicability of family therapy has ensured that it is no longer regarded as simply an additional modality of therapy. Family systems theory has advanced our understanding of psychological dysfunction, and more and more therapists advocate family therapy as the preferred method of treatment for a host of clinical problems. Most training institutions in psychiatry, psychology, and social work include family therapy as an essential component of the curriculum.

REFERENCES & SUGGESTED READINGS

Bateson G et al: Toward a theory of schizophrenia. Behav Sci 1956;1:251.

Bowen M: The use of family therapy in clinical practice. Compr Psychiatry 1966;7:345.

Brown S, Lewis V: *The Alcoholic Family in Recovery.* Guilford, 1998.

de Shazer S, Berg I: Constructing solutions. Fam Ther Networker 1993;12:42.

Dixon L, Lehman F: Family interventions for schizophrenia. Schizophrenia Bull 1995;21:631.

Edwards M, Steinglass P: Family therapy outcomes for alcoholism. J Marital Fam Ther 1995;21:475.

Epstein N, Schlesinger S: Cognitive-behavioral treatment of family problems. In: *Casebook of Cognitive-Behavior Therapy with Children and Adolescents.* Reinecke M, Dattilio F, Freeman A (editors). Guilford, 1996.

Freedman J, Combs G: *Narrative Therapy: The Social Construction of Preferred Realities.* Norton, 1996.

Friedman S (editor): *The New Language of Change.* Guilford, 1993.

Goldner V: The treatment of violence and victimization in intimate relationships. Fam Process 1998;37:263.

Haley J: *Problem Solving Therapy.* Jossey-Bass, 1976.

Holma J, Aaltonen J: Narrative understanding in acute psychosis. Contemp Fam Ther 1998;20:253.

Jackson DD: The study of the family. Fam Process 1965;4:1.

Jacobson N, Gurman A: *Clinical Handbook of Couple Therapy.* Guilford, 1995.

Laird J, Green R (editors): *Lesbians and Gays in Couples and Families: A Handbook for Therapists.* Jossey-Bass, 1996.

Markman H et al: Men and women dealing with conflict in heterosexual relationships. J Social Issues 1993;49:107.

McGoldrick M (editor): *Re-Visioning Family Therapy: Race, Culture, and Gender in Clinical Practice.* Guilford, 1998.

Miller S, Hubble M, Duncan B: *Handbook of Solution-Focused Brief Therapy.* Jossey-Bass, 1996.

Minuchin S, Fishman H: *Family Therapy Techniques.* Harvard University Press, 1981.

Nichols M, Schwartz R: *Family Therapy: Concepts and Methods.* Allyn & Bacon, 1998.

Pinsof W, Wynne L, Hambright A: The outcomes of couple and family therapy: Findings, conclusions & recommendations. Psychotherapy 1996;33:321.

Rolland J: *Helping Families with Chronic and Life-Threatening Disorders.* Basic Books, 1994.

Scharff D, Scharff J: *Object Relations Couple Therapy.* Jason Aronson, 1991.

Scheel M, Ivey D: Neutrality and feminist perspective: Can they co-exist in family therapy? Contemp Fam Ther 1998;20:315.

Schwartz R: *Internal Family Systems Therapy.* Guilford, 1995.

Selvini Palazzoli M et al: *Paradox and Counterparadox.* Jason Aronson, 1978.

Shapiro RJ: Psychoanalytic and systemic models: An overture to a conclusion. In: *International Annals of Adolescent Psychiatry,* Vol 2. Schwartzberg A (editor). University of Chicago Press, 1992.

Singer MT, Wynne LC: Thought disorder and family relations of schizophrenics: Results and implications. Arch Gen Psychiatry 1965;12:201.

Smith C, Nylund D (editors): *Narrative Therapies with Children and Adolescents.* Guilford, 1997.

Snyder M: A gender-informed model of couple and family therapy: Relationship enhanced therapy. Contemp Fam Ther 1992;14:15.

Stewart A et al: *Separating Together: How Divorce Transforms Families.* Guilford, 1997.

Watzlawick P, Weakland J, Fisch R: *Change: Principles of Problem Formation and Problem Resolution.* Norton, 1974.

White M, Epston D: *Narrative Means to Therapeutic Ends.* Norton, 1990.

36 Behavioral Medicine Techniques

Daniel S. Weiss, PhD

Behavioral medicine is a broad field that deals with the application of behavioral science knowledge and techniques to problems related to physical health. Although the field was defined formally only in the 1970s, it includes topics once in the domain of psychosomatic medicine (see Chapter 3). What makes behavioral medicine different is its emphasis on modifying overt behavior contributing to physical (rather than mental) illness and its application of techniques of directed attention to manage both the somatic illness and the adverse effects of somatic treatments. During the past 10 years, cognitive-behavioral techniques have also become a treatment modality (Keefe et al, 1992). Areas such as asthma, human immunodeficiency virus (HIV) status, arthritis, pain management, and smoking cessation are central to behavioral medicine (Blanchard, 1992). In fact, behavioral approaches have advanced to the point that the National Institutes of Health (NIH) have developed a consensus statement (1995).

The principal techniques used in behavioral medicine are relaxation, imagery, hypnosis, and biofeedback. Recently, however, cognitive interventions have begun to be used. Relaxation is both a therapeutic technique in its own right and an important element of the others named. There is increasing awareness in several specialty areas (eg, cardiology) that the techniques of behavioral medicine used in secondary and tertiary prevention may have an important role in primary prevention.

RELAXATION

Probably the most basic technique in behavioral medicine is the systematic induction of a state of relaxation. Psychologically, relaxation reduces arousal and tension, the almost universal concomitants of stress. Physiologically, the "relaxation response" (Benson, 1975) consists of a slowing respiratory rate, reduction of blood pressure, and peripheral vasodilation.

Relaxation therapy has been used with documented success in the management of essential hypertension, chronic pain, and headache. It is probably helpful in a wide variety of clinical conditions associated with stress, whether from threatening external events or pressures or from uncomfortable psychological or physiological states. In addition, relaxation is used to enhance behavior therapy (see Chapter 33) and other techniques of behavioral medicine.

Relaxation training, like any other complex learned behavior, calls for daily practice over a period of time. The beneficial effects of relaxation exercises are realized only through consistent and unswerving use. Audiotaped materials explaining the relaxation exercises and techniques are valuable teaching devices. Tapes are commercially available or may be prepared by the patient or therapist. A tape should include the four elements that Benson (1975) identifies as necessary to elicit the relaxation response: (1) a mental cue that is repeated several times silently during each exhalation; (2) a passive disregard for trying, succeeding, or being distracted, so that attention can be centered on the repetition of the cue; (3) a comfortable position that minimizes muscular activity and tension; and (4) a quiet environment with minimal distractions.

Relaxation can be facilitated by the creative use of words that connote passivity rather than activity and have positive rather than negative association, by proper timing—allowing the individual to move at his or her own pace, and by establishment of specific times and places for practice. Setting aside a special time for relaxation exercises and nothing else may be helpful in its own right. An example of beginning induction follows:

> Close your eyes . . . Let your whole face become comfortably heavy and relaxed. . . . Now . . . slowly breathe in through your nose . . . and allow the air to fill the spaces in your lungs. . . . Feel your chest expand with air. Now . . . hold your breath. . . . Now . . . without pressure or force . . . slowly exhale through your mouth. Feel the air as it passes over your lips. Repeat the breathing cycle . . . inhale . . . hold . . . exhale and relax. Feel your body relaxing. . . . Feel the tension flow out and the calmness and warmth flow in, etc.

IMAGERY

Techniques involving the use of imagery are related to relaxation techniques, and the two are frequently used in conjunction. Visual imagery is most frequently used, but auditory, kinesthetic, olfactory, and gustatory imagery may be used too. Most of what is said about visual imagery and visualization techniques applies to all forms of imagery.

The ability of some people to alter the depth, vividness, and intensity of mental imagery is well documented, and there is anecdotal evidence for a relationship between visualization techniques and creative activity, peak performance, and repair and restoration of physical and mental equilibrium. Like relaxation techniques, visualization techniques take practice. Samuels and Samuels (1975) present an interesting and optimistic account of the history and uses of visualization techniques with and without the use of mind-altering drugs. The Lamaze program for childbirth uses visual imagery to achieve relaxation and reduction of pain.

Some of the techniques used in visualization and other kinds of imagery overlap those used in relaxation and hypnosis. Relaxation is a prerequisite for visualization. Then, depending on whether the imagery is to be guided by a clinician or taught to the patient for future use, the major activity is the intense focus of attention on the image (eg, a warm beach—to promote relaxation—or a strong antibody—to promote healing). As with relaxation, the major obstacle is distraction. The trick is to let distractions enter and flow past rather than trying to resist and overcome them.

As with other techniques of behavioral medicine, the use of visualization should be integrated into an overall treatment program that is acceptable to the patient. Although these techniques may be of use only as adjuncts to other treatments, they may be of use to some patients with medical or psychiatric disorders.

HYPNOSIS

In spite of some lingering antipathy toward the subject, there is no doubt that hypnotic phenomena, induction of trance states, and suggestion can play important roles in the treatment of some types of anxiety and phobias and may even serve the purpose of anesthesia in some individuals. The NIH consensus panel suggests that there is strong evidence that hypnosis can effectively manage the pain associated with some cancers. The discussion of the mechanism of hypnosis that follows is still subject to debate.

As with many of the other techniques of behavioral medicine available to the clinician, hypnosis can be used in the management of a variety of complaints. The technique is particularly valuable for use in children, who are often remarkably responsive to suggestion in situations associated with actual or anticipated pain. Children who acquire a facility for entering the trance state can call on the technique later in life in situations in which hypnoanesthesia might be useful.

Hypnosis should not be offered casually. The patient should give a suitably detailed medical and psychological history, and the therapist should initiate a preinduction discussion during which any anxieties and misconceptions about hypnosis can be verbalized and dealt with. The aim of this phase of the hypnosis experience should be to establish rapport and raise positive expectations in the patient's mind. The therapist may discuss things such as relaxation, attention, the need to trust the hypnotist, the importance of motivation for help, and hypnosis as an experience in itself. The therapist should listen for cues suggesting that certain induction techniques (arm levitation, arm lowering, coin technique) might be resisted. It is better to choose a technique that will be comfortable for the subject than one the therapist happens to prefer.

Once a choice of technique has been made, the therapist gently and progressively suggests that the phenomenon is occurring (eg, the arm is growing heavier, the subject is getting weary holding it up, etc). Instructions for induction are best communicated directly and experientially and are not presented here. However, if induction does not occur promptly, attention may be directed to the opposite of the suggestion in a subtle way. This change of direction may succeed because it now accords with the patient's actual experience (eg, the arm feels lighter, not heavier).

Once induction occurs, several techniques are available for deepening the trance state. All depend on integration of the suggestion with what is already happening: "You will feel your arms growing more relaxed with each breath you take." These deepening procedures allow the patient to become more fully attuned to internal rather than external stimuli and thus strengthen suggestions given during hypnosis.

Termination of the hypnotic session should be done in such a way that the subject gradually reorients awareness outward, notices external stimuli, and reengages with reality. The therapist's cue for signifying that the trance has ended should be chosen to suit the patient. The cues should be clear—many clinicians use a countdown procedure. Even though the therapist may have finished the hypnotic instructions and suggestions and given an instruction to reengage, it may take 10 minutes to fully reengage. During this time, the therapist may usefully review the experience with the patient, noting what was satisfactory and what was unsatisfactory.

BIOFEEDBACK

The most dramatic example of the use of techniques of behavioral medicine in the treatment of somatic complaints is biofeedback. Fuller (1977) has described biofeedback as

the use of instrumentation to mirror psychophysiological processes of which the individual is not normally aware and which may be brought under voluntary control. This means giving a person immediate information about his or her own biological conditions such as: muscle tension, skin surface temperature, brain wave activity, galvanic skin response, blood pressure, and heart rate. This feedback enables the individual to become an active participant in the process of health maintenance.

The process of electronic feedback includes instrumentation that will filter and amplify a psychophysiological signal that is then analyzed and transformed into another kind of signal capable of being "fed back" to the patient in a perceptible and comprehensible way. For example, the patient hears a tone grow louder or sees a light flash more rapidly as muscle tension or heart rate increases. This ability to associate perceived bodily experiences with processes that are ordinarily outside of conscious awareness or experience is the presumed mechanism that initiates voluntary control of the processes.

Biofeedback as a technique for treatment began in 1968, when several lines of pure research led to the discovery that in monkeys and other animals as well as in humans, physiological functions thought to be out of voluntary control were modifiable by appropriate monitoring techniques made perceptible to the subject.

Among the conditions that are now currently treated with biofeedback procedures are migraine headaches, insomnia, Raynaud's disease, enuresis, encopresis, chronic pain, hypertension, muscular tension, irritable bowel syndrome, peptic ulcer, esophageal spasm, fecal incontinence, and many neurological diseases and their sequelae.

Initiation of a biofeedback treatment regimen requires the same careful consideration of diagnosis, etiology, alternative treatments, role of the complaint in the patient's life, and impact of treatment on the patient as is required for any other treatment decision. The patient should be given a clear explanation of the procedure and its rationale.

The basic elements of biofeedback treatment are an initial evaluation session, a baseline session that will introduce the concept of home practice, a goal-setting session that will introduce the feedback part of biofeedback, a series of treatment sessions, a phase of terminal treatment sessions, and a period of follow-up.

The type of instrumentation needed to produce biofeedback depends on the behavioral problem of the patient. The beginning practitioner must learn to identify artifacts in electrophysiological recordings and to distinguish specific physiological events, background levels, and spurious measurements.

The activities in a biofeedback session consist essentially of practice in control of involuntary physiological processes. For example, to teach relaxation of the face and neck muscles to a patient with tension headache, the therapist first attaches the electronic machinery and then develops, with the patient's help, a series of instructions to attain the goals that had been set for that session. Thus, the goal might be to keep a tone below a certain threshold for 15 seconds four distinct times. At the conclusion of each session, specific homework is given, with the results to be reviewed the following session.

SUMMARY

Behavioral medicine has been an outgrowth of a variety of applied and basic science endeavors. The emphasis is on functional analysis of the behavioral aspects of somatic and psychological difficulties. The goal is to enable the patient to control bodily functions and psychological responses.

The practitioner should be aware of the growing scope of behavioral medicine. The techniques are safe and may well play an increasingly importantly role in the prevention and treatment of illness and in the promotion of healthy attitudes and behavior.

REFERENCES & SUGGESTED READINGS

Benson H: *The Relaxation Response.* William Morrow, 1975.

Blanchard EB (editor): Special issue, J Consult Clin Psychol 1992;60:4.

Boudewyns PA, Keefe FJ (editors): *Behavioral Medicine in General Medical Practice.* Addison-Wesley, 1982.

Clark CC: *Enhancing Wellness.* Springer, 1981.

Clarke JC, Jackson JA: *Hypnosis and Behavior Therapy.* Springer, 1983.

Fuller GD: *Biofeedback: Methods and Procedures in Clinical Practice.* Biofeedback Press, 1977.

Gaarder KR, Montgomery PS: *Clinical Biofeedback,* 2nd ed. Williams & Wilkins, 1981.

Keefe PJ, Dunsmore J, Burnett R: Behavioral and cognitive-behavioral approaches to chronic pain: Recent advances and future directions. J Consult Clin Psychol, 1992; 60:528.

National Institutes of Health: Integration of Behavioral and Relaxation Approaches into the Treatment of Chronic Pain and Insomnia. NIH Technol Assess Statement 1995;October 16–18:1.

Samuels M, Samuels N: *Seeing with the Mind's Eye.* Random House, 1975.

Psychiatric Care for the Chronically Ill & Dying Patient

37

Gary M. Rodin, MD

The aim of medical treatment is not only to ensure survival but also to improve the quality of life of patients who are ill. Sensitive and informed primary care providers can manage the psychosocial care of most patients with chronic or terminal illness. However, consultation or treatment provided by a mental health professional is sometimes indicated and helpful. Consideration will be given in this chapter to the psychological and psychiatric aspects of chronic and terminal medical illness, with particular emphasis on psychotherapeutic issues. A more detailed discussion of the psychiatric complications of acute medical illness and of behavioral treatments that may be of value in the medically ill can be found in Chapters 23 and 36, respectively. However, difficulty adjusting to a medical condition is usually not the result of a formal psychiatric disorder.

THE PSYCHOLOGY OF CHRONIC & TERMINAL ILLNESS

The psychological response to a particular illness is variable and depends on multiple factors, such as the characteristics of the medical illness and the personality, life stage, emotional conflicts and vulnerabilities, and cultural and social milieu of the individual affected (Figure 37–1). Because loss and disability are associated with many medical illnesses, severe emotional distress may occur in individuals who would not otherwise be affected. Diseases affecting body parts or regions of great symbolic significance, such as cancer of the breast, head and neck, or testes, may damage self-esteem and alter the sense of personal identity. Conditions such as end-stage renal disease, which require burdensome physical and dietary restrictions and time-consuming treatment, may produce great distress in individuals who value self-sufficiency, independence, or spontaneity. Diseases occurring during adolescence may provoke concerns about physical attractiveness and possible rejection by peers. In the elderly, fears of death or loss of the ability to function autonomously may be prominent (see Chapter 38). Cultural factors also affect the way in which most medical conditions are experienced (see Chapter 7). For example, diseases

such as acquired immune deficiency syndrome (AIDS) still carry a burdensome social stigma everywhere in the world. With other conditions, such as Type 1 diabetes mellitus, illness-related anxiety may be profound but not evident until the first sign of a serious complication, such as retinopathy or nephropathy.

Successful adaptation to a chronic medical illness may be characterized by the preservation of self-esteem; acceptance of the illness such that necessary treatment recommendations can be followed; engagement in vocational, family, and social activities to the extent that is permitted by the illness; and the capacity to tolerate feelings evoked by the illness without persistent anxiety or depression. Although there is no single or predictable pathway of adjustment, some common psychological responses to a serious medical illness can be identified. The initial psychologi-

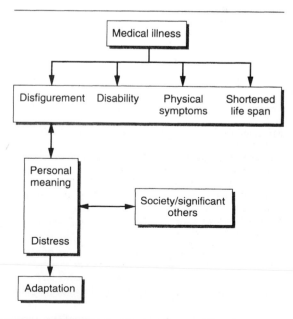

Figure 37–1. The experience of illness.

cal response to a serious or terminal medical condition may resemble a state of grief or mourning. The term *grief* refers to the acute emotional response to the perception of loss whereas *mourning* usually denotes the wider range of feelings evoked by this experience. The term *anticipatory grief* refers to the reaction to anticipated future losses.

Serious medical illness is inevitably associated with multiple losses of both a tangible and symbolic nature. Profound grief reactions may occur following the diagnosis of a potentially ominous condition such as AIDS, the occurrence of a feared complication, such as blindness in Type 1 diabetes mellitus, or the communication to a patient with cancer that further medical treatment is unlikely to halt the progression of the disease. Features of grief that may occur in these circumstances include feelings of shock, disbelief, and emotional numbness. Denial of the objective reality of the illness ("*No, it can't be me*") may be followed by or alternate with unavoidable awareness of the illness. The latter is often associated with anxiety, sadness, anger, somatic distress, and attempts to make sense of what has happened ("*Why me?*"). A 35-year-old man informed of the recurrence of a malignancy demonstrated many of these distressing features of an acute grief reaction. He reported feelings of terror and panic, as if he had entered a "*black hole*," with insomnia, nausea and vomiting, and agitation. He said "*I feel anxious all of the time. I feel overwhelmed, at the mercy of things. I feel shell-shocked. Like I am not part of the world. I have lost all sense of myself.*"

A broad range of feelings related to the illness may be experienced after the initial response to grief, although there are wide individual and cultural differences in this regard. Some individuals never wish to discuss or consider feelings related to their disease. Others welcome the opportunity to communicate their feelings and to find meaning in the experience of illness. Denial has adaptive value in the short term, but adaptation to chronic illness is usually more effective when feelings related to the condition can be acknowledged and expressed. Feelings of sadness and anger are common during the initial psychological adjustment to an illness. Subsequently, a reduction in this dysphoria and sometimes even a process of psychological reorganization and personal growth may occur. The latter may include an increased sense of the value of life and a greater motivation to engage in activities that are personally meaningful. This was expressed by one patient following a remission from her disease. She said "*In spite of my anger, I now get more enjoyment from everything I do. I don't have time to waste. I am looking for meaningful relationships, and I have a hunger to accomplish.*"

Acceptance of the illness often fluctuates and may alternate with what has been referred to as "bargaining" or attempts to postpone the inevitable. Late in the course of a terminal disease, the belief that death is imminent and inevitable may initiate another phase of adjustment. Some individuals review their lives at this time to find meaning in their accomplishments and in their ties to family and to others. Others become preoccupied with their mortality, although many patients with terminal illness continue to focus on the process of living. This commonly involves utilizing active coping mechanisms, maintaining physical activity, and attempting to overcome the complications of the illness. Unfortunately, disturbing feelings of suffering, disappointment, and victimization sometimes persist with the pain and disability of a debilitating illness. This is most likely to occur with those who have suffered from previous traumatic life experiences. Relief from such feelings may not occur until the patient's level of consciousness is altered by the metabolic and neurological complications of the illness and/or by the sedating effects of analgesic medication.

PSYCHIATRIC & PSYCHOSOCIAL INTERVENTIONS IN PATIENTS WITH CHRONIC & TERMINAL ILLNESS

Many emotional disturbances in the medically ill are alleviated by supportive contact with an attending physician. The need to refer a patient to a specialist for psychological treatment depends on a variety of factors, including the severity and nature of the patient's distress, the presence of a psychiatric disorder, the patient's motivation for assistance, and the capacity of the attending physician to deal with such matters. Unfortunately, the rate of detection of emotional disturbances in medical patients is disturbingly low. For example, moderate or severe depression in medical patients may be undetected in more than half of such cases; even when detected, the majority of patients with clinical depression do not receive appropriate antidepressant treatment. A variety of factors may contribute to this low rate of detection and treatment. Many patients are uncomfortable discussing feelings and will refrain from doing so unless the physician specifically indicates a readiness to listen. Some physicians underestimate the significance of emotional disturbances, assuming that it is "natural" for patients who are medically ill to be upset. Too often, when it is "understandable" that a patient is depressed, specific treatments such as psychotherapy or pharmacotherapy are not offered. At the other extreme, premature referral without careful assessment of the patient's emotional state may result when the physician is uncomfortable with emotional issues. In such cases, speedy referral to a psychiatrist or other mental health practitioner may represent an attempt by the physician to avoid the patient's distress. Physicians may recognize that symptoms such as depression are present but do not appreciate that effective treatments are available. The failure to intervene in such cases is unfortunate, since depression is associated with significant disability and distress and medical illness is a risk factor for suicide. The medical profession can play a significant role in suicide prevention; most patients who commit suicide have contacted a physician from a few hours to a few months before death.

PSYCHOTHERAPY FOR PATIENTS WITH CHRONIC OR TERMINAL ILLNESS

A variety of pharmacological and psychosocial interventions are available to treat psychiatric disorders and emotional distress in medically ill patients (see Chapter 39). There are two major psychotherapeutic approaches that can be adopted by a primary care practitioner or by a mental health professional: (1) promotion of active coping strategies and (2) supportive-expressive therapy, to assist with understanding and management of feelings evoked by illness. These two approaches, described below, may be offered on an individual basis or in a group setting.

Promotion of Active Coping Strategies

Serious and disabling medical illness represents a threat to an individual's sense of competence and mastery and may trigger feelings of helplessness, ineffectiveness, and uncertainty. A variety of therapeutic strategies may be employed on an individual, group, or family basis to help patients with such conditions regain a sense of mastery. Techniques that can provide symptomatic relief of illness-related distress include relaxation therapy and mindfulness meditation. The latter refers to techniques to alter attention and awareness as a means of modulating disturbing experience. Education of patients and their families about the medical condition and about steps that can be taken to decrease symptoms, to prolong survival, or to obtain further assistance may diminish feelings of helplessness. These approaches, which can be adapted to specific diseases, are cost efficient, provide peer support, and, when administered in a group setting, may decrease feelings of isolation. Other forms of group therapy, including self-help groups, may facilitate the sharing of experiences and information and reinforce active coping strategies. Behavioral strategies, including relaxation, guided imagery, and hypnosis (see Chapter 36), may help to reduce pain and other distressing symptoms and to prevent demoralization and despair. Cognitive therapy may help to correct cognitive distortions related to medical illness and to replace dysfunctional thoughts with more adaptive ones. Such approaches may be used, together with anxiolytic and analgesic medication, to reduce symptoms and to increase feelings of control over the illness.

Psychodynamic Therapy: Supportive & Expressive

A. Supportive Therapy: The traditional role of the medical practitioner in maintaining a consistent, reliable, empathic relationship with the patient is often the most important psychotherapeutic factor for patients with chronic or terminal illness. Indeed, once the medical treatment plan is established, the relationship with the physician may be one of the most critical factors in maintaining morale and hope. The value of this relationship is too often underestimated by physicians who feel they must respond to a patient's emotional distress by *"doing something"*— prescribing medication, offering advice, ordering further laboratory tests, etc.

The overall aim in supportive psychotherapy is to bolster adaptive and minimize maladaptive coping mechanisms and to decrease adverse psychological reactions such as fear, shame, and self-disparagement. This treatment can often be provided effectively by an interested primary care practitioner who has an ongoing relationship with the patient. Further, a supportive relationship with a medical caregiver may lessen the need for analgesic or psychotropic medication and may reduce the problem of noncompliance with medical treatment. There is no clear boundary between supportive and expressive (insight-oriented) psychotherapy, although there are differences in emphasis (see Chapter 31). In both treatments, the therapist may help the patient to understand the illness experience in a meaningful fashion. However, the objectives in the former are focused more on symptomatic relief and on maintaining psychological equilibrium. This is accomplished by a more structured approach, which is more likely to include interventions such as education, reality testing, reassurance, and advice. Reassurance and advice are most helpful when they are based on a realistic appreciation of the patient's situation. However, the well-intentioned but misguided use of such interventions is common. For example, reassurance that is premature or unrealistic is rarely comforting and may leave patients feeling even more isolated with their distress. Further, although advice may be helpful, particularly when related to management of the illness, it should be given sparingly in personal matters. It is usually best to help patients make their own personal decisions rather than to try to make decisions for them.

B. Expressive (Insight-Oriented) Therapy: The emphasis in expressive psychotherapy is on promoting self-understanding and psychological growth. This treatment, which usually requires referral to a trained psychotherapist, is most suitable for the small minority of medical patients who have identifiable and significant psychological or interpersonal problems, who are motivated to understand their feelings, and who have the ability to form a therapeutic relationship. To begin treatment, some patients need help in overcoming their initial fears of depending on or revealing themselves to another. Expressive psychotherapy may allow medical patients to express their feelings in a safe setting without fears of alienating either their family or their primary caregivers.

Contraindications to expressive psychotherapy in the medically ill include (1) the presence of medical conditions in which emotional arousal may be medically hazardous, eg, recent myocardial infarction; (2) medical crises or other stresses that limit the patient's capacity to tolerate anxiety or emotional disruption; and (3) delirium or dementia caused by cardiovascular, neurological, metabolic, or other disorders. The cognitive impairment associated with these conditions may limit the capacity for verbal expression, and the concomitant emotional lability may increase the vulnerability to states of disorganization and distress when emotional exploration is attempted. The cognitive functions and emotional lability of medical patients should be carefully assessed before insight-oriented psychotherapy is instituted.

Establishing the Focus of Psychological Treatment

The entire spectrum of psychiatric and psychosocial interventions should be considered with medically ill patients who are distressed. Pharmacological and other medical interventions for anxiety, depression, delirium, and pain in medically ill patients are discussed in Chapter 30. Psychosocial interventions involving the family, community agencies, and self-help groups may be of great value in assisting in the process of adjustment. Further, help that is provided by or related to the individual's cultural, ethnic, and religious group may offer emotional support and personal meaning, both of which may alleviate feelings of isolation and despair. Indeed, spiritual and religious issues are important aspects of the illness experience for many medical patients and therapists must be prepared to address these issues explicitly and/or implicitly.

There are many reasons why medical patients seek therapy and there can be an equally wide diversity in its goals. Psychological assistance is most frequently sought to relieve disturbing symptoms of depression or anxiety. Physicians must consider the indications for social, psychological, or pharmacological interventions in such cases. Particularly perplexing to evaluate is the mental state of patients who decide to terminate life-sustaining medical treatment. In such cases, there may be a rational decision to refuse medical treatment or to end life in the face of unbearable suffering. However, such so-called "rational suicides" must be distinguished from other motivations, such as the wish to elicit concern from caregivers, to manage unbearable feelings of helplessness or to be relieved of pain. Also, the decision to stop treatment may be secondary to the effects of depression or organic mental disorders on mental competency, on the ability to form rational intent, or on the ability to remain hopeful about the future. The distinction between a rational decision to stop treatment and a decision that is determined by the hopelessness associated with a depressive disorder is often difficult to make with terminally ill patients. A trial of antidepressant treatment may be indicated in such cases.

Some medical patients seek psychological treatment in the hope that it will improve their health or their chances for long-term survival. This belief has been reinforced in recent years by attention in the media to the role of psychological factors in illness. However, although there is some scientific evidence that links psychological well-being with a favorable medical outcome, unrealistic expectations of benefit from psychological treatment need to be addressed. The desire to modify behavior that is adversely affecting health (eg, noncompliance with a medical treatment regimen), is a valid focus of treatment. However, some patients unrealistically attribute all of their personal difficulties, even preexisting ones, to their illness. Others attempt to deny the significance or even the existence of the illness. The adaptive value of denial should not be underestimated, particularly during the acute phase of an illness. However, when it persists, it may interfere with accepting appropriate treatment or with anticipating and preparing for the personal difficulties that may lie ahead. When such denial should be supported or challenged is a matter of careful clinical judgment. This issue may be illustrated in the following case.

Illustrative Case

A 35-year-old health care worker sought a psychiatric assessment shortly after a routine medical examination revealed a positive human immunodeficiency virus (HIV) blood test. He did not feel in need of current emotional assistance but decided to identify a variety of medical specialists who could provide help that he might subsequently require. He was extremely knowledgeable about the medical aspects of AIDS, both from his medical training and from his personal experience caring for many friends through the terminal stages of their illness. He had also read extensively about the phases of psychological adjustment to a terminal medical illness. He wondered what phase he was in, although he denied any current symptoms of emotional distress. He was extremely concerned about the welfare of others, and he had already made adjustments in his work and personal life to be sure he would not place others at risk. Also, he had bought a large house several years earlier for the express purpose of caring for his friends with AIDS.

When interviewed, the patient was physically wasted and coughed frequently. He was cooperative, articulate, and demonstrated features of mild anxiety. He believed that he had not yet developed any symptoms of AIDS, and he hoped that his recent treatment with protease inhibitors would halt the progression of the disease. However, he reported unexplained increased fatigue and frequent episodes of diarrhea over the past 2 years. When his obvious respiratory symptoms were noted, he became markedly uncomfortable and asserted that he did not believe these symptoms were related to AIDS. His cognitive functions were intact, and his sensorium was clear.

It was evident that the patient had successfully employed active coping strategies to maintain a high level of adjustment both before and after his positive HIV blood test. He demonstrated considerable knowledge about his medical condition and about psychological issues. However, he seemed to deny the apparent progression of his disease or any sense of personal vulnerability. His denial and his active coping strategies were currently adaptive and were not directly challenged. However, ongoing psychotherapeutic contact was arranged to provide support that might be required if his disease progressed further. It was assumed that he might presently be experiencing more distress than he was able to acknowledge and that he was at risk to become more depressed or anxious when the advancement of his disease interfered with his self-sufficient and altruistic stance.

The Process of Therapy in the Medically Ill

Psychotherapy with chronically ill medical patients resembles therapy with patients who are physically well. However, greater flexibility on the part of the therapist is required with the medically ill, because of the adjustments that are necessary when there is an exacerbation of the medical disorder. At such times it may be necessary to shift from insight-oriented therapy to an approach that is more supportive in nature. Further, when a patient is hospitalized, treatment may need to continue in less than optimal circumstances, sometimes at the bedside. Although the patient's right to privacy must be respected, involvement of the therapist through all phases of an illness may be crucial in maintaining the therapeutic alliance. For many patients, the medical illness has already created feelings of isolation from the "normal" or "healthy" world. A therapist who discontinues treatment when the medical condition worsens may heighten these feelings of isolation. In some cases, it may help to continue the therapeutic dialogue by telephone or e-mail when patients cannot travel to appointments.

Countertransference

Medically ill patients may provoke a variety of emotional reactions in the therapist, sometimes referred to as countertransference. Some patients elicit overconcern; others arouse feelings of hostility and rejection. The therapist must identify such feelings to understand the patient better and to maintain an attitude of therapeutic neutrality. Neutrality in this context does not mean indifference but refers to a thera-

peutic stance that is attuned to the patient's feelings and needs. Interventions that arise from the needs of the therapist, even when well intended, may not be useful to the patient. For example, a therapist may become overly supportive to counteract his or her own underlying feelings of frustration and impotence. Such well-meaning interventions may deprive some patients of the opportunity to maintain their sense of autonomy and self-sufficiency or to express their frustration and anger. Hostile feelings in the therapist may also arise and may serve to maintain emotional distance from a patient whose distress threatens to be overwhelming. In other cases, patients with intense anger may hope to achieve a greater sense of control over their feelings by provoking similar feelings in the therapist. To remain constructively involved with the emotional experience of their patients, primary care physicians and therapists who care for the medically ill must learn to be aware of and to tolerate such intense feelings in themselves and in their patients.

Collaboration with the Primary Care Physician

Psychotherapy with medically ill patients places special emotional and practical demands on the therapist. The treatment in such cases often needs to be conducted in collaboration with the primary care physician, who retains responsibility for medical management of the patient. The therapist must remain aware of the patient's current medical status, without assuming direct responsibility for it. Therapists must permit feelings of resentment toward the primary caregivers to emerge, but must be careful not to intervene or to undermine that primary relationship. Attempts by the patient to form special relationships that split the medical staff and create tension among them can be prevented only by frequent communication among all members of the medical team. Because of the need for such communication, it is generally unwise for the therapist to promise absolute confidentiality. Therapists should avoid unnecessary disclosure of personal information about the patient to medical staff, but should be free to communicate about matters that affect the medical course. Some issues regarding collaboration with the medical staff are depicted in the following case.

Illustrative Case

A 21-year-old single diabetic woman was referred for psychiatric consultation during a hospital admission at a time when her vision was deteriorating rapidly. She agreed to the consultation, although she did not feel in need of assistance. In fact, as her vision failed, she resented the increased protectiveness of her family and others and decided to move out of the family home. From the time of onset of her diabetes at age 6 years, she believed that her parents experienced her illness as a burden. She felt unable to rely on them for support and withdrew from emotional contact with them.

The patient began weekly psychotherapy cautiously. Whenever she felt neglected or abused by any of her physicians, she experienced resentment that was generalized to include everyone with whom she was involved, including the therapist. Specifically, she objected to the fact that the medical staff communicated with one another about her and knew that she was seeing a psychiatrist. She was angry that communication between the therapist and the rest of the medical team about her physical status had been established as a condition of her psychotherapy.

Although the patient's concerns about confidentiality were acknowledged to be valid, the importance of the therapist's ongoing contact with the medical staff became increasingly apparent. This collaboration was sometimes necessary to determine the extent to which disturbances in her emotional state were affected by or caused by alterations in her metabolic control. At another point, when the factitious administration of insulin or sedative drugs was suspected, discussion and collaboration with the medical staff were essential. The intimacy and dependency that resulted from the establishment of a therapeutic relationship were frightening to her, and she responded initially with detachment and attempts to split the medical staff. However, this relationship subsequently provided the patient with a limited and restricted means by which she could begin to develop some degree of trust in others. Only later did deep-seated fears of her unacceptability and her potential destructiveness to others emerge.

The Facilitation of Grief & Mourning

Medical patients frequently enter psychotherapy in a state of distress because their usual coping mechanisms have been eroded by the physical and psychological effects of illness. Grief and mourning are commonly related to the anticipated or actual loss of competence and bodily integrity and to the disruption in the expected trajectory of life-span and accomplishments. Oscillations between denying the implications of the illness and feeling overwhelmed by it are common. The first phase of psychotherapy involves listening to the patient and allowing thoughts and feelings related to the illness to emerge in a gradual and tolerable fashion. This may involve providing support and reassurance when patients are flooded with feelings and gentle exploration when feelings have become closed off. The following case illustrates the phases of psychotherapy in a patient who was referred after cancer of the breast was diagnosed.

Illustrative Case

A 32-year-old married woman was referred for psychotherapy after being told that a recent breast biopsy indicated the presence of a malignancy. She reported feeling enraged and hopeless, and refused any medical or surgical treatment for her disease. This refusal reflected her anger, her sense of futility, and her wish to deny the presence of the cancer. She described a dream in which a woman was murdered, which she believed reflected her own experience of being assaulted and potentially destroyed by the illness. She regarded both radiotherapy and surgery as forms of further physical assault.

The initial therapeutic task was to facilitate the gradual expression of feelings related to the illness. The therapist needed to proceed flexibly and to be guided in each session by the patient's willingness and capacity to explore her feelings. During the phase of acute grief, patients are commonly unable to be introspective or to make use of psychological insight. The most important goal at this stage is to provide an environment in which thoughts and feelings related to the illness can be safely discussed. The stabilizing effect of the therapeutic relationship is more beneficial at this stage than are any specific interpretations. The process of understanding cannot begin until the period of acute grief has passed and the patient feels less overwhelmed. The patient described feeling more hopeful after the fifth session and said to the therapist that she had "combined my strength with yours." She also felt able to consider and to proceed with appropriate medical treatment options.

Organization of the Experience of Illness

In the patient just described, the diagnosis of breast cancer revived long-standing feelings of being defective and unacceptable, and undermined her sense of femininity. In the middle phase of therapy, she reported a dream in which she was accepted at a desirable school but then received a notice informing her that she could not attend. For her, this dream represented both the opportunities and plans she felt the illness had stolen from her as well as her feeling of having been damaged and made undesirable to others. The experience of her illness also brought her much closer to underlying feelings of dependency and abandonment. Later in the therapy, she reported a fantasy of being a needy, colicky baby whose mother could not cope with her and for the first time she revealed her belief that her mother never really wanted her.

As therapy progressed, this patient became more able to reflect on her feelings. The therapist could now assist her in integrating and working through the mourning process associated with the illness. Feelings of sadness could be more safely expressed in the presence of a firmly established therapeutic relationship. Providing meaning and organization to her experience in this phase helped to diminish her feelings of helplessness and isolation. This process depended on the empathic involvement of the therapist, whom the patient felt was able to "live the experience with me."

Mastery

Serious medical illness often represents a threat to an individual's sense of competence. An important goal of psychotherapeutic treatment is to restore the sense of competence and mastery. Initial unsuccessful attempts to achieve mastery by denying the illness or by evading its significance may later be replaced by a greater capacity to experience safely a broader range of feelings related to the illness. The patient described above became more able to tolerate feelings of vulnerability without feeling overwhelmed. She now felt motivated to examine her previous tendency to conceal feelings of insecurity and dependency beneath a veneer of self-sufficiency. Although she felt that the illness "removed a crutch," her vulnerabilities were no longer so threatening to her. She felt more able to accept her illness and to consider and select appropriate treatment. She no longer felt the same need to affirm her strength by denying her illness, refusing treatment, or taking her life.

OUTCOME & COST-BENEFIT ANALYSIS OF PSYCHOTHERAPY WITH THE MEDICALLY ILL

The benefit of psychotherapy in improving the quality of life of medical patients is often underestimated by medical practitioners. Some of the clearest evidence of the benefits of psychotherapy has been obtained from studies of the medically ill. The beneficial effects of psychotherapy have been demonstrated not only by improvements in psychological well-being but also by reduced utilization of medical resources. Medical patients who participate in psychotherapy have been shown to require fewer medical investigations and treatments, either because of the effect of psychotherapy on overall health status or because of the more appropriate allocation of medical and psychological resources. There are also reports that psychotherapy may result in prolonged survival in patients with cancer and other serious medical conditions.

SUMMARY

Medical illness is a stressful event in the life of any patient, although the specific meaning of the illness and the psychological response to it may depend on a variety of factors. Treatment of depression or other psychiatric disorders may result in an improvement of the patient's emotional state, an increased ability to engage in a wide range of social and physical activities, and a reduced tendency to utilize health care measures. Psychoeducational approaches and other interventions to support active coping strategies may help maintain morale and quality of life in many medical patients. These may be administered on an individual, family, or group basis. Supportive psychotherapy as an adjunct to treatment may be an important function of the primary care practitioner. A small proportion of medical patients may be suitable for and may benefit from expressive (insight-oriented) psychotherapy conducted by a specially trained psychotherapist. This treatment may diminish the likelihood of persistent depression or of prematurely giving up on the possibilities of life. However, insight-oriented therapy may be contraindicated for some medical patients because of physical debilitation or cognitive impairment.

Psychotherapy may assist medical patients in working through feelings associated with the multiple losses and the possibility or certainty of death related to the illness. Patients grieve for anticipated losses as well as for those that have already occurred. Therapy is often directed toward facilitation of the mourning process and achievement of a sense of competence and mastery related to it. Physical illness may impose realistic limitations that cannot be overcome by psychological treatment. In these and other respects, medical illness may present an ongoing challenge to the sense of competence of the therapist as well as the patient.

Medical complications or hospitalizations may disrupt the therapeutic process. The ability of a patient who is physically unwell to tolerate affective arousal may fluctuate widely, and therapeutic interventions at any point must take this into account. In some cases, the physical condition interferes with the ability of the patient to form a therapeutic relationship. In addition, the therapeutic relationship may be affected by other factors, such as the necessary breach of confidentiality that occurs when therapists work in collaboration with the medical treatment team. Although psychotherapy may in some cases be the most important feature of management of a medically ill patient, psychotherapists more often play a secondary role. The treatment of medical complications is often the most urgent priority.

REFERENCES & SUGGESTED READINGS

Allebeck P, Bolund C: Suicides and suicide attempts in cancer patients. Psychol Med 1991;21:979.

Anderson BL: Psychological interventions for cancer patients to enhance the quality of life. J Consul Clin Psychol 1992;60:552.

Craven J, Rodin G (editors): *Psychiatric Aspects of Organ Transplantation.* Oxford University Press, 1992.

Holland JC, et al (editors): *Psycho-oncology.* Oxford University Press, 1998.

Langer KG: Psychotherapy with the neuropsychologically impaired adult. Am J Psychother 1992;XLVI:620.

Rodin G, Craven J, Littlefield C: *Depression in the Medically Ill: An Integrated Approach.* Brunner/Mazel, 1991.

Spiegel D: Cancer and depression. Brit J Psychiatry 1996; 30(suppl):109.

Starkstein SE, Robinson RG (editors): *Depression in Neurologic Disease.* Johns Hopkins University Press, 1993.

Worden JW: *Grief Counseling and Grief Therapy: A Handbook for the Mental Health Practitioner,* 2nd ed. Springer, 1991.

Geriatric Psychiatry

38

Gary L. Gottlieb, MD, MBA

Long life is desirable if adequate physical function and, particularly, intellectual function can be maintained. Many people face the aging process with apprehension. Fears about cognitive decline are heightened by increasing awareness that pathological processes accompany aging. Older adults are concerned that they will lose their autonomy and personal identity. The aging process may threaten the ability to think, love, and communicate. Early recognition by the physician of behavioral disorders in aging patients may allow rapid treatment of reversible causes and fuller exploitation of retained assets in chronic and deteriorating conditions. Optimization of mental abilities can be expected to favorably influence the outcome of aging-related problems of many kinds and perhaps to avoid the need for long-term custodial or nursing home care.

DEMOGRAPHIC ISSUES

Just 30 years ago, only one of every 11 Americans was over 65 years of age. Today, slightly less than one in eight have reached that age. The elderly population grew by 23% to nearly 31 million during the 1980s. As a result of relatively small depression era birth rates, the older population should grow by about 10% during the 1990s and it is projected to grow by 12% during the first decade of the next century. This rate of growth will yield about 39 million older Americans by 2010 (U.S. Bureau of the Census, 1998). Shortly thereafter, the aging of the post-World War II "baby boom" cohort will cause a dramatic growth in the over-65 population segment. By 2030, about one-fourth of the population—about 66 million people—will be over 65. By the year 2000, 45% of the older population will be at least 75 years old, with the number of those over age 85 growing at a faster rate than any other segment of the population (Soldo and Agree, 1988).

Sex differences in life expectancy and the distribution of minorities among the elderly have important health-related consequences. There are approximately three women for every two men over age 65 and five women for every two men over age 85. Ethnic minorities comprise a growing segment of the older population. In 1997, about 11% of persons over age 65 were nonwhite. By the year 2025, about 15% of the elderly are projected to be members of minority groups (National Center for Health Statistics, 1992). Although life expectancy at birth for whites exceeds that for African-Americans by about 8%, at age 75, mortality rates for the latter are lower than those for whites. However, very old African-Americans have considerably higher rates of poverty and illness than whites in the same age group. Economic and social discrimination and underprivilege associated with minority status are exaggerated by the socioeconomic realities of older age: accrued social and financial resources are limited, barriers to preventive and acute health care are harder to breach, and the need for non-health care governmental services is greater, including housing, transportation, food, and income maintenance. Cultural differences may also affect the expression of illness and the ways in which health care is accessed and delivered.

In 1997, one in eight people over age 65—close to 4 million Americans—had an income below the poverty level. About 10% of the younger population were in that income category. Indigence appears to increase with age: about one-fifth of people who live past the age of 85 have incomes at or below the poverty level. These rates are even more dramatic for women and for minorities. For example, 60% of black women over age 65 not living with their families were below the poverty level in 1997.

ORGAN SYSTEM FUNCTION & AGING

Over the past century, numerous theories have been offered to explain biological aging or the normative decline in the quantity of active metabolic cells and the reduction in cellular function that occur throughout the life cycle (Leventhal, 1996). Some of these theories are partially supported by documented aging changes in cell and tissue structure and function. However, a truly useful and empirically demonstrated theory of the aging process is as yet unavailable.

Diminished reserve and ability to respond to stress and insults reflect a reduction in functional and regenerative capacity. Individual aging can be thought of as the manifestation of a person's genetic vulnerability to disease. Aging affects every organ system. Cells are lost, and enzymatic and messenger systems within cells reach a state of reduced productivity or responsiveness.

Age-related changes in body composition result in a decrease of as much as 80% in total muscle mass and an average increase of 35% in total body fat. Body fat is also redistributed, accumulating within the viscera and diminishing at or near the body surface. In both sexes, the lungs, kidneys, and skin age more rapidly than the heart and liver. Bone mineralization in women after menopause declines 8 to 10 times more rapidly than in men of the same age, which means that women are at risk for osteoporosis-related fractures about 10 years earlier than men. Ovarian function declines in middle age, and production of estrogens and progesterone ceases. This results not only in menopause but in loss of the protective effects of these hormones, increasing the risk of atherosclerotic cardiovascular disease and stroke as well as osteoporosis. In contrast, testicular function and hormonal production and secretion persist in men with little alteration until at least the eighth decade.

The central nervous system undergoes a somewhat selective loss of neurons during aging. Although there is constant cell loss throughout the brain over the life span, total age-related cortical neuronal degeneration is minimal. There is random loss of neurons throughout the cortex and disproportionately greater loss of cells in the locus ceruleus, the substantia nigra, the cerebellum, and the olfactory bulbs.

Brain changes associated with aging could suggest that cognitive decline is also inevitable. However, a growing literature in neuropsychology suggests that aging affects certain aspects of cognition while sparing others and that global decline, such as that seen in dementia, is certainly not normal. Individual factors such as intelligence, education, and environment affect cognitive ability and test performance in aging individuals. Therefore, generalizations regarding changes in cognitive function with aging should be made cautiously.

Memory is the component of cognition that concerns practitioners and patients most. Older adults fear that memory loss will contribute to loss of autonomy. Furthermore, memory loss is the symptom that we most strongly associate with progressive dementia, particularly Alzheimer's disease. Numerous studies have evaluated memory function in older adults compared with younger people. Most of these investigations indicate that there is a decline in the speed with which information is retrieved from memory stores associated with aging and that acquisition and retrieval of new information are most profoundly affected by the aging process. Memory for entrenched learning and personal information does not appear to be affected by aging.

Certain aspects of general intellectual function appear to be unaffected by aging. Knowledge acquired in the course of socialization and development tends to remain stable into older adulthood. However, the abilities required for the solution of complex new problems decline slowly through the life span. Poor physical health and overall loss of personal well-being also affect intellectual function adversely.

MENTAL HEALTH & THE OLDER ADULT

Over 18% of older adults are thought to be suffering from significant mental health problems at any given time (Myers et al, 1984). These people (and their families) depend almost exclusively on primary care physicians to recognize and manage complaints related to intellectual and emotional function—specifically, depression and dementia. Inasmuch as the elderly consume a substantial proportion of general medical services, prevention and early detection of disorders of high prevalence in this population are essential. The subtlety of mental impairment in this population unfortunately limits the ability of many primary care physicians to diagnose and treat the disorders.

Mental function influences all other areas of individual function. Because the ability to interact and communicate with others and to manage one's personal affairs is controlled by higher-order cortical functions, virtually all activities of daily living are adversely influenced by disturbances in cognitive or emotional status.

Similarly, medical well-being and hygienic life style are severely undermined by psychiatric disorders. Compliance with medical regimens is poor among older adults. Older patients with even mild symptoms of depression express a negative perception of their own health status, have more physical complaints, and make more physician visits than do normal elderly patients (Gottlieb, 1996).

Early recognition of mental disorders is important for a number of reasons. Older adults are more vulnerable than others to the central nervous system effects of somatic illnesses and their treatments. For example, urinary tract infections and surgical repair of hip fracture are associated with delirium in the elderly. Similarly, treatment of chronic pain with opioids may impair mood and cognition. The assumption that changes in mental well-being are normal features of the aging process may make the practitioner less aggressive than would be optimal in determining the origin of a change in cognition, affect, or thought content. This may prevent possible improvements in function and quality of life. Numerous studies indicate that between 55% and 80% of elderly depressives will respond to psychotherapeutic or somatic treatments. However, reversibility depends on early recognition and treatment—ie, delayed intervention imposes a risk of chronic deterioration. Improvement in symptoms may prolong productive and autonomous function and postpone or avoid altogether the need for acute or long-term institutionalization.

Mental disorders are the most frequently diagnosed problems in nursing homes. Families report that difficulty in managing the behavior of an impaired older adult is of substantial importance in the decision to seek nursing home placement. Early intervention by the physician can potentially prolong an individual's ability to remain in the less restrictive and more affordable home environment.

Community surveys estimate that severe forms of dementing illness affect more than 5% of people over 65 years of age. Another 10–15% of elderly adults are thought to suffer mild to moderate dementia. Prevalence rates for dementia jump to 23–47% in adults over age 85 (Evans et al, 1989). Nearly 70% of patients who present with evidence of significant cognitive impairment probably have Alzheimer's disease.

The prevalence of symptoms of depression among the elderly is similarly impressive. Prevalence rates of depression in large samples of community-resident elderly of 13–18% have been found (Blazer et al, 1991). Studies of elderly medical patients reveal an even higher prevalence of this disorder (about 27%). Suicide rates among the elderly are disproportionately high. This population comprises only about 12% of the population but accounts for nearly one-fourth of all suicides. For example, although the suicide rate for the general population is approximately 13 per 100,000, the rate for white men in their 80s is close to three times that number (National Center for Health Statistics, 1992). Older people with depression have more somatic symptoms and visit primary care providers more frequently than their nondepressed counterparts, and they rarely are treated by mental health specialists. For that reason, identification and treatment of depression in older adults—or referral for management by a psychiatrist—become a major responsibility of the primary physician.

RISK FACTORS ASSOCIATED WITH AGING

Losses and adverse life events are now recognized as major determinants of psychiatric illness in the elderly. Losses are the price of aging as friends and loved ones die or move away, so that social isolation may replace established support networks. Retirement or loss of primary function in the home, particularly when it is unplanned or unwanted, has been correlated with apathy, involution, and depression. Grief and bereavement are probably the most important threats to emotional well-being of old people. Loss of a child or, more commonly, a spouse is an important risk factor for major depression, hypochondriasis, and decline in function. Although these environmental and psychosocial stressors are unavoidable in the process of normal aging, their identification by the physician is important in preventing morbid outcomes.

The consequences of grief and bereavement can be eased by the establishment of at least one intimate and confiding relationship. The physician who is aware of a recent or impending loss in the life of a patient can help by fostering a relationship with a friend or relative. Family members may need to be instructed about the need for this level of intimacy and support. Isolated elderly people must be repeatedly encouraged to participate in church or community senior activities and, if necessary, support groups for the bereaved. If no network of support or relationship can be established, referral for supportive psychotherapy during the period of acute loss may be necessary.

Retirement is associated with a one-third to one-half reduction in personal income (Gottlieb, 1996; Soldo and Agree, 1988). Role changes will also have direct effects on self-esteem. Many individuals retire in their late 50s or early 60s. Close to 90% of men in their early 50s are in the labor force, whereas only about 50% of men between the ages of 62 and 64 work (Longino and Mittelmark, 1996; US Bureau of the Census, 1997, 1998). The employment rate declines rapidly with advancing age; after age 70, only about 10% of men and 5% of women are still working. Elimination of mandatory retirement and shifting of the American economy from heavy industry to less physically demanding kinds of employment may extend the working longevity of the population in the near future.

The physician should envision retirement as a period of loss in the patient's life history. However, appropriate planning can mitigate its adverse effects. Individuals who undertake retirement with plans to do what they enjoy and value are least likely to become depressed. As soon as the physician is aware of a patient's retirement plans, a process should be put in motion for prevention of adverse consequences. Social workers, activities counselors, and occupational therapists as well as career counselors can, for example, suggest opportunities for skilled volunteer work, part-time employment, and structured recreational activities. Activities planned for the retirement period must be considered meaningful and serve to replace and compensate for the patient's narcissistic investment in work roles.

Functional disability resulting from multiple medical illnesses and orthopedic and neurological disabilities must be perceived as a major loss. However, education about the severity of illness, the prognosis, and the usefulness of medication can allow the patient to maintain control and self-esteem when fears about dependency become dominant. As disability becomes evident, assessment of patient function becomes necessary in two general areas: (1) in the basic activities of daily living (ADL)—eating, bathing and grooming, toileting, ambulation and transportation; and (2) the instrumental activities of daily living (IADL)—functions required to maintain independent community living, including managing finances, using public transportation, shopping, using the telephone, etc. After these assessments, the physician will have adequate data to help the patient improve function while maintaining retained assets.

Sensory function must be assessed carefully, and attempts to correct deficits must be made aggressively. Auditory and visual impairments are common in older adults. These disabilities heighten isolation and may be mistaken for cognitive or emotional disorders. Sensory losses are associated with both paranoid disorders and depression. Paraphrenic disorders (late life paranoia) are highly correlated with hearing loss and, to a lesser extent, with blindness. Audiometric screening and appropriate use of a hearing aid have been shown to reverse some of these symptoms. Deafness may accentuate alienation and discrimination, which may be reversible with the use of an aid. Similarly, cataracts and glaucoma commonly impair vision in the elderly. However, psychiatric symptoms, including confusion, anxiety, fearfulness, and depression, may precede complaints of visual impairment. Improvement of sensory function may eradicate these symptoms without the need for psychiatric intervention.

EVALUATING CLINICAL COMPLAINTS

Although the prevalence of chronic illness peaks in older adulthood, most older people enjoy relatively good health. Even so, older adults consume approximately 30% of all health care resources although they comprise only about 12% of the population. The aging-related challenges and losses described above have been shown to increase somatic symptoms and medical care utilization. Furthermore, older adults are likely to suffer at least mild chronic pain and some alteration in baseline physical health and functional ability. Therefore, it may be difficult to distinguish reality-based complaints and preoccupations from psychiatric symptoms. Similarly, psychiatric and neurological syndromes in geriatric patients are often accompanied by somatic preoccupation.

Preoccupation with physical health and fear of illness cause many older people to describe symptoms for which no organic cause can be found. They may be subjected to uncomfortable, risky, and expensive workups from numerous physicians serially or even simultaneously. Even though aggressive evaluation is essential, and somatic complaints should never be ignored, medical workups may have substantial health risks in frail older patients. Geriatric health care therefore should include communication among all treating physicians and efforts to minimize redundancy and overlap. The care of older patients includes the need to obtain all available records from hospitals, other physicians, and reliable informants.

History Taking

All of the risk factors described in the previous section can be documented in the process of routine medical history taking. The description of medical symptoms and the related systems review form the core of the patient interview. The same rapport required to obtain a good medical history will allow essential psychosocial data to be obtained. However, the interaction of medical and psychiatric disorders in the elderly requires painstaking assessment and special clinical skill to discriminate somatic and behavioral complaints.

Mental Status Examination: Assessing Cognitive Function & Depression

The prevalence of behavioral disorders in the elderly requires that a brief examination of mental status be part of every evaluation. Observation of appearance, affect, mood, psychomotor function (ie, retardation or agitation), speech, and thought processes and content (including suicidal and homicidal ideation) should be part of routine history taking. Attention to these details will improve sensitivity to mood disorders, symptoms of anxiety and panic, paranoid thinking, hallucinosis, other elements of psychosis, and cognitive impairment. The review of systems should garner data about sleep patterns, appetite, concentration, memory, and sexual function.

Retained social skills, the subtlety of findings, and patient and family denial may make routine screening for changes in **cognitive function** a difficult task. The lack of clear age-related norms for intellectual ability hampers efforts to distinguish normal aging from diseases of old people. However, inasmuch as cognitive impairment is highly prevalent in the elderly, and because many conditions that impair cognition can be palliated, it is essential that physicians have the ability to screen rapidly for dysfunction. The Mini-Mental Status Examination (MMSE) (Folstein et al, 1975) is widely used both in clinical research and in practice to screen for problems with orientation, memory, concentration, language, and comprehension. It has been correlated with sophisticated psychometric testing, and cut-off scores for "normal" and impaired function have been established. Orientation, registration, calculating ability (concentration), recall, naming, figure copying, graphic ability, and ability to follow complex commands are superficially screened in only a few minutes. The MMSE is a simple method for determining the need for further evaluation and quickly reassessing cognitive status.

Depression can be difficult to discern in older adults. Older adults with depression often present with complaints of physical illness, and depressive symptoms are easily confused with numerous medical conditions. Subjectively depressed mood, guilt, and suicidal ideation are rarely expressed. Somatic complaints, disturbances of sleep and appetite, anxiety, and apathy often predominate. Patients often insist that their difficulties are physical in origin. Diffuse pain and gastrointestinal discomfort are common. These complaints, as well as apathy, fatigue, and weight loss, are an indication for an extensive workup. Again, aggressive evaluation is necessary to rule out disorders that present with depressed mood, including occult cancer, infections (eg, viral pneumonia or hepatitis), endocrine disorder (eg, hypothyroidism, apathetic hyperthyroidism, Cushing's disease, Addison's disease, panhypopituitarism), central nervous system disease (eg, Parkinson's disease, early Alzheimer's disease), intracranial mass lesions, stroke, major systemic illnesses (eg, congestive heart failure), dehydration, renal disease, and early pulmonary disease. These disorders often affect mood and function and can give rise to symptoms similar to those of major depression. However, even completely negative exhaustive workups rarely convince patients that symptoms are primarily "mental."

Careful scrutiny of patient medication regimens may uncover an iatrogenic origin for changes in function and perceived quality of life. Many drugs given for medical disorders in the elderly have adverse central nervous system side effects. Depressive symptoms are not uncommonly associated with antihypertensives, including reserpine, methyldopa, beta-blockers, and hydralazine. Histamine H_2 antagonists, digoxin, oral hypoglycemics, steroids, and cytotoxic agents may cause depression. Almost any central nervous system depressant, including barbiturates, benzodiazepines, neuroleptics, and alcohol, may also precipitate these symptoms and cognitive changes.

Somatic complaints, vegetative symptoms, apathy, and lethargy often persist even after extensive medical evaluation and changes of drug regimens. Despite the patient's rejection of the diagnosis, major depression is then a likely diagnosis. Similarly, a patient who has recently suffered an acute illness or injury (eg, myocardial infarction, stroke, or hip fracture) who is unable to recover premorbid function should be examined closely. If depression screening and formal mental status examination reveal anorexia, insomnia, fatigue, constricted affect, inability to experience pleasure, hopelessness, and apathy, treatment of depression should be considered.

Many individuals with depression have "good reasons" for being depressed. Support alone, therefore, is unlikely to remedy the situation or induce recovery from the primary medical or surgical illness. Depression and depressive symptoms have been shown to cause disability similar to that imposed by major chronic illnesses. Appropriate treatment of the depression will enhance rehabilitation and permit a prompt return to the premorbid functional level. Accurate diagnosis may prevent the need for supervised care.

Much has been written about cognitive impairment in the presentation of depression in the elderly. The **dementia of depression,** or **pseudodementia,** causes substantial cognitive impairment and can easily be mistaken for parenchymal dementia. Memory impairment associated with major depression in older adults may be partially or completely reversible. Controversy continues while evidence suggests but does not prove that cognitive capacity will recover somewhat with improvement in depression even in patients with mild to moderate organic dementias. Discrimination of dementia of depression from a primary degenerative dementia can be quite difficult. In the dementia of depression, onset of symptoms is usually more sudden, and patients may admit to awareness of impairment, classically responding with "I don't know" rather than confabulating. Psychomotor retardation is prominent, as are constriction of affect and classical vegetative signs. On cognitive screening, disorders of concentration and long-term memory are more prominent than the deficits in recall and registration associated with dementias such as Alzheimer's disease and multi-infarct dementia (MID).

The Workup for Dementia

The prevalence of impairment in intellectual ability among the elderly dictates the importance of appropriate assessment of complaints of memory loss, confusion, and deteriorating functional ability. The purpose of a comprehensive evaluation is to determine the presence of dementia and its potential "reversibility" and to slow deterioration as much as possible. The recommended workup is based on numerous reports that between 10% and 30% of cognitively impaired patients have treatable problems. Equally convincing are data indicating that as many as 30% of geriatric patients, when properly evaluated, may have more than one illness contributing to the dementia. In the early, well-controlled study of Larson et al (1985), treatment of concomitant medical, neurological, and psychiatric disorders provided at least temporary improvement in 27.5% of patients and sustained gains in 14%. Although reversibility was usually not possible, improvement in quality of life was reported by patients and their families.

The evaluation of dementia includes a complete medical and psychiatric history, a review of all medications, a physical examination, a complete neurological examination, and a mental status examination, including rating with an instrument such as the MMSE (see above). Laboratory screening includes a complete blood count, serum electrolytes, liver function tests, rapid plasma reagin, sedimentation rate, serum vitamin B_{12} and folate levels, computed tomographic scan or magnetic resonance imagery of the head, and a chest x-ray. Admittedly, this is a costly workup. However, the cost savings associated with improvement in intellectual ability and prolongation of relative autonomy are estimated to be considerable as well.

In the study by Larson et al (1985), the most common treatable illnesses associated with or causing dementia were drug toxicity, hypothyroidism and other metabolic diseases, and depression. In all, more than 250 medical illnesses were recognized in 60% of the 200 patients studied. Treatment of many of these entities improved outcome.

The vulnerability of older adults to even the rarest toxic effects of medications must be recognized. The sparsest possible drug regimen—particularly the withholding of direct central nervous system toxins—is recommended for all older patients and particularly for those with cognitive impairment. All medications should be considered suspect, and questionably necessary agents should be withdrawn when feasible.

Treatment of other medical illness that may cause or complicate dementia—including thyroid disease, neurosyphilis, vitamin B_{12} or folate deficiencies, azotemia, hypercalcemia, iron deficiency anemia, substance (including alcohol) use disorders, thiamine deficiency, subdural hematoma, central nervous system tumor, normal-pressure hydrocephalus, and depression—should be undertaken in standard fashion but with as much cooperation from caregivers as possible.

Most dementias have irreversible causes. Between 60% and 70% of elderly patients with global cognitive disability suffer from Alzheimer's disease. Another 10–20% probably have multi-infarct dementia (Jorm, 1991). Early recognition of these dementias is important in preventing unnecessary rapid deterioration and in helping families and caregivers to make short- and long-term plans. The clinical diagnosis of Alzheimer's disease requires exclusion of the aforementioned array of other causes of cognitive impairment and correlation with clinical history and presentation. Because of the uncertain nature of the diagnosis and the unpredictable duration of its course, clinicians must be cautious about labeling possibly affected individuals.

Patients with dementia are extremely susceptible to alterations in cognition and function when they become medically ill. Infections, metabolic disturbances, and changes in drug regimens can cause rapid changes in mental status. Any rapid change in function in a patient with a slowly progressive dementia should arouse a suspicion of the presence of a secondary medical process. Aggressive management of medical illnesses is likely to lead to elimination of "excess disability." Similarly, discontinuation of potentially toxic medications can improve function to the patient's baseline level of disability. Examples are anticholinergics, tricyclic antidepressants (anticholinergic effects may cause confusion or delirium), sedative-hypnotics, some antihypertensives and antiarrhythmics, digitalis, antiparkinsonism drugs, analgesics, antineoplastics, and histamine H_2 antagonists.

ISSUES IN PSYCHIATRIC MANAGEMENT OF BEHAVIORAL DISORDERS IN THE ELDERLY

General Issues in Psychotherapy

Psychotherapy is as appropriate for the elderly as it is in younger populations. However, older adults tend to perceive a stigma associated with care from mental health specialists and may for that reason resist referral. Longer-term interventions may not be appropriate in frail populations with chronic and terminal illnesses.

Several types of psychotherapy have been shown to improve mood in older adult depressives. Psychodynamic, behavioral, cognitive, interpersonal, and supportive psychotherapies can be useful in either group or individual settings. As in other populations, therapies must be tailored to individual needs. The major losses and stressors associated with aging are frequently a focus for adaptive strategies. In psychotherapy there is often an attempt to address the major Eriksonian challenge of the final stage of the life cycle: the struggle to maintain ego integrity and hold the line against despair.

Pharmacotherapeutic Issues

Decisions about drug therapy for older adult patients should be made in a spirit of thoughtful conservatism. Although all classes of psychotropics that are useful in younger adults can be used effectively in the elderly, age-related pharmacokinetic and pharmacodynamic changes dictate modifications in the therapeutic approach. Every drug-related decision demands evaluation of potential risks and benefits. The physician must be aware of all prescribed and over-the-counter medications the patient is taking, the patient's history of previous responses and adverse effects, and the potential effects of a medication on overall function. Adverse drug effects may be more important in the older adult than in younger patients. For example, psychotropic use has been shown to be an important risk factor for hip fracture in the elderly. Similarly, constipating effects of anticholinergic drugs may be an inconvenience in a younger person but could cause fecal impaction or even paralytic ileus in an immobilized frail older adult. Therefore, the primary maxim of geriatric pharmacology is always to "start low and go slow."

Although gastric pH and motility and total intestinal surface area and blood flow decrease with age, drug absorption does not appear to be affected by aging in the absence of gastrointestinal disease. Diminished hepatic blood flow and decreased microsomal enzyme activity may slow metabolic pathways in the elderly, causing increased serum levels of some psychotropics and prolonged elimination half-life of others (eg, tertiary amine tricyclic antidepressants and fluoxetine). Drug distribution is affected largely by lipid solubility. Increased proportions of body fat to water in older adults increase the volume of distribution of psychotropics, most of which are highly lipid soluble. Decreases in plasma proteins, including albumin and glycoproteins, can affect protein binding and drug distribution. Decreased renal function reduces clearance of hydrophilic metabolites of tricyclic antidepressants and other psychotropic agents and of lithium in the elderly. Moreover, physical illnesses can alter all aspects of pharmacokinetics, as can interactions with other medications.

Medical illnesses and interactions with other agents alter the therapeutic and toxic effects of psychotropics in the elderly. Changes in neurotransmitters may change the effects of psychotropics, but outcomes have not been well demonstrated. Numerous reports have described the increased vulnerability of the elderly to adverse psychotropic effects, particularly to central nervous system toxicity of these agents. However, systematic scientific studies of changes in pharmacodynamics with age have not been undertaken. Needless to say, suggested treatment with psychotropics is based largely on experience in younger adults. Therefore, cautious titration of dosage is always advised.

Antidepressant pharmacotherapy is the mainstay of treatment for major depression in the elderly. Over the past decade, numerous new antidepressant compounds have been marketed. In spite of only a small number of clinical trials in older adult and frail populations, the favorable side effect profiles of these agents have increased prescription rates for older patients remarkably. The selective serotonin reuptake inhibitors (SSRI), fluoxetine, paroxetine, sertraline, fluvoxamine, and citalopram are well tolerated in even medically compromised older people. Gastrointestinal discomfort, including nausea, vomiting, and diarrhea, agitation, and gait disturbance are the most common side effects. Even with their more benign toxicities, these agents must be used cautiously with older, compromised patients and their propensity for drug-drug interactions must be monitored vigilantly (see Chapter 30).

Unique compounds, including buproprion, venlafaxine, nefazadone, and mirtazapine are also effective and extremely well tolerated. Each of these agents has its own profile of adverse effects and their use should be evaluated in the context of a patient's symptoms and concurrent conditions.

For the past four decades, tricyclic antidepressants have been used extensively and they remain valuable treatments. However, anticholinergic and cardiac side effects, including delayed conduction through the His-Purkinje system and postural hypotension, may limit their utility. Secondary amine tricyclics, particularly desipramine and nortriptyline, are less anticholinergic and less sedating than tertiary amines and they are clearly the preferred agents in this group. These agents should be titrated slowly and serum levels employed to guide dosing and to allow patients to become accustomed to side effects. Similarly, monoamine oxidase inhibitors can be used safely in the elderly. Gradual dose increases and particular attention to hypotensive effects are necessary. Trazodone has little anticholinergic effect and does not prolong cardiac conduction. However, this agent is quite sedating and may cause orthostatic hypotension, premature ventricular contractions, and priapism, all of considerable concern in the elderly. There is evidence that antidepressant efficacy may require longer trials in the elderly. A full 6- to 12-week trial of any agent is recommended.

Anxiolytics and sedative-hypnotics should be used with caution in older adults. Even in relatively low doses, they can cause sedation, cognitive impairment, and ataxia. Although the indications for use of benzodiazepine are similar to those in younger populations, effects on function must always weigh heavily in the decision to treat. Pharmacokinetic and pharmacodynamic changes with aging suggest that short-acting agents with few or no active metabolites (eg, lorazepam, oxazepam, temazepam, triazolam) are superior to long-acting agents with active metabolites (eg, diazepam, flurazepam, chlordiazepoxide). Overall, these agents should be used with extreme caution and only upon clear indications. Short trials and "as needed" dosing are recommended. The use of buspirone, a nonbenzodiazepine with few central nervous system toxic effects that requires chronic dosing, may offer a rational alternative for treatment of anxiety in older adults.

All of the principles of antipsychotic use in younger populations (see Chapter 30) apply, perhaps with greater force, to the elderly. For example, older adults who are treated with neuroleptics appear to be more vulnerable to tardive dyskinesia. Jeste et al (1990) conclude that as many as 40% of older adult inpatients with histories of prolonged neuroleptic exposure have tardive dyskinesia. This risk is even greater in patients with dementia. Treatment with neuroleptics always requires a balancing of the sedative and anticholinergic properties of low-potency agents (eg, thioridazine and chlorpromazine) with the increased risk of extrapyramidal side effects associated with higher-potency drugs (eg, haloperidol and fluphenazine).

Over the past several years, the introduction of several atypical antipsychotic agents offers a seemingly less neurotoxic approach to management of psychosis in older adults. Risperidone, olanzapine, and quetiapine, although each has its own side effect profile (see Chapter 30), are associated with considerably lower incidence rates of acute and long-term movement disorders, have less anticholinergic effects, and have little effect on cardiac function and blood pressure. The use of clozapine should be reserved for older patients with treatment-resistant disorders. Clozapine may provide an important potential benefit for people with preexisting movement disorders who become psychotic. Use of any of these agents in the elderly—and in patients with dementia in particular—requires slow titration and low-dosage regimens.

Psychiatric symptoms often complicate cognitive decline. In the earliest phases of dementia, moderate anxiety and depression are not uncommon. As the illness progresses, paranoia, hallucinosis, agitation, and insomnia may become prominent. These latter symptoms may be the most difficult for families to manage and may serve as an impetus to hospitalization or institutionalization. Any psychiatric symptoms in these patients must be managed holistically. Medical and toxic contributions must be ruled out prior to intervention. Remaining "excess" psychiatric symptoms may respond to drug treatment. Although good studies demonstrating efficacy are sparse, very-low-dose neuroleptic medications can be employed successfully. Benzodiazepines and other sedative hypnotics should be employed only transiently, as they may promote more confusion and even agitation. Other agents, including trazodone, propranolol, valproate, and carbamazepine, have also been suggested for management of agitation in dementia. However, clinical trials demonstrating their safety and efficacy are limited.

Family Issues

The physician is apt to be a most important source of information and support for patients and their families. The physician can be assisted in this task by well-informed nonphysician care providers. People with dementia often deny their symptoms and are unable to "take in" the implications of the diagnosis. Family members and other caregivers can benefit greatly from education about the illness, its possible course, associated symptoms, and available community resources. Appropriate family support can prolong care in noninstitutional settings, protect financial resources, and enhance prevention and early detection of medical or psychiatric illnesses. Family members should be encouraged to attend support groups. Family meetings held by the primary physician or other closely involved providers can educate "en masse" all potential caregivers and provide direction for optimal care. Respite for caregivers should be encouraged.

Community senior adult programs or daycare settings can supplement available family care. Where resources are available, companions and other home health aides may also be employed. Long-term care provided by family caregivers is not without substantial cost. Depending on the level of support necessary, home health and respite care may approach institutionalization in actual dollar costs. Family members may miss days of work, be forced to elect early retirement, and endure stress. Renovations of the home environment and the purchase of medical equipment can be quite expensive. As dementia progresses, these problems must be weighed against the costs of institutionalization.

CONCLUSION

Prevention and early detection of disorders impairing mental function in older adults can be accomplished to a great extent in the primary care setting. The investigative style and personal rapport intrinsic to primary care practice are important tools in screening for risk factors and mental disorder. Treatment of medically and behaviorally complex patients often requires psychiatric consultation or primary psychiatric care.

Geriatric psychiatry is a field whose growth is fueled by the needs and size of the older adult population. Advances in neuroscience, psychotherapy, and psychopharmacology are supporting the development of a specialty that can respond to the enormity of the demands it faces. However, it is the rich experience and wisdom of the older adult, challenged by the attendant changes of the aging process, that make holistic and thoughtful geriatric care exciting and rewarding for the practitioner.

REFERENCES & SUGGESTED READINGS

Alexopoulos GS: Affective disorders. In: *Comprehensive Review of Geriatric Psychiatry (II)*. Sadavoy J, Lazarus LW, Jarvik LF, Grossberg GT (editors). American Psychiatric Press, 1996.

Blazer DG et al: The association of age in depression among the elderly: An epidemiologic exploration. J Gerontol 1991;46:M210.

Covinsky KE et al: Depressive symptoms and 3-year mortality in older hospitalized medical patients. Ann Intern Med 1999;130:563.

Detlefs DR, Myers RJ, Treanor RJ: *1997 Guide to Social Security and Medicare*. William M. Mercer, 1996.

Evans DA et al: Prevalence of Alzheimer's disease in a community population of older persons: Higher than previously reported. JAMA 1989;262:2551.

Finkel SI: The pharmacologic management of agitation in demented nursing home elderly. In: *Psychopharmacotherapy for the Elderly: Research and Clinical Implications*. Bergener M, Belmaker RH, Tropper Meinhardt S (editors). Springer, 1993.

Folstein MF, Folstein SE, McHugh PR: Mini-Mental State: A practical method for grading the cognitive state of patients for the clinician. J Psychiatr Res 1975;12:189.

Garrand J et al: Clinical detection of depression among community-based elderly people with self-reported symptoms of depression. J Gerontol A Biol Sci Med Sci 1998;53:M92.

Gottlieb GL: Financial issues. In: *Comprehensive Review of Geriatric Psychiatry (II)*. Sadavoy J, Lazarus L, Jarvik KL, Grossberg GT (editors). American Psychiatric Press, 1996.

Jeste D, Krull A, Kilbourn K: Tardive dyskinesia: Managing a common side effect. Geriatrics 1990;45(12):49.

Jorm AF: Cross-national comparisons of the occurrence of Alzheimer's disease and other dementias. Eur Arch Psychiatry Clin Neurosci 1991;240:218.

Koenig HG et al: Depressive symptoms in elderly medical-surgical patients hospitalized in community settings. Am J Geriatr Psych 1998;6:14.

Larson EB et al: Diagnostic evaluation of 200 elderly outpatients with suspected dementia. J Gerontol 1985;40:536.

Lazarus LW, Sadavoy J: Individual psychotherapy. In: *Comprehensive Review of Geriatric Psychiatry (II)*. Sadavoy J, Lazarus LW, Jarvik LF, Grossberg GT (editors). American Psychiatric Press, 1996.

Leventhal EA: Biological aspects. In: *Comprehensive Review of Geriatric Psychiatry (II)*. Sadavoy J, Lazarus LW, Jarvik LF, Grossberg GT (editors). American Psychiatric Press, 1996.

Longino CF, Mittelmark MB: Sociodemographic aspects. In: *Comprehensive Review of Geriatric Psychiatry (II)*: Sadavoy J, Lazarus LW, Jarvik LF, Grossberg GT (editors). American Psychiatric Press, 1996.

McKhann G et al: Clinical diagnosis of Alzheimer's disease: Report for the NINCDS-ADRDA work group under the auspices of the Department of Health and Human Services Task Force on Alzheimer's Disease. Neurology 1984;34:939.

Myers JK et al: Six month prevalence of psychiatric disorders in three communities. Arch Gen Psychiatry 1984;41:959.

National Center for Health Statistics: Health United States, 1991. (DHHS Pub. No. [PHS] 92-1232.) US Government Printing Office, 1992.

Newhouse PA: Use of serotonin selective reuptake inhibitors in geriatric depression. J Clin Psychiatry 1996;57(Suppl 5):12.

Reynolds CF et al: Treatment of depression in elderly patients: Guidelines for primary care. In: *Diagnosis and Treatment of Depression in Late Life: Results of the NIH Consensus Development Conference.* Schneider LS, Reynolds CF, Lebowitz BD, Friedhoff AJ (editors). American Psychiatric Press, 1994.

Rothchild AJ: The diagnosis and treatment of late-life depression. J Clin Psychiatry 1996;57(Suppl 5):5.

Rovner BW, Katz IR: Psychiatric disorders in the nursing home: A selective review of studies related to clinical care. Int J Geriatr Psychiatry 1993;8:75.

Soldo BJ, Agree EM: America's elderly population. Population Bull 1988;43:1.

US Bureau of the Census: Current population reports. Health insurance coverage, 1997 and 1998. Government Printing Office, 1997, 1998.

Young RC, Myers BS: Psychopharmacology. In: *Comprehensive Review of Geriatric Psychiatry (II)*. Sadavoy J, Lazarus LW, Jarvik LF, Grossberg GT (editors). American Psychiatric Press, 1996.

39

Consultation Psychiatry in the General Hospital

Richard J. Goldberg, MD, & Craig Van Dyke, MD

Consultation psychiatry is the practical application of psychiatric knowledge and techniques to the care of medical patients in a general hospital. Although it is commonly assumed to be synonymous with psychosomatic medicine, consultation psychiatry is actually more diverse, requiring a knowledge of general psychiatry as well as familiarity with medical and surgical diseases and their treatments, neuroanatomy and neurobehavioral disorders, pharmacology, and systems theory.

As the bridge between psychiatry and medicine, consultation psychiatry has always occupied a strategic position. At present, as psychiatry reenters the mainstream of medicine, this strategic position is more critical than ever. Consultation psychiatry provides scientific understanding and effective management of the emotional and cognitive problems of medical and surgical patients. Consultation psychiatrists participate in the training of medical students, medical residents, and psychiatric residents.

The increased economic pressures on systems to reduce medical costs and length of stay have also created a new recognition of the value of consultation psychiatry, since many of its interventions contribute to more efficient management, reduced length of stay, and more appropriate utilization of medical resources.

THE NEED FOR CONSULTATION

In clinical practice, consultation psychiatrists treat medical and surgical patients with emotional, behavioral, and cognitive problems. Epidemiological studies show that 26% of medical outpatients and a substantial proportion of medical inpatients (Barrett et al, 1988; Mayou et al, 1991) have significant psychiatric symptoms, with the most frequent diagnoses being anxiety, depression, and organic mental disorder. Contributing further to the incidence of psychiatric problems in medical patients is the high rate of physical illness in psychiatric patients (Wells et al, 1989; Sheline, 1990; Knutsen and DuRand, 1991; Anfinson and Kathol, 1992).

With the recent development and application of brief cognitive screening tests (see Chapter 11), there is increasing appreciation that medical and surgical patients have a high rate of cognitive impairments.

For example, about 30% of patients in acute medical inpatient units have cognitive deficits (Lipowski, 1989). The rate may be twice as high on neurology inpatient units. However, since many brief cognitive screening examinations do not systematically assess constructional or language skills, the true prevalence of cognitive impairment in medical populations is probably greater than reported.

Despite a high incidence of emotional and cognitive disturbances, only a small percentage (approximately 2%) of medical and surgical patients are evaluated by a psychiatric consultant (Steinberg et al, 1980; Craig, 1982). The reasons for this are not completely clear, but a number of factors may be at work. If the psychiatric symptoms seem understandable in the context of the patient's illness, the primary physician may feel no need to request a psychiatric consultation. For example, when a patient with cancer develops depressive symptoms, the primary physician may feel the reaction is appropriate and that no treatment is required—or that if treatment is required, the primary physician should be able to provide it. Primary physicians may also believe that a psychiatric consultant might have nothing positive to offer and might even upset the patient. Another critical factor is that in many cases, primary physicians simply fail to recognize emotional and cognitive problems in their patients (Schulberg and Burns, 1988; Ormel et al, 1990).

This chapter focuses on inpatient consultation psychiatry and is intended to enable the primary physician to make better use of these services. Eight common clinical problems for which psychiatric consultation is indicated will be discussed: cognitive disorders (delirium and dementia), depression, patient management problems, symptoms of obscure origin, pain, substance abuse, management of medical and surgical patients with major psychiatric disorders, and forensic issues. The roles of the various professionals that constitute the psychiatric consultation team will then be briefly described.

CONSULTATION PROCEDURE

A primary care physician may request a consultation by making a personal call to the consultant or by written request. Some insurance plans will not pay the consultant unless the referring physician writes an order. Optimally, the patient would be informed of the request for psychiatric consultation and the reason for the request, but in practice this is often not done.

After the primary physician's request for consultation, the consultant's first task is to define as precisely as possible the reasons for the consultation. Sometimes this is quite easy; the patient who has attempted suicide may require evaluation to determine the need for suicide precautions or further psychiatric treatment. At other times the reasons are quite vague—eg, the consultee may believe that the patient's emotional response to the medical illness is inappropriate but is unable to state the problems more precisely. A preliminary discussion with the consultee can sharpen the focus of the consultation. Following this, the consultant reviews the chart to understand the medical context of the problem. Discussion with the nursing staff and the family often provides important supplemental information.

The consultant then interviews the patient, preferably in private. Consultants must initially make it clear that they are psychiatrists and discuss any feelings the patient has about being interviewed by a psychiatrist. Patients are then asked to verbalize their understanding of the medical or surgical problem and the difficulties it has created. During the interview, a formal mental status examination should be performed (Goldberg et al, 1992a). The essence of the consultation process, however, is to gather information about the problems that led to the request for consultation. Although this may seem obvious, it is not uncommon for inexperienced consultants to gather extensive information about the patient's life and psychodynamics without investigating the "chief complaint" identified by the referring physician.

The consultant should then formulate a differential diagnosis and discuss it, along with what has been learned about the specific issues for which the consultation was requested, with the primary physician. These issues should also be discussed with the nursing staff. For example, if a medical patient is depressed with suicidal ideation, the nursing staff needs to understand the context of the patient's depression and the specific precautions to be taken.

The Consultation Note

The consultation note (Garrick and Stotland, 1982) should be brief and specifically labeled as a psychiatric consultation, with date, time, and sources of information. Details of the history and information about the specific problem for which the consultation was requested should be stated. Discretion is called for, since medical records have less protection in terms of privacy than psychiatric records. It is critical to omit superfluous information that may be embarrassing or lead to inappropriate labeling of the patient. The mental status examination should be recorded in detail, since it represents the most objective information in the note. It is particularly helpful as baseline information that can be referred to when the patient is seen later. Finally, a working diagnosis and a differential diagnosis are recorded.

The heart of the consultation note is the recommendations, and these must address the consultee's questions. The recommendations should be stated as specifically as possible. It is not sufficient to indicate that the patient should be evaluated for certain conditions and started on certain medications. Rather, the specific tests recommended and details of the proposed drug regimen should be stated, along with the target symptoms and potential adverse effects. Follow-up examination by the consultant is an integral part of all consultations. This allows the patient, consultee, and consultant to evaluate the impact of the initial recommendations and to make appropriate modifications. Increasing regulation by payers (such as Medicare) has led to very specific documentation requirements for evaluation and management notes, which must be met to support the charge for services.

PSYCHIATRIC CONSULTATION

The eight categories discussed below do not necessarily reflect traditional diagnostic categories, and most are not medical or psychiatric syndromes. All can be considered complex clinical situations that include the interaction of biological, psychological, and social factors. The consultant also needs a working knowledge of how to assess a patient's personality type and how this personality interacts with a particular medical situation to create a behavioral management problem (see Chapter 24). Despite the psychologically traumatic nature of most medical catastrophes, the capacity of people to adjust is remarkably high. Problem patients often have a history of personality or emotional difficulties. As a basic principle of consultation psychiatry, the patient's psychological defenses should be supported whenever possible, and psychotropic medications should be used appropriately when needed. Coping skills and strengths should be discovered and reinforced.

Delirium, Dementia, & Disorders Secondary to a Medical Cause

A significant number of hospital patients have an underlying medical disorder that remains unrecognized or masquerades as some other problem such as depression or noncompliant behavior. A medical etiology should be the first consideration in any evaluation of impaired mood, thought, or behavior. In its most dramatic form, gross delirium is easily recognized by noting the patient's impaired attention, perceptual disturbances, agitation, and disorientation. Visual hallucinations, which many clinicians associate with schizophrenia, are actually more common in organic mental disorders such as delirium tremens and toxic encephalopathy. It is not uncommon for consultees mistakenly to ascribe obvious organic delirium to some psychogenic cause. There are, of course, many less severe cases in which mild delirium or dementia is characterized by impaired intellect, memory deficits, or personality change. In many situations, the consultant will recognize the presence of delirium or dementia only by performing a specific mental status examination (see Chapter 11). Assessment of language and other higher functioning is often neglected but is critical for the detection of aphasia, apraxia, and agnosia.

The recognition of a medical etiology is important because it often has specific treatment. Furthermore, failure to provide treatment may lead to permanent deficits and mislabeling of the patient's symptoms. Specific causes include metabolic derangements, drug toxicity or withdrawal, vascular compromise, infections, intracranial tumors, and neuronal degeneration. The consultant must be prepared to review the medical evaluation of the patient with special emphasis on the presence of neurological findings. The psychiatric consultant must also review all laboratory evaluations and neurodiagnostic tests, such as lumbar puncture, electroencephalography, and cranial computed tomography or magnetic resonance imaging scans and be prepared to make recommendations for further tests. In the hospital setting, most cases of delirium are either partially or entirely reversible. The most frequent cause is metabolic imbalance as a result of alterations in renal, pancreatic, hepatic, cardiovascular, or pulmonary function. A comprehensive drug review is crucial because of the high prevalence of psychiatric symptoms secondary to medication (Abramowicz, 1998). This may be supplemented by toxicology screening and serum levels of potentially psychoactive substances. Although a great many drugs may produce psychiatric symptoms as adverse side effects, the most common offenders are the central nervous system depressants and stimulants, cimetidine, levodopa, corticosteroids, and antihypertensive and cholinergic agents.

Primary treatment of delirium consists of correction of the underlying medical abnormality. In addition, certain adjunctive measures are useful. Neuroleptics in small doses may be useful in controlling the agitation of the confused patient and are often superior to benzodiazepines, which may further confuse patients (Breitbart et al, 1996). Environmental changes can minimize patient confusion. Such manipulations include providing calendars, clocks, night-lights (to minimize "sundowning"), familiar objects from home, and frequent orientation by staff and family. Clear, straightforward, and consistent communication from the staff and family also helps patients organize their experience. Precautions must also be instituted for individuals at risk of hurting themselves (eg, by falling out of bed, getting lost) as a result of their cognitive impairment.

Depression

Depressed mood is probably the most common reason for psychiatric consultations. Unfortunately, although about 40% of hospitalized medically ill older adults experience some form of depression (Koenig et al, 1992), less than 25% of these are recognized and only about 50% of those recognized receive treatment (Koenig et al, 1997). When such depression is a response to the stresses of medical illness, it may respond to improvement in the patient's clinical condition or to reassurance by the primary physician. However, when symptoms become severe and interfere with the patient's activities or participation in treatment, psychiatric evaluation should be requested. Along with depressed mood or crying, the depressed medical patient may be noncompliant with treatment, functioning at a more severely impaired level than is warranted by the medical condition, or preoccupied with somatic symptoms.

There is a tendency to assume that depressed mood in a medical patient represents an understandable adjustment reaction that does not warrant treatment. ("Wouldn't you be depressed if you had cancer?") This may lead to needless suffering, because the depression may respond to treatment of some underlying medical problems or to the use of antidepressant medication.

Although depression is often neglected in the medical setting, it can also be overdiagnosed in medical patients, since its cardinal features may have other causes. For example, sleep disturbances may be secondary to pain, appetite disturbance to nausea, fatigue to anemia, and impaired concentration to the effects of drugs such as theophylline.

As in other settings, the treatment of depression in medically ill patients involves both psychotherapy and antidepressant medications. Supportive psychotherapy assists many patients and their families in coping with the illness. Antidepressant drugs are useful in treating depressed medical patients and can improve mood, appetite, and sleep patterns. Tricyclic agents must be used cautiously in patients with cardiac conduction abnormalities (particularly bundle branch blocks), in patients with delirium or dementia who may become more confused, and in those for whom anticholinergic side effects would be detrimental. Many of these drugs cause orthostatic hypotension and must be used carefully in patients who cannot tolerate a decrease in blood pressure. Monoamine oxidase inhibitors should be used with extreme caution in this population, because they have numerous interactions with food substances and with other drugs. A series of mostly uncontrolled studies has established psychostimulants (methylphenidate or dextroamphetamine) as potentially valuable in the rapid mobilization of depressed elderly medical inpatients (Kraus and Burch, 1992) and in patients with human immunodeficiency virus-related depression (Fernandez et al, 1995). The second generation (nontricyclic) antidepressants appear to have a wide margin of safety and appear well tolerated in medically ill depressed patients (Stoudemire, 1995), although the selective serotonin reuptake inhibitors do have a number of potential medical complications (Goldberg, 1998), such as drug interactions, of which the consultant must be aware.

The evaluation and documentation of suicidal potential (Goldberg, 1987) are major functions of the psychiatric consultant. The possibility of suicide must be evaluated in all depressed medical patients. The consultant must decide whether the patient requires suicide precautions (constant observation, plastic dining utensils, etc) and what type of psychiatric follow-up is indicated after recovery in cases of self-inflicted medical or surgical problems (Goldberg, 1989).

Patient Management Problems

Psychiatric consultation may be requested to assist in management of (1) the agitated, disruptive patient; (2) the patient whose noncompliance may have serious consequences (eg, the patient who insists on leaving the hospital against medical advice); and (3) the patient whose personality problems interfere with clinical management (eg, patients who are excessively demanding, seductive, or paranoid) (see Chapter 24). The psychiatric consultant is not an alternative to the hospital security personnel, though this sometimes seems to be a prevailing expectation. The physically threatening patient is better managed initially by a specially trained team, if available, by calling on properly trained security officers, or, if necessary, by police officers from the community.

The evaluation of patient management problems involves consideration of biological, psychological, and social factors as they interact in a particular clinical setting. Since many patient management problems arise out of some underlying medical process, recognition and correction of that problem are of primary concern. Metabolic imbalance, drug intoxication, and drug withdrawal syndromes are frequent causes of agitation. The consultant should make specific recommendations for immediate management, including the indications and contraindications for use of restraints or medications to control agitation. The consultant should decide whether antipsychotic drugs or benzodiazepines are indicated and in what dosages (Hillard, 1998). The consultant is also expected to offer guidelines regarding the legal implications (if any) of treating such patients (see Chapter 40).

The consultant must assess the extent to which a patient's personality style might be contributing to a dysfunctional response to illness (Goldberg, 1983). At times, brief psychiatric intervention helps the pa-

tient adjust to the situation by identifying specific anxieties concerning illness and hospitalization. Specific issues, if pertinent, should be discussed with the staff along with appropriate management guidelines (eg, limit setting for regressed patients). For many patients, control is a major concern. These patients often engage in power struggles with the staff over their own diagnosis and treatment. Conceding to these patients as much "control" as possible if it does no harm (eg, letting the patient decide which arm the blood is drawn from) minimizes conflict over more critical matters (eg, agreeing to take medications or consent to surgical procedures). Uncontrolled schizophrenia and bipolar affective disorder are, at times, causes of problems in medical patient management.

Social dysfunction contributes to patient management problems in many cases. The psychiatric consultant must often function as a social system consultant by suggesting ways in which medical treatment protocols can be modified to avoid or overcome management problems. When several specialists are involved in the care of the patient, poor communication, diffusion of clinical responsibility, and some mismanagement may result. If patients know that there are conflicting opinions about what should be done for them, they may become anxious, angry, or depressed. One solution is for the psychiatric consultant to suggest that a consensus be reached and executed by the primary physician in charge of the case.

In this section, for the sake of discussion, we have distinguished biological, personality, and social systems. However, it is important to consider how interactions of these factors operate in disruptive or excessively anxious patients. Many instances of abrupt departure against medical advice (and other problems with disruptive patients) emerge through the interplay of an underlying organic mental disorder (eg, drug withdrawal) and dysfunction of the interaction between the patient and the treatment team (Goldberg, 1983). Evaluation and intervention in all three systems are frequently required to resolve such problems without interfering with clinical care.

Symptoms With No Apparent Medical Cause

Psychiatric consultation is often requested for evaluation of patients who have chronic somatic complaints or impaired sensory, motor, or autonomic function for which no medical explanation can be found. The frustration such a patient engenders in the primary clinician is often what prompts the consultation request. The consultant may be asked whether the patient has a conversion disorder. Conversion disorder is characterized by the presence of a psychological conflict, of which the patient is unaware, that produces anxiety, followed by the unconscious "conversion" of this anxiety into a somatic sign or symptom that symbolically expresses and resolves the psychological conflict. Hypnosis or amobarbital interviews may be useful both in evaluating and in treating this condition.

Other categories of psychiatric illness may also lead to physical signs and symptoms with no apparent medical basis. Both depressed and schizophrenic patients may present with somatic preoccupations that are quite confusing until the psychiatric diagnosis is made. Certain patients, usually women, have lifelong patterns of multiple somatic complaints, sometimes called **Briquet's syndrome** or **somatization disorder** (see Chapter 22). Patients with factitious disorders consciously simulate a medical illness or a specific sign or symptom (see Chapter 27). This simulation may represent a lifestyle devoted to simulating medical illness (Munchausen's syndrome or chronic factitious illness). These patients differ from malingerers, who pretend to have medical problems to achieve a specific conscious goal (eg, to obtain narcotics or disability compensation). Recognition of these psychological conditions should alert the staff to withhold invasive diagnostic and therapeutic efforts. Treatment can then be focused on psychosocial issues (Goldberg et al, 1992b).

The consultation psychiatrist should watch for medical illnesses presenting as psychiatric syndromes. Systemic lupus erythematosus, multiple sclerosis, seizure disorders, and degenerative central nervous system diseases (eg, emotional lability associated with multi-infarct dementia) may be puzzling because the somatic signs and symptoms and the associated emotional symptoms are often wrongly attributed to psychiatric illness. Although treatment must be directed first toward the medical condition, it is occasionally necessary to treat the psychiatric symptoms as well (eg, antipsychotic medication for the psychosis associated with systemic lupus erythematosus; Katon et al, 1990).

In the course of psychiatric evaluation of these patients, two recurrent issues need clarification. The first is "secondary gain" (eg, sympathy, or exemption from social expectations or responsibilities). Since all illnesses offer some degree of secondary gain, this mechanism should not be assumed uncritically to "explain" the signs or symptoms. The psychiatric consultant should help the patient and the family prevent secondary gain from impeding recovery.

The second issue is the diagnosis of "histrionic personality disorder" (see Chapter 24). It is not true that patients with this disorder are more likely than others to have conversion disorders. The problem is that these histrionic and seductive patients present their somatic signs and symptoms (which may, in fact, have a medical explanation) in a less-than-believable fashion. Long-term follow-up of patients with the diagnosis of conversion reaction reveals that about 25% have a medical disorder that accounts for the symptoms (Watson and Buranen, 1979). Presumably, the initial presentation of these patients is in the early stages of the medical disease, when it is difficult to make the diagnosis.

Pain

Patients may continue to complain of pain despite analgesic management that is usually effective. This difficult clinical problem may give rise to requests for psychiatric consultation. Such consultation requires an awareness that pain is a complex phenomenon involving an interplay of biological and psychosocial factors. Optimally, the psychiatrist would participate as a member of a multidisciplinary pain assessment team.

The consultant should review these patients with the primary physician, with emphasis on the potential biological basis for the pain and the current treatment strategies. The patient is then evaluated for certain psychiatric disorders that are associated with unusual or refractory pain syndromes. Depression should be considered, since its association with chronic pain may lead to increased preoccupation with the pain and to louder complaints. Other syndromes to consider include schizophrenia, somatoform pain disorder, and factitious disorders (see above).

Psychosocial factors may also play a role in refractory pain syndromes. Pain may have a special meaning for the patient or may be "modeled" after the pain of a person who was emotionally close to the patient. At times it may mimic the pain a close relative experienced in a terminal illness. Cultural background, unresolved mourning, and secondary gain may play a role in the pain syndrome (see Chapter 22).

Patients with chronic pain often increase their demands for pain medication in a way that makes primary physicians uncomfortable. Although it has been estimated that iatrogenic "addiction" is relatively rare in medical patients, physicians often perceive these demands as evidence of drug dependency and therefore request consultation. Because physicians wish to avoid having their patients become "addicted" to opioids, pain is often undertreated (Bernabel et al, 1998). Undermedication often leads to increased protestations of pain. If the patient's complaint has a "dramatic" emphasis, the physician and staff may discount its true nature, so that a vicious cycle may ensue with the patient receiving less and less analgesic medication in spite of increasing complaints. The psychiatric consultant must have a thorough knowledge of analgesic management and be able to recognize pain problems related to undermedication. Cases of "refractory pain" are often adequately managed by simply increasing the analgesic dosage. This is particularly true in the case of acute pain or the pain of terminal cancer. Another mechanism is patient-controlled analgesia, which results in relief of pain often with lower total dosages of opioids.

Over the past few years, techniques for pain control other than opioid analgesics have been developed for chronic pain. Nonsteroidal anti-inflammatory agents are effective alternatives to narcotics for many patients. Tricyclic antidepressants, often in lower doses than used to treat depression, have been effective for chronic pain. The mechanism of their action is unknown, but it appears to be distinct from their antidepressant effects. Supportive psychotherapy, guided imagery, and hypnosis can also be effective for about 25% of patients (see Chapters 21, 33, and 36).

For many years, placebos had a role in the evaluation and treatment of chronic pain, based on the mistaken notion that response to placebos indicated that the pain had a functional (nonorganic) cause. In fact, response to a placebo indicates only that the patient is a placebo responder. Evidence that analgesia produced by placebos can be reversed by the narcotic antagonist naloxone suggests that placebos act at least in part through physiological mechanisms (see Chapter 5).

Substance Abuse

The consultation psychiatrist has a role in the evaluation, treatment, and referral of patients with substance abuse problems who are being treated in a medical setting. Narcotic abusers are not uncommon on surgical wards, where they are usually being treated for abscesses, cellulitis, or injuries. These patients tolerate pain poorly and are quite demanding of the staff's attention. It is helpful to remember that 10–20 mg of methadone twice a day is sufficient to block withdrawal symptoms in most of these patients. After recovery from their medical or surgical problems, referral to a substance abuse treatment facility is indicated.

Withdrawal from alcohol or sedative drugs (particularly barbiturates) is more life-threatening than withdrawal from narcotics. The psychiatric consultant must be prepared to help in the assessment of patients with nonnarcotic substance abuse and to assist in the pharmacological management of delirium tremens and other sedative drug withdrawal syndromes (see Chapter 17).

Inasmuch as patients with alcohol-related medical problems account for up to 25% of admissions to hospitals (Burton et al, 1991; Peteet and Evans, 1991), it is surprising how poorly this problem is evaluated and treated. Other than quantifying the incoming patient's alcohol consumption over the recent past, no other inquiries are usually made. However, it is important to ask about the circumstances at onset or recurrence of drinking, periods of abstinence, attempts at treatment and their outcome, and any history of blackouts or delirium tremens. Referral to alcohol treatment programs should be vigorously pursued.

Management of Other Psychiatric Disorders

A patient with a major psychiatric disorder may be admitted for management of a medical or surgical ill-ness. Since these patients (those with schizophrenia and major affective or anxiety disorders) may be taking a number of psychotropic medications (antipsychotic drugs, antidepressants, lithium carbonate), the psychiatrist should offer consultation on drug interactions and medically relevant side effects. Specific advice on patient management may allow the staff and the patient to become more comfortable with each other. Psychotic patients, for example, need to have reality pointed out to them and their misperceptions corrected (eg, that the antibiotic medication is treating their pneumonia, not poisoning them). The consultant may also act as the liaison between the hospital and other psychiatric referral facilities to provide useful information about the patient's previous psychiatric history and treatment.

Forensic Issues

The psychiatric consultant is often asked to make a judgment about the competence of a patient to refuse or consent to a medical or surgical procedure. Part of this process consists of determining whether the patient has a psychiatric disorder (emotional or cognitive) that impairs judgment (Bostwick and Masterson, 1998; Sullivan and Youngner, 1994). Competence is the ability to give informed consent, ie, to understand the nature, benefits, and risks of treatment and the consequences of refusing it. The standard of competence varies with the risk-to-benefit ratio of the procedure. A patient with moderate organic mental disorder may be competent to consent to a computed tomography scan but not to major surgery. The determination of competence is a judicial decision, though often based on psychiatric opinion.

Most "forensic" cases for which the consultant is called represent patient management problems. For example, the problem of the patient with cancer who refuses chemotherapy can usually be dealt with clinically (through therapy) rather than legally (by seeking to declare the patient incompetent, appointing a guardian, or imposing treatment on an unwilling patient). Patients refusing treatment should be evaluated for the presence of organic mental disorder and depression and asked about concerns regarding their life situation. Court permission is usually required before a patient's medical condition can be treated without consent (beyond provision of emergent, lifesaving measures). The ethical issues in such cases often pose a dilemma for the clinician, usually untrained in ethics or the law.

Although the laws differ in some jurisdictions, commitment is not generally a recourse for patients who refuse medical treatment unless there is a present risk that they will harm themselves or others because of a mental disorder. However, this means being actively suicidal, not simply refusing medical treatment. Even in the rare instance when refusal of medical treatment is an active attempt at suicide, commitment may allow the physicians to treat the mental condition against the patient's will but not the medical condition. Psychiatric consultants should become familiar with the state laws and court decisions in regard to competence, commitment, and obligations regarding the management of dangerous patients.

PSYCHIATRIC CONSULTATION TEAM

Consultation psychiatrists may work alone or in conjunction with other mental health professionals. Although such collaboration is not new, there remains much confusion over the shared and unique contributions of the psychiatrist, psychologist, social worker, and nurse in hospital consultation.

One model that integrates various disciplines involves formation of a multidisciplinary team. The concept of the team, however, implies a coordinated interdisciplinary effort, not four professionals (psychiatrist, psychologist, social worker, and nurse) competing for overlapping territory and role functions. When the contributions to be made by each team member have not been properly identified, there

are strained feelings, competitiveness, political hostility, and confusion—all affecting patient care adversely. It is true that some clinical functions can be performed as well by one professional as another, but it is by understanding the unique contributions of each team member that an effective clinical force is created and directed toward helping patients.

SUMMARY

Consultation psychiatry in the general hospital involves the comprehensive evaluation and treatment of medical and surgical patients. Psychiatrists in this field are in the unique position of being able to consider the interaction of biological, psychological, and social factors. As the primary link between psychiatry and medicine, consultation psychiatrists are playing a major role in the establishment of a biopsychosocial model of medical care. Finally, by identifying and treating psychiatric comorbidity in medical patients, consultation psychiatry may have a positive effect on lowering the cost of medical care (Goldberg and Stoudemire, 1995).

REFERENCES & SUGGESTED READINGS

Abramowicz M (editor): Some drugs that cause psychiatric symptoms. Med Lett 1998;40(1020):21.

Anfinson TJ, Kathol RG: Screening laboratory evaluation in psychiatric patients: A review. Gen Hosp Psychiatry 1992;14:248.

Barrett JE, Barrett JA, Oxman TE, Gerber PD: The prevalence of psychiatric disorders in a primary care practice. Arch Gen Psychiatry 1988;45:1100.

Bernabel R et al: Management of pain in elderly patients with cancer. JAMA 1998;279:1877.

Bostwick JM, Masterson BJ: Psychopharmacological treatment of delirium to restore mental capacity. Psychosomatics 1998;39:112.

Breitbart W et al: A double-blind trial of haloperidol, chlorpromazine, and lorazepam in the treatment of delirium in hospitalized AIDS patients. Am J Psychiatry 1996;153:2.

Burton RW, Lyons JS, Devens M, Larson DB: Psychiatric consultation for psychoactive substance disorders in the general hospital. Gen Hosp Psychiatry 1991;13:83.

Craig TJ: An epidemiological study of a psychiatric liaison service. Gen Hosp Psychiatry 1982;4:131.

Fernandez F et al: Effects of methylphenidate in HIV-related depression: A comparative trial with desipramine. Int J Psychiatry Med 1995;25:53.

Garrick TR, Stotland NL: How to write a psychiatric consultation. Am J Psychiatry 1982;139:849.

Goldberg RJ: Personality types and personality disorders. In: *Psychiatry in the Practice of Medicine.* Leigh H (editor). Addison-Wesley, 1983.

Goldberg RJ: The assessment of suicide risk in the general hospital. Gen Hosp Psychiatry 1987;9:446.

Goldberg RJ: The use of constant observation in general hospitals. Int J Psychiatry Med 1989;19:193.

Goldberg RJ: Selective serotonin reuptake inhibitors, infrequent medical adverse effects. Arch Fam Med 1998;7.

Goldberg RJ, Stoudemire A: The future of consultation-liaison psychiatry and medical-psychiatric units in the era of managed care. Gen Hosp Psychiatry 1995;17:268.

Goldberg RJ, Dubin WR, Fogel BS: Behavioral emergencies: Assessment and psychopharmacologic management. Clin Neuropharmacol 1989;12:233.

Goldberg RJ, Faust D, Novack D: Integrating the cognitive mental status examination into the medical interview. South Med 1992a;85(5):491.

Goldberg RJ, Novack DH, Gask L: The recognition and management of somatization. What is needed in primary care training. Psychosomatics 1992b;33(1):55.

Hilliard JR: Emergency treatment of acute psychosis. J Clin Psychiatry 1998;59(Suppl 1).

Katon W et al: Distressed high utilizers of medical care. DSM-III-R diagnoses and treatment needs. Gen Hosp Psychiatry 1990;12:355.

Knutsen E, DuRand C: Previously unrecognized physical illness in psychiatric patients. Hosp Commun Psychiatry 1991;42:182.

Koenig HG, George LK, Meador KC: Use of antidepressants by nonpsychiatrists in the treatment of medically ill hospitalized depressed elderly patients. Am J Psychiatry 1997;154:10

Krause MF, Burch EA: Methylphenidate hydrochloride as an antidepressant: Controversy, case studies and review. South Med J 1992;85:985.

Lipowski ZJ: Delirium (acute confusional states). JAMA 1987;258:1989.

Mayou R: Comorbidity and use of psychiatric services by general hospital patients. Psychosomatics 1991;32:438.

Mayou R et al: Psychiatric problems among medical admissions. Int J Psychiatry Med 1991;21:71.

Ormel J et al: Recognition, management and outcome of psychosocial disorders in primary care: A naturalistic follow-up study. Psychol Med 1990;20:909.

Peteet JR, Evans KR: Problematic behavior of drug-dependent patients in the general hospital. A clinical and administrative approach to management. Gen Hosp Psychiatry 1991;13:150.

Schulberg HC, Burns BJ: Mental disorders in primary care: Epidemiologic, diagnostic, and treatment research directions. Gen Hosp Psychiatry 1988;10:79.

Sheline Y: High prevalence of physical illness in a geriatric psychiatric inpatient population. Gen Hosp Psychiatry 1990;12:396.

Steinberg H, Torem M, Saravay SM: An analysis of physician resistance to psychiatric consultations. Arch Gen Psychiatry 1980;37:1007.

Stoudemire A: Expanding psychopharmacologic treatment options for the depressed medical patient. Psychosomatics 1995;36:S19.

Sullivan MD, Youngner SJ: Depression, competence, and the right to refuse lifesaving medical treatment. Am J Psychiatry 1994;151:971.

Watson CG, Buranen C: The frequency and identification of false-positive conversion reactions. J Nerv Ment Dis 1979;167:243.

Wells KB, Golding JM, Burnam MA: Chronic medical conditions in a sample of the general population with anxiety, affective, and substance use disorders. Am J Psychiatry 1989;146:1440.

Woods SW et al: Psychostimulant treatment of depressive disorders secondary to medical illness. J Clin Psychiatry 1986;47:12.

40

Forensic Psychiatry

Kenneth L. Appelbaum, MD, & Paul S. Appelbaum, MD

The term "forensic" derives from the Roman "forum," a public place or square where communities conducted their legal and political business. Forensic psychiatry is the medical subspecialty that involves the use of psychiatric expertise to assist in the resolution of legal disputes. As psychiatric knowledge and practice have developed, courts increasingly have called on psychiatrists to help answer legal questions. These requests for psychiatric assistance span a wide range of criminal and civil issues. For example, psychiatric expertise can aid courts in determining the competence or responsibility of criminal defendants and help courts by assessing the capacity of individuals to make medical decisions or manage personal affairs. In addition to conducting clinical evaluations related to specific legal cases, some forensic psychiatrists become involved with the legal regulation of psychiatry, such as legal and professional policies that regulate the scope and standards of psychiatric practice.

The expanding demand for forensic psychiatric services has contributed to the growth and development of the subspecialty. The American Academy of Psychiatry and the Law (AAPL) is the major professional organization of forensic psychiatrists. In 1994 the American Board of Psychiatry and Neurology began examining board-certified general psychiatrists for Added Qualifications in Forensic Psychiatry, and in 1997 the Accreditation Council on Graduate Medical Education began reviewing and accrediting fellowship programs. Many books and journals reflect the burgeoning research and scholarly activities in the field.

THE PSYCHIATRIC EXPERT WITNESS

Courts generally recognize at least two types of witnesses: fact and expert. Fact witnesses may testify about their personal observations of a relevant event. An expert witness, in addition, may be allowed to offer professional inferences or opinions drawn from those facts. The Federal Rules of Evidence, which many states use as a model, declare that "if scientific, technical, or other specialized knowledge will assist the trier of fact to understand the evidence or to determine a fact in issue, a witness qualified as an expert by knowledge, skill, experience, training or education may testify thereto in the form of an opinion or otherwise." Depending on the circumstances, courts may call on psychiatrists to testify as either fact witnesses or expert witnesses.

When a patient becomes involved in court proceedings, a treating psychiatrist may be called as a fact witness. For example, the psychiatrist may be asked to describe the patient's presenting problems, diagnoses, and treatments arising after a personal injury. As a fact witness, however, the psychiatrist generally does not offer opinions about the causal connections, if any, between the injury and the psychiatric disturbance. Testimony derives from the treatment relationship, and the patient is usually the primary source of information.

When functioning as an expert witness, the forensic psychiatrist does not have a traditional doctor-patient relationship with the person being evaluated. The purpose of the evaluation is consultation to the court or referring party, not treatment for the patient. The evaluation involves an impartial assessment related to the legal dispute, and the court expects the psychiatrist to offer inferences and opinions. For example, the psychiatrist may describe the causal connection between an injury and a psychiatric disturbance. In addition to interviews with the injured person, the opinion will often rely heavily on information obtained from third parties, medical records, accident reports, and other sources.

The forensic psychiatrist's involvement with a case typically begins with a referral from an attorney, an insurance company, an administrative agency, or a court. The forensic psychiatrist needs to consider several issues before agreeing to take the case, including clarification of the referral question and a determination of whether the question falls within the psychiatrist's area of expertise. In addition to being asked to provide expert opinions, the forensic psychiatrist may be asked to assist in the preparation of the case. In a 1985 decision, *Ake v Oklahoma*, the United States Supreme Court held that many criminal defendants have a constitutional right to access to a competent psychiatrist who will assist their attorney. This consulting role could involve critiquing the reports of opposing experts and helping the attorney prepare to challenge and cross-examine those experts. Forensic psychiatrists may appropriately serve in the role of either impartial expert or consultant. However, in cases in which the expert is asked to function in both capacities, many commentators, including the Group for the Advancement of Psychiatry (GAP), recommend that the psychiatrist first complete an independent evaluation and formulate a relatively impartial expert opinion prior to becoming involved in the more partisan role of a consultant who assists the attorney in presenting the most favorable case.

The unique aspects of the forensic role, as opposed to the therapeutic role, raise special ethical considerations. In the traditional doctor-patient relationship, the psychiatrist has obligations that include maintaining confidentiality, acting in the patient's best interests, and avoiding harm to the patient. The forensic expert, in contrast, often must reveal sensitive information in reports and testimony and may express opinions that are not in the best interest of the person being evaluated. The forensic psychiatrist has an ethical obligation to inform the evaluee of the limits of confidentiality and of the purpose of the evaluation. Under some circumstances, professional ethics preclude conducting an evaluation. For example, except for evaluations necessary to render emergency care, criminal defendants should not be evaluated prior to access to, or availability of, legal counsel.

After completing the assessment, forensic psychiatrists usually prepare a report detailing their findings and opinions. Sometimes, however, referring attorneys or agencies will ask that reports not be prepared, particularly if the opinions reached are not helpful to their positions. Forensic reports differ from standard clinical reports: all sources of information, including persons interviewed and records reviewed, need to be identified; data are separated from conclusions and are presented in descriptive instead of conclusory terms (eg, a mental status evaluation might describe an evaluee's belief that government agencies control his thoughts through a transmitter implanted in his brain instead of simply concluding that the person has "paranoid delusions"); and jargon and technical terms are either avoided or defined. Reports should explicitly link the data to the evaluator's conclusions and opinions.

Psychiatrists have sometimes been criticized for their involvement in legal proceedings. The contention is that psychiatric assessments lack sufficient reliability to be useful in legal proceedings and that the profession suffers damage to its image when experts take opposing positions in highly publicized cases.

Concerns about reliability are tempered by research indicating that diagnostic reliability for major mental disorders equals or exceeds reliability of other medical diagnoses. Competent psychiatrists also have considerable expertise in human behavior and psychopathology. Forensic psychiatrists have ethical obligations to testify within the limits of their knowledge and expertise.

The impact on the image of psychiatry raises more difficult issues. Some psychiatrists testify on matters outside their areas of expertise or offer opinions that are unsupported by the state of knowledge within the profession. This may cast doubt on whether psychiatrists have any real expertise and has led to suggestions for peer review of psychiatric testimony to improve psychiatrists' performance in court. In other cases, media misrepresentation of psychiatric involvement results in negative public perceptions. The "battle of the experts," however, is not unique to psychiatry. Similar conflicts between opposing experts occur in other branches of medicine and in other fields of science. Divergent opinions and testimony have been given on "objective" issues such as the etiology of birth trauma, the significance of cardiac and other medical symptoms, the interpretation of medical test results, and the causes of structural collapses, airplane crashes, and other accidents. Within psychiatry, experts are more likely to agree on the presence of symptoms and serious mental disorder than on the legal significance of those findings. For example, they might agree on the presence of a mood disorder but disagree on whether the disorder should result in a finding of incompetence or insanity. Psychiatrists, and experts from other professions, need to recognize the distinction between expertise in their fields and nonexpertise on ultimate legal issues.

Despite these criticisms, courts are likely to continue to rely on psychiatric expertise. The profession would abrogate its societal responsibility if it refused to participate appropriately in legal proceedings.

COMPETENCE AS GENERAL CONCEPT

Many forensic evaluations involve questions of competence. Grisso (1986) has described the following elements common to all competence evaluations: functional abilities, contextual demands, causal inferences, and judgmental and dispositional considerations.

Every competence evaluation involves assessing a person's *functional ability* to perform a specific task, and each task places its own unique demands on the person. Except in cases of the most profound incapacity, global determinations of competence or incompetence are meaningless. Thus, the first step in any competence evaluation is to determine whether the person has impairments in those capacities relevant to the specific task. The knowledge and abilities needed to make medical decisions, for example, are not identical to the knowledge and abilities needed by a criminal defendant facing trial. The forensic psychiatrist needs to know the relevant abilities associated with each task at issue.

Contextual demands may differ even within categories of competence-related tasks. For example, the degree of understanding and comprehension needed to consent to high-benefit/low-risk medical interventions such as antibiotics for pneumonia may be lower than that required to consent to low-benefit/high-risk procedures such as experimental brain surgery. Similarly the same range of abilities is not required to stand trial for a minor misdemeanor, such as trespassing, as is required for a serious and complex felony trial. Competence assessments must address these contextual demands in addition to addressing the functional abilities of the individual.

When functional deficits exist, the forensic examiner must make *causal inferences* about their etiology. The significance of functional impairments may vary depending on the cause. Deficits caused by mental disorders, malingering, or simple lack of education can all have different implications for whether evaluees will be permitted to make their own decisions or face the consequences of their behavior. When a mental disorder causes the problems, the forensic psychiatrist may also be asked to address the prognosis and remediability of the impairments.

The final element of all competence assessments involves *judgmental and dispositional determinations.* What is the threshold at which a person should be adjudicated incompetent to perform a task? What severity of functional impairment and how demanding a context are required before a person loses the freedom to make personal decisions? And what should be done with an incompetent person? Should someone else make decisions for that person, and if so, what decision-making standard should that person use? All of these questions involve legal determinations rooted in considerations of justice and morality. Psychiatric training does not confer expertise in legal and moral issues. Psychiatrists have expertise in assessing functional impairments, describing how those impairments will impact a person's performance of certain tasks, and determining the etiology and prognosis of those impairments. Whether someone should be found incompetent and what should happen next are decisions reserved for judges and juries.

CRIMINAL FORENSIC PSYCHIATRY

Confession & Waiver

In the criminal justice system, forensic psychiatrists potentially assess the defendant's behavior from the moment of the crime through arrest, trial, and incarceration. Some criminal suspects choose to make statements or confessions to the police, often before they consult with an attorney. The question that then arises is whether those defendants were competent to confess or to waive *Miranda* rights, such as the right to remain silent. Competent confessions or waivers of rights are generally made in a knowing, intelligent, and voluntary manner. Mental disorders, including mental retardation, can affect those abilities, resulting in incompetence. In the 1986 case *Colorado v Connelly,* the United States Supreme Court held that a criminal suspect's "mental condition" may increase susceptibility to police coercion and impair the voluntariness of a confession or waiver; some official police misconduct, however, is required before the Constitution compels courts to vitiate a waiver or confession as involuntary. Because psychiatrists typically do not participate in police interrogations, competence to confess and to waive *Miranda* rights must be retrospectively assessed, which adds to the difficulty of these evaluations.

Competence to Stand Trial

As a defendant progresses toward trial, other functional abilities become significant. Criminal trials involve adversarial proceedings. To present an adequate defense defendants must have an appreciation of the charges and allegations, an understanding of the roles of courtroom personnel and the nature of trial-related proceedings, and an ability to assist their attorneys. Placing a defendant who lacks these characteristics on trial would violate our sense of fairness, and because an incompetent defendant cannot mount a full defense might also result in an inaccurate verdict. Society has an interest both in convicting the guilty and in acquitting the innocent.

The prevailing standard for determining competence to stand trial derives from the US Supreme Court's decision in *Dusky v US:* whether the defendant has "sufficient present ability to consult with his lawyer with a reasonable degree of rational understanding," and "a rational as well as factual understanding of proceedings against him." Psychiatric disorders can affect these abilities in many ways. For example, a defendant could have a factual understanding of the court process in general but also have delusions that impinge on the capacity to apply that understanding. Paranoid concerns might lead the defendant to view the defense attorney as an enemy instead of an ally. Other delusions could lead a defendant to doubt the neutrality of the judge, to question the motivations of court personnel, or to have false beliefs concerning the purpose and meaning of trial-related events. Similarly, because of clinical depression a defendant might have difficulty mobilizing energy to mount a defense or might actually desire punishment based on depression-induced feelings of guilt. Mental retardation, dementia, thought disorders, and other psychiatric disturbances can also impair understanding, compromise the ability to communicate or testify, and adversely affect other competence-related capacities.

The significance of a defendant's impairments will depend, in part, on the severity of the charges and on the nature of the likely legal proceedings. No absolute threshold exists for determinations of incompetence. The forensic psychiatrist assists the court by describing the defendant's functional impairments, if any, the cause of those impairments, and the prognosis for improvement. If the court adjudicates the defendant as incompetent to stand trial, commitment to a state psychiatric hospital usually follows. In the past, such commitments sometimes resulted in lifetime detention. These untried defendants often were accused of minor crimes and did not necessarily meet civil commitment criteria. In 1972, the US Supreme Court declared these practices unconstitutional in *Jackson v Indiana*. The Court limited commitments of incompetent defendants to "a reasonable period of time necessary to determine whether there is a substantial probability that [the defendant] will attain the capacity [to stand trial] in the foreseeable future." If the defendant is not restorable to competence, "then the state must either institute the customary civil commitment proceedings that would be required to commit indefinitely another citizen or release the defendant." If treatment restores the defendant's competence, the criminal proceedings resume.

Insanity

The insanity defense is one of the most controversial issues for forensic psychiatrists. According to the law, insane defendants lack responsibility for their otherwise criminal acts. A verdict of not guilty by reason of insanity indicates that the defendant was considered unable to control his or her actions and therefore was judged not competent to choose whether to commit the crime. Punishing such offenders would compromise the moral integrity of the criminal justice system.

As with competence to stand trial, insanity is a legal, not a psychiatric, term. The test for insanity has varied over time and in different places. The ancient Greeks and Hebrews and medieval English kings all recognized criminal defenses based on mental disability. Up to the seventeenth and eighteenth centuries, some English jurists endorsed insanity verdicts for defendants who understood "no more than an infant, brute or a wild beast."

The most influential formulation of the standard for insanity in Anglo-American law occurred in 1843 after Daniel M'Naghten killed the private secretary of England's Prime Minister Robert Peel. A jury acquitted M'Naghten by reason of insanity, and the ensuing public outcry led the English House of Lords to formulate the following insanity standard: "At the time of committing the act, the party accused was laboring under such a defect of reason, from disease of the mind, as not to know the nature and quality of the act he was doing; or if he did know it, that he did not know he was doing what was wrong." Roughly a third of the states in the United States use a M'Naghten-type standard for insanity.

The *M'Naghten* standard has been criticized as restrictive and too focused on cognitive understanding, and alternative insanity standards have emerged. The "irresistible impulse" standard arose in the United States soon after M'Naghten. Under this standard, courts would acquit by reason of insanity defendants who lacked the ability to control their behavior. In

1870, New Hampshire adopted the "product test," which was also endorsed in 1954 by the US Court of Appeals for the District of Columbia in *Durham v United States*. The *Durham* decision held that "an accused is not criminally responsible if his unlawful act was the product of mental disease or defect." Supporters of the product standard hoped that it would allow mental health professionals to introduce without restriction all relevant information about the defendant. Opponents saw the standard as vague and subjective. Although New Hampshire retains the product standard, the District of Columbia Court of Appeals overruled the *Durham* decision in 1972, and other states have not endorsed the standard.

A more recent formulation of the insanity standard proposed by the American Law Institute (ALI) combines the irresistible impulse standard with modified elements of the M'Naghten rule. The ALI standard states that "A person is not responsible for criminal conduct if at the time of such conduct as a result of mental disease or defect he lacks substantial capacity either to appreciate the criminality [wrongfulness] of his conduct or to conform his conduct to the requirements of the law." The ALI standard has at least four features worthy of note. First, impairments in either cognition or volition may qualify for an insanity defense. Second, the offender's impairments need only be "substantial," not total. Third, the word "appreciate" implies consideration of a broader range of symptoms, including those associated with disorders of mood or perception, than that implied by the more narrowly cognitive term "know." And fourth, the test allows each jurisdiction to choose between the more restrictive ability to appreciate "criminality" and the more inclusive ability to appreciate "wrongfulness." Most states in the United States use some form of the ALI formulation as their insanity standard.

The ALI standard has also received criticism. Both the American Bar Association and the American Psychiatric Association have questioned the ability of psychiatrists, or other mental health professionals, to assess volitional control. Along with other commentators, these organizations have called for elimination of the prong addressing the ability to conform conduct to the requirements of the law. The US Congress heeded these calls in 1984 with passage of the Insanity Defense Reform Act. Largely in response to the acquittal by reason of insanity of John Hinckley, Jr for the attempted assassination of President Reagan, Congress eliminated the volitional prong and also placed the burden of proving insanity by clear and convincing evidence on the defendant. Although this legislation applies only to federal courts, many states have followed suit.

An additional criticism of the ALI test has led to the development of one more insanity standard. Judge Bazelon, the formulator of the *Durham* "product" test, argued for insanity verdicts for offenders who are "so substantially impaired" that they "cannot justly be held responsible." This test demedicalizes the insanity defense by eliminating the need for a "mental disease or defect." It also provides complete discretion to the judge or jury in determining the type of impairments that warrant exculpation. Perhaps because of its lack of constraints, only one state, Rhode Island, has endorsed the "justly responsible" test, and even then only with additional restrictions.

Regardless of which insanity test a jurisdiction uses, the issue receives more public scrutiny than its practical consequences warrant. This attention probably derives from highly publicized insanity defenses, usually unsuccessful, involving notorious crimes by offenders who often have no other viable defense. Despite the impression created by these cases, fewer than 1% of accused felons resort to the insanity defense, and most acquittals occur after negotiations in which the prosecution agrees not to contest the plea. Most insanity acquittees have psychotic disorders, and unlike other defendants found not guilty, they are not set free. Most states provide for automatic psychiatric confinement of insanity acquittees at least for a period of evaluation. Release criteria tend to be more restrictive for insanity acquittees than for civilly committed patients. The length of hospital confinement for many persons committed after being found not guilty by reason of insanity equals or exceeds the length of incarceration for felons convicted on the same charges. In the 1983 decision *Jones v United States,* the US Supreme Court upheld these procedural differences for many insanity acquittees, even those charged with nonviolent misdemeanors. Popular concern about violent criminals eluding sanctions by feigning insanity appears unwarranted.

An insanity evaluation poses special problems for the forensic psychiatrist. The evaluation requires a reconstruction of the offender's mental status at the time of the crime. Current mental status is relevant only to the extent that it suggests the defendant's likely mental status at the time of the offense. Because the defendant's veracity may be questioned, insanity evaluations often rely heavily on information obtained from third parties. In addition to the defendant's account of events, information may be obtained from victims, witnesses, arresting officers, treating clinicians, family, friends, neighbors, and coworkers. The evaluator may review records pertaining to medical, psychiatric, educational, employment, military, and probation history.

Even if the history confirms the presence of a mental disorder, this finding does not end the inquiry. Persons with serious psychopathology can still be competent to perform certain tasks and be held responsible for their acts. The forensic psychiatrist needs to describe explicitly the linkage, if any, between the defendant's symptoms and behavior in relation to the jurisdiction's insanity test (Table 40–1). This assists the judge or the jury in making the legal determination of sanity or insanity.

Table 40–1. Common standards for trial-related competencies.

I. Competence to confess or to waive *Miranda* rights: The confession or waiver of rights must be made in a knowing, intelligent, and voluntary manner

II. Competence to stand trial: The defendant must have sufficient present ability to consult with his attorney with a reasonable degree of rational understanding and a rational as well as factual understanding of the proceedings against him (*Dusky v United States*)

III. Insanity defense:

  A. *M'Naghten* standard: "[A]t the time of committing the act, the party accused was labouring under such a defect of reason, from disease of the mind, as not to know the nature and quality of the act he was doing; or if he did know it, that he did not know he was doing what was wrong"

  B. Irresistible impulse standard: An accused is not criminally responsible if he lacked the ability to control his behavior

  C. *Durham,* or product, standard: "[A]n accused is not criminally responsible if his unlawful act was the product of mental disease or defect"

  D. American Law Institute (ALI) standard: "A person is not responsible for criminal conduct if at the time of such conduct as a result of mental disease or defect he lacks substantial capacity either to appreciate the criminality [wrongfulness] of his conduct or to conform his conduct to the requirements of the law"

  E. Modified ALI standard: "[A] person is not responsible for criminal conduct if, at the time of such conduct, and as a result of mental disease or defect, that person was unable to appreciate the wrongfulness of such conduct"

  F. Justly responsible standard: An accused is not criminally responsible "if [he] is so substantally impaired that he cannot justly be held responsible"

Guilty But Mentally Ill

Beginning with Michigan in 1975, a number of states have passed statutes establishing the verdict of guilty but mentally ill (GBMI). This verdict can be used for defendants who are found to be mentally ill at the time of the crime but who do not meet the jurisdiction's standard for insanity. Adoption of a GBMI verdict has occurred largely in response to dissatisfaction with some of the more notorious cases in which the insanity defense has been employed, such as the acquittal of John Hinckley, Jr. Many advocates of the GBMI verdict hope that it will reduce the number of successful insanity defenses by providing juries with an alternative verdict. Some also argue that a GBMI finding helps ensure treatment for mentally disordered offenders. Available data tend not to support these assertions.

Most states that have enacted GBMI statutes have not experienced reductions in the incidence of insanity acquittals. The verdict also does little to ensure treatment for offenders. Even in the absence of the GBMI option, every state already has mechanisms to provide treatment for convicts with mental disorders. Other than creating confusion in the minds of the jury, the verdict adds little, if anything, to the available options in criminal proceedings. The American Psychiatric Association, the American Bar Association, and other organizations and commentators have opposed enactment of GBMI legislation.

Presentencing

Courts that want to address the treatment needs of offenders may order psychiatric evaluations after conviction but prior to imposition of the sentence. In addition to a benevolent desire to provide treatment, courts may seek psychiatric information regarding other sentencing goals. The purposes of criminal sentencing typically include considerations of retribution, deterrence, incapacitation, and rehabilitation. An offender's mental condition might not qualify for an insanity defense but still partially mitigate blameworthiness, thus lessening the indicated degree of retribution. Psychiatric conditions can also have relevance to sentencing by affecting the ability of an offender to be deterred from future criminal behavior. If a mental disorder increases the risk of violence and recidivism, a court might impose a longer sentence to confine and incapacitate the offender. And finally, a court might impose conditions of treatment in an attempt to rehabilitate the offender. Although the forensic psychiatrist can provide the court with helpful information, explicit dispositional recommendations (eg, for incarceration or release) are generally inappropriate. In addition to mental condition, legal and moral factors bear on sentencing, and psychiatrists have no special claim to expertise on these.

Correctional Psychiatry

Psychiatric involvement with the criminal justice system does not end with completion of trial-related proceedings. Psychiatrists also provide evaluations and treatment in correctional settings. Although these activities may not be "forensic" in the strict sense of the term, they do require sensitivity to the special issues that arise in providing clinical services in jails and prisons. Correctional inmates have a disproportionate prevalence of mental disorders compared to the general population, but most correctional facilities have a scarcity of resources to meet those needs. In its 1976 decision in *Estelle v Gamble,* the US Supreme Court held that only "deliberate indifference" to prisoners' needs for medical services violated their constitutional rights. As long as minimally adequate services are available, states need not supply the same level of care and services as are found in the community. Nevertheless, psychiatrists who

work in correctional settings often feel compelled to advocate for reasonable services to meet the needs of their incarcerated patients.

CIVIL FORENSIC PSYCHIATRY

Personal Injury

Victims who have suffered psychological or emotional injuries may file tort suits seeking compensation for their damages. A tort is a civil, as opposed to criminal, wrong done to another person. Common examples of tort suits include product liability cases and suits resulting from motor vehicle and other accidents.

Attorneys, courts, and insurance companies often ask forensic psychiatrists to evaluate plaintiffs who allege psychic trauma following a personal injury. These generally complex and extensive evaluations can assist the court in determining the presence, cause, extent, and prognosis of psychic traumas. A central issue in both the legal and psychiatric inquiry involves the question of causation. Victims may receive compensation if an injury results in the development or exacerbation of psychiatric problems. Even victims with prior emotional problems or predispositions may receive compensation if accidents or injuries worsen their problems. Preexisting problems might actually make it easier for plaintiffs to prove their case by helping to explain how relatively minor traumata result in catastrophic responses.

Although the forensic psychiatrist's opinion may be central to the causality inquiry, whether the trauma is the "proximate cause" of the plaintiff's injury remains a decision for the legal fact finder. The legal concept of "proximate" causation assigns liability to the agent(s) judged most responsible for the injury, whether or not their actions contributed most to the injury.

Malpractice

Malpractice suits also fall into the legal category of tort actions. A psychiatrist or other clinician has a duty to act in his or her professional capacity as a reasonable practitioner would act in comparable circumstances. Forensic psychiatrists may be asked to testify about the standard of care at the time that an alleged incident of malpractice occurred and whether the defendant psychiatrist negligently violated that standard through acts of commission or omission.

Plaintiffs need to prove four elements to sustain a claim of malpractice. These can be remembered as the four Ds: duty, dereliction (negligence), damage, and direct or proximate cause. A professional or treatment relationship must exist before a psychiatrist incurs a legal duty to a patient. Once that relationship exists, the psychiatrist must avoid negligent care, which constitutes a dereliction of duty to the patient. If the patient suffers damages, or harm, because of the psychiatrist's negligence, the patient may receive compensation if it can be proved that the psychiatrist's negligence was the proximate cause of that harm.

Psychiatrists are among the least frequently sued of medical specialties, but the incidence of suits against psychiatrists is rising. Although as a general rule anybody can sue anyone for anything at any time, the risk of a successful malpractice suit can be diminished. Sound clinical practice, timely consultation, and adequate documentation can all lessen the likelihood of being sued and increase the likelihood of a successful defense.

Disability & Workers' Compensation

The workers' compensation system established at the beginning of the twentieth century provides no-fault compensation to workers injured on the job while limiting the extent of employer liability for those injuries. Under the system, payment is usually limited to lost earning capacity and circumscribed medical expenses. In its most liberal application, workers' compensation covers mental disabilities resulting from "routine job stress." The claimant need not have experienced a discrete physical or emotional trauma. In addition, at least one state provides coverage as long as the claimant "honestly perceives" that the conditions of employment "aggravated, accelerated, or combined with" an internal predisposition to produce the disability. Disability evaluations performed for the Social Security system or private insurance companies are similar to workers' compensation evaluations except that the cause of the disability does not have to be work related.

When conducting workers' compensation or disability evaluations, psychiatrists may be asked to address issues of psychiatric diagnosis, the causal relationship of the diagnosis to a job-related injury, the claimant's ability to work and whether disability is partial or total, the prognosis for recovery, recommended treatment and the adequacy of the current treatment program, and the estimated date of return to work. Treating psychiatrists, as well as forensic psychiatrists, may be asked for their opinions on these issues.

Testamentary Capacity

Testamentary capacity refers to the mental ability to make a legally valid will. The criteria for competence to execute a will typically include an awareness of the extent of the estate, an appreciation of those heirs who would normally be the recipients of the estate's bounty, an understanding that a will is being executed, and an absence of "insane delusions." Challenges to an individual's testamentary capacity often arise after death. This can create problems for the forensic psychiatrist, who may need to reconstruct the testator's mental condition without the possibility of an examination.

Child-Related Issues

The demand for forensically skilled child psychiatrists has been growing. During child custody disputes, courts may seek psychiatric expertise on parental fitness and on the psychological needs and best interests of the child. In juvenile delinquency proceedings, psychiatrists may comment on the juvenile's amenability to treatment. Courts also may request psychiatric opinions regarding child abuse and neglect and the competence of a child to be a witness in a legal proceeding.

RIGHTS OF PATIENTS & LEGAL ISSUES IN CLINICAL PRACTICE

Civil Commitment

Involuntary hospitalization of people with mental illness dates to colonial times. It is based, in part, on the perception that mental illness frequently impairs the ability of people to recognize the existence of a disorder and seek treatment voluntarily. This paternalistic justification for involuntary commitment is augmented by the recognition that mentally ill people may be led to commit acts that endanger themselves or others. Thus, the state's police functions, which embody the state's powers to protect the populace and maintain order, may also be invoked in the civil commitment process.

Throughout much of our history, people deemed in need of treatment have been subject to commitment, often by procedures that were minimally protective of their rights. This changed in the 1960s and 1970s. States abandoned commitment based solely on a person's need for treatment in favor of a model that requires a finding of being dangerous to self or others. Judicial reviews and procedural protections similar to those afforded criminal defendants were strengthened. In part, these changes were precipitated by public disgust at conditions in state psychiatric facilities. Along with this concern about conditions in public mental institutions, there came a general distrust of the psychiatric profession, which was seen as inappropriately abridging individual liberties based on invalid and unreliable diagnoses. In the 1972 US district court decision *Lessard v Schmidt*, the court epitomized this attitude when it referred to the ambiguity of psychiatric diagnoses and the "devastating . . . deprivations" of liberty that result from civil commitment. This decision, and others, seriously challenged the paternalistic justification for civil commitment.

Today commitment laws typically require that the involuntarily detained person have a mental disorder and pose a risk of harm to self or others. The risk of self-harm can be either from intentional acts or from an inability to meet safely the ordinary demands of life in the community, so-called "grave disability." If safety can be reasonably ensured through options less restrictive than involuntary hospitalization, those options generally must be pursued. Commitment laws typically empower psychiatrists to effect emergency detention without judicial review for periods of a few days to a few weeks. Further detention, however, requires judicial review.

Because it is a legal process, legislatures and courts, not psychiatrists, define the range of mental disorders subject to civil commitment. For example, in *Kansas v Hendricks,* a 1997 decision, the US Supreme Court upheld a Kansas statute allowing civil commitment of persons who due to "mental abnormality" or a "personality disorder" are likely to engage in "predatory acts of sexual violence." The Court rejected arguments made by the American Psychiatric Association in an amicus brief, which contended that the Kansas statute improperly used civil commitment and psychiatric services to address criminal behavior.

Some states have further relaxed criteria for commitment in recent years, for example, allowing hospitalization if the likelihood of deterioration in the near future can be demonstrated. In addition, mechanisms for outpatient commitment have been created in many jurisdictions to facilitate involuntary treatment for persons who may not require hospitalization. Nonetheless, the commitment process remains primarily judicial rather than clinical. Except in emergencies, judges, not psychiatrists, commit patients; they rely largely on testimony of psychiatrists, but the standards they use are legal. Commitment criteria reflect society's compromise between individual liberty and the state's interest in protecting the individual and the general community. Psychiatrists may be asked to testify about the patient's diagnosis, treatment needs, and need for hospitalization. Factors that increase or decrease the risk of future violence may also be identified. Under our current system, however, whether the findings justify the involuntary confinement of the patient ultimately requires a judicial balance of the interest of the patient for liberty against the interest of society for protection. Relevant facts, not merely expert conclusions, are necessary for judges to weigh these competing interests.

Guardianship & Conservatorship

Although our society places a high value on personal autonomy, states may deprive some citizens of the freedom to make their own decisions or to perform certain tasks. These deprivations occur when a court deems persons incompetent and appoints a substitute decision maker or guardian for them. Courts can appoint guardians for both general and specific purposes. General guardians typically have the authority to manage the full range of incompetent persons' affairs: personal, medical, and financial. In other cases, guardians may be appointed to handle only specific tasks. For example, a conservator is a guardian with powers to manage property and finances, and medical guardians make treatment decisions.

Courts do not always specify the legal standard or threshold for competence to manage personal or financial affairs. Clinical commentators, and some courts, have proposed four major standards of competence. The most basic, and least demanding, standard requires the person merely to evidence a choice. Individuals who cannot communicate their choices are not competent. A second standard requires that the person have a factual understanding of information relevant to the decision being made. The third standard examines whether the person can rationally manipulate the relevant information. And the fourth standard requires that the person have a personal appreciation of the situation and the potential consequences of the decision. Patients with psychotic disorders often fail this last test when making treatment-related decisions. For example, they might express choices about taking medications, understand the general risks and benefits of the medications, and be able to manipulate that information rationally as it might apply to other persons. Nevertheless, delusional denial of mental illness can lead them to reject treatment without an appreciation of the personal consequences.

Two standards exist to guide guardians in their substitute decision making. Under a "best interest" standard, the guardian makes a purportedly objective choice based on considerations of what will best meet the needs of the incompetent person. In contrast, when using a "substituted judgment" standard, the guardian attempts to make the decision that the incompetent person would make if competent. Because each approach has its shortcomings, some courts and commentators have adopted a model that combines both. When the previous, competent wishes of the now-incompetent person are known, the guardian follows that choice. In other circumstances, the guardian may make a decision based on a perception of the person's best interests.

Informed Consent & the Right to Refuse Treatment

The concept of informed consent includes three related considerations: ethical obligations, legal rules, and interpersonal processes. As an ethical doctrine, informed consent involves principles of autonomy and patients' rights to self-determination in making medical decisions. Although historically physicians have not always shared information and decisions with their patients, many would agree that patients have the right to make decisions based on access to all available information.

As a legal rule, informed consent first made its appearance in the last half of the twentieth century. Before then, patients could refuse the proposed procedure but had no right to be fully informed prior to making the decision. Failure to obtain the patient's simple consent exposed the doctor to a criminal or civil charge of battery.

Beginning in 1957, a series of court cases rejected the adequacy of simple consent and developed the legal doctrine of informed consent. The leading case in this series, *Canterbury v Spence*, involved a 19-year-old plaintiff who sustained partial paralysis after undergoing a laminectomy for severe back pain. In its 1972 decision, the District of Columbia Court of Appeals upheld the patient's right to an "informed exercise of choice . . . that entails an opportunity to evaluate knowledgeably the options available and the risks attendant upon each."

The core elements of required disclosure include the nature of the patient's condition, the risks and benefits of the proposed treatment, the risks and benefits of alternative treatments, and the likely consequences if the patient remains untreated. When determining how much information the doctor must provide to the patient, courts in most states consider the "materiality" of the particular piece of information to a reasonable patient's decision.

Some exceptions exist to the legal requirement to obtain informed consent. Consent is generally implied in emergencies, when the time spent on disclosure and patient decision making would seriously jeopardize the patient's safety. Patients also may waive their right to an informed consent and give simple consent as long as they do so voluntarily. Under the final exception, "therapeutic privilege," physicians may choose not to disclose information if the disclosure itself would directly harm the patient. Courts tend to limit therapeutic privilege narrowly to prevent it from becoming a loophole that all but vitiates the requirement of informed consent. For example, physicians must discuss side effects even if doing so may result in refusal of treatment.

While maintaining an awareness of the governing legal standards, physicians might best approach informed consent as an interpersonal process integral to good patient care. Ongoing sharing of information and decisions with patients can improve compliance and the therapeutic alliance by engaging patients in the definition of treatment goals and in the selection of treatment.

Confidentiality & Privilege

Psychiatrists have an ethical obligation not to reveal patient information obtained during a treatment relationship. The duty to maintain confidentiality protects the patient's control over personal information. "Testimonial privilege" refers to the patient's right to prevent testimony by a treating psychiatrist in court and some administrative proceedings. In addition to protecting privacy, privilege and confidentiality encourage people to seek treatment with minimal fear of revelation of personal information.

Confidentiality and privilege in psychiatry are like a sterile field in surgery. In their absence, the best treatment often fails. Nevertheless, exceptions to confidentiality and privilege exist. Under some circum-

stances courts can compel psychiatrists to testify over the objections of their patients. For example, the "patient-litigant exception" to privilege occurs when a patient chooses to put his or her mental condition at issue in a judicial proceeding. Other exceptions to privilege may include child custody proceedings, civil commitment and guardianship hearings, and malpractice suits brought by the patient against the psychiatrist. Statutory exceptions to the broader right to confidentiality often include requirements that physicians inform public health authorities of certain communicable diseases and report suspected abuse of children or the elderly. Confidentiality obligations also may yield to competing duties, such as the duty to protect third parties as described below. Psychiatrists need to be familiar with local statutes and case law governing confidentiality and privilege.

Duty to Protect

In its 1976 decision *Tarasoff v Regents of the University of California*, the California Supreme Court articulated an important exception to patient confidentiality. Following a homicide by a student being treated at a university counseling center, the court held that a therapist has a duty to protect identifiable third parties whom the therapist knows, or should know, to be at risk of serious harm from the patient.

Table 40–2. Common standards in civil forensic psychiatry.

I. Elements of malpractice
  A. Duty
  B. Dereliction: negligence in fulfilling a duty
  C. Damage: harm to the patient or third party
  D. Direct causation: the physician's negligence is the legally proximate cause of the harm

II. Generally required findings for civil commitment
  A. Presence of a mental disease or defect
  B. Risk of serious harm
    1. to self
      a. intentional acts
      b. inability to meet safely the ordinary demands of life in the community ("grave disability")
    2. to others
  C. Absence of less restrictive options than involuntary hospitalization

III. Tests of competence to manage personal or financial affairs
  A. Communication of a choice
  B. Factual understanding of information relevant to the decision
  C. Rational manipulation of the relevant information
  D. Appreciation of the situation and the consequences of the decision

IV. Elements of informed consent
  A. Nature of the patient's condition
  B. Risks and benefits of the proposed treatment
  C. Risks and benefits of alternative treatments
  D. Likely consequences if the person remains untreated

V. Duty to protect
  A therapist has a duty to protect third parties whom the therapist knows, or should know, to be at risk of serious harm from a patient

Normally, one person has no obligation to prevent another person from harming a third party, but the court predicated its decision on the "special relationship" between therapists and patients.

Since the California decision, many other states have endorsed the duty to protect in court decisions or statutes. Some states have even expanded the duty to nonidentifiable potential victims, to cases involving dangerous driving, and to threats against property that could unintentionally cause harm to a third party. Although sometimes referred to mistakenly as a "duty to warn," the duty to protect may be fulfilled in ways that do not breach confidentiality. For example, appropriate treatment and hospitalization of the violent patient can often address the risk more effectively and without revealing confidential information.

Dealing with these difficult clinical circumstances requires careful assessment, thoughtful selection of an appropriate intervention, and conscientious implementation of the selected plan (Table 40–2).

CONCLUSION

Forensic psychiatry is a subspecialty area that interacts with philosophy, ethics, morality, and the law. Many cutting-edge issues of individual responsibility, personal rights, and legal regulation of medical practice fall within the field. Knowledgeable forensic psychiatrists can assist courts in the resolution of legal disputes and can influence the development of the standards and regulations that govern their profession.

REFERENCES & SUGGESTED READINGS

American Psychiatric Association: Statement on the insanity defense. Am J Psychiatry 1983;140:681.

American Psychiatric Association: *Guidelines on Confidentiality.* APA, 1987.

American Psychiatric Association: *Task Force Report No. 29: Psychiatric Services in Jails and Prisons.* APA, 1989.

Appelbaum PS: *Almost a Revolution: Mental Health Law and the Limits of Change.* Oxford University Press, 1994.

Appelbaum PS: A theory of ethics for forensic psychiatry. J Am Acad Psychiatry Law 1997;25:233.

Appelbaum PS, Gutheil TG: *Clinical Handbook of Psychiatry and the Law,* 2nd ed. Williams & Wilkins, 1991.

Beck JC (editor): *Confidentiality Versus the Duty to Protect: Foreseeable Harm in the Practice of Psychiatry.* American Psychiatric Press, 1990.

Grisso T: *Evaluating Competencies.* Plenum Press, 1986.

Melton GB et al: *Psychological Evaluations for the Courts: A Handbook for Mental Health Professionals and Lawyers,* 2nd ed. Guilford Press, 1997.

Meyerson AT, Fine T (editors): *Psychiatric Disability: Clinical, Legal and Administrative Dimensions.* American Psychiatric Press, 1987.

Rosner R (editor): *Principles and Practice of Forensic Psychiatry.* Chapman & Hall, 1994.

Schetky D, Benedek E: *Clinical Handbook of Child Psychiatry and the Law.* Williams & Wilkins, 1991.

Simon RI, Sadoff RL: *Psychiatric Malpractice: Cases and Comments for Clinicians.* American Psychiatric Press, 1992.

Steadman HJ et al: *Before and After Hinckley: Evaluating Insanity Defense Reform.* Guilford Press, 1993.

Strasburger LH, Gutheil TG, Brodsky A: On wearing two hats: Role conflict in serving as both psychotherapist and expert witness. Am J Psychiatry 1997;154:448.

Legal Cases

Ake v Oklahoma, 407 US 68, 105 SCt 1087 (1985).

Canterbury v Spence, 150 US App DC 263, 464 F2d 772 (1972).

Colorado v Connelly, 479 US 157, 107 SCt 515 (1986).

Durham v United States, 94 US App DC 228, 214 F2d 862 (1954).

Dusky v United States, 362 US 402, 80 SCt 788 (1960).

Estelle v Gamble, 429 US 97, 97 SCt 285 (1976).

Jackson v Indiana, 406 US 715, 92 SCt 1845 (1972).

Jones v United States, 463 US 354, 103 SCt 3043 (1983).

Kansas v Hendricks, 117 SCt 2072 (1997).

Lessard v Schmidt, 349 FSupp 1078 (ED Wis. 1972).

Tarasoff v Regents of the University of California, 17 Cal 3d 425, 551 P2d 334, 131 Cal Rptr 14 (1976).

41

Emergency Psychiatry

Beth Goldman, MD, MPH

Patients with psychiatric emergencies present in many settings, including emergency rooms, crisis clinics, and physician's offices. There are a broad variety of situations that constitute psychiatric emergencies, including suicidal or homicidal ideation, acute drug overdose or intoxication, recent violent assault or abuse, and acute psychoses. All of these situations require prompt assessment and efficient treatment of disposition. *All* physicians should be familiar with such situations so that they can be alert to their emergent nature, make an appropriate referral, or provide an effective intervention. They should also be familiar with state or local reporting requirements relating to self-injury or injuries to others by means of a weapon.

It is particularly important to note that as funding for treatment on expensive inpatient units decreases, facilities such as emergency rooms and walk-in clinics will be expected to diagnose accurately and treat many patients rather than simply to find them a hospital bed.

This chapter emphasizes actual or attempted suicide and homicide, management of violent patients, acute treatment of victims of rape, abuse, or violence, and treatment of acute drug/alcohol intoxication, withdrawal, and overdose. It is not meant to be a comprehensive guide to the handling of psychiatric and medical emergencies.

SUICIDE

Suicide ranked as the ninth major cause of death in the United States in 1996 with over 30,000 recorded suicides each year. It was the third leading cause of death among 15 to 24 year olds and the fifth leading cause of death for both 5 to 14 year olds and 25 to 44 year olds (Centers for Disease Control, 1996). Conservative estimates indicate that attempted suicide is eight times more frequent than successful suicide. These figures do not include unconsciously motivated fatal "accidents" or other self-destructive behaviors (eg, alcohol abuse).

Those who attempt suicide and succeed differ demographically from those who make unsuccessful attempts. Successful suicide is about three times more common in men than in women and increases with advancing age. Suicide is also more common in persons who are not married and in those who are isolated, uprooted, or lonely. Protestants are more likely to commit suicide than Catholics or Jews, and foreign-born immigrants are at greater risk. Guns are the most commonly used means of successful suicide (50% of men and 25% of women), and men are more likely than women to commit suicide by violent means. Unsuccessful suicide attempts are three times more common in women than in men. They are most common in the 20 to 24 year age group. Unsuccessful attempts commonly involve nonviolent means, such as cutting, poisoning, or carbon monoxide (Table 41–1).

The clinician evaluating the risk of suicide should try to determine whether the patient has formed a definite plan—eg, has the patient made out a will, changed an insurance policy, or decided on the method, time, and place for the act? The clinician must assess previous suicide attempts and obtain a family history of suicide. In evaluating mental status, the clinician should ask about feelings of rejection and uselessness and whether the patient is working. Patients should be asked if they are hearing voices advocating self-harm (command hallucinations). Co-existing depression with associated anxiety or acute worsening of depression is a danger signal, as is a rapid superficial improvement in depression, which may be a sign that a plan for suicide has been devised. Indications for impending suicide or increased risk of suicide among patients include the following: panic disorder and/or agoraphobia; increasing hostility; financial worries (real or imagined) with ideas of impending poverty; painful illnesses, particularly if associated with prolonged sleep disturbance; and a recent history of alcoholism, current intoxication on alcohol, or drug abuse—particularly recent use of cocaine.

Clues to Suicide

People who are contemplating suicide often provide clues that must be carefully assessed.

A. Verbal Clues: The individual may sometimes make direct statements about wanting to die or "end it all." Less direct ways of expressing suicidal ideation are, "It's too much to bear!" "You'd be better off without me!" "I'd be better off dead!" A patient who asks, "How do you leave your body to science?" or who says, "I have a friend who's real

Table 41–1. Risk categories for suicide.[a]

Factor	High-Risk Category	Low-Risk Category
Age	45 years and older	Under 45 years of age
Sex	Male	Female
Race	White	Other races
Marital status	Separated, divorced, widowed	Single, married
Living arrangements	Alone	With others
Employment status[b]	Unemployed, retired	Employed[c]
Physical health	Poor (acute or chronic condition in the 6 months preceding the attempt)	Good[c]
Mental condition	Nervous or mental disorder, mood or behavioral symptoms, including alcoholism	Presumably normal, including brief situational reactions[c]
Medical care (within 6 months)	Yes	No[c]
Method	Hanging, firearms, jumping, drowning	Cutting or piercing, gas or carbon monoxide, poisoning, combination of other methods, other
Season	Warm months (April to September)	Cold months (October to March)
Time of day	6:00 AM to 5:59 PM _Day_	6:00 PM to 5:59 AM _Night_
Where attempt was made	Own or someone else's home	Other type of premises, out of doors
Time interval between attempt and discovery	Almost immediately; reported by person making attempt	Later
Intent to commit suicide (self report)	No[c]	Yes
Suicide note	Yes	No[c]
Previous attempt or threat	Yes	No[c]

[a] Modified and reproduced, with permission, from Tuckman and Youngman (1968).
[b] Does not include homemakers and students.
[c] Includes cases for which information on this factor was not given in the police report.

depressed and talks about suicide a lot" is sending messages in very simple code.

B. Behavioral Clues: A direct behavioral clue is ingestion of a small amount of some potentially lethal drug. Prematurely or inappropriately "putting one's affairs in order," arranging for a casket, and giving away prized possessions are indirect clues.

C. Situational Clues: Situational clues are inherent in life experiences associated with major stress, eg, an impending surgical procedure, a diagnosis of chronic fatal illness, or a recent loss—the death of a loved one, loss of a job, eviction, retirement, etc.

D. Syndromic Clues: Syndromic clues are certain constellations of emotions that are commonly associated with suicide. Depression is the most common, but there are others. Suicide also occurs in people who are not depressed but are disoriented—eg, in acute delirium, suicidal behavior may be an attempt to flee some imagined threat. Individuals with psychotic disorders associated with impaired impulse control may attempt suicide in response to hallucinations commanding them to do so. Suicide also occurs in defiant people, who may view suicide as a means of taking an active, resistive stance in the face of some real or imagined threat to their self-esteem. Suicide by a dependent, dissatisfied individual is of-ten a masked hostile gesture toward some other individual or group perceived as not having fulfilled dependency needs. ("Now you'll feel sorry!")

ASSESSING THE RISK OF SUICIDE

The physician must stay alert to the possibility of suicide in patients presenting for treatment. Most people who attempt suicide have been seen by a physician a few months before, and most successful suicides have signaled their intent to loved ones and others and have expressed a need for help, often in the preceding 24 hours. The physician must regard suicide attempts or verbalized suicidal thoughts as emergencies, since even so-called "hysterical" and "manipulative" patients may succeed in self-destructive acts.

A number of factors influence the assessment of suicide risk: the patient's usual level of functioning, past history of suicide attempts and mental illness, current social and economic circumstances, and cognitive/affective state.

Useful questions that might be considered in any evaluation for suicidal risk can be formulated as follows:

How has the patient reacted to stress in the past, and how effective are his or her typical coping strategies?

Has the patient contemplated or attempted suicide in the past? If so, how frequently and under what circumstances? If the patient has made attempts in the past, how serious were they?

What are the patient's current social and economic circumstances, and how similar are they to past situations when suicide was attempted?

What is the patient's current cognitive state? Hopeless, helpless, powerless? Angry? Oriented, hallucinating, delusional?

Does the patient have somatic manifestations of depression such as constipation, insomnia, fatigue, loss of appetite, diminished libido, anxiety, or menstrual irregularities?

When suicide is suspected, the clinician must ask the patient directly about the nature and extent of suicidal thinking. The following types of suicidal thoughts and the feelings associated with them are discussed in order of increasing risk:

1. **Transient thoughts about dying.** People with transient ideas of death may entertain fantasies such as, "They'll miss me when I'm gone." Such common notions are usually of little significance. Concern and caution are warranted, however, if the patient is an adolescent or an emotionally unstable adult.
2. **Sustained thoughts about dying and recurrent wishes for death.** Sustained ideas about death and recurrent death wishes may function as a painful habit that enables the individual to deal with stress. Suicidal gestures such as superficial wrist cutting or nonlethal ingestion of drugs may occur occasionally.
3. **Frustrated feelings and impulsive behavior.** A patient may have little hope for support from the environment and may feel that most forms of relief have been exhausted. The patient is therefore frustrated and close to anger much of the time. The anger may be turned inward or outward, leading to the possibility of a suicidal or homicidal act.
4. **Court of last resort.** A person may feel depleted of all emotional resources and/or may feel that suicide is the only "escape" from an impossible situation. Such an individual no longer feels rage, frustration, or despair, and death is viewed as a way of avoiding further anguish.
5. **The logical decision to die.** A person may approach suicide from a logical and philosophical point of view. Such a person sees death as inevitable and asks, "So why not now?" This type of individual is at the highest risk of suicide, but the patient's decision rarely comes to the attention of the physician.

If suicide is being seriously considered, the lethality of the method chosen—as well as its availability—must be assessed. A person considering a well-thought-out, concrete plan is at higher risk than one who has no particular plan in mind.

Finally, the nature and extent of the patient's support system must be assessed.

Patients presenting after an unsuccessful suicide attempt must also be assessed. Some patients no longer feel suicidal once they have gotten the message of their distress across by making a suicidal gesture. Again, the lethality of the method as well as the likelihood of intervention and rescue are taken into account when evaluating patients who have "tried to commit suicide."

SUICIDE PREVENTION

The concept that underlies and justifies efforts at suicide prevention is that people contemplating suicide may nonetheless want to be prevented from doing so. Even those who do not want to be "rescued" or dissuaded from their suicidal purpose should be, since proper treatment and environmental adjustments can often restore such people to better health. Astute observation can almost always uncover clues to suicidal intentions. Almost all suicidal behavior stems from a sense of isolation and anguish. The function of suicide is to terminate an existence that has become unbearable. A single significant relationship may be sufficient to sustain an individual in an otherwise intolerable situation.

Except for those in high-risk categories, many persons considered to be at risk for suicide do not require hospitalization. In doubtful cases, the decision about hospitalization is based on the physician's assessment of the adequacy of the patient's external support system and the integrity of the patient's impulse control mechanism. Lack of an effective support system and poor impulse control in patients otherwise at low risk for suicide may call for hospitalization. Conversely, appropriate crisis intervention in the emergency room may obviate the need for hospitalization of some individuals who have presented after making a suicidal gesture.

People with thoughts of suicide should not have access to the means of acting on them. When such a patient is hospitalized with suicide precautions, there should be no access to an unsecured window, stairwell, etc, or to potential instruments of suicide, such as shoelaces, belts, coat hangers, caustic cleansers, and cutlery. Some patients need constant close observation.

Although some general measures apply to the management of all suicidal persons, specific measures depend on the specific underlying diagnosis, since treatment differs depending on whether the patient has a major affective disorder, schizophrenia, delirium, or dysthymic disorder. Appropriate treatment may include psychotherapy, pharmacological therapy, and, in some cases, electroconvulsive therapy.

Illustrative Case 1

A 20-year-old unmarried college student living at home with her parents and younger siblings was brought to the emergency room after a nearly fatal drug overdose. The family had come to the United States from a Middle Eastern country 3 years previously. The patient stated that her suicide attempt was in response to her father's demands that she maintain the cultural values of their native country rather than adopt those of the new culture. She resented his "dictatorial" approach and envied the freedom of her American peers. The patient showed no evidence of psychosis and was felt to be suffering from adjustment disorder.

Treatment centered on several emergency family sessions. The father was approached as the head of the family and was helped to express his concerns and fears about the family's exposure to new cultural attitudes. He was able to see how his attitudes were reflected in his children's conflicts, and he reluctantly agreed to allow them greater freedom. The children learned to view their father not as a tyrant but rather as a man in culture shock still trying to be a good father. After the initial hostility had subsided, an agreement was reached with which both "sides" were able to feel comfortable. The patient was discharged after 1 day in the hospital, and the family was referred to an outpatient psychiatric clinic for further family therapy.

Illustrative Case 2

A 58-year-old divorced surgeon experienced a manic episode. He had a history of depression that began in late adolescence, and his last episode of depression had occurred 10 years before. During the manic episode, he lost all of his hospital affiliations, incurred several malpractice suits, and accumulated huge debts, all in several weeks. He was hospitalized and treated with lithium, and his excitement subsided. He then became suicidally depressed. The depression responded favorably to the addition of tricyclic antidepressant medication to the regimen. After the patient was discharged from the hospital, the dosage of the tricyclic antidepressant was reduced and finally discontinued. Maintenance treatment with lithium alone was subsequently successful.

Illustrative Case 3

A 72-year-old retired married man had experienced the onset of depression 2 years previously. He

was agitated and had regressed, and his wife could not cope with him. Antidepressant medications were tried but had to be stopped because of their side effects. The patient consented to electroconvulsive therapy and underwent a series of nine treatments that resulted in complete remission of symptoms.

SUICIDE IN ADOLESCENTS

The suicide rate among adolescents has risen alarmingly since the middle of the twentieth century. It is the third leading cause of death among 15 to 24 year olds and is the fifth leading cause of death in the 5 to 14 year old age group. Research has indicated that the rise in the suicide rate of adolescents may result in part from changes in our society, including child-rearing practices and loss of stability in the home, as well as increases in the divorce rate. The association between suicide and parental divorce is statistically significant. Other factors associated with suicide in adolescents include antisocial behavior and substance abuse.

Adolescents generally tend to be more impulsive than adults, and the suicidal adolescent is less likely to be suffering from depression than a suicidal adult. Although behavioral changes often precede a suicide attempt, they are less likely to be the classical neurovegetative signs of depression. Symptoms such as social withdrawal, preoccupation with bizarre ideas, or decline in academic performance may precede a suicide attempt in an adolescent suffering from early symptoms of schizophrenia.

Illustrative Case

A 16-year-old boy was admitted to the hospital after swallowing several of his mother's antihypertension pills. The history revealed progressive social withdrawal over the past year, and school records showed a significant decline in academic performance for 2 years. The patient admitted having auditory hallucinations in the form of derogatory voices, and also had ideas of reference. Antipsychotic medications relieved both his hallucinations and his suicidal ideation.

HOMICIDE

Homicide is the killing of one human being by another human being. Murder, as defined by California Penal Code Section 187, is "the unlawful killing of a human being, or a fetus, with malice aforethought." In this discussion, the term "homicide" is used with-

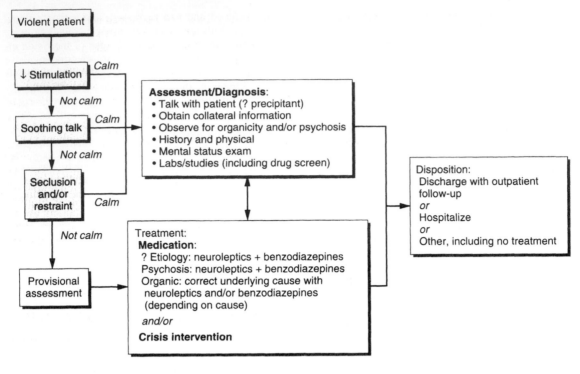

Figure 41–1. Management of the violent patient.

out regard to legal distinctions (justifiable, excusable, with or without malice, etc).

Most homicides occur at night, with the highest incidence between 8:00 PM Saturday and 2:00 AM Sunday. Fifty percent of homicides occur on weekends or holidays; most of them occur in the home; the victim and perpetrator are frequently members of the same family; and the victim may be the perpetrator. Homicide is committed five times more often by men than by women, though in recent years the incidence of homicides perpetrated by women has been increasing.

The risk of homicide is increased in persons with psychosis characterized by persecutory delusions, with the risk particularly high when the delusions have come to focus on one individual. The homicide risk is also increased in individuals with a history of violence, hatred of authority, or antisocial personality traits; any evidence of rivalry, jealousy, or sexual conflicts; a recent history of withdrawal, brooding, and moodiness; and a history of alcoholism or drug abuse.

Most homicidal acts are not premeditated but occur during periods of heightened emotional tension that coincide with the ready availability of some sort of weapon. Anything that impairs impulse control increases the risk of violent assault, eg, "premedicated" murder after the use of alcohol or street drugs by the perpetrator.

Illustrative Case

A 54-year-old municipal employee believed that his supervisor and fellow workers were ridiculing him by making sexual gestures and remarks and creating obstacles to performance of his job. He drank alcohol to excess for many years, and recently began using cocaine. His wife was aware of his misuse of alcohol and street drugs but did not notify his physician. After a negative performance review one day, the patient shot his supervisor and two coworkers. Medical testimony at the patient's trial emphasized impaired judgment resulting from his state of chronic intoxication. He was found guilty of second-degree murder.

GENERAL APPROACH TO VIOLENT OR ACUTELY EXCITED PATIENTS

The physician attempting to deal with a violent patient should use a calm, systematic approach (Figure 41–1). The patient's behavior should be accepted as a symptom of the illness, and no patient should ever be ridiculed. Patients who become violent in the emergency room are often those who have been kept waiting—these patients interpret the wait as a sign that others do not consider them important or do not feel they need immediate treatment. The physician should act promptly and decisively, introduce himself or herself, and explain the plan of treatment: "Mr Allen, I'm Dr Rodriguez of the emergency department staff. I'd like to talk to you for a few minutes and then do a physical examination." The physician should then obtain a history and perform the examination. Information from friends and relatives is often needed to develop an appropriate plan of treatment.

The physician should make sure that backup help is available for management of patients who are obviously psychotic or aggressive. The area should be free of objects that could be used as weapons. The medical staff should never turn their backs or let the patient come between them and the door; the door should be readily accessible to both the patient and the interviewer. If a violent patient escapes security guards, the police should be called immediately.

Threatening calls or letters from patients should never be ignored, since doing so may actually encourage the caller or writer to escalate the activity.

When a violent patient presents in the office or emergency room, it is appropriate to acknowledge realistic fear but not panic. The physician must exercise self-control to control the patient and the situation. Facing the patient at a discreet distance with arms crossed is a nonthreatening stance that nevertheless enables the physician to avoid or deflect blows. The physician should not attempt to deal unaided with a violent patient. Agitated patients confronted with ample force are less likely to become assaultive. Potentially assaultive patients should be discreetly searched for weapons in the emergency room by being asked to change to hospital clothing.

Some patients respond well to nonthreatening, soothing talk. Hostile, ridiculing behavior on the part of the physician may exacerbate the violent situation. Care should be taken never to injure the patient's pride or make insincere promises.

If talk does not soothe the patient, restraints and/or medication may be necessary. If restraints are needed, they should be used promptly and applied as gently as possible. Explanation of the reason for restraints should be given. An early show of authority and control may prevent injuries and property damage and allow treatment and evolution to proceed. It is also important to prevent violence because of the guilt feelings and lowered self-esteem the patient inevitably faces when self-control is restored.

Management of the violent patient depends on the cause of the violence. The patient should be observed for signs of organicity (eg, slurred speech, ataxia). If possible, a physical examination and laboratory testing to rule out intoxication, metabolic imbalance, or trauma should occur. Computed tomography of the head may be necessary if head trauma or brain tumor is suspected. In addition, a history and mental status examination should be performed both to help clarify the circumstances precipitating the violence and to determine if a delirium or functional psychosis might be present.

It is often wise not to medicate the violent patient immediately, as it may confound the diagnosis, particularly if there are side effects. It is particularly wise not to medicate patients who respond to talk or decrease of stimulation. If psychosis is not suspected, an injectable high-potency benzodiazepine, such as lorazepam, may provide adequate sedation. If the patient is believed to be psychotic, a high-potency neuroleptic should be utilized in addition. Many clinicians use a combination of benzodiazepines and neuroleptics if the cause of the violence is not clear. When an organic cause is found, treatment should be directed toward correction of the underlying cause.

VICTIMS OF VIOLENCE &/OR ABUSE

Patients who have been attacked or sexually assaulted are seen in emergency rooms for medical evaluation and treatment. Although such patients do not always present with a psychiatric emergency per se, all should be carefully assessed from a psychological point of view so that proper treatment or referral can be offered.

RAPE

Rape is defined legally as "carnal knowledge of a person by force and against [her] will." Carnal knowledge does not require that emission or complete penetration has occurred. Force includes both physical control over the victim or threatening violence or death.

It is suspected that 90% of rape cases go unreported. A rape occurs about every 2 minutes, and it is estimated that one of three women will be raped at some time during their lives.

Patients may present either immediately after the event (usually for medical attention) or later (often because of psychiatric decompensation). The patient who seeks treatment immediately after the event has a better prognosis than one who delays and may also fare better in court.

The physician treating the rape victim must attend to physical injuries, venereal disease and pregnancy prevention, gynecologic examination, as well as medicolegal documentation and collection of evidence. Details of how to conduct a postrape examination are out of the scope of this text. The patient's psychological needs should be assessed as well.

The typical psychological reaction to rape is classically documented as having an acute phase, lasting several weeks to months, and a longer-term reorganization phase, lasting as long as several years.

Patients presenting just after the rape may appear overwhelmed, labile, anxious, fearful (particularly of men), suspicious, guilty, degraded, or depressed. Derealization, depersonalization, phobias, and exaggerated somatic complaints may occur. Some patients who appear to be calm and coping well just after the rape may simply be "in shock" and are at risk for developing symptoms later.

Long-term effects may include difficulty with relationships, jobs, symptoms of posttraumatic stress disorder, or inappropriate regression and dependency.

Emergency treatment should focus on helping the individual feel protected, safe, and able to regain some sense of control over her own body. Patients, particularly those with psychiatric symptoms, should be assessed to rule out acute psychiatric decompensation such as suicidal ideation or psychosis. Patients should be informed that some of the acute symptoms listed above are to be expected and that long-term psychological recovery from the trauma may take years. The patient should be encouraged to seek psychiatric treatment and informed that it can be very helpful for both management of acute symptoms and integration of the recovery from the experience into the patient's life experiences. Patients should not, however, be pushed to talk about the rape just after the event until or unless they are ready to do so. Legal and psychiatric referrals should be made available to the patient. A few days' supply of benzodiazepines may be offered to extremely anxious or panicky patients who are not known to be substance abusers.

CHILD ABUSE

An estimated 1.5 million cases of child abuse/maltreatment occur annually and 2000–4000 children die each year of abuse and/or neglect. Although it is estimated that only about 5% of actual instances of child abuse get reported, the number of known cases has been increasing. This increase may be a result of improved case finding and reporting as well as a real increase in the actual incidence of child abuse. Increased public awareness may contribute to increased reporting and increasing stress in families and escalating violence in our society may contribute to the rise in the actual incidence of abuse.

Abuse should be suspected when parents repeatedly bring the child in with a variety of injuries or vague complaints, particularly when the explanation for the injury does not make sense or the child appears malnourished or poorly cared for. The child should be examined for unusual lesions and/or evidence of injuries at different ages. Radiological studies may shed light on old trauma. Sexual abuse should be given consideration in very dejected or withdrawn children, and genital areas should be examined.

Physicians and all hospital personnel must report suspected abuse, and in cases in which the child is felt to be at risk, he or she should be hospitalized or temporarily placed out of the home.

Most children will deny abuse out of fear that they or the perpetrator will be punished. All family members should be gently interviewed separately. Since there is usually some ambivalence on the part of both the victim and the perpetrator, direct accusations should not be made. Instead, inquiry could be made about how much stress exists in the household and how it is handled.

Often, longer-term treatment of the parents and child together may result in resolution of the problem.

DOMESTIC VIOLENCE & SPOUSE ABUSE

It is estimated that some form of domestic violence occurs in one out of two homes in the United States at least once a year. Most cases of physical abuse involve the abuse of wives (or female living partners) by men. Such domestic violence crosses all socioeconomic, racial, and cultural lines.

The practice of "wife-beating" has probably occurred since ancient times and has been explicitly and implicitly condoned for most of that time. Early American law permitted it for the purpose of correcting inappropriate behaviors and stipulated that the stick used for such beatings have a circumference no greater than that of the husband's thumb.

The FBI estimates that within the United States a woman is beaten every 18 seconds, and that although almost half of all injuries suffered by women presenting to emergency rooms are the result of battering, only 4% are recognized as such by health care workers. Thirty percent of all women who are murdered are killed by present or former spouses. Furthermore, according to the US Department of Justice, more than 1.7 million people every year confront a spouse with a knife or gun.

Abuse most commonly occurs as part of a chronic maladaptive relationship within the couple. Drug and/or alcohol abuse is commonly involved. Blows are often directed to areas of the body not on "public view," such as the breasts or abdomen, but head trauma is also common. Abuse occurs usually at home and rarely in front of individuals outside the household. Many abusers are possessive, jealous, and intensely dependent on their wives, frequently escalating the abuse when their fears of being abandoned are kindled (eg, when the wife takes a job or focuses attention on the children).

Victims of abuse often blame themselves for the abuse, and those with less healthy ego structures have difficulty leaving the abuser. Abused women frequently present with vague complaints of anxiety, depression, or somatic symptoms and often fail to admit to being battered. Suicidal gestures or attempts are common. As with children, abuse should be suspected in women presenting with repeated injury, particularly when there is a delay between the time of the injury and presentation, with injuries in unusual areas, or with odd explanations for their injuries.

When abuse is suspected, the physician should review old records for evidence of earlier trauma and perform a careful examination, noting all findings in the chart. If possible, photographs should be taken. Care should be taken not to appear overly confrontational or overly judgmental of the husband, or the victim may refuse treatment and flee.

It is important to evaluate the safety of the home, particularly regarding the presence of firearms and other lethal weapons. Emergency shelter should be offered to patients at significant risk for harm if they return home. Suicidal or homicidal patients may require hospitalization. Women not yet ready to leave the abusive situation should be offered treatment when they are ready.

DRUG & ALCOHOL INTOXICATION, WITHDRAWAL, & OVERDOSE

The psychiatrist or other emergency room physician spends considerable time dealing with patients who present with emergencies related to the use and abuse of psychoactive drugs and alcohol.

Although it is not possible to discuss the management of all varieties of such crises fully, the following sections present some general comments on the management of intoxication, withdrawal, and overdose of opiates, stimulants, central nervous system depressants, hallucinogens, phencyclidine, and alcohol.

Any patient presenting in an emergency setting with altered mental status, including confusion, depression, stupor, psychosis, or excitation, should be screened for drugs of abuse. Also, toxicity (possibly related to overdose) from "legitimate" drugs should also be considered. Since patients either may not know or may not be truthful about what they have taken, corroboration from family and friends and from blood and urine samples should be sought. Information on the substance(s) abused, patterns of drug use, date of last use, amount used, extent of prior treatment, nature of the patient's support system, and effects of drug use on the patient's life should be obtained.

OPIATES

Opiates include drugs such as codeine, morphine, hydromorphone, oxycodone, and heroin. Patients who are simply intoxicated may appear drowsy, sometimes euphoric, tranquil, or dulled. Pupillary constriction is a tip-off. Opiate users rarely present for treatment of intoxication per se.

Withdrawal symptoms, though uncomfortable, are not lethal. Anxiety, insomnia, sweating, rhinorrhea, yawning, and lacrimation are early withdrawal signs. Later, abdominal and muscle cramping, chills, diarrhea, and vomiting may occur. About 24 hours after the last dose, pulse, blood pressure, and temperature rise. Symptoms of withdrawal peak at about 48–72 hours after the last dose.

Severe dehydration may require fluid and electrolyte replacement. Patients exhibiting observable, objective signs of withdrawal (eg, elevated vital signs, dilated pupils, sweating) may require inpatient detoxification with methadone and/or alleviation of autonomic instability with clonidine. Some centers perform outpatient detoxification with propoxyphene or acupuncture.

Overdose with opiates constitutes a medical emergency as respiratory depression and coma may result. Induction of emesis (if patient is alert) and reversal of the opiate effect with naloxone (if patient is drowsy or comatose) are standard parts of treatment of opiate overdose. Comatose patients require airway management, possibly including ventilation.

It should be noted that intravenous drug users are at risk for such diseases as endocarditis, hepatitis, and human immunodeficiency virus infection and should be offered appropriate screening.

CENTRAL NERVOUS SYSTEM DEPRESSANTS

Drugs in this category cover a wide gamut, including barbiturates and benzodiazepines, as well as agents such as methaqualone, meprobamate, glutethimide, and ethchlorvynol. Although alcohol is technically in this category, it will be dealt with in a subsequent section.

As in the case of opiates, patients who are intoxicated on these agents rarely seek treatment. Such patients appear drunk, possibly giddy, and disinhibited or violent in early phases of intoxication and uncoordinated and slowed in later stages.

Withdrawal symptoms are characterized by anxiety, restlessness, and gastrointestinal symptoms in the early phases. Later signs of withdrawal include weakness, cramping, tachycardia, autonomic instability, gross tremors, and hyperreflexia. The time of onset of withdrawal symptoms depends on the half-life of the substance abused, as does the time of peak symptoms, when the patient is at highest risk for seizures and delirium.

Treatment of withdrawal consists of medical support and detoxification with a long-acting drug to which the patient is cross-tolerant (particularly a long-acting benzodiazepine or barbiturate). In reliable patients, mild withdrawal may be treated on an outpatient basis using a benzodiazepine.

Treatment of overdose with these agents is mainly supportive (eg, airway protection). Flumazenil may be given to reverse the effects of benzodiazepines, but it must be used with caution, as patients who are physically dependent on benzodiazepines may develop seizures following the use of this agent.

CENTRAL NERVOUS SYSTEM STIMULANTS

Unlike the case for opiates and central nervous system depressants, both intoxication and withdrawal symptoms may require emergency treatment. Cocaine and amphetamines have similar effects.

Mild intoxication includes euphoria and feelings of increased ability and self-confidence. Dilated pupils and adrenergic stimulation occur. Severe intoxication may result in psychotic behavior, such as repetitive motions, paranoia, ideas of reference, and hallucinations. Formication, irritability, emotional lability, and violence may be seen. Autonomic hyperactivity, resulting in extremely elevated pulse and blood pressure, may be life threatening. Seizures may also occur, with the risk of death.

Treatment is directed toward managing the effects of adrenergic stimulation (eg, ice for fevers, propranolol for tachycardia), seizures, and psychotic symptoms (decreasing stimulation and/or use of neuroleptics).

Patients coming off of central nervous system stimulants may develop extreme fatigue, hyperphagia, and hypersomnia. Severe depression and suicidal ideation are common, and such patients should be evaluated and protected if necessary.

HALLUCINOGENS

Patients who take hallucinogens such as lysergic acid diethylamide (LSD) most commonly seek treatment for "bad trips," confusional states, psychosis, or flashbacks.

Individuals having a "bad trip" become frightened of the disorganization and sense of loss of control engendered by the drug, fearing that they are losing their mind. These patients should not be left alone, should be allowed to rest in a quiet environment, and should be reassured that the strange experiences they are having are the temporary result of the drug. In severe cases, a benzodiazepine may help the patient to relax. Antipsychotic agents should be avoided.

Occasional users develop an acute confusional state or a delirium, sometimes including paranoia or other delusions, which may endanger the patient or others. These patients require close observation and sometimes restraints until the drug is eliminated. Drugs with anticholinergic properties (eg, thorazine) should be avoided because they can add to the delirium.

Some patients, usually those with underlying psychiatric disorders, continue to display psychotic symptoms after the drug has been cleared from the body. They may require hospitalization and treatment with psychotropic agents. Other patients have "flashbacks" or brief periods of perceptual distortion or depersonalization that mirror the drug experience. Treatment consists of reassurance that if the patient refrains from drug use, flashbacks will not persist.

PHENCYCLIDINE

Phencyclidine (PCP) is a special case in that the drug may mimic depressants, stimulants, hallucinogens, or analgesics, depending on the drug dose. Patients may be brought in because of bizarre behavior such as posturing or staring into space. Nystagmus, hypertension, and drooling in a patient presenting bizarrely should suggest PCP. Patients who have ingested high doses may become psychotic, unstable, and violent. Unlike those on LSD, patients on PCP often cannot be "talked down" and usually require isolation. Use of psychotropic drugs is controversial. Autonomic instability and seizures may also occur with PCP, so patients require frequent observation with measurements of vital signs to ensure that immediate medical management can occur. Some clinicians also recommend acidification of the urine.

Some individuals develop a prolonged psychosis after ingesting PCP. Such patients require hospitalization, as the phenomenon may last weeks to months.

ALCOHOL

Because 4% of Americans suffer from alcohol abuse and 25% of all hospitalized patients have problems related to alcohol, the emergency room physician must become familiar with a variety of alcohol-related crises.

Patients who abuse alcohol present to emergency rooms in various stages of intoxication and for a variety of reasons. Patients may require treatment for alcohol-related illness (eg, pancreatitis), for symptoms of withdrawal, and for alcohol-related mood and behavioral disturbances (eg, violence, suicidal depression), or because they request assistance in quitting.

Behavioral manifestations of alcohol intoxication

vary with the blood alcohol level. However, as tolerance develops, more alcohol is required to produce signs of intoxication. Intolerant persons will show signs of intoxication (eg, ataxia, slowing) at 100 mg/dL, but behavioral and mood changes can occur at lower levels. Levels of 400 mg/dL or higher may lead to coma, depending on the degree of tolerance.

Intoxicated patients should be screened for suicidal and homicidal ideation, and belligerent individuals should be handled as described above. All intoxicated patients must be detained in the emergency room until they are no longer legally drunk. Patients must be observed for signs and symptoms of withdrawal.

Signs of withdrawal include tremor, anxiety, sleeplessness, restlessness, sleep disturbances, and elevation of pulse and blood pressure. Symptoms usually begin within the first 24 hours of abstinence. Note that withdrawal is precipitated by a *decrease* in alcohol consumption and may be delayed by concomitant use of benzodiazepines, barbiturates, and general anesthesia (all cross-tolerant with alcohol). The syndrome, if untreated, may progress to delirium tremens, a life-threatening illness characterized by autonomic instability with hyperpyrexia, delirium, and seizures (see Chapter 17).

All alcohol patients who present to the emergency room should be given thiamine, 100 mg, before any glucose is given to prevent Wernicke-Korsakoff syndrome (see Chapter 16). Patients with signs of withdrawal usually require admission for detoxification with benzodiazepines or barbiturates. Reliable patients with mild symptoms and good support systems may be detoxified on an outpatient basis.

As with any central nervous system depressant, respiratory depression and coma may occur with an overdose (intentional or unintentional), particularly if other sedative-hypnotic drugs have been ingested. Management is supportive.

Note that anyone with depleted glycogen stores (patients with liver disease or in a fasting state) may develop delirium from hypoglycemia with ingestion of even small amounts of alcohol. This is because alcohol suppresses gluconeogenesis. A stat blood sugar should be checked on anyone presenting with altered mental status.

GENERAL COMMENTS

Because many patients use a variety of drugs, clinical pictures of intoxication, withdrawal, and overdose may be complicated. Comatose patients who have ingested unknown substances are usually treated with a protocol involving airway management, lavage, opiate and sometimes benzodiazepine reversal, and cardiac monitoring for arrhythmia caused by agents such as tricyclic antidepressants or cocaine.

Many patients present to the emergency room

wishing to receive help in becoming abstinent. The decision to admit to a 24-hour facility is based on many factors, including presence or absence of withdrawal symptoms and/or level of intoxication, medical complications, history of prior treatment for substance abuse, level of support available to the patient, presence or absence of suicidal or homicidal ideation and psychosis, assessment of the patient's prognosis, and, finally, availability of resources in the community.

OTHER PSYCHIATRIC EMERGENCIES

ACUTE NONPSYCHOTIC DISORDERS

Emergencies may occur in three types of nonpsychotic disorders: anxiety disorders, including panic attacks and conversion reactions of a dissociative type, as well as fugue states; personality disorders; and antisocial states, in which aggressive behavior occurs frequently (see Chapters 21, 22, and 24).

Illustrative Case 1

An 18-year-old man was brought to the emergency room after threatening his mother with a knife when she refused to give him money. He had a long history of depression and antisocial behavior—theft, assault, robbery—and had been incarcerated in juvenile facilities several times. He was released after a brief period of observation, since his mother refused to press charges and he was neither psychotic nor depressed.

Illustrative Case 2

A 22-year-old male college student was brought to the emergency room for evaluation after a sudden onset of paralysis and aphonia following a motor vehicle accident. The other driver had been tailgating him for a mile and then smashed his car from behind. After medical examination failed to account for the symptoms, thiopental sodium was administered intravenously, the patient was encouraged to recall the events of the accident, and the symptoms quickly disappeared. The patient then related that just before the onset of paralysis and aphonia, he had experienced a feeling of murderous rage toward the other driver.

DELIRIUM

Delirium is common in patients presenting to emergency rooms, particularly in association with alcohol or drug intoxication. Any stimulant or depressant drug may cause delirium when taken in sufficient quantities. Of special importance is phencyclidine psychosis, since individuals who have ingested this drug often exhibit episodes of extreme violence, and the reaction lasts longer than reactions caused by other hallucinogens (see Chapter 17). Delirium may also be caused by factors such as head trauma, cardiovascular disorders, metabolic disorders, prescription drugs, and infections (see Chapters 16 and 39).

Illustrative Case

A 68-year-old woman was brought to the hospital by her brother, who had been called by the manager of her apartment building. She had been wandering the halls and bothering other tenants and had not been caring for herself. Laboratory studies revealed severe hypothyroidism. Thyroid hormone replacement therapy led to gradual improvement in the patient's mental status.

DEMENTIA

Persons suffering from dementia are usually not highly aggressive. They do have a lowered threshold of emotional control, however, and may become assaultive when they find themselves in situations they do not understand.

Illustrative Case

An 86-year-old man was admitted to the hospital after he assaulted his 89-year-old sister. She reported that over the past several years, he had shown progressive deterioration in intellectual function. He completely denied his failing abilities and became assaultive when his sister tried to help him prepare a meal. Examination revealed senile dementia.

ACUTE PSYCHOTIC DISORDERS

Impulse control may be tenuous in individuals experiencing an acute psychotic episode, and loss of control may make them extremely assaultive. The paranoid delusions associated with paranoid schizophrenia and other paranoid psychotic disorders may lead patients to act out; there is special cause for concern if patients believe a specific person in the environment is the source of their persecution.

The excitement that may erupt during a catatonic episode occurs less frequently than agitation caused by paranoid delusions, but it is unpredictable and is usually associated with extreme violence.

Illustrative Case 1

A 40-year-old single man with a long history of paranoid schizophrenia made an appointment at a medical clinic for evaluation of chronic urologic complaints. After the examination, he was told that there were no physical abnormalities. A few minutes later, the patient thought he heard the doctor discussing his case in a demeaning way with a group of nurses. In a rage, he pulled out a gun and shot the physician.

Individuals in the manic phase of bipolar disorder may be assaultive if they feel someone is interfering with their activities. Manic patients are not always jovial and humorous and may in fact be extremely agitated and aggressive. Aggressive behavior may also occur during episodes of depression; in fact, psychotically depressed people may be homicidal. The victim is often a loved one with whom the patient has identified and onto whom the patient's misery is projected. ("You're just like me, and we're both miserable. I'll kill you and then myself, and then we'll both be free from all of this.") The act is committed to save the other person from "a life of misery."

Illustrative Case 2

During a recurrent manic attack, a 31-year-old man became impatient while waiting for a bus. He approached a car stopped at an intersection, pulled the driver out, drove off at high speed, and hit another vehicle. In the emergency room, he had to be physically restrained while the physician treated him for severe lacerations.

Illustrative Case 3

A 42-year-old woman who had been married for some time became pregnant for the first time. Three months after delivery of a healthy child, she experienced severe depression with suicidal ideation. In her state of hopelessness, she drowned the child in the bathtub and then slashed her wrists.

UNTOWARD CONSEQUENCES OF PSYCHOTROPIC MEDICATION

Emergencies may arise from both intentional and unintentional overdose as well as side effects of psychiatric medications.

Patients who attempt suicide overdose on a variety of substances, often "cleaning out the medicine cabinet." They should be searched for empty pill containers, family members should be asked what medications might be available to the patient, and, of course, blood and urine should be taken for screening. Such patients are managed supportively as described above.

Management of **tricyclic antidepressant** (TCA) overdose includes administration of fluids and, if necessary, pressor agents to counteract hypotension as well as continuous monitoring for cardiac arrhythmias. Patients who manifest delirium secondary to the anticholinergic effects of tricyclic antidepressants may require physostigmine. Patients must also be monitored for seizures. Patients who have ingested large amounts of tricyclic antidepressants usually require admission to an intensive care unit. Forced diuresis or dialysis is of no value in TCA overdose. Patients on therapeutic doses of TCAs may also present with medical emergencies such as urinary retention, paralytic ileus, and delirium resulting from the anticholinergic actions of the drugs.

Overdose on **selective serotonin reuptake inhibitors (SSRIs)** produces less severe complications than overdose on TCAs. The few deaths that have been associated with these drugs involved multiple agents or alcohol or ingestion of massive amounts of the drug. Although seizures occur in about a third of overdose cases involving **bupropion,** most patients have recovered unscathed.

Management of **lithium** toxicity and/or overdose is directed toward removing lithium from the body as rapidly as possible. Patients presenting with mild or moderate symptoms of lithium toxicity (eg, tremor, mild confusion, gastrointestinal distress) and serum levels below 3 mEq/L may usually be managed by withholding lithium and administering saline, monitoring urine output, and checking levels frequently. Higher levels, presence of renal disease, more advanced signs of toxicity (stupor, seizures), and failure to respond to diuresis usually require dialysis.

Neuroleptic agents rarely cause death if taken alone in overdose. Although coma and hypotension may occur, cardiac arrhythmias are rare. Management of overdose includes the usual supportive measures. Patients on neuroleptics may present in crisis as a result of the extrapyramidal effects of neuroleptics and may be treated acutely with diphenhydramine or benztropine given intramuscularly or intravenously. Neuroleptic malignant syndrome, a medical emergency, should be considered in a patient with fever, rigidity, and autonomic instability. Elevated creatine phosphokinase is a hallmark of the condition (see Chapter 18).

Monoamine oxidase inhibitors (MAOIs) may cause sympathomimetic overstimulation (hypertensive crisis) if taken with tyramine-containing foods and/or sympathomimetic drugs. Symptoms include headache, diaphoresis, mydriasis, muscular rigidity, and extreme hypertension. For mild crisis, chlorpromazine may be given. For severe symptoms, phentolamine (*not* a beta blocker) is used. Hypotension, particularly postural, is also associated with MAOI use and is dose related. Treatment consists of placing the patient in a Trendelenburg position, intravenous hydration, and, in cases in which these measures are not effective, careful use of pressor agents in extremely low doses (as hypertensive rebound may occur). Acidification of urine and/or dialysis may be necessary if the patient who has overdosed continues to deteriorate.

ADJUSTMENT DISORDER & POSTTRAUMATIC STRESS DISORDER

Adjustment disorder represents a transient response to overwhelming environmental stress in individuals without apparent underlying psychiatric illness. Adjustment disorder is characterized by impaired social or vocational functioning and by symptoms that exceed the normally expected reaction. Such symptoms may develop in persons who suffer a major loss or in those who are victims of violence (eg, rape, spouse beating, or child abuse).

Posttraumatic stress disorder (stress response syndrome) is a reaction to an identifiable stress outside the normal range of experience (eg, car crash, natural disaster). The pattern of response consists of an initial outcry (an emotional response that is almost a reflex), followed by denial (emotional numbing, avoidance of ideas connected with the stressor, and behavioral constriction), an intrusive phase (unbidden ideas and feelings that are difficult to dispel), and a phase of working through and completion.

In both adjustment disorder and posttraumatic stress disorder, prompt crisis intervention may facilitate resolution of symptoms and prevent development of a more chronic psychiatric disorder (see Chapters 21 and 23).

SUMMARY

Dealing with psychiatric emergencies requires considerable knowledge and skill. The physician must be able to reach an accurate diagnosis quickly and begin appropriate treatment without delay. The crisis should be resolved promptly and in a way that eases the transition to the next phase of treatment. How the physician behaves during the emergency phase will strongly influence what happens later.

REFERENCES & SUGGESTED READINGS

Centers for Disease Control and Prevention/National Center for Health Statistics: Monthly Vital Statistics Report. Vol. 46, No. 1, Supplement, 1996.

Dubin W, Weiss K: Emergency psychiatry. In: *Psychiatry,* revised edition. Michels R (editor). JB Lippincott, 1996/7.

Garza-Trevino ES et al: Efficacy of combination of intramuscular antipsychotics and sedative-hypnotics for control of psychotic agitation. Am J Psychiatry 1989; 146:1598.

Hillard JR: Emergency treatment of acute psychosis. J Clin Psychiatry 1998;59(Suppl 1):57.

Hyman S: *Manual of Psychiatric Emergencies,* 3rd ed. Little, Brown, 1994.

Mann J (editor) Suicide. Psychiatric Clin North Am 1997;20 [entire issue].

Maris, RW: Social and familial risk factors in suicide behavior. Psychiatric Clin North Am 1997;20:519.

Murphy GE: Suicide and attempted suicide. In *Psychiatry,* revised edition. Michels R (editor). JB Lippincott, 1996/7.

Salzman C et al: Parenteral lorazepam versus parenteral haloperidol for the control of psychotic disruptive behavior. J Clin Psychiatry 1991;52:177.

Tardiff K (editor): The violent patient. Psychiatr Clin North Am 1988;11(4):1.

Tuckman J, Youngman WF: A scale for assessing suicide risk of attempted suicides. J Clin Psychol 1968;24:17.

Index

NOTE: Entries in bold face type are defined in the glossary in Chapter 8. Page numbers in bold face type indicate a major discussion. A *t* following a page number indicates tabular material and an *f* following a page number indicates a figure. Drugs are listed under their generic names. When a drug trade name is listed, the reader is referred to the generic name.